QUICK REFERENCE TO KEY FEATURES

EMPOWERING THE FAMILY BOXES

Quick Reference to Key Features continues on page xxix.

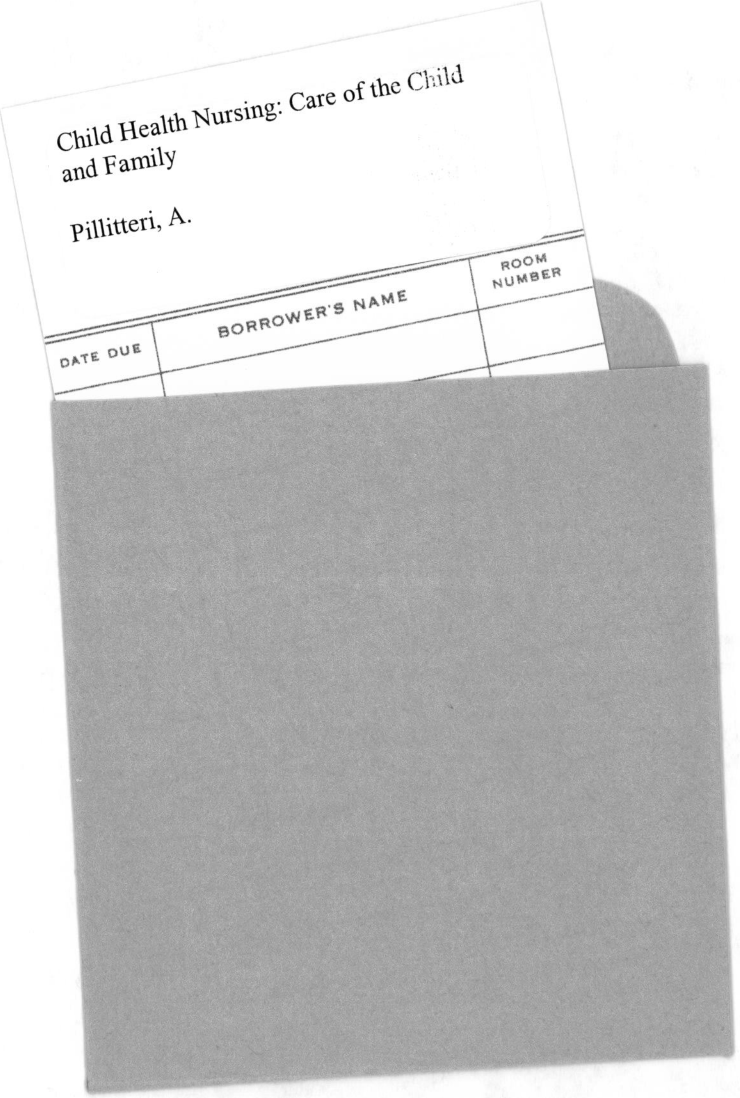

CHILD HEALTH NURSING

Care of the Child and Family

CHILD HEALTH NURSING

Care of the Child and Family

Adele PILLITTERI, PhD, RN, PNP

Chairperson
Department of Nursing
University of Southern California
Los Angeles, California

Lippincott
Philadelphia • New York • Baltimore

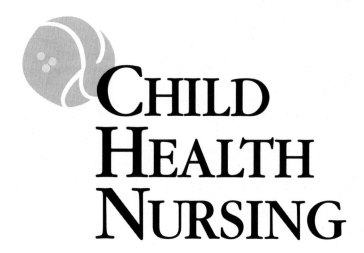

Acquisitions Editor: Jennifer E. Brogan
Coordinating Editorial Assistant: Susan Barta Rainey
Project Editor: Tom Gibbons
Senior Production Manager: Helen Ewan
Senior Production Coordinator: Nannette Winski
Design Coordinator: Brett MacNaughton
Indexer: Maria Coughlin

Printed in the United States of America. For information write Lippincott Williams & Wilkins, 227 East Washington Square, Philadelphia, PA 19106.

Library of Congress Cataloging in Publications Data

Pillitteri, Adele.
Child health nursing : care of the child and family / by Adele Pillitteri.
p. cm.
Includes bibliographical references and index.
ISBN 0-7817-1624-1 (cloth : alk. paper)
1. Pediatric nursing. 2. Child care. I. Title.
[DNLM: 1. Nursing Care—in infancy & childhood. 2. Pediatric Nursing—methods 3. Maternal-Child Nursing—methods. 4. Family Health nurses' instruction. WY 159.P641c 1999]
RJ245.P538 1999
610.73'62—dc21
DNLM/DLC
for Library of Congress 98-51353
CIP

Care has been taken to confirm the accuracy of the information presented and to describe generally accepted practices. However, the authors, editors, and publisher are not responsible for errors or omissions or for any consequences from application of the information in this book and make no warranty, express or implied, with respect to the contents of the publication.

The authors, editors and publisher have exerted every effort to ensure that drug selection and dosage set forth in this text are in accordance with current recommendations and practice at the time of publication. However, in view of ongoing research, changes in government regulations, and the constant flow of information relating to drug therapy and drug reactions, the reader is urged to check the package insert for each drug for any change in indications and dosage and for added warnings and precautions. This is particularly important when the recommended agent is a new or infrequently employed drug.

Some drugs and medical devices presented in this publication have Food and Drug Administration (FDA) clearance for limited use in restricted research settings. It is the responsibility of the health care provider to ascertain the FDA status of each drug or device planned for use in their clinical practice.

9 8 7 6 5 4 3 2 1

To my family:
Joseph, Rusty, Dawn, Bill, Heather, J.J. and Lynn
with love

REVIEWERS

Helene Berman, RN, PhD
University of Western Ontario
School of Nursing
Health Sciences Addition
London, Ontario, Canada

Theresa Krauss Cotton, MSN, CRNP, NNP
Neonatal Nurse Practitioner Program
University of Pennsylvania
Newborn Pediatrics
Pennsylvania Hospital
Kencrest: High Risk Follow-Up Program
Allegheny University Health Systems
Philadelphia, Pennsylvania

Claire Cowan
University of Toronto
Faculty of Nursing
Toronto, Ontario, Canada

Kit Devine, RNC, MSN
Women's Health Nurse Practitioner
Fertility and Endocrine Associates
Adjunct Faculty
Bellarmine College
Louisville, Kentucky

Susan Dudek, RD, CDN,BS
Part-Time Assistant Professor
Dietetic Technology Program
Erie Community College
Williamsville, New York
Consultant Dietitian
Chaffee Hospital and Home
Springville, New York

Sharon Ferrante, MS, RNC
Faculty Member
Muhlenberg Regional Medical Center
School of Nursing
Plainfield, New Jersey

Marcia L. Gasper, RNC, MSN, EdD Candidate
Associate Professor of Nursing
Division of Allied Health and Nursing
Westmoreland County Community College
Youngwood, Pennsylvania

Regina Grazel, RNC, MSN, CNSC
Perinatal Clinical Nurse Specialist
Our Lady of Lourdes Medical Center
Camden, New Jersey
Clinical Instructor, Maternal Child Nursing
Villanova University
Villanova, Pennsylvania

Mona Harris, EdS, MS, BSN, AA, RN
Lead Instructor, Family Nursing
Labette Community College
Parsons, Kansas

Shaun Hartford, MSN, RN, CPN
Nursing Instructor
Baptist Memorial Hospital Systems
School of Professional Nursing
San Antonio, Texas

Dawn Hughes, MS, RNC
Assistant Professor
Mt. Carmel College of Nursing
Columbus, Ohio

M. Katherine Hutchinson, RNC, MS, PhD
Assistant Professor, Department of Nursing
Rutgers, The State University of New Jersey
Camden, New Jersey

M. Regina Jennette, EdD, RN
Director of Nursing Program
West Virginia Northern Community College
Wheeling, West Virginia

Laurie Kaudewitz, BSN, MSN, RNC
Assistant Professor
East Tennessee State University
Johnson City, Tennessee

Celesta Kirk, RN, CS, MSN, MA, FNP
Associate Professor
East Tennessee State University
Johnson City, Tennessee

Barbara W. Law, MSN, RN, CCRN
Family Nurse Practitioner
Medical-Surgical Clinical Specialist
Associate Professor of Nursing
Washington State Community College
Marietta, Ohio

Kim A. Luciano, RN, NPC
Pediatric Nurse Practitioner
Newark Beth Israel Medical Center
Newark, New Jersey

Linda McIntosh-Liptok, RN, MSN
Clinical Instructor
Kent State University, Tuscarawas Campus
New Philadelphia, Ohio

Mary Muscari, PhD, RN, CRNP, CS
Assistant Professor
University of Scranton
Scranton, Pennsylvania

Estelle B. Resnick, RN, BSN, MA
Professor
Capital Community Technical College
Hartford, Connecticut

Cheryl Sams, BSCN, MSN
Clinical Nurse Specialist
Hospital for Sick Children
Faculty
Ontario Nurse Practitioner Program
Ryerson Polytechnic University
Toronto, Ontario, Canada

Lori Elizabeth Steffen, RN, BSN, CPNP
St. Cloud Hospital
Pediatrics and Neonatal Intensive Care Unit
St. Cloud, Minnesota

Rosemary Theroux, RNC, MS
Private Nurse Practitioner Practice
Medway, Massachusetts
Clinical Instructor
Northeastern University
Boston, Massachusetts

Roselena Thorpe, RN, PhD
Professor and Chairperson
Nursing Department
CCAC, Allegheny Campus
Pittsburgh, Pennsylvania

Catherine Ultrino, RN, MSN, OCN
Nurse Manager, Oncology Unit/Oncology Clinic
Boston Regional Medical Center
Stoneham, Massachusetts

Donna Wilsker, RN, BSN, MSN
Assistant Professor
Department of Nursing
Lamar University
Beaumont, Texas

PREFACE

Child health nursing is an expanding area as a result of the broadening scope of practice within the nursing profession and the recognized need for better preventive and restorative care in this area. The importance of this need is reflected in the fact that many of the year 2000 health goals for the nation focus on the nursing care of children. At the same time that the information in this area of nursing is increasing, less time is available in nursing programs to cover it.

Child Health Nursing is written with this challenge in mind. It views child healthcare as a continuum of knowledge from the prenatal period through adolescence. It is designed to present the content comprehensively yet efficiently. It is based on a philosophy of nursing care that respects children as individuals yet views them as part of families and the society.

This book is developed for undergraduate student use in a child health course or for a curriculum in which concepts of child care are integrated throughout the program. It provides a comprehensive, in-depth discussion of the many facets of child health nursing, while promoting a sensitive, holistic outlook on nursing practice. As such, the book is also useful for graduate students who are interested in reviewing or expanding their knowledge in these areas.

Basic themes that are integrated into this text include the experience of wellness and illness as family-centered events; the importance of knowledge of child development in the planning of nursing care; the emphasis of child health promotion as a building block for a lifetime of healthy living; and the significance of the physical and emotional effects of illness on the child. Also included are themes reflective of changes in healthcare delivery and the importance of meeting the needs of a culturally diverse population.

THE CHANGING HEALTHCARE SCENE

Managed care has drastically changed the healthcare delivery system, increasing the role of the nurse from a minor to a major player. Educational changes have to keep pace with healthcare reform so that nurses are prepared for this new level of responsibility. An increasingly multicultural population will continue to be reflected among both nurses and their clients, necessitating fine tuning of culturally sensitive care.

New nursing curricula that are in keeping with this spirit of change emphasize outcomes, a greater emphasis on communication, therapeutic interventions, critical thinking, and the nursing process.

Nursing issues that grow out of the current climate of change include the following:

- **The importance of health teaching with families as a cornerstone of nursing responsibilities.** The teaching role of the nurse has greater significance in the new healthcare milieu as the emphasis on preventive care and short stays in the acute care setting creates the need for families to be better educated in their own care. *Empowering the Family* displays throughout the text address this issue.
- **An emphasis on National Health Goals.** As a way to focus care and research, National Health Goals have gained wider attention at a time when there is a greater need than ever to be wise in the choice of how dollars are spent. Students can familiarize themselves with these goals by referring to the *Focus on National Health Goals* displays that appear at the beginning of each chapter.
- **The importance of individualizing care according to sociocultural uniqueness.** This is a reflection of both greater cultural sensitivity and an increasingly diverse population of caregivers and care recipients. Greater emphasis is being placed on the implications of multiple sociocultural factors in terms of how they affect the patient's response. *Focus on Cultural Competence* displays throughout the text show how cultural factors can be given greater consideration in the planning of care.
- **Changing areas of practice.** The variety of new care settings, as well as the diversity of roles in which workers can practice, is reflected both in the proliferation of community-based nursing facilities and in the increase in the numbers of pediatric and neonatal nurse practitioners. This text places emphasis on the specific needs of clients related to the various healthcare settings in which they find themselves today.

ORGANIZATION OF THE TEXT

Child Health Nursing follows the family and child from the prenatal period through adolescence. Coverage includes ambulatory and in-patient care and focuses on primary as well as secondary and tertiary care.

The book is organized in five units:

Unit I provides an introduction to child health nursing. A framework for practice is presented, as well as current trends and the importance of considering childrearing within a family and sociocultural context.

Unit II examines the nursing role in health promotion for the childbearing family. A separate chapter details the role of the nurse as a genetic counselor and an advocate for fetal health. Additional chapters discuss the care of the newborn and family and the changing role when a complication for the newborn develops. The remaining chapters cover principles of growth and development and care of the child from infancy through adolescence, including child health assessment and health teaching with children and families.

Unit III presents the nursing role in supporting the health of children and their families. The effects of illness on children and their families, diagnostic and therapeutic procedures, and pain management are addressed, with respect to care of the child and family in hospital, home, and ambulatory settings.

Unit IV examines the nursing role in restoring and maintaining the health of children and families when illness occurs. Disorders are presented according to body systems so that students have a ready orientation for locating content.

Unit V discusses the nursing role in restoring and maintaining the mental health of children and families. Separate chapters discuss the role of the nurse with child abuse and when mental, long-term, or fatal illness is present.

PEDAGOGIC FEATURES

Each chapter in the text is organized to provide a complete learning experience for the student. Numerous pedagogic features help the student understand and increase retention. Important elements include the following:

- **Vibrant Full-Color Design.** This striking design has been implemented to highlight all the boxes, tables, illustrations and photos.
- **Chapter Objectives.** Learning objectives are included at the beginning of each chapter to identify the outcomes expected after the material in the chapter has been mastered.
- **Key Terms.** Terms that would be new to the student are listed at the beginning of each chapter in a ready reference list. The terms first appear in boldface type to draw the student's attention to them and are defined as they are used.
- **Tables and Displays.** Numerous tables and displays summarize important information and provide detail on some topics so that the student has a ready reference.
- **Clinical Vignettes.** Short scenarios appear at the beginning of each chapter. These vignettes provide a taste of what is to come in the chapter, preparing the learner for the material to be presented and applying information that was covered previously. At the end of the chapter, critical thinking questions related to the scenario bring the chapter full circle.
- **Checkpoint Questions.** Throughout the text, Checkpoint Questions appear to help the reader check his or her progress and remain focused on the topic at hand. They ask the reader to use the knowledge just gained in the last few pages, thus helping the reader remember this information.
- **"What If" Questions.** What If questions also appear periodically throughout the text. They require further thought than the checkpoint questions, as they ask the reader to apply the information just acquired in an "actual" situation. The reader must process the information and apply it to the new situation, thus maximizing learning and emphasizing critical thinking.
- **Key Points.** A review of important points is highlighted at the end of the chapter in a list, to help the student monitor his or her own comprehension of each chapter.
- **Critical Thinking Exercises.** To involve the student in the decision-making realities of the clinical setting, several questions are posed at the end of each chapter. They can also serve to form a basis for conference or class discussion.

• **References and Suggested Readings.** These provide the student with the information needed to do more in-depth reading of the sources noted in the text, as well as other relevant articles on the topics included in the chapter.

• **Appendices.** Appendices provide another quick reference to laboratory values, growth charts, vital sign parameters, and drugs safe for use during pregnancy and lactation.

NURSING PROCESS

The nursing process format found throughout this text provides a strong theoretical underpinning for this important concept and helps student understand how to use the nursing process in clinical practice.

• **Nursing Process Overview.** Each chapter begins with a review of nursing process in which specific suggestions, such as examples of nursing diagnoses and outcome criteria helpful to modifying care in the area under discussion, are given. These reviews improve students' preparation in clinical areas so they can focus their care planning and apply principles to practice.

• **Nursing Diagnoses and Related Interventions.** A consistent format highlights the nursing diagnosis and related interventions throughout the text. A special heading draws the student's attention to these sections where individual nursing diagnoses, outcome identification, and outcome evaluation are detailed for the major conditions and disorders discussed.

• **Nursing Care Plans.** Nursing care plans are written for specific clients, to stress the importance of individualized care planning. The care plans are written with an emphasis on aiding the student to apply theory to practice and to make use of critical thinking skills.

RECURRING FEATURES

Child Health Nursing includes several special features to help the student meet the challenges of a dynamic healthcare environment. These features, which appear throughout the text, help the student focus on important information or provide additional insights.

• **Focus on National Health Goals.** To emphasize the nursing role in accomplishing the healthcare goals of our nation, these displays state specific ways in which child health nursing can provide better outcomes for both the child and family. They help the student to appreciate the importance of national health planning and the influence that nurses can have in creating a healthier nation.

• **Focus on Nursing Research.** These displays summarize research carried out by nurses on topics related to child health nursing. They appear throughout the text to accentuate the use of research as the basis for nursing care.

• **Focus on Cultural Competence.** These displays serve to broaden the student's perspective on the many specific cultural influences that can affect the nursing goals and interventions that nurses provide in the child health setting. They stress the need for nursing care to be modified to meet individualized needs.

• **Nursing Procedures.** Techniques of procedures specific to child healthcare are boxed in an easy-to-follow two-column format and often enhanced with color figures.

• **Assessing the Client.** These visual guides provide head-to-toe assessment information for overall health status or specific disorders or conditions.

• **Empowering the Family.** These boxes present detailed health teaching information for the family, emphasizing the importance of a partnership between nurses and clients in the management of health and illness.

• **Enhancing Communication.** This feature presents case examples of adequate communication and better communication, illustrating for the student how being aware of communication can improve the patient's understanding and positively impact outcomes.

• **Managing and Delegating Unlicensed Assistive Personnel.** In response to a changing healthcare environment, these boxes present practical information to help the nurse manage and delegate appropriate responsibilities to unlicensed assistive personnel.

• **Drug Highlight.** These boxes provide quick reference for medications that are commonly used for the health problems described in the text. They list the drug name (brand and generic, if applicable), dosage, pregnancy category, side effects, and nursing implications.

ANCILLARY PACKAGE

A complete learning and teaching package includes the following:

- **Free Interactive Self-Study CD-ROM** (stored on the inside back cover of each book). Multiple-choice NCLEX-style questions challenge the student's comprehension and application of important material. Feedback is provided for each answer.
- **Instructor's Manual.** The perfect complement to classroom teaching strategies, this resource contains useful discussion topics, case studies, and critical thinking exercises.
- **Computerized Test Bank.** Multiple-choice NCLEX-style questions include rationales for each question.
- **Overhead Transparencies.** Full-color acetate transparencies illustrating important material enhance student understanding and facilitate classroom discussion.
- **Study Guide.** This companion to the text challenges the student's retention of key concepts and encourages critical thinking and application of information to real nursing situations.

Adele Pillitteri, PhD, RN, PNP

ACKNOWLEDGMENTS

I would like to express my sincere appreciation to: Developmental Editors Danielle DiPalma and Maryann Foley; Jennifer Brogan, Editor; Susan Barta Rainey, Editorial Assistant; Melissa Olson, Art Editor; Helen Ewan, Production Manager; Tom Gibbons, Project Editor; Nannette Winski, Production Coordinator; and all the members of the Production Services Group involved with this text for their assistance and guidance throughout the project; photographers Caroline Brown and Barbara Proud; and the countless nursing reviewers who generously added their expertise to this new edition.

—A.P.

CONTENTS

(continued from inside cover)

DRUG HIGHLIGHT BOXES

ENHANCING COMMUNICATION BOXES

FOCUS ON CULTURAL COMPETENCE BOXES

(continued from page xxix)

NURSING CARE PLANS

ASSESSMENT BOXES

CHILD HEALTH NURSING

Care of the Child and Family

UNIT

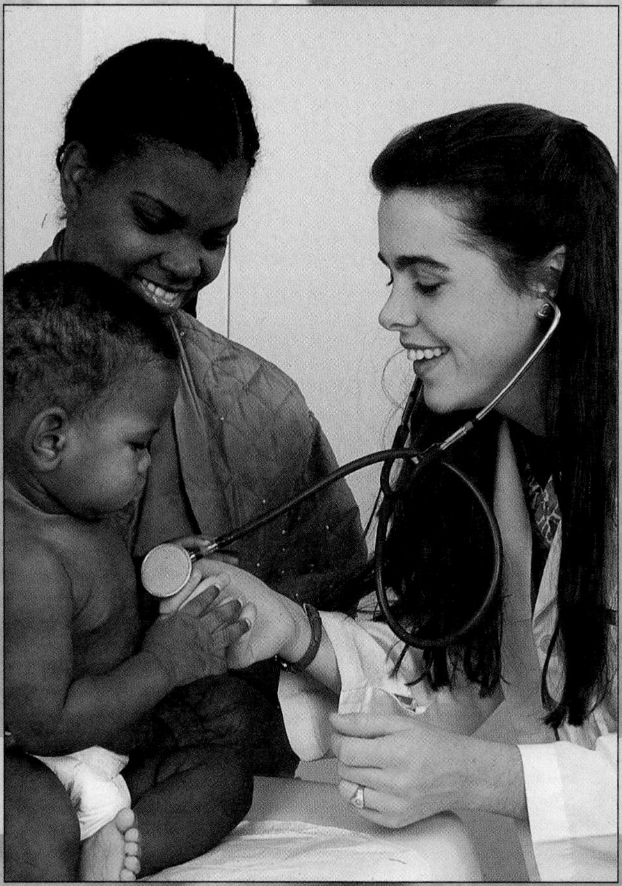

1

CHILD HEALTH NURSING PRACTICE

A Framework for Child Health Nursing

CHAPTER 1

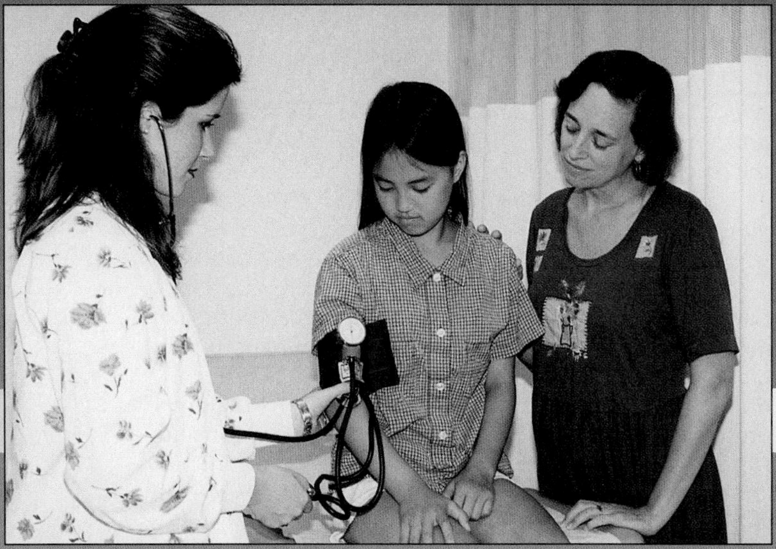

Key Terms

- clinical nurse specialist
- family centered
- family nurse practitioner
- child health nursing
- mortality rate
- neonatal nurse practitioner
- neonate
- nursing research
- pediatric nurse practitioner
- scope of practice
- rooming in

Objectives

After mastering the contents of this chapter, you should be able to:

1. Identify the goals and philosophy of child health nursing.
2. Describe the evolution, scope, and professional roles of child health nursing.
3. Define common statistical terms used in the field, such as *infant mortality* and *neonatal death rate.*
4. Discuss common standards of child health nursing and the health goals for the nation in terms of their implications for child health nursing.
5. Discuss the interplay of nursing process, nursing research, and nursing theory as they relate to the future of child health nursing practice.
6. Use critical thinking to identify areas of care that could benefit from additional nursing research.
7. Integrate knowledge of trends in child health care with the nursing process to achieve an understanding of quality child health nursing care.

Anna Melendez is a newborn with respiratory distress who must be transported to the regional center for care about 30 miles from the local hospital. Her parents, Melissa and Roberto, have many concerns. They don't want to be so far from their daughter, and they don't know how they will pay for her special care. Also, they are aksing many questions about what's wrong with their daughter and who will be taking care of her. Their son, Miguel, now 6 years old, is scared he will never see Anna again. What are some health care issues evident in this scenario? What trends in child health care delivery have affected this family?

In this chapter you'll learn about standards and philosophies of child health care and how these standards and philosophies affect care. After you've studied the chapter, turn to the critical thinking exercises at the end of the chapter to help sharpen your skills and test your knowledge.

Care of childrearing families is a major focus of nursing practice. To have healthy children, it is important to promote the health of the family from the time before children are born until they reach adulthood. As children grow, the family needs continued health supervision and support. As children reach maturity, a new cycle begins and new support becomes necessary. The nurse's role in all these phases focuses on promoting healthy growth and development of the child and family in health and in illness (Figure 1-1).

GOALS AND PHILOSOPHIES OF CHILD HEALTH NURSING

The primary goal of **child health nursing** care can be stated simply as the promotion and maintenance of optimal family health to ensure cycles of optimal childrearing. Major philosophical assumptions about child health nursing are listed in Box 1-1. The goals of child health nursing care are necessarily broad because the scope of practice is so broad. The range of practice includes:

- Care of children during the perinatal period (6 weeks before conception to 6 weeks after birth)
- Care of children from infancy through adolescence
- Care in settings as varied as ambulatory clinics, pediatric intensive care units, and the home

In all settings and types of care, keeping the family at the center of care delivery is an essential goal. Child health nursing is always **family centered,** which means the family is considered the primary unit of care. The level of family functioning impacts the health status of individuals. If the family's level of functioning is low, the emotional, physical, and social health and potential of individuals in that family can be adversely affected. A healthy family, on the other hand, establishes an environment conducive to growth and health-promoting behaviors that sustain family members during crises. Similarly, the health of individuals and the ability to function strongly influences the health of family members and overall family functioning. Thus, a family-centered approach enables the nurse to better understand an individual and, in turn, provide holistic care. Box 1-2 provides

BOX 1.1

PHILOSOPHY OF CHILD HEALTH NURSING

1. Child health nursing is family centered; assessment data must include family as well as individual assessment.
2. Child health nursing is community centered; the health of families both depends on and influences the health of communities.
3. Child health nursing is research oriented because research is the means whereby critical knowledge increases.
4. Nursing theory provides a foundation for nursing care.
5. A child health nurse serves as an advocate to protect the rights of all family members.
6. Child health nursing uses a high degree of independent nursing functions because teaching and counseling are so frequently required.
7. Promoting health is an important nursing role because this protects the health of the next generation.
8. Childhood illnesses can be stressful. They can alter family life in both subtle and extensive ways.
9. Personal, cultural, and religious attitudes and beliefs influence the meaning of illness and its impact on the family. Circumstances such as illness or pregnancy are meaningful only in the context of a total life.
10. Child health nursing is a challenging role for the nurse and is a major factor in promoting high-level wellness in families.

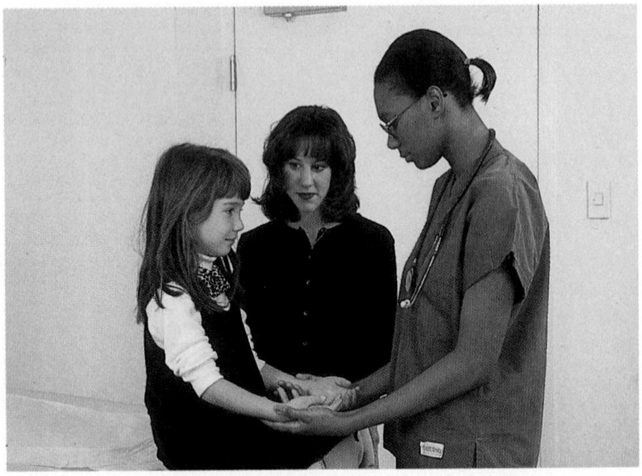

FIGURE 1.1 Child health nursing includes care of the family. During a health maintenance visit, a child health nurse assesses a pediatric client with her mother present.

BOX 1.2

COMMON MEASURES TO ENSURE FAMILY-CENTERED CHILD HEALTH CARE

Principle	*Nursing Interventions*
1. The family is the basic unit of society.	Encourage families to use community services so that family members are not separated by care needs. Encourage rooming-in in child health hospital settings. Participate in early discharge programs to reunite families as soon as possible. Encourage family and sibling visiting in hospitals to promote family contacts.
2. Families represent racial, ethnic, cultural and socioeconomic diversity.	Assess families for strengths and specific needs. Respect diversity in families as a special richness of that family.
3. Children grow both individually and as part of a family.	Include developmental stimulation in care. Encourage families to give care to an ill child. Share or initiate information on health planning with family members so care is family oriented.

a summary of key measures for the delivery of family-centered child health care.

STANDARDS OF CHILD HEALTH NURSING PRACTICE

The importance a society places on caring can best be measured by the concern it places on its most vulnerable members or its elderly, disadvantaged, and young citizens. Specialty organizations develop standards of care to promote consistency and ensure quality nursing care in their areas of nursing practice. In child health, standards were developed in the 1980s by the Division of Maternal Child Health Nursing Practice of the American Nurses' Association to provide important guidelines for planning care and devising outcome criteria for the evaluation of nursing care. Recently updated in connection with the Society of Pediatric Nurses, these standards are shown in Box 1-3.

✔ CHECKPOINT QUESTIONS

1. What is the primary goal of child health nursing?
2. Why is child health nursing family centered?

A FRAMEWORK FOR CHILD HEALTH NURSING CARE

Child health nursing can be visualized within a framework in which nursing, using nursing process, nursing theory, and nursing research, acts to care for families during childrearing years through four phases of health care:

- Health promotion
- Health maintenance
- Health restoration
- Health rehabilitation

Examples of these phases of health care as they relate to child health are shown in Table 1-1.

The Nursing Process

Nursing care, at its best, is designed and implemented in a thorough manner, using an organized series of steps, to ensure quality and consistency of care. The nursing process, a proven form of problem solving based on the scientific method, serves as the basis for assessing, planning, and organizing care. That the nursing process is applicable to all health care settings from the ambulatory and health maintenance clinic to the pediatric intensive care unit is proof that the method is broad enough to serve as the basis for all of nursing care (Carpenito, 1996).

The nursing process consists of five steps:

1. Assessment
2. Nursing diagnosis
3. Outcome identification and planning
4. Implementation
5. Outcome evaluation

All subsequent chapters in this book begin with a Nursing Process Overview that summarizes the major nursing concerns in each step of the process for the content of that particular chapter. Nursing care plans or care pathways throughout demonstrate the use of the nursing process for a selected client, provide examples of critical thinking in nursing, and clarify nursing care for specific client needs.

Nursing Research

Research is the controlled investigation of a problem using a scientific method. Bodies of professional knowledge grow and expand to the extent that people in that profession plan and carry out research. **Nursing research** is the controlled investigation of problems that have impli-

BOX 1.3

AMERICAN NURSES ASSOCIATION/SOCIETY OF PEDIATRIC NURSES STANDARDS OF CARE AND PROFESSIONAL PERFORMANCE

STANDARDS OF CARE

Comprehensive pediatric nursing care focuses on helping children and their families and communities achieve their optimum health potentials. This is best achieved within the framework of family-centered care and the nursing process, including primary, secondary and tertiary care coordinated across health care and community settings.

Standard I: Assessment
The pediatric nurse collects health data.

Standard II: Diagnosis
The pediatric nurse analyzes the assessment data in determining diagnoses.

Standard III: Outcome Identification
The pediatric nurse identifies expected outcomes individualized to the client.

Standard IV: Planning
The pediatric nurse develops a plan of care that prescribes interventions to obtain expected outcomes.

Standard V: Implementation
The pediatric nurse implements the interventions identified in the plan of care.

Standard VI: Evaluation
The pediatric nurse evaluates the child's and family's progress toward attainment of outcomes.

STANDARDS OF PROFESSIONAL PERFORMANCE

Standard I: Quality of Care
The pediatric nurse systematically evaluates the quality and effectiveness of pediatric nursing practice.

Standard II: Performance Appraisal
The pediatric nurse evaluates his or her own nursing practice in relation to professional practice standards and relevant statutes and regulations.

Standard III: Education
The pediatric nurse acquires and maintains current knowledge in pediatric nursing practice.

Standard IV: Collegiality
The pediatric nurse contributes to the professional development of peers, colleagues, and others.

Standard V: Ethics
The pediatric nurse's decisions and actions on behalf of children and their families are determined in an ethical manner.

Standard VI: Collaboration
The pediatric nurse collaborates with the child, family, and health care provider in providing client care.

Standard VII: Research
The pediatric nurse uses research findings in practice.

Standard VIII: Resource Utilization
The pediatric nurse considers factors related to safety, effectiveness and cost in planning and delivering care.

From the American Nurses Association and the Society of Pediatric Nurses. (1996). *Statement on the scope and standards of pediatric clinical practice.* Washington, DC: American Nurses Publishing House.

cations for nursing practice. It is the method by which the foundation of nursing grows, expands, and improves.

Some current examples of questions that warrant nursing investigation in the area of child health nursing are:

- What is the best stimulus to encourage parents to bring children for health maintenance care?
- What is the best use of unlicensed assistive personnel in child health care settings?
- What are the special needs of a child and his family discharged from a same day ambulatory surgery setting?
- How much self-care should a preschooler be expected (or encouraged) to provide during illness?
- What is the effect of managed care on the quality of nursing care?
- What active measures can nurses take to reduce the incidence of child abuse?
- What are the effects of long-term home care on parents' or children's mental health?
- How is high self-esteem maintained in children with a disability?

Focus on Nursing Research boxes found in chapters throughout this text contain summaries of current child health nursing research. It is hoped that the content of these boxes will assist students in developing a question-

TABLE 1.1 Definitions and Examples of Phases of Health Care

TERM	DEFINITION	EXAMPLES
Health promotion	Educating clients to be aware of good health through teaching and role modeling	Teaching children the importance of practices such as thorough tooth brushing or safer sex practices
Health maintenance	Intervening to maintain health when risk of illness is present	Teaching parents the importance of safeguarding their home by childproofing it against poisoning
Health restoration	Prompt diagnosis and treatment of illness using interventions that will return client to wellness most rapidly	Caring for a child during a respiratory illness
Health rehabilitation	Preventing further complications from an illness; bringing ill client back to optimal state of wellness or helping client to accept inevitable death	Helping a child with chronic renal disease to continue to attend school

ing attitude regarding current nursing practice and in thinking of ways to incorporate research findings into care.

Nursing Theory

One of the requirements of a profession (together with other critical determinants, such as member self-set standards, monitoring of practice quality, and participation in research) is that the concentration of a discipline's knowledge flows from a base of established theory.

Nursing theorists offer helpful ways to view clients and nurses so nursing activities can best meet client needs (e.g., by seeing the client not simply as a physical form but as a dynamic force with important psychosocial needs). In child health nursing, it is vital to view clients as extensions or active members of a family as well as holistic beings. Only with this broad focus can nurses appreciate the significant effect of a child's illness or of the introduction of a new member on a family.

Another issue most nursing theorists address is how nurses should be viewed or what should be the goals of nursing care. At one time, the goal of nursing care could have been stated as providing care and comfort to injured and ill people; currently, most nurses would perceive this view as a limited one, because they are equipped to do much more. Extensive changes in the scope of child health nursing have occurred as health promotion or keeping parents and children well becomes more important.

A third issue addressed by nurse theorists concerns the activities of nursing care; as goals become broader, so do activities. For example, when the primary goal of nursing was considered to be caring for ill people, nursing actions were limited to bathing, feeding, and providing comfort. Currently, with the promotion of health as a major nursing goal, teaching, counseling, supporting, and advocacy are also common roles. With new technologies available, nurses are caring for clients who are more ill than ever before. Because care of children during their developing years helps protect not only current health but the health of the next generation, child health nurses fill these expanded roles to a unique and special degree.

Table 1-2 summarizes the tenets of a number of common nursing theorists and suggests ways these could be applied to child health care through the situation of one child. The third column of the table ("Emphasis of Care") demonstrates that, although the theoretical bases of these theories differ, the result of any one of them is to provide a higher level of care. These different theories, therefore, are not contradictory, but rather complement each other in the planning and implementation of holistic nursing care.

CHILD HEALTH NURSING TODAY

At the beginning of the 20th century, the infant mortality rate (the number of infants per 1000 births who die during the first year of life) was over 100 per 1000. In response to efforts to lower this rate, health care shifted from a treatment focus to a preventive one, dramatically changing the scope of child health nursing. Research on the benefits of early prenatal care led to the first major national effort to provide prenatal care to all pregnant women through prenatal nursing services (home visits) and clinics. Today, thanks to these and other community health measures (such as efforts to encourage breastfeeding, increased immunization and injury prevention) as well as many technological advances, the infant mortality rate has fallen from 100 per 1000 to 6.9 per 1000 (National Center for Health Statistics [NCHS], 1998).

Medical technology has contributed to a number of important advances in child health: childhood diseases such as measles and poliomyelitis are almost eradicated; specific genetic markers and genes responsible for many inherited diseases have been identified and will revolutionize medical therapy in the coming years; and the ability to improve life for high risk infants has grown substantially. In addition, a growing trend toward health care consumerism, or self-care, has made many childrearing families active participants in their own health monitoring and care. Health care consumerism has also moved care from hospital to community sites and from long-term hospital stays to overnight surgical and ambulatory settings.

But there is still much more to be done. National health care goals established in 1990 for the year 2000 continue to stress the importance of child health to overall community health (Department of Health and Human Services [DHHS], 1995) and although health care may be more advanced, it is still not accessible to everyone. These and other social changes and trends have expanded the roles of nurses in child health care and, at the same time, have made the delivery of quality child health nursing care a continuing challenge.

calls and snapshots, and encourage the family to visit as soon as possible.

When regionalization concepts of newborn care first became accepted, transporting the ill or premature newborn to the regional care facility was the method of choice (Figure 1-4). Today, however, when it is known in advance that a child may be born with a life-threatening condition, it may be safer to transport the mother to the regional center during pregnancy, because the uterus has advantages as a transport incubator that far exceed any commercial incubator yet designed.

An important argument against regionalization for pediatric care is that children will feel homesick in strange settings, overwhelmed by the number of sick children they see, and frightened because they are miles from home. These are definitely important considerations. Because nurses more than any other health care group set the tone for hospitals, it is their responsibility to see that clients and families feel as welcome in the regional centers as they would have been in a small hospital. Staffing should be adequate enough to allow sufficient time for nurses to comfort frightened children, prepare them for new experiences, and offer support to the family. Documenting the importance of such actions allows them to be incorporated in critical pathways and preserve the importance of the role.

Increased Reliance on Comprehensive Care Settings

Comprehensive health care is designed to meet all of a child's needs in one setting. In the past, care of children tended to be specialized. For example, a child with a congenital anomaly such as myelomeningocele or cerebral palsy might have been followed by a team of specialists for each facet of the problem. Such a team might include a neurologist, a physical therapist, an occupational therapist, a psychologist for intelligence quotient testing, speech therapist, orthopedic surgeon, and finally, a special education teacher. The parents might need to find a special dentist who would accept multihandicapped clients. Each specialist would look only at one area of the child's needs rather than the whole child's development. Without extra guidance, parents would find themselves lost in a maze of visits to different health care personnel. If they were not receiving financial support for their child's care, they might not have been able to afford all the necessary services at one time. It might have been difficult to decide which of the child's problems needed to be treated immediately and which could be left untreated, without worsening and developing into permanent disability. Although specialists are still important to a child's care, a trusted primary care provider to help parents in the coordination of a child's specialized services is essential due to today's managed care environment. In many settings, this primary care provider who follows the child through all phases of care is an advanced practice nurse such as a family nurse practitioner or pediatric nurse practitioner (Cohen & Juszczak, 1997). Nurses can be helpful in seeing that both parents and children have all their needs met by a primary health care provider in this way. The family must become empowered to seek out a family-centered setting that will be best for their health (see Empowering the Family box).

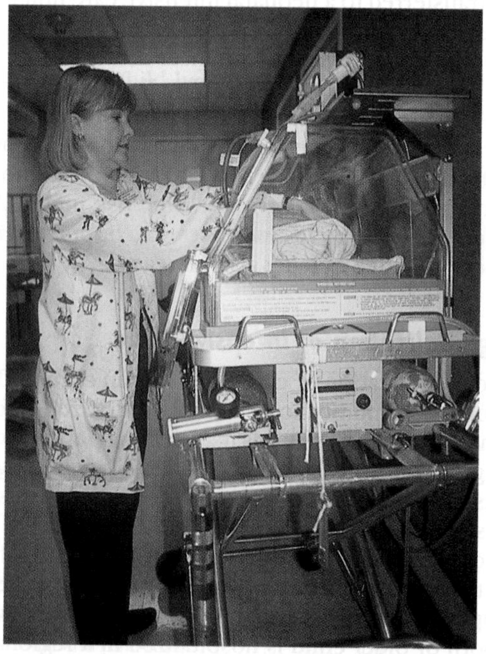

FIGURE 1.4 An infant transport incubator is prepared to move a premature infant to a regional hospital. Helping with safe movement of ill newborns to regional centers is an important nursing responsibility.

Increased Use of Alternative Treatment Modalities

There is a growing tendency for families to consult providers of alternative forms of therapy such as acupuncture or therapeutic touch in addition to, or instead of, traditional health care providers. Nurses have an increasing obligation to be aware of alternative therapies, which have the potential to enhance or detract from the effectiveness of traditional therapy (see Focus on Cultural Competence box).

In addition, the health care team who is unaware of the existence of some alternative forms of therapy may lose an important opportunity to capitalize on the positive features of that particular therapy. For instance, it would be important to know that an adolescent who is about to undergo a painful procedure is experienced at meditation. Asking the adolescent if she wanted to meditate before the procedure could help her relax. Not only could this decrease the child's discomfort, but it could also offer the child a feeling of control over a difficult situation.

Increased Reliance on Home Care

Early hospital discharge has resulted in many children returning home before they are fully ready to care for themselves. Ill children may choose to remain at home for care rather than be hospitalized. This has created a "second system" of care and requires many additional care providers. Nurses are instrumental in assessing children and their fam-

EMPOWERING THE FAMILY: Tips on Selecting a Health Care Setting

1. Can it be reached easily (going for preventive care when well or for care when ill should not be chores)?
2. Will the staff provide continuity of care so you'll always see the same primary care provider if possible?
3. Does the physical set-up of the facility provide for a sense of privacy yet a sense that health care providers share pertinent information so you do not have to repeat your history at each visit?
4. Is the cost of care and the number of referrals to specialists explained clearly?
5. Is preventive care and health education stressed (keeping well is as important as recovering from illness)?
6. Do health care providers respect your opinion and ask for your input on health care decisions?
7. Do health care providers show a personal interest in you?
8. Is health education done at your learning level?
9. Is the facility handicapped accessible?

ilies on hospital discharge to help plan the best type of continuing care; devising and modifying procedures for home care; and sustaining the clients' morale and interest in health care during such situations as home monitoring to control asthma. Because home care is a unique and expanding area in child health nursing, it is discussed in Chapter 15.

Increased Use of Technology

The use of technology is increasing in all health care settings. Learning to do computer charting and to seek information on the Internet are examples of this. In addition to learning these technologies, it is important for child health nurses to be able to explain technology use and advantages to clients. Otherwise, clients can find new technology more frightening than helpful to them.

WHAT IF? What if an infant is to remain hospitalized after surgery in the intensive care unit? How would you address the needs of the child and the family to provide family centered care?

FOCUS ON CULTURAL COMPETENCE

The term *alternative health care practices* refers to therapy such as acupuncture, homeopathy, therapeutic touch, herbalism, and chiropractic care or nontraditional sources of health care such as tribal medicine or *yerberos* or *curanderos.* Some people seek out these types of therapy or alternative providers before consulting a traditional health care provider; others consult them after what they perceive to be inadequate care by a traditional provider.

Respecting these forms of care can be instrumental in showing families that their sociocultural traditions and needs are important. Assessing what nontraditional measures are being used is important because the action can interfere with prescribed medications. For instance, the consumption of traditional ethnic remedies such as Jin Bu Huan, a Chinese herbal medicine to relieve pain, can cause adverse effects such as life-threatening bradycardia and respiratory depression. Lead poisoning has resulted from ingestion of "greta," a traditional Mexican remedy employed as a laxative.

Health Care Concerns and Attitudes

The 1980s brought about considerable change in the health care system and particularly in child health. As we approach the year 2000, there are likely to be even more changes as the United States actively works toward effective health goals and guaranteed health care for all citizens (Nesbitt, 1996).

Increasing Concern Regarding Health Care Costs

The advent of managed care has concentrated efforts on reducing the cost of health care. This has direct implications for child health nursing because nurses must become more aware of the costs of supplies and services. Helping to reduce costs while maintaining quality care has become a major nursing challenge.

Increasing Emphasis on Preventive Care

A generally accepted theory is that it is better to keep individuals well than to restore health after they have become ill. Counseling parents on ways to keep their homes safe for children is an important form of illness prevention in child health nursing. The facts that accidents are still a major cause of death in children is a testament to the need for much more anticipatory guidance in this area (Wegman, 1996).

Increasing Emphasis on Family-Centered Care

Health promotion with families during childrearing is a family-centered event, because teaching health awareness and good health habits is accomplished chiefly by role modeling. Illness in a child is automatically a family-centered event, because parents have to adjust work schedules to allow one of them to stay with the ill child; siblings may have to sacrifice an activity such as a birthday party or having a parent watch their school play; family finances may have to be readjusted to pay for hospital and medical bills. A family may feel drawn together by the fright and concern of an acute illness; unfortunately, when an illness becomes chronic, it may pull a family apart or destroy it.

In recent years, the US government has recognized that the care of individual family members is a family-centered event. The Family Medical Leave Act (FMLA) of 1993 is a federal law that requires employers with 50 or more employees to provide a minimum of 12 weeks of unpaid, job-protected leave to employees under four circumstance crucial to family life:

1. Upon the birth of the employee's child
2. Upon the adoption or foster placement of a child with the employee
3. When the employee is needed to care for a parent, spouse, or child with a serious health condition
4. Whenever the employee is unable to perform his or her functions because of a serious health condition (29 CFR 825.11)

A "serious health condition is an illness, injury, impairment, or physical or mental condition involving such circumstances as inpatient care or incapacity requiring 3 workdays' absence. Illness must be documented by a health care provider." Nurse pracitioners are specifically listed as those who can document a health condition (McGovern & Cossi, 1995).

By adopting a view of a new child or illness as a family event, nurses are well equipped to provide family-centered care. Nurses can be instrumental in including family members in events from which they were once totally excluded, such as an unplanned emergency surgery. They can help child health care to be family centered by consulting with family members about a plan of care and providing clear health teaching so family members can monitor their own care (Figure 1-5). Nurses play an active role in both health promotion teaching and sustaining families through a child's illness. Nurses can educate families about the Family Medical Leave Act; many people are still not aware that they can take time off to spend with a new baby, to care for a child with a serious health condition or to tend to a personal health crisis. Nurse practitioners can help ensure that the criteria of the FMLA are met by appropiately documenting a client's health condition.

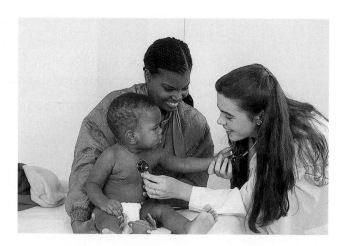

FIGURE 1.5 Family-centered care: The nurse involves the family in the care of the child.

Increasing Concern for the Quality of Life

In the past, health care of children was centered on maintaining physical health. More recently, however, a growing awareness that the quality of life is as important as physical health has expanded the scope of health care to include the assessment of psychosocial facets of life in such areas as self-esteem and independence. Good interviewing skills are necessary to elicit this information at health care visits. Nurses can be instrumental not only in assessing for such information but also in planning ways to improve the quality of life in the areas the client considers most important.

One way in which the quality of life is being improved for children with chronic illness is the national mandate to allow them to attend regular school; they are guaranteed entrance despite severe illness or use of medical equipment such as a ventilator (Public Law 99-452). Nurses, serving as school nurses or consultants to schools, play important roles in making these efforts possible.

Increasing Awareness of the Individuality of Clients

Children today do not fit readily into any set category. Varying family structures, cultural backgrounds, socioeconomic statuses and individual circumstances lead to unique and diverse clients. As a result of advancements in research and treatments, children who previously would not have survived are now growing and thriving. Individuals with mental and physical disabilities are also establishing families and rearing children. Many families who have come from foreign countries enter the US health care system for the first time with a sick child. This requires a greater sensitivity in the health care provider to the sociocultural aspects of care. As the level of violence in the world increases, more and more families are exposed to living in potentially violent communities (Campbell & Schwarz, 1996). The incidence of abused children is also increasing. All of these concerns require increased nursing concern.

Empowerment of Health Care Consumers

Due in part to the influence of managed care and a strengthened focus on health promotion and disease prevention, individuals and families have recently begun to take increased responsibility for their own health. This begins with learning preventive measures to stay well. For some families, it means following a more nutritious diet and planning regular exercise; for others, it can mean an entire change in lifestyle. When a family member is ill, empowerment means learning more about the illness, participation in the treatment plan, and preventing the ilness from returning. Families are very interested in participating in decision making regarding their options. Parents want to accompany their ill children into the hospital for overnight stays. They are eager for information about their child's health and want to contribute to the decision-making process. They may question treatments or care plans that they feel are not in their child's best interest. When health care providers do not provide answers to a client's questions or are insensitive to needs, many health care consumers are willing to take their business to another health care setting.

Nurses can be instrumental in promoting empowerment of parents and children by respecting views and concerns, addressing clients by name, and by regarding parents as important participants in their child's health—keeping them informed and helping them to make decisions about their child's care. Although the nurse may have seen 25 clients already in a particular day, he or she can make each client feel as important as the first by showing a warm manner and keen interest. Empowering the Family displays are presented throughout the text to provide insight into ways in which the nurse may help empower the family.

✔ CHECKPOINT QUESTIONS

7. How does the Family Medical Leave Act support family-centered care?
8. Why has empowerment of the health care consumer become increasingly important?

ADVANCED PRACTICE ROLES FOR NURSES IN CHILD HEALTH CARE

As trends in child health care change, so do the roles. All child health nurses function in a variety of settings as caregivers, client advocates, researchers, case managers, and educators.

Family Nurse Practitioner

A **family nurse practitioner** (FNP) is an advanced practice role, which provides health care all persons throughout the age span working in conjunction with a physician. The FNP takes the health and pregnancy history, performs physical examinations, orders appropriate diagnostic and laboratory tests, and plans continued care through pregnancy and for the family afterward. FNPs then follow the family indefinitely to promote health and optimal family functioning.

Neonatal Nurse Practitioner

The **neonatal nurse practitioner** (NNP) is skilled in the care of the newborn, both well and ill. NNPs may work in level I, II or III newborn nurseries, neonatal intensive care units, neonatal follow-up clinics, physician groups, or in transporting the ill infant. The NNP's responsibilities include managing patient care in an intensive care unit, conducting normal newborn assessments and physical examinations, and providing high-risk follow-up discharge planning (Britton, 1997).

Pediatric Nurse Practitioner

A **pediatric nurse practitioner** (PNP) is a nurse prepared with extensive skills in physical assessment, interviewing, and well-child counseling and care. In this role, a nurse interviews parents as part of an extensive health history and performs a physical assessment of the child. If the nurse's diagnosis is that the child is well, he or she discusses with the parents any childrearing problems mentioned in the interview; gives any immunizations needed; offers necessary anticipatory guidance (based on the nursing plan); and arranges a return appointment for the next well-child checkup. The nurse serves as a primary health caregiver or as the sole health care person the parents and child see at all visits.

The PNP who determines that a child has a common illness (e.g., iron deficiency anemia) orders the necessary laboratory tests and prescribes appropriate drugs for therapy (Figure 1-6). If the PNP determines that the child has a major illness (e.g., congenital subluxated hip, kidney disease, or heart disease), he or she consults with an associated pediatrician; together, they decide what further care is necessary. Nurse practitioners may also work in inpatient or specialty settings providing continuity of care to hospitalized children. As school nurse practitioners, they provide care to all children in a given community or school setting (Jones & Clark, 1997).

Clinical Nurse Specialists

Clinical nurse specialists are nurses prepared at the master's degree level who are capable of acting as consultants in their area of expertise, as well as serving as role models, researchers, and teachers of quality nursing care. Examples of areas of specialization in child health care are neonatal and child and adolescent health care.

Consider, for example, how a clinical nurse specialist might intervene to help in the care of a 4-year-old child with diabetes mellitus who has been admitted to the hos-

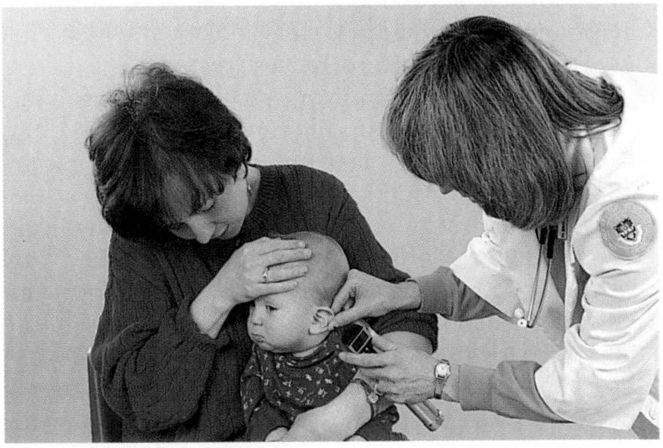

FIGURE 1.6 Pediatric nurse practitioner is an extended role for nurses.

pital. The child is difficult to care for because he is so fearful of hospitalization and perplexed because his parents are having difficulty accepting his diagnosis. A clinical nurse specialist could be instrumental in helping a primary nurse organize care and meet with the parents to help them accept what is happening. Neonatal clinicians manage infant's care at birth and in intensive care settings; they provide home follow-up care to ensure the newborn remains well.

Case Manager

A Case Manager is a graduate level nurse who supervises a group of patients from the time they enter a health care setting until they are discharged from the setting, monitoring the effectiveness and cost and satisfaction of their health care. Case management can be a vastly satisfying type of nursing role because if the health care setting is one with "seamless walls" or follows people both during an illness and on their return to the community, it involves long-term contacts and lasting relationships.

CHECKPOINT QUESTIONS

9. Why have family nurse practitioners become a popular advanced practice role?
10. In what roles does a pediatric nurse practitioner function?

LEGAL CONSIDERATIONS OF PRACTICE

Legal concerns arise in all areas of health care. Child health nursing carries some legal concerns that extend above and beyond other areas of nursing, because care is often given to clients who are not of legal age for giving consent for medical procedures. Nurses are legally responsible for protecting the rights of their clients and accountable for the quality of their individual nursing care and that of other health care team members. Understanding the **scope of practice** (the range of services and care that may be provided by the nurse based on state requirements) and standards of care can help nurses practice within appropriate legal parameters.

Informing clients about their rights and responsibilites is helpful in protecting them. In a society in which child abuse is of national concern, nurses are becoming increasingly responsible for identifying and reporting each incident of suspected abuse in children (Pillitteri et al, 1993).

Documentation is essential in protecting the nurse and justifying his or her actions. This concern is long lasting, because children who feel they were wronged by health care personnel can bring a lawsuit at the time they reach legal age. This means that a nursing note written today may need to be defended as many as 20 years in the future. Nurses need to be conscientious about obtaining informed consent for invasive procedures and in determining that parents are aware of any risks to the child involved with a procedure or test. In divorced or blended families (those in which two adults with children from previous relationships now live together), it is important to establish who has the right to give consent for health care. Personal liability insurance is strongly recommended for all nurses so they do not incur great financial losses during a malpractice or professional negligence suit.

If a nurse knows that the care provided by another practitioner was inappropriate or insufficient, he or she is legally responsible for reporting the incident. Failure to do so can lead to a charge of negligence or breach of duty.

The exact legal ramifications of procedures or care are discussed in further chapters with procedures or treatment modalities.

ETHICAL CONSIDERATIONS OF PRACTICE

Ethical issues are increasing in frequency in health care today (Pappas, 1997). Some of the most difficult decisions in health care settings are those that involve children and their families. Just a few of the major potential conflicts include:

- Abortion, particularly partial-birth abortions
- Resuscitation (how long should it be continued?)
- How many procedures or how much pain should a child be asked to endure to achieve a degree of better health?
- What should be the balance between modern technology and quality of life?

Legal and ethical aspects of issues are often intertwined, which makes the decision-making process complex. Because child health nursing is so strongly family centered, it is common to encounter some situations in which the interests of one family member are in conflict with those of another. It is not unusual for the values of a family to not match those of a health care provider. For example, when a child's condition is considered to be terminal, the family must make a decision about further treatment and life-support measures. The circumstances are usually not clear-cut and the decisions that need to be made are difficult. The nurse is certain to discover many different issues in the course of practice and can do much to aid clients when they reach such decision-making impasses by providing factual information and supportive listening and by aiding the family in clarification of values.

The United Nations Declaration of Rights of the Child (see Appendix A) provides guidelines for determining the rights of clients in regards to health care.

KEY POINTS

Standards of child health nursing practice have been formulated by the ANA in conjunction with the Society of Pediatric Nurses to serve as guides for practice.

Nursing theory and nursing research are methods by which child health nursing expands and improves.

The most significant measure of child health is the infant mortality rate. It is the number of deaths in infants from birth to 1 year per 1000 live births. This rate is declining steadily, but in the United States is still higher than 20 other nations.

Trends in child health nursing include changes in the settings of care, increased concern about health care costs, increased preventive care and family-centered care.

Advanced practice roles in child health nursing include family, neonatal, and pediatric nurse practitioners; clinical nurse specialists; and case managers. All of these expanded roles contribute to making child health care an important area of nursing and health care.

Child health care has both legal and ethical considerations over and above other areas of practice.

CRITICAL THINKING EXERCISES

1. How might family-centered care help the Melendez family described in the beginning of the chapter? How can you empower the family to better care for Anna?
2. Canada has a health care delivery system based not on profit but on provision of care for all citizens through a tax-supported program. The infant mortality rate in Canada is lower than in the United States. What are some reasons that might contribute to this? How do sociocultural aspects affect infant mortality rate?
3. Interview a pediatric nurse practitioner. Prepare a presentation for your fellow students about the roles, functions, and responsibilities of this advanced practice role.

REFERENCES

American Nurses Association and the Society of Pediatric Nurses. (1996). *Statement of the scope and standards of pediatric clinical practice.* Washington, D.C. American Nurses Publishing House.

Britton, J.R. (1997). Neonatal nurse practitioner and physician use on a newborn resuscitation team in a community hospital. *Journal of Pediatric Health Care, 11*(2), 61.

Campbell, C., & Schwarz, D.F. (1996). Prevalence and impact of exposure to interpersonal violence among suburban and urban middle school students. *Pediatrics, 98*(3.1), 396.

Carpenito, L.J. (1996). *Nursing diagnosis: Application to clinical practice* (5th ed.). Philadelphia: Lippincott-Raven.

Centers for Disease Control (1998).Guidelines for treatment of sexually transmitted diseases. *MMWR, 47*(RR-1), 10.

Cohen, S.S., & Juszczak, L. (1997). Promoting the nurse practitioner role in managed care. *Journal of Pediatric Health Care, 11*(1), 3.

Department of Health and Human Services (1995). *Healthy people 2000: Midcourse review.* Washington, D.C.: Public Health Service.

Department of Health and Human Services (1997). Births, marriages, divorces, and deaths for 1996. *Monthly Vital Statistics Report, 45*(12), 5.

Gazmararian, J.A., et al. (1997). Maternity experiences in a managed care organization. *Health Affairs, 16*(3), 198.

Guyer, B. (1997). Annual summary of vital statistics. *Pediatrics, 100*(6), 905.

Hickson, G.B. (1997). Pediatric practice and liability risk in a managed care environment. *Pediatric Annals, 26*(3), 179.

Jones, M.E., & Clark, D. (1997). Increasing access to health care: A study of pediatric nurse practitioner outcomes in a school-based clinic. *Journal of Nursing Care Quality, 11*(4), 53.

Katz, D.A. (1997). The profile of HIV infection in women: A challenge to the profession. *Social Work in Health Care, 24*(3), 127.

Kerfoot, K. (1997). The health care organization and patterns of nursing care delivery. In J. Zerwekh & J.C. Claborn (eds.). *Nursing today: Transition and trends.* Philadelphia: W.B. Saunders.

McGovern, P.M., & Cossi, D.A. (1995). The Family Medical Leave Act. *AAOHN Journal, 43*(10), 508.

National Center for Health Statistics (1998). Trends and current status in childhood mortality. *Vital and Health Statistics, 42,* 21.

National Center for Health Statistics (1998). Births, marriages, divorces and deaths. *Monthly Vital Statistics Report, 46*(7), 4.

Nesbitt, T.S. (1996). Rural maternity care: New models of access. *Birth, 23*(3), 161.

Pappas, A. (1997). Ethical issues. In J. Zerwekh & J.C. Claborn (eds.). *Nursing today: Transition and trends.* Philadelphia: W.B. Saunders.

Pillitteri, A., et al. (1993). Parent gender, victim gender and family socioeconomic influences on the reporting of child abuse by nurses. *Issues in Comprehensive Pediatric Nursing, 16,* 287.

Ryan, S., Jones, M., & Weitzman, M. (1996). School based health services. *Current Opinion in Pediatrics, 8*(5), 453.

Walton, J.C. & Waszkiewicz, M. (1997). Managing unlicensed assistive personnel. *MEDSURG Nursing Journal, 6*(1), 24.

Wegman, M.E. (1996). Infant mortality: Some international comparisons. *Pediatrics, 98*(6.1), 1020.

SUGGESTED READINGS

Brindis, C.D., & Sanghvi, R.V. (1997). School-based health clinics: Remaining viable in a changing health care delivery system. *Annual Review of Public Health, 18,* 567.

Gascoigne, G.B. (1997). The 1996 U.S. Preventive Services Task Force Report: What's no longer worth doing? *Clinical Pediatrics, 36*(5), 273.

Meerabeau, L. (1998). Consumerism and healthcare. *Journal of Advanced Nursing, 27*(4), 721.

Neill, S.J., & Muir, J. (1997). Educating the new community children's nurses: Challenges and opportunities? *Nurse Education Today, 17*(1), 7.

Reinhard, C., Paul, W.S., & McAuley, J.B. (1997). Epidemiology of pediatric tuberculosis in Chicago, 1974 to 1994: A continuing public health problem. *American Journal of the Medical Sciences, 313*(6), 336.

The Childrearing Family

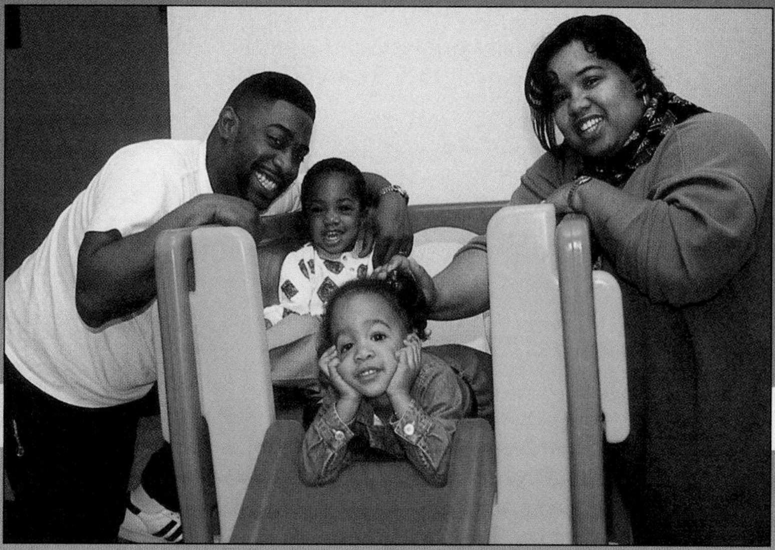

2
CHAPTER

Key Terms

- community
- ecomap
- family
- family nursing
- family of orientation
- family of procreation
- family theory
- genogram

Objectives

After mastering the contents of this chapter, you should be able to:

1. Describe family structure, function, and family roles.
2. Assess a family for structure and health.
3. Formulate nursing diagnoses related to family health.
4. Develop outcomes to assist a family achieve optimal health.
5. Plan nursing health teaching strategies, such as helping a family modify its lifestyle to accommodate an ill child.
6. Implement nursing care, such as teaching a family more effective wellness behaviors.
7. Evaluate outcomes for achievement and effectiveness of nursing care to be certain that goals have been achieved.
8. Identify National Health Goals related to the family and specific ways that nurses can help the nation achieve these goals.
9. Identify areas of care related to family nursing that could benefit from additional nursing research.
10. Use critical thinking to analyze additional ways that nursing care can be family centered or that client care can better include family members.
11. Integrate knowledge of family nursing with nursing process to promote quality child health nursing care.

Marlo Hanavan is a 32-year-old bookkeeper and the mother of two small children, ages one month and 2 years. Her 2 year old daughter has just been diagnosed by their family practitioner as having cerebral palsy. She needs long-term physical therapy and attends a special school. Mr. Hanavan is unemployed because of an accident at work. He has some income from selling woodworking products at craft shows. Mrs. Hanavan states that on many weeks she doesn't have enough money to pay bills; she is forced to choose between health care and groceries. Is the Hanavan family a well family?

In the previous chapter, you learned about the philosophy of child health nursing and the roles that nurses play in this area. In this chapter, you'll add information about families that helps to ensure a healthy outcome for children. This is important information because inadequate parenting because of a dysfunctional family structure can be responsible for poor childrearing practices.

After you've studied the chapter, turn to the Critical Thinking Exercises at the end of the chapter to sharpen your skills and test your knowledge.

No social group has the potential to provide the same level of support and long-lasting emotional ties as one's family. Maintaining healthy family life is so important that a number of National Health Goals speak directly to maintaining healthy family life (see the Focus on National Health Goals box). Because of the importance of the family to the individual, family-centered care has become a focus of modern nursing practice. **Family nursing,** a distinct specialty area that sees the family rather than the individual as its client, is based on concepts about family behavior (Kirschling et al, 1994). **Family theory** is a set of perspectives *from the family's point of view* that helps the nurse address the important health issues of the childrearing family. The strain on a family can be tremendous when a child is ill or passing through a difficult developmental period such as adolescence.It is important that family structures and roles be flexible enough to adjust to the changes. The roles individuals assume in the family and the general family structure can also influence a family's perception of their child's illness, as well as their ability to adjust to these situations and positively influence their outcome.

For all these reasons, family-centered child health nursing considers the strengths, vulnerabilities, and patterns of family functioning in order to support families through the passages of childrearing and to encourage healthy coping mechanisms within families facing a crisis. This means that health assessment and intervention planning should include consideration of social, emotional, spiritual, and financial resources, as well as the physical condition of the home and the community environment.

This chapter defines the concept of family and describes family types, family functions, and variations that affect family life. With these elements in mind, it then addresses family assessment and the family's place as part of the community.

FOCUS ON NATIONAL HEALTH GOALS

A number of National Health Goals speak directly to achieving healthy family and community life. The following goals are representative:

- Lower the current baseline of 25.2 children per 1000 who are younger than age 18 who are maltreated.
- Reduce the prevalence of blood lead levels exceeding 15 µg/dL in children aged 6 months to 5 years to no more than 500,000 from a current baseline of 3,000,000 (DHHS, 1995).

Nurses can be instrumental in helping to see that goals such as these for more healthy family living are met by assessing families and their environment to identify families at risk, assisting with counseling or further testing, and maintaining contact with families to ensure long-term measures for care can be instituted. Family violence is further discussed in Chapter 33; lead poisoning from excessive lead in the environment is discussed in Chapter 31.

NURSING PROCESS OVERVIEW

for Promotion of Family Health

Assessment

Family assessment provides information on the meaning of a current health situation to family members and the emotional support that can be expected to be offered to an individual from the family. It is vital to understanding what childhood illness means to the family. Family structure and function are both considered (see Managing and Delegating Unlicensed Assistive Personnel).

Nursing Diagnosis

Nursing diagnoses used in connection with families generally relate to the family's ability to handle stress

MANAGING AND DELEGATING UNLICENSED ASSISTIVE PERSONNEL

Unlicensed assistive personnel have many opportunities to interact with families in waiting rooms at ambulatory health care visits, in emergency rooms, or when families are waiting for a member to return from surgery. Teach unlicensed assistive personnel to use these occasions, not for simple chatting but to observe family interactions. Families often relate easily with such people and share information with them that they do not share with professional health care providers (perceiving health care providers as too busy to have time to listen).

and to provide a positive environment for individual growth and development. Examples include:

- Parental role conflict related to prolonged separation from child during a long hospitalization
- Altered family processes related to emergency hospital admission of oldest child
- Ineffective family coping related to inability to adjust to child's illness
- Family coping: Potential for growth related to improved perceptions of child's capabilities
- Health-seeking behaviors related to lack of knowledge to foster the child's growth and development.

Altered parenting and Parental role conflict are diagnoses that suggest that parents need additional help with the parenting role. The first coping diagnosis (Ineffective family coping) indicates that a family is not functioning at an optimum level; the second (Potential for growth) is used for a well family or one that is exhibiting enhanced growth with regard to a specific event, such as the sudden diagnosis of illness in a child. Potential for enhanced parenting and Health-seeking behaviors are diagnoses that apply to families actively investigating more effective ways to manage stress and improve family functioning.

Outcome Identification and Planning

Planning for nursing care must include a design that is appropriate and desired by the majority of family members. This type of family-centered goal setting is important in promoting compliance. The plan of care must also consider community environment; for example, it is not helpful to suggest that a family take regular walks together to improve their relating skills if their neighborhood is unsafe; a regular outing at the local YWCA in a family gym class might be more practical. Urging family members to plan together not only encourages shared decisions but promotes improved family communication.

Implementation

A plan for improving family health can be implemented easily if family members have agreed on it out of support for one another. It may be necessary in some instances to encourage family members to agree on a plan or to abide by a chosen plan; otherwise, they may expend needless energy carrying out an activity that is counterproductive or in direct opposition to the major goal.

Outcome Evaluation

Evaluation should reveal not only that a goal was achieved but that the family feels more cohesive after working together toward the goal. If evaluation does not reveal these two factors, reassessment is needed to determine whether further interventions are still required. Examples of outcome criteria that might be established are:

- Family members state they are adapting well to the presence of a newborn.
- Mother states she feels prepared to manage home care of her ill child.
- Father states he has arranged the family financial resources to accommodate health care expenses for the family.

THE FAMILY

How well a family works together and meets any crisis depends on its structure (family composition) and function (activities or roles family members carry out) and how well the family can organize itself against potential threats.

Defining the Concept of Family

A **family** is defined by the U.S. Census Bureau as "a group of people related by blood, marriage, or adoption living together" (U.S. Bureau of the Census, 1997). This definition is workable for gathering comparative statistics but is necessarily limited when assessing a family for health concerns or support people available because, in reality, families can and do occur between unmarried couples. Spradley & Allender (1996) define the family in a much broader context as "two or more people who live in the same household (usually), share a common emotional bond, and perform certain interrelated social tasks." This is a better definition for health care providers because it addresses the broad range of types of families health care providers encounter. Like individuals, families manifest both wellness behaviors and illness behaviors. Box 2-1 lists generally accepted characteristics of a "well" or functioning family. Wellness behaviors may decrease during

BOX 2.1

TWELVE BEHAVIORS INDICATING A WELL FAMILY

1. The ability to provide for the physical, emotional, and spiritual needs of family members.
2. The ability to be sensitive to the needs of family members.
3. The ability to communicate thoughts and feelings effectively.
4. The ability to provide support, security, and encouragement.
5. The ability to initiate and maintain growth-producing relationships.
6. The capacity to maintain and create constructive and responsible community relationships.
7. The ability to grow with and through children.
8. The ability to perform family roles flexibly.
9. The ability to help oneself and to accept help when appropriate.
10. The capacity for mutual respect for the individuality of family members.
11. The ability to use a crisis experience as a means of growth.
12. A concern for family unity, loyalty, and interfamily cooperation.

Reprinted from Otto, H. (1963). Criteria for assessing family strengths. *Family Process, 2,* 329, with permission.

periods of heightened stress. Assessing families for these characteristics is helpful in establishing the extent of wellness or illness behavior and empowering a family to move toward reality behaviors (Bushy, 1997).

Family Types

Many types of families exist and a family type may change over time as it is affected by birth, work, death, divorce, and the growth of family members. For the purposes of description of family in child health nursing, two basic family structures can be described:

- **Family of orientation** (the family one is born into; or oneself, mother, father, and siblings, if any)
- **Family of procreation** (a family one establishes; or oneself, spouse, and children)

More specific descriptions vary greatly depending on family roles, generational issues, means of family support, and sociocultural influences (see the Focus on Cultural Competence box). Although the traditional household of a married couple with children makes up 74% of the total families of children, this number represents a decline compared to previous years. Increasing in incidence is the single-headed family (an increase from 10% of all families in 1960 to nearly 26% in 1997) (NCHS, 1998).

The Nuclear Family

The traditional nuclear family structure is composed of a husband, wife, and children. As young people move away from their parents when they marry or establish independent housekeeping, more and more families today are nuclear in structure (no grandparents, aunts, or uncles live in the home). After World War II, the nuclear family became the most common family structure as young, married people began to move away from their parents. Today, the number of nuclear families in the United States is declining due to the increase in divorce, single-parenthood, and remarriage; the acceptance of alternative lifestyles; and greater disparity. An advantage of a nuclear family is its ability to provide support to family members because people feel genuine affection for each other. Although a person receives strong support from such a family structure, the nuclear family may offer limited support in time of illness or other crisis (there are fewer family members to share the burden and offer support).

> **FOCUS ON CULTURAL COMPETENCE**
>
> Families tend to display characteristics of their culture and community. Knowing some of the basic norms and taboos of different cultural groups is an important part of the nurse's knowledge base. This basic knowledge of a family's cultural background helps the nurse to understand the family's value system and the degree of support family members have available.
>
> The types of families that live in communities tend to be culturally determined: some cultures enjoy extended families; others consist of single-parent families. Some cultures respect elderly family members and depend on them for advice; others are more oriented in the present. Whether families are headed by males or females is also culturally determined.
>
> Remember that poverty is a major problem for many nondominant ethnic groups. Characteristic responses that are sometimes described as cultural limitations are actually the consequences of poverty, for example, parents seeking medical care for their child late in the course of an illness. Solving some problems may be a question of locating adequate financial resources rather than overcoming cultural influences.

The Extended (Multigenerational) Family

The extended family includes not only the nuclear family but other family members such as grandmothers, grandfathers, aunts, uncles, cousins, and grandchildren. An advantage of such a family is that it offers more people to serve as resources during crises and provides more role models for behavior and learning values. A possible disadvantage of an extended family is that family resources must be stretched to accommodate all members. In an extended family, a person's strongest support person or a child's primary caregiver may not be the mother or father. The grandmother or an aunt, for example, may provide the largest amount of child care, even though the child's mother is also present every day.

The Single-Parent Family

In as many as 50% to 60% of families with school-age children today, only one parent lives in the home. This increase in single-parent families is due both to the high rate of divorce and to the increasingly common practice in the United States of women raising children outside marriage (Guyer, 1997). A health problem in a single-parent family is almost always compounded, because if the parent is ill there is no back-up person for child care. If a child is ill, there is no close support person to give reassurance or a second opinion on whether the child's health is improving.

Low income is often an additional problem encountered by single-parent families, because the parent is most often a woman (single-father households account for only 4% of parent–child households). Low income occurs because women's incomes are lower than men's by about 40%. Single parents also may have difficulty with role modeling or identifying their own role in the family (they must provide financial support as well as child care). Trying to fulfill several central roles is not only time consuming but mentally and physically exhausting, and, in many instances, dissatisfying. Such a parent may have low self-esteem (if a spouse left or if the other parent refuses to help with child support). Single-parent fathers may have difficulty with home management or child care if they had little experience with these roles. This interferes with decision making and can impede effective daily functioning (Figure 2-1).

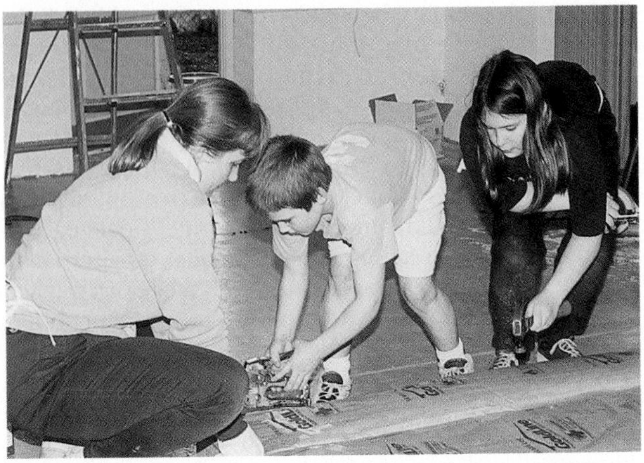

FIGURE 2.1 Working together as a family instills a sense of family pride.

A single-parent family has the advantage of offering a child a special parent–child relationship and increased opportunities for self-reliance and independence. If there has been a divorce, one parent may have been given legal custody of the children or both parents may have joint custody. Either way, both parents often participate in decision making. At a time of illness, both may be active in visiting a hospitalized child and anxious to receive reports of the child's progress. Identifying who is the custodial parent is important when consent forms for care are signed.

The Blended Family

In a blended family or "remarriage" or "reconstituted family," a divorced or widowed person with children marries someone who also has children of his or her own. Advantages of blended families are increased security and resources. Another benefit is that the children of blended families are exposed to different ways of life and may become more adaptable to new situations.

Childrearing problems may arise in this type of family from rivalry among the children for the attention of a parent or competition with the stepparent for the love of the biologic parent. In addition, each spouse may encounter difficulties helping to rear the other's children. Often stepparents believe they are thrust into a limited or challenged role of authority. Children may not welcome a stepparent because they have not yet resolved their feelings about the separation of their biologic parents (either through divorce or death); the stepparent may differ from their biologic parents, particularly in terms of discipline and caregiving; or they may believe that the stepparent threatens their relationship with their biologic parent. They may also become distressed at seeing their other biologic parent move into another home and become a stepparent to other children.

Moreover, financial difficulties can be severe for a number of reasons. One parent may be obligated to pay child support for children from a previous marriage while supporting children of the current marriage. Economic disparity between biologic parents can create conflicts and distorted expectations. Nurses can be instrumental in offering emotional support to members of a remarriage family until the adjustments for mutual living have been made.

The Communal Family

Communes are comprised of groups of people who have chosen to live together as an extended family group; their relationship to each other is motivated by social value or interest rather than by kinship. The values of commune members are often religiously or spiritually based and may be more freedom and free-choice oriented than those of a traditional family structure. Because of the number of people present, members may have few set traditional family roles. Some commune communities are described as cults or are composed of a group of people who follow a charismatic leader.

People with this philosophy may have difficulty conforming with health care regimens (health care may be seen as an established system that they are rejecting). On the other hand, people who reject traditional values may be the most creative people in a community and the most interested in participating in their own care and thus may have the best outcomes from therapy.

The Cohabitation Family

Cohabitation families comprise couples who are living together but remain unmarried. They may be heterosexual or homosexual. Such people can offer as much psychological comfort to each other as those who are formally married. Although such a relationship may be temporary, it may also be as long lasting and as meaningful as a more traditional alliance. Long-term cohabitation alliances are growing in number because of pressure to adhere to a monogamous relationship to avoid contracting human immunodeficiency virus (HIV) or other sexually transmitted diseases, an increased fear of divorce and its effects, and a more widespread acceptance of cohabitation.

The Single Alliance Family

Many single young adults live together in shared apartments, dormitories or homes for companionship and financial security while completing school or beginning their careers. Although these relationships are often temporary, they have the same characteristics as cohabitation families.

The Gay or Lesbian Family

In homosexual unions, individuals of the same sex live together as partners for companionship and sexual fulfillment. Such a relationship offers support in times of crisis comparable with that offered by a traditional nuclear or a cohabitation family. Some lesbian and gay families include children because of previous heterosexual marriages or through the use of artificial insemination or adoption (Brewaeys & van Hall, 1997). Laws governing homosexual partners can affect health care if homosexual partners are not covered by health insurance policies. Lack of understanding by health care providers can further impede health care (Harrison & Silenzio, 1996, Perrin & Kulkin, 1996).

The Foster Family

Children whose parents are unable to care for them may be placed in a foster or substitute home by a child protection agency (Carlson, 1996). Foster parents receive remuneration for their care. They may or may not have children of their own or other foster children. Foster home placement is theoretically temporary until children can be returned to their own parents. If return is impossible or is not imminent, children may be raised to adulthood in foster care. Such children may feel insecure in such settings, concerned that soon they will have to move again. They may have some emotional difficulties related to the reason they were removed from their original home.

When caring for children from foster homes, it is important to ascertain who has legal responsibility to sign for health care for the child (a foster parent may or may not have this responsibility; Gitlitz & Kuehne, 1997). Most foster parents are as concerned with health care as biologic parents and can be depended on to follow health care instructions conscientiously.

CHECKPOINT QUESTIONS

1. Why has the number of nuclear families in the United States decreased?
2. What is the strength of a single-parent family?
3. How do the laws governing homosexual partners affect gay or lesbian families?

Family Function and Roles

A family is a small community group, and, as a group, it must designate certain people to complete certain tasks. Otherwise, work is duplicated or never completed. The majority of roles that people view as appropriate are the roles they saw their own parents fulfilling. Each new generation takes on the values of the previous generation, passing traditions and culture from generation to generation.

An important part of family assessment is to identify the roles that family members assume. Most families can identify an individual who serves as a financial manager, a problem solver, a decision maker, a nurturer, a health manager, and a gatekeeper who allows information into and out of the family. Knowing who fulfills these roles in a family helps you to work effectively with the family. If a hospitalized child will need continued care after he or she returns home, for example, then it would be important to identify and contact the nurturing member of the family because it will probably be this person who will supervise or give the needed care at home. Take care not to make assumptions about role fulfillment based on gender or stereotyping, because every family operates differently. For example, although nurturing has typically been thought of as a female characteristic, many men are just as nurturing as women and in some families fulfill this role.

If a pregnancy will cause a major change in lifestyle for the family, it would be good to identify and contact the person in the family who is the decision maker or the person who is the problem solver (not necessarily the same). If the child's illness will involve increased family expense, then identifying and contacting the wage earner for the family would be important.

Knowledge of who is a family's safety and health officer is important before contacting a family for discharge planning. The gatekeeper for a family is the person who allows information into the family and releases information from it. It is important to identify this family member before attempting to introduce a change such as a new pattern of nutrition into a family. Identifying the family's emotional support person helps evaluate the family's ability to cope with stress, such as the care of an ill family member (Baker, 1994).

Family Tasks

Duvall and Miller (1990) have identified eight tasks that are essential for a family to perform to survive as a unit. These tasks differ in degree from family to family and depend on the growth stage of the family, but are usually present to some extent in all families.

- *Physical maintenance.* A healthy family provides food, shelter, clothing, and health care for its members. Being certain that a family has ample resources to provide for a new member is important in child health nursing.
- *Socialization of family members.* This task involves preparation of children to live in the community and interact with people outside the family. A family that is located in a community with a culture or values different from its own may find this a very difficult task.
- *Allocation of resources.* Determining which family needs will be met and their order of priority is called allocation of resources. In healthy families, there is justification, consistency, and fairness in the distribution. Resources include not only financial wealth but material goods, affection, and space. In some families, resources are limited, so no one has new shoes. A danger sign would be a family in which one child has $100 sneakers while others are barefoot.
- *Maintenance of order.* This task includes opening an effective means of communication between family members, establishing family values, and enforcing common regulations for all family members (see the Empowering the Family box). Determining the place of a new infant and what rules he or she will need to follow may be an important task for a developing family. In healthy families, members know the family rules and respect and follow them without difficulty.
- *Division of labor.* The issue here is who will fulfill certain roles such as family provider, who will be the children's caregiver, and who will be the home manager. Pregnancy or an illness of a child may change this familial arrangement and cause the family to rethink this task.
- *Reproduction, recruitment, and release of family members.* Often not a great deal of thought is given

EMPOWERING THE FAMILY: Suggestions for Keeping Family Members in Touch With One Another

Traditionally, families gathered for an evening meal and this allowed for a set time period each day for interaction and problem solving while the problems were still small enough to be solvable. If this isn't possible, suggestions for better communication might be:

- Set up a bulletin board or chalk board family members check each day for messages.
- Use a telephone answering tape or video camera to leave messages.
- Plan an earlier wake-up time so all family members can have breakfast together every morning.
- Reserve one night a week as "family night" when the family plans a special activity to do together.
- Join in other's activities (if one is playing in a ball game, all come and watch).

to this task: who lives in a family often happens more by changing circumstances than by true choice. Having to accept a child with a disability into an already crowded household may make this a less-than-welcome event or cause reworking of this task.

- *Placement of members into the larger society.* This task consists of selecting community activities, such as school, religious affiliation, or a political group, that correlate with the family's beliefs and values. Selecting a health maintenance facility or choosing a hospital or hospice setting is part of this task.
- *Maintenance of motivation and morale.* A sense of pride in the family group, when created, helps members serve as support people to each other during crises. Assessing to see whether this feeling is present helps in care planning.

Family Life Cycles

Families, like individuals, pass through predictable developmental stages (Duvall & Miller, 1990). To predict the likelihood of a family using health promotion activities, therefore, it is helpful to assess its developmental stage. The age of the oldest child marks the stage. Because families are delaying the age at which they have a first child and parents are living longer, the length of stages 1, 7, and 8 is growing.

Stage 1: Marriage and the Family

Although Duvall referred to this stage as marriage, what occurs during it is applicable to couples forming cohabitation, lesbian, gay, or single alliances when formal marriage does not occur. During this first stage of family development, members work to achieve three separate identifiable tasks:

- Establish a mutually satisfying relationship
- Learn to relate well to their families of orientation
- If applicable, engage in reproductive life planning

Establishing a mutually satisfying relationship includes merging a couple's values brought into the relationship from the families of orientation. This means not only adjusting to each other in terms of routines (e.g., sleeping, eating, or housecleaning) but also sexual and economic aspects. This first stage of family development is a tenuous one, as evidenced by the high rate of divorce or separation of partners at this stage. Illness of a member at this stage may be enough to destroy the still lightly formed bonds of partners if the partners do not receive support from their former family members or from alert health care providers.

Stage 2: The Early Childbearing Family

The birth or adoption of a first baby is usually an exciting yet stressful event, which requires economic and social role changes. An important nursing role during this period is health education about well-child care and how to integrate a new member into a family. It is a further developmental step to change from being able to care for a well baby to caring for an ill baby. One way of determining whether a parent has made this change is to ask what the new parent has tried to do to solve a childrearing or health problem. Even if what the person answers is not therapeutic or the best solution to the problem, as long as it is sensible (not "I don't do anything when the baby's sick; I just take her right to my mother" but "I've been trying to give her a little water and keep her warm"), it probably means the parent has mastered this developmental step. Parents who have difficulty with this step need a great deal of support and counseling from health care providers to be able to care for an ill child at home or to give care to the child during a hospitalization.

Stage 3: The Family With Preschool Children

A family with preschool children is a busy family because children at this age demand a great deal of time related to growth and developmental needs and safety considerations as accidents become a major health concern. If a child is hospitalized because of an accident, parents may have difficulty facing the injury because they feel they should have done more to prevent the accident. It may be difficult for parents to visit the hospital because they must care for other young children at home. If the child returns home for further care, a family in this stage may need continued support and help from a community health nurse to provide necessary health care for the ill member.

Stage 4: The Family With School-Age Children

Parents of school-age children have the important responsibility of preparing their children to be able to function in a complex world while at the same time maintaining their own satisfying marriage relationship. For many families, this is a trying time. Illness imposed at this stage adds to the burdens already present and may be enough to dissolve the marriage. Support systems within a family may be deceptive in that family members may be physically present but provide little or no emotional support, if internal tension exists. Many families during this period will need to turn to a tertiary level (e.g., friends, church organizations, or counseling) for adequate support.

Important nursing concerns during this family stage are monitoring children's health in terms of immunization, dental care, and health care assessments; monitoring child safety related to electrical or automobile accidents; and encouraging a meaningful school experience that will make learning a lifetime concern, not to be abandoned after a mere 12 years.

Stage 5: The Family With Adolescent Children

The primary goal for a family with teenagers differs considerably from the goal of the family in previous stages, which was to strengthen family ties and maintain family unity. Now the family must loosen family ties to allow adolescents more freedom and prepare them for life on their own. As technology advances at a rapid rate, the gap between generations increases; life when the parents were young was different from what it is for their teenagers. This makes stage 5 a trying stage for both children and adults.

Violence—accidents, homicide, and suicide—is the major cause of death in adolescents. The incidence of deaths from HIV infection is growing (Department of Health and Human Services [DHHS], 1997). The nurse working with families at this stage, therefore, needs to spend time counseling members on safety (driving defensively and not under the influence of alcohol); proper care and respect for firearms; the dangers of drug abuse; and safer sex practices. If a generation gap exists between parents and children, children are unable to talk to parents about these problems, particularly those of a controversial nature such as sexual responsibility. A community health nurse is a neutral person who can assist families at this stage when communication difficulties exist.

Stage 6: The Launching Center Family

For many families, the stage at which children leave to establish their own households is the most difficult stage, because it appears to represent the breaking up of the family. Parental roles change from those of mother or father to once-removed support people or *guideposts.* The stage may represent a loss of self-esteem for parents, who feel themselves being replaced by other people in their children's lives. They may feel old for the first time and less able to cope with responsibilities. Illness imposed on a family at this stage may be detrimental to the family structure, breaking up an already disorganized and noncohesive group.

A nurse, again, serves as a counselor to such a family. He or she can help the parents gain a better perspective to see that what their children are doing is what they have spent a long time preparing them to do, or that leaving home is a positive, not a negative, step.

Stage 7: The Family of Middle Years

When a family returns to a two-partner nuclear unit, as it was before childbearing, the partners may view this stage either as the prime time of their lives (with opportunity to travel, economic independence, or time to spend on hobbies) or as a period of gradual decline (lacking the constant activity and stimulation of children in the home, finding life boring without them, or experiencing an "empty nest" syndrome). Because the family has returned to a two-partner union, support people may not be as plentiful as they were before. Having a baby at this point in life may be viewed as exciting or worrisome, depending on individual circumstances.

Stage 8: The Family in Retirement or Older Age

The number of families of retirement age is approximately 15% to 20% of the population. As a group, family members in retirement or older age are more apt to suffer from chronic and disabling conditions than members in younger age groups. Although families at this stage are not having children, they remain an important family type in reference to maternal and child health nursing because they often offer a great deal of support to the young adult who is just beginning a family and needs child care advice; many grandparents are full-time child care providers for grandchildren while the parents are at work.

> WHAT IF? What if a family had a school-age child and a newborn baby? In what family stage would they be? What type of stressors might jeopardize the family's well-being?

Changing Patterns of Family Life

Family life has changed significantly in the United States over the last 50 years. This is due to many complex and interrelated factors, such as increased mobility, the increase in the number of two wage-earner families, and an increase in the number of one-parent families. Understanding the impact these changes have on family structures and family life can help you create plans of care that are realistic and better meet the needs of today's families (see Enhancing Communication box).

Mobility Patterns

Population movement has an important influence on the quality of family life. During the 20th century, vast num-

ENHANCING COMMUNICATION

The Bennett family is composed of Ms. Bennett and her three children: Mark, 4; Bryan, 2; and Deanne, 2 months. You are concerned because the family has missed so many health maintenance visits the children are underimmunized.

Less Effective Communication

Nurse: It's good to see you here today, Ms. Bennett. I know money is a problem, but you've got to start coming more often until your children get caught up with their immunizations.
Ms. Bennett: It's hard with three children—
Nurse: I can't tell you enough how important immunizations are. Mark, you know, won't be able to start school if he isn't immunized.
Ms. Bennett: It's hard—
Nurse: Babies, you know, have almost no natural immunity. That's why they need immunizations.
Ms. Bennett: It's hard—
Nurse: Immunizations are the most important thing you can do for your children. There's no reason important enough not to get them immunized.
Ms. Bennett: I'll do better. I promise.

More Effective Communication

Nurse: It's good to see you here today, Ms. Bennett. I know money is a problem, but you've got to start coming more often until your children get caught up with their immunizations.
Ms. Bennett: It's hard with three children—
Nurse: I can't tell you enough how important immunizations are. Mark, you know, won't be able to start school if he isn't immunized.
Ms. Bennett: It's hard—
Nurse: What could I do to make coming to the clinic easier for you?
Ms. Bennett: I only have two car seats so I can only bring two kids at one time.
Nurse: Let me give you the number of an agency to call to borrow an extra seat, not only so you can come to the clinic but so you can take them out safely other times.

In our zeal to educate people about good health practices, it is easy to rush in and teach without first assessing what are the family's most important needs. Unless these needs are met, people may agree to comply with a better health regimen, but then not be able to do so because their needs were not met.

bers of rural families have moved to urban communities; many urban families have moved to the suburbs. This pattern of mobility is expected to continue in the future. This means that an area with many child health care facilities may find itself with few children or families to use them; areas with many children or families may have few facilities specific for their care. Parents will travel a great distance to obtain health care for an ill child, but they are less apt to do so for health maintenance or health promotion care. Thus, if this circumstance goes unrecognized, goals such as routine immunization may be neglected. Families need to be asked if convenient health care is available.

Families of migrant farm workers are a particular group who have difficulty finding consistent health care because of their constant movement (Bechtel, 1995) Children from these families have been identified as being at high risk for intestinal parasites, low socioeconomic status and lack of immunizations.

New immigrant families have the problem of adjusting not only to a new country but also to a different health care system (Norton et al, 1996). Ensuring their access to health care may require a great deal of education and community outreach. Restrictive laws on health care not being available to illegal aliens limit access. Nurses can be instrumental in seeing that health care organizations consider these issues and institute innovative measures such as providing transportation to facilities, changing locales or services so facilities and needs remain balanced, or setting up outreach and translator programs so non-English speaking residents can receive adequate health care.

Poverty

Although the United States is a large and wealthy country, extreme poverty still exists and, in some areas, seems to be growing. As many as 20% of all children and 10% of families have incomes that fall below the poverty line. Poverty places children and families at risk for a variety of health care problems. A child living in poverty, for example is less likely to receive routine health maintenance care; nutrition may be inadequate to meet the needs for optimal growth and development.

A family who, in a given week, must choose between groceries and a child's immunizations will obviously buy groceries; the child's immunizations must wait until another time. If the family is forced to make this same choice week after week, the child could grow up without protection against a number of potentially lethal diseases. Poverty allows acute illness to become chronic, forces families to live in high crime neighborhoods, and, because of the high stress level always present, may increase domestic violence.

Nurses can be instrumental in helping families secure benefits such as food stamps or funding from Women, Infants, and Children Special Supplemental Food Program (WIC) and referring them to free or scaled-payment health care programs so a healthy environment and health care can be provided despite limited financial resources (Figure 2-2). New laws restrict the number of families eligible for federal assistance. Some families who ordinarily would not qualify for Medicaid funding will qualify if the mother is pregnant.

The Homeless Family

It is estimated that more than 3 million people in the United States today are homeless. Although there is diversity in homeless families as in all others, they share a number of common characteristics. Many homeless families are headed by a female, and an increasing number are headed by pregnant and parenting adolescents. Such families do

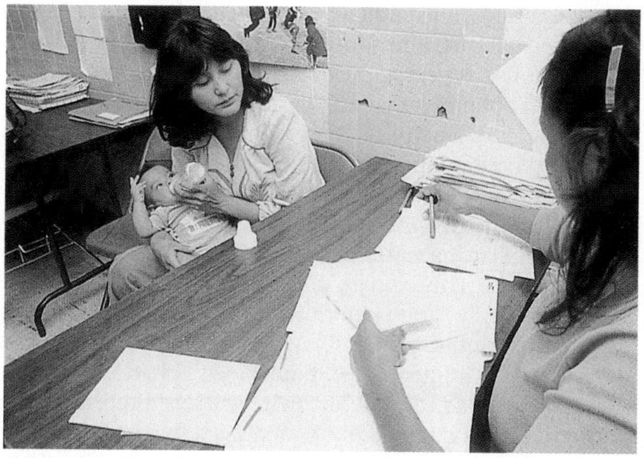

FIGURE 2.2 This community health nurse helps a mother gain access to area programs and provides guidelines for governmental services to promote her infant's health.

not use health care providers or community agencies as effectively as other families (Hatton, 1997). Many mothers of homeless families have a childhood history of physical abuse and of battering as an adult (Clarke et al, 1995). The frequency of drug, alcohol, and severe psychiatric problems is greater in these families than in nonhomeless families.

At least half of homeless children are under 5 years of age. Such children tend to perform less well than others on standard screening tests such as the Denver II. This is probably due to decreased environmental stimulation and lack of exposure to normal play activities. They have more physical illnesses, such as anemia, pneumonia, and dental problems. They may have inadequate growth.

When caring for homeless families, it is important to remember that they lack effective support people. This means they may need a health care provider to serve in this capacity during times of stress or illness (see Focus on Nursing Research box).

Increasing Number of One-Parent Families

One-parent families are increasing in number because of the high divorce rate and the number of women having children outside marriage. An increasing number of children are being raised by a male single parent.

Nurses can be instrumental in helping single parents strengthen new occupation or parenting skills and to be available to provide a second opinion on a course of action or care to prevent parenting responsibilities from becoming overwhelming (Sachs et al, 1997).

Increasing Divorce

Divorce is rarely easy for the people involved. Because they are so emotionally involved and their perceptions of their roles are changing so drastically, parents may be unable to give their children the support they need during a divorce. This can leave marked negative effects on children (Delaney, 1995). For children, the loss of a parent through divorce may be little different from loss of a parent through death. Severing ties with grandparents is also difficult.

Children may manifest grief with physical symptoms such as nausea or fatigue as a response to divorce. Their performance in school may suffer. Boys have been identified as generally having more emotional trauma from divorce than girls, probably because they lose their gender role model if the mother becomes the parent with custody.

Although divorce is a stressful time for children, a redeeming feature may be that the period following a divorce may be less stressful to children than living in a home where there was a high level of conflict between parents. Children need an explanation of why the divorce has occurred and assurance that it was not their fault. The parent who will now be raising them may need help in not assuming the role of the injured party and portraying the other partner as dishonorable. Although a person was not a good marriage partner, he or she may have been a good parent and may be well loved by the children.

Children may have difficulty thinking of themselves as good people if they believe that one of their parents is bad or they were responsible for the divorce. They may need time to discuss how they feel about their parents so they do not think of one parent as kind and loving and the other one as selfish and unreliable.

FOCUS ON NURSING RESEARCH

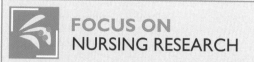

How Well Do Women in Homeless Shelters Manage Health Problems?

For this study, a nurse researcher interviewed 30 women living in a transitional shelter as to how they managed health problems. Typically, women reported they managed health problems by overcoming them alone, rather than seeking help from either friends or health care professionals. The researcher concluded that nursing interventions to supply information on health care and eligibility for services could improve health outcomes among families in shelters.

Hatton, D.C. (1997). Managing health problems among homeless women with children in a transitional shelter. *Image: the Journal of Nursing Scholarship, 29* (1): 33.

Decreasing Family Size

The birth rate in the United States has declined steadily from 1900 to the present. Because the United States is remaining at a point below zero population growth, fewer infants are being born in a year than people are dying (Guyer, 1997). Although small families have fewer child care requirements for parents, they also limit parent experience in childrearing; thus, the amount of counseling time per parent may increase.

Dual-Parent Employment

As many as 60% of women of childbearing age work at a full-time job outside their home today; as many as 90% work at least part time. The implication of this trend for health care providers is that health care facilities must schedule times when parents are free to come or bring children to the facilities (parents will choose to miss work for an ill care visit but not necessarily for a health maintenance one). It means that instructions on how to take medicine must not be "three times a day" but at times when a parent will be home to supervise the administration (e.g., before breakfast, after a parent returns from work, and at bedtime). Dual parent employment has increased the number of children in day care centers or after school programs. This may complicate child care because there is an increased incidence of infection such as acute diarrhea in children in day care. Nurses can be helpful in aiding parents to choose a quality care center that takes the necessary precautions against infection. School-age children often return home from school before parents return from work. Helping parents prevent loneliness in these "latch-key" children and helping children make good use of their time is a nursing responsibility.

Increased Family Responsibility for Health Monitoring

In the past, parents relied on health care providers to be the monitors of their child's health. They accepted health care advice with few questions or expressed opinions. Today, the majority of parents expect to take (and should be encouraged to take) an active role in monitoring their child's health and being participants in planning and goal setting. Changes in healthcare, such as shortened length of hospital stays and a increased focus on health promotion and maintenance, have added to the increased responsibilities and health monitoring of families.

This increased consumer awareness puts increased responsibility on nurses to include parents and children in health care decisions. Using nursing process for planning helps to accomplish this because the goal setting encourages parent participation. Health teaching such as reducing smoking in the home or increasing the fiber content in meals becomes an important aspect with interested learners. The severity of upper respiratory illnesses and inflammatory bowel disease in children is reduced in the home when parents do not smoke.

Increased Abuse in Families

An alarming statistic in relation to family nursing is that the number of instances of domestic abuse is increasing yearly. This is apparently related to an increased stress level in the population as a whole as well as better reporting of abuse. Detecting abuse begins with the awareness that it does occur; careful screening for the possibility at family contacts is essential (Poirier, 1997; Attala, 1996).

UNIQUE CONCERNS OF THE ADOPTING FAMILY

Adoption brings a number of challenges to the adopting parents and the adopted child, as well as to other children in the family, if any (Peterson, 1997). It is helpful if parents of an adopted child visit a health care facility shortly after the child is placed in their home, so that a base of health information can be obtained, potential problems discussed, and possible solutions explored. If the birth mother of an adopted child consumed an inadequate diet and received little prenatal care, the adopted child may be at higher risk for abnormal neurologic development than others. Children from countries that are wartorn have a greater risk of having illnesses such as hepatitis B and intestinal parasites and growth retardation, because health supervision has not been adequate (Mitchell & Jenista, 1997).

It is important when assessing a family with a newly adopted child to ascertain the stage of parenting the parents have reached. The average parents have 9 months to prepare physically and emotionally for a coming baby. Although adoptive parents may have been planning on a baby for much longer than 9 months, the actual appearance of a child can occur suddenly. In a few days' time, adoptive parents are asked to make the mental steps toward parenthood that biologic parents make over 9 months. They may need a great deal of "talk time" at health care visits to explore their feelings about this change in their life and their feelings about being parents. They may be having difficulty trying to preserve a child's native culture if the child was adopted from another country. Adoptive parents may have low self-esteem because they were unable to conceive or have married a partner who is unable to conceive. To bolster this, they may need frequent assurance that they are functioning well as parents.

It is also necessary to assess sibling responses to the adopted child. Biologic children (whether born before or after the adoption) may sometimes feel inferior to the adopted child, because they were not "chosen" or superior because they are the "real" children of the parents. Other adopted children or older biologic children may fear that the parents are dissatisfied with them. Siblings need talk time to voice their feelings about having an adopted child as a sibling.

It is generally accepted that adopted children should be told early that they are adopted. Knowing from early childhood that they are adopted is not nearly as stressful as accidentally stumbling onto the information when they are school-age or adolescents. By age 3 years, children are old enough to understand the story of their adoption: they grew inside the tummy of another woman, but because the woman could not care for them after birth, the woman gave them to the adopting parents to raise and love. It is important for parents not to criticize the birth mother as part of the explanation. Children need to know for their own self-esteem that their birth mothers were good people and that they were capable of being loved by them.

By the time children are 6 years old, they are definitely ready to be told about adoption. When children are first told about their adoption, they may exhibit "honeymoon behavior" or may try to behave absolutely perfectly for fear of being given away again. Following this "honeymoon," children may deliberately annoy parents, testing them to see whether, despite their behavior, parents will still keep them. A child may say things such as "I don't have to listen to you—you're not my real mother." It helps parents put these comments in perspective if they are reminded that it may happen and that nonadoptive children use the same ploys ("Daddy lets me do it" to mother).

As adopted children enter puberty and begin to think about having children of their own, they may need some talk time to express their feelings about being adopted. Some adopted children of this age have difficulty establishing a sense of identity because they do not know who their birth parents were. It is common for them to spend time tracing records and trying to locate their birth parents. Counsel adopting parents that this is not a rejection of them, but a normal consequence of being adopted. Children seek out their birth parents not because they do not love their adoptive parents, but because they need that information to know where they fit into the eternal scheme of the world.

Counseling an adopted child or forming a relationship with one as a health care provider carries an additional responsibility, that of making certain that the relationship with an adoptive child is not ended abruptly or thoughtlessly. The person who will continue health supervision should be introduced to an adopted child so he or she doesn't feel abandoned. When hospitalized, all preschoolers worry about being abandoned and left in the hospital. Preschoolers who have just been told that they are adopted, that they were chosen by their adoptive parents "from all the babies in the hospital nursery," may be terribly afraid that they are now being returned to the hospital to be given back. Parents of an adopted child may need help in preparing the child for this experience and also encouragement to stay with the child in the hospital as much as possible to reduce fear.

✔ CHECKPOINT QUESTIONS

4. How does smaller family size affect parenting?
5. What are common health problems of children adopted from foreign countries?
6. How have shortened hospital stays increased family responsibilities for monitoring health care?

ASSESSMENT OF FAMILY STRUCTURE AND FUNCTION

Assessment of family health can be carried out on a variety of levels and in varying degrees of detail. There are many different ways to collect data on the family; the method chosen should match the way in which the assessment data will be used.

General characteristics of family type and functioning can be assessed using observation and general history questions (Table 2-1). When more detailed information about family environment and roles is required, using an assessment tool specifically developed for that purpose is most effective.

The Well Family

Assessment of psychosocial family wellness requires measurement of how the family relates and interacts as a unit, including communication patterns, bonding, roles and role relationships, division of tasks and activities, governance of the family structure, decision making and problem solving, and leadership within the family unit. Assessment also looks at how the family relates to the outside community.

The Family APGAR (Smilkstein, 1978) is a screening tool of the family environment (Figure 2-3). A family APGAR form is administered to each family member, and their scores are compared. The tool is easy to use and can complement history taking (Sprusinska, 1994).

The **genogram,** a diagram that details family structure, provides information about a family's history and roles of various family members over time, usually through several generations (Figure 2-4). The genogram provides a basis for discussion and analysis of family interactions (Friedman, 1997).

TABLE 2.1 Family Assessment

AREA OF ASSESSMENT	QUESTIONS TO ASK
Type of family	Who lives in the home? Is the family nuclear, extended, or other?
Family finances	Are finances adequate? Is money divided evenly among family members?
Safety	Is the home safe from fire or accidents?
Health	Does the family eat a nutritious diet? Do they receive adequate sleep? Are immunizations current? Is there a balance between work and recreation? Can they cope with problems adequately?
Emotional support	
Within family	Do members eat together or spend an equal amount of time with each other daily? Do they band together to defend each other from outsiders?
Outside family	Is the family active in community organizations or activities? Do they visit (or are they visited by) friends and relatives? Can the family name one outside person they can always rely on for help in a time of crisis?
Family roles	
Nurturing figure	Who is the primary caregiver to children or any disabled member?
Provider	Who is the main family provider?
Decision maker	Who makes decisions, particularly in the area of finances and leisure time?
Problem solver	Who does the family depend on to provide the solution for problems?
Health manager	Who ensures that family members keep return health appointments, immunizations are kept current, and preventive care such as a mammogram for the mother is scheduled?
Gatekeeper	Who determines what information will be released from the family or what new information can be introduced?

The Family in Crisis

Nursing assessment of the family often occurs when the family is in crisis. The way families react to a crisis situation depends largely on the particular crisis affecting them, their past experiences with problem solving, their perception of the event (whether they can clearly see what is the problem), and the resources available to them to help with problem solving. McCubbin and McCubbin (1993) have suggested that assessing these factors is vital to predicting the probable extent of the crisis for the family. The effect of a crisis on a family changes perceptions and resources available. Renewed assessment is therefore necessary in light of a crisis to see if the family is weathering the impact (a double ABCX model of assessment; Figure 2-5). To use this model, first assess what is the stressor affecting the family. A stressor is an event or transition that has the potential to influence the family's

The Family APGAR Questionnaire

	Almost always	Some of the time	Hardly ever
I am satisfied with the help that I receive from my family* when something is troubling me.	_____	_____	_____
I am satisfied with the way my family discusses items of common interest and shares problem solving with me.	_____	_____	_____
I find that my family accepts my wishes to take on new activities or make changes in my lifestyle.	_____	_____	_____
I am satisfied with the way my family expresses affection and responds to my feelings such as anger, sorrow and love.	_____	_____	_____
I am satisfied with the way my family and I spend time together.	_____	_____	_____

SCORING

Scoring: The patient checks one of three choices, which are scored as follows: 2 points for "Almost always," 1 point for "Some of the time" and 0 for "Hardly ever." The scores for each of the five questions are the totaled. A score of 7 to 10 suggests a highly functional family. A score of 4 to 6 suggests a moderately dysfunctional family. A score of 0 to 3 suggests a severely dysfunctional family.

WHAT IS MEASURED

Adaptation — How resources are shared, or the member's satisfaction with the assistance received when family resources are needed.

Partnership — How decisions are shared, or the member's satisfaction with mutuality in family communication and problem solving.

Growth — How nurturing is shared, or the member's satisfaction with the freedom available within the family to change roles and attain physical and emotional growth or maturation.

Affection — How emotional experiences are shared, or the member's satisfaction with the intimacy and emotional interaction within the family.

Resolve — How time* is shared, or the member's satisfaction with the time commitment that has been made to the family by its members.

*Besides sharing time, family members usually have a commitment to share space and money. Because of its primacy, time was the only item included in the Family APGAR; however, the nurse who is concerned with family function will enlarge understanding of the family's resolve by inquiring about family member's satisfaction with shared space and money.

FIGURE 2.3 The Family APGAR Questionnaire. (From Smilkstein, G. [1978]. The Family APGAR. *Journal of Family Practice*, 6, 1231.)

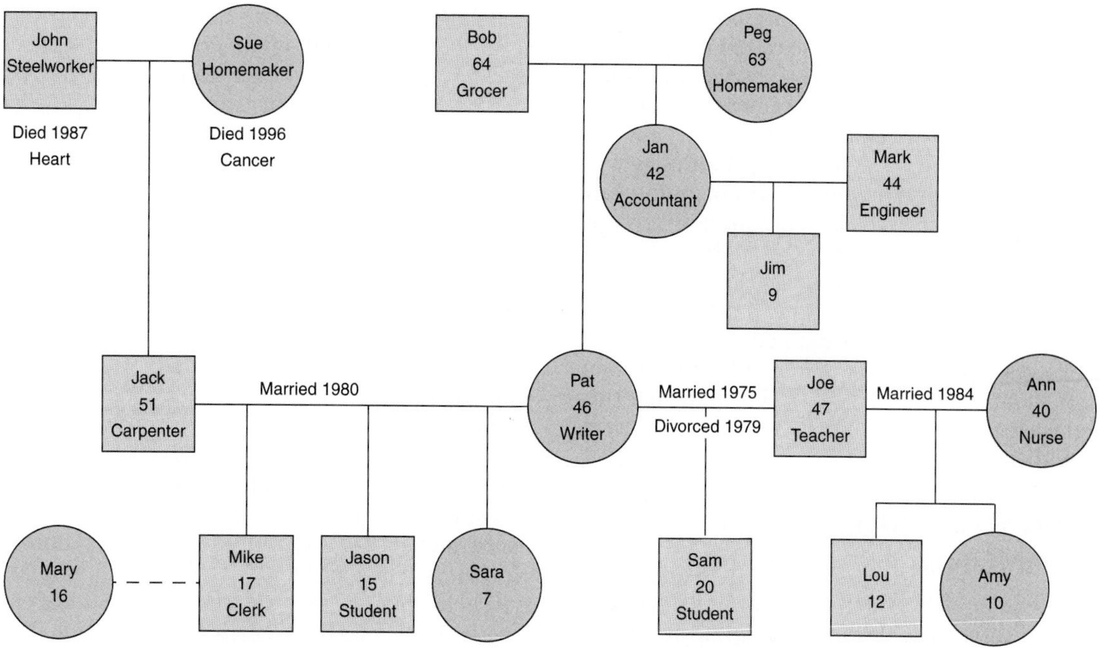

FIGURE 2.4 A family genogram showing three generations. Males are depicted by squares, females by circles. Each family member's name, age, and occupation is supplied.

dynamics. A house fire would be an example. Next, assess the family's perception of the stressor. If the family states that they had adequate home insurance so everything can be replaced, for example, the stressor may have little effect. If they feel overwhelmed by the loss of their home and possessions, it is having a major effect. For a third step, evaluate the resources that are available to the family, both internal and external. What is the family type; what are their vulnerabilities, do they have friends who can help replace possessions; do they belong to a church or synagogue that will help, for examples. Every family will make some kind of adjustment to a problem. This adjustment and then the family's changed perception of the event lead to a need for further assessment.

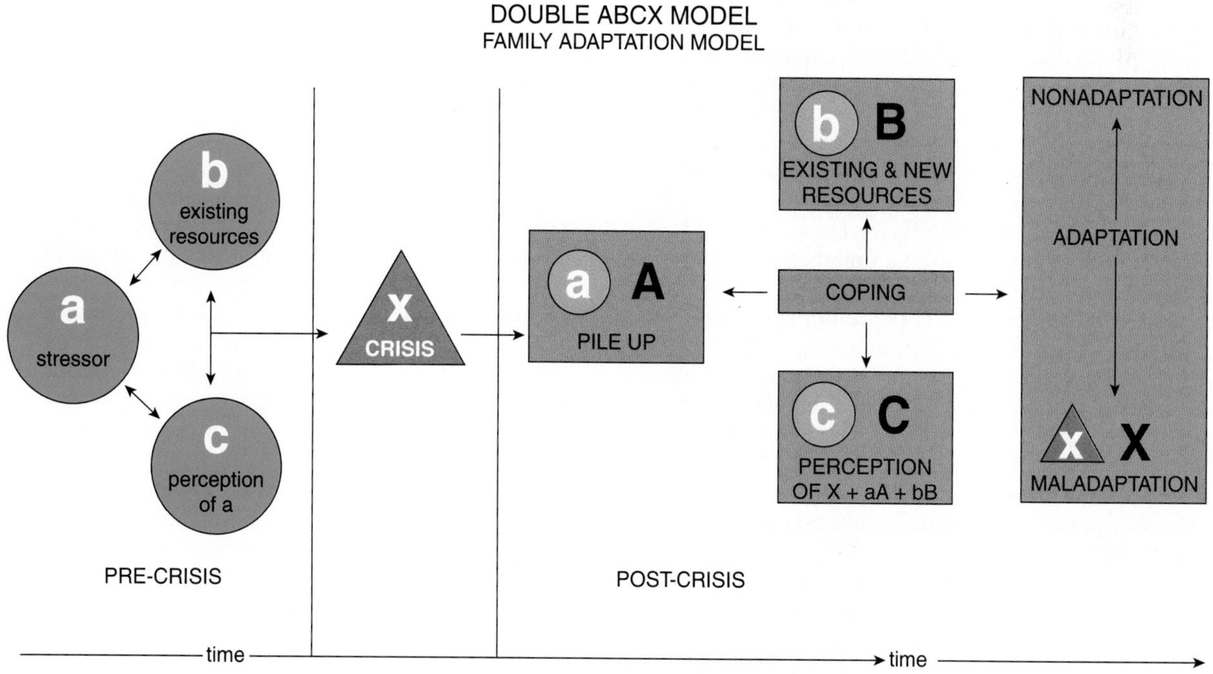

FIGURE 2.5 The ABCX System for Family Assessment. (McCubbin, H.I., & Patterson, J. [1983]. Family stress adapation to crises: a double ABCX model of family behavior. In McCubbin, H., Sussman, M., & Patterson, J. [eds.]. *Social stresses and the family: Advances and developments in family stress theory and research.* New York: Haworth Press.)

This is a useful model for family assessment because it does not assume that because A (a stressor) happens, an automatic outcome will occur. It respects the individuality of families, an important factor to remember in family assessment (McCubbin & McCubbin, 1993).

Listing a family's strengths and coping abilities as well as its areas of vulnerability not only aids in planning care but also the actual process of identifying strengths by and with the family members themselves strengthens the family. Family assessment carried out with the family together in this way will bring out these sorts of insights and better prepare family members to cope with the current level of stress and difficult decision making that may be ahead for them. The Empowering the Family box provides practical suggestions to help families enduring a crisis to deal with stress.

THE FAMILY AS PART OF A COMMUNITY

Community can be defined in many ways, but it is generally accepted to refer to a limited geographic area in which the residents relate to and interact among themselves. When asked what community they are from, therefore, people may mention an entire city; a school district; a geographic district ("the east side"); a street name ("Pine Street area"); or a natural marking ("the lower creek area").

Because the health of individuals is influenced by the health of their community, it is important to become acquainted with the community in which you practice (Bryan et al, 1997). If you are caring for a client from a community unknown to you, then assess that community to see if there are aspects about it that contributed to an illness (and therefore need to be corrected) and to determine whether the person will be able to return to such a community without extra help and counseling from a health care provider (Figure 2-6).

Community assessment consists of examining the various systems that are present in almost all communities to see if they are functioning adequately (Thomas, 1997). Knowing the individual aspects of families or community may help you understand why some children reach the illness level they do before parents bring them in for health

EMPOWERING THE FAMILY: Suggestions for Managing Family Stress

1. Recognize individual stress levels, a level that differs from person to person. Because one person is not upset by some condition does not mean that another person will not be annoyed or upset. On the other hand, if a situation does not annoy a person, that person should not feel that he or she has to react to it just because someone else does.
2. Learn to change those things you cannot accept and accept those things you cannot change. Trial and error is often required to determine the difference between the two categories.
3. Often a total change is unnecessary; a modification will be ample to make the difference.
4. Verbalize personal reactions to stress. Almost nothing limits the extent of a threat more than being able to accurately describe it.
5. Reach out for support. People under stress are often so involved in their problems that they do not realize that people around them want to help. Sometimes the people closest to the person feeling stress are under a similar threat and so are no longer able to offer support. When this happens, the person must then call on second- or third-level support persons (family or community people) for help.
6. Develop a habit of reaching out to give support when others are in threat (to network). Survival is a collaborative function of social groups; a favor offered now can be called in when the person is in need at a later date.
7. Face a situation as honestly as possible. As a rule, knowing the exact nature of a threat is less stressful than a "shadow-haunting, something-is-out-there" feeling. On the other hand, do not feel compelled to face intense threats, such as a serious complication of a disorder or a fatal illness in a child until you have had time to mobilize your defenses, or you may be overwhelmed.
8. Do not rush decisions or make final adaptive outcomes to a stress situation. As a rule, major decisions should be delayed at least 6 weeks after an event; 6 months is an even better time interval.
9. Anticipate life events and plan for them to the extent possible. Anticipatory guidance will not totally prepare you for a coming event but will at least serve notice that distress over the situation is normal.
10. Remember that accidents increase when people are under stress. A person worrying about a complication of a disorder, for example, is more apt to have an automobile accident than a person who is stress free. Children are more apt to poison themselves when the family is under stress than during a nonstress time.
11. Action feels good during stress because doing something brings a sense of control over feelings of helplessness and disorganization. Action often is so satisfying that people do things such as write threatening letters or make harmful remarks that they later regret. Channel your energy into therapeutic action (such as going for a long walk) instead.

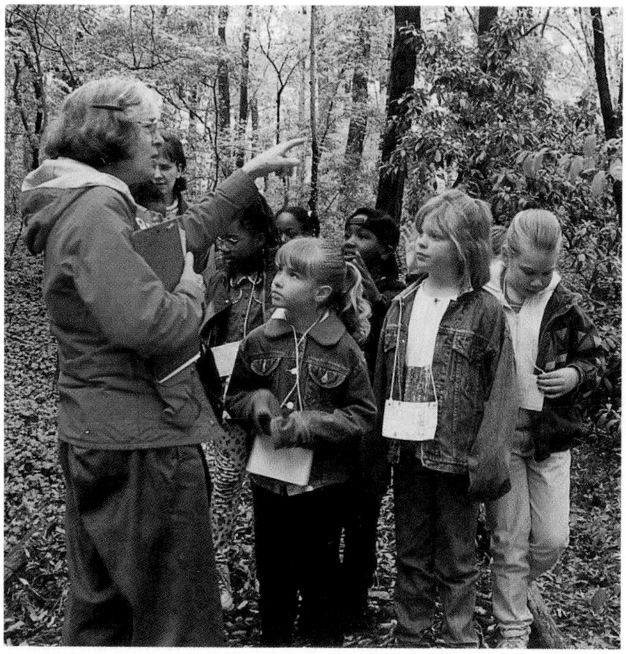

FIGURE 2.6 Community experiences can be a rich source of learning for children. Here a naturalist guides children on a walk through a community park.

care. In addition, such knowledge can set the stage for care (e.g., a mother and child living alone in a city has no transportation available to her until her partner comes home from work, so she cannot bring the child in for routine health maintenance care; a 5-year-old child develops measles because there are no free immunization services in the community). It is easier for a nurse to prepare a child for return to a community after a hospitalization if, for example, he or she knows the specific features of the community where the family lives. (Does the Pine Street area have well or city water? How many flights of stairs does someone from the Stevens Plaza area have to walk to reach an apartment? Is there public transportation so the child can return for follow-up care?) Table 2-2 summarizes areas of community assessment to use in discharge planning (Weiss, 1997).

A second aspect of community assessment is to determine health problems in particular communities and the relationship of the family to the community. This is done by means of an **ecomap**, a diagram of family and community relationships (Figure 2-7). Such a "map" helps to assess the emotional support available to a family from the community. A family whom you assess as having few connecting lines between its members and community contacts may need increased nursing contact and support in order to remain a well family. The Nursing Care Plan demonstrates both family and community assessment.

✔ CHECKPOINT QUESTIONS

7. How does a genogram differ from an ecomap?
8. What is a family APGAR?
9. Why is assessing transportation in a community important in regards to health care?

(text continues on page 40)

TABLE 2.2 Community Assessment

AREA OF ASSESSMENT	QUESTIONS
Age span	Is the family within the usual age span of the community and thereby assured of support people?
Education	If the person is school age, is there provision for schooling? Is there a public library for self-education? Is there easy access to such places if the person is disabled? If a special program such as diet counseling is needed, does it exist?
Environment	Are environmental risks present such as air pollution? Busy highways? Train yards? Pools or water where frequent drownings occur? Will hypothermia be a problem?
Finances, occupation	Is there a high rate of unemployment in the community? What is the average occupation? Will this family have adequate finances to manage comfortably? Are supplemental aid programs available?
Health care delivery	Is there a health care agency the family can use for comprehensive care? Is it convenient in terms of finances and time?
Housing	Are houses mainly privately owned or apartments? Are homes close enough together to afford easy contact? Are they in good repair? Is upkeep such as constant repair or extensive lawn mowing a problem?
Political	Is the community active politically? Can adults reach a local polling place to vote or do they know how to apply for absentee ballots?
Recreational	Are recreational activities of interest available? Are they economically feasible?
Religion	Is there a facility where the family can worship as they choose? Is there easy transportation to it?
Safety, protection	Is there adequate protection so family members can feel safe to leave home or remain home alone? Do they know about available "hot lines" and local police and fire department numbers? Is the home safe from fire?
Sociocultural	What is the dominant culture in the community? Does the family fit into this environment? Are foods that are culturally significant available?
Transportation	Is there public transportation? Will family members have access to it if they are disabled?

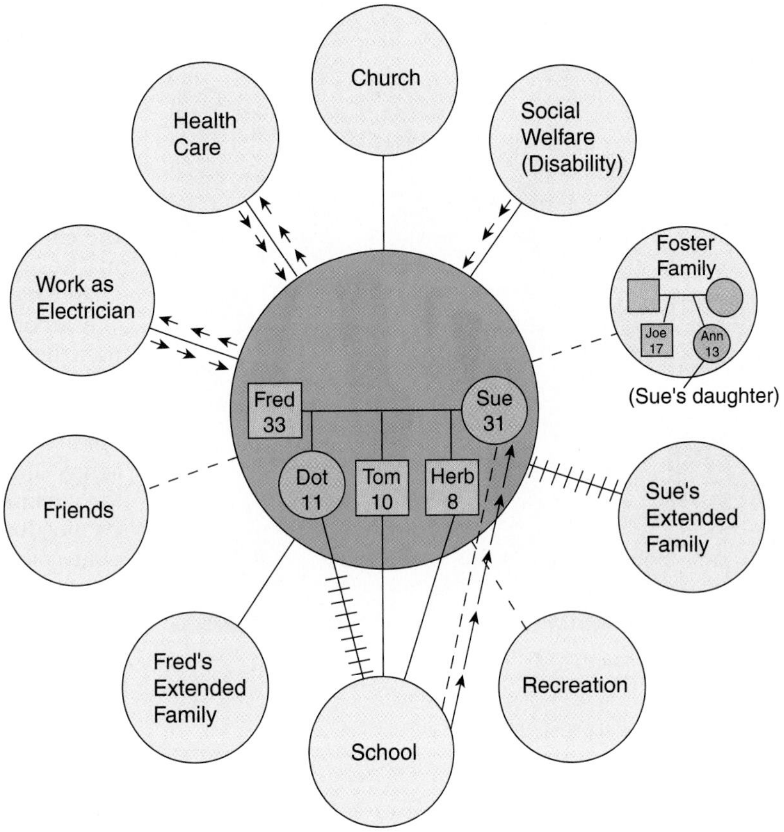

FIGURE 2.7 Ecomap of a family's relationship to its environment. The family members and their ages are shown in the center circle; the outer circles show community contacts. Lines indicate types of connections: solid line, strong; dotted line, tenuous; line with cross bars, stressful. Arrows signify energy or resource flow, and absence of lines indicates no connection.

Nursing Care Plan

THE FAMILY WITH AN ILL CHILD

A 12-year-old male with cystic fibrosis is brought to the child development clinic for evaluation. His parents state, "He's been acting out in school quite a bit and he doesn't always take his medicines or do his treatments like he's supposed to." Client states, "Everybody's so busy, nobody has time for me. I'm not like the other kids, I'm always sick. Things will even get worse when the new baby comes."

Assessment: Blended family. Client oldest child with one stepsister, age 8 years; middle-class family living in modest 3-bedroom home in the suburbs. Father works two jobs and does not participate in community activities. "Who has time?" Mother currently attending college full time with financial aid; 5 months pregnant and active in local government. Family involved in weekly trips to the local high school pool for swimming. Client refuses to go. Daily household chores done primarily by client with some help from sister. Client home alone after school until dinner time. Client and family with few close friends. Two neighbors available in case of an emergency. Numerous community activities available for children and parents.

Client's respiratory rate 26; thin and pale. Productive cough with tenacious sputum. Last medications taken yesterday morning. Lungs with fine bilateral rales.

Nursing Diagnosis: Altered family processes related to impact of child's illness and situational stressors

Outcome Identification: Family will verbalize improved family functioning and interaction by 3 months' time

Outcome Evaluation: Family states participation in at least one group activity per week; family reports sitting down to a family meal at least twice a week; family demonstrates positive methods of communication.

(continued)

Interventions	Rationale
1. Meet with family to identify areas of needed support. Encourage family members to verbalize needs and feelings.	1. Expression of feelings provides a safe outlet for emotions and helps to increase other family members' awareness of the needs.
2. Complete a family APGAR and genogram. Prioritize needs for each family member.	2. Family APGAR provides information about how families relate and interact. A genogram details family structure and roles. Priority setting promotes more focused, directed care for outcome achievement.
3. Develop strategies to assist each family member in meeting priority needs. Instruct in measures such as communication, relaxation, time management, and contracting.	3. Use of therapeutic measures assists in clarifying the needs and expectations and helps reduce stress.
4. Ascertain a common activity enjoyed by all members. Encourage participation in this activity, initially once a month, then twice a month, then weekly.	4. Participation in a common group activity fosters bonding. Gradually increasing the frequency of the activity promotes integration into the family routine.
5. Encourage joint cooperation in meal planning and cleanup at least once per week.	5. Working together with a common task fosters interaction, communication, and trust.
6. Investigate possible outside community resources available. Encourage the family to use the services.	6. Community resources provide additional support in areas of need.

Nursing Diagnosis: Social isolation related to illness and family stressors

Outcome Identification: Client will demonstrate participation in outside activities.

Outcome Evaluation: Client reports joining a local youth organization; states a friend visits after school at least once a week.

Interventions	Rationale
1. Explore with client about outside activities that he might like or dislike. Develop a list of activities that he would be willing to participate in.	1. Exploration of likes and dislikes provides a baseline from which to build future suggestions.
2. Evaluate family's ecomap. Contact local community organizations with client and set up a visit. Enlist the aid of the school nurse and guidance counselor in providing contacts.	2. Ecomapping helps to assess the emotional support available to the family. Contacting the organization with the client offers support and helps reduce his possible anxiety with new situations. School personnel provide additional support and reassurance.
3. Encourage client to participate in outside activities chosen.	3. Participation with others diminishes feelings of loneliness and isolation.

Nursing Diagnosis: Ineffective management of therapeutic regimen related to family stressors and feelings of being different

Outcome Identification: The client will demonstrate adherence to prescribed treatment program.

Outcome Evaluation: The client takes medications as prescribed; performs respiratory treatments as scheduled; demonstrates behaviors to reduce the risk of complications and exacerbations of cystic fibrosis. Respiratory rate within age-acceptable parameters; absence of cough; lungs clear or with minimal rales; sputum clear.

(*continued*)

Interventions	Rationale
1. Listen to client's concerns about being sick and different from others.	1. Listening provides clues to understanding client's motivation for behavior.
2. Provide explanations of illness and rationale for treatment based on client's knowledge base.	2. Building on a client's knowledge base facilitates teaching and learning and minimizes repetition.
3. Review medication regimen and procedures for respiratory treatments. Demonstrate procedures, if necessary, and have client return demonstrate. Look for ways to incorporate treatment regimen into client's usual routine.	3. Review and redemonstration helps to reinforce measures and ensure client is doing them correctly. Incorporation of regimen within client's routine helps to promote positive adjustment and decrease feelings of being different.
4. Enlist the aid of parents and sister in regimen. Encourage each to assist with one aspect of the treatment program.	4. Family participation helps to increase client cooperation and promote positive adjustment to the experience. Family involvement in one aspect divides the responsibility so as not to overwhelm them, thus minimizing the risk of added stress on the family system.
5. Assess respiratory status for changes.	5. Follow-up assessment provides clues about the effectiveness of and client's adherence to treatment.
6. Encourage client and family participation in cystic fibrosis support groups.	6. Support groups help to minimize the feeling of being alone and different.

KEY POINTS

A family is a group of people who share a common emotional bond and perform certain interrelated social tasks.

Common types of families encountered are nuclear, extended, single-parent, blended, cohabitation, single alliance, gay, lesbian, and foster families.

Common family tasks are physical maintenance, socialization of family members, allocation of resources, maintenance of order, division of labor, reproduction, recruitment and release of members, placement of members into the larger society, and maintenance of motivation and morale.

Common life stages of families are marriage, early childbearing, families with preschool, school-age, and adolescent children, launching center and middle-years families, and the family in retirement.

Changes in patterns of family life that are occurring are increased mobility, one-parent families, dual-parent employment, divorce, social problems such as abuse and decreased socioeconomic level, and family size.

Considering a family as a unit (a single client) helps to plan nursing care that meets the family's total needs.

Families exist within communities; assessment of the community and the family's place within the community yields further information on family functioning.

Families are not always functioning at their highest level during periods of crisis; reassessing them during a period of stability may reveal a stronger family than on first assessment.

Because families work as a unit, unmet needs of any member can spread to become unmet needs of all family members.

CRITICAL THINKING EXERCISES

1. The Hanovans are a family you met at the beginning of the chapter. Why is this a particularly unfortunate time for the Hanavans to have to choose between health care and groceries?
2. Analyze your family type and structure. What family stage according to Duvall has your family reached? What would a genogram of your family look like? An ecomap?

REFERENCES

Attala, J. M. (1996). Detecting abuse against women in the home. *Home Care Provider, 1* (1), 12.

Baker, N. A. (1994). Avoiding collisions with challenging families. *MCN: American Journal of Maternal Child Nursing, 19,* 97.

Bechtel, G. A. (1995). Community health nursing in migrant farm camps. *Nurse Educator, 20* (4), 15.

Brewaeys, A. & van Hall, E. V. (1997). Lesbian motherhood: the impact on child development and family functioning. *Journal of Psychosomatic Obstetrics and Gynecology, 18*(1), 1.

Bryan, Y. E., et al. (1997). Preparing to change from acute to community-based care. *Journal of Nursing Administration, 27* (5), 35.

Bushy, A. (1997). Empowering initiatives to improve a community's health status. *Journal of Nursing Care Quality, 11* (4), 32.

Carlson, K. L. (1996). Providing health care for children in foster care: a role for advanced practice nurses. *Pediatric Nursing, 22* (5): 418.

Clarke, P. N., et al. (1995). Health and life problems of homeless men and women in the southeast. *Journal of Community Health Nursing, 12* (2): 101.

Delaney, S. E. (1995). Divorce mediation and children's adjustment to parental divorce. *Pediatric Nursing, 21* (5): 434.

Department of Health and Human Services. (1995). *Healthy people 2000: midcourse review.* Washington, DC: DHHS.

Department of Health and Human Services. (1997). Births, marriages, divorces, and deaths for 1996. *Monthly Vital Statistics Report, 45* (12), 5.

Duvall, E. M. & Miller, B. (1990). *Marriage and family development.* Philadelphia: J. B. Lippincott.

Friedman, L. C. (1997). *Family nursing* (4th ed.). New York: Prentice-Hall.

Gitlitz, B., & Kuehne E. (1997). Caring for children in foster care. *Journal of Pediatric Health Care, 11* (3), 127.

Guyer, B., et al. (1997). Annual summary of vital statistics—1996. *Pediatrics, 100* (6), 905.

Harrison, A. E., & Silenzio, V. M. (1996). Comprehensive care of lesbian and gay patients and families. *Primary Care Clinics in Office Practice, 23* (1), 31.

Hatton, D. C. (1997). Managing health problems among homeless women with children in a transitional shelter. *Image: The Journal of Nursing Scholarship, 29* (1), 33.

Kirschling, J. M., et al. (1994). "Success" in family nursing: experts describe phenomena. *Nursing and Health Care, 15* (4), 186.

McCubbin, M. A., & McCubbin, H. I. (1993). Family coping with health crises: the resiliency model of family stress, adjustment and adaptation. In Danielson, C., Hamel-Bissil, B., & Winstead-Fry, P. (Eds.) *Families, health and illness.* New York: Mosby.

Mitchell, M. A., & Jenista, J. A. (1997). Health care of the internationally adopted child: chronic care long-term medical issues. *Journal of Pediatric Health Care, 11* (3), 117.

National Center for Health Statistics. (1998). Births, marriages, divorces, and deaths. *Monthly Vital Statistics Report, 46*(7), 3.

Norton, S. A., Kenney, G. M., & Ellwood, M. R. (1996). Medicaid coverage of maternity care for aliens in California. *Family Planning Perspectives, 28* (3), 108.

Otto, H. (1963). Criteria for assessing family strengths. *Family Process*. 2, 329.

Percy, M. A. (1995). Children from homeless families describe what is special in their lives. *Holistic Nursing Practice, 9* (4), 24.

Perrin, E. C., & Kulkin, H. (1996). Pediatric care for children whose parents are gay or lesbian. *Pediatrics, 97* (5), 629.

Peterson, E. A. (1997). Supporting the adoptive family: a developmental approach. *MCN: American Journal of Maternal Child Nursing, 22* (3), 14.

Poirier, L. (1997). The importance of screening for domestic violence in all women. *Nurse Practitioner, 22* (5), 105.

Sachs, B., Pietrukowicz, M., & Hall, L. A. (1997). Parenting attitudes and behaviors of low-income single mothers with young children. *Journal of Pediatric Nursing, 12* (2), 67.

Smilkstein, G. (1978). The family APGAR. *Journal of Family Practice, 6,* 1231.

Spradley, B. W., & Allender, J. A. (1996). *Community health nursing: concepts and practice.* (4th ed.). Philadelphia: J. B. Lippincott.

Sprusinska, E. (1994). The family APGAR index: study on relationship between family function, social support, global stress and mental health perception in women. *International Journal of Occupational Medicine and Evironmental Health, 7* (1), 23.

Thomas, E. (1997). Community nursing profiles: their role in needs assessment. *Nursing Standard, 11* (37), 39.

United States Census. (1997). *Statistical abstract of the U.S.* Washington, DC: U.S. Department of Commerce.

Weiss, M. (1997). The quality evolution in managed care organizations: shifting the focus to community health. *Journal of Nursing Care Quality, 22* (4), 27.

SUGGESTED READINGS

Anderson, J. M. (1996). Empowering patients: issues and strategies. *Social Science and Medicine, 43* (5), 697.

Barrett, D., & Beckett, W. (1996). Child prostitution: reaching out to children who sell sex to survive. *British Journal of Nursing, 5* (18), 1120.

Blatt, S. D., et al. (1997). A comprehensive multidisciplinary approach to providing health care for children in out-of-home care. *Child Welfare, 76* (2), 331.

Fishbein, E. G. & Burggraf, E. (1998). Early postpartum discharge: how are mothers managing? *Journal of Obstetrics, Gynecologic and Neonatal Nursing, 27*(2), 142.

Ford-Gilboe, M., & Campbell, J. (1996). The mother-headed single-parent family: a feminist critique of the nursing literature. *Nursing Outlook, 44* (4), 173.

James, J., & Underwood, A. (1997). Poverty initiatives to protect children from its effects. *Practitioner, 241* (1573), 222.

Swanwick, M. (1996). Child-rearing across cultures. *Pediatric Nursing, 8* (7), 13.

Wagner, J. D., et al. (1995). What is known about the health of rural homeless families? *Public Health Nursing, 12* (6), 400.

Wayland, J., & Rawllins, R. (1997). African American teen mothers' perceptions of parenting. *Journal of Pediatric Nursing, 12* (1), 13.

Sociocultural Aspects of Child Health Nursing

3

CHAPTER

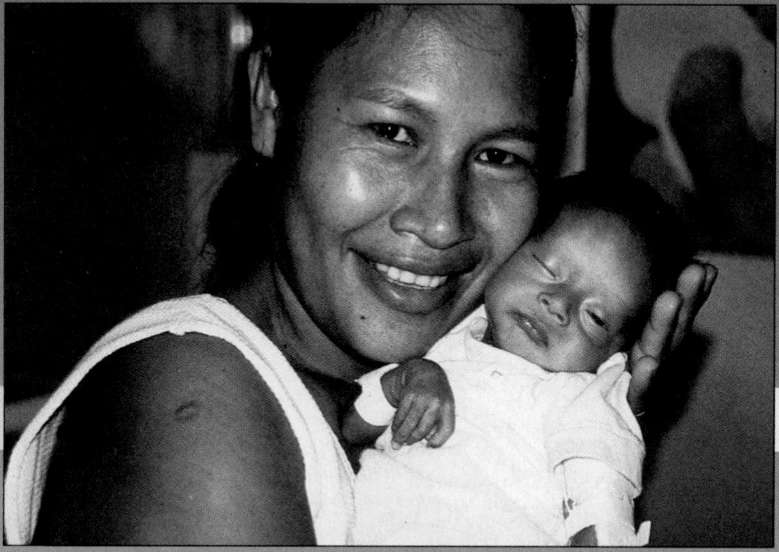

Key Terms

- acculturation
- assimilation
- cultural competence
- cultural values
- culture
- ethnicity
- ethnocentrism
- mores
- norms
- pain threshold
- pain tolerance
- stereotyping
- taboos
- threshold sensation
- transcultural nursing

Objectives

After mastering the contents of this chapter, you should be able to:

1. Describe ways that sociocultural influences affect child nursing care.
2. Assess a family for sociocultural influences that might influence the way it responds to childrearing.
3. Formulate nursing diagnoses related to culturally appropriate aspects of nursing care.
4. Develop outcomes to assist families who have specific cultural needs to thrive in their community.
5. Plan and implement nursing care that respects sociocultural needs and wishes of families.
6. Evaluate outcome criteria to be certain that goals of care related to sociocultural aspects have been achieved.
7. Identify National Health Goals related to sociocultural considerations that nurses could be instrumental in helping the nation to achieve.
8. Identify areas of care related to sociocultural considerations that could benefit from additional nursing research.
9. Use critical thinking to analyze how the sociocultural aspects of care affect family functioning and develop ways to make nursing care more family centered.
10. Integrate sociocultural aspects of care with nursing process to achieve quality child health nursing care.

Anna Rodriques is a 12-year-old child who is hospitalized for surgical repair of a broken tibia. She has a cast on her right leg and will be on bedrest for 3 days, then gradually she will be allowed to learn crutch walking.

In planning care for her, you assume that because her culture is Hispanic, her family orientation will be male dominated, her time focus will be on the present rather than the future, and nutrition preferences will be Mexican American. Based on this, you concentrate on talking mainly about her current problem (bedrest) rather than future care at home. You speak to the dietitian about avoiding milk because lactase deficiency is present in many Mexican Americans. You consult with Anna's father regarding the major aspects of her care.

You are surprised to hear Anna complain on the second day of her hospitalization that she feels like a second-class person because her father has been asked for more input about her care than she has. She says she is particularly concerned that bone healing will not take place because she has had little milk to drink. She doesn't feel bedrest is a problem. She is more concerned about being prepared to play soccer by next month.

In previous chapters, you learned about the standards and philosophy of child health and family structure. In this chapter, you'll add information about how to care for people from diverse cultures during their childrearing years. This is important information because it can help protect the health of both children and families.

After you've studied the chapter, turn to the Critical Thinking Exercises at the end of the chapter to sharpen your skills and test your knowledge.

To understand why people respond the way they do to preventive health measures or illness, it is necessary to assess their socioeconomic status and their cultural beliefs, because these factors can strongly influence their responses (Ling, 1997).

People's **ethnicity** refers to the cultural group into which they were born, although the term is sometimes used in a narrower context to mean only race. **Culture** is a view of the world and a set of traditions that a specific social group use and transmit to the next generation. **Cultural values** are preferred ways of acting based on those traditions. To understand why people react to health care in differing ways, it is important to understand their background and cultural values (Leininger, 1995).

Cultural values often arise from environmental conditions (in a country where water is scarce, daily bathing is not practiced; in a country where meat is scarce, ethnic recipes use little meat). Such values influence people's view of themselves and their approach or lack of approach to situations such as health care. The usual values of a group are termed **mores** or **norms.** Expecting families to seek care when a child is ill or parents to bring children for immunizations are examples of norms in the United States. Actions that are not acceptable to a culture are called **taboos.** Three taboos that are almost universal are murder, incest, and cannibalism. Issues such as abortion and child abuse are controversial because these are taboos only to some, not all people.

Cultural values influence the manner in which people carry out childrearing, and respond to health and illness. In a culture in which the male is the authority figure, for example, it might be expected that the father rather than the mother answers questions about an ill child; if you are from a culture in which females are expected to provide all child care, you might find it annoying to hear a man taking over the responses at a health interview. A nurse who has been culturally influenced to believe that stoic behavior is the "proper" response to pain may be impatient with a family or chld who has been influenced to believe that expressing discomfort is "proper." Nurses need to be certain to include all cultural groups in nursing research samples so more is learned about cultural preferences in relation to nursing interventions and care.

Cultural differences occur across not only different ethnic backgrounds but also different lifestyles. Adolescents, urban city youth, the hearing impaired, and gays or lesbians have separate cultures from the mainstream. A parent who has been deaf since birth, for example, expects her deaf culture to be respected by having health care professionals attempt to communicate with her in her language.

The United States is a country of such varied cultural groups and socioeconomic conditions that under any given circumstance you are likely to see a wide range of behaviors exhibited (Figure 3-1). Given the wide range of the cultural mix, almost any behavior can be considered appropriate for some individuals at some time and place. Nursing care that is guided by cultural aspects and respects individual differences is termed **transcultural nursing** (Leininger, 1997).

Stereotyping consists of expecting people to act in characteristic manners without regard to individual characteristics; it is generally derogatory in nature. Statements such as "Men never diaper infants well" or "Japanese women are never assertive" are examples of stereotyping. Stereotyping occurs largely because of lack of exposure to enough people in a particular group and, consequently, a lack of understanding of the wide range of differences among people. In the above examples, the first

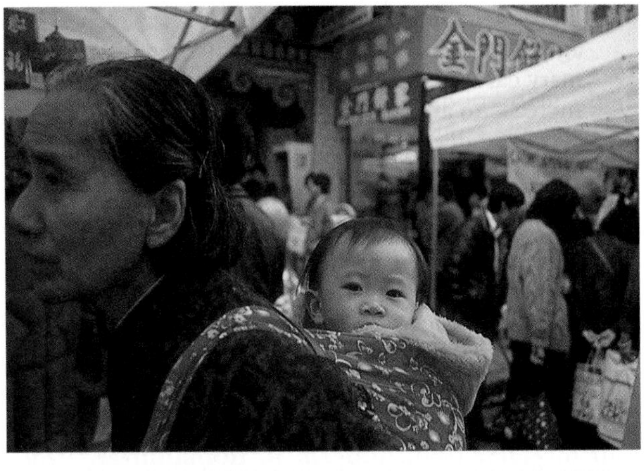

FIGURE 3.1 Various cultural preferences are evident in childrearing. In some cultures extended family members, such as grandparents, take an active part in caring for the child. Learning about different ways is important in care planning.

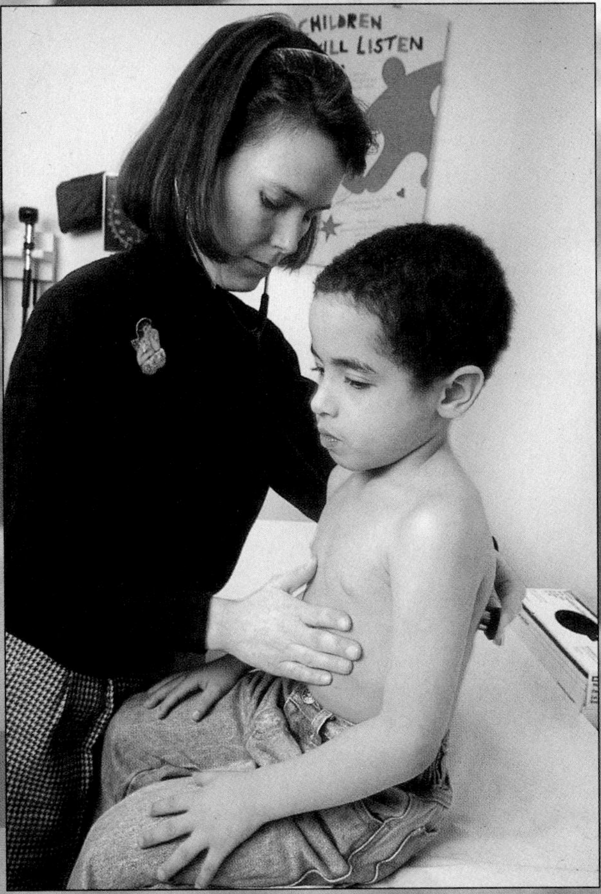

UNIT

2

The Nursing Role in Health Promotion for the Childrearing Family

Fetal Development, Environmental Influences, and Genetic Assessment and Counseling

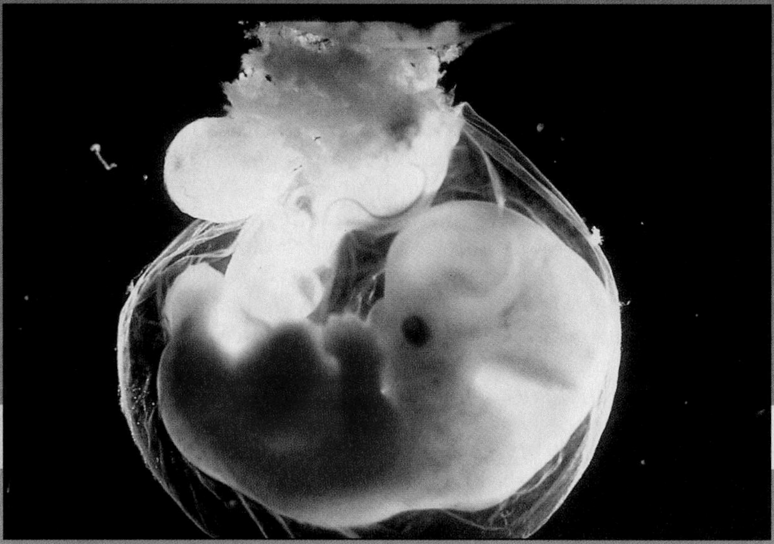

4

CHAPTER

Key Terms

- alleles
- amniotic cavity
- blastocyst
- capacitation
- cephalocaudal
- chorionic villi
- chromosomes
- decidua
- ductus arteriosus
- ductus venosus
- ectoderm
- embryo
- entoderm
- fertilization
- foramen ovale
- genes
- genetics
- genome
- genotype
- gestational age
- heterozygous
- homozygous
- implantation
- imprinting
- karyotyping
- mesoderm
- morula
- organogenesis
- phenotype
- surfactant
- teratogen
- trophoblast
- umbilical cord
- yolk sac
- zygote

Objectives

After mastering the contents of this chapter, you should be able to:

1. Trace the development of the fetus from fertilization through birth.
2. Identify possible environmental influences that may impact fetal growth and development.
3. Describe the nature of inheritance, patterns of recessive and dominant mendelian inheritance, and common chromosomal aberrations such as nondisjunction syndromes.
4. Assess a family for the probability of inheriting a genetic disorder.
5. Formulate nursing diagnoses related to genetic disorders and the needs of the developing fetus.
6. Establish outcomes that meet the needs of the family undergoing genetic assessment and counseling and those of the developing fetus.
7. Plan nursing care related to a genetic alteration and to maintenance of healthy fetal growth and development.
8. Implement nursing care measures to identify or counsel families facing a genetic disorder and to promote optimal fetal growth and development within a safe fetal environment.
9. Evaluate outcomes for achievement and effectiveness of nursing care.
10. Identify National Health Goals and specific measures related to genetic disorders, fetal growth and development, and fetal teratogens that nurses can take to help the nation achieve these goals.
11. Identify areas related to genetic assessment, fetal growth and development, and fetal teratogens that could benefit from additional nursing research.
12. Use critical thinking to analyze ways that nurses can contribute to health education to promote fetal development and counseling for parents facing genetic issues.
13. Integrate knowledge of genetic inheritance, fetal growth, and development and environmental influences on the fetus with nursing process to achieve quality child health nursing care.

Mrs. Alvarez is a woman you meet at a clinic. She was adopted as a newborn and never felt a need to locate her birth parents because her adoptive parents provided a "close to perfect" childhood for her. After college, she married the most eligible bachelor in her hometown. Both friends and family hurried to assure her they would make a perfect couple. Mrs. Alvarez is now pregnant with their first child. She has quit smoking approximately 2 months ago, but her husband and other family members continue to smoke. At 15 weeks into the pregnancy, she has been advised her child may have a chromosomal abnormality. She asks you, "How can this be happening? There's no disease in either of our families. Could it be from the beer I drank a few months ago at a family reunion? Or is it from secondary smoke?" How would you answer her?

In previous chapters, you learned about caring for childrearing families. In this chapter, you'll add information about the care of the family with a possible genetic disorder and typical fetal growth and development, including possible environmental influences that can affect the fetus. This is important information because it can influence the health of a family for generations to come.

After you've studied the chapter, turn to the Critical Thinking Exercises at the end of the chapter to sharpen your skills and test your knowledge.

Crucial to the care of the childrearing family is a solid foundation prior to the child's birth. This foundation involves ensuring the optimal safe environment for fetal growth and development. Circumstances such as genetic alterations or environmental influences can interfere with this, thus affecting the overall health of the family.

The possibility of a genetic disorder crosses the minds of many parents and families whether or not there is any family history of genetic disorders. Many couples will ask health care providers about their chances of having a child with a genetic disorder and about genetic testing. Advances in genetic screening have made genetic testing more common.

Routinely, most women are offered screening to evaluate for possible neural tube or chromosome defects during pregnancy. Additional tests may be offered if the woman is over age 35 because certain genetic disorders, such as Down syndrome, increase with increasing maternal age. Couples who already know of the existence of a genetic disorder in their family or those who have had a previous child born with a congenital anomaly often require additional, more extensive testing. If the results indicate a genetic disorder, families will almost certainly undergo an emotional period of decision making. Informative and sensitive genetic counseling by health care providers educated in the specialty of genetics is essential. Because most screening takes place in an ambulatory setting, the nurse plays a vital role as educator, supporter, and communicator for the family (Guralnick, 1998).

Through advancements in medical research and photography, there is now a clear idea of what the fetus looks like from the moment of fertilization until birth. The fetus grows and develops steadily at predictable stages. These stages provide a guide for determining the well being of an individual fetus. Knowledge about fetal growth and development can provide an important frame of reference, allowing family members to begin thinking about and accepting the newest family member even before the child actually arrives.

For optimal fetal growth and development, a safe environment is essential. However, outside influences, such as maternal infections, use of drugs, alcohol or nicotine, and exposure to chemicals may interfere with this safe fetal environment, placing the fetus at risk for problems. In addition, exposure to certain substances, such as radiation or drugs, have been linked to some genetic disorders.

Because the ultimate goal is a healthy newborn, National Health Goals have been established to address the issues of genetics and fetal growth. These are shown in the Focus on National Health Goals.

NURSING PROCESS OVERVIEW

for Genetic Counseling and Fetal Development

Assessment

Assessment is a crucial step in any nursing intervention, but it plays an especially vital role in genetic counseling and fetal development. Assessment measures

FOCUS ON NATIONAL HEALTH GOALS

National Health Goals address genetic disorders, and screening and fetal growth. These are:

- Increase to at least 90% the proportion of women who are offered screening and counseling for prenatal detection of fetal abnormalities.
- Increase to at least 95% the proportion of newborns screened by state-sponsored programs for genetic disorders and other disabling conditions and to 90% the proportion of newborns testing positive for disease who receive appropriate treatment.
- Reduce the fetal death rate (death below 20 or more weeks of gestation) to no more than 5 per 1000 live births from a baseline of 7.6/1000.
- Reduce low birth weight to an incidence of no more than 5% of live births and very low birth weight to no more than 1% of live births from baselines of 6.9 and 1.2% (DHHS, 1995).

Nurses can be instrumental in helping the nation achieve these goals by being sensitive to the need for genetic screening, counseling and education in all settings. Nursing research in such areas as determining when people are responsive to genetic counseling, the effect on bonding of learning alpha-fetoprotein level during pregnancy, and how soon women make lifestyle changes during pregnancy to more healthy actions could lead to increased success for meeting these goals.

include a detailed family history; client health history; such as lifestyle patterns and environment; physical examination; and a series of laboratory tests that may demand equally varied techniques for obtaining maternal, fetal, and cell samples for analysis. Using the stages of fetal development, the expected date of birth of the fetus can be predicted more accurately. Nurses serve as members of genetic assessment and counseling teams in many roles, especially to help obtain the initial family history, assist with the preliminary physical examination, obtain blood serum for analysis, or assist with procedures, such as amniocentesis.

Nursing Diagnosis

Typical nursing diagnoses related to the area of genetic disorders and fetal development may include:

- Health-seeking behaviors related to knowledge of fetal growth and developmental milestones
- Knowledge deficit related to effects of exposure of teratogens on the fetus
- Risk for fetal injury related to lack of information about teratogenicity of alcohol, drugs, and cigarettes
- Decisional conflict related to testing for an untreatable genetic disorder
- Fear related to outcome of genetic screening tests
- Situational low self-esteem related to identified chromosomal abnormality
- Knowledge deficit related to inheritance pattern of a genetic disorder
- Health-seeking behaviors related to potential for genetic transmission of disease
- Altered sexuality pattern related to fear of conceiving a child with a genetic disorder

Outcome Identification and Planning

Goals and outcome criteria established for teaching about fetal growth should be realistic and based on the parents' knowledge and desire for information. When additional assessment measures are necessary, be sure to include this material in the teaching plan, explaining why further assessment is necessary and what the parents can expect.

Often, helping a family, but more specifically the woman, plan to avoid teratogens may be difficult because a total change in lifestyle, such as not smoking, not drinking alcohol, or changing a work environment, may be involved. Fortunately, most families are highly motivated to complete a pregnancy satisfactorily. With this level of motivation, planning becomes the task of determining the best route to achieve a goal rather than educating about the need for goal achievement.

Try to turn long-term goals into more manageable, short-term ones. For example, to *reduce* smoking in pregnancy or to stop smoking just for the duration of the pregnancy may be more realistic than a goal to *stop* smoking altogether. Eliminating the pressure of making a major permanent lifestyle change may help the family concentrate their efforts on themselves and the fetus over the next several months. Continued reinforcement of their progress may help to continue reducing smoking or not smoking after the baby is born, providing a smoke-free environment for the child.

Outcome identification and planning for families involved with genetic assessment differ according to the type of assessments performed and the results. It may include determining what information the couple needs before testing or helping couples to arrange for further assessment measures during a pregnancy. Goals must be realistic and consistent with the couple's or family's lifestyle.

Implementation

Nurses play a key role in conveying findings about fetal growth and development in as much detail as parents request and also in educating clients and families about health promotion practicies to minimize environmental risks to the fetus. Teaching parents about fetal growth and development helps them to visualize the fetus at each stage of development. This, in turn, helps them to understand the importance of implementing healthy behaviors, such as avoiding substances that may be dangerous to the fetus. Role model health-promotion behaviors to maximize the teaching.

Parental reaction to the knowledge that their child has a possible genetic disorder or to the birth of a child with a genetically inherited disorder usually is similar to those of parents whose child dies at birth. Often both experience grief and must work through stages of shock and denial ("This cannot be true"), anger ("It's not fair this happened to us"), bargaining ("If only this would go away"), to reorganization and acceptance ("It has happened to us and it is all right"). In the newborn period, if they have not finished working though these stages of grief, intervening may be difficult.

As a rule, concentrate on short-term actions. For example: What are the immediate needs of the family, fetus, and newborn? What kind of continued follow-up will be necessary? After the birth, will the baby need to be hospitalized for immediate surgical correction of accompanying congenital anomalies? Will the parents take the baby home, or will he or she be placed temporarily in foster care?

Identifying support people who can be helpful to the parents during the time of disorganization and shock is also important. These may be the usual family resource people, such as grandparents or other family members. In some families, these people may be as disturbed by the diagnosis as the parents and so cannot offer their usual support. Secondary support sources that may be helpful include organizations such as the following:

- March of Dimes Birth Defects Foundation
  1275 Mamaroneck Avenue
  White Plains, NY 10605
- Klinefelter Syndrome and Associates
  PO Box 119
  Roseville, CA 95678-0119

- Fragile X Foundation
  441 York Street, Suite 215
  Denver, CO 80206
- Association for Children with Down Syndrome
  2616 Martin Avenue
  Bellmore, NY 11710
- Turner's Syndrome Society
  15500 Wayzata Boulevard
  Wayzata, MN 55391

Be aware that not all parents are ready to talk to members of such organizations at the time of diagnosis. To join the organization makes the diagnosis "real" or moves them out of denial before they may be ready.

Identifying health care personnel with whom the parents will need to maintain contact during the next few months offers additional support. Consistent, clear communication among all health care team members is essential. At some point, decisions may need to be made about the future, such as schooling, surgical procedures, behavior problems, or future development. Ensure that the parents have health care providers where they know they can turn to at all times, especially when they are moving out of denial.

Outcome Evaluation

Examples of outcome criteria may include:

- Fetus demonstrates achievement of appropriate milestones for gestational age.
- Parents describe a smoke-free home environment.
- Couple states they feel capable of coping no matter what the outcome of genetic testing.
- Couple accurately states the chances of genetic disorder occurring in their next child.
- Couple states they have resolved their feelings of low self-esteem related to birth of child with genetic disorder.

FETAL DEVELOPMENT

In just 38 weeks, a fertilized egg matures from a single cell carrying all the necessary genetic material to a fully developed fetus ready to be born.

Fetal growth and development is typically divided into three periods: pre-embryonic (first 2 weeks beginning with fertilization), embryonic (from weeks 3 through 8), and fetal (from week 8 through birth).

Fertilization: The Beginning of Pregnancy

Fertilization is the union of the ovum and a spermatozoon. Usually, only one ovum reaches maturity each month. Because the functional life of spermatozoa is about 48 hours, possibly as long as 72 hours, the total critical timespan during which fertilization may occur is about 72 hours (48 hours preceding ovulation plus 24 hours afterward).

Normally, an ejaculation of semen averages 2.5 mL of fluid containing 50 to 200 million spermatozoa per milliliter, or an average of 400 million per ejaculation. At the time of ovulation, there is a reduction in the viscosity (thickness) of cervical mucus, making it easier for spermatozoa to penetrate it. Sperm transport is so efficient close to ovulation that spermatozoa deposited in the vagina during intercourse generally reach the cervix within 90 seconds and the outer end of a fallopian tube within 5 minutes after deposition.

Spermatozoa move by means of their *flagella* (tails) and uterine contractions through the cervix, the body of the uterus, and into the fallopian tubes toward the waiting ovum. Sperm undergo **capacitation** (changes in the plasma membrane of the sperm head, which reveals the sperm-binding receptor sites) to be ready for fertilization.

All the spermatozoa that achieve capacitation reach the ovum and cluster around the protective layer of cells. Hyaluronidase (a proteolytic enzyme) is apparently released by the spermatozoa and acts to dissolve the layer of cells protecting the ovum. It is believed that the large numbers of sperm contained in an ejaculation provide enough enzymes to dissolve the corona cells. Under ordinary circumstances, only one spermatozoon is able to penetrate the cell membrane of the ovum. Once it effectively penetrates the zona pellucida, the cell membrane becomes impervious to other spermatozoa.

Immediately after penetration of the ovum, the chromosomal material of the ovum and spermatozoon fuse, forming a **zygote.** Because the spermatozoon and ovum each carried 23 chromosomes (22 autosomes and 1 sex chromosome), a fertilized ovum has 46 chromosomes. If an X-carrying spermatozoon enters the ovum, the resulting child will have two X chromosomes and will be female (XX). If a Y-carrying spermatozoon fertilizes the ovum, the resulting child will have an X and a Y chromosome and will be male (XY).

From the fertilized ovum (the zygote) the future child and also the accessory structures needed for support during intrauterine life, such as the placenta, the fetal membranes, the amniotic fluid, and the umbilical cord, are formed.

Implantation

Once fertilization is complete, the zygote migrates toward the body of the uterus. It is propelled along the near fallopian tube by currents initiated by the *fimbriae,* the fine, hairlike structures that line the openings of the fallopian tubes. Peristaltic action of the tube and movement of the tube cilia help propel the ovum along the length of the tube. During the 3 to 4 days before the zygote reaches the body of the uterus, mitotic cell division, or *cleavage,* begins. The first cleavage occurs at about 24 hours; cleavage divisions continue to occur at a rate of one about every 22 hours. By the time the zygote reaches the body of the uterus, it consists of 16 to 50 cells. At this stage, because of its bumpy outward appearance, it is termed a **morula** (from the Latin word *morus,* meaning "mulberry").

The morula continues to multiply as it floats free in the uterine cavity for 3 or 4 more days. Large cells tend to collect at the periphery of the ball, leaving a fluid space surrounding an inner cell mass. At this stage, the structure is termed a **blastocyst.** It is this structure that attaches to the uterine endometrium. The cells in the outer ring are known as **trophoblast** cells. They are the part of the structure that will later form the placenta and membranes. The inner cell mass (embryoblast cells) is the portion of the structure that will later form the embryo.

Implantation, or contact between the growing structure and the uterine endometrium, occurs approximately 8 to 10 days after fertilization. The blastocyst brushes against the rich uterine endometrium (in the second [secretory] phase of the menstrual cycle), a process termed *apposition.* It attaches to the surface of the endometrium (*adhesion*) and settles down into its soft folds (*invasion*). Stages to this point are depleted in Figure 4-1. Implantation is an important step in pregnancy because as many as 50% of zygotes never achieve it. Once implanted, the zygote is called an **embryo** (Sadler, 1995).

> **CHECKPOINT QUESTIONS**
>
> 1. When does implantation occur?
> 2. What term is used to refer to the implanted fertilized ovum?

Embryonic and Fetal Structures

The Decidua

After fertilization, the corpus luteum in the ovary continues to function rather than to atrophy because of the influence of human chorionic gonadotropin (HCG) hormone secreted by the trophoblast cells. Thus, the uterine endometrium continues to grow in thickness and vascularity. The endometrium is now termed **decidua** (the Latin word for "falling off") because it will be discarded after the birth of the child. The decidua has three separate areas:

1. *Decidua basalis,* or the part of the endometrium lying directly under the embryo (or the portion where the trophoblast cells are establishing communication with maternal blood vessels)
2. *Decidua capsularis,* or the portion of the endometrium that stretches or encapsulates the surface of the trophoblast
3. *Decidua vera,* or the remaining portion of the uterine lining

As the embryo continues to grow, it pushes the decidua capsularis before it like a blanket, eventually bringing the structure into contact with the opposite uterine wall and fusing with the endometrium of the opposite wall.

Chorionic Villi

Once implantation is achieved, the trophoblastic layer of cells of the blastocyst begins to mature rapidly. As early as the 11th or 12th day, miniature villi, or probing "fingers," termed **chorionic villi,** reach out from the single layer of cells into the uterine endometrium.

Chorionic villi have a central core of loose connective tissue surrounded by a double layer of trophoblast cells. The central core of connective tissue contains fetal capillaries. The outer layer of cells is instrumental in the pro-

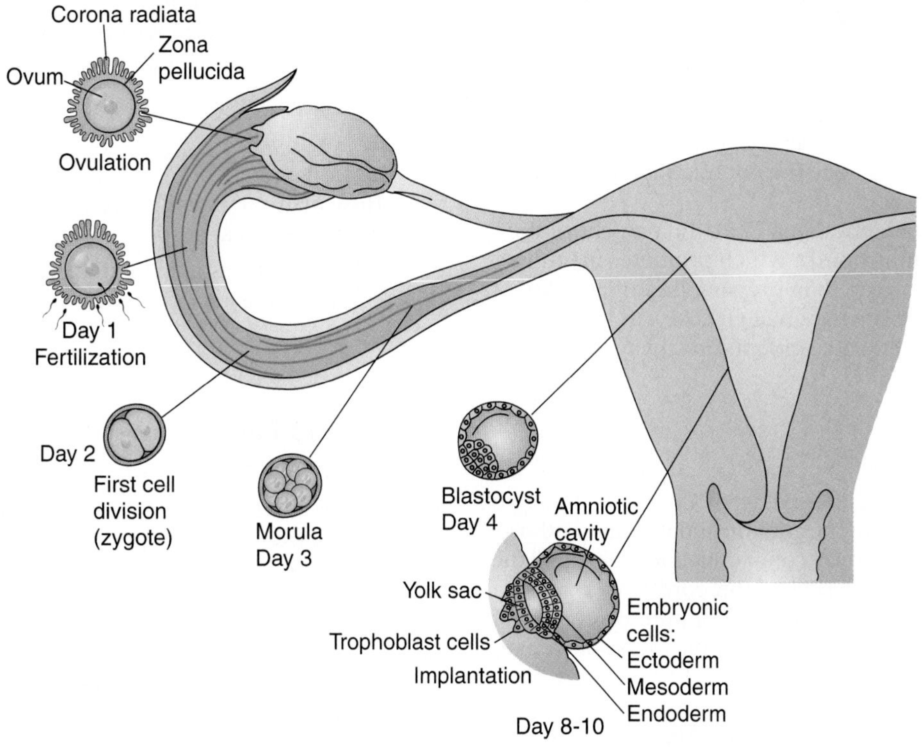

FIGURE 4.1 Schema of ovulation, fertilization, and implantation. At the time of implantation, the blastocyst is already differentiated into germ layers (ectoderm, mesoderm, and entoderm). Cells at the periphery of the structure are trophoblast cells that mature into the placenta.

duction of various placental hormones, such as HCG, somatomammotropin (human placental lactogen [HPL]), estrogen, and progesterone. The inner layer appears to function early in pregnancy, protecting the growing embryo and fetus from certain infectious organisms such as the spirochete of syphilis. However, this layer of cells disappears between the 20th and 24th week. This is why syphilis is considered to have a high potential for fetal damage late in pregnancy, when cytotrophoblast cells are no longer present. Unfortunately, the layer appears to offer little protection against viral invasion at any point.

The Placenta

The placenta, Latin for "pancake," which is descriptive of its size and appearance at term, arises out of trophoblast tissue. It serves as the fetal lungs, kidneys, and gastrointestinal tract and as a separate endocrine organ. Its growth parallels that of the fetus, covering about half the surface area of the internal uterus.

Aside from serving as the source of oxygen and nutrients for the fetus, the placenta is a separate, important hormone-producing system. Hormones produced include:

- Human chorionic gonadotropin (HCG), which is the first hormone to be produced, acts as a fail-safe measure to ensure continued production of progesterone and estrogen; also may play a role in suppressing the maternal immunologic response to prevent placental tissue rejection; exerts an effect on the fetal testes (if fetus is male) to begin testosterone production, causing the maturation of the male reproductive tract
- Estrogen (primarily estriol), which contributes to the mother's mammary gland development in preparation for lactation and stimulates uterine growth to accommodate the developing fetus
- Progesterone, which is necessary to maintain the endometrial lining of the uterus during pregnancy; also appears to reduce the contractility of the uterine musculature
- Human placental lactogen (HPL [human chorionic somatomammotropin]), which promotes mammary gland (breast) growth in preparation for lactation and helps regulate maternal glucose, protein, and fat levels so adequate amounts are always available to the fetus

The Umbilical Cord

The **umbilical cord,** consisting of one vein and two arteries, is formed from the amnion and chorion and provides a circulatory pathway connecting the embryo to the chorionic villi. The function of the cord is to transport oxygen and nutrients to the fetus from the placenta and to return waste products from the fetus to the placenta.

The Membranes and Amniotic Fluid

The chorionic villi on the medial surface of the trophoblast (those that are not involved in implantation because they do not touch the endometrium) gradually thin and leave the medial surface of the structure smooth (the *chorion laeve,* or *smooth chorion*). The smooth chorion eventually becomes the *chorionic membrane*, the outermost fetal membrane. Once it becomes smooth, it offers support to the sac that contains the amniotic fluid. A second membrane lining the chorionic membrane, the *amniotic membrane* or amnion, forms beneath the chorion. These membranes cover the fetal surface of the placenta and give that surface its typical shiny appearance.

Unlike the chorionic membrane, the amniotic membrane not only offers support to amniotic fluid but actually produces the fluid. In addition, it produces a phospholipid that initiates the formation of prostaglandins, which cause uterine contractions and may be the "trigger" that initiates labor.

Amniotic fluid is constantly being newly formed and reabsorbed, so it is never stagnant within the membranes. Because the fetus continually swallows the fluid, it is absorbed across the fetal intestine into the fetal bloodstream. From there, the umbilical arteries exchange it across the placenta. Some fluid is probably absorbed by direct contact with the fetal surface of the placenta.

Amniotic fluid is an important protective mechanism for the fetus because it:

- Shields against pressure or a blow to the mother's abdomen
- Protects the fetus from changes in temperature (liquid changes temperature more slowly than air)
- Probably aids muscular development (allows the fetus freedom to move)
- Protects the umbilical cord from pressure, protecting fetal oxygenation

Even if the membranes rupture before birth and the bulk of the amniotic fluid is lost, some will always surround the fetus in utero because new fluid is constantly being formed. Amniotic fluid is slightly alkaline with a pH of about 7.2.

✓ CHECKPOINT QUESTIONS

3. How many arteries and veins are usually found in the umbilical cord?
4. What structures give the fetal surface of the placenta its shiny appearance?

Origin and Development of Organ Systems

From the beginning of fetal growth, development proceeds in a **cephalocaudal** (head-to-tail) direction, that is, head development occurs first and is followed by development of the middle and, finally, lower body parts. This pattern of development continues after birth, evidenced by newborns lifting up their head approximately a year before walking. As a fetus grows, body organ systems develop from specific tissue layers called germ layers.

Primary Germ Layers

At the time of implantation, the blastocyst already has differentiated to a point at which two separate cavities appear in the inner structure: (1) a large one, the **amniotic cavity,** which is lined with a distinctive layer of cells, the **ectoderm** and (2) a smaller cavity, the **yolk sac,** which is lined with **entoderm** cells.

Between the amniotic cavity and the yolk sac, a third layer of primary cells, the **mesoderm,** forms. The embryo will begin to develop (from an *embryonic shield*) at the point where the three cell layers (ectoderm, entoderm, mesoderm) meet. Each germ layer of primary tissue develops into specific body systems Table 4-1). Knowing which structures rise from each germ layer is important because coexisting congenital defects found in newborns usually arise from the same layer. For example, a tracheoesophageal fistula (both organs arising from the entoderm) is a common birth anomaly. Heart and kidney defects (both organs arising from the mesoderm) are also commonly seen together.

Knowing the origins of body structures also helps to explain why certain screening procedures are ordered for newborns with congenital malformations. A kidney x-ray examination, for example, may be ordered for a child born with a heart defect. A child with a malformation of the urinary tract is often investigated for reproductive abnormalities as well.

All organ systems are complete, at least in a rudimentary form, at 8 weeks' gestation. During this early time of **organogenesis** (organ formation), the growing structure is most vulnerable to invasion by teratogens (see discussion later in the chapter). Figure 4-2 illustrates critical periods of fetal growth.

TABLE 4.1 Origin of Body Tissue

GERM LAYER	BODY PORTIONS FORMED
Ectoderm	• Central nervous system (brain and spinal cord) • Peripheral nervous system • Skin, hair, and nails • Sebaceous glands • Sense organs • Mucous membranes of the anus, mouth and nose • Tooth enamel • Mammary glands
Mesoderm	• Supporting structures of the body (connective tissue, bones, cartilage, muscle, ligaments and tendons) • Dentin of teeth • Upper portion of the urinary system (kidneys and ureters) • Reproductive system • Heart • Circulatory system • Blood cells • Lymph vessels
Entoderm	• Lining of pericardial, pleura, and peritoneal cavities • Lining of the gastrointestinal tract, respiratory tract, tonsils, parathyroid, thyroid, thymus glands • Lower urinary system (bladder and urethra)

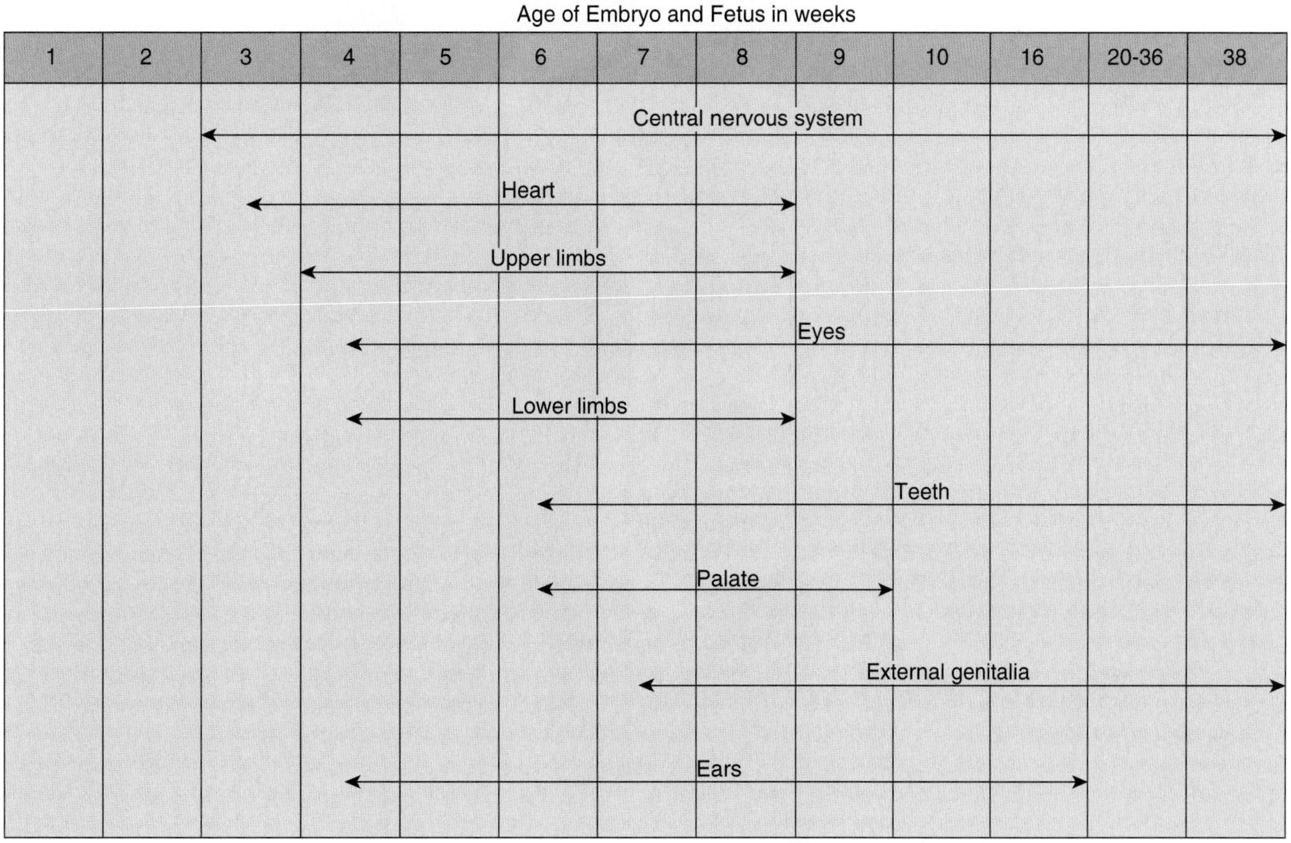

FIGURE 4.2 Critical periods of fetal growth.

Cardiovascular System

The cardiovascular system is one of the first systems to become functional in intrauterine life. Simple blood cells joined to the walls of the yolk sac progress to a network of blood vessels, and to a single heart tube forming as early as the 16th day of life, beating as early as the 24th day. The septum that divides the heart into chambers develops during the 6th or 7th week. Heart valves begin to develop in the 7th week. The heart beat may be heard with a Doppler as early as the 10th to 12th week of pregnancy. An electrocardiogram (ECG) may be recorded on a fetus as early as the 11th week, although the accuracy of such ECGs is in doubt until about the 20th week of pregnancy when conduction is more regulated.

The heart rate of a fetus is affected by fetal oxygen level, body activity, and circulating blood volume just as in adult life. After the 28th week of pregnancy, when the sympathetic nervous system has matured, the heart rate will begin to show a baseline variability of about 5 beats per minute on a fetal heart rate rhythm strip.

Fetal Circulation. As early as the 3rd week of intrauterine life, fetal blood has begun to exchange nutrients with the maternal circulation across the chorionic villi. Fetal circulation (Figure 4-3) differs from extrauterine circulation in several respects. During intrauterine life, the fetus derives its oxygen and excretes carbon dioxide not from oxygen exchange in the lungs but from the placenta. Blood does enter the lungs while the child is in utero, but this blood flow is to supply the cells of the lungs themselves, not for oxygen exchange. Specialized structures present in the fetus shunt blood flow to supply the most important organs, the brain, liver, heart, and kidneys.

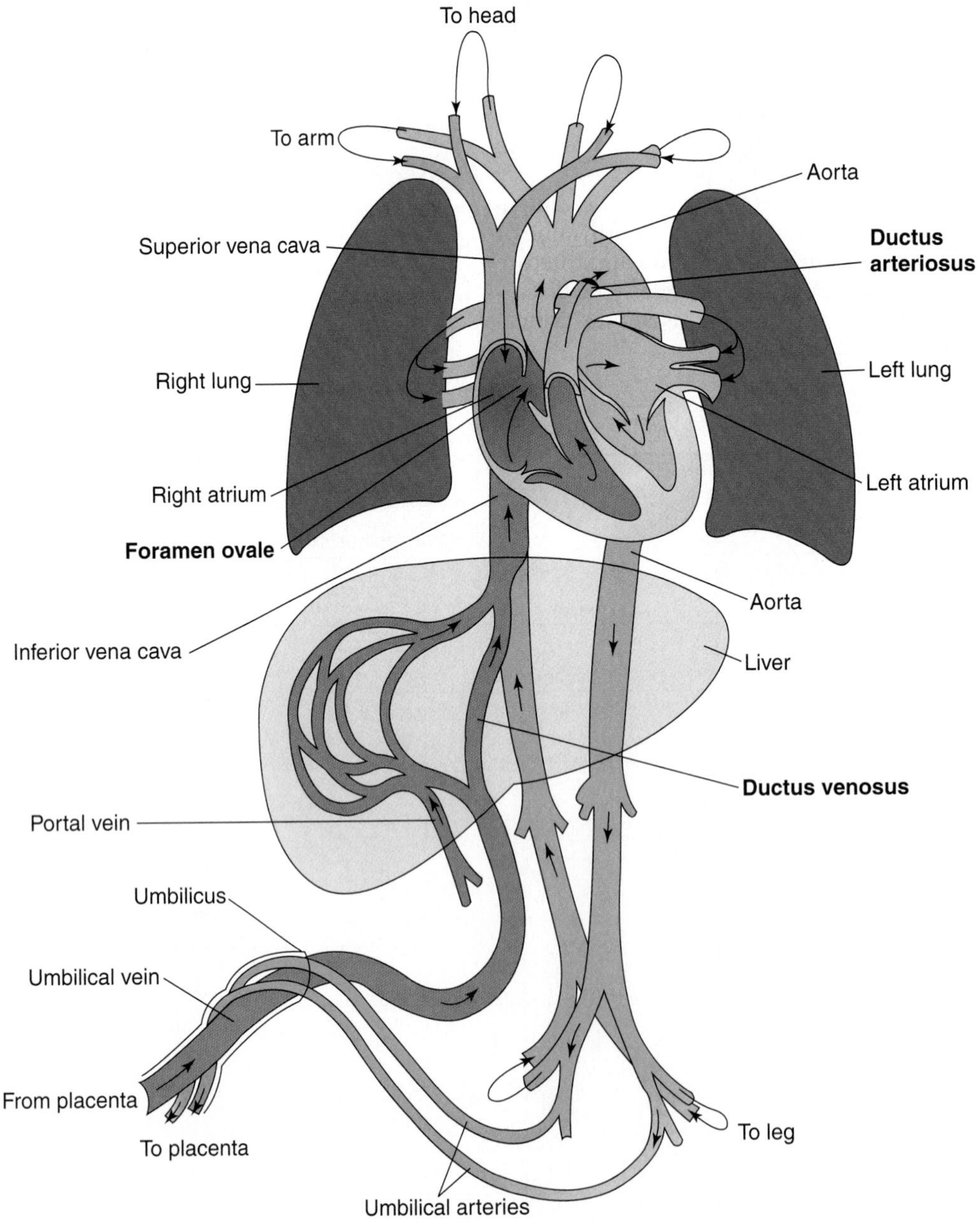

FIGURE 4.3 Fetal circulation.

Blood arriving at the fetus from the placenta is highly oxygenated. This blood enters the fetus through the umbilical vein (called a vein even though it carries oxygenated blood, because the direction of the blood is toward the fetal heart). The umbilical vein carries the blood to the inferior vena cava through an accessory structure, the **ductus venosus.** The ductus venosus receives most of the oxygenated blood from the umbilical vein to supply the fetal liver. It then empties into the inferior vena cava. From the inferior vena cava, blood is carried to the right side of the heart. As the blood enters the right atrium, the bulk of it is shunted into the left atrium through an opening in the atrial septum, the **foramen ovale.** From the left atrium, it follows the course of normal circulation into the left ventricle and into the aorta.

Blood from the arms and head is returned to the heart by the superior vena cava. The blood enters the right atrium and leaves it by the normal circulatory route, that is, through the tricuspid valve into the right ventricle, then through the pulmonary artery in the normal manner. A small portion of this blood flow services the lung tissue. However, the larger portion is shunted away from the lungs, through an additional structure, the **ductus arteriosus,** directly into the aorta and then into the descending aorta.

Most of the blood flow from the descending aorta is transported by the umbilical arteries (called arteries even though they are now transporting deoxygenated blood, because they are carrying blood away from the fetal heart) back through the umbilical cord to the placental villi, where new oxygen exchange takes place.

The blood oxygen saturation level of the fetus is about 80% of the newborn's saturation level. The rapid fetal heart rate during pregnancy (120 to 160 beats per minute) is necessary to supply oxygen to cells when red blood cells are never fully saturated. Despite a low blood oxygen saturation level, carbon dioxide does not accumulate in the fetal system because of its rapid diffusion into maternal blood across a favorable placental pressure gradient.

Fetal Hemoglobin. Fetal hemoglobin differs from adult hemoglobin in several ways:

- Different composition (two alpha and two gamma chains as compared with two alpha and two beta chains of adult hemoglobin)
- Greater oxygen affinity (increases its efficiency)
- More concentrated (at birth, a newborn's hemoglobin level is about 17.1 g/100 mL compared with an adult's normal level of 11 g/100 mL; a newborn's hematocrit is about 53% compared with an adult's normal level of 45%)

The change from fetal to adult hemoglobin levels begins before birth and accelerates after birth.

Respiratory System

At the 3rd week of intrauterine life, the respiratory and digestive tracts exist as a single tube. Like all body tubes, initially it is a solid structure, which then canalizes (hollows out). By the end of the 4th week, a septum begins to divide the esophagus from the trachea. At the same time, lung buds appear on the trachea.

Until the 7th week of life, the diaphragm does not completely divide the thoracic cavity from the abdomen. During the 6th week of life, lung buds may extend down into the abdomen, reentering the chest only as the chest's longitudinal dimension increases and the diaphragm becomes complete (at the end of the 7th week). If the diaphragm fails to close completely, the stomach, spleen, liver, or intestines may enter the thoracic cavity. The child may be born with a diaphragmatic hernia, compromising the lungs and perhaps displacing the heart.

Important respiratory development milestones include the following:

- Alveoli and capillaries begin to form between the 24th and 28th weeks. Both capillary and alveoli development must be complete before gas exchange can occur in the fetal lungs.
- Spontaneous respiratory movements begin as early as 3 months of pregnancy, continuing throughout pregnancy.
- Specific lung fluid with a low surface tension and low viscosity forms in alveoli to aid in expansion of alveoli at birth; it is rapidly absorbed after birth.
- **Surfactant,** a phospholipid substance, is formed and excreted by the alveolar cells at about the 24th week of pregnancy. This decreases alveolar surface tension on expiration, preventing alveolar collapse and improving the infant's ability to maintain respirations in the outside environment. Surfactant has two components: *lecithin* and *sphingomyelin.* Early in the formation of surfactant, sphingomyelin is the chief component. At about 35 weeks, there is a surge in the production of lecithin. This then becomes the chief component by a ratio of 2:1. With fetal lung movements, surfactant mixes with amniotic fluid. Analysis of the lecithin/sphingomyelin (L/S) ratio by an amniocentesis technique is one of the primary tests of fetal maturity. Lack of surfactant is a factor associated with the development of respiratory distress syndrome (see Chapter 6). Any interference with the blood supply to the fetus appears to enhance surfactant development. This type of stress probably increases steroid levels in the fetus. Increased steroid levels are associated with alveolar maturation (Cunningham et al, 1997).

Nervous System

Like the circulatory system, the nervous system begins to develop extremely early in pregnancy. During the 3rd and 4th weeks of life, active formation of the nervous system and sense organs has already begun.

- A *neural plate* (a thickened portion of the ectoderm) is apparent by the 3rd week of gestation. Its top portion differentiates into the neural tube, which will form the central nervous system (brain and spinal cord), and the neural crest, which will develop into the peripheral nervous system.
- Brain waves can be detected on electroencephalogram (EEG) by the 8th week.

- All parts of the brain (cerebrum, cerebellum, pons, and medulla oblongata) form in utero, although they are not completely mature at birth. Growth continues to occur rapidly during the 1st year and continues at high levels until 5 or 6 years of age.
- The eye and inner ear develop as projections of the original neural tube.
- By 24 weeks, the ear is capable of responding to sound; the eyes exhibit a pupillary reaction, indicating sight is present.

The neurologic system seems particularly prone to insult during the early weeks of the embryonic period. All during pregnancy and at birth, the system is vulnerable to damage from anoxia.

Endocrine System

As soon as endocrine organs mature in intrauterine life, function begins, including the following:

- The fetal adrenal glands supply a precursor for estrogen synthesis by the placenta.
- The fetal pancreas produces the insulin needed by the fetus. (Insulin does not cross the placenta.)
- The thyroid and parathyroid glands play vital roles in metabolic function and calcium balance.

Digestive System

The digestive tract is separated from the respiratory tract at about the 4th week. After this time, the intestinal tract grows extremely rapidly. Initially solid, the tubes canalize (hollow out) to become patent. Later, the endothelial cells of the gastrointestinal tract proliferate extensively, occluding the lumens once more. They have to canalize again. Atresia or stenosis can develop if either the first or second canalization does not occur. The proliferation of cells shed in the second recanalization forms the basis for meconium (see below).

Because the abdomen becomes too small to contain the intestine, a portion of the intestine, guided by the vitelline membrane (a part of the yolk sac) enters the base of the umbilical cord during the 6th week of intrauterine life. Intestine remains in the base of the cord until about the 10th week. At this time, the fetal trunk has extended and enlarged the abdominal cavity so it is large enough to accommodate all the intestinal mass. As the intestine returns to the abdominal cavity, it must rotate 180 degrees. Failure to do so can result in inadequate mesentery attachments, possibly leading to volvulus of the intestine. If any intestinal coils remain outside the abdomen, in the base of the cord, a congenital anomaly, *omphalocele,* develops. A similar defect, gastroschisis, occurs when the original midline fusion that occurred at the early cell stage is incomplete. If the vitelline duct does not atrophy after return of the intestines, a Meckel's diverticulum (a pouch of intestinal tissue) or an opening between the intestine and the umbilicus can result.

Meconium, consisting of cellular wastes, bile, fats, mucoproteins, mucopolysaccharides, and portions of the vernix caseosa, the lubricating substance that forms on the fetal skin, forms in the intestines as early as the 16th week. Meconium is black or dark green (obtaining its color from bile pigment) and sticky.

The gastrointestinal tract is sterile before birth. Because vitamin K is synthesized by the action of bacteria in the intestines, this can cause vitamin K levels to be low in the newborn infant. In addition, sucking and swallowing reflexes are not mature until the fetus is about 32 weeks or the fetus weighs 1500 g.

The ability of the gastrointestinal tract to secrete enzymes essential to carbohydrate and protein digestion is mature at 36 weeks. However, *amylase,* an enzyme found in saliva and necessary for digestion of complex starches, is not mature until 3 months after birth. Many newborns have not yet developed *lipase,* an enzyme needed for fat digestion.

The liver is active throughout gestation, functioning as a filter between the incoming blood and the fetal circulation and a deposit for fetal stores such as iron and glycogen. However, it is still immature at birth, possibly leading to hypoglycemia and hyperbilirubinemia, two serious problems in the first 24 hours after birth.

Musculoskeletal System

The fetus can be seen to move as early as the 11th week, although this movement is not felt until nearly 20 weeks. In the first 2 weeks of fetal life, cartilage prototypes provide position and support. Ossification of bone tissue begins about the 12th week. The ossification process continues all through fetal life and actually until adulthood. Carpals, tarsals, and sternal bones generally do not ossify until birth is imminent.

Reproductive System

A child's sex is determined at the moment of conception by a spermatozoon carrying an X or a Y chromosome and can be determined as early as 8 weeks by chromosomal analysis. At about the 6th week of life, the gonads (ovaries or testes) form.

- If testes form, testosterone is secreted, apparently influencing the sexually neutral genital duct to form other male organs.
- In the absence of testosterone secretion, female organs will form.

Normally, testes descend from the pelvic cavity, where they first form into the scrotal sac late in intrauterine life, at the 34th to 38th week.

Urinary System

Although rudimentary kidneys are present as early as the end of the 4th week, they do not appear to be essential for life before birth. Urine is formed by the 12th week and is excreted into the amniotic fluid by the 16th week of gestation. At term, fetal urine is being excreted at the rate of 500 mL/day. An amount of amniotic fluid that is less than normal (oligohydramnios) suggests that fetal kidneys are not secreting adequate urine.

The complex structure of the kidneys gradually develops during gestation and for months afterward. The loop of Henle, for example, is not fully differentiated until the child is born. Glomerular filtration and concentration of urine in the newborn are not efficient because the kidneys are not fully mature even by birth.

Early in the embryonic stage of urinary system development, the bladder extends to the umbilical region. On rare occasions, an open lumen between the urinary bladder and the umbilicus fails to close. Termed a *patent urachus,* this is discovered at birth by the persistent drainage of a clear, acid-pH fluid (urine) from the umbilicus.

Integumentary System

The skin of a fetus appears thin and almost translucent until subcutaneous fat begins to be deposited at about 36 weeks. Skin is covered by soft, downy hairs (lanugo) and a cream cheese-like substance, vernix caseosa, important for lubrication and for keeping skin from macerating.

Immune System

IgG maternal antibodies cross the placenta into the fetus primarily during the third trimester of pregnancy, giving a fetus temporary passive immunity against diseases for which the mother has antibodies. These often include poliomyelitis, rubella (German measles), rubeola (regular measles), diphtheria, tetanus, infectious parotitis (mumps), and pertussis (whooping cough). Little or no immunity to the herpes virus (the virus of cold sores and genital herpes) is transferred to the fetus; thus, the average newborn is potentially susceptible to this disease.

The level of passive IgG immunoglobulins peaks at birth and then decreases over the next 9 months while infants begin to build up their own stores of IgG as well as IgA and IgM. Because the passive immunity received by the newborn has already declined substantially by about 2 months, immunization against diphtheria, tetanus, pertussis, and poliomyelitis is typically started. Passive antibodies to measles have been demonstrated to last over a year. Consequently, the immunization for measles is not given until 15 months' extrauterine age.

It has been shown that a fetus is capable of active antibody production late in a pregnancy. Generally, this is not necessary, however, because antibodies are manufactured only when stimulated by an invading antigen, and antigens rarely invade the intrauterine space. However, infants whose mothers have had an infection such as rubella during pregnancy typically have IgM antibodies to rubella in their blood serum at birth. Because IgA and IgM antibodies cannot cross the placenta, their presence in a newborn is proof that the fetus has been exposed to the disease.

> **CHECKPOINT QUESTIONS**
>
> 5. When does surfactant excretion by alveolar cells begin?
> 6. Which immunoglobulin crosses the placenta?

Milestones of Fetal Growth and Development

Parents often have many questions about their baby's appearance and age during gestation. Figure 4-4 illustrates the comparative size and appearance of human embryos and fetuses at different stages. Fetal developmental milestones based on **gestational age** (measured from the first day of the mother's last menstrual period) are highighted in Table 4-2.

Determination of Estimated Birth Date

It is impossible to predict the day of birth with a high degree of accuracy. Traditionally, this date has been referred to as the EDC, for estimated date of confinement. However, since women are no longer confined after

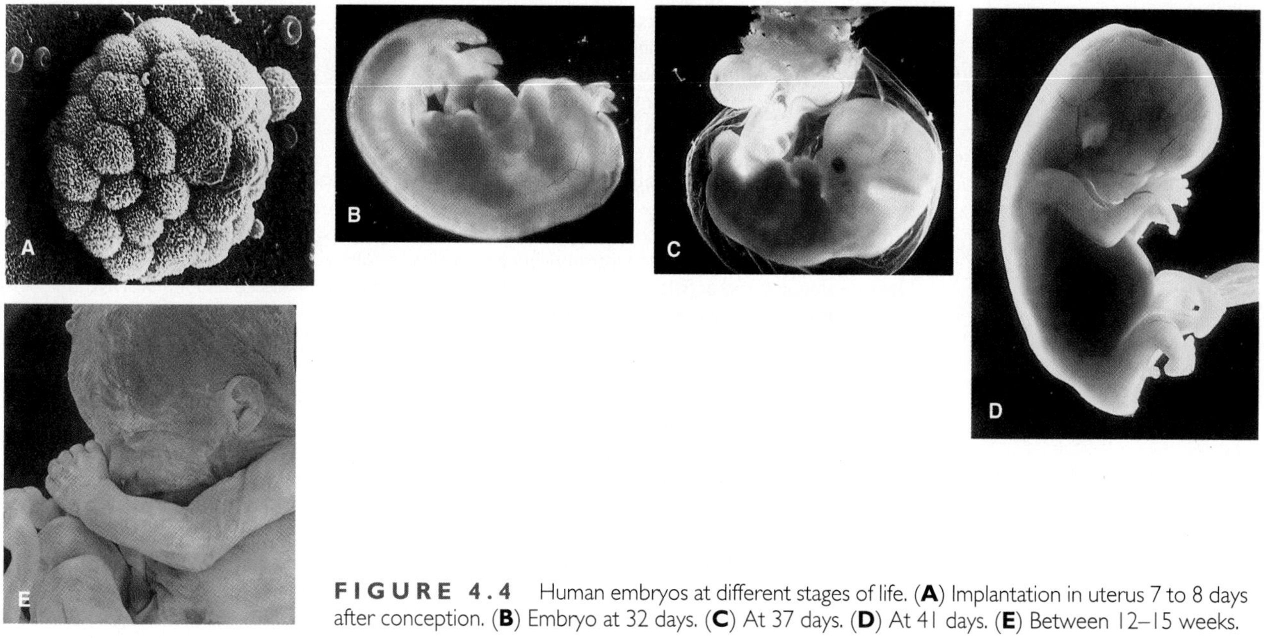

FIGURE 4.4 Human embryos at different stages of life. (**A**) Implantation in uterus 7 to 8 days after conception. (**B**) Embryo at 32 days. (**C**) At 37 days. (**D**) At 41 days. (**E**) Between 12–15 weeks.

TABLE 4.2 Fetal Developmental Milestones

GESTATIONAL AGE	MILESTONES
End of 4 Gestation Weeks	• Length is 0.75 to 1 cm. • Weight is 400 mg. • The spinal cord is formed and fused at the midpoint. • Lateral wings that will form the body are folded forward to fuse at the midline. • Head folds forward, becoming prominent, composing about one third of the entire structure. • The back is bent so the head almost touches the tip of the tail. • The rudimentary heart appears as a prominent bulge on the anterior surface. • Arms and legs are budlike structures. • Rudimentary eyes, ears, and nose are discernible.
End of 8 Gestation Weeks	• Length is 2.5 cm (1 in). • Weight is 20 g. • Organogenesis is complete. • The heart with a septum and valves is beating rhythmically. • Facial features are definitely discernible. • Extremities have developed. • External genitalia are present, but sex is not distinguishable by simple observation. • The primitive tail is regressing. • Abdomen appears large as the fetal intestine is growing rapidly. • Sonogram shows a gestational sac, diagnostic of pregnancy
End of 12 Gestation Weeks (First Trimester)	• Length is 7 to 9 cm. • Weight is 45 g. • Nail beds are forming on fingers and toes. • Spontaneous movements are possible, although usually too faint to be felt by the mother. • Some reflexes, such as Babinski reflex, are present. • Bone ossification centers are forming. • Tooth buds are present. • Sex is distinguishable by outward appearance. • Kidney secretion has begun, although urine may not yet be evident in amniotic fluid. • Heart beat is audible by a Doppler.
End of 16 Gestation Weeks	• Length is 10 to 17 cm. • Weight is 55 to 120 g. • Fetal heart sounds are audible with an ordinary stethoscope. • Lanugo (the fine, downy hair on the back and arms of newborns, apparently serving as a source of insulation for body heat) is well formed. • Liver and pancreas are functioning. • Fetus actively swallows amniotic fluid, demonstrating an intact but uncoordinated swallowing reflex.
End of 20 Gestation Weeks	• Length is 25 cm. • Weight is 223 g. • Spontaneous fetal movements can be sensed by the mother. • Antibody production is possible. • Hair forms, extending to include eyebrows and hair on the head. • Meconium is present in the upper intestine. • Brown fat, a special fat that will aid in temperature regulation at birth, begins to be formed behind the kidneys, sternum, and posterior neck. • Fetal heart beat is strong enough to be audible through the abdomen with an ordinary stethoscope. • *Vernix caseosa,* a cream cheese–like substance produced by the sebaceous glands that serves as a protective skin covering during intrauterine life, begins to form. • Definite sleeping and activity patterns are distinguishable (the fetus has developed biorhythms that will guide sleep–wake patterns throughout life).
End of 24 Gestation Weeks (Second Trimester)	• Length is 28 to 36 cm. • Weight is 550 g. • Passive antibody transfer from mother to fetus probably begins as early as the 20th week of gestation, certainly by the 24th week of gestation. Infants born before antibody transfer has taken place have no natural immunity and need more than the usual protection against infectious disease in the newborn period until the infant's own store of immunoglobulins can build up. • Meconium is present as far as the rectum. • Active production of lung surfactant begins.

(continued)

TABLE 4.2 Fetal Developmental Milestones *(Continued)*

GESTATIONAL AGE	MILESTONES
	• Eyebrows and eyelashes are well defined. • Eyelids, previously fused since the 12th week, now open. • Pupils are capable of reacting to light. • When fetuses reach 24 weeks, or 601 g, they have achieved a practical low-end age of viability if they are cared for after birth in a modern intensive care facility.
End of 28 Gestation Weeks	• Length is 35 to 38 cm. • Weight is 1200 g. • Lung alveoli begin to mature, and surfactant can be demonstrated in amniotic fluid. • Testes begin to descend into the scrotal sac from the lower abdominal cavity in males. • The blood vessels of the retina are extremely susceptible to damage from high oxygen concentrations (an important consideration when caring for preterm infants who need oxygen).
End of 32 Gestation Weeks	• Length is 38 to 43 cm. • Weight is 1600 g. • Subcutaneous fat begins to be deposited (the former stringy, "little-old man" appearance is lost). • Fetus is aware of sounds outside the mother's body. • Active Moro reflex is present. • Delivery position (vertex or breech) may be assumed. • Iron stores that provide iron for the time during which the neonate will ingest only milk after birth are beginning to be developed. • Fingernails grow to reach the end of fingertips.
End of 36 Gestation Weeks	• Length is 42 to 49 cm. • Weight is 1900 to 2700 g (5 to 6 lb). • Body stores of glycogen, iron, carbohydrate, and calcium are augmented. • Additional amounts of subcutaneous fat are deposited. • Sole of the foot has only one or two crisscross creases compared with the full crisscross pattern that will be evident at term. • Amount of lanugo present begins to diminish. • Most babies turn into a vertex or head-down presentation during this month.
End of 40 Gestation Weeks (Third Trimester)	• Length is 48 to 52 cm; crown to rump is 35 to 37 cm. • Weight is 3000 g (7 to 7½ lb). • Fetus kicks actively—hard enough to cause the mother considerable discomfort. • Fetal hemoglobin begins its conversion to adult hemoglobin. The conversion is so rapid that, at birth, about 20% of hemoglobin will be adult in character. • Vernix caseosa is fully formed. • Fingernails extend over the fingertips. • Creases on the soles of the feet cover at least two thirds of the surface. • Fetus often sinks into the birth canal during last 2 weeks (in primiparas [women having their first babies]).

childbirth, EDB (estimated date of birth) or EDD (estimated date of delivery) is more commonly used today.

Nagele's rule, the standard method used to predict the length of a pregnancy, is shown in Box 4-1. Gestation age wheels or birth date calculators, which can be used to predict a birth date, are also available.

If fertilization occurs early in a menstrual cycle, the pregnancy will probably end "early"; if ovulation and fertilization occur later in the cycle, the pregnancy will end "late." Because of these normal variations, a pregnancy ending 2 weeks before or 2 weeks after the estimated calculated date of birth is considered well within the normal limit (a pregnancy of 38 to 42 weeks in length).

WHAT IF? A couple first comes to the clinic on August 5th. What if the woman tells you she had her last menstrual period March 13th to March 19th? What would be the estimated date of birth?

PREVENTION OF FETAL EXPOSURE TO TERATOGENS

A **teratogen** is any factor, chemical or physical, that adversely affects the fertilized ovum, embryo, or fetus. To reach maturity in optimal health, a fetus needs sound genes and a healthy intrauterine environment that pro-

BOX 4.1

NAGELE'S RULE

To calculate the date of birth by this rule, count backward 3 calendar months from the first day of the last menstrual period and add 7 days. For example, if the last menstrual period began May 15, you would count back 3 months (April 15, March 15, February 15) and add 7 days, to arrive at a date of birth of February 22.

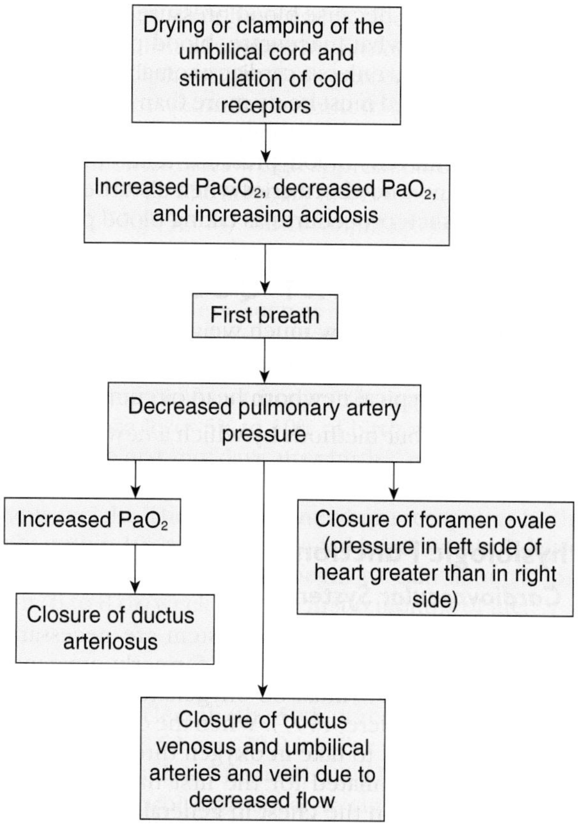

FIGURE 5.2 Circulatory events at birth.

- Elevated white blood cell count, about 15,000 to 30,000 cells/mm^3, possibly as high as 40,000 cells/mm^3 if birth was stressful; predominantly polymorphonuclear cells (neutrophils) initially, then predominantly lymphocytes by end of first month

Keep in mind that capillary heel sticks may reveal a false high hematocrit or hemoglobin value because of sluggish peripheral circulation. Warm the extremity before the blood drawing to improve the accuracy of this value by increasing circulation movement. Also, remember that leukocytosis is a response to the trauma of birth and is nonpathogenic; an increased white blood cell count should not be taken as evidence of infection. However, infection must not be dismissed as a possibility if other signs of infection (e.g., pallor, respiratory difficulty, or cyanosis) are present (Polinski, 1996).

Blood Coagulation. Most newborns are born with a prolonged coagulation or prothrombin time, because their blood levels of vitamin K are lower than normal. Vitamin K is synthesized through the action of intestinal flora and is necessary for the formation of factor II (prothrombin), factor VII (proconvertin), factor IX (plasma thromboplastin component), and factor X (Stuart-Prower factor). A newborn intestine is sterile at birth unless membranes were ruptured more than 24 hours before birth. Therefore, it takes about 24 hours for flora to accumulate and for vitamin K to be synthesized. Because almost all newborns can be predicted to have a diminished blood coagulation ability, vitamin K (Aquamephyton, for example) is administered intramuscularly into the lateral anterior thigh, the preferred site for all injections in the newborn immediately after birth.

Respiratory System

The first breath of a newborn is initiated by a combination of cold receptors, a lowered PaO_2 (PaO_2 falls from 80 mm Hg to as low as 15 mm Hg), and an increased $PaCO_2$ ($PaCO_2$ rises as high as 70 mm Hg). A first breath requires a tremendous amount of pressure (about 40 to 70 cm H_2O). The presence of fluid in the lungs eases the surface tension on alveolar walls and makes a first breath easier. This allows the alveoli to inflate more easily than if the lung walls were dry. About a third of this fluid is forced out of the lungs by the pressure of vaginal birth. Additional fluid is quickly absorbed by lung blood vessels and lymphatics after the first breath.

Once the alveoli have been inflated initially, breathing becomes much easier for the baby, requiring only about 6 to 8 cm H_2O pressure. Within 10 minutes of birth, a newborn has established a good residual volume. By 10 to 12 hours of age, vital capacity is established at newborn proportions. The heart in a newborn takes up proportionately more space than in an adult, so the amount of lung expansion space available is proportionately limited.

A baby born by cesarean birth does not have as much lung fluid expelled at birth as one born vaginally, and so may have more difficulty with establishing effective respiration (excessive fluid blocks air exchange space). Newborns who are immature and whose alveoli collapse each time they exhale (because of the lack of pulmonary surfactant) have trouble in establishing effective residual capacity and respirations. If the alveoli do not open well, a newborn's cardiac system is compromised, because closure of the foramen ovale and ductus arteriosus depends on free blood flow through the pulmonary artery and good oxygenation of blood. A newborn who has difficulty establishing respirations at birth should be examined closely in the postpartal period for a cardiac murmur or indication that he or she still has patent cardiac structures, especially a patent ductus arteriosus.

Gastrointestinal System

Although the gastrointestinal tract is usually sterile at birth, bacteria may be cultured from the intestinal tract in most babies within 5 hours after birth, from all babies at 24 hours of life. Bacteria enter the tract through the newborn's mouth. Some mouth bacteria are airborne. Others may come from vaginal secretions at the time of birth, from hospital bedding, and from contact at the breast. Accumulation of bacteria in the gastrointestinal tract is necessary for digestion and for the synthesis of vitamin K. Because milk, the infant's main diet for the first year, is low in vitamin K, this intestinal synthesis is necessary for blood coagulation.

Although a newborn's stomach holds about 60 to 90 mL, a newborn has limited ability to digest fat and starch because the pancreatic enzymes, lipase and amylase, are deficient for the first few months of life. The newborn regurgitates easily because of an immature cardiac sphincter between the stomach and esophagus. Immature liver functions may lead to lowered glucose and protein serum levels.

Stools. The first stool of the newborn is usually passed within 24 hours after birth. It consists of **meconium**, a sticky, tarlike, blackish-green, odorless material formed from mucus, vernix, lanugo, hormones, and carbohydrates that accumulated during intrauterine life. A newborn who does not pass a meconium stool by 24 to 48 hours after birth should be examined for the possibility of meconium ileus, imperforate anus, or bowel obstruction.

About the 2nd or 3rd day of life, the newborn stool changes in color and consistency, becoming green and loose. This is termed a **transitional stool**, which may resemble diarrhea to the untrained eye. By the 4th day of life, breastfed babies pass three or four light yellow, sweet-smelling stools per day. A formula fed newborn usually passes two or three bright yellow stools a day with a slightly more noticeable odor.

Urinary System

The average newborn usually voids within 24 hours after birth. A newborn who does not take in much fluid for the first 24 hours may void later than this, but the 24-hour cutoff point is a good rule of thumb. Newborns who do not void within this time should be examined. Possible causes are urethral stenosis or absent kidneys or ureters.

Males should void with enough force to produce a small projected arc; females should produce a steady stream, not just continuous dribbling.

The kidneys of newborns do not concentrate urine well. Urine is usually light in color and odorless. The infant is about 6 weeks of age before much control over reabsorption of fluid in tubules and concentration of urine are evident.

A single voiding in a newborn is only about 15 mL and may be easily missed in a thick diaper. Specific gravity is 1.008 to 1.010. The daily urinary output for the first 1 or 2 days is about 30 to 60 mL total, rising to about 300 mL by week 1. The first voiding may be pink or dusky because of uric acid crystals that were formed in the bladder in utero. This is an innocent finding. A small amount of protein may be normally present in voidings for the first few days of life until kidney glomeruli are more fully mature. Typically, the number of voids is documented. Diapers can be weighed to determine the amount.

Autoimmune System

The newborn has difficulty forming antibodies against invading antigens up to 2 months of age and so is prone to infection during this time (Askin, 1995). For this reason, most immunizations against childhood diseases are not given to babies younger than 2 months. The infant at birth, however, has passive antibodies (IgG) from the mother that crossed the placenta—in most instances, antibodies against poliomyelitis, measles, diphtheria, pertussis, chickenpox, rubella, and tetanus. There is little natural immunity transmitted against herpes simplex, so exposure to it must be prevented because without antibody protection in the infant, herpes simplex infections can become systemic or create a rapidly fatal form of the disease in the newborn (Jones, 1996). Newborns are routinely administered hepatitis B vaccine during the first 12 hours after birth.

Neuromuscular System

Mature newborns demonstrate general neuromuscular function by moving their extremities and attempting to control head movement. Limpness or total absence of a muscular response to manipulation is never normal and suggests narcosis, shock, or cerebral injury. A newborn occasionally makes twitching or flailing movements of extremities in the absence of a stimulus because of the immaturity of the nervous system. A number of reflexes can be tested with consistency by using simple maneuvers.

Blink Reflex. A blink reflex in a newborn serves the same purpose as it does in an adult, that is, to protect the eye from any object coming near it by rapid eyelid closure. It may be elicited by shining a strong light such as a flashlight or otoscope light on the eye. It can rarely be elicited by a sudden movement toward the eye.

Rooting Reflex. If a newborn's cheek is brushed or stroked near the corner of the mouth, the child will turn the head in that direction. This reflex serves to help the baby find food. The reflex disappears at about the 6th week of life. At about this time, the eyes focus steadily and a food source can be seen. Thus, the reflex is no longer needed.

Sucking Reflex. When a newborn's lips are touched, the baby makes a sucking motion. The sucking reflex begins to diminish at about 6 months of age. It disappears immediately if it is never stimulated—for example, in a newborn with a tracheoesophageal fistula who is not allowed to take oral fluids. It can be maintained in such an infant by offering the child a non-nutritive sucking object such as a pacifier (after the fistula has been corrected by surgery and until oral feedings can be given).

Swallowing Reflex. The swallowing reflex in the newborn is the same as in the adult. Food that reaches the posterior portion of the tongue is automatically swallowed. Gag, cough, and sneeze reflexes also are present to maintain a clear airway in the event that normal swallowing does not keep the pharynx free of obstructing mucus.

Extrusion Reflex. A newborn will extrude any substance that is placed on the anterior portion of the tongue. This protective reflex prevents the swallowing of inedible substances, disappearing at about 4 months of age. Until then, an infant may seem to be spitting out or refusing solid food placed in the mouth.

Palmar Grasp Reflex. Newborns will grasp an object placed in their palm by closing their fingers on it (Figure 5-3A). It is a primitive reflex apparently from a time newborns clung to their mother for safety. The reflex disappears at about age 6 weeks to 3 months. A baby begins to grasp meaningfully at about 3 months of age.

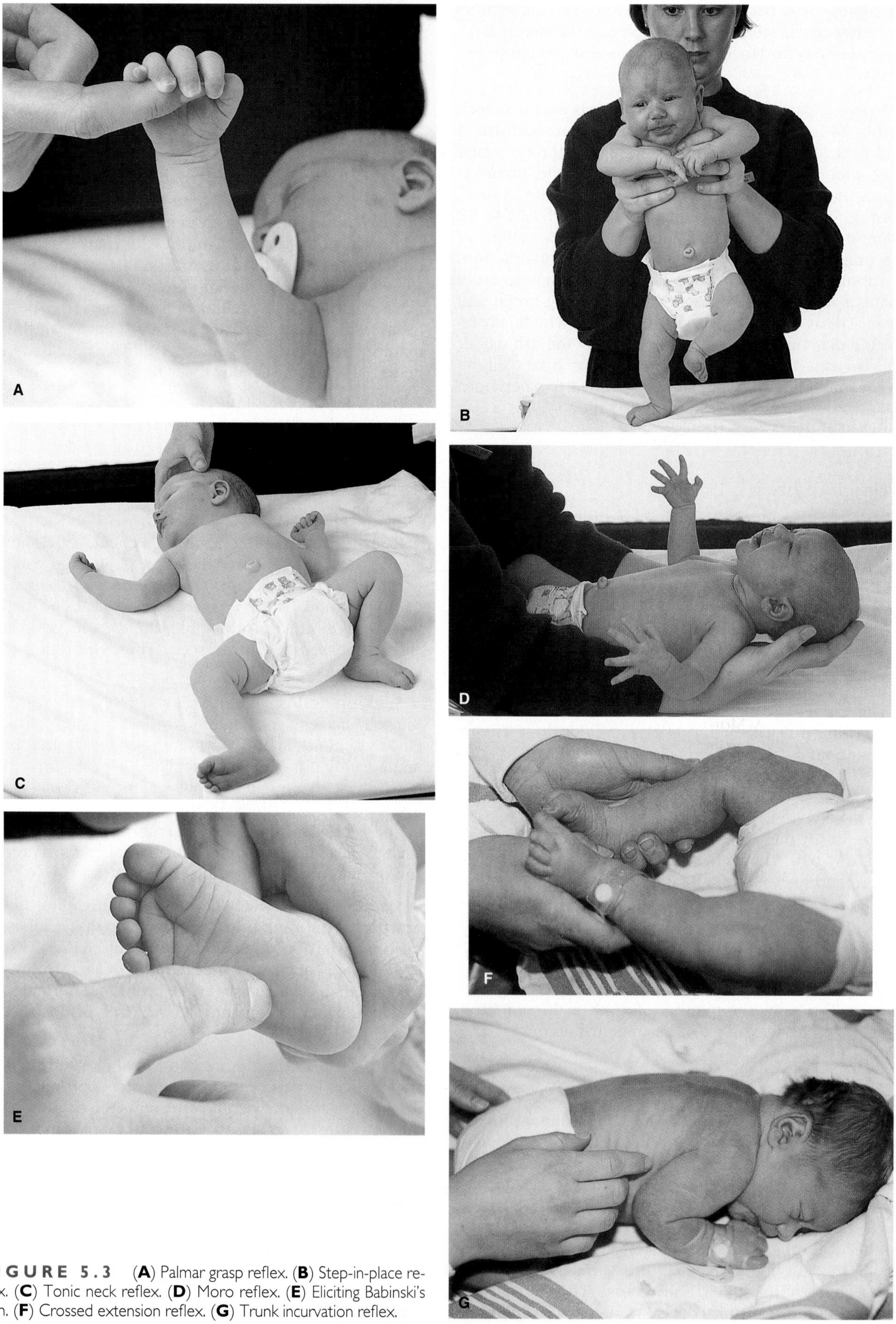

FIGURE 5.3 (**A**) Palmar grasp reflex. (**B**) Step-in-place reflex. (**C**) Tonic neck reflex. (**D**) Moro reflex. (**E**) Eliciting Babinski's sign. (**F**) Crossed extension reflex. (**G**) Trunk incurvation reflex.

Step (Walk)-in-Place Reflex. Newborns who are held in a vertical position with their feet touching a hard surface will take a few quick, alternating steps (Figure 5-3*B*). This reflex disappears by 3 months of age. By 4 months, babies can bear a good portion of their weight unhindered by this reflex.

Placing Reflex. The placing reflex is similar to the step-in-place reflex, except it is elicited by touching the anterior surface of a newborn's leg against the edge of a bassinet or table. A newborn will make a few quick lifting motions as if to step onto the table.

Plantar Grasp Reflex. When an object touches the sole of a newborn's foot at the base of the toes, the toes grasp in the same manner as the fingers do. The reflex disappears at about 8 to 9 months of age in preparation for walking. However, it may be present during sleep for a longer period of time.

Tonic Neck Reflex. When newborns lie on their backs, their heads usually turn to one side or the other. The arm and the leg on the side to which the head turns extend, and the opposite arm and leg contract (Figure 5-3*C*). If you turn a newborn's head to the opposite side, he or she will often change the extension and contraction of legs and arms accordingly. It is also called a boxer or *fencing reflex,* because the newborn's position simulates that of someone preparing to box or fence. Unlike many other reflexes, the tonic neck reflex does not appear to have a function. It does stimulate eye coordination, however, because the extended arm moves in front of the face. It may signify handedness. The reflex disappears between the 2nd and 3rd months of life.

Moro Reflex. A Moro (startle) reflex (Figure 5-3*D*) can be initiated by startling the newborn by a loud noise or by jarring the bassinet. The most accurate method of eliciting the reflex is to hold newborns in a supine position and allow their heads to drop backward an inch or so. They abduct and extend their arms and legs. Their fingers assume a typical "C" position. They then bring their arms into an embrace position and pull up their legs against their abdomen (adduction). The reflex simulates the action of someone trying to ward off an attacker, then covering up to protect himself. It is strong for the first 8 weeks of life and fades by the end of the 4th or 5th month, when the infant can roll away from danger.

Babinski Reflex. When the side of the sole of the foot is stroked in an inverted "J" curve from the heel upward, the newborn fans the toes (positive Babinski sign; Figure 5-3*E*). This is in contrast to the adult, who flexes the toes. This reaction occurs because of the immaturity of nervous system development. It remains positive (toes fan) until at least 3 months of age, when it is supplanted by the down-turning or flexing adult response.

Magnet Reflex. If pressure is applied to the soles of the feet of a newborn lying in a supine position, she pushes back against the pressure. This and the two following reflexes are tests of spinal cord integrity.

Crossed Extension Reflex. One leg of a newborn lying supine is extended and the sole of that foot is irritated by being rubbed with a sharp object, such as a thumbnail. This causes the newborn to raise the other leg and extend it as if trying to push away the hand irritating the first leg (Figure 5-3*F*).

Trunk Incurvation Reflex. When newborns lie in a prone position and are touched along the paravertebral area by a probing finger, they will flex their trunk and swing their pelvis toward the touch (Figure 5-3*G*).

Landau Reflex. A newborn who is held in a prone position with a hand underneath supporting the trunk should demonstrate some muscle tone. Babies may not be able to lift their head or arch their back (as they will at 3 months of age) in this position, but neither should they sag into an inverted "U" position. The latter response indicates extremely poor muscle tone, the cause of which should be investigated.

Deep Tendon Reflexes. A patellar reflex can be elicited in a newborn by tapping the patellar tendon with the tip of the finger. The lower leg will move perceptibly if the infant has an intact reflex. To elicit a biceps reflex, place the thumb of your left hand on the tendon of the biceps muscle on the inner surface of the elbow. Tap the thumb as it rests on the tendon. You are more likely to feel the tendon contract than to observe movement. A biceps reflex is a test for spinal nerves C5 and C6; a patellar reflex is a test for spinal nerves L2 through L4.

The Senses

The senses in newborns appear to be much better developed than previously believed.

Hearing. A fetus is able to hear in utero. As soon as amniotic fluid drains or is absorbed from the middle ear by way of the eustachian tube—within hours after birth—hearing in newborns becomes acute. However, they appear to have difficulty locating sound, but respond with generalized activity to a sound.

Vision. Newborns see as soon as they are born and possibly have been "seeing" light and dark in utero for the last few months of pregnancy as the uterus and the abdominal wall were stretched thin. Newborns demonstrate sight at birth by blinking at a strong light (blink reflex) or following a bright light or toy a short distance with their eyes, but they cannot follow the image past the midline of vision. They focus best on black and white objects at a distance of 9 to 12 in. A pupillary reflex is present from birth.

Touch. The sense of touch is well developed at birth. Newborns demonstrate this by quieting at a soothing touch and by positive sucking and rooting reflexes, which are elicited by touch. They also react to painful stimuli.

Taste. A newborn has the ability to discriminate taste because taste buds are developed and functioning before birth. A newborn turns away from a bitter taste such as salt but readily accepts the sweet taste of milk or glucose water (Cunningham et al, 1997).

Smell. The sense of smell is present in newborns as soon as the nose is clear of mucus and amniotic fluid.

Newborns turn toward their mothers' breasts partly out of recognition of the smell of breast milk and partly as a manifestation of the rooting reflex. Their ability to respond to odors can be used to document alertness.

✔ CHECKPOINT QUESTIONS

4. What factors are responsible for initiating the newborn's first breath?
5. A Moro reflex is the best single assessment of neurologic ability in a newborn. What is the best way to test this reflex?

Physiologic Adjustment to Extrauterine Life

All newborns seem to move through periods of irregular adjustment in the first 6 hours of life before their body systems stabilize. These periods were first described by Desmond in 1963 and are termed periods of reactivity (Nelson, 1997b). These are summarized in Table 5-1. Newborns who are ill or who had difficulty at birth may not pass through these typical stages. Signs of this typical reactivity pattern, therefore, is an indication that the baby is healthy and adjusting well to extrauterine life. The transition from one period to another is an important indicator of neurologic status.

APPEARANCE OF THE NEWBORN

Skin

General inspection of the newborn's skin reveals many characteristic findings.

Color

Most term newborns have a ruddy complexion because of the increased concentration of red blood cells in blood vessels and a decrease in the amount of subcutaneous fat, which makes the blood vessels more visible. This ruddiness fades slightly over the 1st month.

Cyanosis. The newborn's lips, hands, and feet are likely to appear cyanotic from immature peripheral circulation. Acrocyanosis is so prominent in some newborns that it appears as if a line is drawn across the wrist or ankle, with pink skin on one side and blue on the other, as if some stricture were cutting off circulation. This is a normal phenomenon in the first 24 to 48 hours after birth.

Generalized mottling of the skin is common. **Central cyanosis**, or cyanosis of the trunk, however, is always a cause for concern. Central cyanosis indicates decreased oxygenation. It may be the result of a temporary respiratory obstruction or an underlying disease state.

Hyperbilirubinemia. Hyperbilirubinemia leads to **jaundice**, or yellowing of the skin (Sater, 1995). This occurs on the 2nd or 3rd day of life in about 50% of all newborns as a result of the breakdown of fetal red blood cells **(physiologic jaundice)**. The infant's skin and sclera of the eyes appear noticeably yellow. This occurs as the high red blood cell count built up in utero is destroyed. Many newborns have such immature liver function that indirect bilirubin, a breakdown product of heme, cannot be converted to the direct form and excreted. As long as the bilirubin remains in the circulatory system, the red of the blood cells obscures its color. When the level of this indirect bilirubin rises above 7 mg/100 mL, however, bilirubin permeates the tissue outside the circulatory system and causes the infant to appear jaundiced.

TABLE 5.1 Periods of Reactivity: Normal Adjustment to Extrauterine Life

ASSESSMENT	FIRST PERIOD (FIRST 15–30 MIN)	RESTING PERIOD (30–120 MIN)	SECOND PERIOD (2–6 H)
Color	Acrocyanosis	Color stabilizing; pink all over	Quick color changes occur with movement or crying
Temperature	Temperature begins to fall from intrauterine temperature of about 100.6°F	Temperature stabilizes at about 99°F	Temperature increases to 99.8°F
Heart rate	Rapid, as much as 180 bpm while crying	Slowing to between 120 and 140 bpm	Wide swings in rate with activity
Respirations	Irregular; 30–90 breaths per min while crying; some nasal flaring, occasional retraction may be present	Slows to 30–50 breaths per min; barreling of chest occurs	Respirations become irregular again with activity
Activity	Alert; watching	Sleeps	Awakes
Ability to respond to stimulation	Reacts vigorously	Difficult to arouse	Becoming responsive again
Mucus	Visible in mouth	Small amount present while sleeping	Mouth full of mucus, causing gagging
Bowel sounds	Able to be heard after first 15 min	Present	Often has first meconium stool

From Desmond, M. N., et al. (1963). The clinical behavior of the newly born; the term baby. *Journal of Pediatrics, 62*, 307; with permission.

Bruising at birth leads to hemorrhage of blood into the subcutaneous tissue or skin. This blood is removed as bruising heals by the breakdown of blood components. As the red blood cells are hemolyzed, additional indirect bilirubin is released. **Cephalhematoma,** a collection of blood under the periosteum of the skull bone, can lead to the same phenomenon (Tan & Lim, 1995).

If intestinal obstruction is present and stool is not being evacuated, intestinal flora may break down bile into its basic components and release indirect bilirubin into the bloodstream again. Early feeding of newborns promotes intestinal movement and excretion of meconium and helps prevent indirect bilirubin buildup from this source.

There is no set level at which indirect serum bilirubin requires treatment. If the level rises above 10 to 12 mg/100 mL, treatment will usually be considered although other factors such as age, maturity and breastfeeding will be considered. At about 20 mg/100 mL, enough indirect bilirubin has left the bloodstream that it could interfere with the chemical synthesis of brain cells and cause permanent cell damage, a condition termed **kernicterus**. If this occurs, it could leave permanent neurologic effects including cognitive impairment. Treatment for physiologic jaundice in newborns is rarely necessary except for measures such as early feeding (to speed passage of feces through the intestine and prevent reabsorption of bilirubin from the bowel). Phototherapy (exposure of the infant to light to initiate maturation of liver enzymes) may be used (see Chapter 6).

Pallor. Pallor in newborns is usually the result of anemia. Anemia may be caused by (1) excessive blood loss at the time the cord was cut; (2) inadequate flow of blood from the cord into the infant at birth; (3) fetal–maternal transfusion; (4) low iron stores caused by poor maternal nutrition during pregnancy; or (5) blood incompatibility in which a large number of red blood cells were hemolyzed in utero. It may be the result of internal bleeding (the baby should be watched closely for signs of blood in stool or vomitus). Infants with central nervous system damage may appear pale as well as cyanotic. A gray color in newborns is generally indicative of infection. Twins may be born with a twin transfusion phenomenon, in which one twin is larger and has good color and the smaller twin has pallor (Thigpen, 1996).

Harlequin Sign. Occasionally, because of immature circulation, a newborn who has been lying on his or her side will appear red on the dependent side of the body and pale on the upper side, as if a line had been drawn down the center of the body. This is a transient phenomenon and, although startling, of no clinical significance. The odd coloring fades immediately if the infant's position is changed or the baby kicks or cries vigorously.

Birthmarks

A number of commonly occurring birthmarks can be identified in newborns. It is important to differentiate the various types of hemangiomas so you neither give false reassurance to parents nor worry them unnecessarily about these lesions.

Hemangiomas. The **hemangiomas** are vascular tumors of the skin. Three types are found.

- **Nevus flammeus** (Figure 5-4*A*): a macular purple or dark red lesion (sometimes called a *port-wine stain* because of its deep color) present at birth, generally appearing on the face but also possibly on the thighs. Those above the bridge of the nose tend to fade; the others are less likely to. May also occur as lighter, pink patches at the nape of the neck (*stork's beak marks;* Figure 5-4*B*), which do not fade either but are covered by the hairline and so are of no consequence (more common in females).
- **Strawberry hemangiomas**: elevated areas formed by immature capillaries and endothelial cells associated with high maternal estrogen levels (Figure 5-4*C*); most present at birth in the term neonate, but may appear up to 2 weeks after birth, possibly continuing up to 1 year of age. Usually absorbed and shrink in size after the first year, with 50% to 75% of these lesions disappearing by age 7 years (Esterly, 1996). Typically not present in the preterm infant because of epidermal immaturity. Laser therapy may be helpful (Achauer et al, 1998). Application of cortisone ointment may speed their disappearance by interfering with the binding of estrogen to its receptor sites.

  It is important for parents to understand that the mark may grow. Otherwise, they may confuse it with cancer (a skin lesion increasing in size is one of the seven danger signals of cancer). Surgery to remove strawberry hemangiomas is rarely recommended because it may lead to secondary infection, resulting in scarring and permanent disfigurement.
- **Cavernous hemangiomas** (Figure 5-4*D*): dilated vascular spaces, usually raised and resembling a strawberry hemangioma but do not disappear with time. Subcutaneous infusions of interferon alpha-2a can be used to reduce these in size (Castello et al, 1997), or they can be removed surgically. Children who have a skin lesion may have additional ones on internal organs. Blows to the abdomen, such as those from childhood games, can cause bleeding from internal hemangiomas. Children who have cavernous hemangiomas are usually assessed at health maintenance visits for hematocrit level to determine possible internal blood loss.

Mongolian Spots. Mongolian spots, collections of pigment cells (melanocytes), are slate-gray patches across the sacrum or buttocks and possibly the arms and legs. They tend to occur in children of Asian, Southern European, or African extraction. They disappear by school age without treatment. Parents can be assured that they are not bruises or they may worry that the baby sustained a birth injury.

Vernix Caseosa

Vernix caseosa, a white, cream cheese–like substance that serves as a skin lubricant, is usually noticeable on a newborn's skin, at least in the skin folds, at birth in a term neonate. Its color reflects the color of the amniotic fluid. If it is yellow, the amniotic fluid was yellow from bilirubin. If it is green, meconium was present in the amniotic fluid.

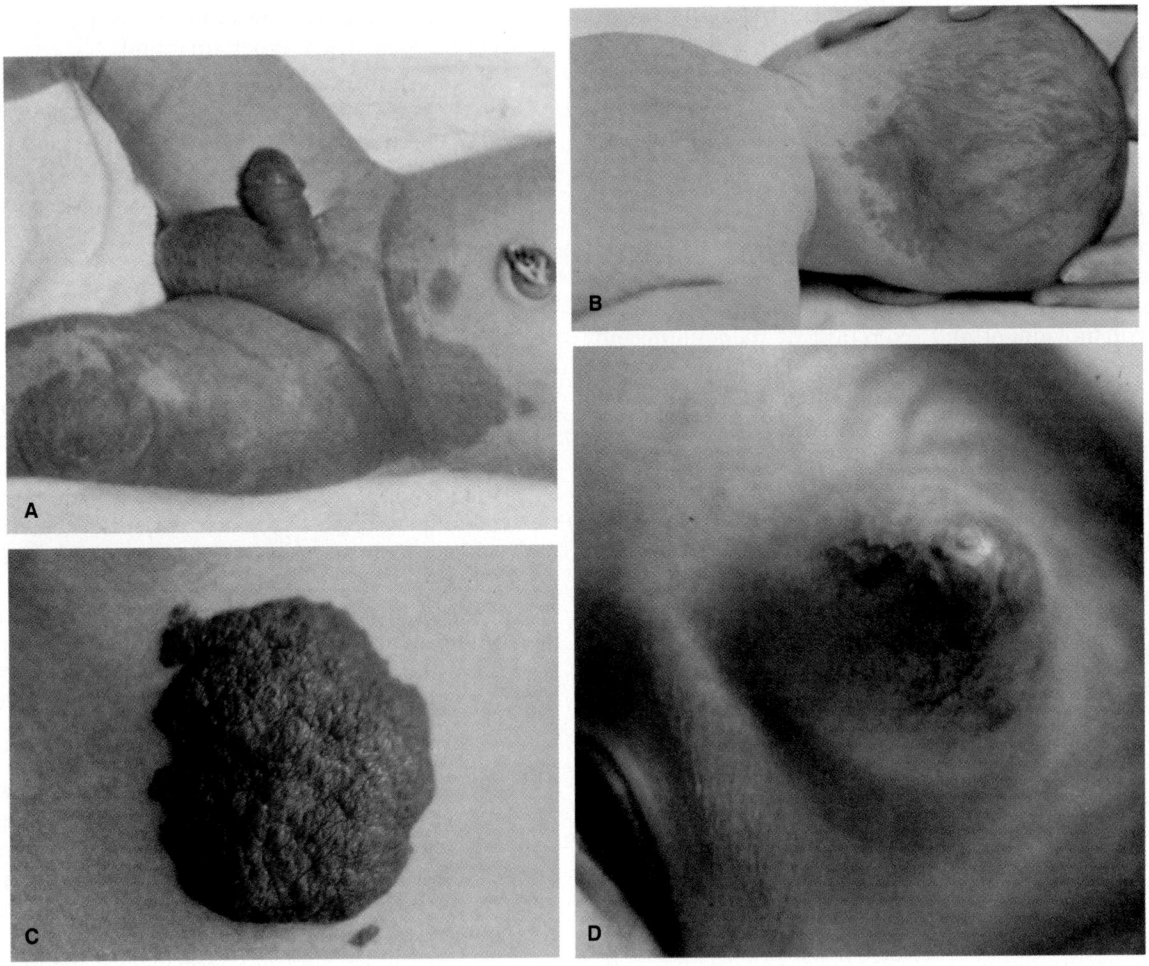

FIGURE 5.4 Types of hemangiomas found on the newborn. (**A**) Nevus flammeus (port-wine stain) formed of a plexus of newly formed capillaries in the papillary layer of the corium. It is deep red to purple, does not blanch on pressure, and does not fade with age. (**B**) Stork's beak mark, commonly occurring on nape of neck. It blanches on pressure; although it does not fade, it is not noticeable as it becomes covered by hair. (**C**) Strawberry hemangiomas consist of dilated capillaries in entire dermal and subdermal layers. They continue to enlarge after birth but usually disappear by age 10 years.(**D**) Cavernous hemangiomas consist of a communicating network of venules in subcutaneous tissue and do not fade with age.

Handle newborns with gloves to protect yourself from exposure to body fluids until the first bath when vernix is washed away. Harsh rubbing should never be employed to wash away vernix. The newborn's skin is tender, and breaks in the skin from too vigorous attempts at removal may open portals of entry for bacteria.

Lanugo

Lanugo is the fine, downy hair that covers a newborn's shoulders, back, and upper arms. It may be found also on the forehead and ears. The newborn of 37 to 39 weeks' gestational age has more lanugo than the 40-week-old infant. Postmature infants (over 42 weeks) rarely have lanugo. Lanugo is rubbed away by the friction of bedding and clothes against the newborn's skin. By age 2 weeks, it has disappeared.

Desquamation

Within 24 hours of birth, the skin of most newborns has become extremely dry. The dryness is particularly evident on the palms of the hands and the soles of the feet. It may result in areas of peeling similar to those after a sunburn. This is normal and needs no treatment. Parents may apply hand lotion to prevent excessive dryness if they wish.

Newborns who are postmature and have suffered intrauterine malnutrition have extremely dry skin with a leathery appearance and cracks in the skin folds. This should be differentiated from normal desquamation.

Milia

Newborn sebaceous glands are immature. At least one pinpoint white papule (a plugged or unopened sebaceous gland) can be found on the cheek or across the bridge of the nose of every newborn. Such lesions, termed **milia** (Figure 5-5), disappear by 2 to 4 weeks of age as the sebaceous glands mature and drain. Parents should be instructed to avoid scratching or squeezing the papules to prevent secondary infection.

Erythema Toxicum

In most normal mature infants, a newborn rash called **erythema toxicum** is observed (Figure 5-6). It usually ap-

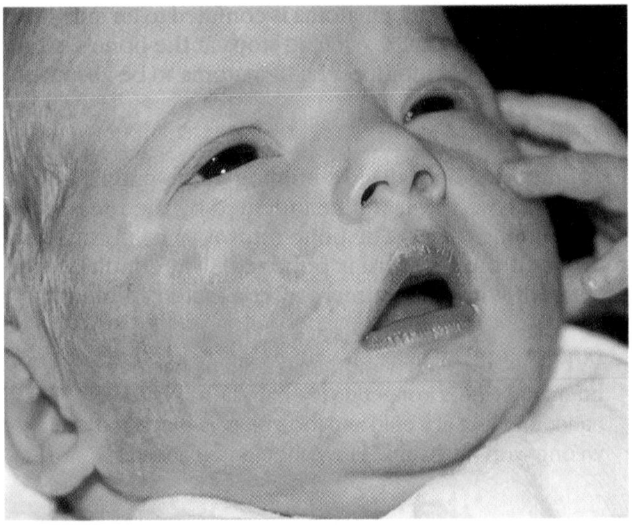

FIGURE 5.5 Milia are unopened sebaceous glands frequently found on the nose, chin, or cheeks of a newborn. One is evident here on the right check.

pears in the 1st to 4th day of life but may appear up to 2 weeks of age, beginning as a papule, increasing in severity to become erythema by the 2nd day, then disappearing by the 3rd day. It is sometimes called a *flea-bite rash* because the lesions are so minuscule. One of the chief characteristics of the rash is its lack of pattern. It occurs sporadically and unpredictably as to time and place on skin surfaces. It may last a matter of hours rather than days.

Forceps Marks

If forceps were used for birth, there may be a circular or linear contusion matching the rim of the blade of the forceps on the infant's cheek (Figure 5-7). This mark disappears in 1 to 2 days along with the edema that accompanies it. Closely assess the facial nerve while the newborn is at rest and during crying episodes to detect any potential facial nerve compression requiring further evaluation.

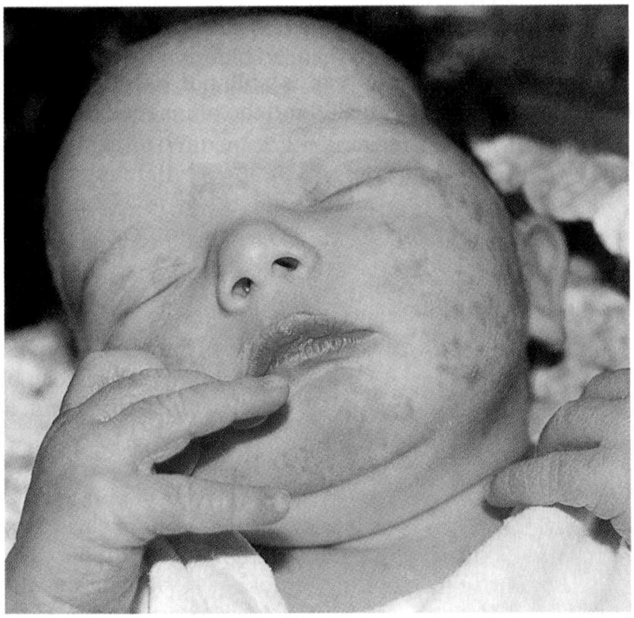

FIGURE 5.6 Erythema toxicum is found on almost all newborns. The reddish rash consists of sporadic pinpoint papules on an erythematous base. It fades spontaneously in a few days.

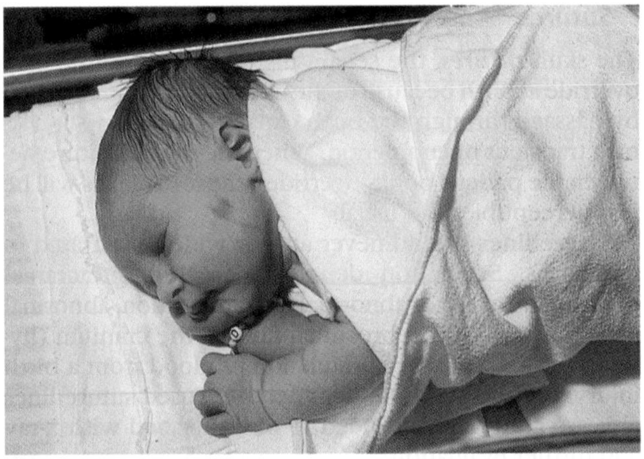

FIGURE 5.7 Forceps marks are commonly found in newborns delivered by forceps. Such marks are transient and disappear in a day or two.

Skin Turgor

Newborn skin should feel resilient if the underlying tissue is well hydrated. If a fold of the skin is grasped between the thumb and fingers, it should feel elastic. When it is released, it should fall back to form a smooth surface. If severe dehydration is present, the skin will not smooth out again but will remain in an elevated ridge. Poor turgor is seen in newborns who suffered malnutrition in utero, who have difficulty sucking at birth, or who have certain metabolic disorders, such as adrenogenital syndrome.

Head

A newborn's head appears disproportionately large because it is about one fourth of the total length; in an adult, the head is one eighth of total height. The forehead of the newborn is large and prominent. The chin appears to be receding, and it quivers easily if the infant is startled or cries. Well-nourished newborns have full-bodied hair; poorly nourished or preterm infants have stringy, lifeless hair.

Fontanelles

The fontanelles are the spaces or openings where the skull bones join. The anterior fontanelle is at the junction of the two parietal bones and the two fused frontal bones. It is diamond shaped and measures 2 to 3 cm (0.8 to 1.2 inch) in width and 3 to 4 cm (1.2 to 1.6 inch) in length. The posterior fontanelle is at the junction of the parietal bones and the occipital bone. It is triangular and measures about 1 cm (0.4 inch) in length.

The anterior fontanelle will be felt as a soft spot. The posterior fontanelle is so small in some newborns that it cannot be palpated readily. The anterior fontanelle normally closes at 12 to 18 months of age. The posterior fontanelle closes by the end of the 2nd month.

6. A new mother has chosen to bottle feed her newborn. The baby's grandmother tells you she used to prepare homemade formula using evaporated milk and honey. She also says that at 3 months, babies were changed to skim milk to keep them from gaining too much weight. How would you explain to the new mother and grandmother the reasons why the formula she described is no longer recommended?

REFERENCES

Achauer, B. M. et al. (1998). Intralesional bare fiber laser treatment of hemangioma of infancy. *Plastic and Reconsructive Surgery, 101* (5), 1212.

American Academy of Pediatrics: Committee on Injury and Poison Prevention. (1996). Selecting and using the most appropriate car safety seats for growing children: guidelines for counseling parents. *Pediatrics, 97*(5), 761.

American Academy of Pediatrics: Task Force on Infant Positioning and SIDS. (1996). Positioning and sudden infant death syndrome (SIDS): update. *Pediatrics, 98*(6), 1216.

American Academy of Pediatrics: Committee on Nutrition. (1976). Iron supplementation for infants. *Pediatrics, 57,* 278.

American Academy of Pediatrics: Committee on Nutrition. (1980). Vitamin and mineral supplement needs in normal children in the United States. *Pediatrics, 66,* 1015.

Andrews, M. M., & Boyle, J. S. (1996). *Transcultural concepts in nursing care.* Philadelphia: Lippincott.

Apgar, V., et al. (1958). Evaluation of the newborn infant: second report. *Journal of the American Medical Association, 168,* 1985.

Askin, D. F. (1995). Bacterial and fungal infections in the neonate. *Journal of Obstetric, Gynecologic and Neonatal Nursing, 24*(7), 635.

Ballard, J. L., et al. (1991). The new Ballard Scale. *Journal of Pediatrics, 119,* 417.

Brazelton, T. B. (1973). Neonatal behavior assessment scale. *Clinics in Developmental Medicine, 50,* 1.

Brooks, C. (1997). Neonatal hypoglycemia. *Neonatal Network, 16*(2), 15.

Castello, M. A. et al. (1997). Successful management with interferon alpha-Za after therapy failure in an infant with a giant cavernous hemangioma. *Medical and Pediatric Oncology, 28*(3), 213.

Cunningham, F. G., et al. (1997). *Williams' obstetrics.* Stamford, CT: Appleton & Lange.

Das-Eiden, R., & Reifman, A. (1996). Effects of Brazelton demonstrations on later parenting: a meta-analysis. *Journal of Pediatric Psychology, 21*(6), 857.

Department of Health and Human Services. (1995). *Healthy people 2000: midcourse review.* Washington, DC: DHHS.

Desmond, M. N., et al. (1963). The clinical behavior of the newly born: the term infant. *Journal of Pediatrics, 62,* 307.

Dubowitz, L., et al. (1970). Clinical assessment of gestational age in the newborn infant. *Journal of Pediatrics, 77,* 1.

Esterly, N. B. (1996). Cutaneous hemangiomas, vascular stains and malformations, and associated syndromes. *Current Problems in Pediatrics, 26*(1), 3.

Gibson, E., et al. (1995). Infant sleep position following new AAP guidelines. *Pediatrics, 96*(1), 69.

Greiner, T. (1996). The concept of weaning: definitions and their implications. *Journal of Human Lactation, 12*(2), 123.

Guyer, B. et al. (1997). Annual summary of vital statistics. *Pediatrics, 100*(6), 905.

Johnson, K. B., & Oski, F. A. (1997). *Oski's essential pediatrics.* Philadelphia: Lippincott.

Jones, C. L. (1996). Herpes simplex virus infection in the neonate: clinical presentation and management. *Neonatal Network, 15*(9), 11.

Kaminski, J., & Hall, W. (1996). The effect of soothing music on neonatal behavioral states in the hospital newborn nursery. *Neonatal Network 15*(1), 45.

Keefe, M. R., Froese-Fretz, A., & Kotzer, A. M. (1997). The REST regimen: an individualized nursing intervention for infant irritability. *MCN: American Journal of Maternal Child Nursing, 22*(1), 1620.

Lawrence, R. A. (1998). *Breastfeeding: a guide for the medical profession* (5th ed.). St. Louis: Mosby.

Letko, M. D. (1996). Understanding the Apgar Score. *Journal of Obstetric, Gynecologic and Neonatal Nursing, 25*(4), 299.

Lopez-Alarcon, M., Villalpando, S., & Fajardo, A. (1997). Breastfeeding lowers the frequency and duration of acute respiratory infection and diarrhea in infants under six months of age. *Journal of Nutrition, 127*(3), 435.

Luzuriaga, K. et al. (1998). Combination treatment with zidovudine, didanosine, and nevirapine in infants with human immunodeficiency virus type 1 infection. *New England Journal of Medicine, 336*(19), 1343.

McQueen, D. A. (1997). The nutritional adequacy of mineral content of formulas. *Pediatrics in Review, 18*(2), 67.

Nelson, N. M. (1997b). Recovery period. In Hoekelman, R. A., et al. *Primary pediatric care* (3rd ed.). St. Louis: Mosby, p. 500.

Nelson, N. M. (1997a). Physiological status of the healthy infant. In Hoekelman, R. A., et al. *Primary pediatric care* (3rd ed.). St. Louis: Mosby, p. 497.

Pascale, J. A., et al. (1996). Breastfeeding, dehydration, and shorter maternity stays. *Neonatal Network, 15*(7), 37.

Polinski, C. (1996). The value of the white blood cell count and differential in the prediction of neonatal sepsis. *Neonatal Network, 15*(7), 13.

Saadeh, R., & Akre, J. (1996). Ten steps to successful breastfeeding: a summary of the rationale and scientific evidence. *Birth, 23*(3), 154.

Sansoucie, D. A., & Cavaliere, T. A. (1997). Transition from fetal to extrauterine circulation. *Neonatal Network, 16*(2), 5.

Sater, K. J. (1995). Color me yellow: caring for the infant with hyperbilirubinemia. *Journal of Intravenous Nursing, 18*(6), 317.

Silverman, W. A., & Anderson, D. H. (1956). A controlled clinical trial of effects of water mist on obstructive respiratory signs, death rate and necroscopy findings among premature infants. *Pediatrics, 17,* 1.

Tan, K. L., & Lim, G. C. (1995). Phototherapy for neonatal jaundice in infants with cephalhematomas. *Clinical Pediatrics, 34*(1), 7.

Thigpen, J. (1996). Discordant twins: a case report. *Neonatal Network, 15*(8), 35.

Tin, W., Wariyar, U. K., & Hey, E. N. (1997). Selection biases invalidate current low birthweight weight-for-gestation standards. *British Journal of Obstetrics and Gynaecology, 104*(2), 180.

Usher, R., et al. (1966). Judgment of fetal age. *Pediatric Clinics of North America, 13,* 835.

Vecchi, C. J., et al. (1996). Neonatal individualized predictive pathway: a discharge planning tool for parents. *Neonatal Network, 14*(4), 7.

Wright, A., Rice, S., & Wells, S. (1996). Changing hospital practices to increase the duration of breastfeeding. *Pediatrics, 97*(5), 669.

SUGGESTED READINGS

American Academy of Pediatrics: Committee on Injury and Poison Prevention/Committee on Fetus and Newborn. (1996). Safe transportation of premature and low birth weight infants. *Pediatrics, 97*(5), 758.

Baird, P. B. (1996). Neonatal glucose screening. *Neonatal Network,* 15(6), 63.

Buchko, B. L., et al. (1994). Comfort measures in breastfeeding, primiparous women. *Journal of Obstetric, Gynecologic, and Neonatal Nursing, 23*(1), 46.

Garland, J., et al. (1996). Clinical utility of a glucose reflectance meter for screening neonates for hypoglycemia. *Journal of Perinatology, 16*(4), 250.

Howard, C. R. et al. (1998). Neonatal circumcision and pain relief: current training practices. *Pediatrics, 101*(3.1), 423.

Kotagal, U. R., et al. (1997). Use of hospital-based services in the first three months of life: impact of an early discharge program. *Journal of Pediatrics, 130*(2), 250.

Levitt, C. A., et al. (1996). Breast-feeding policies and practices in Canadian hospitals providing maternity care. *Canadian Medical Association Journal, 155*(2), 181.

Lutes, L. (1996). Bedding twins/multiples together. *Neonatal Network, 15*(7), 61.

MacKeith, N. (1995). Who should examine the 'normal' neonate? *Nursing Times, 91*(14), 34.

Malloy-McDonald, M. B. (1995). Skin care for high-risk neonates. *Journal of Wound, Ostomy and Continence Nursing, 22*(4), 177.

Maxon, A. B., Vohr, B. R., & White, K. R. (1996). Newborn hearing screening: comparison of a simplified otoacoustic emissions device. *Early Human Development, 45*(1), 171.

Montgomery, D. L., & Splett, P. L. (1997). Economic benefit of breast-feeding infants enrolled in WIC. *Journal of the American Dietetic Association, 97*(4), 379.

Morley, R. (1996). The influence of early diet on later development. *Journal of Biosocial Science, 28*(4), 481.

Shore, C. (1996). Successful breastfeeding. *Paediatric Nursing, 8*(9), 32.

Stashwick, C. A. (1994). Overcoming obstacles to breastfeeding. *Patient Care, 28,* 88.

Yang, W. T., et al. (1997). Sonographic features of head and neck hemangiomas and vascular malformations; review of 23 patients. *Journal of Ultrasound in Medicine, 16*(1), 39.

Yip, E., Lee, J., & Sheehy, Y. (1996). Breast-feeding in neonatal intensive care. *Journal of Paediatrics and Child Health, 32*(4), 296.

The Family With a High-Risk Newborn

6

CHAPTER

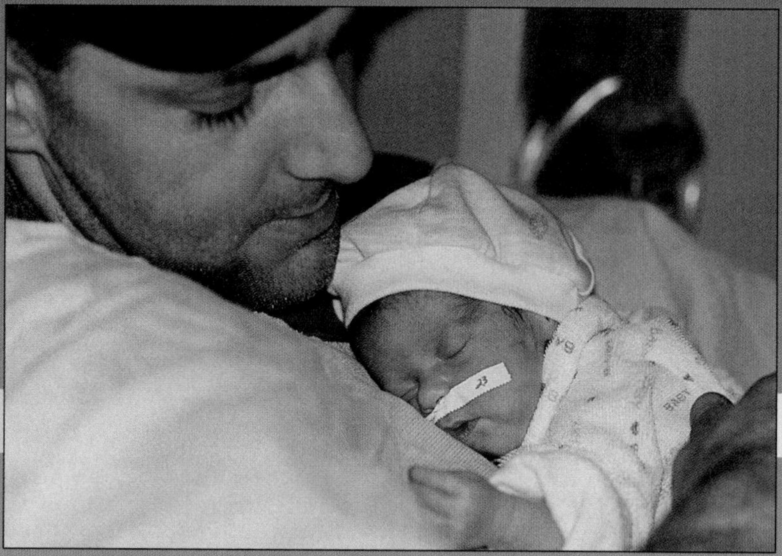

Key Terms

- apnea
- apparent life-threatening event
- appropriate for gestational age
- azotemia
- brown fat
- caudal regression syndrome
- developmental care
- extracorporeal membrane oxygenation (ECMO)
- extremely-very-low-birth-weight infant
- gestational age
- hemorrhagic disease of the newborn
- hydrops fetalis
- hyperbilirubinemia
- hyperglycemia
- hypocalcemia
- hypoglycemia
- intrauterine growth retardation
- kernicterus
- large-for-gestational-age infant
- low-birth-weight infant
- macrosomia
- ophthalmia neonatorum
- periodic respirations
- periventricular leukomalacia
- postterm infant
- postterm syndrome
- preterm infant
- primary apnea
- retinopathy of prematurity
- secondary apnea
- small-for-gestational-age infant
- term infant
- very-low-birth-weight infant

Objectives

After mastering the contents of this chapter, you should be able to:

1. Define the terms *small-for-gestational-age infant, term infant, large-for-gestational-age infant, preterm infant,* and *postterm infant* and describe common illnesses that occur in these high-risk newborns.
2. Assess a high-risk newborn to determine if safe transition to extrauterine life occurs.
3. List nursing diagnoses related to the high-risk newborn and family.
4. Identify appropriate outcomes for the high-risk newborn and family.
5. Plan nursing care focusing on priorities to stabilize the high-risk newborn's body systems.
6. Implement nursing care for the high-risk newborn and family.
7. Evaluate established outcomes to determine achievement and effectiveness of care.
8. Identify National Health Goals related to high-risk newborns and their families that nurses could be instrumental in helping the nation to achieve.
9. Identify areas related to the care of high-risk newborns that could benefit from additional nursing research.
10. Use critical thinking to analyze the special crisis imposed on families when alterations of newborn development, gestational age, or neonatal illness occur.
11. Integrate knowledge of the needs of the high-risk infant and family with nursing process to achieve quality child health nursing care.

Mr. and Mrs. Atkins had a 36-week-old, 2-lb baby boy last night after a short, 4-hour labor. The baby took a few gasping respirations at birth but then stopped breathing. He was resuscitated by the neonatal nurse practitioner and respiratory therapist and then transported to the intensive care nursery. Mr. Atkins was not present for the birth because he was out of town on business. You notice Mrs. Atkins has not visited the intensive care nursery to see her son. She also refused to sign the birth certificate because she could not decide on a name. She said, "I don't want to give him our favorite name because he might die." Mr. Atkins telephoned early this morning and acted more upset that the baby was born than relieved the baby was receiving intensive care. You heard him asking his wife, "What did you do to cause this?" What type of help do the Atkins need to better accept what has happened?

In previous chapters, you learned about the child-rearing family and caring for the family with a newborn who is well at birth. In this chapter, you'll add information about how to care for the newborn who is ill or has a significant variation in gestational age or weight. This is important information because learning to recognize these infants at birth and organizing care for them can be instrumental in helping protect both their present and future health.

After you've studied the chapter, turn to the Critical Thinking Exercises at the end of the chapter to sharpen your skills and test your knowledge of this nursing care area.

Certain risk factors involving the newborn's mother such as maternal age (very young or older than average); concurrent disease conditions (e.g., diabetes); pregnancy complications (such as placenta previa); and an unhealthy maternal lifestyle (such as drug abuse) place the newborn at high risk. In addition, the infant who is born postterm or under- or overweight for gestational age is also at risk for complications at birth and in the first few days of life. However, not all instances of high risk can be predicted. Even the newborn from a "perfect" pregnancy may require specialized care or may develop a problem over the first few days of life necessitating special interventions. With shorter hospital lengths of stay for newborns, parents need thorough education because these problems may require rehospitalization or additional follow-up at home. National Health Goals related to the high-risk newborn and family are shown in Focus on National Health Goals.

Being able to predict that an infant is high risk allows for advanced preparation, arranging for specialized skilled health care personnel to be present at the child's birth and perform necessary interventions, such as resuscitating the newborn who has difficulty establishing respirations. Immediate, skilled handling of any problems that occur may help to save the newborn's life and also prevent future problems, such as neurologic disorders.

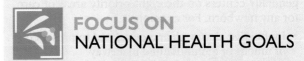

FOCUS ON NATIONAL HEALTH GOALS

Preterm birth has the potential for leading to so many complications in newborns that a National Health Goal was written specifically concerning it:

- Reduce low birth weight to an incidence of no more than 5% of live births and very low birth weight to an incidence of no more than 1% of live births from baselines of 6.9% and 1.2%, respectively (DHHS, 1995).

Nurses can be instrumental in helping the nation achieve this goal being prepared for resuscitation of preterm infants and by planning developmental care that can help prevent conditions such as apnea, intraventricular hemorrhage, and periventricular leukomalacia.

Further research is needed as to how best to position infants to promote development and prevent fatigue, what measures can best prevent conditions such as intraventricular hemorrhage, and what measures can make parents feel most comfortable and allow them to interact with their infants best in neonatal intensive care units.

NURSING PROCESS OVERVIEW

for Care of the Family With a High Risk Newborn

Assessment

All infants are assessed at birth for obvious congenital anomalies and **gestational age** (number of weeks they remained in utero). Both determinations can be done by the nurse who first inspects the infant. These assessments are made with the infant under a prewarmed radiant heat warmer to safeguard against heat loss.

Continuing assessment of high-risk infants involves the use of instrumentation such as cardiac, apnea, and blood pressure monitoring. However, no matter how many monitors are used, they never replace the role of commonsense observation. Carefully evaluate comments from fellow nurses that an infant "isn't himself" or "looks funny." These comments, although not scientific, are the same observations that a parent who knows his or her baby well reports at health visits. A nurse who knows an infant well from having cared for the child consistently over time often senses changes before a monitor or other equipment begins to put a quantitative measurement on the factor.

Nursing Diagnosis

To establish nursing diagnoses for high-risk infants, it is important to be aware of the normal assessment parameters of this population. Nursing diagnosis

continue for up to 24 hours of life, possibly causing rebound hypoglycemia.

NURSING DIAGNOSES AND RELATED INTERVENTIONS

Nursing Diagnosis: Ineffective breathing pattern related to possible birth trauma in large-for-gestational-age newborn

Outcome Identification: Newborn will initiate and maintain respirations at birth.

Outcome Evaluation: Newborn initiates breathing at birth; maintains normal newborn respiratory rate of 30 to 60 breaths per minute.

Some large-for-gestational-age infants have difficulty establishing respirations at birth because of birth trauma. Increased intracranial pressure from birth of the larger-than-usual head may lead to pressure on the respiratory center. This, in turn, causes a decrease in respiratory function. A diaphragmatic paralysis may occur due to cervical nerve trauma as the head is bent laterally to allow for birth of the large shoulders. This prevents active lung motion on the affected side. If the infant had to be delivered by cesarean birth, transient fluid can remain in the lungs and interfere with effective gas exchange. Careful observation will detect these conditions. Care of the infant with these disorders is discussed in Chapter 19.

Nursing Diagnosis: Risk for altered nutrition; less than body requirements related to additional nutrients needed to maintain weight and prevent hypoglycemia

Outcome Identification: Infant will ingest adequate fluid and nutrients for growth during neonatal period.

Outcome Evaluation: Infant's weight follows percentile growth curve; skin turgor is good; specific gravity of urine is 1.003 to 1.030; serum glucose is above 45 mg/dL.

As a rule, the large-for-gestational-age infant needs to be breastfed immediately to prevent hypoglycemia. The infant may need supplemental formula feedings after breastfeeding to supply enough fluid and glucose for the larger than normal size for the first few days. Newborns who are offered bottles often have more difficulty than others learning to breastfeed. Offer support and instructions to overcome this hurdle.

It is important not to overestimate this infant's ability to feed at birth. The infant may seem as if he or she should do well with breastfeeding because the baby is already the size of a 2-month-old infant. However, the infant is an inexperienced newborn, so sucking may not be effective enough for the infant to obtain an adequate supply of milk.

Nursing Diagnosis: Risk for altered parenting related to high-risk status of large-for-gestational-age infant

Outcome Identification: Parents demonstrate adequate bonding behavior during neonatal period.

Outcome Evaluation: Parents hold infant; speak of the child in positive terms; state accurately why the infant needs to be closely observed in postnatal period.

Parents may underestimate this infant's needs because of the child's excessive size. He or she seems so large and healthy. Parents may be confused about why the infant needs careful watching. They may read more into the child's condition than is present (he or she must be sick in some way that they are not being told about) and so bonding does not happen as instinctively as it might.

A large-for-gestational-age infant needs the same developmental care that all other infants need. Singing or talking to the baby, stroking the child's back, and rocking the baby are all important. Encourage parents to treat their baby as a fragile newborn who needs warm nurturing, not as a tough "big boy or girl" who has grown past that stage. Also remind the parents that the infant's birth weight is not a correlation of the child's projected adult size. Parents may fear that the infant may grow to be a larger than normal adult.

CHECKPOINT QUESTIONS

12. Why might a LGA newborn have difficulty establishing respirations at birth?
13. Why may breastfeeding be difficult for a LGA newborn?

The Preterm Infant

A preterm infant is usually defined as a live-born infant born before the end of week 37 of gestation; another criterion used is a weight of less than 2500 g (5 lb, 8 oz) at birth. Infants born after the 37th week are term. Infants who are born weighing 1500 to 2500 g are considered low-birth-weight (LBW) infants; those born weighing 1000 to 1500 g are considered very-low-birth-weight (VLBW) infants. Those born 500 to 1000 g are considered **extremely-very-low-birth-weight (EVLBW) infants.** All such infants need neonatal intensive care from the moment of birth to give them their best chance of survival without neurologic after effects. A lack of lung surfactant makes them extremely vulnerable to respiratory distress syndrome (Scanlon, 1997).

The maturity of a newborn is determined by physical findings such as sole creases, skull firmness, ear cartilage, and neurologic findings that reveal gestational age, as well as the mother's report of the date of her last menstrual period and sonographic estimations of gestational age.

Preterm babies of *every* weight need to be differentiated at birth from small-for-gestational-age babies (who also may have a low birth weight). Each of the two conditions results from different situations and therefore will cause different problems of adjustment to extrauterine life. A preterm infant is immature and small but well proportioned for age. Unlike the small-for-gestational-age infant, this baby appears to have been doing well in utero. For an unexplained reason, the "trigger" that initiates labor was activated too early and birth has resulted even though the baby is immature. Premature infants are invariably low-birth-weight infants. Differentiating characteristics of small-for-gestational-age and preterm infants are compared in Table 6-2.

TABLE 6.2 Differences Between Small-for-Gestational-Age and Preterm Infants

CHARACTERISTIC	SMALL-FOR-GESTATIONAL-AGE INFANT	PRETERM INFANT
Gestational age	24–44 wk	Younger than 37 wk
Birth weight	Under 10th percentile	Normal for age
Congenital malformations	Strong possibility	Possibility
Pulmonary problems	Meconium aspiration, pulmonary hemorrhage, pneumothorax	Respiratory distress syndrome
Hyperbilirubinemia	Possibility	Very strong possibility
Hypoglycemia	Very strong possibility	Possibility
Intracranial hemorrhage	Strong possibility	Possibility
Apnea episodes	Possibility	Very strong possibility
Feeding problems	Most likely to be due to accompanying problem such as hypoglycemia	Small stomach capacity; immature sucking reflex
Weight gain in nursery	Rapid	Slow
Future retarded growth	May always be under 10th percentile due to poor organ development	Not likely to be restricted in growth as "catch-up" growth occurs

Incidence

Preterm birth occurs in approximately 7% of live births of Caucasian infants. In African-American infants, the rate is doubled to approximately 14% (Cunningham et al, 1997).

When a preterm infant is recognized by a gestational-age assessment and health care personnel, watch for the specific problems of prematurity such as respiratory distress syndrome, hypoglycemia, and intracranial hemorrhage.

Causes

Preterm infant deaths account for 80% to 90% of the infant mortality in the first year of life. Infant mortality could be reduced dramatically if the causes could be discovered and corrected. However, the exact cause of early birth is rarely known (Givens & Moore, 1995).

Assessment

Appearance. On gross inspection, a preterm infant appears small and underdeveloped (Figure 6-5). The head is disproportionately large (3 cm or more greater than chest size). The skin is generally unusually ruddy because the infant has little subcutaneous fat beneath it; veins are easily noticeable, and a high degree of acrocyanosis may be present. The preterm neonate, 24 to 36 weeks, typically is covered with vernix caseosa. However, in very preterm newborns less than 25 weeks' gestation, vernix is absent because it has not formed yet. Lanugo is usually extensive, covering the back, forearms, forehead, and sides of the face. Both anterior and posterior fontanelles are small. There are few or no creases on the soles of the feet.

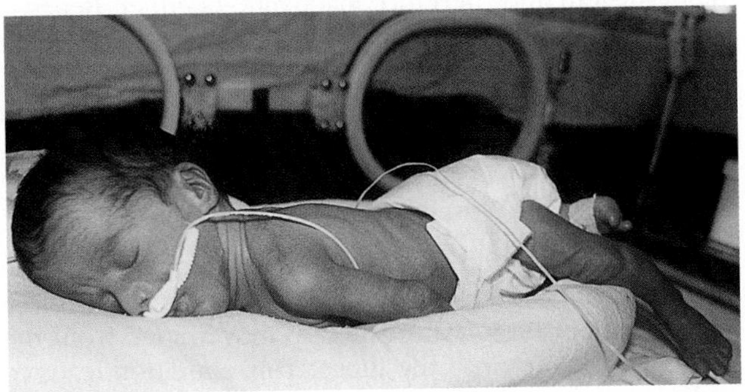

FIGURE 6.5 An immature infant. Notice the lax position of limbs due to immature muscle development.

Physical findings and reflex testing are used to differentiate between term and preterm newborns. These are illustrated in Figure 6-6. The eyes of most preterm infants appear small. Although difficult to elicit, pupillary reaction is present. Ophthalmoscopic examination is extremely difficult and often unrewarding, because the vitreous humor may be hazy. The preterm infant has varying degrees of myopia (near-sightedness) because of lack of eye globe depth.

The cartilage of the ear is immature and allows the pinna to fall forward. The ears appear large in relation to the head. The level of the ears should be carefully inspected to rule out chromosomal abnormalities (Figure 6-6*H*).

Neurologic function in the preterm child is often difficult to evaluate. The observation of spontaneous movement and provoked movements may yield findings as important as reflex testing. If tested, reflexes such as sucking and swallowing will be absent if the infant's age is below 33 weeks; deep tendon reflexes such as the Achilles tendon reflex are markedly diminished (see Figure 6-6*A* through *E*) During an examination, a preterm infant is much less active than a mature infant and rarely cries. If the infant does cry, the cry is weak and high pitched.

Potential Complications

Anemia of Prematurity. Many preterm infants develop a normochromic, normocytic anemia. Blood cells may be fragmented or irregularly shaped. The reticulocyte count is also low, because the bone marrow doesn't

A

Premature Infant **Full-term Infant**

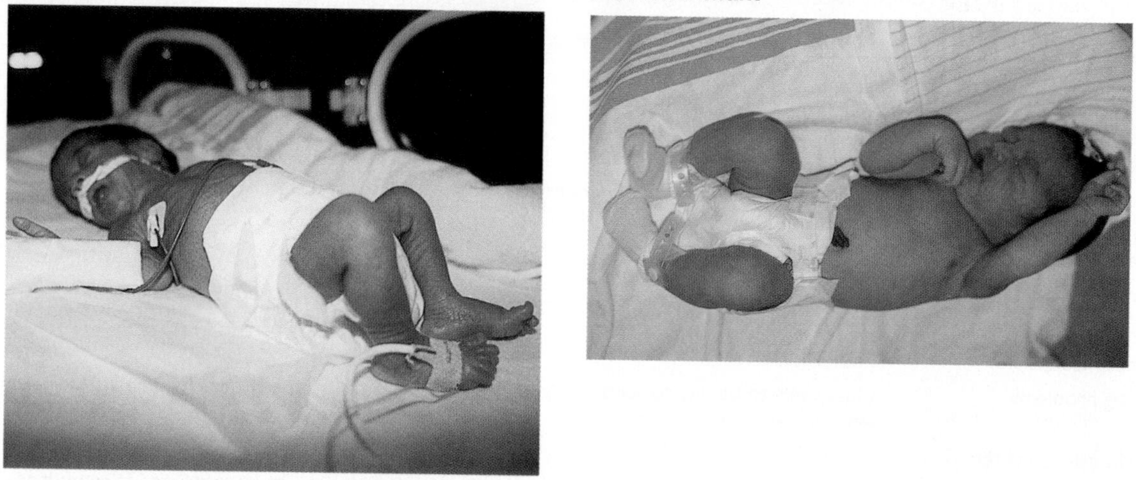

RESTING POSTURE *The premature infant is characterized by very little, if any, flexion in the upper extremities and only partial flexion of the lower extremities. The full-term infant exhibits flexion in all four extremities.*

B

Premature Infant, 28–32 Weeks **Full-term Infant**

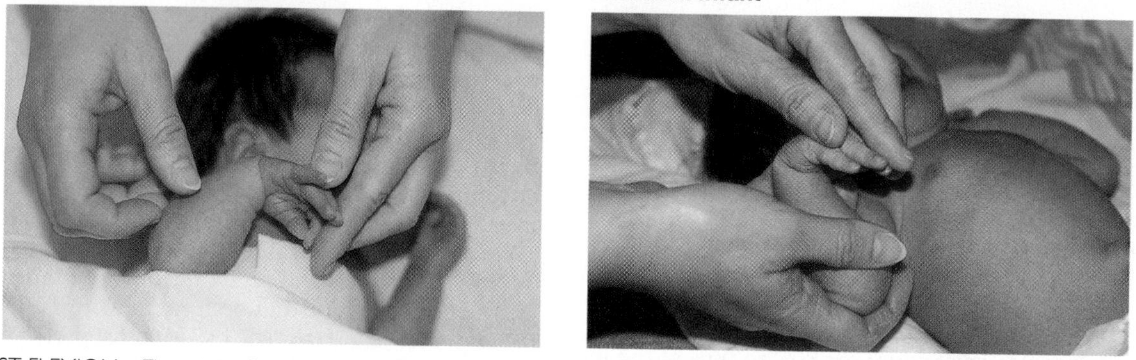

WRIST FLEXION *The wrist is flexed, applying enough pressure to get the hand as close to the forearm as possible. The angle between the hypothenar eminence and the ventral aspect of the forearm is measured. (Care must be taken not to rotate the infant's wrist.) The premature infant at 28–32 weeks' gestation will exhibit a 90° angle. With the full-term infant it is possible to flex the hand onto the arm.*

FIGURE 6.6 Examples of physical examination findings and reflex tests used to judge gestational age. (**A**) Resting posture. (**B**) Wrist flexion. (*Figure continues.*)

increase its production until approximately 32 weeks. The infant will appear pale, may be lethargic and anorectic, and will generally fail to thrive. The fault appears to be immaturity of the hematopoietic system combined with destruction of red blood cells due to low levels of vitamin E, which normally protects red blood cells against destruction. Excessive blood drawing for electrolyte or blood gas analysis can potentiate the problem. For this reason, records of the amount of blood drawn for analysis must be kept on preterm infants.

Anemia of prematurity will improve with administration of vitamin E. Red blood cell production can be stimulated by the administration of DNA recombinant erythropoietin. In addition, the infant may need blood transfusions to supply needed red blood cells.

Kernicterus. Kernicterus is destruction of brain cells by invasion of indirect bilirubin. This invasion results from the high concentrations of indirect bilirubin in the blood from excessive breakdown of red blood cells. Preterm infants are more prone to the condition than term infants, because with acidosis that occurs from poor respiratory exchange, brain cells are more susceptible to the effect of indirect bilirubin than normally. Preterm infants also have less serum albumin available to bind indirect bilirubin and therefore inactivate its effect. Because of this, kernicterus may occur at lower levels (as low as 12 mg per 100 mL of indirect bilirubin) in these infants. It is important to monitor indirect bilirubin levels in preterm infants. If jaundice occurs, phototherapy or exchange transfusion can be started to prevent excessively high indirect bilirubin levels.

Persistent Patent Ductus Arteriosus. Because preterm infants lack surfactant, their lungs are noncompliant. It is more difficult for them to move blood from the pulmonary artery into the lungs. This condition leads to pulmonary artery hypertension, which may interfere with closure of the ductus arteriosus. Administer intravenous therapy cautiously to avoid increasing blood pressure and

C

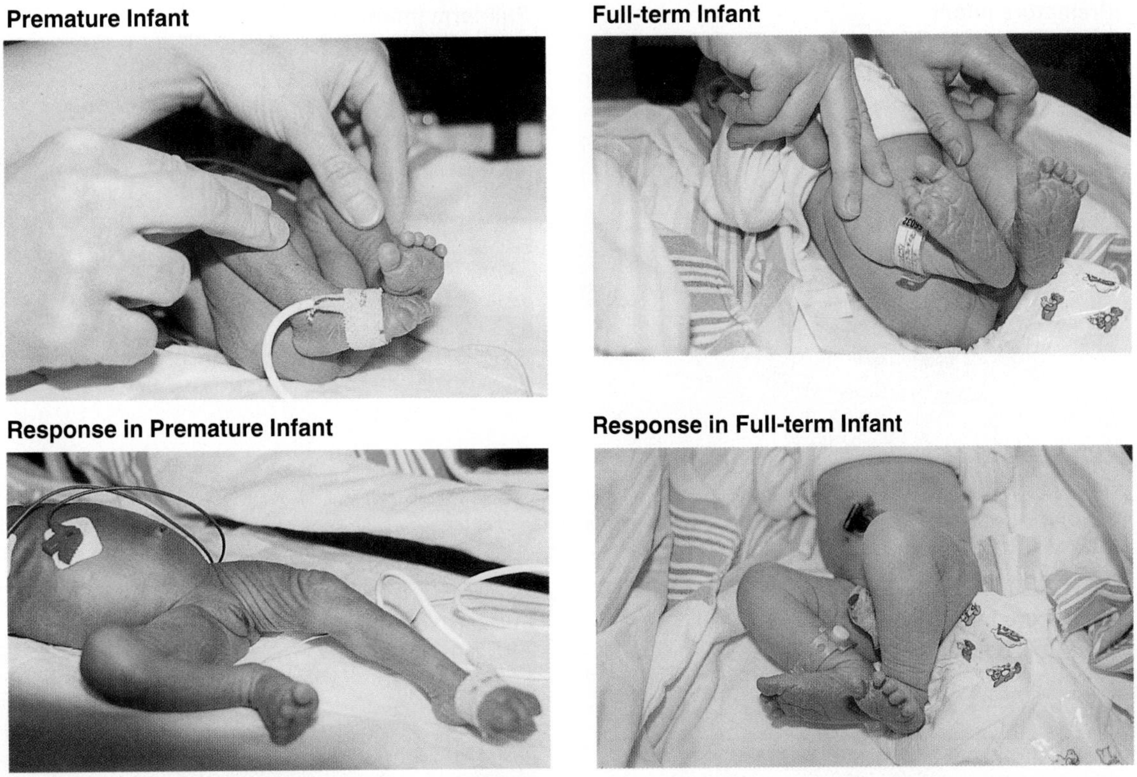

RECOIL OF EXTREMITIES *Place the infant supine. To test recoil of the legs (1) flex the legs and knees fully and hold for 5 seconds (shown in top photos). (2) extend the legs fully by pulling on the feet, (3) release. To test the arms, flex forearms and follow same procedure. In the premature infant response is minimal or absent (bottom left); in the full-term infant extremities return briskly to full flexion (bottom right).*

D

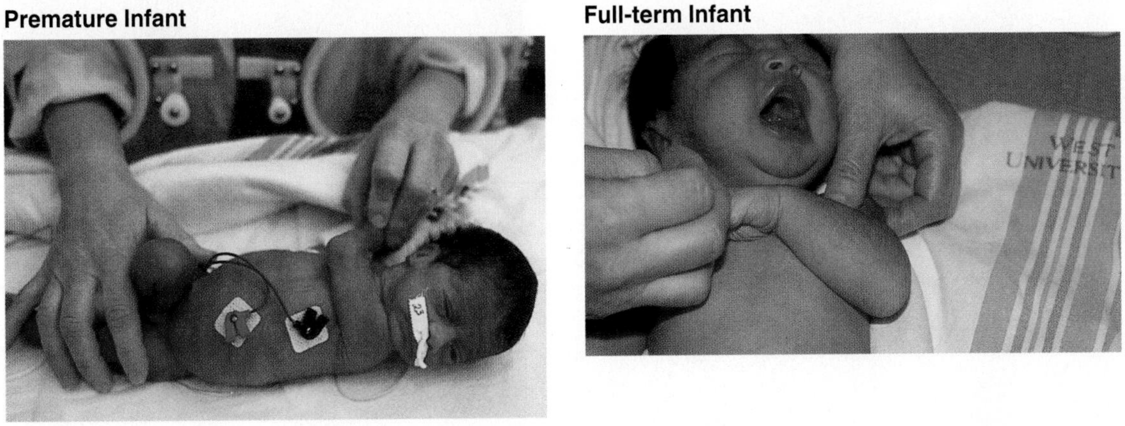

SCARF SIGN *Hold the baby supine, take the hand, and try to place it around the neck and above the opposite shoulder as far posteriorly as possible. Assist this maneuver by lifting the elbow across the body. See how far across the chest the elbow will go. In the premature infant the elbow will reach near or across the midline. In the full-term infant the elbow will not reach the midline.*

FIGURE 6.6 *(Continued)*
(**C**) Recoil of extremities (legs): (1) flex and hold; (2) extend. (**D**) Scarf sign.

compounding this problem. Indomethacin may be administered to initiate closure of the patent ductus arteriosus.

Periventricular/Intraventricular Hemorrhage. Preterm infants are particularly prone to periventricular hemorrhage (bleeding into the tissue surrounding the ventricles) or intraventricular hemorrhage (bleeding into the ventricles). These conditions occur in as many as 50% of infants of very low birth weight. Preterm infants have fragile capillaries and immature cerebral vascular development, increasing their susceptibility. With a rapid change in cerebral blood pressure, such as with hypoxia, intravenous infusion, ventilation, and pneumothorax, the capillaries rupture. The

(text continues on page 148)

E

Premature Infant

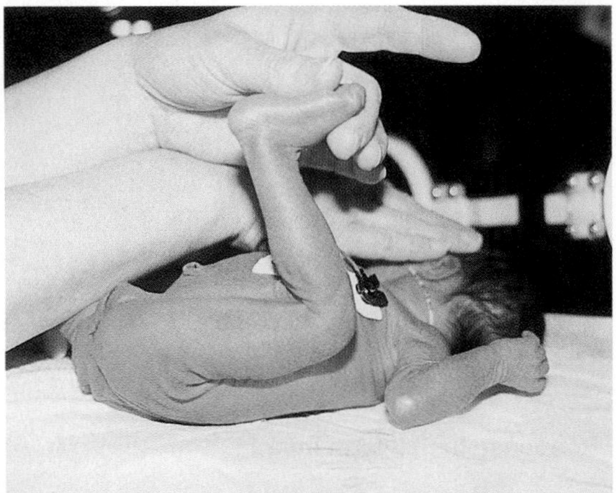

Full-term Infant

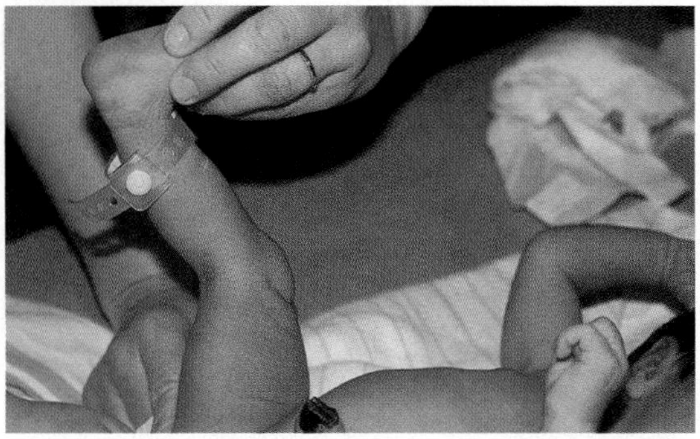

HEEL TO EAR *With the baby supine and the hips positioned flat on the bed, draw the baby's foot as near to the ear as it will go without forcing it. Observe the distance between the foot and head as well as the degree of extension at the knee. In the premature infant very little resistance will be met. In the full-term infant there will be marked resistance; it will be impossible to draw the baby's foot to the ear.*

F

Premature Infant

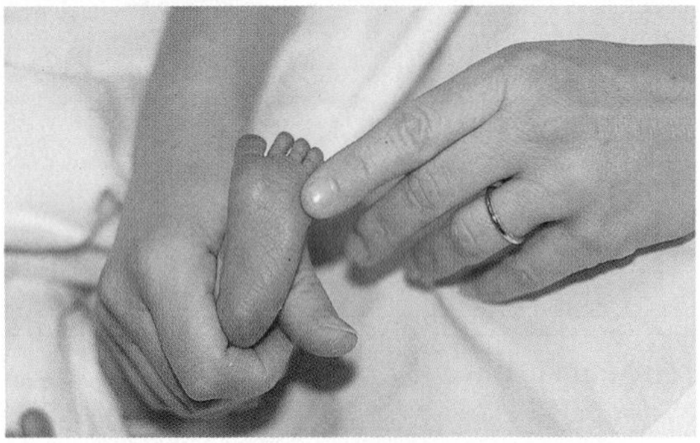

Full-term Infant

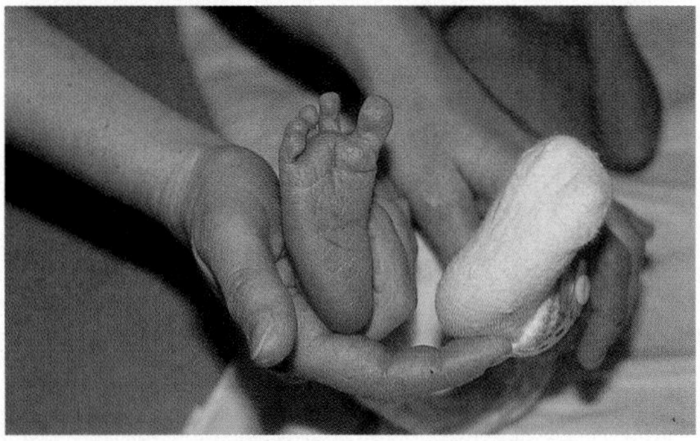

SOLE (PLANTAR) CREASES *The sole of the premature infant has very few or no creases. With the increasing gestation age, the number and depth of sole creases multiply, so that the full-term baby has creases involving the heel. (Wrinkles that occur after 24 hours of age can sometimes be confused with true creases.)*

G

Premature Infant

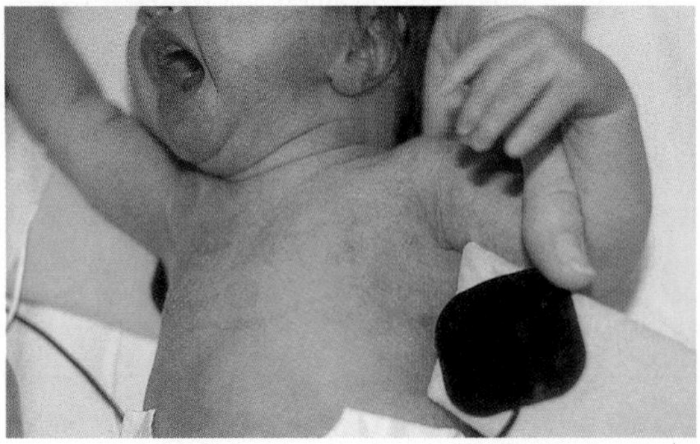

Full-term Infant

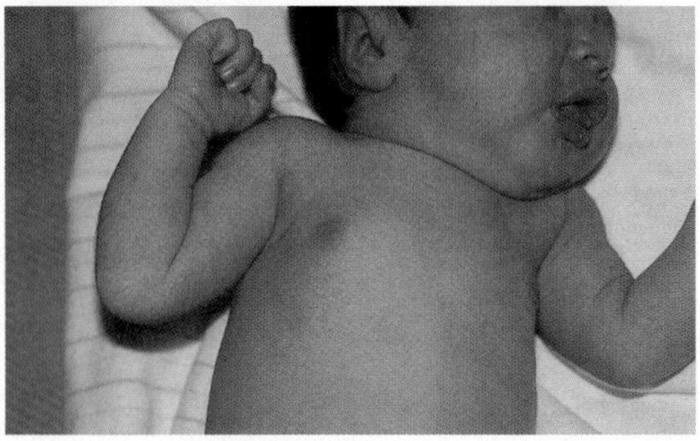

BREAST TISSUE *In infants younger than 34 weeks' gestation the areola and nipple are barely visible. After 34 weeks the areola becomes raised. Also, the infant of less than 36 weeks' gestation has no breast tissue. Breast tissue arises with increasing gestational age due to maternal hormonal stimulation. Thus, an infant of 39 to 40 weeks will have 5 to 6 mm of breast tissue, and this amount will increase with age.*

FIGURE 6.6 *(Continued)*
(**E**) Heel to ear. (**F**) Plantar creases. (**G**) Breast tissue.

H

Premature Infant, 34–36 Weeks

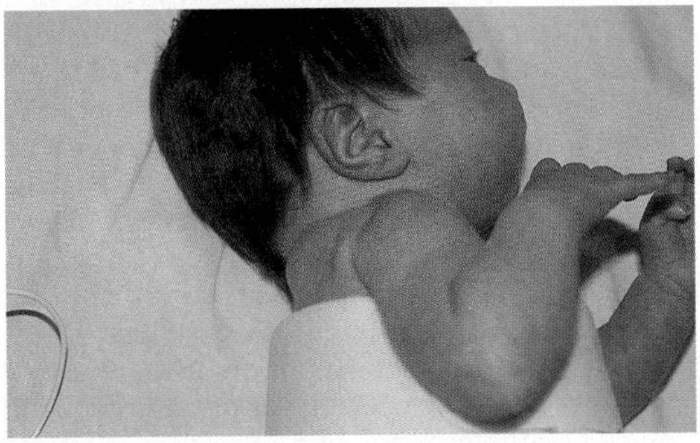

Full-term Infant

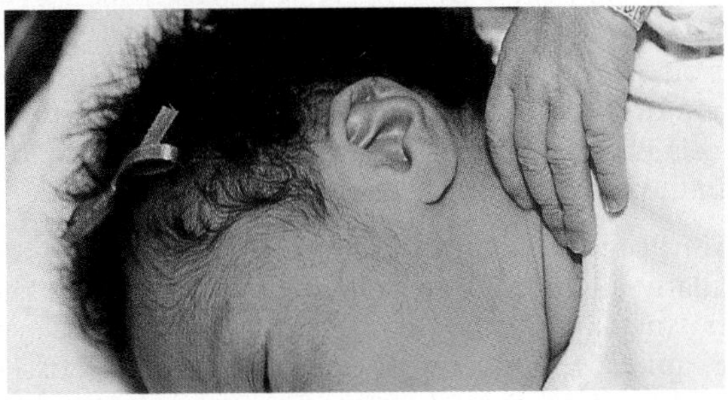

EARS *At fewer than 34 weeks' gestation infants have very flat, relatively shapeless ears. Shape develops over time so that an infant between 34 and 36 weeks has a slight incurving of the superior part of the ear; the term infant is characterized by incurving of two thirds of the pinna; and in an infant older than 39 weeks the incurving continues to the lobe. If the extremely premature infant's ear is folded over, it will stay folded. Cartilage begins to appear at approximately 32 weeks so that the ear returns slowly to its original position. In an infant of more than 40 weeks' gestation, there is enough ear cartilage so that the ear stands erect away from the head and returns quickly when folded. (When folding the ear over during examination be certain that the surrounding area is wiped clean or the ear may adhere to the vernix.)*

I

Premature Male

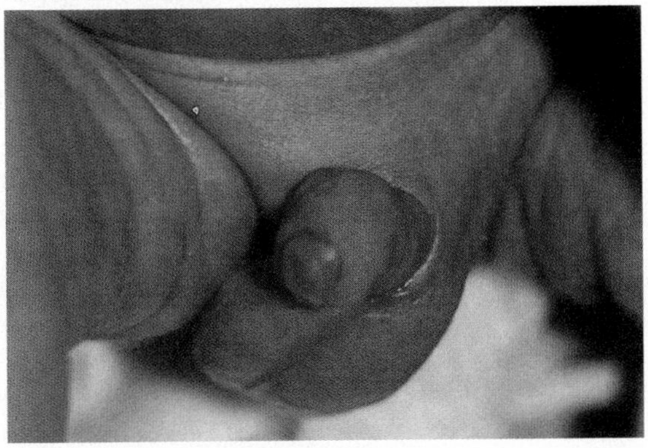

Full-term Male

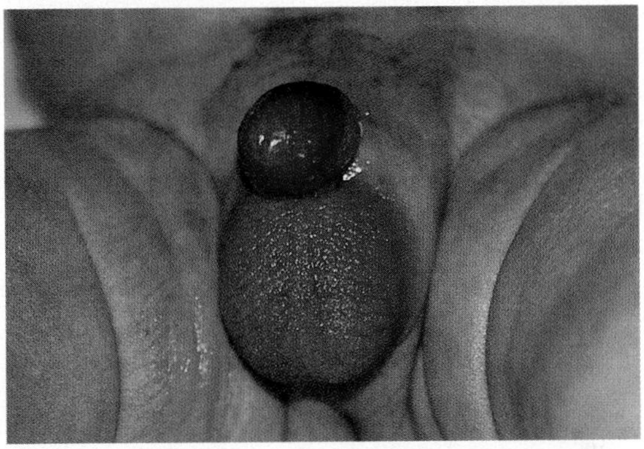

MALE GENITALIA *In the premature male the testes are very high in the inguinal canal and there are very few rugae on the scrotum. The full-term infant's testes are lower in the scrotum and many rugae have developed.*

J

Premature Female

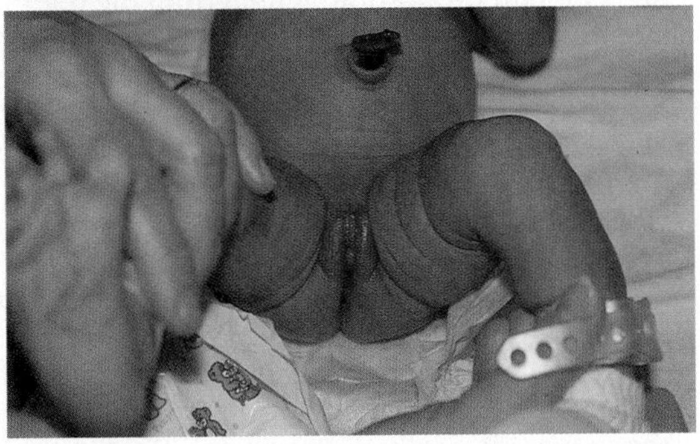

Full-term Female

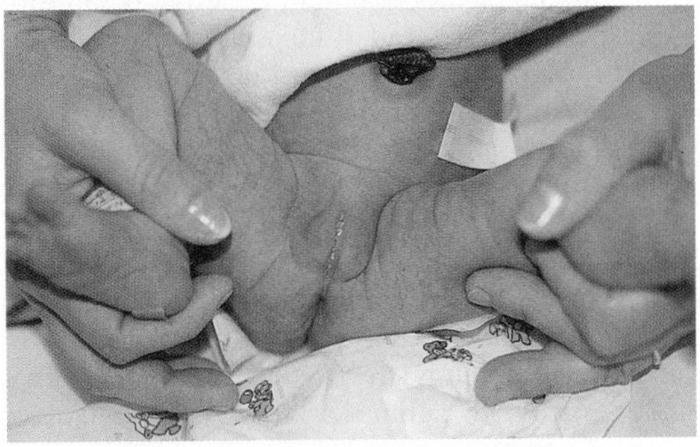

FEMALE GENITALIA *When the premature female is positioned on her back with hips abducted, the clitoris is very prominent and the labia majora are very small and widely separated. The labia minora and the clitoris are covered by the labia majora in the full-term infant.*

FIGURE 6.6 *(Continued)*
(**H**) Ear. (**I**) Male genitalia. (**J**) Female genitalia.

infant experiences brain anoxia beyond the rupture. Hydrocephalus may occur from bleeding into the aqueduct of Sylvius with resulting obstruction of the aqueduct. Preterm infants often have a cranial ultrasound done after the first few days of life to detect if a hemorrhage has occurred. Prognosis is guarded until it can be shown that development in the infant is normal after an intracranial bleed.

Other Potential Complications. Preterm infants are particularly susceptible to a number of illnesses in the early postnatal period, including respiratory distress syndrome, apnea, retinopathy of prematurity (all discussed later in this chapter), and necrotizing enterocolitis (discussed in Chapter 24).

NURSING DIAGNOSES AND RELATED INTERVENTIONS

Because a preterm infant has few body resources, both physiologic and psychological stress must be reduced as much as possible and interventions initiated gently to prevent depletion of resources. Close observation and analysis of findings are essential to managing problems quickly.

Nursing Diagnosis: Impaired gas exchange related to immature pulmonary functioning

Outcome Identification: Newborn will initiate and maintain respirations after surfactant therapy.

Outcome Evaluation: Newborn initiates breathing at birth after resuscitation; maintains normal newborn respirations of 30 to 60 breaths per minute free of assisted ventilation; exhibits oxygen saturation levels of at least 90% as evidenced by arterial blood gases (ABGs).

Preterm infants have great difficulty initiating respirations at birth because the pulmonary capillary bed is immature and lung surfactant may be deficient, requiring the infant to use maximum strength to inflate the alveoli each time. Infants cannot maintain effective respirations under these conditions. And, if meconium aspiration occurs, the respiratory problem is further compromised.

Because the preterm infant is unable to initiate effective respirations as quickly as the mature infant, he or she is prone to irreversible acidosis. To prevent this, the infant must be resuscitated within 2 minutes after birth and be kept warm during resuscitation procedures so he or she is not expending extra energy to increase the metabolic rate to maintain body temperature. All procedures must be carried out gently; the preterm infant's tissues are extremely sensitive to trauma and can easily be damaged or bruised. When blood from bruising is reabsorbed, this can lead to hyperbilirubinemia, yet another problem.

Giving 100% oxygen to preterm infants during resuscitation or to maintain respirations presents the danger of pulmonary edema and retinopathy of prematurity (blindness of prematurity; see discussion later in this chapter). The development of both of these conditions depends on saturation of the blood with oxygen (a PaO_2 of more than 100 mm Hg, which usually occurs when oxygen is administered at a concentration over 70%). As long as an infant is cyanotic, the blood saturation level of oxygen is likely to be low.

The preterm infant may need continued oxygen administration after resuscitation, because he or she often has difficulty maintaining respirations. The soft rib cartilage of the preterm infant tends to create respiratory problems because it collapses on expiration. The accessory muscles of respiration may be underdeveloped as well, leaving the preterm infant with no backup muscles to use when he or she becomes fatigued from trying to maintain respirations. Many preterm infants may have higher PaO_2 levels when placed prone than when supine, because this increases lung effectiveness.

Many preterm babies, particularly those under 32 weeks of age, have an irregular respiratory pattern (a few quick breaths, a period of 5 seconds to 10 seconds without respiratory effort, a few quick breaths again, and so on). There is no bradycardia with this irregular pattern (sometimes termed **periodic respirations**). Although the pattern is seen in term infants as well, the pattern seems to be intensified by immaturity and uncoordinated respiratory efforts. With true apnea, the pause in respirations is more than 20 seconds and bradycardia does occur. True apnea is discussed in more detail later in this chapter.

Nursing Diagnosis: Risk for fluid volume deficit related to insensible water loss at birth and small stomach capacity

Outcome Identification: Newborn will demonstrate intake of adequate fluid and electrolytes to meet body needs.

Outcome Evaluation: Plasma glucose is between 40 and 60 mg per 100 mL; specific gravity of urine is maintained at 1.003 to 1.030; urine output is maintained at 1 mL/kg/h; electrolyte levels are within normal limits.

The preterm newborn has a high insensible water loss due to the large body surface as compared with total body weight. The infant also is unable to concentrate urine well because of immature kidney function and thus excretes a high proportion of fluid from the body. All these factors make it important that the preterm baby receive up to 160 to 200 mL of fluid per kilogram of body weight daily (higher than the term infant).

Intravenous fluid administration typically begins within hours after birth to fulfill this fluid requirement and provide glucose to prevent hypoglycemia. Intravenous fluid should be given via a continuous infusion pump to ensure a constant infusion rate and prevent accidental fluid overload. Intravenous sites must be checked conscientiously, because the lack of subcutaneous tissue places the preterm newborn at risk for infiltration, which damages the tissues. Specially designed no. 27 gauge needles are available for use on small veins. However, many preterm infants lack adequately sized peripheral veins for even this small a needle. Therefore, they need to receive intravenous fluid by an umbilical venous catheter.

Monitor the baby's weight, specific gravity and amount of urine, and serum electrolytes to ensure adequate fluid intake. Too little fluid and calories may lead to dehydration and starvation, acidosis, and weight loss. Overhydration may lead to non-nutritional weight gain, pulmonary edema, and heart failure.

Measure urine output by weighing diapers rather than urine collection bags because disposable collection bags may lead to skin irritation and breakdown from frequent changing and leaking. The range of urine output for the first few days of life in preterm babies is high in comparison with that of the term baby—40 to 100 mL per kg per 24 hours, compared with 10 to 20 mL per kg per 24 hours. The specific gravity is low, rarely more than 1.012 (normal term babies may concentrate urine up to 1.030). Also, test urine for glucose and ketones. Hyperglycemia caused by the glucose infusion may lead to glucose spillage into the urine and an accompanying diuresis. If the glucose being supplied is too low and body cells are using protein for metabolism, ketone bodies will appear in urine.

Blood glucose determinations, such as with Dextrostix every 4 to 6 hours, helps to determine hypoglycemia (decreased serum glucose) or **hyperglycemia** (increased serum glucose). The blood glucose range should be between 40 mg/mL and 60 mg/mL. Because of the numerous blood tests performed, be certain to keep a record of all blood drawn so the child does not become hypovolemic from the amount drawn. Check for blood in the stools to evaluate for possible bleeding from the intestinal tract. This is helpful in determining the possible cause of hypovolemia if it occurs.

Nursing Diagnosis: Risk for altered nutrition, less than body requirements related to additional nutrients needed for maintenance of rapid growth, possible sucking difficulty, and small stomach

Outcome Identification: Infant will receive adequate fluid and nutrients for growth during hospitalization.

Outcome Evaluation: Infant's weight follows percentile growth curve; skin turgor is good; specific gravity of urine is maintained between 1.003 to 1.030; infant has no more than 15% weight loss in first 3 days of life and continues to gain weight after this point.

Nutrition problems arise with the preterm infant because the body is attempting to continue to maintain the rapid rate of intrauterine growth. Therefore, the preterm newborn requires a larger amount of nutrients in the diet than the mature infant. If these nutrients are not supplied, the infant will develop **hypocalcemia** (decreased serum calcium) or **azotemia** (low protein level in blood). Delayed feeding and resultant decrease in intestinal motility may also add to hyperbilirubinemia, a problem the infant already is at high risk of developing when fetal red blood cells begin to be destroyed.

Nutrition problems are compounded by the preterm infant's immature reflexes, which make swallowing and sucking difficult. In addition, small stomach capacity may affect nutrition, because a distended stomach may cause the infant respiratory distress. Increased activity necessitated by ineffective sucking may increase the metabolic rate and oxygen requirements. This increases the caloric requirements even more. An immature cardiac sphincter (between the stomach and esophagus) allows regurgitation to occur readily. The lack of a cough reflex may lead the infant to aspirate regurgitated formula. Digestion and absorption of nutrients in the stomach and intestine may also be immature.

Feeding Schedule. With the early administration of intravenous fluid to prevent hypoglycemia and supply fluid, feedings may be safely delayed until the infant has stabilized his or her respiratory effort from birth. Preterm infants may be fed by total parenteral nutrition until they are stable enough for other means. Feedings by breast, gavage or bottle are begun as soon as the infant is able to tolerate them to prevent deterioration of the intestinal villi. Most preterm infants have a chest x-ray before a first feeding. The presence of air in the stomach shows that the route to the stomach is clear.

The preterm infant needs 115 to 140 cal per kilogram body weight per day, compared with 100 to 110 cal per kilogram body weight per day needed by the term infant. Protein requirements are 3 to 3.5 g per kilogram body weight, compared with 2.0 to 2.5 g per kilogram body weight for a term newborn. Because preterm infants have a small stomach capacity, they cannot take large feedings. They must be fed more frequently with smaller amounts than the mature infant. Formulas containing as many as 80 cal/oz may be used (Berry et al., 1997). Feedings may be as small as 1 or 2 mL every 2 to 3 hours. Vitamin E, vitamin A, and calcium supplements may be necessary. As soon as the newborn reaches term age, iron supplements are recommended (Fletcher, 1997).

Gavage Feeding. The gag reflex is not intact until an infant is 32 weeks' gestation. Although a sucking reflex is present earlier, the ability to coordinate sucking and swallowing is inconsistent until approximately 34 weeks of gestation. Thus, infants born before 32 to 34 weeks of gestation are usually started on gavage feedings. Bottle or breastfeeding is gradually introduced as they mature. To avoid tiring, preterm nipples that are softer than regular nipples are used (Figure 6-7).

Preterm infants must be observed closely after both oral and gavage feeding to be certain that the filled stomach is not causing them respiratory distress. Offering a pacifier will help to strengthen this reflex, better prepare an infant for bottle feeding, and provide oral satisfaction. In addition, initiating and maintaining non-nutritive sucking help the newborn remember how to suck.

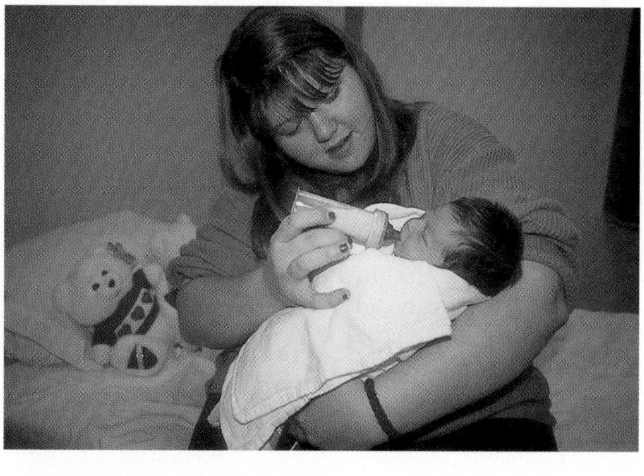

FIGURE 6.7 Feeding a preterm infant. Notice the small nipple and bottle used.

Gavage feedings may be given intermittently every few hours or continuously. Infants may be fed by continuous drip feedings at about 1 mL/h. This can be helpful for infants on ventilators or those who experience oxygen deprivation with handling. As long as the infant is being gavage fed, stomach secretions are usually aspirated, measured, and replaced before the feeding. An infant who has a stomach content of more than 2 mL just before a feeding is receiving more formula than he or she can digest in the time allowed. Feedings should not be increased but possibly even cut back to ensure better digestion and decrease the possibility of regurgitation and aspiration. Inability to digest this way is also a symptom of necrotizing enterocolitis (see Chapter 24).

Formula. The caloric concentration of formulas used for preterm infants is usually 24 cal/oz compared with 20 cal/oz for a term baby. Supplementing minerals such as calcium and phosphorus and electrolytes such as sodium, potassium, and chloride may be necessary, depending on the newborn's blood studies. Vitamin K should be administered at birth, same as with a term baby, except that the amount is more often 0.5 mL instead of 1 mL because of the infant's small size. Vitamin A is important in improving healing and possibly reducing the incidence of lung disease. Vitamin E seems to be important in preventing hemolytic anemia in preterm infants. Iron supplements interfere with the absorption of vitamin E and so are not added to formula until the infant has gained an average birth weight.

Parents may be confused about the lack of an iron supplement. They need an explanation of the particular blood problem that must be prevented and that iron supplements most likely will be started on discharge from the hospital or at least by age 3 months. Again, parents should have an explanation of what is happening. By the time of discharge, their infant has reached term maturity, and iron deficiency anemia due to low iron stores then becomes the infant's chief health risk.

Breast Milk. There is increasing evidence that, although preterm infants grow well on the increased caloric distribution of commercial formulas, the best milk for them is breast milk. The immunologic properties of breast milk apparently play a major role in preventing neonatal necrotizing enterocolitis, a destructive intestinal disorder that often occurs in preterm babies.

Manually expressed breast milk may be used for infant gavage feedings. It can be frozen for safe transport and storage. It is best if infants receive their own mother's breast milk rather than banked milk, as this contains more sodium; higher sodium levels are necessary for fluid retention in a preterm infant.

Nursing Diagnosis: Ineffective thermoregulation related to immaturity

Outcome Identification: Infant will maintain body temperature within normal limits until term age.

Outcome Evaluation: Infant's temperature is 97.6°F (36.5°C) axillary.

A preterm baby has a great deal of difficulty maintaining body temperature, because he or she has a relatively large surface area per pound of body weight. In addition, because the infant does not flex the body well but remains in an extended position, rapid cooling from evaporation is more likely to occur.

The preterm infant has little subcutaneous fat for insulation, and poor muscular development does not allow the child to move as actively as the older infant to produce body heat. The preterm infant also has a limited amount of **brown fat,** the special tissue present in newborns to maintain body temperature. The infant is unable to shiver, a useful mechanism to increase body temperature; on the other hand, the child is unable to sweat and thereby reduce body temperature because of an immature central nervous system and hypothalamic control. Thus, the infant depends on the environmental temperature provided for him or her. The infant must be kept under a radiant heat warmer or Isolette.

Even weighing should be delayed until the infant is placed in the warmth of an Isolette or under a radiant warmer with a Servocontrol.

During any transport, keeping the newborn warm is crucial. Remember that infants lose heat by radiation. If a warmed Isolette is placed near a cold window or air conditioner, the infant will lose heat to the distant source. Also, keep this in mind when transporting an infant on a cold day. The vehicle and transporting Isolette need to prewarmed. An additional heat shield or plastic wrap may be placed over an infant on a radiant warmer to help conserve heat.

Nursing Diagnosis: Risk for infection related to immature immune defenses in preterm infant

Outcome Identification: Infant will remain free of infection during hospital stay.

Outcome Evaluation: Temperature instability decreasing, being maintained at 97.6°F (36.5°C) axillary; absence of further signs and symptoms of infection such as poor growth or a reduced temperature.

The skin of the preterm baby is easily traumatized and therefore offers less resistance to infection than the skin and mucous membranes of the mature baby. In addition, the preterm infant has a lowered resistance to infection. The infant has difficulty producing phagocytes to localize infection and has a deficiency of IgM antibodies because of insufficient production. Linen and equipment used with the preterm infant must be clean to reduce the chances of infection. Staff members must be free of infection, and handwashing and gowning regulations must be strictly enforced.

✔ CHECKPOINT QUESTIONS

14. Why does acidosis clear quickly in the term newborn, but may cause irreversible problems in the preterm newborn?
15. During the first few days of life, how much urine should the preterm neonate produce?
16. How many calories are required by the preterm newborn daily?

Nursing Diagnosis: Risk for altered parenting related to interference with parent–infant attachment resulting from hospitalization of infant at birth

Outcome Identification: Parents demonstrate adequate bonding behavior by the time of infant's discharge from hospital.

Outcome Evaluation: Parents visit frequently and hold infant; speak of him or her in positive terms.

The first and second periods of reactivity normally observed in newborns at 1 hour and 4 hours of life (see Chapter 5) are delayed in the preterm infant. In some infants, no period of increased activity or tachycardia may appear until 12 to 18 hours of age. If the purpose of a period of reactivity is to stimulate respiratory function, this places the preterm infant in even greater threat of respiratory failure, because respiratory efforts may not be stimulated. A second consequence of a delayed period of reactivity is the loss of an opportunity for early interaction between parents and the newborn.

Currently it is recognized that, although it is extremely important to conserve the preterm infant's strength by reducing sensory stimulation as much as possible and handling the infant gently, the child needs as much loving attention as possible. Rocking the infant, singing and talking to him, and gentle holding are measures to help the infant develop a sense of trust in people, which will enable the child to relate satisfactorily to them in the future. Holding the baby using kangaroo care (holding the infant with skin-to-skin contact) is yet another way to increase bonding. Encourage the parents to begin interacting with the infant in as normal a manner as possible (see Empowering the Family).

Before effective bonding can be established, parents may need time to come to terms with their feelings of disappointment and guilt. A nurse can be instrumental in helping them air these feelings, and develop a more positive attitude toward their preterm infant (Coffman et al., 1995).

If the infant cannot be removed from an Isolette or radiant heat warmer, the child can still be held using kangaroo care or handled and stroked in the Isolette or warmer. Because parents are not psychologically ready for birth when the preterm baby is born, it may be more difficult for them to believe they have a child than if the baby were born at term. Encourage breast milk expression for use by the infant if the child is too young to nurse. If the infant is not breast fed, encourage parents to come into the hospital and hold the baby before and after gavage feedings or to give bottle feedings. By feeding their baby or providing breast milk for the feedings, the parents and family are directly participating in the care and taking on responsibility for the infant's welfare.

On the days they cannot visit, parents can still stay in touch by telephone. By the time the baby is ready for discharge, the parents should be able to feel that they are taking home "their" baby, one that they know and are ready to love.

Parents visiting a high-risk nursery often need a great deal of attention and support from nursing personnel. Remember that, although radiant warmers, Isolettes, ventilators, and monitors are familiar equipment to nurses, they are unusual and frightening equipment to parents. A parent may want very much to touch an infant but be so afraid that touching might set off an alarm that he or she stands back with arms folded instead (Figure 6-8).

Making parents and the baby's siblings welcome in a high-risk nursery is a major role for the nurse of high-risk infants (see Enhancing Communication). Be aware of any possible restrictions in sibling visitation because of infections, such as colds or fever. It is also important to make

EMPOWERING THE FAMILY: Guidelines for Parents of a Newborn in Intensive Care

- Learn the name of your infant's primary nurse or care manager and physician. Make a point of talking to them when you visit so the information you receive is consistent and these people can grow to know you.
- Discuss with your infant's care manager or primary nurse the time you will usually visit so she or he can reserve this time for you. It also helps them to schedule the baby's procedures and rest times so there is time during your visits for you to hold your infant and interact with him.
- Ask for explanations of any equipment or medications being used with your infant so you understand the plan of care. Insist on being included in care decisions.
- If you cannot visit on any day, feel free to telephone the nursery and ask to talk to your infant's primary care nurse or physician. Such telephone calls are not viewed as a bother but are welcomed as the mark of a concerned parent.
- If you planned to breastfeed, ask if you can supply expressed breast milk for your infant as soon as feedings are started. This may help to give you a feeling of having a greater part in your baby's care.
- Supply a tape recording of your family's voices so your baby can learn to recognize them and a small toy for your baby's bed. These actions not only supply auditory and visual stimulation for your child but also help to give you a more "normal" feeling toward infant care.
- Use your baby's name when you talk about him or her (not "the baby") to help you gain a firm feeling that this is your baby, not the nursery's.
- If your child is hospitalized a distance from home, ask if transfer to a local hospital in a less technical environment at a later date will be possible.

To help prevent episodes of apnea:

- Maintain a thermal neutral environment
- Use gentle handling to avoid excessive fatigue
- Always suction gently to minimize nasopharyngeal irritation (may cause bradycardia due to vagal stimulation)
- Use indwelling nasogastric tubes rather than intermittent ones(reduces amount of vagal stimulation)
- Burp and observe an infant carefully after feeding (full stomach can put pressure on the diaphragm)
- Never take rectal temperatures in infants prone to apnea (resulting vagal stimulation can cause bradycardia leading to apnea)

Theophylline or caffeine sodium benzoate may be administered to stimulate respirations. The mechanism by which these drugs reduce the incidence of apneic episodes is unclear, but they appear to increase an infant's sensitivity to carbon dioxide, ensuring better respiratory function. Those infants who have had an apneic episode severe enough to require resuscitation are at high risk for sudden infant death syndrome (SIDS). Such infants may be discharged home with a monitoring device to be used for 2 to 6 months.

CHECKPOINT QUESTIONS

21. By when does transient tachypnea of the newborn typically resolve?
22. What measures could be used initially to stimulate the infant with apnea?

Sudden Infant Death Syndrome

Sudden Infant Death Syndrome (SIDS) is sudden unexplained death in infancy (David, 1997). It tends to occur at a higher than usual rate in the infants of adolescent mothers, infants of closely spaced pregnancies, and underweight infants and preterm infants. Also prone to SIDS are infants with bronchopulmonary dysplasia as well as preterm infants, twins, siblings of another child with SIDS, Native American infants, Alaskan native infants, economically disadvantaged black infants, and infants of narcotic-dependent mothers. The peak ages of incidence are between 2 weeks and 1 year of age.

Although the cause of SIDS is unknown, a number of theories about its cause have been postulated. In addition to prolonged but unexplained apnea, other possible contributing factors may include:

- Viral respiratory or botulism infection
- Distorted familial breathing patterns
- Possible lack of surfactant in alveoli
- Sleeping prone rather than on the side or back

Typically affected infants are well nourished. Parents report that the infant may have had a slight head cold. After being put to bed at night or for a nap, the infant is found dead a few hours later. Infants who die this way do not appear to make any sound as they die, which indicates that they die with laryngospasm. Although many infants are found with blood-flecked sputum or vomitus in their mouths or on the bedclothes, this seems to occur as the result of death, not as its cause. An autopsy often reveals petechiae in the lungs and mild inflammation and congestion in the respiratory tract. However, these symptoms are not severe enough to cause sudden death. It is clear that these children do not suffocate from bedclothes or choke from overfeeding, underfeeding, or crying. Since the American Academy of Pediatrics recommendation to always put newborns to sleep on their back or side, the incidence of SIDS has declined dramatically (AAP, 1996).

Parents have a difficult time accepting the death of a child. This is especially true when it happens so suddenly. In discussing the child, they often use both the past and present tense as if they are not yet aware of the death. Many parents experience a period of somatic symptoms that occur with acute grief, such as nausea, stomach pain, or vertigo. Parents should be counseled by a nurse or someone else trained in counseling at the time of the infant's death; it helps if they can talk to this same person periodically for however long it takes to resolve their grief. Supportive organizations are available for help. Organizations that may be helpful for referral are:

- Sudden Infant Death Alliance
10500 Little Patuxent Parkway
Suite 420
Columbia, MD 21044
- National SIDS Resource Center
8201 Greensboro Drive, Suite 600
McLean, VA 22102

The Sudden Infant Death Syndrome Alliance has chapters in most large cities offering support to parents and helping them to understand that the feelings they are experiencing are not unique.

The SIDS Alliance suggests that mandatory autopsies be performed on all children who die from SIDS in the hope that the cause of the phenomenon can be identified. Autopsy reports should be given to parents as soon as they are available (if toxicology tests are included in the autopsy, results will not be available for weeks). Reading the report that their child died an unexplained death can help to reassure them that the death was not their fault. They need this assurance if they are to plan for other children. If there are older children in the family, they also need assurance that SIDS is a disease of infants and that the strange phenomenon that invaded their home and killed a younger brother or sister will not also kill them. If they wished the infant dead, as all children wish siblings were dead on some days, reassure them that their wishes are not that powerful and that they did not cause the baby's death.

When another child is born, the parents can be expected to become extremely frightened at any sign of illness in the child. They need support to see them through the first few months of the second child's life, particularly past the point at which the first child died. Some parents need support to view a second child as an individual child and not as a replacement for the one who died.

Often, the sibling of a SIDS infant is screened using a sleep study as a precaution within the first 2 weeks of life. Depending on the parents' level of anxiety, the sibling may receive this screening before discharge. In addition, the sibling may also be placed on apnea monitoring pending the results of the sleep study.

Apparent Life-Threatening Event (ALTE)

Some infants have been discovered cyanotic and limp in their beds but have survived after mouth-to-mouth resuscitation by parents. An episode of this kind is called an **apparent life-threatening event** (ALTE). For these children as well as for preterm infants with a tendency toward apnea or the siblings of a child who died from SIDS, apnea monitoring is available. An alarm sounds when the neonate experiences a period of apnea of 20 seconds or more or a decreased heart rate below 80 bpm occurs (Figure 6-9). If parents are going to use an apnea monitor at home, make certain they will be able to hear it in most parts of the house or apartment. Usually the alarm is not loud enough to be heard in the basement from an upstairs bedroom. Caution them about household noises such as a loud television, radio, vacuum cleaner, or hair dryer that may interfere with hearing the alarm. Be sure they know how to apply and reposition the leads and that they are comfortable enough with the monitor to see past it to the child. In addition, parents of high-risk infants should be taught cardiopulmonary resuscitation before the infant is discharged from the hospital (Figure 6-10).

Caring for a child at home on an apnea monitor may be extremely stressful for the parents and their relationship. Finding a competent babysitter is often described by parents as a major problem. Most parents of a baby with a home apnea monitor can benefit from a community or home care referral, so they have a second opinion as to how well they are managing as well as a listening ear to discuss the strain of having always to be alert for a sound that means their infant has stopped breathing. Having someone periodically review with them what steps to take should the alarm sound (jiggle the baby, begin mouth-to-mouth resuscitation, call the emergency squad) can be very comforting. These parents are under a tremendous strain. This may be accentuated by a lack of sleep at night because many parents report that they are always listening for an alarm. Because SIDS is a baffling disease, these parents may live in fear of it until their child reaches at least 1 year of age.

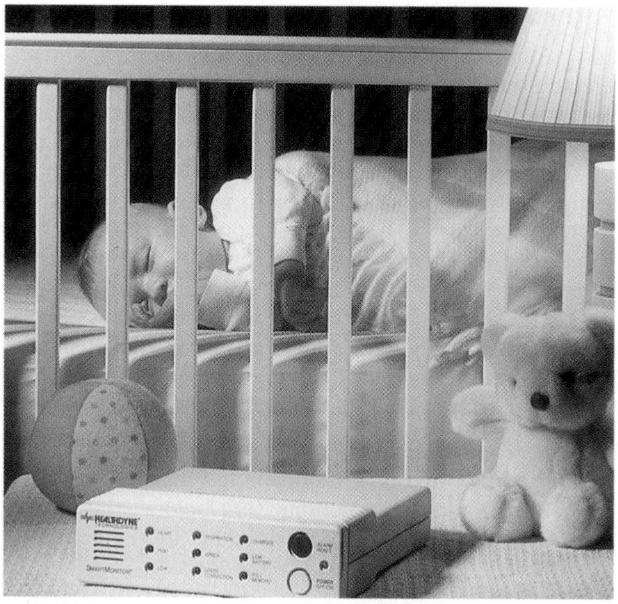

FIGURE 6.9 An apnea monitor for home monitoring.

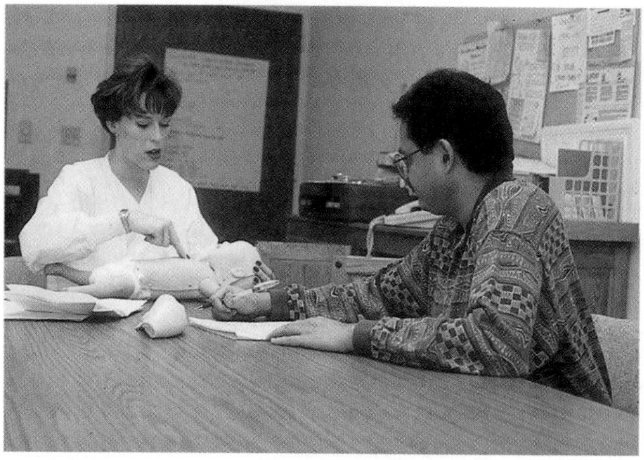

FIGURE 6.10 Parents of infants with ALTE need to learn resuscitation before the infant is discharged from the hospital. Here a nurse teaches the technique using a doll.

Periventricular Leukomalacia

Periventricular leukomalacia (PVL) is abnormal formation of the white matter of the brain. It is caused by an ischemic episode, which interferes with circulation to a portion of the brain. Phagocytes and macrophages invade the area to clear away necrotic tissue, and what is left is an area in the white matter of the brain that is revealed on sonogram as a hollow space. PVL occurs most frequently in preterm infants who experience cerebral ischemia. Once the condition has occurred, there is no therapy for PVL. Infants may die from the original insult; they may be left with long-term effects such as learning disabilities. Any action to reduce environmental stimuli or sudden shifts in cerebral blood flow, such as avoiding rapid fluid infusions or sudden noises, is important to preventing PVL and limiting the long-term effects of prematurity.

> **✓ CHECKPOINT QUESTIONS**
>
> 23. What is the peak age of incidence for SIDS?
> 24. When does the alarm sound on an apnea monitor?

Hemolytic Disease of the Newborn

The term *hemolytic* is Latin for destruction (lysis) of red blood cells. In the past, hemolytic disease of the newborn was most often caused by an Rh blood type incompatibility. Because prevention of Rh antibody formation has been available for more than 20 years, the disorder is now most often caused by an ABO incompatibility. In both instances, the mother builds antibodies against the infant's red blood cells, leading to hemolysis (destruction) of the cells. The destruction of red blood cells causes severe anemia and hyperbilirubinemia.

Rh Incompatibility

Theoretically, no direct connection exists between the fetal and maternal circulation, and no fetal blood cells enter the maternal circulation. In actuality, occasional placental villi break and a drop or two of fetal blood does enter maternal circulation. If the mother's blood type is Rh (D) negative and the fetal blood type is Rh positive (contains the D antigen), the introduction of fetal blood causes sensitization to occur, and the mother begins to form antibodies against the D antigen. Few antibodies form this way, however. Most form in the mother's bloodstream in the first 72 hours after birth, because there is an active exchange of fetal–maternal blood as placental villi loosen and the placenta is delivered. After this sensitization, in a second pregnancy, there will be a high level of antibody D circulating in the mother's bloodstream, which acts to destroy the fetal red blood cells early if the fetus is Rh positive. By the end of the second pregnancy, the fetus can be severely compromised by the action of these antibodies crossing the placenta and destroying red blood cells. Some infants require intrauterine transfusions to combat red cell destruction. Preterm labor may be induced to remove the fetus from the destructive maternal environment.

ABO Incompatibility

In most instances of ABO incompatibility, the maternal blood type is O and the fetal blood type is A; it may also occur when the fetus has type B or AB blood. A reaction in an infant with type B blood is often the most serious.

Hemolysis can become a problem with a first pregnancy in which there is an ABO incompatibility. The antibodies to A and B cell types are naturally occurring antibodies, which are present from birth in individuals whose red cells lack these antigens. Unlike the antibodies formed against the Rh D factor, these antibodies are large (IgM) class and do not cross the placenta. The infant of an ABO incompatibility, therefore, is not born anemic, as is the Rh-sensitized child. Hemolysis of the blood begins with birth, when blood and antibodies are exchanged during the mixing of maternal and fetal blood as the placenta is loosened and may continue for up to 2 weeks of age.

Assessment

Interestingly, preterm infants do not seem to be affected by ABO incompatibility. This may be because the receptor sites for anti-A or anti-B antibodies do not appear on red cells until late in fetal life. Even in the mature newborn, the direct Coombs' test may only be weakly positive because of the few anti-A or anti-B sites present. The reticulocyte count (immature or newly formed red blood cells) is usually elevated as the infant attempts to replace destroyed cells.

With Rh incompatibility, the infant may not appear pale at birth despite the red cell destruction that has occurred in utero. This is because the accelerated production of red cells during the last few months in utero compensates to some degree for the destruction. The liver and spleen may be enlarged from an attempt to produce new blood cells. If the number of red cells has decreased, the blood in the vascular circulation may be hypotonic to interstitial fluid; fluid shifts from the lower to higher isotonic pressure by the law of osmosis, causing extreme edema. Finally, the severe anemia results in heart failure.

Hydrops fetalis is an old term for the appearance of a severely involved infant at birth. *Hydrops* refers to the edema, and *fetalis* refers to the lethal state. The infant does not appear jaundiced because the maternal circulation has evacuated the rising indirect bilirubin level. With birth, progressive jaundice, usually occurring within the first 24 hours of life, reveals in both Rh and ABO incompatibility that a hemolytic process is at work. The indirect bilirubin level rises rapidly as red blood cells are destroyed and indirect bilirubin is released. Indirect bilirubin is fat soluble and cannot be excreted from the body. Under normal circumstances, the liver enzyme glucuronyl transferase converts indirect bilirubin to direct bilirubin. Direct bilirubin is water soluble and combines with bile for excretion from the body with feces. In preterm infants or those with extreme hemolysis, the liver is unable to convert bilirubin, which is the reason jaundice becomes so extreme.

Normally, cord blood has an indirect bilirubin level of 0 to 3 mg/100 mL. An increasing indirect bilirubin level is dangerous because if the level rises above 20 mg/dL in a term or 12 mg/dL in a preterm infant, brain damage from kernicterus can occur. Meanwhile the infant needs to use body stores to maintain metabolism in the presence of anemia. This causes a progressive hypoglycemia with Rh hemolytic disease in at least 20% of infants, compounding their initial problem. A decrease in hemoglobin during the first week of life to a level less than that of cord blood is a later indication of blood loss or hemolysis.

Therapeutic Management

Initiation of early feeding, use of phototherapy, and exchange transfusion all may be immediate measures necessary to reduce indirect bilirubin levels in the infant affected by ABO or Rh incompatibility. In addition, because of the newborn's critical status, breastfeeding may be temporarily suspended. In newborns with severe hemolytic disease, the hemoglobin concentration may continue to drop during the first 6 months of life or their bone marrow may fail to increase production of erythrocytes in response to continuing hemolysis. If this occurs, the infant may need an additional blood transfusion to correct this late anemia. Therapy with erythropoietin to stimulate red blood cell production is also possible.

Initiation of Early Feeding. Bilirubin is removed from the body by being incorporated into feces. Therefore, the sooner bowel elimination begins, the sooner bilirubin removal begins. Early feeding, therefore, stimulates bowel peristalsis and accomplishes this.

Suspension of Breastfeeding. Pregnanediol, the breakdown product of progesterone, interferes with the conjugation of indirect bilirubin. It is excreted in breast milk for the first 24 to 48 hours. Breastfed babies, therefore, may evidence more jaundice than bottle-fed babies. Although rare, temporary suspension of breastfeeding for 24 hours may be necessary to reduce an accumulating indirect bilirubin level in some infants.

Phototherapy. An infant's liver processes little bilirubin in utero because the mother's circulation does this for the infant. With birth, exposure to light apparently "triggers" the liver to assume this function. Additional light appears to speed the conversion potential of the liver. Phototherapy is the light technique that is most often used. In phototherapy, the infant is continuously exposed to specialized light such as quartz halogen, cool white daylight, or special blue fluorescent light. The lights are placed 12 to 30 inches above the newborn. Specialized fiberoptic light systems incorporated into a fiberoptic blanket also have been developed. The infant is undressed except for the diaper, so that as much skin surface as possible is exposed to the light (Figure 6-11).

Continuous exposure to bright lights this way may be harmful to the newborn's retina, so the infant's eyes must always be covered while under bilirubin lights. Eye dressings or cotton balls can be firmly secured in place by an additional dressing. The infant must be checked frequently to be certain the dressings have not slipped or are causing corneal irritation. A constant concern is that suffocation from eye patches could occur.

The stools of an infant under bilirubin lights are often bright green because of the excessive bilirubin that is excreted as the result of the therapy. They are also frequently loose and may be irritating to skin. Urine may be dark colored from urobilinogen formation. Assess skin turgor and intake and output to ensure that dehydration is not occurring. Monitor axillary temperature to prevent the infant from overheating under the bright lights.

An infant under phototherapy should be removed for feeding so that he or she continues to have interaction with the parents. In addition, supplemental feedings with additional formula may be recommended to prevent dehydration. Formula appears to bind most effectively with bilirubin. The eye patches should be removed during this time to give the infant a period of visual stimulation. To prevent a lengthy hospitalization, infants may be discharged and continue therapy at home.

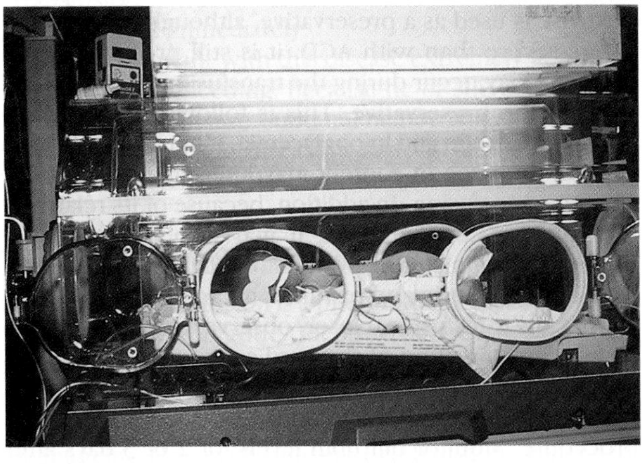

FIGURE 6.11 A newborn receiving phototherapy is undressed except for a diaper so that he receives maximum exposure to the lights. His eyes are covered snugly to protect them from the bright light.

Parents need an explanation of the rationale for phototherapy. Isolettes are automatically associated with seriously ill infants. At the same time, the use of lights does not seem scientific (almost a home remedy). Parents can easily be confused by the two interventions, one seemingly serious and the other seemingly not serious at all.

Home Phototherapy. Home phototherapy allows for uninterrupted contact between the parents and the newborn and therefore has the potential to aid bonding. Important considerations are that the lights are set so that they are a full 12 inches away from the infant to prevent burning and that the infant continuously wears eye patches and a diaper during phototherapy to protect the retinas of the eyes and the ovaries or testes.

The infant should have the eye patches removed when away from the lights for feeding for a period of visual stimulation and interaction. The point at which infants are most apt to dislodge eye patches is when they cry as they wake for a feeding. Urge parents not to allow an infant under bilirubin lights to cry for a sustained period to avoid having this happen.

The infant's progress can be measured daily by a transcutaneous bilirubinometer, a hand-held fiberoptic light that is placed against the infant's skin. The intensity of the yellow color of the skin is measured by the meter, and a numerical level of bilirubin is calculated (Dai et al, 1997).

A newer innovation for hyperbilirubinemia management is the phototherapy blanket, a fiberoptic blanket that is wrapped around the baby. Light generated by the blanket has the same effect on bilirubin levels as banks of overhead lights. The advantages of a blanket are that the infant can be held for long periods without an interruption in the phototherapy, and eye patches are unnecessary (see Empowering the Family).

Exchange Transfusion. Intensive phototherapy in conjunction with hydration and close monitoring of serum bilirubin levels is the preferred method of treatment. However, despite these measures, if bilirubin levels are rapidly rising, exchange transfusion may be necessary. The procedure involves alternatively withdrawing small amounts (2 to 10 mL) of the infant's blood and then replacing it with equal amounts of donor blood. The blood is exchanged slowly to prevent alternating hypovolemia and hypervolemia. Exchange transfusion may need to be repeated because additional unconjugated bilirubin from tissue moves into the circulation after the initial exchange.

The therapy may be used for any condition that leads to hyperbilirubinemia or polycythemia. When used as therapy for blood incompatibility, it removes approximately 85% of sensitized red cells. It reduces the serum concentration of indirect bilirubin and often prevents heart failure in infants. Because indirect bilirubin levels rise at relatively predictable levels, standards for performing exchange transfusion depend on the indirect bilirubin concentration and transfusion is used when this level exceeds:

mother's circulation is no longer supplying him or her. The overproduction of insulin causes the development of severe hypoglycemia. Hyperbilirubinemia also may occur in these infants because, if immature, they are unable to effectively clear bilirubin from their system. Hypocalcemia also frequently develops because parathyroid hormone is lower in these infants due to hypomagnesemia from excessive renal losses of magnesium.

The infant born to a woman with Class D diabetes or beyond will be small for gestational age because of poor placental perfusion. The problems of hypoglycemia, hypocalcemia, and hyperbilirubinemia remain the same.

Therapeutic Management

To prevent serum glucose from falling too low, IDM infants are fed early with formula or administered a continuous infusion of glucose. It is important that the child not be given only a bolus of glucose. Otherwise, rebound hypoglycemia (accentuating the problem) may occur. Some IDM infants have a small left colon, apparently another effect of intrauterine hyperglycemia, which limits the amount of oral feedings they can take in their first days of life. Signs of a small colon would include vomiting or abdominal distention after the first few feedings.

The Infant of a Drug-Dependent Mother

Infants of drug-dependent women tend to be small for gestational age. The infant will show withdrawal symptoms (neonatal abstinence syndrome) shortly after birth if the mother is dependent on a drug (see Assessing the Newborn of a Drug-Addicted Mother). These include:

- Irritability
- Disturbed sleep patterns
- Constant movement possibly leading to abrasions on their elbows, knees, or nose
- Tremors
- Frequent sneezing
- Shrill, high-pitched cry
- Possible hyperreflexia and clonus (neuromuscular irritability)
- Convulsions
- Tachypnea (rapid respirations) possibly so severe that it leads to to hyperventilation and alkalosis
- Vomiting and diarrhea leading to large fluid losses and secondary dehydration

Specific tools may be used to quantify and assess the infant's status. These tools are often called Neonatal Abstinence Scoring (NAS) tools.

ASSESSING the Newborn of a Drug-Addicted Mother

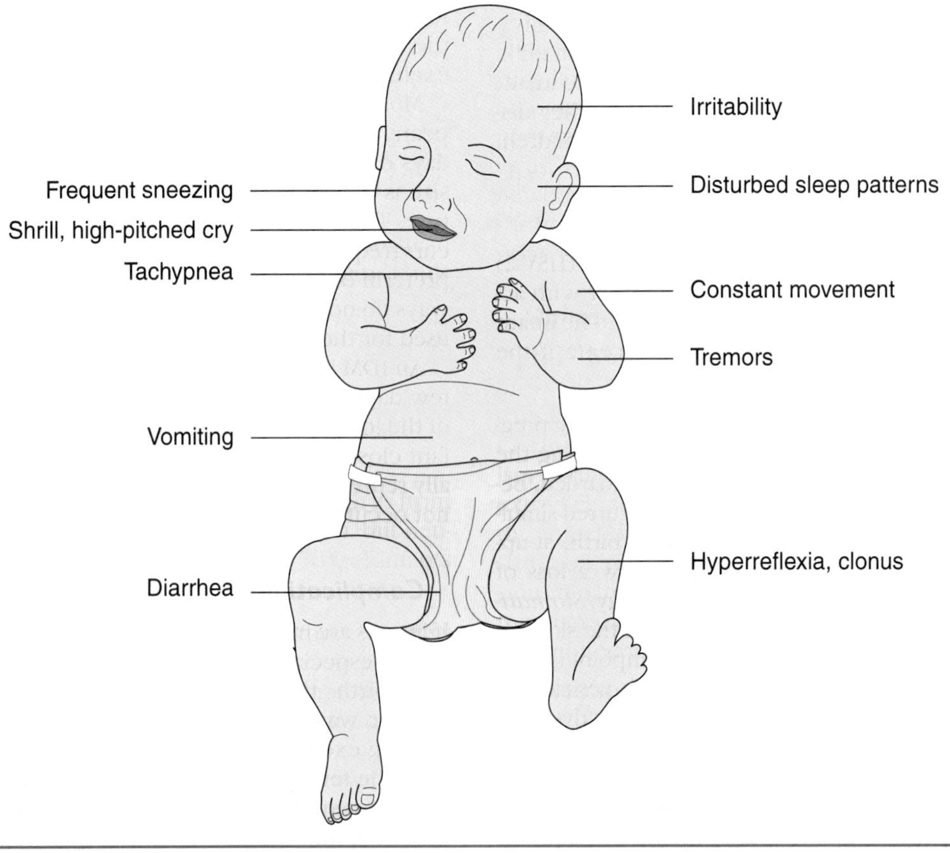

In newborns experiencing opiate withdrawal, symptoms usually begin 24 to 48 hours after birth. However, in some cases, they may not appear for up to 10 days. Generally, they last approximately 2 weeks. In some infants, mild symptoms may appear for up to 6 months.

In heroin-addicted neonates, the symptoms begin within the first 2 weeks of life, with an average onset of approximately 72 hours. The symptoms may last 8 to 16 weeks or longer.

In methadone-addicted newborns, withdrawal begins later and lasts longer than heroin withdrawal. The onset varies. The newborn may exhibit signs and symptoms early, beginning at 24 to 48 hours; the newborn may have early symptoms, improve, then have these symptoms reappear at 2 to 4 weeks of age; or the newborn may exhibit no signs and symptoms until he is 2 to 3 weeks old.

There is no predictable withdrawal sequence noted for the cocaine-addicted neonate. Research is being done to determine if withdrawal actually occurs or whether the signs and symptoms the newborn exhibits are the direct result of the cocaine effect.

Narcotic metabolites or quinine (heroin is often mixed with quinine) may be obtained from an infant's urine in the first hour after birth. These products are quickly cleared from the body, however, so by the time symptoms become severe, detection of narcotic substances may no longer be possible (Ostrea et al, 1997).

Infants of drug-dependent women usually seem most comfortable when firmly swaddled. They should be kept in an environment free from excessive stimuli (a small isolation nursery, not a large, noisy one). Some quiet best if the room is darkened. Many infants of heroin-addicted women suck vigorously and continuously and seem to find comfort and quiet if given a pacifier. Infants of methadone- and cocaine-addicted women may have extremely poor sucking ability and may have difficulty getting enough fluid intake unless gavage fed.

Specific therapy for an infant is individualized according to the nature and severity of the symptoms. Maintenance of electrolyte and fluid balance is essential. If the infant has vomiting or diarrhea, intravenous fluid administration may be indicated. The drugs used to counteract withdrawal symptoms include paregoric, phenobarbital, methadone, chlorpromazine (Thorazine), and diazepam (Valium). These are typically used if the neonatal abstinence scoring system average score is high on three successive scores and nursing interventions do not reduce the score. An infant should not be breastfed to avoid passing narcotics in breast milk to the child.

Evaluation is necessary to determine before discharge whether an environment that allowed for drug abuse will be safe for an infant. Infants who are exposed to drugs in utero may have long-term neurologic problems.

The Infant With Fetal Alcohol Syndrome (FAS)

Alcohol crosses the placenta in the same concentration as is present in the maternal bloodstream. Fetal alcohol syndrome appears in 2 per 1000 newborns (Ostrea et al, 1997). Because it is unknown if there is a safe threshold of alcohol ingestion during pregnancy, alcohol intake should be avoided to prevent any teratogenic effects on the newborn.

The newborn with fetal alcohol syndrome has a number of possible problems at birth. Characteristics that mark the syndrome are: pre- and postnatal growth retardation; central nervous system involvement such as cognitive impairment, microcephaly, and cerebral palsy; and facial features such as short palpebral fissures and a thin upper lip. During the neonatal period, the infant may be tremulous, fidgety, irritable, and may demonstrate a weak sucking reflex. Sleep disturbances are common, with the baby either tending to be always awake or always asleep, depending on the mother's alcohol level close to birth.

Native American and socioeconomically deprived black infants are those most apt to be affected. The most serious long-term effect is cognitive impairment. Behavior problems such as hyperactivity may occur in school-age children. Growth deficiencies may remain through life. The infant needs follow-up so any future problems can be discovered.

CHECKPOINT QUESTIONS

31. Why are infants of diabetic mothers fed early?
32. What is the average time of onset for withdrawal symptoms for the heroin-addicted neonate?
33. Name two characteristic facial features of the neonate with fetal alcohol syndrome.

KEY POINTS

Priorities for infants born with special needs such as the preterm or postterm infant are the same priorities of care as with term infants: initiation and maintenance of respirations, establishment of extrauterine circulation, control of body temperature, intake of adequate nourishment, establishment of waste elimination, establishment of an infant–parent relationship, prevention of infection, and provision of developmental care for mental and social development.

Many high-risk infants need resuscitation at birth. Prompt action with such measures as warmth, oxygen, intubation and suctioning are needed.

A small-for-gestational-age (SGA) infant is one whose birth weight is below the 10th percentile on an intrauterine growth curve for that age infant. The infant could be preterm, term, or postterm.

Small-for-gestational-age infants have difficulty maintaining body warmth because of low fat stores and may develop hypoglycemia from low nutritional stores.

A large-for-gestational-age (LGA) infant is one whose birth weight is above the 90th percentile on an intrauterine growth chart for that gestational age.

The infant could be born preterm, term, or postterm. Large-for-gestational-age infants tend to be infants of diabetic mothers; they are particularly prone to hypoglycemia or birth trauma.

A preterm infant is one born before 37 weeks of gestation. Preterm infants have particular problems with respiratory function, anemia, jaundice, persistent patent ductus arteriosus, and intracranial hemorrhage. Infants who are born weighing 1500 to 2500 g are also termed low-birth-weight (LBW) infants; those born weighing 1000 to 1500 g are very-low-birth-weight (VLBW) infants; those born weighing between 500 and 1000 g are extremely-very-low-birth-weight (EVLBW) infants. All such infants need intensive care from the moment of birth to give them their best chance of survival without neurologic after effects caused by their being so critically close to the age of viability.

A postterm infant is one who has remained in utero past week 42 of pregnancy. Postterm infants have particular problems with establishing respirations, meconium aspiration, hypoglycemia, temperature regulation, and polycythemia.

Respiratory distress syndrome (RDS) commonly occurs in preterm infants from a deficiency or lack of surfactant in alveoli. Without surfactant, alveoli collapse on expiration and require extreme force for reinflation. Primary therapy is synthetic surfactant replacement followed by oxygen and ventilatory support.

Transient tachypnea of the newborn is a temporary condition caused by slow absorption of lung fluid at birth. Close observation of the infant is necessary until the fluid is absorbed and respirations slow to a normal rate.

Meconium aspiration syndrome occurs from the infant inhaling meconium-stained amniotic fluid during birth. Meconium is irritating to the airway and may lead to both airway spasm and pneumonia. Infants need oxygen, ventilatory support, and possibly an antibiotic until the effects of the insult to the airway subside. It is important that they are suctioned before oxygen administration under pressure to prevent meconium being forced further into their lungs.

Apnea is a pause in respirations longer than 20 seconds with accompanying bradycardia. It tends to occur in preterm infants who have secondary stresses such as infection, hyperbilirubinemia, hypoglycemia, or hypothermia. Apnea monitors are used to detect the incidence, and infants who are high risks for this return home on a home monitoring apnea program.

Sudden infant death syndrome (SIDS) is the sudden, unexplained death of an infant. It is associated with infants sleeping on their stomachs (prone) and infants who were born preterm. An important preventive measure may be advising parents to position their infant on the side or back for sleeping.

Hemolytic disease of the newborn is destruction of red blood cells from Rh or ABO incompatibility. Affected infants are jaundiced from release of bilirubin from injured red blood cells. Phototherapy or exchange transfusion is used to prevent kernicterus.

Hemorrhagic disease of the newborn is a lack of clotting ability resulting from a deficiency of vitamin K at birth. Prevention is by injection of vitamin K to all infants at birth.

Retinopathy of prematurity is destruction of the retina due to exposure of immature retinal capillaries to oxygen. Monitoring oxygen saturation via arterial blood gases is an important preventive measure.

Severe infections that may be seen in newborns include streptococcal group B pneumonia, hepatitis B infection, ophthalmia neonatorum (gonococcal and chlamydial conjunctivitis), and herpesvirus infection.

Infants of diabetic women and those of drug-abusing women are high risk at birth for further complications. Both need careful assessment for respiratory distress and hypoglycemia.

CRITICAL THINKING EXERCISES

1. The Atkins are the family you met at the beginning of the chapter. Mrs. Atkins doesn't want to visit or "waste her favorite name" on her new baby because the baby might die. How would you advise her?
2. Retinopathy of prematurity is an example of a disease that is caused by the therapy given the infant. Elaborate on the measures a nurse can take to safeguard infants against this disorder.
3. Infants who are cared for in neonatal nurseries may need either reduced stimulation because they fatigue so easily or increased stimulation because their stay in the nursery will be so extended. Develop a plan for each instance to demonstrate your understanding of the effects of sensory deprivation and stimulation in this situation.

REFERENCES

American Academy of Pediatrics Committee on Injury and Poison Prevention. (1996). Safe transportation of premature and low birth weight infants. *Pediatrics, 97*(5), 758.

American Heart Association. (1992). Pediatric basic life support. *Journal of the American Medical Association, 268*(12), 2251.

Beckmann, C. A. (1997). Use of neonatal boundaries to improve outcomes. *Journal of Holistic Nursing, 15*(1), 54.

Bell, R. P., & McGrath, J. M. (1996). Implementing a research-based kangaroo care program in the NICU. *Nursing Clinics of North America, 31*(2), 287.

Berry, M. A., Abrahamowicz, M., & Usher, R. H. (1997). Factors associated with growth of extremely premature infants during initial hospitalization. *Pediatrics, 100*(4), 640.

Blanchette, V., et al. (1997). Hematology. In Avery, G., et al. *Neonatology.* Philadelphia: J. B. Lippincott.

Bremer, D. L. et al. (1998). Cryotherapy for retinopathy of prematurity. *Archives of Ophthalmology, 116*(3), 329.

Coffman, S., et al. (1995). Infant-mother attachment: relationships to maternal responsiveness and infant temperament. *Journal of Pediatric Nursing, 10*(1), 9.

Crouse, D. T., & Cassady, G. (1997). The small for gestation age infant. In Avery, G., et al. *Neonatology.* Philadelphia: J. B. Lippincott.

Cunningham, F. G. et al. (1997). *Williams obstetrics.* Stamford, CT: Appleton & Lange.

Dai, J., Parry, D., Krahn, J. (1997). Transcutaneous bilirubinometry: its role in the assessment of neonatal jaundice. *Clinical Biochemistry, 30*(1), 1.

David, C. M. (1997). Sudden infant death syndrome: a hypothesis. *Medical Hypotheses, 49*(1), 61.

Department of Health and Human Services. (1995). *Healthy people 2000: midcourse review.* Washington, DC: DHHS.

Fletcher, A. B. (1997). Nutrition. In Avery, et al. *Neonatology.* Philadelphia: J. B. Lippincott.

Freij, B. J., & McCracken, G. H. (1997). Acute infections. In Avery, G., et al. *Neonatology.* Philadelphia: J. B. Lippincott.

Freij, B. J., & Sever, J. L. (1997). Chronic infections. In Avery, G., et al. *Neonatology.* Philadelphia: J. B. Lippincott.

Gibbins, S. A., & Chapman, J. S. (1996). Holding on: parents' perceptions of premature infants: transfers. *Journal of Obstetric, Gynecologic and Neonatal Nursing, 25*(2), 147.

Givens, S. R., & Moore, M. L. (1995). Status report on maternal and child health indicators. *Journal of Perinatal and Neonatal Nursing, 9*(1), 818.

Griffin, T., et al. (1997). Parental evaluation of a tour of the neonatal intensive care unit during a high-risk pregnancy. *Journal of Obstetric, Gynecologic, and Neonatal Nursing, 26*(1), 59.

Karch, A. M. (1997). *Lippincott's nursing drug guide* Philadelphia: Lippincott.

Kinneer, J. D., & Browns, J. V. (1997). Developmental care in advanced practice neonatal nursing education. *Journal of Nursing Education, 36*(2), 79.

Kirsten, D. (1995). Patent ductus arteriosus in the preterm infant. *Neonatal Network, 15*(2), 19.

Lederhaas, G. (1997). Pediatric pain management. *Journal of the Florida Medical Association, 84*(1), 37.

Malloy-McDonald, M. B. (1995). Skin care for high-risk neonates. *Journal of Wound, Ostomy, and Continence Nursing, 22*(4), 177.

May, K. M. (1997). Searching for normalcy: mothers' caregiving for low birth weight infants. *Pediatric Nursing, 23*(1), 17.

McGrath, J. M., & Conliffe-Torres, S. (1996). Integrating family-centered developmental assessment and intervention into routine care in the neonatal intensive care unit. *Nursing Clinics of North America, 31*(2), 357.

Ogata, E. S. (1997). Carbohydrate homeostasis. In Avery, G., et al. *Neonatology.* Philadelphia: J. B. Lippincott.

Ostrea, E. M., et al. (1997). The infant of the drug dependent mother. In Avery, G., et al. *Neonatology.* Philadelphia: J. B. Lippincott.

Phibbs, R. H. (1997). Delivery room management. In Avery, G., et al. *Neonatology.* Philadelphia: J. B. Lippincott.

Pokorni, J. L., & Stanga, J. (1996). Caregiving strategies for young infants born to women with a history of substance abuse and other risk factors. *Pediatric Nursing, 22*(6), 540.

Revenis, M. E., & Johnson, L. A. (1997). Multiple gestations. In Avery, G., et al. *Neonatology.* Philadelphia: J. B. Lippincott.

Scanlon, J. W. (1997). The very-low-birth-weight infant. In Avery, G., et al. *Neonatology.* Philadelphia: J. B. Lippincott.

Shea, K. M. et al. (1998). Postterm delivery: a challenge for epidemiology research. *Epidemiology, 9*(2), 199.

Singh, N. C., Ouellette, Y. I., & Jochelson, P. (1997). Lower airway disease. In Singh, N. C. *Manual of pediatric critical care.* Philadelphia: Saunders.

Sweeney, M. M. (1997). The value of a family-centered approach in the NICU and PICU: one family's perspective. *Pediatric Nursing, 23*(1), 64.

Whitsett, J. A., et al. (1997). Acute respiratory disorders. In Avery, G., et al. *Neonatology.* Philadelphia: J. B. Lippincott.

Wyatt, T. H. (1995). Pneumothorax in the neonate. *Journal of Obstetric, Gynecologic and Neonatal Nursing, 24*(3), 211.

SUGGESTED READINGS

Arlotti, J. P. et al. (1998). Breastfeeding among low-income women with or without peer support. *Journal of Community Health Nursing, 15*(3), 163.

Braveman, P., et al. (1995). Problems associated with early discharge of newborn infants. *Pediatrics, 96*(4.1), 716.

Britton, J. R. (1997). Neonatal nurse practitioner and physician use on a newborn resuscitation team in a community hospital. *Journal of Pediatric Health Care, 11*(2), 61.

Floyd, A. M. (1997). An NICU infant stress reduction QI team: applying research findings to clinical care. *Joint Commission Journal on Quality Improvement, 23*(2), 93.

Hamelin, K., & Overly, B. (1996). Premature infants and car seat safety. *Canadian Nurse, 92*(4), 31.

Martin, S., et al. (1997). Comparison of two methods of bedside blood glucose screening in the NICU: evaluation of accuracy and reliability. *Neonatal Network, 16*(2), 39.

O'Connor, M. A. (1997). Fetal maternal case management. *Nursing Care Management, 2*(2), 55.

Pickler, R. H., & Reyna, B. A. (1996). Advanced practice nursing in the care of the high-risk infant. *Journal of Perinatal and Neonatal Nursing, 10*(1), 46.

Stevens, B., et al. (1996). Developmental versus conventional care: a comparison of clinical outcomes for very low birth weight infants. *Canadian Journal of Nursing Research, 28*(4), 97.

Principles of Growth and Development

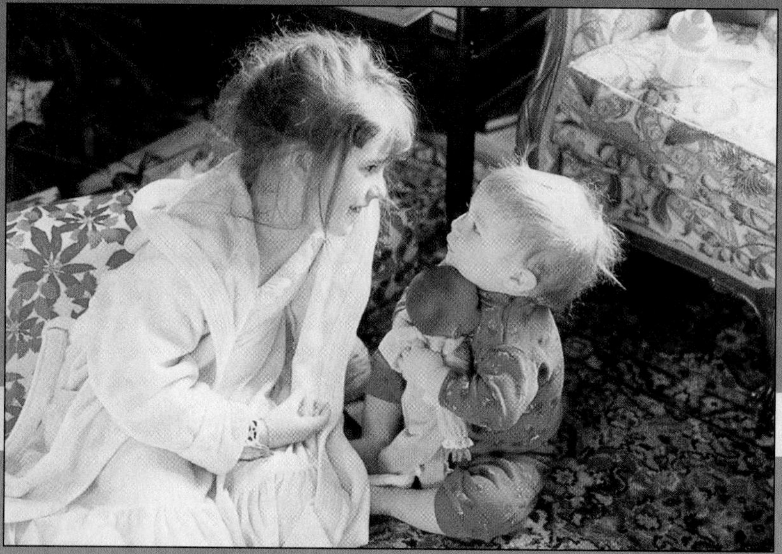

7

CHAPTER

Key Terms

- abstract thought
- accommodation
- adaptability
- approach
- assimilation
- attention span
- autonomy versus shame
- centering
- cognitive development
- concrete operational thought
- conservation
- conventional development
- development
- developmental milestone
- developmental task
- distractibility
- egocentrism
- formal operational thought
- growth
- identity versus role confusion
- industry versus inferiority
- initiative versus guilt
- intuitive thought
- libido
- macronutrient
- maturation
- micronutrient
- mood quality
- permanence
- postconventional development
- preoperational thought
- prereligious stage
- reversibility
- rhythmicity
- role fantasy
- schema
- sensorimotor stage
- temperament
- threshold of response
- trust versus mistrust

Objectives

After mastering the contents of this chapter, you should be able to:

1. Describe principles of growth and development and developmental stages according to major theorists.
2. Assess a child to determine the stage of development the child has reached.
3. Formulate nursing diagnoses that address wellness as well as both a potential for and an actual delay in growth and development.
4. Identify appropriate outcomes for nursing goals for a growing child.
5. Plan nursing interventions to assist a child in achieving and maintaining normal growth and development.
6. Implement nursing actions such as providing age appropriate play materials to support normal growth and development patterns.
7. Evaluate outcome criteria to be certain that nursing goals related to growth and development have been achieved.
8. Identify National Health Goals related to growth and development that nurses can be instrumental in helping the nation to achieve.
9. Identify areas of nursing care related to growth and development that could benefit from additional nursing research.
10. Use critical thinking to analyze factors that influence growth and development and ways to strengthen paths to achieving a new developmental stage.
11. Integrate knowledge of growth and development with nursing process to achieve quality child health nursing care.

John Olson is a 4-year-old boy you see at an ambulatory care visit. At 4 months of age, John was taken away from his mother because she was not caring for him adequately. He was then moved back and forth among 12 different foster homes until he was finally adopted at age 3½. His adoptive parents, who have cared for him for 6 months, tell you they find him cold and unloving, unable to respond to them. They ask you what they can do to change this.

How has John's background contributed to his behavior? What stage of psychosocial development does he not seem to have achieved? How could his parents help him at this point in time?

In previous chapters, you learned about childbearing and what an important year this can be in a child's life. In this chapter, you'll add information about growth and development that is important for all the continuing years of the child's life. This is important information because nurses are directly responsible for assessing growth and development of children.

After you've studied the chapter, turn to the Critical Thinking Exercises at the end of the chapter to sharpen your skills and test your knowledge.

All children pass through predictable stages of growth and development as they mature. Understanding the stage of development a child has reached is important, because parents often will ask a nurse what to expect from their child regarding developmental progress. Health care visits provide the opportunity to assess present growth and development and to supply anticipatory guidance on the topic (Modrcin-McCarthy & Dalton, 1996).

For these reasons, learning about growth and development is essential to the establishment of complete and effective nursing care plans for children. This chapter addresses the most important factors to assess for each age group. Later chapters supply detailed descriptions of individual age groups. National Health Goals related to growth and development are presented in Focus on National Health Goals.

FOCUS ON NATIONAL HEALTH GOALS

National Health Goals that address growth or development of children include the following:

- Reduce to less than 10% the prevalence of mental disorders among children and adolescents from a baseline of 12%.
- Reduce growth retardation among low-income children aged 5 and younger to less than 10% from a baseline of 16%. Growth retardation is defined as height-for-age below the fifth percentile on a standard growth chart.
- Reduce dietary fat intake to an average of 30% of calories or less and average saturated fat intake to less than 10% of calories among children age 2 and older (DHHS, 1995).

Recognizing normal growth and development patterns for children helps in determining if children are following normal development and when referrals are needed. The following are nursing research topics that could shed more information in this area: Are there differences between urban and rural children in the way they approach childhood problems? How do characteristics of temperament affect the way children respond to hospitalization? How does the environment of children influence health?

NURSING PROCESS OVERVIEW

for Promotion of Normal Growth and Development

Assessment

Height and weight should be measured and plotted on a standard growth chart for children at all health care visits. History taking and observation should focus on whether **developmental milestones** (major markers of normal development) have been met. A 24-hour recall history for nutritional intake and a description of school and play behaviors should also be documented. Periodic screening tests (i.e., the Denver II, vision tests, and audiometry screening) should be scheduled at standard times, as discussed in Chapter 13. For the most accurate assessment, be certain to account for illness, sleepiness, fatigue, or "bad days" (a day on which the child did not test well). The developmental stage that a child has reached is assessed through observation and careful listening to how the child describes himself or herself, how the parents describe the child, and what specific activities the child can accomplish (Figure 7-1).

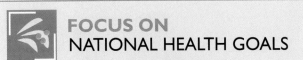

Nursing Diagnosis

When assessment is completed, a child profile is devised. Based on this profile, needs and problems are identified. Nursing diagnoses most frequently used in this area include:

- Risk for altered growth and development related to lack of age-appropriate toys and activities
- Altered growth and development related to prolonged illness
- Family coping: potential for growth related to parent's seeking information about child's growth and development
- Health-seeking behaviors related to appropriate stimulation for infants
- Altered nutrition, less than body requirements related to parental knowledge deficit regarding child's protein need
- Knowledge deficit related to potential long-term effects of obesity in school-age child

Outcome Identification and Planning

To provide holistic nursing care, consider all aspects of the child's health—physical, emotional, cultural, cog-

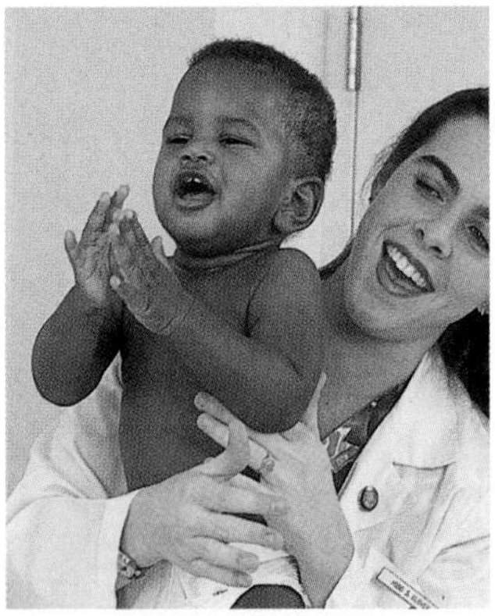

FIGURE 7.1 Growth and development are assessed by both observation and specific testing. Here a 12-month-old demonstrates mastery of well-coordinated and intentional hand movements.

nitive, spiritual, nutritional, and social—and remember that each child's developmental progress is unique. A child cannot be forced to achieve milestones faster than that child's own timetable will allow. Through anticipatory guidance, a child, however, can be encouraged to reach his or her maximum developmental potential. Nurses can play an important role in offering guidance to both the child and family toward this end.

Planning includes the child's family even when the child is no longer completely dependent, however, privacy issues must be considered for adolescents. To develop psychosocially, a child continues to need emotional support from loved ones, just as he or she needs nutritional support to grow physically. Parents of a child with a developmental delay may use denial as a protective mechanism for a long time; this means that planning may have to be centered on helping parents accept what is happening; plans for the child may be delayed until the parents are convinced that a problem truly exists.

Implementation

Interventions to foster growth and development include encouraging age-appropriate self-care in the child and suggesting age-appropriate toys or activities to parents. It may be necessary to help parents accept a child's delayed growth or motivate a child to reach his or her upper limits. Role modeling is an important ongoing intervention with children and families. Modeling, for example, can demonstrate that problem solving is a more effective approach to life's challenges than acting out.

Outcome Evaluation

Evaluation for specific growth and developmental milestones (see Chapters 8 through 12) must be ongoing to be accurate and useful, because many children do not test well until school age. Ongoing evaluation provides an opportunity for early detection of various problems. If a child has difficulty achieving one developmental task, he or she may have difficulty with the next as well. Evaluation must also be comprehensive. If a developmental task involves only gross motor function, it may not be apparent that something is wrong with the child's fine motor function until he or she is in school and is asked to perform fine motor tasks. The following are examples of outcome criteria that might be developed:

- A child, who is 5 years old, expresses less negativism by next clinic visit.
- At a 9-month checkup, parents describe how they have made a safe space in their home for their infant to crawl so he is not confined to the playpen.
- Parents list tasks they believe are appropriate for a 6-year-old child by next office visit.
- Parents state they are beginning to phase out high-carbohydrate, non-nutritive snacks for their preschooler.

IMPORTANCE OF KNOWLEDGE ABOUT GROWTH AND DEVELOPMENT TO THE ROLE OF THE NURSE

Information about growth and development is important in all phases of child care.

Health Promotion and Illness Prevention

Determining a child's developmental stage is often the primary focus of a health interview. For instance, during her child's 24-month checkup, a mother might ask if it is normal that her 3-year-old child cannot yet pedal a tricycle. This question or any other questions about a child's developmental progress cannot be answered without a full understanding of the average ranges.

In addition to reassurance that their child is doing well, parents also need periodic anticipatory guidance regarding their child's development (Colson & Dworkin, 1997). For example, it would be important to discuss additional home safety with a parent when a child is approaching the age for creeping. Parents should be cautioned to think about fencing open stairways and clearing cleaning compounds out of bottom cupboards. Parents of a child who is almost 1 year old will appreciate being cautioned that the child's appetite may decrease during the coming year. With this caution, they will not see a rejection of food as the beginning of a feeding problem but as a usual step of development. The parent of a child approaching puberty generally welcomes a discussion on how to prepare a child for this growth phase (Whitener et al, 1998).

It is important that anticipatory guidance be offered at the appropriate time, or it will be useless. Information given too early is forgotten by the time it is needed. If it is given too late, the parents may have already addressed (or ignored) the issues, possibly not in the most growth-enhancing way for the child. To be able to supply anticipatory guidance this way at the appropriate time or plan nursing care to meet the needs of children and their families, it is necessary to recognize the predictable stages of growth and development, from newborn to young adult, through which each child passes.

Health Restoration and Maintenance

It is also essential to consider developmental stages when caring for a sick child or one having surgery (Lancaster, 1997; Noble et al, 1997). It is terribly awkward to prepare a 5-year-old child for surgery without being sensitive to how much a 5-year-old child can be expected to comprehend. Will the child understand that an anesthetic is a gas? What a surgeon is? What stitches are? Understanding the child's developmental stage helps in choosing the right words. It would be equally frustrating to offer tablet-form medicine to a child to swallow when he or she is too young to coordinate tongue and throat muscles well enough to swallow pills.

Physical growth is another important factor to consider. Disease affects children differently at various stages of growth. A 12-year-old child who has fractured a long bone, for example, has a potentially more serious fracture than an 8-year-old child who fractures the identical bone. The 8-year-old child must metabolize enough calcium to meet two major needs: healing the fracture site and maintaining healthy bone cells. The 12-year-old child, who is undergoing a period of rapid growth, must meet three needs: his or her body must supply not only enough calcium for healing and maintaining existing healthy bone cells but also an additional amount for rapid bone growth. If the child does not take in adequate calcium during the healing period to supply the extra amount for growth, the affected limb may be left shorter than its mate. Members of a health care team must recognize this danger and, if necessary, supply extra calcium so no permanent disability will result.

PRINCIPLES OF GROWTH AND DEVELOPMENT

Growing up is a complex phenomenon because of the many interrelated facets involved. Children do not merely grow taller and heavier as they get older. Maturing also involves growth in ability to perform skills, to think, to relate to people, and to trust or have confidence in oneself.

The terms *growth* and *development* are occasionally used interchangeably but they are different. **Growth** is generally used to denote an increase in physical size or a quantitative change. Growth in weight is measured in pounds or kilograms; growth in height is measured in inches or centimeters.

Development is used to denote an increase in skill or the ability to function (a qualitative change). Development can be measured by observing a child's ability to perform specific tasks (e.g., how well the child picks up small objects such as raisins), by recording the parent's description of the child's progress, or by using standardized tests such as the Denver II Screening Test. **Maturation** is a synonym for development.

Psychosexual development is a specific type of development that refers to developing instincts or sensual pleasure (Freudian theory). Psychosocial development refers to Erikson's stages of personality development. Moral development is the ability to grow to know right from wrong.

Cognitive development refers to the ability to learn or understand from experience, to acquire and retain knowledge, to respond to a new situation, and to solve problems (intelligence; see section on Piaget's Theory of Cognitive Development). It is measured by intelligence tests and by observing the child's ability to function effectively in his or her environment.

Patterns

Neither physical growth nor aspects of maturation occur haphazardly. Several principles govern this process (Box 7-1). As shown in Figure 7-2, general growth (i.e., growth of respiratory, digestive, renal, musculoskeletal, and circulatory tissue) proceeds fairly smoothly during childhood. Certain body tissues, however, mature more rapidly than others. Neurologic tissue (spinal cord and brain) grows so rapidly the first 2 years that brain growth reaches mature proportions by 2 to 5 years. Lymphoid tissue (e.g., spleen, thymus, lymph nodes, and tonsillar tissue) also grows rapidly during infancy and childhood to provide protection to the child against infection. The spleen is usually palpable 1 or 2 cm in preschool children, and in 5-year-old children, tonsillar tissue has already reached its peak size (about twice that of an adult). On assessment, younger school-age children will appear to have large tonsils and thymus glands because of this early growth of lymphoid tissue (the back of their throat seems to be "all tonsils"). In contrast, the reproductive organs (i.e., genital tissue) show little growth until puberty (Buckler, 1997).

CHECKPOINT QUESTIONS

1. What is the difference between the terms *growth* and *development?*
2. Which body systems grow most rapidly during early childhood?

FACTORS INFLUENCING GROWTH AND DEVELOPMENT

Genetic inheritance and environmental influences are the two primary factors in determining a child's pattern of growth and development. Temperament is an example of genetic influence. Nutrition is an environmental influence. A unique combination of these factors determines how each child grows and matures.

Genetics

From the moment of conception when a sperm and ovum fuse, the basic genetic makeup of an individual is cast. In addition to physical characteristics such as eye color and height potential, inheritance determines other characteristics such as learning style and temperament. Although each child is unique, certain gender-related characteristics influence normal growth and development. An individual may also inherit a genetic defect or defects, which may result in disability or illness at birth or later in life.

Gender

On the average, females are born weighing less (by an ounce or two) and measuring less in length (by an inch or

permanent and continue to exist even though they are out of sight or changed in some way. For example:

- Infants will search for a block hidden by a blanket, knowing the block still exists.
- Infants will know that a parent remains the same person whether dressed in a robe and slippers or pants and a T-shirt.
- Infants learn that they are a separate entity from objects. They learn where their body stops and their bed, playthings, or parent begins.

A great deal of the mouthing and handling of objects by infants and the delight of watching a caregiver appear is part of primary and secondary schema and discovering **permanence**. The world begins to make sense and the developmental task of achieving trust falls into place when the concept of permanence has been learned (infants know their parents exist and will return to them). Gaining a concept of permanence also contributes to "eighth-month anxiety," a stage in which infants continue to cry for their parents because they know their parents still exist even when out of sight.

During the final phase of the infant year (coordination of secondary reactions), infants begin to demonstrate goal-directed behavior. After noticing that hitting a mobile makes it move, infants then reach for and hit a music box nearby, in this way actively seeking new experiences. It is important that infants have enough stimulating objects around for exploring so that experimenting and learning can proceed in this way.

Toddler

The toddler period is one of transition as children complete the final stages of the sensorimotor period (defined in Table 7-6 as tertiary circular reaction and invention of new means) and begin to develop some cognitive skills of the preoperative period, such as symbolic thought and egocentric thinking. In the *tertiary circular reaction schema,* children use trial and error to discover new characteristics of objects and events. Toddlers sitting in a high chair and dropping objects over the edge of the tray are exploring both permanence and the different actions of toys. During the schema of "invention of new means," children are able to think through actions or mentally project the solution to a problem. If given a box, children will investigate how the top of the box can be removed; if given a second box, even one that varies in shape, children can foresee how the top can be removed. Toddlers following a ball that has rolled under a coffee table no longer have to follow the ball's path to retrieve it but can project where it rolled and walk around the coffee table to find it again.

During the period of **preoperational thought,** children relearn on a conceptual level some of the lessons they mastered as infants at the sensorimotor level, before having language. Now, children are able to use symbols to represent objects. However, they are unable to view one object as necessarily being different from another. On a walk through a department store, for example, children do not know whether they are seeing a succession of toys or if the same ones keep reappearing. They draw conclusions only from obvious facts they see: Daddy is shaving; therefore he must be going to work, because he went to work after he shaved yesterday. This type of faulty reasoning (prelogical reasoning) will lead children to wrong conclusions and will make their judgment faulty as well. How children think has many implications for nursing. If a nurse made John's bed yesterday and then he went to surgery, he may cry at the sight of you approaching with clean sheets today, thinking he will have to go to surgery again.

Preschooler

Piaget sees preschool children as moving on to a substage of preoperational thought termed **intuitive thought.** During this time, children have a tendency to look at an object and see only one of its characteristics (referred to as **centering**). For example, they see that a banana is yellow but do not notice that it is also long. Centering is noticeable when children are learning about medicine (they observe that it tastes bitter, but cannot understand that it is also good for them).

Centering contributes to the preschooler's lack of **conservation** (the ability to discern truth, even though physical properties change) or **reversibility** (ability to retrace steps). For example, if preschoolers see beads being poured from one glass into another glass that is taller and thinner, they will only notice one changing characteristic. They might say that there are now more beads in the second glass (because the level has risen), or that there are fewer beads (because the second glass is narrower), even when told that no beads have been added or removed. When the beads are poured back into the first glass, they still will not understand that the number of beads is unchanged. This immature perception leads children, as it did during the toddler period, to make faulty conclusions. It takes more years of development for children to learn that when thought processes (i.e., they *know* the number of beads did not change) and perceptions conflict, thought processes are more trustworthy.

Preschool thinking is also influenced by **role fantasy,** or how children would like something to turn out. Children use **assimilation** (taking in information and changing it to fit their existing ideas). For example, because a child wants to go outside and play, he or she says that the outside wants him or her to come and play. Children believe that wishes are as real as facts, that dreams are as real as daytime happenings. They perceive animals and even inanimate objects as being capable of thought and feeling (saying that the dog took the doll because the dog was feeling sad). This is often called magical thinking. Later, children learn **accommodation** (i.e., they change their ideas to fit reality rather than the reverse). **Egocentrism,** or perceiving that one's thoughts and needs are better or more important than those of others, is also strong during this period. Preschoolers are unable to believe that not everyone knows facts they know, and if asked "What is your name?" may reply "Don't you know my name?" Children define objects mainly in relation to themselves, so that a spoon is "what I eat with," not just a curved metal object.

School-Age Child

Piaget viewed school age as a period during which **concrete operational thought** begins. School-age children are able to discover concrete solutions to everyday problems and recognize cause-and-effect relationships. By understanding that beads do not change in number just because they are poured from one glass to another, children have grasped the concept of conservation. Conservation of numbers is learned as early as age 7 years, conservation of quantity at age 7 or 8 years, conservation of weight at age 9 years, and conservation of volume at age 11 years. Reasoning during school age tends to be inductive, proceeding from specific to general. Thus, school-age children can reason that a toy they are holding is broken, that the toy is made of plastic, and that all plastic toys break easily.

Adolescent

Piaget sees adolescence as the time when cognition achieves its final form, that of **formal operational thought.** When this stage is reached, adolescents are capable of thinking in terms of possibility—what could be—rather than being limited to thinking about what already is (**abstract thought**). This makes it possible for adolescents to use scientific reasoning.

Criticisms of Piaget's Theory

Piaget has been criticized because he used only a small sample of subjects (his own children) to develop his theory. Because children today begin activities to learn reading much earlier than they did at the time the theory was devised, the age groups and "norms" may no longer be relevant. Learning computer use at an early age may change both the rate and type of cognitive development.

Kohlberg's Theory of Moral Development

Lawrence Kohlberg (1927–1987), a psychologist, studied the reasoning ability of boys and, based on Piaget's development stages, developed a theory on moral reasoning or the way that children gain knowledge of right and wrong.

Children pass through stages of moral development as well as cognitive and psychosocial development. These stages have been described by Kohlberg (1984) and are summarized in Table 7-7. Recognizing these stages can help identify how a child may feel about an illness (e.g., whether the child thinks of it as "bad"). Recognizing moral reasoning also helps in determining whether the child can be depended on to carry out self-care activities such as self-administered medicine, that is, whether the child has internalized standards of conduct so he or she does not "cheat" when away from external control. Moral stages closely approximate cognitive stages of development, because a child must be able to think abstractly (be able to conceptualize an idea without a concrete picture) before being able to understand how rules apply to him or her, even when no one is there to enforce them.

Infant

The infant period is a **prereligious stage.** Infants have little concept of any motivating force beyond that of their parents. Infants learn that when they do certain actions, parents give affection and approval; for other actions, parents scold and label the behavior as "bad." To support this stage of development, it is important for caregivers to praise the

TABLE 7.7 Kohlberg's Stages of Moral Development

AGE (YEAR)	STAGE	DESCRIPTION	NURSING IMPLICATIONS
Preconventional (Level I)			
2–3	1	Punishment/obedience orientation ("heteronomous morality"). Child does right because a parent tells him or her to and to avoid punishment.	Child needs help to determine what are right actions. Give clear instructions to avoid confusion.
4–7	2	Individualism. Instrumental purpose and exchange. Carries out actions to satisfy own needs rather than society's. Will do something for another if that person does something for the child.	Child is unable to recognize that like situations require like actions. Unable to take responsibility for self-care, because meeting own needs interferes with this.
Conventional (Level II)			
7–10	3	Orientation to interpersonal relations of mutuality. Child follows rules because of a need to be a "good" person in own eyes and eyes of others.	Child enjoys helping others because this is "nice" behavior. Allow child to help with bed making and other like activities. Praise for desired behavior such as sharing.
10–12	4	Maintenance of social order, fixed rules and authority. Child finds following rules satisfying. Follows rules of authority figures as well as parents in an effort to keep the "system" working.	Child often asks what are the rules and is something "right." May have difficulty modifying a procedure because one method may not be "right." Follows self-care measures only if someone is there to enforce them.
Postconventional (Level III)			
Older than 12	5	Social contract, utilitarian law-making perspectives. Follows standards of society for the good of all people.	An adolescent can be responsible for self-care because he or she views this as a standard of adult behavior.
	6	Universal ethical principle orientation. Follows internalized standards of conduct.	Many adults do not reach this level of moral development.

From Kohlberg, L. (1984). *The psychology of moral development.* New York: Harper & Row, with permission.

infant for doing as asked. Caregivers should also know that the average infant is trying hard to please; if he or she falls short of doing this it is probably due to immature development rather than any effort to displease.

The development of trust is important in moral development, because infants who have developed a sound sense of trust are better able to develop a spiritual orientation in future years and thus be bound by a moral conscience (they can trust in a spiritual being as well as humans around them).

Toddler

Toddlers begin to formulate a sense of right and wrong, but their reason for doing right is centered most strongly in "mother or father says so" rather than in any spiritual or societal motivation. Kohlberg refers to this as a punishment obedience orientation (the child is good because a parent says the child must be, not because it is "right" to be good).

Toddlers may not obey requests from people other than their parents because they do not view their authority as being at the same level as their parents' authority. While providing nursing care, it might be necessary to ask a parent to reinforce instructions to be certain the toddler will follow them.

Preschooler

Preschoolers tend to do good out of self-interest rather than out of true intent to do good or because of a strong spiritual motivation. When asked why it is wrong to steal from a neighbor, for example, the preschooler will answer, "Because my mother says it's wrong." Children at this age imitate what they see, so if they see less-than-perfect role modeling, they may copy those wrong actions and assume those actions are correct. Preschoolers have great difficulty handling new situations, because they are unable to judge whether a previously learned principle of right or wrong can be applied to this new situation. Because of egocentrism, a preschooler will do things for others only in return for things done for him or her. This means it may be necessary to remind the child of actions taken on his or her behalf or trade off actions (e.g., "Lie still now for me while I change your dressing and I'll read you a story when I'm through").

School-Age Child

School-age children enter a stage of moral development termed **conventional development,** the level at which many adults function. Young school-age children adhere to a phase of development termed the *nice girl, nice boy* stage. Children engage in actions that are "nice" rather than necessarily right. Sharing, for example, is "nice." Stealing is not. Young school-age children may lie about their actions to disguise that they have been involved in an action that is not "nice."

When asked why it is wrong to steal from a neighbor, the school-age child most often answers, "Because it's not nice" or "The police will arrest you." School-age children may have difficulty following self-care measures reliably when out of a nurse's or parent's sight, because they feel it is necessary to obey rules only when the rules can be clearly enforced.

Adolescent

As adolescents become capable of abstract thought, they are capable of internalizing standards of conduct (they do what they think is right regardless of whether they have social rules). This is termed **postconventional development.** In this stage, if asked why it is wrong to steal from a neighbor, the adolescent will answer, "Because it deprives the neighbor of possessions he or she has earned." Adolescents are capable of carrying out self-care measures even when someone else is not present, because they are capable of understanding not only the importance of the measures to themselves but also the principle that certain things should be done simply because they are right. Many adolescents do not enter this phase of development, however, and as adults they continue to act like school-age children, doing right things only when obvious authority or set rules are present.

Criticisms of Kohlberg's Theory

Kohlberg's theory is currently being challenged as being male-oriented because his original research was conducted entirely with boys. Carol Gilligan (1982) suggests that girls do not score well on Kohlberg's scale because, being more concerned with relationships than men, they make moral decisions differently.

✔ CHECKPOINT QUESTIONS

7. If a preschool child tells you that his broken leg wants to get better, what type of thinking is he using?
8. Suppose the same child tells you that he knows all nurses wear white and because you are not wearing white, you cannot be a nurse. What type of thought process is he using?
9. Why is the stage of moral reasoning of the school-age child often termed the "nice" stage?
10. What is a common criticism of Kohlberg's theory of moral development?

KEY POINTS

Knowledge of growth and development is important in health promotion and illness prevention because it lays the basis for assessment and anticipatory guidance.

Genetic factors that influence growth and development are gender, race and nationality, intelligence, and health. Environmental influences include quality of nutrition, socioeconomic level, parent–child relationship, ordinal position in the family, and environmental health.

To meet growth and development needs, children need to follow basic guidelines for a healthy diet, such as eating a variety of foods; maintaining ideal weight; avoiding too much saturated fat and cholesterol; eating foods with adequate starch and fiber; and avoiding too much sugar, the same as adults.

Temperament is a child's characteristic manner of thinking, behaving, or reacting. Chess and Thomas (1985) described an "easy to care for child" and a "difficult child" based on temperament. Helping parents understand the effect of temperament is a nursing role.

Common theories of development are Freud's psychoanalytic theory and Erikson's theory of psychosocial development. Both of these theories describe specific tasks, which children complete at each stage of development in order to mature to a well-adapted adult.

Piaget's theory of cognitive development describes ways that children learn. Kohlberg advanced a theory of moral development or how children use moral reasoning to solve problems they face.

Although growth and development occur in known patterns, their rate varies from child to child. Caution parents not to be concerned because two siblings are different as long as they both fit within usual parameters.

CRITICAL THINKING EXERCISES

1. John is the 4-year-old boy you met at the beginning of the chapter. He had been moved many times from his own home to foster homes before he was recently adopted. His parents stated that they found him cold and unloving. What developmental task was John unable to complete because of these frequent moves at such a young age? What are actions his new parents could take to try and strengthen this developmental task at this point?
2. A mother describes her two children as "totally different." One is shy and quiet and agreeable, and one is aggressive and persistent. What characteristic is she describing? Which child does she probably view as easier to care for? What anticipatory guidance could you give her to help her better understand these differences in her children?
3. The parents of a 2-year-old child express that they want their child to achieve well in life. They ask you what specific steps they should take to foster high achievement in their child. What advice would you give them?
4. Children who are hospitalized for long periods may fall behind in development. What specific measures could you take to promote developmental growth and encourage a sense of autonomy in a hospitalized 2-year-old child? To promote a sense of industry in a hospitalized 10-year-old child?

REFERENCES

Beck, C. T. (1996). A meta-analysis of the relationship between postpartum depression and infant temperament. *Nursing Research, 45*(4), 225.

Buckler, J. M. H. (1997). *A reference manual of growth and development.* Oxford: Cambridge, MA: Blackwell Science.

Carey, W. B., & McDevitt, S. C. (1994). *Prevention and early intervention: individual differences as risk factors for the mental health of children.* New York: Brunner/Mazel.

Chess, S., & Thomas, A. (1985). Temperamental differences: a critical concept in child health care. *Pediatric Nursing, 11*(2), 167.

Colizza, D. F., & Colvin, S. (1995). Food choices of healthy school-age children. *Journal of School Nursing, 11*(4), 17.

Colson, E. R., & Dworkin, P. H. (1997). Toddler development. *Pediatrics in Review, 18*(8), 255.

Department of Health and Human Services. (1995). *Healthy people 2000: midcourse review.* Washington, DC: DHHS.

Dudek, S. G. (1997). *Nutrition handbook for nursing practice.* Philadelphia: Lippincott.

Erikson, E. H. (1985). *Childhood and society.* New York: W. W. Norton.

Gallo, A. M. (1996). Building strong bones in childhood and adolescence; reducing the risk of fractures in later life. *Pediatric Nursing, 22*(5), 369.

Gilligan, C. (1982). *In a different voice: psychological theory and women's development.* Cambridge, MA: Harvard University Press.

Harrell, J. S., et al. (1996). Effects of a school-based intervention to reduce cardiovascular disease risk factors in elementary school children: the Cardiovascular Health in Children Study. *Journal of Pediatrics, 128*(6), 797.

Kagan, J. (1997). Temperament and the reactions to unfamiliarity. *Child Development, 68*(1), 139.

Kleinman, R. E., et al. (1996). Dietary guidelines for children: US recommendations. *Journal of Nutrition, 126*(4s), 1028s.

Kohlberg, L. (1984). *The psychology of moral development.* New York: Harper & Row.

Lancaster, K. A. (1997). Care of the pediatric patient in ambulatory surgery. *Nursing Clinics of North America, 32*(2), 441.

Lawson, K. D., Middleon, S. J., & Hassall, C. C. (1997). Olestra, a nonabsorbed, noncaloric replacement for dietary fat: a review. *Drug Metabolism Reviews, 19*(3), 651.

Mitchell, M. A., & Jenista, J. A. (1997). Health care of the internationally adopted child. *Journal of Pediatric Health Care, 11*(3), 117.

Modrcin-McCarthy, M. A., & Dalton, M. M. (1996). Responding to Healthy People 2000: depression in our youth, common yet misunderstood. *Issues in Comprehensive Pediatric Nursing, 19*(4), 275.

Noble, R. R., et al. (1997). Special considerations for the pediatric perioperative patient: a developmental approach. *Nursing Clinics of North America, 32*(1), 1.

Philbin, M. K. (1996). Some implications of early auditory development for the environment of hospitalized preterm infants. *Neonatal Network, 15*(8), 71.

Robinson, P. (1993). *Freud and his critics.* Berkeley: University of California Press.

Satter, E. (1995). Feeding dynamics: helping children to eat well. *Journal of Pediatric Health Care, 9*(4), 178.

Schwartz, R., & Abegglen, J. A. (1996). Failure to thrive: an ambulatory approach. *Nurse Practitioner, 21*(5), 12.

Wadsworth, B. J. (1989). *Piaget's theory of cognitive and affective development.* (4th ed.). New York: Longman.

Whitener, L. M. et al. (1998). Use of theory to guide nurses in the design of health messages for children. *ANS: Advances in Nursing Science, 20*(3), 21.

SUGGESTED READINGS

Alsop-Shields, L., & Alexander, H. (1997). A study of errors that can occur when weighing infants. *Journal of Advanced Nursing, 25*(3), 587.

Carr, K. (1995). Using Orem's model in the care of adolescents. *Nursing Times, 91*(25), 35.

Frederick, C., & Reining, K. M. (1995). Essential components of growth and development. *Journal of Post Anesthesia Nursing, 10*(1), 12.

Grace, J. T. (1995). Families and nurses: building partnerships for growth and health. *Journal of Obstetric, Gynecologic and Neonatal Nursing, 24*(4), 298.

Guidelines for school health programs to promote lifelong healthy eating. (1997). *Journal of School Health, 67*(1), 9.

Keller, C., & Stevens, K. R. (1996). Childhood obesity: measurement and risk assessment. *Pediatric Nursing, 22*(5), 494.

MacDonald, A. (1997). Know your vitamins and minerals. *Nursing Times, 93*(21), 72.

Miles, M. S. et al. (1998). Maternal concerns about parenting prematurely born children. *MCN: American Journal of Maternal Child Nursing, 23*(2), 70.

Purdy, K. S., et al. (1996). You are what you eat: healthy food choices, nutrition, and the child with juvenile rheumatoid arthritis. *Pediatric Nursing, 22*(5), 391.

Reiser, D. J. (1996). Developmental care: first things first. *Neonatal Network, 15*(3), 61.

Watts, P., et al. (1996). Environmental factors and nutritional status of rural children. *Nursing Connections, 9*(2), 43.

The Family With an Infant

8

CHAPTER

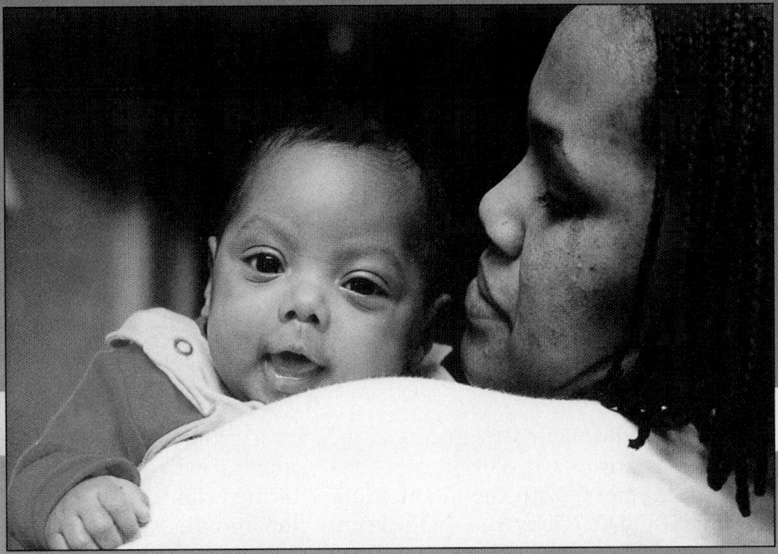

Key Terms

- adipocytes
- baby-bottle syndrome
- binocular vision
- coordination of secondary schema
- deciduous teeth
- eighth-month anxiety
- extrusion reflex
- fine motor development
- gross motor development
- hand regard
- Landau reflex
- natal teeth
- neck-righting reflex
- neonatal teeth
- object permanence
- parachute reaction
- pincer grasp
- prehensile ability
- primary circular reaction
- seborrhea
- secondary circular reaction
- social smile
- stranger anxiety
- thumb opposition
- ventral suspension

Objectives

After mastering the contents of this chapter, you should be able to:

1. Describe normal infant growth and development and associated parental concerns.
2. Assess an infant for normal growth and development milestones.
3. Formulate nursing diagnoses related to infant growth and development and associated parental concerns.
4. Identify appropriate outcomes to promote optimal infant growth and development and health.
5. Plan nursing care to meet the infant's growth and development needs.
6. Implement nursing care related to normal growth and development of the infant.
7. Evaluate outcomes for achievement of optimal growth and development and effectiveness of care.
8. Identify National Health Goals related to infant growth and development that nurses can be instrumental in helping the nation achieve.
9. Identify areas related to nursing care of the infant that could benefit from additional nursing research.
10. Use critical thinking to analyze methods of care for the infant to be certain care is family centered.
11. Integrate knowledge of infant growth and development with nursing process to achieve quality child health nursing care.

You meet Mrs. Simpson at a pediatric clinic when she brings in her 2-month-old son, Bryan. She looks tired. She tells you that she feels exhausted because her baby "is awake all night, crying constantly." She stopped breastfeeding and changed him to formula to see if that would help, but it didn't. She tells you his bowel movements are normal. When you weigh Bryan, you find that he is gaining weight well. When you talk to him, he demonstrates a social smile.

What condition, common to early infancy, is Mrs. Simpson describing? What suggestions could you make to her to help her enjoy caring for Bryan more?

In previous chapters, you learned about the newborn and the capabilities with which children are born. In this chapter, you'll add information about the dramatic changes, both physical and psychosocial, that occur during the first year. This is important information because it builds a base for care and health teaching for the age group.

After you've studied the chapter, turn to the Critical Thinking Exercises at the end of the chapter to sharpen your skills and test your knowledge.

Infancy is traditionally designated as the period from 1 month to 1 year of age. This year is one of rapid growth and development, with the infant tripling birth weight and increasing length by 50%. In these important months, the infant undergoes such rapid development that parents sometimes believe their baby looks different and demonstrates new abilities each day. During this period, the baby's senses sharpen and, with the process of attachment to primary caregivers, forms his or her first social relationships. Because of the growth and learning potential, this first year is a crucial one. Without proper nutrition, the baby will not grow and physically thrive, and without the proper stimulation and nurturing care by consistent caregivers, the infant may not develop a healthy interest in life or a feeling of security essential for future development. Because it is so important, infant health promotion has been the subject of much concern. The Focus on National Health Goals box lists National Health Goals related to the infant year.

Infants are usually seen at health care facilities for health maintenance at least six times during the first year. Although infant health care visits are scheduled less frequently than formerly, a standard schedule is for 2-week, 2-month, 4-month, 6-month, 9-month, and 12-month visits. These visits are as important for the parents as they are for the infants because they provide an opportunity for parents to ask questions about their child's growth pattern and developmental progress. They also provide opportunities for health care providers to assess for potential problems. Anticipatory guidance offered at these visits can help parents prepare for the rapid changes that mark the first year of life. When appropriate, encouraging parents to join clubs or networking groups helps to increase their knowledge base and confidence level. Table 8-1 details usual procedures at infant maintenance visits including immunizations (AAP, 1997). First-year immunizations and any risks associated with these are discussed in Chapter 22.

FOCUS ON NATIONAL HEALTH GOALS

A number of National Health Goals focus on promotion of health during the infant year. These are:

- Increase to at least 75% the proportion of parents and caregivers who use feeding practices that prevent baby bottle tooth decay. Special target population: parents and caregivers with less than high school educations.
- Reduce drowning deaths to no more than 2.3/100,000 for children aged 4 years and younger from a baseline of 4.2/100,000.
- Increase the use of occupant protection systems, such as child automotive safety seats, to 95% from a baseline of 84%.
- Reduce the prevalence of blood lead levels exceeding 15 μg/dL among children aged 6 months through 5 years to no more than 500,000.
- Increase to at least 90% the proportion of babies aged 18 months and younger who receive recommended primary care services at appropriate intervals (DHHS, 1995).

Nurses can be instrumental in helping the nation achieve these goals by educating parents about the importance of not putting an infant to bed with a bottle of milk or juice, the use of infant care seats, and using lead-free paint. A number of areas related to these topics that could benefit from additional nursing research are effective ways that mothers are able to comfort infants while in car seats without removing the infants from the seats; characteristics of programs that were successful for community lead removal; and effective ways to teach cardiopulmonary techniques to parents to prevent fatal outcomes from childhood drownings.

NURSING PROCESS OVERVIEW

for Healthy Development of the Infant

Assessment

Nursing assessment of the infant should begin by interviewing the primary caregiver. Important areas to discuss are nutrition, growth patterns, and development. The infant's height, weight, and head circumference are important indicators of growth and should be measured and plotted on standard growth charts. These charts represent average growth and are used to determine if that individual baby's growth is falling within the same relative percentile with each health checkup. For more information about typical assessment findings, see Assessing the Average Infant.

Physical assessment of the infant must be done quickly yet thoroughly because the baby can tire or become hungry, making it difficult to judge overall

TABLE 8.1 Health Maintenance Schedule, Infant Period

AREA OF FOCUS	METHODS	FREQUENCY
Assessment		
Developmental milestones	History, observation Formal Denver Developmental Screening Test (DDST II)	Every visit At 3 months and 1 year
Growth milestones	Height, weight, head circumference plotted on standard growth chart; physical examination	Every visit
Nutritional adequacy	History, observation; height/weight information	Every visit
Parent–child relationship	History, observation	Every visit
Vision and hearing defects	Grossly, by observation and history	Every visit
Dental health	History, physical examination	Every visit after teeth erupt
Anemia	Hematocrit	9-month visit
Lead screening	Whole blood lead level	9-month visit
Tuberculosis screening	Tine test	12-month visit
Sickle cell anemia	Sickledex or hemoglobin electrophoresis	9-month visit (if not tested at birth)
Immunizations		
Diphtheria, pertussis, and tetanus (DPT) and *Haemophilus influenzae* type B (HiB)	Check history and past records; inform caregiver about any risks and side effects; administer immunization in accordance with health care agency policies	2-, 4-, and 6-month visits 2-, 4-, and possibly 6-month visit depending on brand of vaccine
Trivalent oral poliomyelitis		2- and 4-month visits Optional 6-month visit
Hepatitis B (HPVcV)		Birth, 1–2 month; 12-month visit
Varicella		12-month visit
Measles, mumps, rubella (MMR)		12-month visit
Anticipatory Guidance		
Infant care	Active listening and health teaching	Every visit
Expected growth before next visit	Health teaching	Every visit
Expected developmental milestones before next visit	Health teaching	Every visit
Problem Solving		
Any problems expressed by caregiver during the course of the visit	Active listening and health teaching	Every visit

behavior and temperament. The primary caregiver should be present to make the child comfortable. Using a calm, unhurried approach helps the infant feel safe enough to accept your interventions.

Nursing Diagnosis

Much of your assessment of the infant and family will focus on basic needs such as sleep, nutrition, activity, and parents' adjustment to their new role. Possible nursing diagnoses might include:

- Ineffective breastfeeding related to maternal fatigue
- Knowledge deficit related to normal infant growth and development
- Altered nutrition, less than body requirements, related to difficulty sucking
- Health-seeking behaviors related to adjusting to parenthood
- Altered growth and development related to lack of stimulating environment
- Risk for altered parenting related to long hospitalization of infant
- Family coping: potential for growth related to increased financial support
- Maternal sleep pattern disturbance related to baby's need to nurse every 2 hours
- Maternal social isolation related to stress of caring for infant and lack of adequate social support
- Altered role performance related to new responsibilities within the family

Outcome Identification and Planning

It is important to establish goals for infant care that are realistic. Parents of infants, especially first-time parents, must do a lot of adjusting, and this takes time. Try to suggest activities that can be easily incorporated

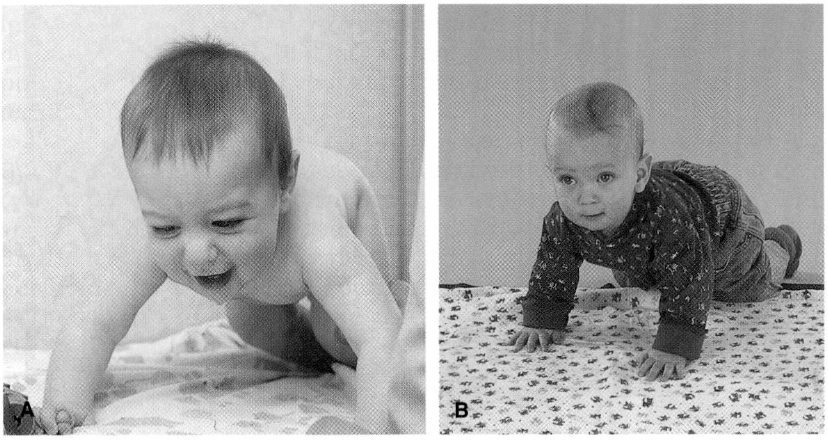

FIGURE 8.3 (**A**) Hitching. The infant moves backward in a modified sitting position. (**B**) Creeping. The older infant moves forward, carrying his torso above and parallel to the floor.

A 7-month-old child sits alone, but only when the hands are held forward for balance (Figure 8-6). An 8-month-old child is able to sit securely without additional support. This is a major milestone in development that should always be considered in assessment. Children with delayed mental or motor development may not accomplish this step at this time.

At 9 months, infants sit so steadily that they can lean forward and regain their balance. They may still lose their balance if they lean sideways, a skill that is not achieved for another month.

Standing Position. A stepping reflex can still be demonstrated at 1 month of age. In a standing position, the infant's knees and hips flex rather than support more than momentary weight. A 2-month-old child, when held in a standing position, holds his or her head up with the same show of support as in a sitting position. The stepping reflex is still present. At 3 months, infants begin to try to support part of their weight. The stepping reflex begins to fade.

At 4 months, infants make an attempt to sustain their weight actively on their legs. They are successful at doing this because the stepping reflex has faded.

The 5-month-old child continues the ability to sustain a portion of his or her weight. The tonic neck reflex should be extinguished, and the Moro reflex is fading. By 6 months, infants support nearly their full weight when in a standing position. A 7-month-old child bounces with enjoyment in a standing position.

The 9-month-old child can stand holding onto the coffee table if he or she is placed in that position. Some 9-month-old children can pull up to that position. The 10-month-old child can pull herself to a standing position by holding onto the side of a playpen or a low table; she cannot let herself down again as yet.

At around 11 months, the child learns to "cruise" or move about the crib or room by holding onto objects such as the crib rails, chairs, walls, and low tables (Figure 8-7). At 12 months, a child stands alone at least momentarily. Some parents expect their child to walk at this time and are disappointed to see him or her not moving but merely

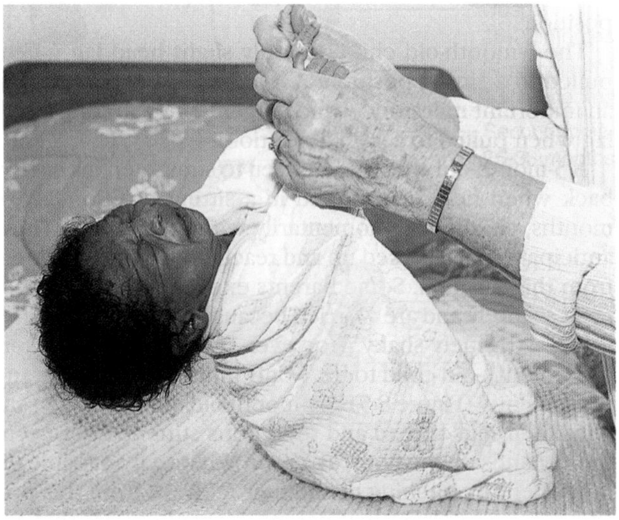

FIGURE 8.4 An infant is pulled to a sitting position to demonstrate head lag. Notice how evident this is in the very young infant.

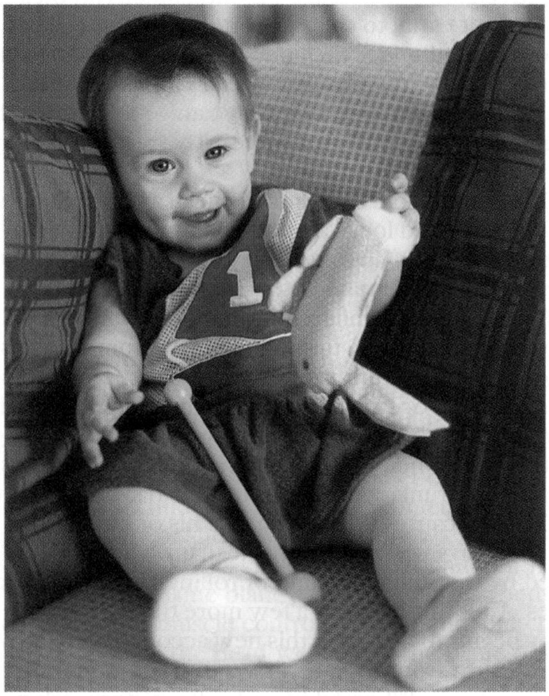

FIGURE 8.5 A 6-month-old infant sitting. Notice how she is propped with pillows to maintain the position.

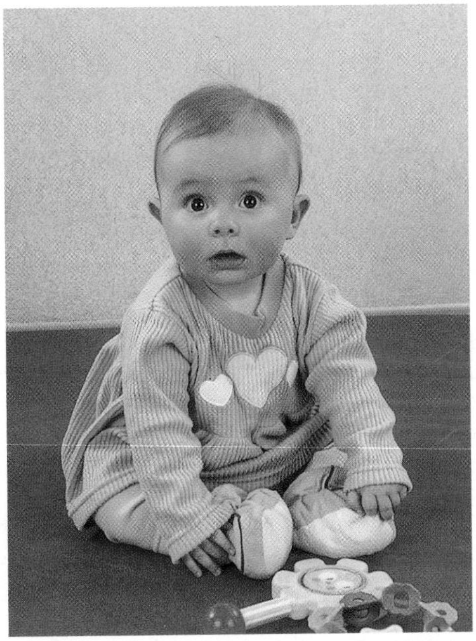

FIGURE 8.6 At 7 months the infant sits independently.

standing. A child has until about 22 months of age to walk and still be within the normal limit, however (Figure 8-8).

CHECKPOINT QUESTIONS

3. What four positions are used to evaluate gross motor development?
4. At what age would you expect an infant to sit securely without support?

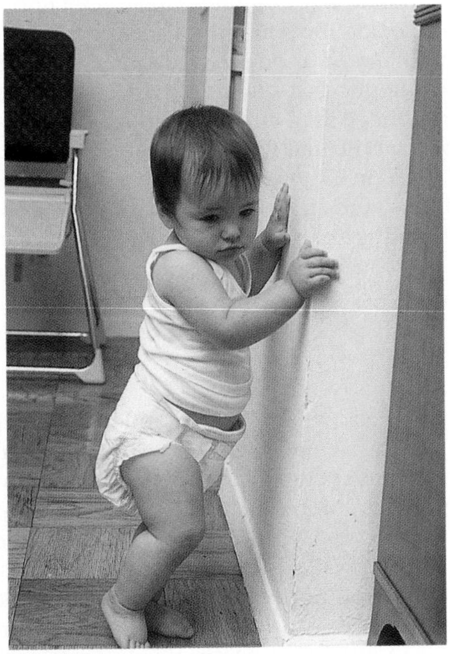

FIGURE 8.7 An 11-month-old child cruising along the walls. Further childproofing of the house will be necessary to keep the infant safe.

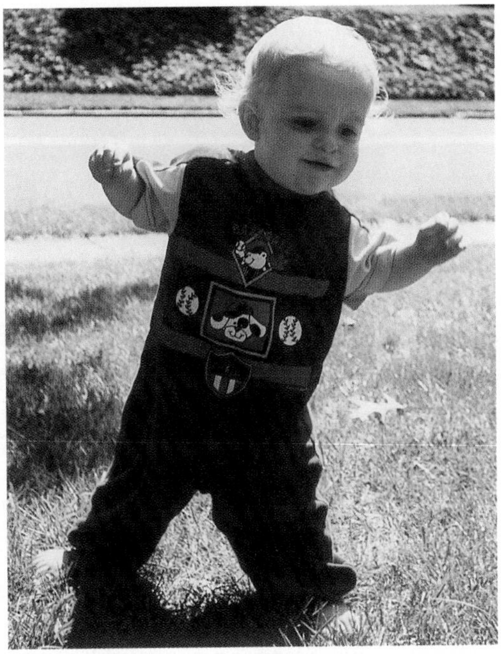

FIGURE 8.8 There is a wide variation in the age at which walking is first accomplished, typically ranging from 8 to 15 months. Here a child has mastered it by 1 year.

Fine Motor Development

One-month-old infants still have a strong grasp reflex and so hold their hands in fists so tightly it is difficult to extend the fingers. As the grasp reflex begins to fade, the 2-month-old child will hold an object for a few minutes before dropping it. The hands are held open, not fisted.

At 3 months, infants reach for attractive objects in front of them. Their grasp is unpracticed, however, and so they usually miss them. Inform parents that this is part of normal development. Otherwise, they may think the child is nearsighted or farsighted, or has poor coordination.

By 4 months, infants bring their hands together and pull at their clothes. They will shake a rattle placed in their hand for a long time. **Thumb opposition** (ability to bring the thumb and fingers together) is beginning, but the motion is a scooping or raking one, not a picking-up one, and is not very accurate. The infant is limited to handling large objects (Figure 8-9). Palmar and plantar grasp reflexes have disappeared.

The 5-month-old child can accept an object that is handed to him or her and grasp it with the whole hand. He or she can reach and pick up an object without its being offered and often plays with his or her toes as objects. Fisting that persists beyond 5 months suggests a delay in motor development. Unilateral fisting suggests hemiparesis or paralysis on that side.

By 6 months, grasping has advanced to a point where the child can hold objects in both hands. Infants at this age will drop one toy when a second one is offered for the same hand. They can hold a spoon and start to feed themselves (with much spilling). Moro, palmar grasp, and the tonic neck reflex have completely faded. A Moro reflex that persists beyond this point should arouse grave suspicion of neurologic disease.

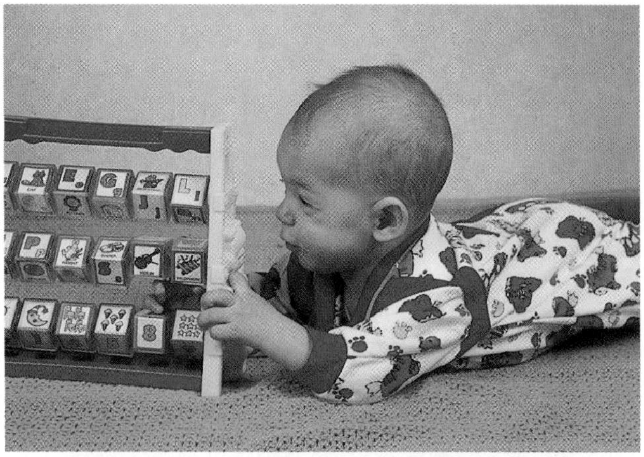

FIGURE 8.9 By age 4 months, the infant is able to manipulate large objects.

The 7-month-old child can transfer a toy from one hand to the other. He or she holds a first object when a second one is offered. By 8 months, random reaching and ineffective grasping have disappeared as a result of advanced eye–hand coordination.

A major milestone of 10 months is the ability to bring the thumb and first finger together in a **pincer grasp** (Figure 8-10). This enables the child to pick up small objects such as crumbs or pieces of cereal from a highchair tray. The infant uses one finger to point to objects. He or she offers toys to people but then cannot release them (Deloian, 1996).

At 12 months, infants can draw a semistraight line with a crayon. They enjoy putting objects such as small blocks in containers and taking them out again. They can hold a cup and spoon to feed themselves fairly well (if they have been allowed to practice) and can take off socks and push their hands into sleeves (again, if they have been allowed to practice). They can offer toys and release them.

WHAT IF? What if a 10-month-old child can pick up very small articles such as marbles? What does this mean in terms of infant safety?

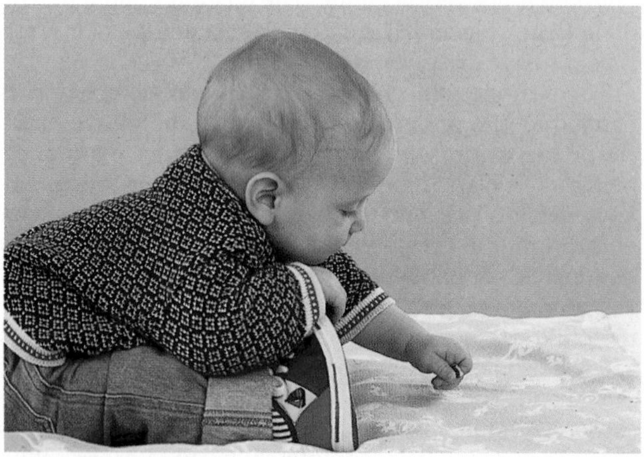

FIGURE 8.10 An infant almost ready to demonstrate a pincer grasp.

Developmental Milestones

In addition to gross and fine motor skills that are developing at this time, language and play behavior also mark major milestones in the first year of life. Motor and cognitive development and play throughout this year are summarized in Table 8-2.

Language Development

A child begins to make small, cooing (dovelike) sounds by the end of the first month. The 2-month-old child differentiates a cry. For example, caregivers can distinguish a cry that means hungry from one that means wet or from one that means lonely. This is an important milestone in development for an infant and in marking how far a parent has progressed in the task of learning the infant's cues. A first-time parent has more difficulty making the distinction in crying than one who has experienced this before. The infant's ability to make throaty, gurgling, or cooing sounds also increases at this time.

In response to a nodding, smiling face or a friendly tone of voice, the 3-month-old child will squeal with pleasure. This is an important step in development because the baby becomes even more fun to be with. Parents spend increased time with the infant not just to care for him or her but because they enjoy his or her company.

By 4 months, an infant is very "talkative," cooing, babbling, and gurgling when spoken to. He or she definitely laughs out loud.

By 5 months, the infant says some simple vowel sounds, for example, *goo-goo* and *gah-gah.*

At 6 months, infants learn the art of imitating. They may imitate a parent's cough, for example, or say "Oh!" as a way of attracting attention.

The amount of talking infants do increases at 7 months. They can imitate vowel sounds well, for example, *oh-oh, ah-ah,* and *oo-oo.* By 9 months, the infant usually speaks a first word: *da-da* or *ba-ba.* Occasionally a mother may need reassurance that *da-da* for daddy is an easier syllable to pronounce than *ma-ma* for mother. German mothers report that the first word their babies say is *da,* which means "here" in German. By 10 months, the infant masters another word such as *bye-bye* or *no.*

At 12 months, infants can generally say two words besides *ma-ma* and *da-da;* they use those two words with meaning.

Play

Parents often ask what toy their child would enjoy. Because they can fix their eyes on an object, 1-month-old children are interested in watching a mobile over their crib or playpen. Mobiles should be black and white or brightly colored and light enough in weight so they move when someone walks by them. They should face down toward the infant, not sideways toward the adults standing beside the crib. Musical mobiles provide extra stimulation. One-month-old children spend a great deal of time watching the parent's face, appearing to enjoy this activity so much that the face may become their favorite "toy." Help parents to appreciate not worrying that they are

TABLE 8.2 Summary of Infant Growth and Development

MONTH	MOTOR DEVELOPMENT	FINE MOTOR DEVELOPMENT	SOCIALIZATION AND LANGUAGE	PLAY
0–1	Largely reflex	Keeps hands fisted; able to follow object to midline		Enjoys watching face of primary caregiver, listening to soothing sounds
2	Holds head up when prone	Has social smile	Makes cooing sounds; differentiates cry	Enjoys bright-colored mobiles
3	Holds head and chest up when prone Reflexes: grasp, stepping, tonic neck are fading	Follows object past midline	Laughs out loud	Spends time looking at hands or uses them as toy during the month (hand regard)
4	Turns front to back; no longer has head lag when pulled upright; bears partial weight on feet when held upright			Needs space to turn
5	Turns both ways; Moro reflex fading			Handles rattles well
6	Reaches out in anticipation of being picked up; first tooth (central incisor) erupts; sits unsteadily (still needs support)	Uses palmar grasp	May say vowel sounds (*oh-oh*)	Enjoys bathtub toys, rubber ring for teething
7		Transfers objects hand to hand	Beginning fear of strangers	Likes objects that are good size for transferring
8	Sits securely without support		Fear of strangers (ability to tell known from unknown people) reaches peak	Enjoys manipulation, rattles and toys of different textures
9	Creeps or crawls (abdomen off floor)		Says first word (*da-da*)	Needs space for creeping
10	Pulls self to standing	Uses pincer grasp (thumb and finger) to pick up small objects		Plays games like patty-cake and peek-a-boo
11	"Cruises" (walks with support)			"Cruises"
12	Stands alone; some infants take first step	Holds cup and spoon well; helps to dress (pushes arm into sleeve)	Says two words plus *ma-ma* and *da-da*	Likes toys that fit inside each other (pots and pans); nursery rhymes; will like pull-toys as soon as walking

spoiling their baby by sitting and holding him or her for long periods of time. They will enjoy recalling such calm moments later, when they are stacking blocks, winding up toys, or playing table games with their growing child.

Hearing is a second sense that is a source of pleasure for the child in early infancy. Even a newborn "listens" to the sound of a music box or a musical rattle. He or she stirs and seems apprehensive at the sound of a raucous rattle.

A 2-month-old child will hold a light, small rattle for a short period of time and then drop it. He or she is very attuned to mobiles or a cradle gym strung across the crib. The infant continues to spend a great deal of time just watching the people around him or her.

Three-month-old children can handle small blocks or small rattles. Four-month-old children need a playpen or a sheet spread on the floor so they have an opportunity to exercise their new skill of rolling over. Rolling over is so intriguing it may serve as a "toy" for the entire month.

A 5-month-old child is ready for a variety of objects to handle such as plastic rings, blocks, squeeze toys, clothespins, rattles, plastic keys. All these should be small enough that the infant can lift them with one hand, yet big enough that he or she cannot possibly swallow them.

A 6-month-old child can sit steadily enough to be ready for bathtub toys such as rubber ducks or plastic boats. Because they are starting to teethe, infants enjoy a teething ring to chew on at this time.

Because 7-month-old children can transfer toys, they are interested in items, such as blocks, rattles, or plastic keys, small enough to do this. As their mobility increases, they begin to be more interested in brightly colored balls or toys that previously rolled out of reach.

Eight-month-old children are sensitive to differences in texture. They enjoy having toys that have different feels to them, such as velvet, fur, fuzzy, smooth, or rough items.

The 9-month-old child needs the experience of creeping. This means time out of a playpen so he or she has room to maneuver. Many 9-month-old children begin to enjoy toys that go inside one another, such as a nest of blocks or rings of assorted sizes that fit on a center post. Some are more interested in pots and pans than toys.

At 10 months, infants are ready for peek-a-boo and will spend a long time playing the game with their hands or with a cloth over their head that they can reach and remove. They can clap and are also ready to play patty-cake. These games have a positive value, just as laughing out loud did for the 3-month-old child. They make the baby feel like an active part of the household. A family feeling begins to grow as the baby is able to participate in active games.

The 11-month-old child has learned to cruise. They often find this so absorbing that they spend little time doing anything else during the month.

The 12-month-old child enjoys putting things in and taking things out of containers. They like little boxes that fit inside one another or dropping objects such as blocks into a cardboard box. As soon as they are able to walk, they will be interested in pull toys. A lot of time may be spent listening to someone saying nursery rhymes or listening to music.

CHECKPOINT QUESTIONS

5. At what month should an infant be able to pick up small objects using a pincer grasp?
6. How many words should a 12-month-old child use?

Development of Senses

Sensory development proceeds step by step during the infant year.

Vision

A 1-month-old child regards an object in the midline of vision (directly in front of himself or herself) as it is brought into close proximity, about 18 in (46 cm) away. The infant follows it a short distance, but not across the midline as yet. He or she studies or regards a human face with a fixed stare. The 2-month-old child focuses well (from about age 6 weeks) and follows objects with the eyes (although still not past the midline). This ability is a major milestone in development, indicating that the infant has achieved **binocular vision,** or the ability to fuse two images into one (Figure 8-11).

Three-month-old children typically hold their hands in front of their face and study their fingers for long periods of time **(hand regard)**. Blind children also demonstrate this phenomenon, however, so it may not be so much a test of vision as of cognitive or exploratory development.

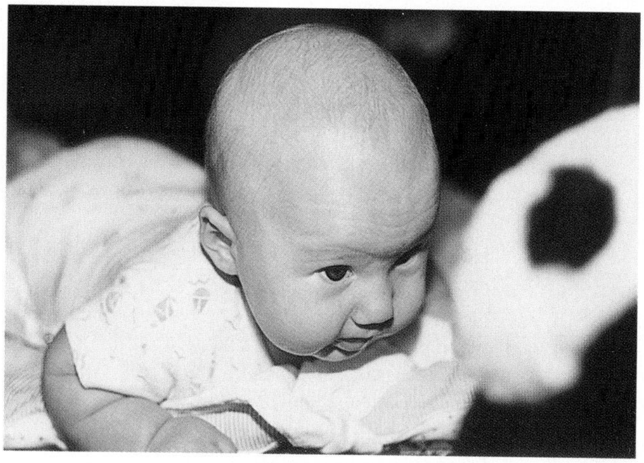

FIGURE 8.11 The 2-month old infant focuses steadily and lifts her head up while prone. Note her interest in the stuffed panda bear.

Four month-old children recognize familiar objects, such as a frequently seen bottle, rattle or toy animal. They follow their parents' movements with their eyes eagerly. At 6 months, infants are capable of organized depth perception. This increases the accuracy of their reach for objects as they begin to perceive distances accurately. Up until 6 months of age, the newborn may experience normal difficulty in establishing eye coordination. After this age, however, an infant whose eyes still "cross" should be examined by a physician.

Seven-month-old children pat their image in a mirror. Their depth perception has matured to the extent that they can perform such tasks as transferring toys from hand to hand. By 10 months, the infant looks under a towel or around a corner for a concealed object (beginning of **object permanence**).

Hearing

Hearing is demonstrated by the 1-month-old child who quiets momentarily at a distinctive sound such as a bell or a squeaky rubber toy. Hearing awareness becomes so acute by 2 months of age that the infant will listen or stop an activity at the sound of spoken words. Many 3-month-old children will turn their heads to attempt to locate a sound. When the 4-month-old child hears a distinctive sound, he or she will turn toward the sound and look in that direction.

At 5 months of age, the infant demonstrates that he or she can localize a sound downward and to the side, by turning the head and looking down. A 6-month-old has progressed to being able to locate a sound made above him or her. By 10 months, the infant can recognize his or her name and listen acutely when spoken to. By 12 months, the infant can easily locate a sound in any direction and turn toward it. A vocabulary of two words plus *ma-ma* and *da-da* also demonstrates that he or she can hear.

Emotional Development

Socialization, or learning how to interact with others, is an extended phenomenon. One month-old children show

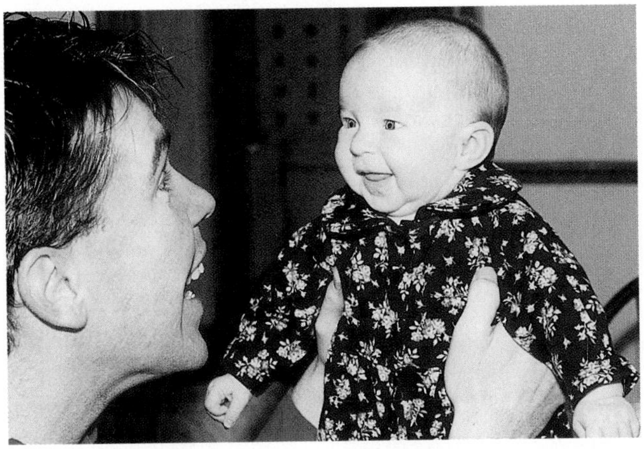

FIGURE 8.12 A 3-month-old smiles delightedly at her father's happy face. This indicates that the child has developed increased social awareness.

they can differentiate between a face and other objects by studying a face or the picture of a face longer than other objects. They quiet best and eat best for the person who has been their primary caregiver.

When an interested person nods and smiles at a 6-week-old infant, he or she smiles in return. This is a **social smile** and is a definite response to the interaction, not the faint, quick "smile" that younger infants, even newborns, demonstrate. It is a major milestone for assessing a number of areas, most notably vision, motor control, and intelligence. Cognitively challenged children or children with spasticity may not demonstrate a social smile until much later.

At 3 months, the infant demonstrates increased social awareness by readily smiling at the sight of a parent's face (Figure 8-12). Many three-month-old children laugh out loud at the sight of a funny face.

By 4 months, when a person who has been playing with and entertaining an infant leaves, the infant is likely to cry to show he or she enjoyed the interaction. Infants at this age recognize their primary caregiver and prefer that person's presence to others. By 5 months, a baby may show displeasure when an object is taken away from him or her. This is a step beyond showing displeasure when a person leaves. The baby can be counted on to laugh at seeing a funny face.

At 6 months, infants are increasingly aware of the difference between people who regularly care for them and strangers. They may begin to draw back from unfamiliar people.

Seven-month-old children show obvious fear of strangers. They may cry when taken from their parent, attempt to cling to him or her, and reach out to be taken back. Parents may view this as a bad trait or a regression in socialization. It is actually a big step forward, because it shows the infant is able to differentiate persons, to know the difference between those he or she trusts and those he or she does not know.

Fear of strangers appears to reach its height during the eighth month, so much so that this phenomenon is often termed **eighth-month anxiety,** or **stranger anxiety.** An infant at the height of this phase will not go willingly from a parent's arms to a nurse's. Taking a few minutes to talk to the child and parent first is time well spent (Dacey & Travers, 1997).

The 9-month-old child is very aware of changes in tone of voice. They will cry when scolded, not because they understand what is being said, but because they sense their parent's displeasure.

By 12 months, most children have overcome their fear of strangers and are alert and responsive again when approached. They like to play interactive nursery rhymes and rhythm games, and "dance" with others. They like being at the table for meals and joining in family activities.

> **✔ CHECKPOINT QUESTIONS**
>
> 7. What does the ability to focus and follow objects with the eyes indicate?
> 8. At what age do infants demonstrate a social smile?

Cognitive Development

In the first month of life, an infant mainly uses simple reflex activity. There is little evidence that infants at this age see themselves as separate from their environment. However, this does not mean they are unable to respond actively or interact with people. They are very people oriented from within moments after birth.

Primary Circular Reaction

By the third month of life, the child enters a cognitive stage identified by Piaget (1966) as **primary circular reaction.** During this time, he or she explores objects by grasping them with the hands or by mouthing them (Figure 8-13). At this stage, the infant appears to be unaware of what actions he or she can cause or what actions occur independently. For example, if an infant's hand

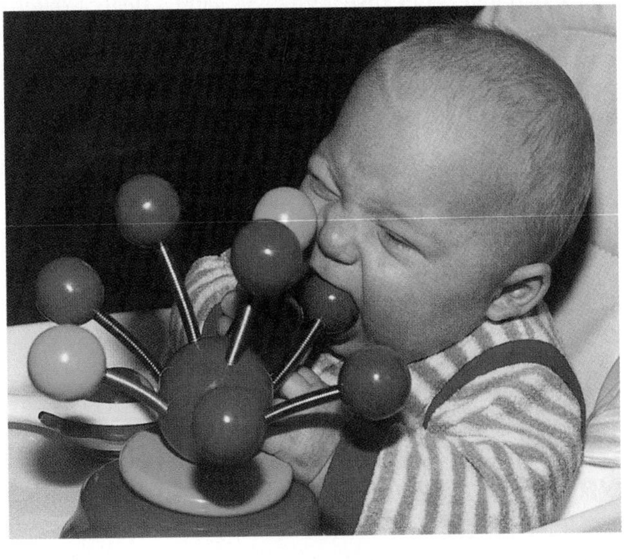

FIGURE 8.13 Mouthing of objects or fingers is a method by which an infant explores the world. This also helps the infant to separate self from environment.

should accidentally strike a mobile across the crib, the infant appears to enjoy watching the brightly colored birds move in front of him, but makes no attempt to hit the mobile again, not realizing that his hand caused the movement.

Secondary Circular Reaction

At about 6 months of age (cognitive development has wide variation), the child passes into a stage that Piaget (1966) called **secondary circular reaction.** During this time, the infant is able to realize that his or her actions can initiate pleasurable sensations. The infant reaches for a mobile above the crib, hits it, watches it move, realizes that his hand initiated the motion, and hits it again.

The infant is still unaware of the permanence of objects. For example, if an object is hidden from vision (a baby drops it from her hand or it is hidden by a blanket), the infant will not search for it. Gone is gone. If any part of the object is exposed, the infant is able to visualize the whole object and will reach to obtain it.

Coordination of Secondary Schema

An infant of 10 months discovers object permanence or realizes that an object out of sight still exists. Infants are ready for peek-a-boo once they have gained the concept of permanence. They know their parent still exists even when hiding behind a hand or blanket. Waiting for the parent to reappear is exciting. If a baby drops a piece of breakfast cereal or a spoon from her highchair tray, although it is out of sight, she knows it still exists and will reach for it. Piaget (1966) called this stage of cognitive development **coordination of secondary schema.**

As infants reach 1 year of age, they are capable of reproducing interesting events (she accidentally hits a mobile once; it moves; she hits it again) and producing new events. He drops objects from a highchair or playpen and watches where they fall or roll. This is a frustrating activity for caregivers because it involves a great deal of reaching and picking up. It is an important activity for infants, however, because it contributes to their awareness of the permanence of objects and how they are able to control events in their world.

> **✔ CHECKPOINT QUESTIONS**
>
> 9. When does an infant typically exhibit stranger anxiety?
> 10. When would an infant be ready to play peek-a-boo?

THE NURSING ROLE IN HEALTH PROMOTION OF THE INFANT AND FAMILY

The nursing role with infants is wide-ranging because infants are so dependent on their caregivers for safety, learning, and emotional development.

Promoting Infant Safety

Accidents are a leading cause of death in children from 1 month through 24 years of age. They are second only to acute infections as a cause of acute morbidity and physician visits.

Most accidents in infancy occur because parents either underestimate or overestimate the child's ability. Nursing interventions that help parents become sensitive to their infant's developmental progress help to establish sound parent–child relationships and provide anticipatory guidance for the child's safety (see Empowering the Family).

Preventing Aspiration

The accident that leads to the greatest number of infant deaths is aspiration. Round, cylindrical objects are more dangerous than square or flexible objects in this regard. A 1¼-in (3.2-cm) cylinder, such as a carrot or hot dog, is particularly dangerous because it can totally obstruct the infant's airway. An inflated balloon when bitten, can be sucked back into their mouth, obstructing the airway in the same way. Parents who feed an infant formula should be advised not to prop bottles. By doing this, they are overestimating their infant's ability to push the bottle away, sit up, turn the head to the side, cough, and clear the airway if milk should flow too rapidly into the mouth and the infant begins to aspirate.

Other incidents of aspiration occur because parents underestimate the baby's ability to grasp and place objects in the mouth. Newborns' grasp and sucking reflexes automatically cause them to react this way. Parents must be certain that nothing comes within the child's reach that would not be safe to put into the mouth. Parents should buy clothing without decorative buttons, and check toys and rattles to ensure that they have no small parts that will snap off or fall out. A test of whether a toy could be dangerous if the infant puts it inside the mouth is whether it fits inside a toilet paper roll. If it does, it is small enough to be aspirated. Even a newborn can wiggle to a new position to reach an attractive object such as a teddy bear with small button eyes. When solid foods are introduced, parents must be careful to offer small pieces of hot dogs or grapes, not large chunks. Children under about 5 years should not be offered popcorn or peanuts because of the danger of aspiration.

As the infant becomes more adept at handling toys, toys must be checked for loose pieces or parts such as button eyes on stuffed toys that could be grasped and pulled off. If parents are going to offer an infant a pacifier, they should be certain that it is a one-piece construction and has a flange large enough to keep the object from completely entering the child's mouth (Figure 8-14).

Preventing Falls

Falls are a second major cause of infant accidents. No infant, beginning with the newborn, should be left unattended on a raised surface. Normal wiggling can bring a baby to the edge of a bed, couch, or table top, resulting in a fall.

EMPOWERING THE FAMILY: **Accident Prevention Measures for Infants**

POTENTIAL ACCIDENT	PREVENTION MEASURE
Aspiration	Be certain any object that an infant can grasp and bring to the mouth is either safe to eat or too big to fit in the mouth. Do not feed an infant foods such as popcorn or peanuts, because these are easily aspirated.
	Store baby products such as powder out of infant's reach; powder is high risk for aspiration.
	Inspect toys and pacifiers for small parts that could be aspirated if broken off; don't make homemade pacifiers.
Falls	Never leave the infant on an unprotected surface, such as a bed or couch, even if the child is in an infant seat.
	Place a gate at the top and bottom of stairways; do not allow an infant to walk with a sharp object in the hands or mouth (it could pierce the throat in a fall).
	Raise crib rails and make sure they are locked before walking away from crib.
	Do not leave a child unattended in a highchair; avoid using an infant walker.
Motor vehicle	Never transport unless the infant under 20 lb is buckled into a rear-facing infant seat in the back seat of the car. Don't place an infant seat in the passenger side if the car has an air bag. Be aware of the proper technique for placing an infant in a car seat.
	Do not be distracted by an infant while driving.
	Do not leave an infant unattended in a parked car (can become dehydrated from excess heat, move gear shift, or be abducted).
Suffocation	Allow no plastic bags near infant's reach.
	Do not use pillows in a crib.
	Store unused appliances such as refrigerators or stoves with the doors removed.
	Buy a crib that is approved for safety (spacing of rails is not over 2⅜ in [6 cm] apart).
	Remove constricting clothing such as a bib from neck at bedtime.
Drowning	Do not leave infants alone in a bathtub or unsupervised near water (even buckets of cleaning water).
Animal bites	Do not allow the infant to approach a strange dog; supervise play with family pets.
Poisoning	Never present medication as a candy.
	Buy medications in containers with safety caps; put away immediately after use.
	Never take medication in front of infants.
	Place all medication and poisons in locked cabinets or overhead shelves.
	Never leave medication in a pocket or handbag.
	Use no lead-based paint in any area of the home.
	Hang plants or set on high surfaces.
	Post telephone number of the poison control center by the telephone.
	Provide syrup of ipecac with proper instructions for first-aid supply boxes.
Burns	Test warmth of formula and food before feeding (use extra precaution with microwave warming).
	Do not smoke or drink hot liquids while holding or caring for infant.
	Buy flame-retardant clothing for infants.
	Use a sunscreen on a child over 6 months when out in direct or indirect sunlight; limit the child's sun exposure to less than ½ h at a time.
	Turn handles of pans toward back of stove.
	Use a cool-mist, not a hot-mist, vaporizer; remain in room to monitor so child cannot reach vaporizer.
	Keep a screen in front of a fireplace or heater.
	Monitor infants carefully near candles.
	Do not leave infants unsupervised near hot-water faucets.
	Do not allow infants to blow out matches (don't teach children that fire is fun).
	Keep electric wires and cords out of reach; cover electrical outlets with safety plugs.
General	Know the whereabouts of infants at all times.
	Be aware that the frequency of accidents is increased when parents are under stress. Take special precautions at these times.
	Choose babysitters carefully and explain and enforce all precautions when sitters are in charge.

Constipation

Breastfed infants are rarely constipated because their stools tend to be loose. Constipation may occur in formula-fed infants if their diet is deficient in fluid. This can be corrected with the addition of more fluid.

Some parents misinterpret the normal pushing movements of a newborn to be constipation. When defecating, infants' faces do turn red, and they grimace and grunt. As long as stools are not hard and contain no evidence of fresh blood (as might occur with a rectal fissure), this is normal infant behavior.

If constipation persists beyond 5 or 6 months of age, encourage parents to check with the infant's health care provider about possible measures to relieve this. Adding foods with bulk, such as fruits or vegetables, and increasing fluid intake even more generally relieves the problem. Apple juice (3 or 4 oz) or prune juice (0.5 to 1 oz daily) may be given as a temporary measure.

All infants with a history of constipation for more than 1 week should be examined for an anal fissure or tight anal sphincter. Softening stools and thereby relieving the pain of defecation often solves the problem and helps the fissure to heal. If an unusually tight anal sphincter exists, parents will be given instructions to manually dilate the sphincter two or three times daily until it dilates sufficiently. Hirschsprung's disease (aganglionic megacolon or lack of nerve innervation to a portion of the colon) may be manifested early in life as constipation. If no stool is present in the rectum of a constipated infant on rectal examination, the possibility of this disease is suggested. A careful history must then be taken to assess whether the infant manifests other symptoms of Hirschsprung's disease: ribbonlike stools, bouts of diarrhea, and a distended abdomen (see Chapter 24).

Chronic constipation also may occur in children with congenital hypothyroidism (decreased functioning of the thyroid gland). Therefore, an infant with constipation also should be carefully observed for characteristic symptoms of hypothyroidism, such as lethargy, protruding tongue, and failure to meet developmental milestones (see Chapter 27). Infants with either Hirschsprung's disease or hypothyroidism need therapy to correct the disorder.

Loose Stools

Many first-time parents are unfamiliar with the loose consistency or color of normal newborn stools, so they mistakenly report normal stooling as diarrhea. Stools of breastfed infants are generally softer than those of formula-fed infants. If a mother takes a laxative while breastfeeding, its effect may be demonstrated as very loose stools in the infant. The infant who is formula fed may have loose stools if the formula is not mixed properly.

Occasionally, loose stools may begin with the introduction of solid food, such as fruit. Malabsorption syndrome (celiac disease), or inability to digest fat, may manifest itself first by loose stools and a distended abdomen and deficiency of fat-soluble vitamins (see Chapter 24).

When talking to a parent about this problem, inquire about the duration of the loose stools, the number of stools per day, their color and consistency, and whether there is any mucus or blood in them. Is there associated fever, cramping, or vomiting? Is the infant wetting at least six diapers daily? Does the infant continue to eat well? Appear well? Seem to be thriving?

Infants with associated symptoms such as fever, cramping, vomiting, loss of appetite, a decrease in voiding, and weight loss should be examined by a health care provider because this implies an infectious process. Dehydration occurs rapidly in a small infant who is not eating and is losing body fluid through loose stools.

Colic

Colic is paroxysmal abdominal pain that generally occurs in infants under 3 months of age (Berkowitz, 1997). The infant cries loudly and pulls the legs up against the abdomen. The infant's face becomes red and flushed, the fists clench, and the abdomen is tense. If offered a bottle, the infant will suck vigorously for a few minutes as if starved, then stop as another wave of intestinal pain occurs.

The cause of colic is unclear. It may occur in susceptible infants from overfeeding, from swallowing too much air while feeding, or from a formula too high in carbohydrate. Formula-fed babies are more likely to have colic than breastfed babies possibly because they swallow more air while drinking (see Focus on Nursing Research).

Although infants continue to thrive despite colic, the condition should not be dismissed as unimportant. It is a distressing and frightening problem for parents because the infant not only appears to be in acute pain, but the distress persists for hours, usually into the middle of the night so that no one in the family gets adequate rest. This is a difficult beginning to a parent–child relationship, which needs to be strong and binding for the parents to enjoy parenting and for the infant to thrive in their care.

FOCUS ON NURSING RESEARCH

Does Infant Temperament Play a Role in Colic?

To answer this question, 25 infants, between 4 and 8 months of age, who had colic were compared to 30 infants of similar age who did not have colic. Infant temperament was rated by their mothers, and the degree of bother the mother experienced in relationship to the infant's temperament was examined. Results of the study showed that more mothers of infants with colic rated the infant's temperament as difficult than did the mothers of infants who did not have colic.

This is an interesting study because it helps reveal how detrimental colic can be to the parent–infant relationship. It is interesting to ask whether the infants with colic were viewed as more "difficult" because they had colic or whether infants with "difficult" temperaments actually have more colic.

Jacobson, D., & Melvin, N. (1995). A comparison of temperament and maternal bother in infants with and without colic. *Journal of Pediatric Nursing, 10*(3), 181.

Take a thorough history of infants with colic symptoms, because intestinal obstruction or infection may mimic an attack of colic and be misinterpreted by the casual interviewer. Ask parents about the duration of the problem and its frequency—it usually lasts up to 3 hours a day and occurs at least 3 days every week. Ask for a description of what happens just before the attack (e.g., if it occurs after feeding) and a description of the attack itself and associated symptoms. Document the number and type of bowel movements because bowel movements are not abnormal with colic. Constipation, narrow, ribbonlike stools, and the presence of blood or mucus in the stool suggest other complicating problems. A family medical history is important to obtain because allergy to milk may simulate colic.

Determine the baby's feeding pattern: breastfed or bottle fed; if bottle fed, ask about the type of formula and how it is prepared. Explore with parents how they are feeding the baby and whether they are burping the infant adequately after feeding. Are they holding the baby firmly upright so air bubbles can rise? For the breastfed baby, a change in maternal diet (e.g., avoiding "gassy" foods) can reduce or limit colicky periods. It may be helpful to recommend that both breast- and formula-fed infants receive small, frequent feedings to prevent distention and discomfort. Offering a pacifier may be comforting. Sugar water may be helpful (Markestad, 1997).

Some persons recommend placing a hot water bottle on the infant's stomach for comfort, but this should be discouraged. A basic rule for any abdominal discomfort is to avoid heat in case appendicitis is developing. This is highly unlikely in so young an infant, but parents will remember they once used heat and may use it again when the child is older. Hot water bottles and heating pads should also not be used because they might burn the delicate skin of infants.

Changing the formula bottle to the type with disposable bags that collapse as the baby sucks may help minimize the amount of air swallowed. Taking the infant for a ride in the car is often reported as being helpful in soothing colicky babies. Commercial manufacturers produce music boxes that simulate the sound of a heart beat, which also may be helpful.

Occasionally, an antiflatulent, such as simethicone, is required to alleviate attacks and give both the parents and the child some rest. Caution parents to check with their primary health care provider before giving any medication to help avoid overdosing (Myers et al, 1997). It is important to think of colic as a family problem or else a vicious circle may gradually begin. The infant cries and the parents become tense and unsure of themselves. The infant senses the tension and develops more colic. Help parents plan relief time from infant care to relieve their stress level.

In most infants, colic disappears almost magically at 3 months of age, probably because it becomes easier to digest food and the infant maintains a more upright position by this time, which allows less gas to form (see the Nursing Care Plan).

Spitting Up

Almost all infants spit up, although formula-fed babies appear to do it more than breastfed babies. Parents who did not handle their infant much in the health care facility where the child was born may discover that an infant spits up only after they take the baby home. They may interpret this as vomiting or think the infant is developing an infection. Ask them to describe carefully what they mean by "spitting up." How long has the baby been doing it? How frequently? What is the appearance of the spit-up milk? Almost all milk that is spit up smells at least faintly sour, but it should not contain blood or bile.

The baby who spits up a mouthful of milk (rolling down the chin) two or three times a day (or sometimes after every meal) is experiencing normal, early-infancy spitting up. Associated symptoms such as diarrhea, abdominal cramps, fever, cough, cold, or loss of activity, are indicative of illness. If the infant is spitting up so forcefully that the milk is projected 3 or 4 feet away, it may be beginning pyloric stenosis (an abnormally tight valve between the stomach and duodenum) that requires surgical intervention. If the spitting up is a large amount with each feeding, parents may be describing gastroesophageal reflux in which a lax cardiac sphincter and esophagus allow regurgitation of gastric contents into the esophagus. This also requires medical attention (see Chapter 24).

Burping the baby thoroughly after a feeding often helps limit spitting up. Parents may try sitting the infant in an infant chair for half an hour after feeding. Changing formulas generally is of little value or effectiveness. Reassure parents that spitting up decreases in amount as the baby becomes better at coordinating swallowing and digestive processes (the cardiac sphincter matures). In the meantime, a bib can protect the baby's clothing and the parent. After a few months, the child will naturally stay in an upright position longer and gravity will help to correct the problem.

Diaper Dermatitis

Some infants have such sensitive skin that diaper dermatitis (diaper rash) is a problem from the first few days of life. It occurs for a number of reasons.

When parents do not change their children's diapers frequently, feces is left in contact with skin and irritation may result in the perianal area. Urine that is left in diapers too long breaks down into ammonia, a chemical that is extremely irritating to infant skin. Ammonia dermatitis of this type is generally a problem in the second half of the first year of life when the infant is producing a larger quantity of urine than before. For some infants, it is a problem from the first week.

Frequent diaper changing, applying petroleum jelly or A & D or Desitin ointment, and exposing the diaper area to air may relieve the problem. Some infants may have to sleep without diapers at night to control the problem.

Whenever the entire diaper area is erythematous and irritated so that the outline of the diaper on the skin can be identified, one must suspect an allergy to the material in the diaper or to laundry products if a commercially washed or home-washed diaper is being used. Changing the brand or type of diaper or washing solution usually alleviates the problem.

If a diaper area is covered with lesions that are bright red, with or without oozing, last longer than 3 days and

Nursing Care Plan

THE INFANT WITH COLIC

The parents bring their 2-month-old son in for a routine health maintenance visit. Their major concern is what to do about his crying at night.

Assessment: Well-proportioned 2-month-old male infant. Height and weight at 50th percentile on growth chart. Bottle feeding with intake of approximately 4 oz of commercial formula every 4 hours. Experiencing 2 to 3 soft yellow bowel movements daily. "He's been crying every night lately from about 6 P.M. till 2 A.M. His face gets red, and he pulls his legs up against his belly. I give him a bottle, he sucks for a few minutes like he's starving, and then stops and starts to cry, pulling his legs up again. We've tried everything but my husband and I are exhausted. We're at the end of our rope." Physical examination within normal limits. Diagnosis of colic is made.

Nursing Diagnosis: Ineffective family coping, compromised related to difficulty managing infant crying episodes

Outcome Identification: Parents will demonstrate positive coping measures by the end of 1 week.

Outcome Evaluation: Parents state increased feelings of control over situation; identify measures for stress reduction.

Interventions	Rationale
1. Educate the parents about the common characteristics of colic, including duration, timing, and intensity of crying, and bottle feeding as a possible factor in the presence of normal stool passage.	1. Education promotes better understanding of the problem, alleviating some of the stress and anxiety associated with it.
2. Reassure parents that they are not the cause of the child's discomfort.	2. Parents may feel guilty if they are unable to soothe their child. Reassurance that the problem is not their fault can aid in objective problem solving.
3. Caution parents that crying in infants produces frustration in adults. Help the parents plan constructive ways to deal with the crying.	3. Acknowledging their frustration helps to validate their feelings. A plan of action provides opportunities to regain some control over the situation.
4. Help the parents devise some respite time.	4. Time away can help relieve feelings of frustration and tension.
5. Urge the parents to call the health care provider for suggestions if they need further help. Explain that colic generally resolves by 3 months of age.	5. Support from health care providers can aid in coping. Knowing that colic is usually a time-limited problem provides the parents with the knowledge that there is an end in sight.

Nursing Diagnosis: Health-seeking behaviors related to appropriate measures for colic relief

Outcome Identification: Parents will verbalize increased confidence in caring for infant within 1 week.

Outcome Evaluation: Parents state that infant appears playful after feeding; sleeps at least for some period between 6 P.M. and 2 A.M.

Interventions	Rationale
1. Support parents in attempts to allow infant to cry for short periods (e.g., 5 to 10 minutes) before comforting.	1. Infants can learn self-quieting abilities to comfort themselves.
2. Have parents relate steps used to prepare formula and demonstrate bottle feeding and burping techniques. Review methods for proper formula preparation, bottle holding, and burping.	2. Proper techniques can minimize the amount of air swallowed during feeding and possible subsequent development of intestinal gas.

(continued)

3. Advise parents to feed the infant in a quiet environment.	3. Quiet environmental surroundings are soothing to the infant.
4. Recommend small, frequent feedings.	4. Small, frequent feedings prevent distention and discomfort.
5. Instruct parents to place the infant in an infant seat or upright position for ½ hour after feeding, gently rock or rub the infant's back or abdomen, use music boxes, or take the infant for a ride in the car.	5. An upright position prevents distention. The other measures provide comfort and are soothing to the infant.
6. Suggest the use of a pacifier.	6. Sucking on a pacifier may increase peristalsis and promote passage of gas through the intestine.
7. Advise parents to contact the health care provider if these measures are ineffective. Anticipate the need for possible drug therapy with simethicone.	7. Simethicone, an antiflatulent, should only be given to an infant under the direction of a health care provider.

appear as red pinpoint lesions, suspect a fungus (monilial or candidiasis) infection. This is discussed in Chapter 22.

Miliaria

Miliaria, or prickly heat rash, occurs most often in warm weather or when babies are overdressed or sleep in overheated rooms. The symptoms are clusters of pinpoint, reddened papules with occasional vesicles and pustules surrounded by erythema. They usually appear on the neck first and may spread upward to around the ear and onto the face or down onto the trunk.

Bathing the infant twice a day during hot weather, particularly if a small amount of baking soda is added to the bathwater, may improve the rash. Eliminating sweating by reducing the amount of clothing on the infant or lowering the room temperature should bring about almost immediate improvement and prevent further eruption.

Baby-Bottle Syndrome

Putting an infant to bed with a bottle can result in aspiration or decay of all the upper teeth and the lower posterior teeth (VonBurg, Sanders & Weddell, 1995; Figure 8-21).

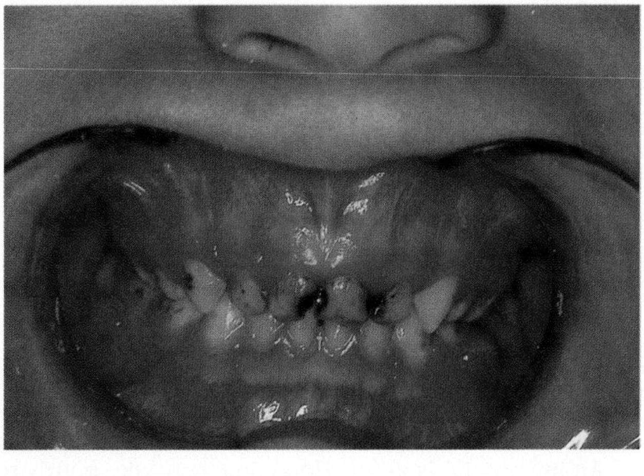

FIGURE 8.21 Baby-bottle syndrome. Notice the extensive decay in the upper teeth.

Decay occurs because while the infant sleeps, liquid from the propped bottle continuously soaks the upper front teeth and lower back teeth (the lower front teeth are protected by the tongue). The problem, called **baby-bottle syndrome,** is most serious when the bottle is filled with sugar water, formula, milk, or fruit juice. The carbohydrate in these solutions ferments to organic acids that demineralize the tooth enamel until it decays.

To prevent this problem, advise parents never to put their baby to bed with a bottle. If parents insist that the bottle is necessary, encourage them to fill it with water and use a nipple with a smaller hole to prevent the baby from receiving a large amount of fluid. If the baby refuses to drink anything but milk, the parents might dilute the milk with water more and more each night until the bottle is down to water only.

Obesity in Infants

Obesity in infants is defined as a weight greater than the 90th to 95th percentile on a standardized height/weight chart. Obesity occurs when there is an increase in the number of fat cells due to excessive calorie intake. It is important that obesity be prevented in infants, because the extra fat cells formed at this time are likely to remain through childhood and even into adulthood. If the child becomes obese because of overingesting milk, iron deficiency anemia may also be present because of the low iron content of both breast and commercial milk. Once infant obesity begins, it is difficult to reverse. Prevention is the key.

Overfeeding in infancy often occurs because parents were taught to eat everything on their plate, and they continue to instill this concept in their children. This appears to be the case most often with formula-fed infants whose parents have urged them to empty their bottle or finish a cereal serving. It can occur any time parents automatically feed an infant when the child cries, rather than investigating what the cry might really mean. An infant should take no more than 32 oz of formula daily, so that when solid food is introduced, a bottle of water can be substituted for formula at one feeding. All commercial infant formula contains 20 cal/mL. Advance, a formula fortified with iron for older infants and toddlers, is an example of a formula that contains 20% fewer calories than other formulas and therefore can be used to prevent extra weight gain. Skim milk should not be given, because it contains so little fat that essential fatty acid requirements may not be sufficient to ensure cell growth.

Another way to help prevent obesity is to add a source of fiber, such as whole grain cereal and raw fruit to the infant's diet. These prolong stomach emptying time and can thus help reduce food intake. Caution parents about giving obese infants foods with high amounts of refined sugars such as pudding, cake, cookies, and candy. Encourage parents to learn more about balanced diets and to provide them for their entire family.

CHECKPOINT QUESTIONS

18. What is the cause of colic?
19. What is baby-bottle syndrome?

Unique Concerns of the Family With a Disabled or Chronically Ill Infant

A child who is born with an illness or disability is usually hospitalized immediately after birth for diagnosis and treatment. This may result in delayed bonding because the child is separated from the parents during this time. If such an infant is hospitalized, encourage parents to visit regularly to help in forming a strong parent–child attachment. If parents cannot visit, make certain that they know they can telephone the hospital to inquire about their child's well-being. In addition, encourage nurses to supply instant photographs of the infant for parents to take home with them.

Many of the developmental events of the infant year (social smile, laughing out loud, reaching for an object, uttering the first word, sitting, talking) are activities that encourage parent–child interaction because they make an infant fun to be with and naturally make a parent want to spend a great deal of time with the child. The child who is mentally disabled may not reach these milestones. A child with physical limitations may be unable to meet them as well if he or she is unable to reach up and pat a mother's face or hold out arms to be picked up by a father. If the child cannot interact with the parents in these ways, the parents may find themselves equally unable to interact with the child. If an infant leaves the hospital with a cast or other equipment such as a ventilator for care, parents may be so concerned with these items that they are unable to initiate the normal everyday singing and playing activities with their child.

To encourage parents' relationship with a child, point out the positive things the infant can do. Perhaps the child's facial expression says, "Pick me up," even though he doesn't reach up with his hands; perhaps his eyes follow his mother's actions even though he can't yet call to her.

Helping parents to interact more fully with their infants helps to build a sense of trust in the infant. Without a sense of trust, children have difficulty expressing themselves to others; they do not believe that they are lovable or that people would want to interact with them. Physically disabled individuals—no matter what their ages—need people around them to give them help at whatever point they are unable to meet their own needs. It is unfortunate when a physically disabled child is unable to reach out for help because of a lack of a sense of trust.

Remember also that disabled or chronically ill infants experience the same health and growth problems as other infants. Parents may be reluctant to bring up these concerns at health care visits because they believe such problems pale in comparison to the child's primary disease or disability. When taking the health histories of children with chronic or longstanding medical problems, be sure to ask the parents about secondary concerns. "What about everyday things? Any problems there?" Treat these concerns seriously, so parents can feel confident about bringing them to your attention. Also be sure to mention that they are part of normal infant development so parents can begin to view their child apart from his or her illness or disability.

Teething pain, discomfort from diaper rash, and colic are all potential problems in infancy and may occur even more frequently in babies with other illnesses. For instance, parents may not want to "bother" an ill infant with physical care as often as they would a well child (e.g., before homes were well-heated, bathing an ill infant could cause extensive chilling, and many people still believe that bathing is not appropriate for ill children). Colic may occur because parents are reluctant to tire ill infants by burping them after a feeding. Parents' attention may be so focused on the primary health problem rather than on everyday concerns, such as diaper care, that diaper dermatitis occurs. The bowel movements of physically disabled or chronically ill children may be looser than normal because of a liquid diet or medicine. Their urine may be more concentrated because of reduced intake. These conditions may lead to diaper rashes. Offering anticipatory guidance to parents can go a long way toward helping them meet the needs of infants with unique needs.

Nutrition and the Disabled Infant

Nutrition is often a concern for the infant who is born with a disability or who is ill at birth. The infant who has an elevated temperature because of illness may have increased metabolic needs and require more calories than normal. To compound the problem, the child may become too fatigued to be able to take adequate feedings. If any degree of neurologic involvement is present, sucking and swallowing reflexes may not be coordinated. With gastrointestinal involvement, feeding may be impossible.

To ensure adequate calorie and protein intake, the infant may be maintained on nasogastric tube or gastrostomy feedings or total parenteral nutrition. These methods reduce the amount of opportunity for sucking. Because sucking provides pleasure as well as satisfies thirst, this is a major loss. Provide the infant with nonnutritive sucking experiences if possible.

An infant who is ill for a long time may take poorly to solid foods once they are introduced, because he or she is not hungry enough to be interested in a new eating method. Children who have had esophageal tracheal surgery can reach 2 years of age without ever having tasted solid food. Help parents to experiment with different foods to find a taste that does appeal to the child or teach them to limit foods to only those the child appears to like most from all five pyramid food groups.

KEY POINTS

The infant period is from 1 month to 12 months. Children typically double their weight at 4 to 6 months and triple it at 1 year.

Infants develop their first tooth at about 6 months; by 12 months, they have six to eight teeth.

Important gross motor milestones during the infant year are lifting chest off a bed at 2 months, sitting at 6 to 8 months, creeping at 9 months, "cruising" at 10 to 11 months, and walking at 12 months.

Important fine motor accomplishments are the ability to pass an object from one hand to the other (7 months) and a pincer grasp (10 months).

Important milestones of language development during the first year are differentiating a cry (2 months), making simple vowel sounds (5 to 6 months), and saying two words besides ma-ma and da-da (12 months). The more infants are spoken to, the easier language is to acquire.

Providing infants with proper toys for play helps development. All infant toys need to be checked to be sure they are not small enough to be aspirated.

Important milestones of vision development are ability to follow a moving object past the midline (3 months), and ability to focus securely without eyes crossing (6 months).

According to Erikson, the developmental task of the infant year is the development of a sense of trust versus mistrust.

Infants must be protected from aspiration of small objects and falls. Be aware that a skill an infant cannot accomplish one day, such as crawling, may be accomplished the next.

Solid food is generally introduced into the infant's diet at 5 to 6 months of age. Before infants can eat solid food effectively, they must lose their extrusion reflex.

Common concerns related to infant development are teething, thumb sucking, use of pacifiers, sleep problems, constipation, colic, diaper dermatitis, baby-bottle syndrome (syndrome of decayed teeth from infants sucking on a bottle of formula while they sleep) and obesity. Nurses play a key role in teaching parents about these problems and measures to deal with them.

Remember that parent–infant attachment is critical to mental health. Urge parents to continue to give as much care as possible to sick infants to maintain this important relationship.

CRITICAL THINKING EXERCISES

1. Bryan, the 2-month-old boy you met at the beginning of the chapter, was diagnosed as having colic. What are common suggestions you could make to his parents to help reduce his discomfort and the amount of crying?
2. A 3-month-old child will be hospitalized for several months out of state because of severe burns. As her nurse, what steps could you take to foster a sense of trust in her in light of this extensive parental separation?
3. The mother of a 10-month-old child tells you that her baby is "into everything." At a well-child assessment, formulate specific questions you would want to ask in order to feel confident that the infant's house is safe for him. Develop a teaching plan for the parents that addresses this 10-month-old child's safety needs.
4. A 1-month-old infant is going to be followed in your health maintenance setting. Describe the immunization schedule you would discuss with her father as recommended for the first year.
5. The father of a 4-month-old child tells you his son spits out all the solid food he tries to feed him. What advice would you give him?

REFERENCES

American Academy of Pediatrics. (1997). Air bag safety issues examined. *AAP News, 13*(1), 1.

American Academy of Pediatrics Committee on Infectious Diseases. (1997). Recommended childhood immunization schedule—United States. *Pediatrics, 99*(1), 136.

American Academy of Pediatrics Committee on Injury and Poison Prevention. (1995). Injuries associated with infant walkers. *Pediatrics, 95*(5), 778.

American Academy of Pediatrics Committee on Nutrition. (1995). Fluoride supplementation for children. *Pediatrics, 95*(5), 777.

Berkowitz, C. D. (1997). Management of the colicky infant. *Comprehensive Therapy, 23*(4), 277.

Dacey, J. S., & Travers, J. R. (1997). Physical and cognitive development in infancy. In Dacey, J. S., & Travers, J. R. *Human development across the age span* (3rd ed.). Chicago: Brown & Benchmark.

Deloian, B. J. (1996). Developmental management of infants. In Burns, C. E., et al. *Pediatric primary care: a hand-book for nurse practitioners.* Philadelphia: Saunders.

Department of Health and Human Services. (1995). *Healthy people 2000: midcourse review.* Washington, DC: DHHS.

Erikson, E. (1986). *Childhood and society* (3rd ed.). New York: W. W. Norton.

Jacobson, D., & Melvin, N. (1995). A comparison of temperament and maternal bother in infants with and without colic. *Journal of Pediatric Nursing, 10*(3), 181.

Markestad, T. (1997). Use of sucrose as a treatment for infant colic. *Archives of Disease in Childhood, 76*(4), 356.

McLoyd, V. C. (1998). Socioeconomic disadvantage and child development. *American Psychologist, 53*(2), 185.

Myers, J. H. Moro-Sutherland, D., & Shook, J. E. (1997). Anticholinergic poisoning in colicky infants treated with hyoscyamine sulfate. *American Journal of Emergency Medicine, 15*(5), 532.

Oyen, N. et al. (1997). Combined effects of sleeping position and prenatal risk factors in sudden infant death syndrome: the Nordic Epidemiological SIDS Study. *Pediatrics, 100*(4), 613.

Piaget, J. (1996). *The origins of intelligence in children*. New York: International Universities Press.

Skinner, J. D. et al. (1997). Transitions in infant feeding during the first year of life. *Journal of the American College of Nutrition, 15*(3), 209.

Von Burg, M. M., Sanders, B. J., & Weddell, J. A. (1995). Baby bottle tooth decay: a concern for all mothers. *Pediatric Nursing, 2*(6), 515.

SUGGESTED READINGS

Berkowitz, D., Naveh, Y., & Berant, M. (1997). Infantile colic as the sole manifestation of gastroesophageal reflex. *Journal of Pediatric Gastroenterology and Nutrition, 24*(2), 231.

Bordman, H. B., & Holzman, I. R. (1996). Infant care knowledge of primiparous urban mothers. *Journal of Perinatology, 16*(2.1), 107.

Boswell, W. C., et al. (1996). Prevention of pediatric mortality from trauma: are current measures adequate? *Southern Medical Journal, 89*(2), 218.

Cohen, L. R., et al. (1997). Pediatric injury prevention counseling priorities. *Pediatrics, 99*(5), 704.

Crowcroft, N. S., & Strachan, D. P. (1997). The social origins of infantile colic: questionnaire study covering 76,747 infants. *BMJ, 314*(7090), 1325.

Curry, D. M., & Duby, J. C. (1994). Developmental surveillance by pediatric nurses. *Pediatric Nursing, 20*(5), 40.

Lawrence, R. (1995). The clinician's role in teaching proper infant feeding techniques. *Journal of Pediatrics, 126*(6), 5112.

McQueen, D. A. (1997). The nutritional adequacy of mineral content of formulas. *Pediatrics in Review, 18*(2), 67.

Parish, A. R. (1997). Sudden infant death syndrome: a proposed discovery. *Medical Hypotheses, 49*(2), 177.

Ramey, C. T., & Ramey, S. L. (1998). Early intervention and early experience. *American Psychologist, 53*(2), 109.

Sharber, J. (1997). The efficacy of tepid sponge bathing to reduce fever in young children. *American Journal of Emergency Medicine, 15*(2), 188.

The Family With a Toddler

9

CHAPTER

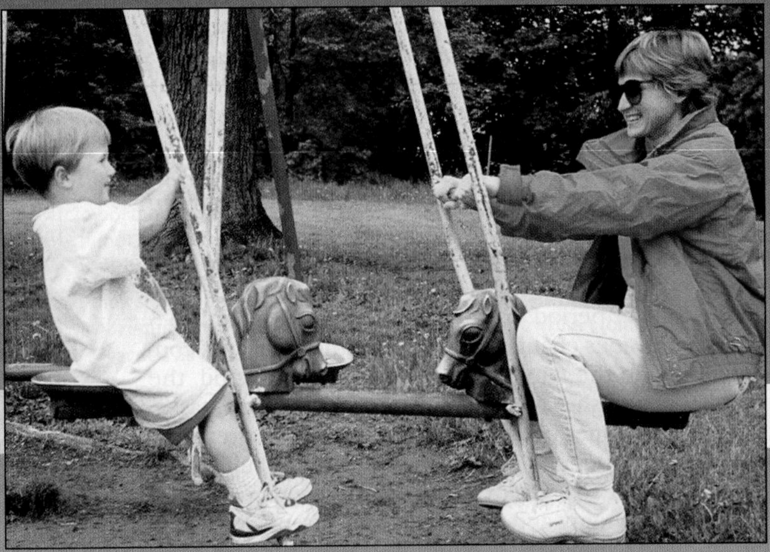

Key Terms

- assimilation
- autonomy
- deferred imitation
- discipline
- lordosis
- parallel play
- preoperational thought
- punishment
- tertiary circular reaction stage

Objectives

After mastering the contents of this chapter, you should be able to:

1. Describe normal growth and development of the toddler period and common parental concerns.
2. Assess a toddler for normal growth and development milestones.
3. Formulate nursing diagnoses related to toddler growth and development or parental concerns regarding development.
4. Identify appropriate outcomes for nursing care of the toddler.
5. Plan nursing care to meet the toddler's growth and development needs such as anticipatory guidance to prevent problems such as sleep disturbances, temper tantrums, or inappropriate toilet training practices.
6. Implement nursing care to promote normal growth and development of the toddler such as discussing toddler developmental milestones with parents.
7. Evaluate goal outcomes established for care to be certain nursing goals associated with growth and development have been achieved.
8. Identify National Health Goals related to the toddler age group that nurses can be instrumental in helping the nation to achieve.
9. Identify areas related to care of the toddler that could benefit from additional nursing research.
10. Use critical thinking to analyze methods of care for the toddler to be certain care is family centered.
11. Integrate knowledge of toddler growth and development with nursing process to achieve quality child health nursing care.

anteroposterior and transverse diameters of the chest reach adult proportions. Pulse rate decreases to about 85 bpm; blood pressure holds at about 100/60 mm Hg.

The bladder is easily palpable above the symphysis pubis; voiding is frequent enough (9 to 10 times a day) that play is interrupted and accidents may occur if the child becomes absorbed in an activity.

The child who earlier in life had an indeterminant longitudinal arch in the foot generally demonstrates a well-formed arch now. Muscles are noticeably stronger and make activities such as gymnastics possible. Many children this age exhibit **genu valgus** (knock-knees), which disappears with skeletal growth.

Weight, Height, and Head Circumference

Weight gain is slight during the preschool years. The average child gains only about 4.5 lb (2 kg) a year. Appetite remains as it was during the toddler years, which is considerably less than some parents would like or expect. Parents may bring their preschooler to the health care facility because they fear their child is losing weight. When the child's weight is plotted on a growth chart, however, it becomes evident that he or she is indeed putting on some weight; what parents were noticing was the age-appropriate change in body shape from rounded to slim.

Height gain is also minimal during this period; only 2 to 3.5 inches (6 to 8 cm) a year on average. Head circumference is not routinely measured at physical assessments on children over 2 years of age (see Appendix E for averages).

Teeth

Children generally have all 20 of their deciduous teeth by 3 years of age. Rarely do new teeth erupt during the preschool period.

CHECKPOINT QUESTIONS

1. Are height and weight gain dramatic during the preschool period?
2. How many new teeth usually develop during this time?

Developmental Milestones

Each year during the preschool period marks a major step forward in gross motor, fine motor, and language development. Play activities change focus as the preschooler learns new skills and understands more about his or her world (Figure 10-1). Table 10-1 summarizes the major milestones of the period.

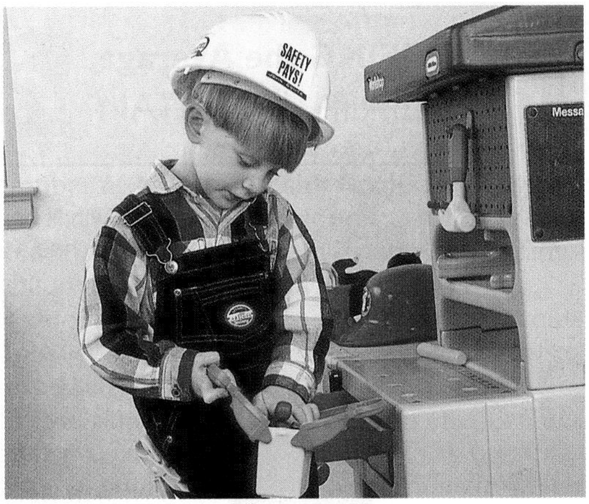

FIGURE 10.1 Preschoolers enjoy meaningful play and like to imitate the roles of adults, as they learn about the world around them.

Language Development

A 3-year-old child has a vocabulary of about 900 words. They are used to ask questions constantly, mostly "how" and "why" questions, such as "Why is snow cold? Does the dog sleep at night? What does your tongue do?" A child needs simple answers so curiosity, vocabulary building, and questioning are encouraged and also because the depth of the child's understanding is often deceptive. For example, if a parent tells a child that shoes should go on with the buckles on the outside, the child may seem to understand, but he or she may return in a few minutes to ask, "Why do I have to go outside to put on my shoes?" Words with double and triple meanings can be truly confounding to children of this age. Four- and 5-year-old children continue to ask many questions. They enjoy participating in mealtime conversation and are able to describe something from their day in great detail (see Focus on Cultural Competence).

Preschoolers are egocentric, so they define objects in relation to themselves (a key is not a metal object but "what I use to open a door," and a car is not a means of transportation but "what Mom uses to take me to school").

TABLE 10.1 Summary of Preschool Growth and Development

AGE (YR)	FINE MOTOR	GROSS MOTOR	LANGUAGE	PLAY
3	Undresses self; stacks tower of blocks; draws a cross	Runs; alternates feet on stairs; rides tricycle; stands on one foot	Vocabulary of 900 words	Able to take turns; very imaginative
4	Can do simple buttons	Constantly in motion; jumps; skips	Vocabulary of 1500 words	Pretending is major activity
5	Draws a 6-part man; can lace shoes	Throws overhand	Vocabulary of 2100 words	Likes games with numbers or letters

FOCUS ON CULTURAL COMPETENCE

Whether children are allowed to ask questions or not is culturally determined. In a society in which children are expected to be seen and not heard, a preschool child may not have the same expressive vocabulary as a child who has been encouraged to ask questions. Recognition that differences among cultures can affect levels of development means that assessment must be individualized, that is, meaningful in terms of the cultural milieu.

Play

Preschoolers do not need many toys. Their imaginations are keener than they will be at any other time in their lives. They enjoy games that use imitation, such as playing house. They imitate what they see parents doing: eating meals, mowing the lawn, cleaning house, arguing, and so forth. They pretend to be teachers, cowboys, firefighters and store clerks. Many preschoolers have imaginary friends as a normal part of having an active imagination. These often exist until children formally begin school.

Four- and 5-year-old children divide their time between rough-housing and imitative play. Five-year-old children are also interested in group games that they have learned in a kindergarten or preschool group.

Emotional Development

Children change a great deal in their ability to understand the world and how they relate to people during the preschool years.

Developmental Task: Initiative Versus Guilt

The developmental task for the preschool-age child is to achieve a sense of initiative (Erikson, 1986). The child with a well-developed sense of initiative has discovered that learning about new things is fun.

If children are criticized or punished for attempts at initiative, they develop a sense of guilt for wanting to try new activities or have new experiences. Those who leave the preschool period with guilt may carry it with them into new situations, such as starting elementary school. They may even have difficulty later in life making decisions about everything from changing jobs to choosing an apartment, because they cannot envision that they are capable of solving associated problems.

Preschoolers need exposure to a wide variety of experiences and play materials so they can learn as much about the world as possible. They are ready to reach outside their homes for new experiences, such as a trip to the zoo or an amusement park (Figure 10-2). They are interested in seeing new places, and especially enjoy going with the family on vacation. These types of experiences lead to increased vocabulary; preschoolers not only learn

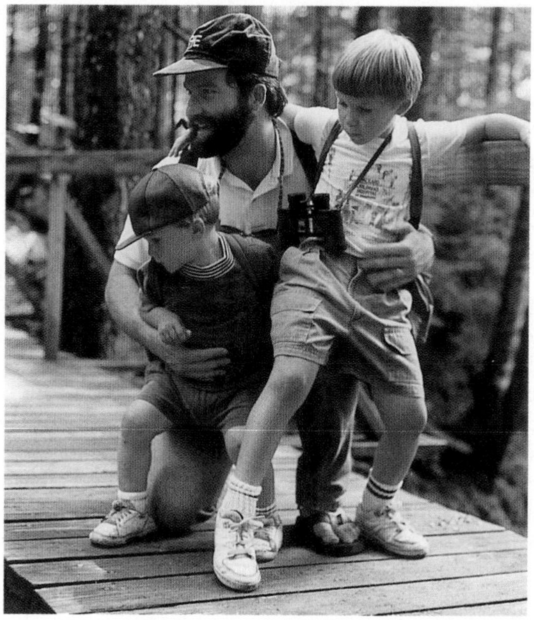

FIGURE 10.2 Preschoolers like exposure to new events and places. Here a 3-year-old is eager to explore the woods during a hike with the family.

words, such as *giraffe, elephant,* and *bear,* but they learn to transfer them from abstract concepts to the objects to which they relate.

Preschoolers should have exposure to play materials such as:

- Finger paints
- Soapy water to splash or blow into bubbles
- Mud to make pies
- Sand to build castles
- Modeling clay or homemade dough to mold into figures and make into pretend cookies

These are messy activities, and many parents are not able to let a child indulge in them more than once a week, but any experience with free-form play is helpful.

Preschoolers have such active imaginations that they need little guidance in play. They smear both hands into clay or finger paint and create instinctively. Urge parents to support this kind of play and not try to take it over. If a parent draws a tree with finger paint, for example, and says, "Now you draw one," a child may decide it is no fun to finger paint. He knows that his tree will not look as good as his parent's. As he is not ready for competition, he will drop out of the activity rather than be shown up as inferior.

Preschoolers may make nothing recognizable out of clay or finger paint, preferring simply to handle the medium. As long as they enjoy the feel of the material, they do not need to make anything. Pressure to make things is not fun and can discourage their interest in learning.

Imitation. Preschoolers need free rein to imitate the roles of the people around them. Again, role play should be fun and does not have to be accurate. If a child is a police officer and is busy putting out fires, or a firefighter and is stopping playmates from speeding, the fact that he is freely imitating a role is more important than the fact that he is absolutely certain of the adult role. If a parent is concerned that the child should separate these two roles accurately, it is usually best not to stop the play to do so. Rather, the next time they are driving past the fire station, the parent could explain that this is where firefighters work who put out fires or that the police station is where people work who make certain that other people drive safely.

Children generally imitate activities they see their parents performing at home. A young girl will set the table for breakfast, eat with her "husband," help clean off the table, and leave for work. A young boy might cook, pretend to feed a doll, and put the doll to bed as he has seen his father do with a younger sister. Many aspects of life today prevent children from imitating adult roles. The pace of life is faster than ever before; parents find their weekend schedules so full with home projects that they overlook the need to take a preschooler to visit their work environment. Such visits are recommended, when possible, because they provide a visual context for the parent's job and let the child give form to such words as *photocopier, cash register,* and *fax machine.* Another difficulty arises when a parent works in the city but lives in the suburbs or country an hour's train ride away. Taking the child to see the store or office then becomes a problem of scheduling and logistics.

Today, as many as 90% of mothers of childbearing age work outside the home at least part time. Remind a mother to introduce her preschooler to her "other" self—lawyer, secretary, or telephone repair person—in the same way the child is exposed to the father's work side.

Fantasy. Toddlers cannot differentiate between fantasy and reality (they believe cartoon characters are real). Preschoolers begin to make this differentiation. They may become so intense about a fantasy role, however, that they are afraid they have lost their own identity—that they have become "stuck" in their fantasies. Such intense involvement in play is part of "magical thinking" or believing that thoughts and wishes come true.

Parents sometimes strengthen this feeling without realizing it: they (and you) must be careful in this regard. A preschooler, for example, may pretend that she is a white rabbit delivering Easter eggs. Her mother walks into the room, is aware of the game, and decides to participate. She says, "That's strange, I don't see Cindy anywhere. All I see is a white rabbit." Then she leaves the room. Cindy may be frightened that she has actually become a white rabbit. She worries that her mother will not fix dinner for her or will not want her to live in the house any more.

A better response for the mother would be to support the imitation—this is age-appropriate behavior and a good way of exploring roles—but help the child maintain a difference between pretend and real. She might say, "What a nice white rabbit you're pretending to be," thus supporting the fantasy and yet reassuring the child that she is still herself.

In a health care setting, it is particularly important that you let children know they are still recognizable. When examining the ears of a girl who thinks she is a rabbit, you can comment that her ears are all better again, rather than play to the make-believe with remarks about long, furry (rabbit) ears.

Oedipus and Electra Complexes

Although the development of Oedipus and Electra complexes may have been overstated by Freud because of gender biases, many children do appear to manifest such behavior. **Oedipus complex** refers to the strong emotional attachment of a preschool boy to his mother; **Electra complex** is the attachment of a preschool girl to her father. Each child competes with the same-sex parent for the love and attention of the other parent. Parents who are not prepared for this behavior may feel hurt or rejected. For example, a daughter prefers to sit beside her father at the table or in the car; she asks her father to tuck her in at night. She is "Daddy's girl." The mother may feel left out of the family interaction when this happens. On the other hand, a boy will ask his mother for favors. He wants to sit beside her, to have her read to him, and to tuck him in for the night, and the father may feel left out.

Parents can be reassured that this phenomenon of competition and romance in preschoolers is normal. Parents may need help in handling feelings of jealousy and anger, particularly if the child is vocal in expressing feelings toward a parent. It is difficult for a mother to reply calmly to a 3-year-old daughter who is shouting at her, "I hate you! I only love Daddy!" By understanding the motivation behind such a statement, the parent may be able to calmly react by stating, "Well, I don't like to be shouted at, but I still love you."

Gender Roles

Preschoolers need exposure to an adult of the opposite gender so they can become familiar with opposite gender roles. Single parents should plan opportunities for their children to spend some time with adults other than themselves, such as a grandparent, an aunt or an uncle, for this exposure. A nursery school teacher may serve as this person. Because most nursery school teachers are women, the mother may have to look elsewhere to find an adult male role model. If the child is hospitalized during the preschool period, a male nurse could help fill this role.

Children's gender-typical actions are strengthened by parents, strangers, nursery school teachers, other family members, and other children. Parents who do not want their child to grow up as they did, with a fixed role as a result of gender stereotyping, should be aware that they reinforce such attitudes by their actions as well as by their words. For example, a father may tell his son that it is important for both boys and girls to do housework, but if the father will not do dishes no matter how many pile up in the kitchen he is teaching the child that managing a household is not a man's job.

Socialization

Because 3-year-old children are capable of sharing, they play with other children their age much more agreeably than do toddlers, which is a reason why the preschool period is a sensitive and critical time for socialization. Children who are exposed to other playmates have an easier time learning to relate to people than those, for instance, who are raised in an environment where they never see other children of the same age (Figure 10-3).

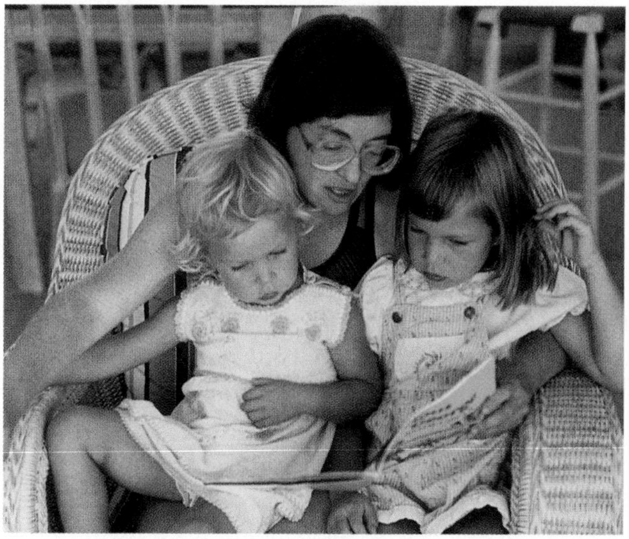

FIGURE 10.3 Preschoolers are interested in sharing activites with other children, such as listening to a story.

Although 4-year-old children continue to enjoy play groups, they may become involved in arguments more, especially as they become more certain of their role in the group. This development, like so many others, may make parents worry that a child is regressing. However, it is really forward movement, involving some testing and identification of their group role.

The 5-year-old child begins to develop "best" friendships, perhaps on the basis of who he walks to school with or who lives closest to him or her. The elementary rule that an odd number of children don't play well together pertains to children at this age. Two or four will play; three or five will quarrel.

Cognitive Development

At age 3 years, cognitive development according to Piaget is still preoperational (Piaget, 1969). Although children at this period do enter a second phase called **intuitional thought,** they lack the insight to view themselves as others see them or put themselves in another's place. The preschooler is unable to make this kind of mental substitution; therefore he feels he is always right. He argues with the forcefulness that comes from believing he is 100% correct. This is an important point for you to remember when explaining procedures to a preschooler. He cannot see your side of the situation; he cannot hurry because you must have something done by 10 o'clock; he cannot sit still just because you want him to.

Also, preschoolers are not yet aware of the property of **conservation.** This means that if they have two balls of clay of equal size, but one is squashed flatter and wider than the other, preschoolers will insist that the flatter one is bigger (because it is wider) or that the intact one is bigger (because it is taller). They are unable to see that only the form, not the amount, has changed. This inability to appreciate conservation has implications for working with preschoolers. Using the same theory, you will find that the preschooler cannot comprehend that a procedure done two separate ways is the same procedure. Thus, if the nurse before you told a child to turn on his right side and then his left side while his bed was made, you may have to allow him to turn these same ways, too.

> **CHECKPOINT QUESTIONS**
>
> 3. How many words does a 3-year-old child typically have in his or her vocabulary?
> 4. How might children who do not develop a sense of initiative react in a new situation?

Moral and Spiritual Development

Children of preschool age determine right from wrong based on their parents' rules. They have little understanding of the rationale for these rules or even whether the rules are consistent. If asked the question, "Why is it wrong for you to steal from your neighbor's house?" the average preschooler answers, "Because my mother says it's wrong." When pressed further, the preschooler justifies that conviction with, "It just is, that's all."

Because preschoolers depend on parents to supply rules for them, when faced with a new situation they have difficulty seeing that the rules they know may also apply to a new situation.

> WHAT IF? What if a preschooler understands the rule "Don't steal from stores"? Would he also understand "Don't steal from a hospital"?

Preschoolers begin to have an elemental concept of God if they have been provided some form of religious training. Belief in an outside force aids the development of conscience (Kohlberg, 1981); however, preschoolers tend to do good out of self-interest rather than because of strong spiritual motivation. Children this age enjoy the security of religious holidays, prayers, and grace said before meals, because these rituals can offer them the same reassurance that a familiar nursery rhyme read over and over does.

PLANNING AND IMPLEMENTATION FOR HEALTH PROMOTION OF THE PRESCHOOLER AND FAMILY

Preschoolers are old enough to begin to take responsibility for their own actions. Preschooler safety, nutritional health, daily activities and family functioning are all impacted by this increased responsibility.

Promoting Preschooler Safety

As preschoolers broaden their horizons, safety issues grow. By age 4, children may project an attitude of independence and the ability to take care of their own needs. Part of this is pseudo-independence; they still need supervision to be certain they do not injure themselves or other children while roughhousing and to ensure they do not stray too far from home. Their interest in learning adult roles may lead them into exploring the blades of a

EMPOWERING THE FAMILY: Common Safety Measures to Prevent Accidents During the Preschool Years

Possible Accident	*Prevention Measure*
Motor vehicles	Maintain child in car seat; do not be distracted by child while driving.
	Do not allow preschooler to play outside unsupervised.
	Do not allow preschooler to operate electronic garage door.
	Teach safety with tricycle (look before crossing driveways; do not cross streets).
	Teach child to always hold hands with a grownup before crossing a street.
	Teach parking lot safety (hold hands with grownup; do not run behind cars that are backing up).
	Children should wear helmets when riding bicycles.
Falls	Supervise preschooler at playgrounds.
	Help child to judge safe distances for jumping or safe heights for climbing.
Drowning	Do not leave child alone in bathtub or near water.
	Teach beginning swimming.
Animal bites	Do not allow child to approach strange dogs.
	Supervise child's play with family pets.
Poisoning	Never present medication as a candy.
	Never take medication in front of a child.
	Never store food or substances in containers other than their own.
	Post telephone number of local poison control center by the telephone.
	Stock each first-aid box with syrup of ipecac, with proper instructions for administering.
	Teach child that medication is a serious substance and not for play.
Burns	Buy flame-retardant clothing.
	Turn handles of saucepans toward back of stove.
	Store matches in closed containers.
	Do not allow preschooler to help light birthday candles, fireplaces, etc. (fire is not fun or a "treat").
	Keep screen in front of a fireplace or heater.
Community safety	Teach preschooler that not all people are friends. ("Do not talk to strangers or take candy from strangers").
	Define a stranger as someone child does not know, not someone odd looking.
	Teach child to say "no" to people whose touching he does not enjoy, including family members. (When a child is sexually abused, the offender is usually a family member or close family friend.)
General	Know whereabouts of preschooler at all times.
	Be aware that frequency of accidents is increased when parents are under stress. Special precautions must be taken at these times.
	Some children are more active, curious, and impulsive and therefore more vulnerable to accidents than others.

lawn mover or an electric saw. They must be reminded repeatedly of automobile safety. A preschooler's thought "I want to play with Mary across the street" can be so quick and so intense that he or she will run into the middle of the street before remembering "Watch out for cars" or "Don't cross the street."

Because preschoolers imitate adult roles so well, they may imitate taking medicine if they see family members doing so. A good rule for parents is never to take medicine in front of children. Safety points for the preschool period are summarized in Empowering the Family. (See also Focus on Nursing Research.)

Keeping Children Safe, Strong, and Free. The preschool years are not too early a time to educate children about the potential threat of harm from strangers or

FOCUS ON NURSING RESEARCH

What Preschool Children are Most Apt to Suffer a Serious Injury?

This is an important question because, if such children could be identified, health education to prevent injury could be directed at those families. To answer the question, the birth certificate of children born during a 10-year time period in Tennessee were analyzed as to maternal age, race, education, neighborhood income, parity, use of prenatal care, residence location, infant's gender and gestational age. Death certificates were then examined to see which children had suffered a mortal injury. The results showed that in the group studied there were 803 deaths from injury. Children had at least a 50% increased risk of fatal injury if they were born to a mother who (1) had less than a high school education, (2) was less than 20 years of age at the time of the child's birth, and (3) had two or more children compared with no other children. Neither race nor income was significantly associated with childhood injury mortality.

This is an important study for nurses because it helps identify types of parents who could benefit from additional counseling about childhood safety. When time for health teaching is limited, making sure you reach the parents who need it most in that limited time period becomes an important consideration in care.

Scholer, S. J., Mitchel, E. F., Jr., & Ray, W. A. (1997). Predictors of injury mortality in early childhood. *Pediatrics, 100*(3.1):342.

even how to address bullying behavior from people (children or adults) they know. This includes:

- Warning a child never to talk with or accept rides from strangers.
- Teaching a child how to call for help in an emergency (yelling or running to a designated neighbor's house if outside, or dialing 911 if near a phone).
- Describing what police officers look like and expressing that police officers can help in an emergency situation.
- Explaining that if children or adults ask them to keep secrets about anything that has made them uncomfortable, they should tell their parents or another trusted adult, even if they have promised to keep the secret.

It is often difficult for parents to impart this type of information to a preschooler, because parents can't imagine their children will ever be in such situations, nor do they want to terrify their children about the world around them. However, if discussed in a calm yet serious manner, children can begin to use the information to build safe habits that will help them later when they are old enough to walk home from school alone or play with their friends, unsupervised, at the playground. Playground injuries are a frequent type of injury in this age child (Mack et al, 1997).

WHAT IF? What if a preschooler tells you she knows not to leave preschool with anyone who is strange? Is that the same as knowing not to leave with a stranger?

Motor Vehicle and Bicycle Safety. With more and more cars being equipped with front seat air bags, parents need to make sure their children are safely buckled into a car seat when riding in the car. Children this age should not be seated in the front seat if the car has a passenger side air bag (AAP, 1996). Many preschoolers outgrow their car seats during this period (when they reach 40 lb), but they may still be too small for regular seat belts. The shoulder harness should be carefully positioned so it does not go across the child's face or throat. During this stage and until the child is large enough for the shoulder harness to fit properly, a booster seat is the safest method for restraining the child. Preschoolers are able to unhook seat belts without difficulty. Parents must stress their important role in preventing injury in accidents (Niemcryk et al, 1997).

This is also the right age to promote bicycle safety. Head injuries are a major cause of death and injury to preschoolers, and bicycle accidents are among the major causes of such injuries. Some parents may have already purchased a helmet for the child when he or she was a toddler and riding in a bicycle seat. Once the child begins riding independently, however, he or she definitely needs a safety helmet approved for children his age and size. (ANSI and Snell Memorial Foundation are two organizations that have set safety standards for bicycle helmets; Powell et al, 1997). Encourage parents who ride bicycles to demonstrate safe riding habits by wearing helmets as well. A parent who routinely wears a helmet may well prove to be the most compelling reason for the preschooler to wear one.

Promoting Nutritional Health of the Preschooler

Like the toddler period, the preschool years are not a time of fast growth, so the child is not likely to have a ravenous appetite. Offering small servings of food is still a good idea, so the child is not overwhelmed and is allowed the successful feeling of cleaning a plate and asking for more.

Most children are hungry after preschool and enjoy a snack when they arrive home. Because sugary foods may dull a child's appetite for dinner, urge parents to make the snack nutritious: fruit, cheese, juice, or milk, rather than cookies and a soft drink.

Teach parents to make every attempt to make mealtime a happy and enjoyable part of the day for everyone. Some preschool children learn to eat as quickly as possible (and thus incompletely) to escape from the table before something unpleasant happens, such as an argument that they know is brewing. Initiative, or learning how to do things, can be strengthened by allowing a child to prepare simple foods, such as making a sandwich or spreading jelly on toast.

Recommended Daily Dietary Allowances

Parents need to select food for a preschooler based on the food pyramid. The mineral most apt to be deficient in a preschool diet is iron because the age group may not eat a great deal of meat (Zive et al, 1995). Many parents ask whether their preschooler needs to take supplementary vitamins. As long as the child is eating foods from all pyramid food groups and meets the criteria for a healthy child (i.e., alert and active, with height and weight within normal averages), additional vitamins are unnecessary.

If parents do give vitamins, they must remember that the child will undoubtedly view the vitamin as candy rather than medicine because of the attractive shapes and colors of preschool vitamins. Vitamins must be stored out of reach with other medicines. Caution parents not to give more than the recommended daily amount or else poisoning from high doses of fat-soluble vitamins and iron can result. Poisoning from excessive ingestion is an increasing problem among toddlers and preschoolers.

Promoting Nutritional Health With a Vegetarian Diet

A vegetarian diet is usually colorful and therefore appeals to the preschooler. Many vegetables, fruits, and grains are also good snack foods and so are convenient for the child who eats frequently during the day.

If the diet is deficient in any aspect, it is usually calcium, vitamin B_{12} and vitamin D. Check to see that the child is ingesting a variety of calcium sources (green leafy vegetables; milk products). Vitamin D is found in fortified cereals and milk. Vitamin B_{12} is found almost exclusively in animal products so the child may need a supplemental source of this (Sanders, 1995).

> **✔ CHECKPOINT QUESTIONS**
>
> 5. When do preschoolers outgrow their car seats? What is the best safety method to follow for preschoolers who no longer use a car seat?
> 6. Are preschool vitamin supplements necessary for all children?

Promoting Development of the Preschooler in Daily Activities

The preschooler has often mastered the basic skills needed for most self-care activities, including self-feeding, dressing, washing (with supervision), and toothbrushing (again, with supervision).

Dressing

Many 3-year-old children and most 4-year-old children are able to dress themselves except for difficult buttons, although there may be a conflict over what the child will wear. Preschoolers prefer bright colors or prints and may select items that do not match. As with other preschool activities, however, children need the experience of choosing their own clothes. One way for parents to solve the problem of mismatching is to fold together shirts and pants that go together so the child sees them as a set rather than individual pieces. If children insist on wearing mismatched clothes, parents should make no apologies for their appearance. A simple statement, such as "Mark chose his own clothes today," explains the situation. Anyone who understands preschoolers knows that the experience children gain in being able to select their own clothing is worth more than perfect appearance by adult standards.

Sleep

Many toddlers going through a negative phase resist naps no matter how tired they are. Preschoolers, on the other hand, are more aware of their needs; when they are tired, they often curl up on a couch or soft chair and fall asleep. Many preschoolers, particularly those who attend afternoon day care or preschool, give up afternoon naps. Encourage parents to learn whether the school requires children to take a nap. If they rest there, the child may have some difficulty getting to sleep at the usual bedtime established at home.

Children in this age group continue to have problems with refusing to go to sleep. Night waking from nightmares or night terrors reaches its peak (Atkinson, 1995; King et al, 1997). Preschoolers may have difficulty sleeping in a dark room and may need a night light, whereas they did not need one before. A helpful suggestion for parents is to maintain enjoyable activities and continue bedtime routines to reduce stress before bedtime.

Exercise

The preschool period is an active phase during which the child receives a great deal of exercise. Roughhousing is a good way of getting rid of tension and should be allowed as long as it does not become destructive or harmful. Also, preschoolers love time-honored games such as ring-around-the-rosy, London Bridge, or other more structured games that they were not ready for as toddlers.

Bathing

Although preschoolers certainly sit well in the bathtub, they should still not be left unsupervised at bathtime. They may decide to add more hot water and scald themselves or to practice swimming and slip and be unable to get their head out of the water. Most preschoolers enjoy soaking in the bathtub to get clean and enjoy having a bubble bath or playing with soap crayons. Some girls develop vulvar irritation (and perhaps bladder infection) from exposure to these products, however, so parents must use common sense in using them. Preschoolers do not clean their fingernails or ears well, so these areas often need "touching up" by a parent or older sibling.

Hair washing can be a problem. The preschooler is too heavy for a parent to hold over the sink to rinse hair. Children are also unable to close their eyes well enough or long enough (because they insist on opening them to see

EMPOWERING THE FAMILY: Tips to Make Hairwashing a More Pleasant Experience

- Try washing hair in the tub and asking your child to look at a toy hung from the ceiling while hair is rinsed.
- Use a shampoo that does not sting the eyes.
- If that doesn't help, purchase a soap guard (plastic visor) to keep shampoo out of the eyes.
- Remember, patience with this in-between age is your greatest help.

whether the parent is finished) to keep soap out while they have their hair rinsed in an upright position. For tips on hair washing, see Empowering the Family.

Because preschoolers like to imitate adults, they begin to be interested in taking showers rather than baths as they see their parents doing. Although children may not get too clean the few times they try showering, parents do not usually have to be concerned because most preschoolers shower only a few times, then return to tub soaking, which allows them to play with bath toys.

Preschoolers can wash and dry their hands perfectly adequately if the water faucet is regulated for them (again, so they do not scald themselves with hot water). Children this age are not paragons of neatness, however, and may clean hands at the expense of a bathroom towel. When possible, parents should turn down the temperature of the water heater to under 120°F.

Care of Teeth

If independent toothbrushing was not started as a daily practice during the infant or toddler years, it should be started during the preschool years. The child should continue to drink fluoridated water or receive a prescribed oral fluoride supplement if this is not provided in the water supply (AAP, 1995).

One good toothbrushing period a day, with parents helping them use dental floss to clean between the teeth, is often more effective than more frequent half-hearted brushings. Although many preschoolers do well brushing their own teeth, parents must check that all tooth surfaces are cleaned. They should floss the teeth, because this is a skill beyond a preschooler's motor ability.

Toothbrushing is generally well accepted by preschoolers because it imitates adults. Electric or battery-operated toothbrushes are favorites because of the adult responsibility involved in handling them. Children must be supervised when using an electric toothbrush and must be taught not to use it or any other electrical appliance near a basin of water.

Encouraging children to eat apples, carrots, celery, chicken, or cheese for snack foods rather than candy or sweets is yet another way to attempt to prevent tooth decay. When a child is introduced to chewing gum, it should be the sugar-free variety.

Children should have made a first visit to a dentist by 2½ years of age for evaluation of tooth formation. Because this age usually shows no cavities, this should have been a pain-free visit; fear of the dentist should not be present (Poulton et al, 1997) and the idea that dentists like to help rather than hurt should have been implanted. If parents did not take the child for this previously, it should be done during the preschool period.

It is important that deciduous teeth be preserved to protect the dental arch. If teeth are pulled as a result of disease, the permanent teeth can drift out of position or the jaw may not grow enough to accommodate them.

Night Grinding. Bruxism, or grinding the teeth at night (usually during sleep) is a habit of many young children. Teeth grinding may be a way of "letting go," similar to body rocking, that children do for a short time each night to release tensions and allow themselves to fall asleep. Children who grind their teeth extensively may have anxiety of a greater degree than the average child. Children with cerebral palsy may do it because of spasticity of jaw muscles. If the grinding is extensive, the crowns of the teeth can become abraded. It is possible for the condition to advance to such an extent that the tooth nerves are exposed. If the problem seems to stem from anxiety, identifying and relieving the source of the anxiety are essential for treatment. If some damage is evident, refer families to a pedodontist so the teeth can be evaluated, repaired (capped), and conserved.

Promoting Healthy Family Functioning

Some parents who enjoyed maintaining a rhythm of care for an infant and allowed for ritualistic behavior of a toddler may have difficulty being the parents of a pre-schooler, because more flexibility and creativity are required. Others come into their own as the parents of a preschooler. They delight in encouraging imaginative games and play.

A major parental role during this time is to encourage vocabulary development. One way to do this is to read aloud to the child; another is to answer questions so the child sees language as an organized system of communication. Answering a preschooler's questions is often difficult because the questions are frequently philosophical, for example, "Why is grass green?" The child may listen to an explanation of chlorophyll but then repeat the question, regardless of the clarity of the explanation, because the parent underestimated the extent of the question. The child did not want to know what makes grass green, but why, philosophically, it is not red or blue or yellow. The obvious answer to that is "I don't know." Many parents, however, have trouble making such an admission to a child. Those who are confident can give this answer without feeling threatened. Parents who are less sure of themselves may feel extremely uncomfortable when they do not know the answers to a 4-year-old child's questions (see Enhancing Communication).

Discipline

Preschoolers have definite opinions on things such as what they want to eat, where they want to go, and what they want to wear. This may bring them into opposition with their parents' opinions of what they should eat or wear, or where they should go. It is important for parents to guide a child through these struggles without discouraging the child's right to have an opinion. "Timeout" is a good technique to correct behavior for parents to continue through the preschool years (see Chapter 9). The technique of timeout allows parents to discipline without using physical punishment. It allows the child to learn a new way of behavior without extreme stress.

ENHANCING COMMUNICATION

Mr. Edwards is the father of a preschooler, Darryl. You overhear him talking to his son while they wait for a well-child visit.

Less Effective Communication

Darryl: Why are we waiting?
Mr. Edwards: It's how things work here.
Darryl: Why?
Mr. Edwards: I have no idea.
Darryl: Why is that girl here? Is she sick?
Mr. Edwards: I really don't know.
Darryl: When are we going home?
Mr. Edwards: I couldn't tell you.
Darryl: What's that girl's name?
Mr. Edwards: I have no idea.

More Effective Communication

Darryl: Why are we waiting?
Mr. Edwards: It's how things work here.
Darryl: Why?
Mr. Edwards: People have to take turns. We're waiting for our turn.
Darryl: Why is that girl here? Is she sick?
Mr. Edwards: She might be. Some children are here because they're sick and some are just in for a checkup like you.
Darryl: When are we going home?
Mr. Edwards: As soon as the nurse practitioner checks you over.
Darryl: What's that girl's name?
Mr. Edwards: I don't know. Do you want to ask her?

Preschoolers ask 300 to 400 questions a day as they explore their world. In the first scenario, Mr. Edwards tries to discourage questions by offering almost no answers. In the second scenario, when he tries to answer the child's questions, the father is not only supplying information, he is also helping the child build vocabulary. Because preschoolers ask so many questions, you may have to encourage parents to continue to answer questions this way. Otherwise, discouraging questions can become the method of interaction.

Parental Concerns Associated With the Preschool Period

Common Health Problems of the Preschooler

The mortality of children during the preschool years is low and becoming increasingly lower every year as more infectious diseases are preventable. The major cause of death is automobile accidents, followed by poisoning and falls (DHHS, 1997).

In contrast, the number of minor illnesses, such as colds, ear infections and flu symptoms, in preschoolers is exceptionally high, more than that of any other age. Children who live in homes in which parents smoke have a higher incidence of ear (otitis media) and respiratory infections than others. Children who attend day care or preschool programs also have an increased incidence of respiratory infections and gastrointestinal disturbances (such as vomiting and diarrhea).

This may be the parents' first experience with other than a transient illness in their child. Many parents may find it difficult to cope with constant minor colds. Thus, stress may arise between parent and child, an almost monthly battle of "Stay indoors until your cold is better," conflict over day care, or frequent whining and clinging behavior because the child's stomach is upset. Such illnesses may cause parents to perceive a child as sickly or not able to cope with everyday life. Whereas parents encouraged independence before, they may now begin to overprotect, to shelter to too great a degree. They need reassurance that frequent minor illnesses are common in preschoolers. As they become more experienced in handling these conditions, their perception of whether an illness is a problem will change.

Table 10-2 shows the usual health maintenance schedule for preschoolers. Table 10-3 lists problems that parents may have in evaluating a preschooler's illness.

Common Fears of the Preschooler

Because preschool imagination is so active, it can lead to a number of fears. Fears of the dark, mutilation, and separation or abandonment are all very real to the preschooler.

Fear of the Dark. The tendency to fear the dark is an example of a fear heightened by the child's vivid imagination: a stuffed toy by daylight becomes a threatening monster in the dark. Children may awaken screaming if they are roused by a nightmare. They may be reluctant to go to bed or to go to sleep by themselves unless a light is on.

If parents are prepared for this fear and understand that it is a phase of growth, they will be better able to cope with it. It is generally helpful if they monitor the stimuli their children are exposed to, especially around bedtime. This includes television, adult discussions, and frightening stories. Parents are sometimes reluctant to leave a child's light on at night because they do not want to cater

TABLE 10.2 Health Maintenance Schedule, Preschool Period

AREA OF FOCUS	METHODS	FREQUENCY
Assessment		
Developmental milestones	History, observation	Every visit
	Formal Denver Developmental Screening Test (DDST II)	Before start of school
Growth milestones	Height, weight plotted on standard growth chart; physical examination	Every visit
Hypertension	Blood pressure	Every visit
Nutrition	History, observation; height/weight information	Every visit
Parent–child relationship	History, observation	Every visit
Behavior problems	History, observation	Every visit
Vision and hearing defects	History, observation	Every visit
	Formal Preschool E and audiometer testing	Before start of school
Dental health	History, physical examination	Every visit
Tuberculosis	Tine test	Before start of school
Immunizations		
Diphtheria, pertussis, and tetanus; trivalent oral poliomyelitis	Check history and past records; inform caregiver about any risks and side-effects; administer immunization in accordance with health care agency policies	Before start of school
MMR		Before start of school
Anticipatory Guidance		
Preschool care	Active listening and health teaching	Every visit
Expected growth and developmental milestones before next visit	Active listening and health teaching	Every visit
Accident prevention	Counseling about street and personal safety	Every visit
Problem Solving		
Any problems expressed by caregiver during course of the visit	Active listening and health teaching regarding temper tantrums, toilet training	Every visit

TABLE 10.3 Parental Difficulties Evaluating Illness in the Preschool Child

DIFFICULTY	HELPFUL SUGGESTIONS FOR PARENTS
Evaluating seriousness of illness or condition	Preschoolers are eager to please and tend to answer all questions such as, "Does your stomach hurt?" with a yes. Observing the child for signs of illness—refusing to eat, holding an arm stiffly, having to go to the bathroom frequently—is often more productive as an evaluation technique.
Evaluating bowel and bladder problems	Preschoolers are independent in toilet habits for the first time, so parents do not have diaper contents to evaluate. Frequent trips to the bathroom, rubbing the abdomen, and holding genitals are the usual signs of bowel or bladder dysfunction.
Evaluating nutritional intake	Preschoolers begin to eat away from home at friends' houses or at day care, or to stay overnight with grandparents, so parents do not observe daily food intake as accurately as before. Observing whether the child is growing and active is better than monitoring any one day's food intake.
Evaluating bedwetting	Many preschoolers continue to have occasional enuresis at night until school age. If other signs are present—pain, low-grade fever, listlessness—the child should have a urine culture, as persistent bed wetting can indicate a low-grade urinary tract infection.
Evaluating activity vs hyperactivity	Many lay magazines have articles on hyperactivity in children. Parents often wonder whether their active child is truly hyperactive. As a rule of thumb, if a child can sit through a meal (when he is hungry), watch a half-hour television show (that is his favorite), or sit still while his favorite story is read to him, he is not hyperactive.
Age-specific diseases to be aware of	Preschool age is a time for vision and hearing assessment. For the first time, the child is able to be tested by a standard chart or by audiometry.
	Urinary tract infections tend to occur with a high frequency in preschool-age girls.
	Language assessment should be done if the child is not able to make his wants known by complete, articulated sentences by age 3 (exceptions are transposing *w* for *r* and broken fluency: "I want-want-want to go").

and decided to use them. Correction should be unemotional, for example, "That's not a word we like to hear you use. When you're angry, why don't you say 'fudge' (or whatever)." The correcting is no different from that involved when the child uses poor grammar. If parents become emotional, the child realizes the value of such words and may continue using them to get attention.

Unique Concerns of the Family With a Disabled or Chronically Ill Preschooler

Learning how to do things when you have physical limitations can be frustrating. Being unable to understand how to do things because of physical or mental limitations can be even more so. To learn problem solving, however, is part of developing a sense of initiative. A preschooler with a disability such as cerebral palsy has a greater need for problem-solving skills than the average child, because even simple procedures such as eating or getting dressed can be difficult if a physical handicap limits the options.

Preschoolers with a handicap or chronic illness should attend a preschool program if at all possible. Many of the learning activities that preschoolers enjoy, such as playing with paint, clay, or soap bubbles, are messy. If the child must remain in bed, the parents may not offer these types of experiences. A large tray of dry oatmeal or other breakfast cereal with sand shovels or cars and trucks is a good substitute activity for such a child. Although not necessarily neat, these substances (which are available even in a hospital setting) can be swept away easily at the finish of play. Table 10-5 lists the nursing actions that aid a disabled or chronically ill child to solve problems and develop a sense of initiative.

Nutrition and the Disabled or Chronically Ill Preschooler

Experiences with eating help to reinforce in preschoolers a sense of initiative. Chronically ill or disabled preschoolers who are limited in the foods they can eat (e.g., they have to maintain a diet of soft foods) or in their ability to help with food preparation may miss this reinforcement. If their appetite is diminished because of illness to the point where they take little or nothing orally, it is still important that they continue to join the family at meals. In most households, this is a time for socialization, and preschoolers are ripe for the learning that goes with this type of daily interaction. Encourage parents to include the disabled or ill child in family meals and in other social occasions whenever possible.

CHECKPOINT QUESTIONS

11. How should parents react to their preschooler if he begins to masturbate while watching television?
12. What types of illness are frequent in preschoolers attending a child care center?
13. Is broken fluency true stuttering?

KEY POINTS

Although preschoolers grow only slightly and gain just a little weight, they seem much taller than when they were toddlers because their contour changes to more childlike proportions.

Erikson's developmental task for the preschool period is to gain a sense of initiative or learn how to do things. Play materials ideal for this age group are those that stimulate creativity such as modeling clay or colored markers.

Promoting childhood safety is a major role, because preschoolers' active imaginations can lead them into dangerous situations.

Appetite is not large because this is not a rapid growth time. Preschoolers are interested in helping with food preparation.

Common parental concerns during the preschool period are with "broken fluency," imaginary friends, difficulty sharing, and sibling rivalry.

Preschool is often the time when a new sibling is born. Good preparation for this is necessary to prevent intense sibling rivalry.

Preschoolers have a number of universal fears, including fear of the dark, mutilation, and abandonment. All care provided for this age group must include active measures to reduce these fears as much as possible.

Preschoolers are still operating at a cognitive level that prevents them from understanding conservation (objects have not changed substance although they have changed appearance). This means they need an explanation, for example, of how they will be the same person postoperatively as they were preoperatively.

Preschoolers are self-centered (egocentric). This makes it difficult for them to share and view someone else's side of a problem. They need good explanations of how a procedure will benefit them before they can agree to it.

Many preschoolers begin preschool programs or day care. Late in the preschool period, they may be enrolled in kindergarten. Parents often appreciate guidance in how to orient their children to these new experiences.

Preschoolers who are disabled or who have chronic illnesses may have difficulty achieving a sense of initiative, because they may be limited in their ability to participate in activities that stimulate initiative. They may need special play times set aside for stimulation and learning.

CRITICAL THINKING EXERCISES

1. Terry is the 3-year-old girl you met at the beginning of the chapter. Terry's mother was concerned because Terry told exaggerated stories about events at her preschool site. How would you recommend her mother handle this?
2. Many children these days are raised as vegetarians. Is this an adequate diet for a preschooler? What are simple foods preschoolers can help prepare to build a sense of initiative and interest in food?
3. A 3-year-old child is starting day care because his mother is returning to work. Specify the suggestions you could make to his mother about choosing a safe setting. How should she prepare her child for the experience?
4. The parents of a preschooler tell you that their daughter keeps the entire family awake at night because she is so afraid of the dark. Formulate a plan of action to enable her family to help her sleep.
5. The mother of a 4-year-old boy who you see in a well-child conference tells you she cannot stand messy activities. Explain the activities you could suggest to the mother that would stimulate a sense of initiative but not be messy.

REFERENCES

American Academy of Pediatrics Committee on Injury and Poison Prevention. (1996). Selecting and using the most appropriate car seat safety seats for growing children. *Pediatrics, 97*(5), 761.

American Academy of Pediatrics Committee on Nutrition. (1995). Fluoride supplementation for children. *Pediatrics, 95*(5), 777.

Atkinson, E., et al. (1995). Sleep disruption in young children. *Child Care Health Development, 21*(4), 233.

Chiocca, E. M. (1998). Language development in bilingual children. *Pediatric Nursing, 24*(1), 43.

Department of Health and Human Services. (1997). Death rates by age and sex: United States. *Monthly Vital Statistics Report,* No. 44, 2.

Department of Health and Human Services. (1995). *Healthy people 2000: midcourse review.* Washington, DC: DHHS.

Erikson, E. H. (1986). *Childhood and society.* New York: W. W. Norton.

King, N., et al. (1997). Children's nighttime fears. *Clinical Psychology Review, 17*(4), 431.

Kohlberg, L. (1981). *The philosophy of moral development, moral states and the idea of justice.* New York: Harper & Row.

Mack, M. G., et al. (1997). A descriptive analysis of children's playground injuries in the United States 1990–1994. *Injury Prevention, 3*(2), 100.

Niemcryk, S. J., et al. (1997). Motor vehicle crashes, restraint use, and severity of injury in children in Nevada. *American Journal of Preventive Medicine, 13*(2), 109.

Piaget, J. (1969). *The theory of stages in cognitive development.* New York: McGraw-Hill.

Poulton, R., et al. (1997). Good teeth, bad teeth and fear of the dentist. *Behavior Research and Therapy, 35*(4), 327.

Powell, E. C., Tanz, R. R., & DiScala, C. (1997). Bicycle-related injuries among preschool children. *Annals of Emergency Medicine, 30*(3), 260.

Sanders, T. A. (1995). Vegetarian diets and children. *Pediatric Clinics of North America, 42*(4), 955.

Sawicki, J. A. (1997). Sibling rivalry and the new baby: anticipatory guidance and management strategies. *Pediatric Nursing, 23*(3), 298.

Scholer, S. J., Mitchel, E. F., Jr., & Ray, W. A. (1997). Predictors of injury mortality in early childhood. *Pediatrics, 100*(3.1), 342.

Ulione, M. S., & Dooling, M. (1997). Preschool injuries in child care centers: nursing strategies for prevention. *Journal of Pediatric Health Care, 11*(3), 111.

Yairi, E., et al. (1996). Predictive factors of persistence and recovery: pathways of childhood stuttering. *Journal of Communication Disorders, 29*(1), 51.

Zive, M. M., et al. (1995). Vitamin and mineral intakes of Anglo-American and Mexican-American preschoolers. *Journal of the American Dietetic Association, 95*(3), 329.

SUGGESTED READINGS

Brayden, R. M., & Poole, S. R. (1995). Common behavioral problems in infants and children. *Primary Care Clinics in Office Practice, 22*(1), 81.

Dahl, E. K. (1996). The concept of penis envy revisited: a child analyst listens to adult women. *Psychoanalytic Study of the Child, 51,* 303.

Frederick, C., & Reining, K. M. (1995). Essential components of growth and development. *Journal of Post Anesthesia Nursing, 10*(1), 12.

Kagan, J. (1997). Temperament and the reactions to unfamiliarity. *Child Development, 68*(1), 139.

Lancaster, K. A. (1997). Care of the pediatric patient in ambulatory surgery. *Nursing Clinics of North America, 32*(2), 441.

Mansfield, R. T. (1997). Head injuries in children and adults. *Critical Care Clinics, 13*(3), 611.

Noble, R. R., et al. (1997). Special considerations for the pediatric perioperative patient: a developmental approach. *Nursing Clinics of North America, 32*(1), 1.

Swick, D. (1997). Submersion injuries in children. *International Journal of Trauma Nursing, 3*(2), 59.

Thomas, R. M. (1996). *Comparing theories of child development* (4th ed.). Pacific Grove, CA: Brooks-Cole.

Whitener, L. M. et al. (1998). Use of theory to guide nurses in the design of health messages for children. *ANS: Advances in Nursing Science, 20*(3), 21.

The Family With a School-Age Child

11

CHAPTER

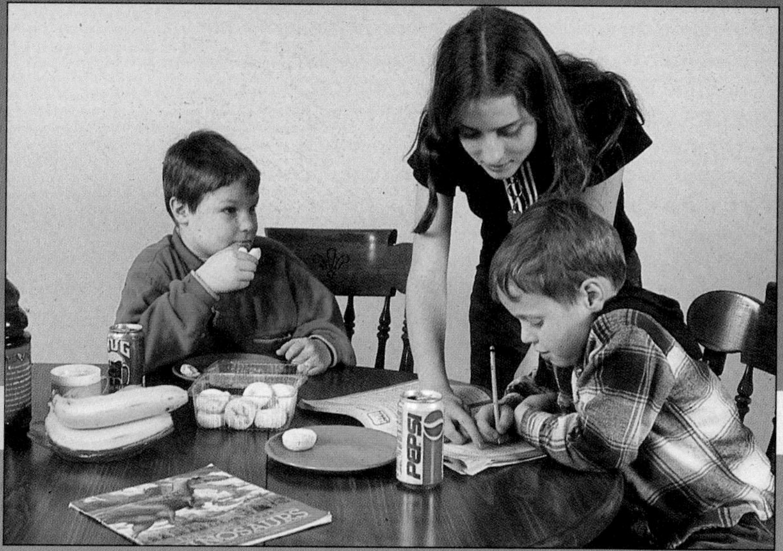

Key Terms

- accommodation
- caries
- class inclusion
- conservation
- decenter
- inclusion
- latchkey child
- malocclusion
- nocturnal emissions
- preconventional reasoning

Objectives

After mastering the contents of this chapter, you should be able to:

1. Describe the normal growth and development pattern and common parental concerns of the school-age period.
2. Assess a school-age child for normal growth and development milestones.
3. Formulate nursing diagnoses for the family of a school-age child.
4. Identify appropriate outcomes based on health assessment findings.
5. Plan anticipatory guidance to prevent problems of growth and development in the school-age child (e.g., teaching about normal puberty).
6. Implement nursing care to help achieve normal growth and development of the school-age child, such as counseling parents about helping their child adjust to a new school.
7. Evaluate outcome criteria to be certain that goals of care have been achieved.
8. Identify National Health Goals related to the school-age child that nurses can be instrumental in helping the nation achieve.
9. Identify areas related to care of school-age children that could benefit from additional nursing research.
10. Use critical thinking to analyze ways in which the care of the school-age child can be more family centered.
11. Integrate knowledge of school-age growth and development with the nursing process to achieve quality child health nursing care.

Shelly Lewis is a 6-year-old girl who recently started first grade. Her mother tells you that, although Shelly says she likes school, she has developed a lot of nervous habits such as nail biting since she started. Her mother asks you if this is normal. How would you advise her mother?

In the previous chapter, you learned about the preschooler and the capabilities children develop in these years. In this chapter, you'll add information about the dramatic changes, both physical and psychosocial, that occur during the school-age years. This is important information because it builds a base for care and health teaching for the age group.

After you've studied the chapter, turn to the Critical Thinking Exercises at the end of the chapter to sharpen your skills and test your knowledge.

In this chapter, the term *school age* refers to children between the ages of 6 and 12. Although the school-age years represent a time of slow physical growth, cognitive and developmental growth proceed at rapid rates. Because of this, there are many differences among children from one year to the next. Seven- and 10-year-old children have very different needs and outlooks, as do 11- and 12-year-old children. It is important to assess all children as individuals and try to understand the particular developmental needs of each child based on his or her own developmental status, not based on where you think he or she should be.

The school-age period is usually the first time that children begin to make truly independent judgments. This may create some conflicts with parents if they are not prepared for this. Unlike the infant or toddler, whose progress is marked by obvious new abilities and skills (e.g., ability to sit up or roll over; ability to speak a full sentence), the development of the school-age child is more subtle. Progress may, in fact, be marked by mood swings; what the child enjoys on one occasion may not be acceptable on another. For instance, a child may ask parents for a guitar and lessons, and then after the family has invested in these, the child quickly loses interest. The child of school age is also more influenced by the attitudes of his friends than previously. He or she may choose not to do something that was previously enjoyable because no friends are interested in that activity. Parents who make too much of these likes and dislikes may find themselves engaged in unnecessary conflicts with their child. Focus on National Health Goals lists National Health Goals related to the school-age period.

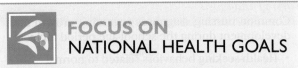

FOCUS ON NATIONAL HEALTH GOALS

A number of National Health Goals address the health of the school-age population, including these three:

- Increase to at least 30% the proportion of people age 6 and older who engage regularly, preferably daily, in light to moderate physical activity for at least 30 minutes per day.
- Reduce deaths caused by motor vehicle accidents to no more than 5.5 per 100,000 children age 14 years and younger.
- Reduce dental caries so that the proportion of children with one or more caries (in permanent or primary teeth) is no more than 35% among children ages 6 through 8 years (DHHS, 1995).

Nurses can be instrumental in helping the nation achieve these goals by such actions as urging children to begin and maintain a consistent exercise program, brush teeth and go for dental checkups regularly, and follow safety rules both in and around automobiles. Additional nursing research is needed to strengthen knowledge about the following: What is the ideal exercise program that is interesting enough to children that it will hold their attention for a long span of time? What are effective ways to teach street safety to children in the early school years? What strategies are most effective in helping school-age children to brush teeth daily?

NURSING PROCESS OVERVIEW

For Healthy Development of the School-Age Child

Assessment

Growth and development of the school-age child should be assessed with both a history and physical examination. Be certain that the history includes an account of school activities and progress. School-age children are interested and able to contribute to their own health history; it is useful to interview children 10 years or older, at least in part, without their parents being present. During the physical examination, show your respect for the fact that modesty is at an adult level by having children use a cover gown.

Parents often mention behavioral issues or conflicts during yearly health visits for the school-age child. Some parents feel they are losing contact with their children during these years and so may misinterpret a normal change in behavior, especially if they are not prepared for what to expect from their child.

When problems are discussed in the health care setting, it is important not only to take the history from the parent but also to allow the child to express the problem by him- or herself. Parents may consider a child who behaves differently from siblings as "abnormal" when he is just expressing his own personality. It may be necessary to obtain the opinion of school personnel regarding the problem or even just determine whether they feel a problem exists. In some instances, a counselor's opinion may be sought. If the problem is related to a medical condition, its effect on the family should also be assessed, because the illness of a child will certainly affect the functioning of the family unit.

EMPOWERING THE FAMILY: Common Safety Measures to Prevent Accidents During the School Years

Accident	*Preventive Measure*
Motor vehicle accidents	Encourage children to use seat belts in a car; role model their use.
	Teach street-crossing safety; stress that streets are no place for roughhousing, pushing, or shoving.
	Teach bicycle safety, including advice not to take "passengers" on a bicycle and to use a helmet.
	Teach parking lot and school bus safety (do not walk in back of parked cars, wait for crossing guard, etc.).
Community	Teach to avoid areas specifically unsafe, such as train yards, grain silos, back alleys. Teach not to go with strangers (parents can establish a code word with child; child does not leave school with anyone who does not know the word).
	Teach to say "no" to anyone who touches them whom they do not wish to do so, including family members (most sexual abuse is by a family member, not a stranger).
Burns	Teach safety with candles, matches, campfires—fire is not fun. Teach safety with beginning cooking skills (remember to include microwave oven safety, such as closing firmly before turning on oven; not using metal containers). Teach safety with sun exposure—use sun block.
	Teach not to climb electric poles.
Falls	Teach that roughhousing on fences, climbing on roofs, etc., is hazardous.
	Teach skateboard safety.
Sports injuries	Wearing appropriate equipment for sports (face masks for hockey; mouthpiece and cup for football; helmet for bicycle riding, skateboarding or in-line skating; batting helmets for baseball) is not babyish but smart.
	Teach not to play to a point of exhaustion or in a sport beyond physical capability (pitching baseball or toe ballet for a grade-school child).
	Teach to use trampolines only with adult supervision to avoid serious neck injury.
Sex	Teach rules of safer sex (use of condoms; inspecting partner, etc.).
Drowning	Children should learn how to swim; dares and roughhousing when diving or swimming are not appropriate.
	Teach not to swim beyond limits of capabilities.
Drugs	Teach to avoid all recreational drugs and to take prescription medicine only as directed. Avoid tobacco and alcohol.
Firearms	Teach safe firearm use. Parents should keep firearms in locked cabinets with bullets separate from gun.
General	Teach school-age children to keep adults informed as to where they are and what they are doing.
	Be aware that the frequency of accidents increases when parents are under stress and therefore less attentive. Special precautions must be taken at these times.
	Some children are more active, curious, and impulsive and therefore more vulnerable to accidents than others.

wiches. They may eat meals that they have planned or prepared more willingly than ones that are just set in front of them.

Most parents would like children to develop better table manners. Because they are in a hurry to finish eating, school-age children tend to gulp their food. Many meals are interrupted by spilled milk. As children become teenagers and are more aware of the impression they make on others, manners often improve dramatically. It is some comfort for parents to know that a child usually displays better table manners in other people's homes than in his or her own.

Recommended Daily Dietary Allowances

Nutrition is a major area of focus for health promotion of the school-age child. Although parents may have less to say about what the school-age child eats, it is important that the increasing energy requirements that come with

BOX 11.1

TEACHING POINTS TO HELP CHILDREN AVOID SEXUAL ABUSE

1. Your body is your property and you can decide who looks at it or touches it.
2. Secrets are fun things to keep. If a person asks you not to tell about something that was done to you that you didn't like, it's not a secret. It's all right to tell about it.
3. Don't go anywhere with a stranger (a stranger is someone you do not know, not someone "strange"). Don't be fooled by people asking you to show them directions or to go with them because your mother is sick or hurt.
4. Being touched by someone you like is a good feeling. You don't have to allow anyone to touch you in a way you don't like. Don't allow yourself to be left alone with a person you are uncomfortable with because he or she touches you in a way you don't like.
5. A "private part" is the part of you a bathing suit touches. If anyone asks you to show them a private part or touches a private part, tell them to stop, and tell someone else.
6. If the person you tell doesn't believe you, keep telling people until someone believes you.

this age (often in spurts) are met daily with foods of high nutritional value.

During the late school years, the recommended daily dietary allowances begin to be separated into categories for girls and boys because boys require more calories and other nutrients at this time. Both girls and boys require more iron in prepuberty than they did between the ages of 7 years and 10 years. Adequate calcium and fluoride intake remains important to ensure good teeth.

Because school-age children typically dislike vegetables, their intake may be deficient in fiber. A good rule for how much fiber they need is their age plus 5 g (Dwyer, 1995).

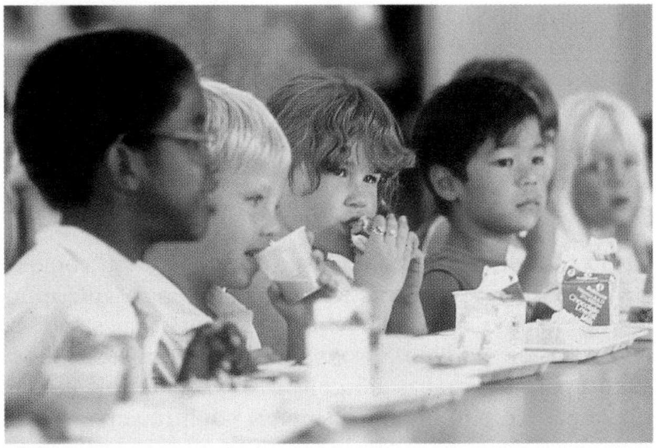

FIGURE 11.7 School lunch programs provide nutritious meals to help school-age children meet recommended daily allowances.

Promoting Nutritional Health With a Vegetarian Diet

School-age children who are raised in vegetarian homes must be taught aspects of vegetarian nutrition if they are going to eat in a school cafeteria. Unfortunately, many school lunch programs offer mainly milk and meat or cheese foods, such as sloppy joe sandwiches, macaroni and cheese, or pizza. This forces children who are vegetarian to carry packed lunches to maintain their diet. These could consist of cucumber, tomato, or peanut butter sandwiches on whole-grain bread; hot soups; salads; vegetable sticks; and fruit.

School-age children often eat at other children's houses and attend parties. Those who are vegetarians need to be educated to notify a host that they eat a special diet or to choose correctly from foods they are served.

A potential problem to assess with vegetarian school-age children is whether they are obtaining enough protein and calcium so they are prepared for the rapid growth spurt of puberty. Foods high in calcium are green, leafy vegetables (e.g., spinach and turnip greens), prunes, nuts, enriched bread, and cereals. Soybeans, legumes, nuts, grains, and immature seeds (e.g., green beans, lima beans, and corn) are relatively high in protein. As with any individual on a vegetarian diet, children may need a vitamin B_{12} supplement. Encourage outside activities for sun exposure to increase vitamin D. Iron may need to be supplemented, especially if girls have heavy menstrual flows (Nathan et al, 1996).

Promoting Development of the School-Age Child in Daily Activities

With life centered on school activities and friends, the school-age child still needs parental guidance for most activities of daily life. Habits and lifestyle patterns gained during this period can form the basis for healthy (or unhealthy) patterns of living later in life.

In addition to nutritional needs, areas of concern for the school-age child and family include sleep needs, dressing, exercise, hygiene, and dental care.

Dress

Although school-age children are capable of fully dressing themselves, they are not capable of taking care of their clothes until later in the school-age years—clothes taken off are dropped on the floor rather than placed in a hamper or a drawer. This is the right age (if not started already) to teach children the importance of caring for their own belongings. School-age children have definite opinions about style of clothing, often based on the likes of their friends rather than the preferences of their parents. Insisting that a child dress differently from classmates is unfair and even cruel. A child who wears different clothing may become the object of exclusion from a school club or group. In schools with a gang culture, children may not be able to wear a certain color or style or will be mistaken for a gang member. Many schools are requiring uniforms to avoid this problem.

Sleep

Sleep needs vary among individual children. Younger school-age children generally require 10 to 12 hours of sleep each night, and older ones require about 8 to 10 hours. Most 6-year-old children are too old for naps but do require a quiet time after school to get them through the remainder of the day. Nighttime terrors may continue during the early school years and may actually increase during the first-grade year, as the child reacts to the stress of beginning school.

During the early school years, many children enjoy a quiet talk or a reading time at bedtime. At about age 9, when friends become more important, children generally are ready to give up nighttime talks with parents. Some parents react strongly to this change and feel rejected. They may need some help to take at face value their child's statement, "I'm tired. I'd rather go to sleep."

Exercise

School-age children need daily exercise. Although they go to school all day, they do not automatically receive daily exercise. School is basically a sit-down activity. Children who are bused to and from school may therefore return home without having spent much time in active exercise.

Exercise need not involve organized sports. It can come from neighborhood games, walking with parents, or from bicycle riding. As children enter preadolescence, those with poor coordination may become reluctant to exercise. They should be stimulated to participate in some daily exercise, or else obesity, which is a preteen problem, can result.

Hygiene

Children of 6 or 7 years of age still need help in regulating bath water temperature and in cleaning ears and fingernails. By age 8, children are generally capable of bathing themselves, but may not do it well because they are too busy to take the time or because they do not find bathing as important as their parents do.

Both boys and girls become interested in showering as they approach their teens. This can be encouraged as perspiration increases with puberty along with sebaceous gland activity. When girls begin to menstruate, they may be afraid to take baths or wash their hair during their period if they have heard stories that this is not safe. They need information on the importance and safety of good hygiene during their menses. Boys who are uncircumcised may develop inflammation under the foreskin from increased secretions, if they do not wash regularly.

Care of Teeth

With proper dental care, the average child today can expect to grow up cavity free. To ensure that this happens, school-age children should visit a dentist at least twice yearly for a checkup, cleaning, and possibly a fluoride treatment to strengthen and harden the tooth enamel (Figure 11-8). Some children develop a fear of dentists and, if the dentist hurts them, want to avoid going at all. The advantage of frequent visits is that if cavities are filled when they are small, the drilling required is minimal and little pain is involved. If cavities are not treated promptly in this way but are allowed to grow large, the drilling hurts, causing these children to refuse to go back to the dentist. More large cavities then grow, and a vicious circle develops. Pedodontists specialize in caring for children's teeth and understand the developmental level of their patients. Children who tend to develop caries might be encouraged to visit a pedodontist if one is available and affordable.

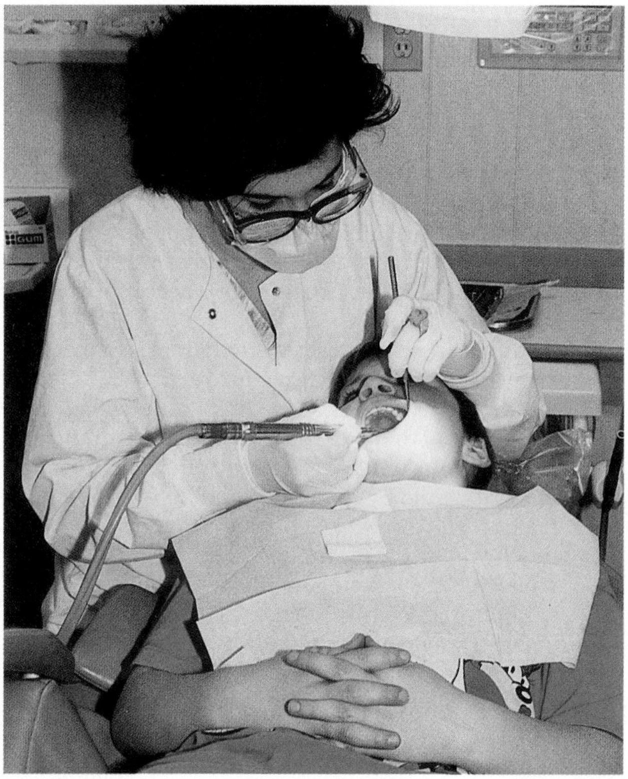

FIGURE 11.8 Dental caries are the number-one health problem in school-age children. Children need to be taught dental health measures and encouraged to visit a dentist twice a year.

School-age children have to be reminded to brush their teeth daily. If brushing becomes an area of conflict for the family, brushing well once a day may be more effective than brushing more often but doing an inadequate job. For effective brushing, the child should use a soft toothbrush, fluoride-based toothpaste, and dental floss to clean between teeth to help remove all plaque with each brushing.

Between-meal snacks are best limited to high-protein foods such as chicken and cheese, rather than snacks such as candy. Fruits, vegetables, and cereals, which are fortified with minerals and vitamins, can all be fun after-school snacks for this age group. If the child does eat candy, a type that is eaten quickly and dissolves quickly, such as a plain chocolate bar, is better than slowly dissolving or sticky candy, which stays in contact with the teeth longer.

Promoting Healthy Family Functioning

At 6 years of age, most children have passed through a preschool phase of attraction for the parent of the opposite sex and identify again with the parent of the same sex (Freud, 1962). Children from one-parent homes, or those with a parent who has difficulty being a good role model, may need help in finding a suitable adult to serve as this important person in their life.

To their parents' annoyance, many children often quote their teacher as the final authority on all subjects.

This may be the first time the parents see someone surpassing them in their child's eyes, and accepting the situation can be painful. Children also cite their friends as guides for behavior: "Mary Jane doesn't have to go to bed until 10 o'clock," or "Billy's mother lets him go to the movies every Saturday." Parents may require help to realize that these remarks are a normal consequence of being exposed to other adults and children. A simple "There are all kinds of ways of doing things, but in our house, the rule is this" shows no criticism of Billy's or Mary Jane's or Miss Smith's way of life, yet conveys a special "our house" feeling and offers security to the child.

Parents often must be reminded that even the simplest tasks of everyday life require repeated practice before they can be accomplished well, and that good manners and grammar are not instinctive and must be learned in the same way as other tasks. The way parents correct children as they learn simple tasks can influence the childrens' opinions of themselves and their ability to continue learning new tasks. "Putting all the silverware in a pile is one way of putting them away; another way would be to divide spoons, forks, and knives separately" is always preferable to "What a silly way to put away silverware!" Comments such as "Can't you do anything right?" or "Why don't you ever do what I say?" should always be avoided, because children will rise only to the level expected of them. A child who is constantly told that he or she is stupid or thoughtless, bad or ill behaved may begin to act that way to conform to the parents' expectations.

If parents have difficulty telling what a child's completed project is supposed to be, the time-honored "Tell me about it" is preferable to "What is it?" It is good for parents to find a redeeming characteristic in a project, no matter how shakily put together it is: "I like the bright color you painted it" or "That must have been fun to make" does this. Actively displaying and using their gifts are part of having school-age children in a family. A finger painting hung on the refrigerator door will enhance, not detract from, the most elegant home. The best-dressed woman looks even more radiant wearing her child's necklace made of macaroni on a string. Both examples are gestures of love, a gesture that goes well with everything.

In talking to parents of school-age children, the following are good questions for you to ask to estimate the degree of interaction that occurs in the home and whether the parents are strengthening the child's sense of accomplishment:

- How do you correct John when he does something such as show poor manners at the table? ("It looks better to swallow food before you talk" or "Don't you ever do anything right? Swallow before you talk.")
- Do you hang up his drawings?
- Does he have chores that are his to accomplish?

CHECKPOINT QUESTIONS

9. A type A school lunch supplies what portion of a child's RDA?
10. If children attend school every day, do they need additional exercise?

Common Health Problems of the School-Age Period

Children in their early school years have one of the lowest rates of death and serious illness of any age group. The two leading causes of death that do occur are accidents and cancer. Minor illnesses are largely due to dental caries, gastrointestinal disturbances, and respiratory disorders, usually of an infectious origin.

Table 11-3 shows the usual health maintenance pattern for these children. Table 11-4 lists problems that parents may have in evaluating illness in the school-age child. Many communities are establishing school-based community health care clinics to improve the health care available for school-age children.

Dental Caries

Caries (cavities) are progressive, destructive lesions or decalcification of the tooth enamel and dentine. When the pH of the tooth surface drops to 5.6 or below (which happens after children eat readily fermented carbohydrates, such as sucrose), acid microorganisms (acidogenic lactobacilli and aciduric streptococci) found in dental plaque attack the organic cementing medium of teeth and destroy it. Plaque tends to accumulate in deep grooves of the teeth and contact areas between teeth, making these areas most susceptible to dental decay. The enamel on primary teeth is thinner than on permanent teeth, making them more susceptible to destruction. The distance from the enamel to the pulp is shorter also, so destruction of the tooth nerve can occur quickly. Neglected caries result in poor chewing and, therefore, poor digestion, abscess and pain, and, sometimes, osteomyelitis (bone infection).

As stated earlier, dental caries are largely preventable with proper brushing and use of fluoridated water or fluoride application. When caries do occur, it is important that they be treated quickly and that the child's dental hygiene practices are evaluated and improved, if that is deemed necessary. Most important, the child must believe that he has a stake in the health or disease of his teeth, so he willingly undertakes the self-care measures necessary to ensure healthy teeth, with parental support rather than parental command.

Malocclusion

The upper jaw in children matures rapidly in early childhood along with skull growth; the lower jaw forms more slowly, which forces teeth to make a prolonged series of changes until they reach their final adult alignment and position. Good tooth occlusion, in which the upper teeth overlap the lower teeth by a small amount and teeth are evenly spaced and in good alignment, is necessary for optimum formation of teeth, health of the supporting tissue, optimum speech development, and what most people view as a pleasant physical appearance for high self-esteem. **Malocclusion** (a deviation from the normal) may be congenital and related to conditions such as cleft palate, a small lower jaw, or familial traits tending toward malocclusion. The condition can result from constant

TABLE 11.3 Health Maintenance Schedule, School-Age Period

AREA OF FOCUS	METHODS	FREQUENCY
Assessment		
Developmental milestones	History, observation	Every visit
Growth milestones	Height, weight plotted on standard growth chart; physical examination	Every visit
Hypertension	Blood pressure	Every visit
Nutrition	History, observation; height/weight information	Every visit
Parent–child relationship	History, observation	Every visit
Behavior or school problems	History, observation	Every visit
Vision and hearing disorders	History, observation	Every visit
	Formal Snellen or Titmus testing	At 7–8 yr and 10–12 yr
	Audiometer testing	At 6 yr and 10–12 yr
Dental health	History, physical examination	Every visit
Scoliosis	Physical examination	Yearly after age 8 yr
Thyroid	Physical examination, history	Every visit after age 10 yr
Tuberculosis	Tine test	Depending on prevalence of tuberculosis in community
Bacteriuria	Clean-catch urine	At 6–7 and 10–12 yr
Anemia	Hematocrit	At 11–12 yr
Immunizations		
Rubeola, mumps, and rubella	Check history and past records; inform caregiver about any risks and side-effects; administer immunization in accordance with health care agency policies.	At 12 yr
Hepatitis B		At 11–12 yr or in older adolescence, if not administered in infancy or three injections were not completed.
Td		At 11–12 yr if at least 5 yr have elapsed since last DTP, DTaP, DT
Varicella		At any age after 1 yr if not previously immunized or at 11–12 yr if lacking reliable history of chickenpox
Anticipatory Guidance		
School-age care	Active listening and health teaching	Every visit
Expected growth and developmental milestones before next visit	Active listening and health teaching	Every visit
Accident prevention	Counseling about street and personal safety	Every visit
Problem Solving		
Any problems expressed by caregiver during course of the visit	Active listening and health teaching regarding cigarette smoking, drug abuse, school adjustment	Every visit

mouth breathing or abnormal tongue position (tongue thrusting). Thumb sucking appears to have little role in malocclusion as long as the thumb sucking does not persist past the time of eruption of the permanent front teeth (6 to 7 years). The loss of teeth due to extraction or accident may lead to malocclusion if not properly treated to maintain alignment.

Malocclusion may be either crossbite (sideways) or anterior or posterior. Children with a malocclusion should be evaluated by an orthodontist to see if braces or other orthodontic work is necessary. The time to begin correction varies with the extent of the malocclusion and the jaw size. Teeth braces are not only expensive, but they also cause pain for children when they are first applied and at periodic visits when they are tightened to maintain pressure for further straightening. Some children develop mild, shallow ulcerations (canker sores) of the buccal membrane from friction of a metal wire. Rubbing the offending wire with dental wax dulls the surface and gives relief. Ora-Jel (an over-the-counter drug) rubbed on the ulceration also gives relief. Children who wear braces need to have their teeth assessed frequently to see that they are

TABLE 11.4 Parental Difficulties Evaluating Illness in the School-Age Child

DIFFICULTY	HELPFUL SUGGESTIONS FOR PARENTS
Evaluating seriousness of illness	For the first time, a school-age child may view illness as a way to avoid unpleasant activities (school, a coach who asks too much, household chores). Evaluating whether the child has symptoms when he is asked to do something he likes to do often reveals the difference between exaggeration and an ill child (too sick to eat spinach, not too sick to eat ice cream; too sick to go to school, not too sick to go ice skating). If the child uses symptoms of illness as a means of avoiding situations, parents must evaluate what it is that the child wants so badly to avoid and see if some change should be made in expectations.
Evaluating nutritional intake	Many school-age children eat lunch at school; they may spend weekends away from home and weeks away at camp. As with all ages, noting whether they are growing and active is better than monitoring any one day's food intake.
Evaluating puberty changes	There is a wide variation in the time that secondary sex characteristics occur (9–17 yr for girls; 10–18 yr for boys). Children should be examined if and when they or their parents are concerned that pubertal changes are delayed.
Age-specific diseases to be aware of	School age is a time to evaluate vision; children normally develop vision changes as maturity of the eye globe increases. Squinting, rubbing eyes, or poor marks in school may be signs of poor vision. Streptococcal sore throats occur with a high frequency in early-school-age children. Those with sore throats should be examined by a health care provider to prevent complications, such as glomerulonephritis or rheumatic fever, from developing. Girls, in particular, must be evaluated for scoliosis (curvature of the spine). Parents detect this by noticing that the girl's skirts hang unevenly or bra straps are uneven. Parents may need to be cautioned that vomiting or headache in the morning that passes fairly quickly (at about the same time the school bus leaves) may be a symptom of school phobia, but physical examination is in order because these are also symptoms of other conditions. Absence seizures, a neurologic condition that typically arises in school-age years, can be confused with behavior problems if observation is not thorough. Attention deficit disorder (see Chapter 54) can also lead to behavior or inattention disorders.

brushing properly around the braces (a Water Pik is often recommended for thorough cleaning) and that they are using dental floss to remove plaque from around wires.

After the removal of braces, many children must wear retainers to maintain the correction the braces achieved. Although braces are wired into place, retainers are not. Wearing a retainer can prove troublesome for the child, because it must be removed when eating (e.g., in the school cafeteria or in a restaurant). Show appropriate sympathy and help the child problem solve if he or she is bothered by the appearance of braces or wearing a retainer. For instance, if removing the retainer in front of friends is truly embarrassing for the child, perhaps he or she could remove the retainer in the bathroom before going to the cafeteria each day. Braces and retainers have become a common feature of life for children of school age. Most children will find some comfort in not being the only one to suffer this indignity and, once used to their own appliances, will experience little reluctance in letting their classmates see them.

Concerns and Problems of the School-Age Period

One of the most important disorders of the school age period is attention deficit disorder (ADD) because it interferes so dramatically with school progress. This is discussed in Chapter 34. Focus on Nursing Research cites some concerns of preadolescents.

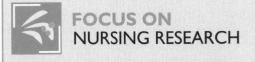

FOCUS ON NURSING RESEARCH

What Are the Concerns of Preadolescents?

To answer this question, four focus groups of 9- to 12-year-old African-American and Hispanic girls were organized and queried about their feelings regarding puberty and the transition to adolescence. Among the factors these girls named as being appealing about growing up were increasing independence from parents, widening social relations with same- and opposite-sex friends, and an increase in decision making regarding clothes and activities. Things they did not like were an increase in peer pressure, high parental expectations, and having to take more responsibility for their own actions at home and school.

This is an important study for nurses because it documents that the prepubertal period is a stressful time. It can alert health care providers to be aware that some children will need counseling because of the stress of the period.

Doswell, W. M., & Vandestienne, G. (1996). The use of focus groups to examine pubertal concerns in preteen girls: initial findings and implications for practice and research. *Issues in Comprehensive Pediatric Nursing, 19*(2), 103–120.

NURSING DIAGNOSES AND RELATED INTERVENTIONS

Nursing Diagnosis: Parental anxiety related to behavior of school-age child

Outcome Identification: Parent will voice that he feels less anxious by next health supervision visit.

Outcome Evaluation: Parent states that undesired behavior has decreased in frequency; parent feels less stress about child's health or future.

Problems Associated With Language Development

The common speech problem of the preschool years is broken fluency. The most common problem of the school-age child is articulation. The child has difficulty pronouncing *s, z, th, l, r,* and *w* or substitutes *w* for *r* ("west" instead of "rest") or *r* for *l* ("radies" instead of "ladies"). This is most noticeable during the first and second grades; it usually disappears by the third grade. Speech therapy for this normal developmental stage is not necessary.

Common Fears and Anxieties of the School-Age Child

Anxiety Related to Beginning School. Adjusting to grade school is a big task for a 6-year-old child. Even if he or she attended preschool, this is different. The rules are firmer, and the elective feeling ("If he doesn't like it, we'll take him out of it") is gone. School is for keeps until age 16 or longer, a time span that is difficult for the child to imagine. Whereas preschool learning was carried out through fun activities, part of every day in grade school involves obvious work (see the Nursing Care Plan).

Because school is an adjustment, a health assessment of all school-age children should include an inquiry about progress in school. You can obtain information by asking the parent, "How is Susan doing in school?" followed by a second question, "How does her teacher say she is doing?" If there is a discrepancy between the answers, the situation bears study. The answer to the first question reveals the parent's attitude toward the child's progress. The answer to the second may indicate that the child is having trouble adjusting to a structured school environment. Some parents have to alter their expectations to conform with their child's actual ability. This can be difficult.

One of the biggest tasks of the first year of school is learning to read. It is best if parents have prepared their child for this by reading to him since infancy, pointing to the words and pictures as they went along. This helps children to realize that sentences flow from left to right and that the words, not the pictures, tell the story. Empowering the Family offers some useful hints to help parents encourage reading in their young school-age child.

Many first-grade children are capable of mature action at school but appear less mature when they return home. Their pseudo-sophistication of the day is gone. They may bite their nails, suck their thumb, or talk baby talk. Some develop tics (irregular movements of isolated muscle groups), such as:

- Wrinkling the forehead
- Shrugging the shoulders
- Twisting the mouth
- Coughing
- Clearing the throat
- Frequently blinking or rolling the eyes

Such movements may occasionally be confused with seizure activity. Tics, however, disappear during sleep and occur mainly when the child is subjected to stress or anxiety. Scolding, nagging, threatening, or punishing does not stop either tics or nail biting; it invariably makes these problems worse. Methods such as using bad-flavored clear nail polish and restraining the child's hands to prevent nail biting are also ineffective.

To stop these behaviors, the underlying stress should be discovered and alleviated. Urge parents to spend some time with the child after school or in the evening, so he or she continues to feel secure in the family and does not feel pushed out by being sent to school. If such behavior manifestations persist despite attempts to eliminate their cause, the child may need to be referred for counseling.

School Phobia. *School phobia* is fear of attending school. It is a type of "social phobia" similar to agoraphobia (fear of going outside the home). Children who resist attending school this way may develop physical signs of illness, such as vomiting, diarrhea, headache, or abdominal pain on school days. This lasts until after the school bus has left or the child is allowed to stay home for the day. The cause of resistance to school must be determined before it can be cured. In some instances, it may be fear of separation from the parents. The child may be overdependent on the parents or may be reluctant to leave home because he or she feels that younger siblings will usurp the parents' affection while he or she is at school. The anxiety of separation may also result because the parent is overprotective of the child.

The child may also be reacting to a particular teacher or to a particular situation, such as a test or having to shower in gym class. If this is so, the parents should investigate the matter. The child's fear may be well grounded. Counseling may help the child accept the situation. If not, parents should attempt to have the child transferred to another classroom or perhaps excused from a disliked situation such as showering. Because the problem of school phobia is usually only partly the child's, the entire family generally requires counseling to resolve the issue. As a rule, the child should continue to attend school once it has been established that he or she is free of any illness that would prevent this. Firmness on the part of parents should prevent the development of problems such as school failure, peer ridicule, or a pattern of avoiding difficulties. The child may benefit from a drug such as citalopram to reduce panic attacks (Lepola et al, 1996) and a gradual program of school involvement, such as walking to school but not going in, then going to school but staying for only 1 hour, staying for half a day, and so on, until he or she can stay all day every day. Parents should treat the illness matter of factly (a great deal of reassurance that these symptoms are not major will be necessary) and take him or her firmly to the bus or to the classroom.

Nursing Care Plan

THE SCHOOL-AGED CHILD STARTING KINDERGARTEN

A 6-year-old girl is brought to the clinic for a checkup in preparation for starting school in the fall.

Assessment: 6-year-old female within normal limits for height, weight, and development. Currently attending afternoon nursery school 5 days a week. Her mother states, "She's been attending this school for the last 2 years. In the fall, she'll be going to a new school for a full day." Child observed to be restless in chair during conversation with mother about the new school. When asked, child says, "I don't want to go to a new school. I want to stay in my old school with all my friends."

Nursing Diagnosis: Anxiety related to beginning a new school in the fall

Outcome Identification: The child will exhibit signs of increased comfort about new school experience.

Outcome Evaluation: Child verbalizes positive statements about new school; voices desire to visit school and meet teachers; exhibits age-appropriate coping behaviors.

Interventions	Rationale
1. Assess the child for her thoughts and feelings about current nursery school routine, including teachers, friends, and activities.	1. Assessment provides information about the child's school experience and possible clues for the child's anxiety, providing a baseline for future strategies and teaching.
2. Explore with the child's mother her views on the child's experiences in her current school and expectations for the new school.	2. Exploration with the mother provides additional clues to understanding the child's anxieties and serves as a means for identifying possible stressors that may be impacting on the child.
3. Talk with the child about what she thinks the new school will be like, acknowledging her anxieties and providing feedback to clarify any misconceptions.	3. Talking with the child allows her to share feelings and concerns openly and safely, possibly increasing the child's awareness of them and their impact on her. Acknowledging the child's anxiety validates her feelings. Providing feedback helps to correct any misinformation.
4. Encourage the mother to contact the school district to arrange for a visit to the school with her daughter.	4. Visiting the school provides the child with exposure to the new environment, preparing her for the actual experience.
5. Have the mother arrange for a follow-up visit to the school with her daughter to meet the teachers and spend time observing and being part of the classroom experience.	5. Follow-up visit and spending time with the teachers and class allows the child to actively participate in the experience, helping to alleviate feelings of the unknown and to increase feelings of control.
6. Urge the mother to contact the parents of another child who is currently attending the school to act as the daughter's "buddy."	6. Having a buddy helps to minimize the feelings of isolation and loneliness.
7. Arrange for a follow-up clinic appointment within 1 month with the mother and daughter.	7. A return visit aids in evaluating the child's level of anxiety and in determining the effectiveness of the suggestions.

Handling school phobia requires coordination among the school, school nurse, and health care provider who diagnoses the problem. A nurse is the ideal person to coordinate such efforts and to help the parents allow the child some independence not only in going to school but in other activities. Counseling may be necessary to help parents realize that this is partly their problem and that they need to allow the child to develop some independence. A few children require psychiatric therapy to resolve their difficulties with school.

EMPOWERING THE FAMILY: Tips to Help Make Reading More Enjoyable for Your Child

- Set an example by being seen reading, so your child associates learning to read with adult activity. If you spend most of your free time watching television, your child will think reading is mainly for children and assume that it is not important.
- Make reading more fun by encouraging the practical use of reading. Ask your child to read recipes while you cook or to read road signs during a car trip.
- Play a treasure hunt game in which you hide a small object, such as a favorite toy, then write simple clues on slips of paper—"Look under a lamp," then, under the lamp, "Look in a book," and so on until your child has been led to the hidden object. Such games help your child see reading as an important means of obtaining information. Your child can develop writing skills by playing the same game for you to follow.

Latchkey Children

Latchkey children are school children who are without adult supervision for a part of each weekday. The term alludes to the fact that they generally carry a key so they can let themselves into their home after school.

Latchkey children have become a prominent concern because in as many as 90% of families today, both parents work at least part-time outside the home. Few parents have work hours so flexible that they can always be at home when the child leaves for or returns from school. Extended family members who once watched children after school are often working as well or may no longer be close at hand; many communities are no longer close-knit enough to have neighbors who can be depended on to help out with informal child care.

A major concern is that latchkey children can feel lonely and have an increased tendency to have accidents, delinquent behavior, and decreased school performance from lack of homework supervision. They are also more prone to alcohol and beginning drug use (Mulhall et al, 1996). For those children who feel safe in their community, however, a short period of independence every day may actually be beneficial, because it encourages problem solving in self-care.

A number of helpful suggestions for parents whose children must spend time alone before or after school are shown in Box 11-2. Many communities offer special after-school programs for such children. Nurses are in a position to educate parents about such services so their children can feel both safe and stimulated creatively during this time. Boy Scouts of America and the Council of Campfire Girls are examples of organizations that offer programs to help children adjust to being home alone. Many communities are organizing hotline numbers that a child who is alone can call if a problem arises. At health visits, assess whether parents or the child appears to have a problem with, or is uncomfortable about, after-school arrangements. For the child who is extremely fearful or impulsive or who finds problem solving difficult, time alone after school may not be appropriate. Determine the individual circumstances, and recommend changes when possible.

✓ CHECKPOINT QUESTIONS

11. If children eat candy, what is the best type for them to eat in terms of preventing caries?
12. Should children with school (social) phobia be encouraged to attend school?

Sex Education

It is important that school-age children be educated about pubertal changes and responsible sexual practices (McGrory, 1995). Preteenagers should have adults they can turn to for answers to questions about sex. Ideally, this should be their parents, but because sex is an emotionally charged topic, some parents may be extremely uncomfortable discussing it with their children. As a result, health care personnel often become resource persons for this (Swenson et al, 1995).

The American Academy of Pediatrics recommends that sex education be incorporated into health education throughout the school years in a manner that is appropriate to age and development (AAP, 1990). Topics to teach and discuss in a sex education course for both preadolescent boys and girls include:

- Reproductive organ function
- Secondary sexual characteristics so children will know what is going on in their bodies
- Physiology of reproduction so they understand what menstruation is and why it occurs
- Male sexual functioning, including why the production of increased amounts of seminal fluid leads to nocturnal emissions
- Explanation of the physiology of pregnancy and the possibility that comes with sexual maturity for starting unplanned or unwanted pregnancies
- Birth control measures and the principles of safer sex
- Social and moral implications of sexual maturity

A sex education course that includes films and discussions is helpful but never answers all of a preteen's questions. (Most youngsters would rather avoid asking a ques-

BOX 11.2

TIPS FOR LATCHKEY CHILDREN AND PARENTS

Safety Teaching for the Child

Always to lock doors and never to show keys to others or indicate that he or she stays home alone.

To answer the telephone and say a parent is busy, not absent from home.

What to do in event he or she loses key (stay with a neighbor, etc.).

Not to go into the house if the door is open or a window is broken.

Fire safety (practice a fire drill from all rooms of the house).

To check in with parents by telephone when he or she first arrives home from school.

To identify a caller before opening the door. Agree on a secret code word; child should not open the door or go with a person unless the person knows the word.

How to change light bulbs safely if it will be dark before parents return home. If appropriate, teach child how to change fuses or reset circuit-breaker switches.

How to report a fire and telephone police (practice this with the child).

Safety Responsibilities of Parents

Prepare a safety kit and keep it filled; include a flashlight in case of a power failure so the child does not need to light candles.

Plan after-school snacks that do not require cooking to prevent burns.

Keep firearms locked with the key in a place unknown to child. Instruct in firearm safety.

Keep a list of emergency telephone numbers (including parents' work numbers) by the telephone.

Arrange with a neighbor who is usually home during the late afternoon for the child to stay there in an emergency.

If an older child will be watching a younger one, be certain both children understand the rules laid down and the degree of responsibility expected.

Be certain the child understands that rules that apply during other times (never swim alone; do not play by the railroad tracks) also apply during independent time.

Parental Actions to Prevent Loneliness

Urge the child to telephone either parent every day to touch base (be sure the child has work telephone numbers).

Be certain to make additional time available at home after work so the child is able to describe his or her day.

Each morning help the child plan an activity for that day so he or she has something purposeful to look forward to during time alone.

Allow special privileges such as listening to music that other members of the family do not like as well; allow extra television hours during this time.

Consider a pet. Even a caged animal, such as a hamster or a bird, offers companionship in a quiet house.

Call the child if there will be a delay in arriving home; unexpected time alone is very frightening to a child.

Leave messages on the refrigerator or in the bathroom that just say hi.

Leave a tape or video recorded message for the child to play (make sure it is not full of tasks to do, but is a welcoming message).

Encourage the child to read; fictional characters serve as friends as well as help to pass time.

Urge the child to network with other latchkey children as to how they use time effectively; talking on the telephone to another child reduces loneliness for both.

Parental Actions to Increase Socialization

Help the child plan after-school activities such as joining a science club for one afternoon a week.

Explore sports programs at school or in the community, as these often are held after school.

Explore latchkey groups at the school the child attends, a public library, or a church.

Network with other parents (nurse can help) or ask for flex time so child supervision can be alternated after school.

Be sure the child socializes with friends on weekends or on days when either parent is home.

Parental Actions to Increase Self-Esteem

Praise the child for the ability to take care of himself or herself for short time intervals (rather than scold that there are cracker crumbs on the carpet).

Walk with the child through the empty house and together identify sounds (the click of the furnace turning on, the refrigerator starting to defrost, etc.), so he or she can problem solve the cause of sounds when home alone.

Help the child to view quiet time as beneficial time in which he or she can do some things more efficiently than at noisy times (e.g., homework).

Do not allow child to use the latchkey role to provoke parental guilt. Allow the child to have some say in family spending and thus see how his or her time alone (which allows both parents to work) contributes to family unity and progress.

American Academy of Pediatrics, Committee on Injury and Poison Prevention. (1995b). Skateboard injuries. *Pediatrics 95*(4), 611.

Coppens, N. M., & Koziara, D. M. (1997). Children's perceptions concerning school injuries. *Journal of School Nursing, 13*(3), 14.

Cunningham, F. G. et al. (1997). *Williams obstetrics* (20th ed.). Norwalk, CT: Appleton & Lange.

Department of Health and Human Services. (1995). *Healthy people 2000: midcourse review.* Washington, DC: DHHS.

Doswell, W. M., & Vandestienne, G. (1996). The use of focus groups to examine pubertal concerns in preteen girls: initial findings and implications for practice and research. *Issues in Comprehensive Pediatric Nursing, 19*(2), 103.

Dwyer, J. T. (1995). Dietary fiber for children: how much? *Pediatrics, 96*(5.2), 1019.

Erikson, E. H. (1986). *Childhood and society.* New York: W. W. Norton.

Freud, S. (1962). *Three essays on the theory of sexuality.* New York: Hearst Corporation.

Johnson, E. O., et al. (1995). Inhalants to heroin; a prospective analysis from adolescence to adulthood. *Drug and Alcohol Dependence, 40*(2), 159.

Kohlberg, L. (1981). *The philosophy of moral development: moral stages and the idea of justice.* New York: Harper & Row.

Lepola, U., et al. (1996). Citalopram in the treatment of early-onset panic disorder and school phobia. *Pharmacopsychiatry, 29*(1), 30.

MacDonald, A. (1997). Know your vitamins and minerals. *Nursing Times, 93*(21), 72.

McGrory, A. (1995). Education for the menarche. *Pediatric Nursing, 21*(5), 439.

Mulhall, P. F., Stone, D., & Stone, B. (1996). Home alone: is it a risk factor for middle school youth and drug use? *Journal of Drug Education, 26*(1), 39.

Nathan, I., et al. (1996). The dietary intake of a group of vegetarian children aged 7-11 years compared with matched omnivores. *British Journal of Nutrition, 75*(4), 533.

Neumark-Sztainer, D., et al. (1997). Adolescent vegetarians: a behavioral profile of a school-based population in Minnesota. *Archives of Pediatrics and Adolescent Medicine, 151*(8), 833.

Piaget, J., & Infelder, B. (1969). *The psychology of the child.* New York: Basic Books.

Roberts, A. (1996). Systems of life: hormones and sexual puberty. *Nursing Times, 92*(11), 35.

Swenson, I. E., Foster, B., & Assay, M. (1995). Menstruation, menarche, and sexuality in the public school curriculum; school nurses' perceptions. *Adolescence, 30*(119), 677.

Westhoff, W. W. et al. (1996). Acquisition of high-risk behaviors by African-American, Latino and Caucasian middle-school students. *Psychological Reports, 79*(3.1), 787.

Yarnold, B. M. (1996). Use of inhalants among Miami's public school students, 1992. *Psychological Reports, 79*(3.2), 1155.

SUGGESTED READINGS

Chiocca, E. M. (1998). Language development in bilingual children. *Pediatric Nursing, 24*(1), 43.

Dashiff, C. J., & Buchanan, L. A. (1995). Menstrual attitudes among black and white premenarcheal girls. *Journal of Child and Adolescent Psychiatric Nursing, 8*(3), 5.

Flakierska-Praquin, N., et al. (1997). School phobia with separation anxiety disorder: a comparative 20 to 29 year follow-up study of 35 school refusers. *Comprehensive Psychiatry, 38*(1), 17.

Holaday, B., et al. (1994). Chronically ill latch key children. *Clinical Pediatrics, 33*(5), 303.

Hockenberry-Eaton, M., et al. (1996). Mother and adolescent knowledge of sexual development: the effects of gender, age, and sexual experience. *Adolescence, 31*(121), 35.

McConnochie, K. M., et al. (1997). Ensuring high-quality alternatives while ending pediatric inpatient care as we know it. *Archives of Pediatrics and Adolescent Medicine, 151*(4), 341.

Roberts, A. (1996). Systems of life: abnormalities of puberty. *Nursing Times, 92*(15), 31.

Simko, L. C. (1997). Water fluoridation: time to reexamine the issue. *Pediatric Nursing, 23*(2), 155.

Whitener, L. M. et al. (1998). Use of theory to guide nurses in the design of health messages for children. *ANS: Advances in Nursing Science, 20*(3), 21.

The Family With an Adolescent

12

CHAPTER

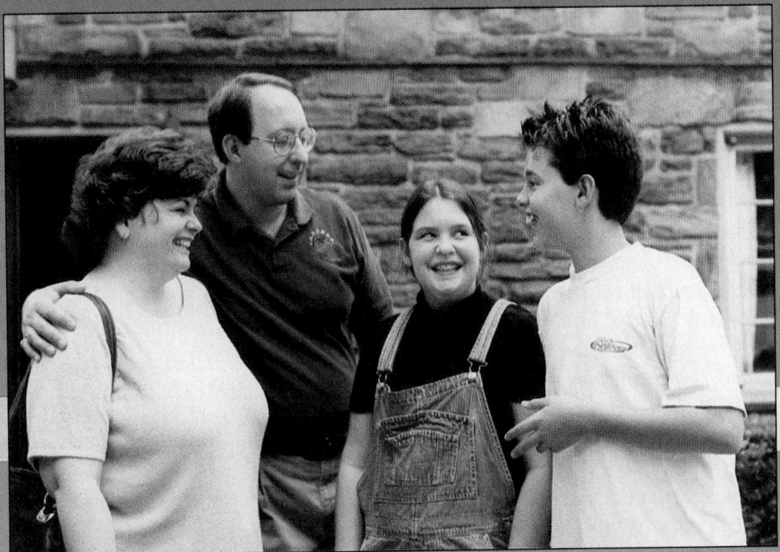

Key Terms

- abstinence
- adolescence
- androgenic hormones
- adrenarche
- comedones
- contraceptive
- elective termination of pregnancy
- emancipated minor
- formal operations
- glycogen loading
- identity
- menarche
- menstrual cycle
- puberty
- reproductive life planning
- role confusion
- sexuality
- substance abuse
- thelarche

Objectives

After mastering the contents of this chapter, you should be able to:

1. Describe the normal growth and development pattern and common parental concerns of the adolescent period.
2. Assess adolescents for normal growth and development milestones.
3. Formulate nursing diagnoses for the family of an adolescent.
4. Identify appropriate outcomes based on health assessment findings.
5. Plan nursing care related to growth and development concerns of the adolescent, such as planning health teaching necessary to accept pubertal changes.
6. Implement nursing care related to growth and development or special needs of the adolescent, such as organizing a discussion group on ways to prevent drug abuse.
7. Evaluate outcome criteria to be certain that nursing goals were achieved.
8. Identify National Health Goals related to the adolescent that nurses could be instrumental in helping the nation to achieve.
9. Identify areas related to care of adolescents that could benefit from additional nursing research.
10. Use critical thinking to analyze ways in which care of the adolescent could be more family centered.
11. Integrate knowledge of adolescent growth and development with nursing process to achieve quality child health nursing care.

Raul is a 16-year-old boy you see at an adolescent clinic. His chief concern is a head cold. His parents tell you Raul seemed depressed for a long time after he lost a girlfriend but now seems happy again. They are pleased because he recently gave away his collection of baseball cards to a young neighbor. They see this as a sign he is maturing. You mention to Raul that a decongestant would probably make him feel better. He asks you how many pills it would take to kill someone, then jokes that he was kidding. His parents tell you Raul has been joking about killing himself a lot lately.

The physician in the clinic prescribes a decongestant and suggests Raul return in 6 months. Did Raul have some needs that were not met by his clinic?

In the previous chapter, you learned about the school-age child and the capabilities children develop during that time period. In this chapter, you'll add to your knowledge base information about the changes, both physical and psychosocial, that occur during the adolescent years. This is important information because it builds a base for care and health teaching for the age group.

After you've studied the chapter, turn to the Critical Thinking Exercises at the end of the chapter to sharpen your skills and test your knowledge.

Adolescence is the time period between 13 years and 18 to 20 years, which serves as a transition period between childhood and adulthood. It can be divided into an early period (13 to 14 years), a middle period (15 to 16 years), and a late period (17 to 20 years). However, adolescence is defined not so much by chronologic age as by physiologic, psychological, and sociologic factors. The drastic change in physical appearance and the change in expectations of others (especially parents) may lead to both emotional and physical health problems.

Adolescents invariably feel a sense of pressure throughout this period. They are mature in some respects but still young in others. For example, the adolescent's sexual interests are awakening, yet personal or parental pressures often discourage sexual exploration. This duality causes a major dilemma for the adolescent leading to many growth and developmental concerns of the age.

Sexuality, in particular, is a major area of concern for adolescents and their families. The nurse who cares for childrearing families can be asked a variety of detailed questions about sexuality. One of the biggest contributions nurses can make is to encourage clients to ask questions about sexual and reproductive functioning. With this attitude, problems of sexuality and reproduction are brought out into the open and made as resolvable as other health concerns or problems.

There is such a strong adolescent subculture today that parents may feel that the minute their child enters the teenage years, all communication stops. Parents may expect difficulty controlling the child or understanding teenage values, as though entering this period locks the adolescent into a shell or pulls down a curtain between child and parents. This can become a self-fulfilling prophecy, whereby the parents actually cause the communication breakdown. At other times, of course, a communication problem can begin when a teenager refuses to respect parents' opinions and stops asking for them. Many of the problems adolescents bring to health care personnel arise from this communication impasse, no matter how it started. They often come to health care facilities with many misconceptions, seeking adult help and guidance. National Health Goals related to adolescence are shown in Focus on National Health Goals.

NURSING PROCESS OVERVIEW

for Healthy Development of the Adolescent

Assessment

Parents rarely bring adolescents for health maintenance visits, and adolescents generally don't come to health care facilities on their own unless they are ill.

FOCUS ON NATIONAL HEALTH GOALS

Health teaching in the adolescent years is important, because healthy habits begun at this time can influence health over a lifetime. For this reason, a number of National Health Goals relate to adolescent health:

- Reduce the proportion of adolescents who have engaged in sexual intercourse to no more than 15% by age 15 from a baseline of 27% of girls and 33% of boys.
- Reduce the number of overweight adolescents to a prevalence of no more than 1.5% among adolescents ages 12 through 19 from a baseline of 15%.
- Reduce smokeless tobacco use by males ages 12 through 24 to a prevalence of no more than 4% from a baseline of 8.9% in males; 6.6% in females.
- Reduce deaths caused by alcohol-related motor vehicle accidents to no more than 18% among people ages 15 to 24 from a baseline of 21.5%.
- Reduce suicide to no more than 8.2 per 100,000 youths ages 15 to 19 from a baseline of 10.3 per 100,000.
- Increase to 30% the proportion of adolescents who exercise regularly from a baseline of 22% (DHHS, 1995).

Nurses can be instrumental in helping the nation achieve these goals by educating adolescents about sexual activity, abstinence and refusal skills, safer sex practices and avoiding cigarettes, smokeless tobacco, alcohol, drug abuse, and violence and by acting as support people for adolescents during times of crisis to help prevent suicide. Areas in which additional knowledge is needed that could benefit from additional nursing research are identifying effective programs that reduce the use of smokeless tobacco or cigarette smoking, documenting the best actions for nurses to take in emergency rooms when adolescents are admitted following rape or suicide attempts, and constructing rapid surveys to identify adolescents who are abusing drugs.

Unless adolescents need a physical examination for athletic clearance, these children are usually not seen for health assessments as often as they were when younger. When adolescents are accompanied by their parents at health visits, it is best to obtain their health history separately from parents to promote independence and responsibility for self-care. When performing physical examinations on adolescents, be aware that they may be very self-conscious. They also need health assurance and appreciate comments such as "Your hair has a nice, healthy feel" or "This is an accessory nipple. Have you ever wondered about it?" (see Focus on Cultural Competence).

Nursing Diagnosis

Frequent nursing diagnoses related to adolescents and their families are:

- Health-seeking behaviors related to normal growth and development
- Self-esteem disturbance related to facial acne
- Anxiety related to concerns about normal growth and development
- Pain related to uterine cramping from menstruation
- Disturbance in body image related to early development of secondary sex characteristics
- Anxiety related to fear of contracting sexually transmitted disease
- Health-seeking behaviors related to responsible sexual practices
- Risk for altered nutrition, less than body requirements related to combined needs of adoloscence and pregnancy
- Risk for injury related to peer pressure to use alcohol and drugs
- Potential for enhanced parenting related to increased knowledge of teenage years

Outcome Identification and Planning

When planning with adolescents, respect the fact that they have a desire to exert independence and do things their own way. They are not likely to adhere to a plan of care that disrupts their lifestyle or makes them appear different from others their age. Including them in planning is essential so that the plan will be accepted. Establishing a contract (i.e., the adolescent agrees to take medication daily) may be the most effective means to reach a goal.

A major part of nursing care in this area is to empower adolescents to feel control over their bodies. Thus, health teaching should be planned to provide the client with knowledge about the reproductive system and specific information about ways to alleviate discomfort or prevent reproductive disease. It may also be important to plan interventions to strengthen a person's gender identity.

The pregnancy rate in adolescents is high. A major problem encountered with the pregnant adolescent during planning is that she may have difficulty accepting the pregnancy. As a result, she may have difficulty pursuing prenatal care.

Adolescents are very present-oriented; a program that provides immediate results, such as focusing on short-term goals such as increased respiratory function, will be carried out well. Conversely, a regimen oriented toward the future, with long-term goals such as preventing hypertension, may not be as successful. This is not to say that it is not important to teach adolescents about the necessity for maintaining a healthy lifestyle—eating well, *not* smoking, and generally taking care of their bodies—but that information should be geared as much as possible to specific, short-term benefits to their health.

Teaching by peers can be an effective way to motivate teens. Organizing peer support groups this way can be a major activity of school nurses.

Implementation

Adolescents do poorly with tasks that someone else tells them they *must* do. If they help to plan tasks, however, they can carry them out successfully and implementation goes smoothly. Adolescents have little patience with adults who do not demonstrate the behavior they are being asked to achieve; a parent or nurse who smokes and asks an adolescent not to smoke may not get very far. Evaluate how an intervention appears from the adolescent's standpoint before initiating instructions.

To help adolescents understand reproductive functioning and sexual health throughout their life, specific teaching might include:

- Explaining to a young boy that nocturnal emissions are normal
- Teaching an adolescent girl what is normal and abnormal in relation to menstrual function
- Teaching an adolescent safer sex practices

Teaching is often enhanced by the use of illustrations from books or journals, clips from videos or compact disks, or models of internal and external reproductive systems. Nursing interventions in this area, however, include much more than education. For example, empathy for a young woman's concern of increased tension before menstruation may help

FOCUS ON CULTURAL COMPETENCE

In the United States, as in most developed countries, adolescence covers a long time span. In developing countries, in contrast, adolescence tends to be much shorter because adolescents must take full-time jobs to help support their families. Socioeconomic factors definitely influence the length of adolescence across all cultures. Recognizing that adolescents may have differing responsibilities and life experiences based on cultural expectations can be useful to the nurse when making an assessment. In a family in which an adolescent is expected to begin working full-time or to marry at an early age, the nurse may need to make a broader health assessment. Factors to consider include occupational hazards or the effects of job, family, and financial stress on the adolescent. Readiness for childbearing is also important.

validate her concern. Role modeling can also be a valuable intervention. Discussing the subject of reproduction in a matter-of-fact way, or treating menstruation as a positive sign of growth, rather than as a burden, may help clients assume a positive attitude about these subjects from the start.

Interventions that strengthen an individual's sense of maleness or femaleness may improve a client's gender identity. For example, a young woman who feels that a female role is to be assertive needs opportunities in her care plan for decision making and self-care; a hospitalized adolescent who views a man's role as being a person who watches Monday night football needs time structured for this activity at the same priority level as other activities. Adolescents who are pregnant need help to enroll in prenatal care and follow healthy recommendations for care and activity during pregnancy.

These organizations address some of the concerns of adolescence and may be of use for possible referral.

- American Association of Suicidology
  2459 S. Ash Street
  Denver, CO 80222
- Partnership for a Drug-Free America
  405 Lexington Avenue
  New York, NY 10174
- Children of Alcoholic Parents
  23425 N. W. Highway
  Southfield, MI 46075
- Planned Parenthood Federation of America, Inc.
  810 Seventh Avenue
  New York, NY 10019
- Sexual Information and Education Council of the United States (SIECUS)
  130 W. 42nd Street, Suite 2500
  New York, NY 10036
- Tough Love
  P. O. Box 1069
  Doylestown, PA 18901

Outcome Evaluation

Evaluation of goals should include not only whether desired outcomes have been achieved but whether adolescents are pleased with their accomplishments. Individuals will have difficulty accomplishing desired goals as adults unless they have high self-esteem that includes feeling secure in body image.

How people, including adolescents, feel about themselves sexually has a great deal to do with how quickly they recover from an illness or even how well motivated they are to do those things necessary to remain well. Evaluating whether goals related to sexuality have been achieved is important in being certain that the person will be able to accomplish activities in other life phases that depend on being sure of sexuality or gender role. The following are examples of outcome criteria that might be established:

- Client states she is able to feel good about herself even though she is the shortest girl in her class.
- Client states he is no longer fearful of contracting a sexually transmitted disease.
- Client states she is better able to control symptoms of premenstrual syndrome.
- Client consistently uses chosen method of contraception.
- Adolescent reports intake of appropriate nutrients during prenatal care in light of frequent meals at fast-food restaurants.
- Client states he has not ingested alcohol for 2 weeks.
- Parents voice that they feel more confident about their ability to parent an adolescent.
- Client states she feels high self-esteem despite persistent facial acne.

NURSING ASSESSMENT OF GROWTH AND DEVELOPMENT OF THE ADOLESCENT

Physical Growth

The major milestones of development in the adolescent period are the onset of puberty and the cessation of body growth. Between these milestones, physiologic growth is rapid and the development of adult coordination is slow. At first, the gain in physical growth is mostly in weight, leading to the stocky, slightly obese appearance of prepubescence; later comes the thin, gangly appearance of late adolescence.

Most girls are 1 to 2 inches (2.4 to 5 cm) taller than boys coming into adolescence and generally stop growing within 3 years from menarche. Thus, those girls who start menstruating at 10 years of age may reach their adult height by age 13.

Boys grow about 4 to 12 inches (10 to 30 cm) in height and gain 15 to 65 lb (7 to 30 kg) during adolescence. Girls grow 2 to 8 inches (5 to 20 cm) in height and gain 15 to 55 lb (7 to 25 kg). Growth stops with closure of the epiphyseal lines of long bones. This occurs at about 16 or 17 years in females and about 18 to 20 years in males.

The increase in body size does not occur in all organ systems at the same rate. For example, the skeletal system grows faster than the muscles, and muscle mass increases more rapidly than heart size. These differences in growth rates lead to lack of coordination and possibly to poor posture. It makes adolescents appear long-legged and awkward during a rapid growth spurt, because their extremities elongate first, followed by trunk growth. Both sexes may lack coordination. The 13-year-old child, for example, typically reaches to pick up a glass of milk at the dinner table and spills it, having reached beyond it because the arm is longer than the child realized.

Because the heart and lungs increase in size more slowly than the rest of the body, blood flow and oxygen supply are reduced. Thus, adolescents may have insufficient energy and become fatigued trying to do the various activities that interest them. Pulse rate and respiratory rate decrease slightly (to 70 bpm and 20 breaths/min, respectively), and blood pressure increases slightly (to 120/70 mm Hg), reaching adult levels by late adolescence. With adulthood, blood pressure becomes slightly higher in males than females because more force is necessary to distribute blood to the larger male body mass.

EMPOWERING THE
Teaching Adolescent

Exercise
It is good to continue moderate exercise
Excessive exercise can cause amenorrhea

Sexual relations
Intercourse is not contraindicated during
blood). Heightened or decreased sexual
menstrual flow.

Activities of daily living
Nothing is contraindicated (many people
harmful).

Pain relief
Any mild analgesic is helpful. Prostagland
pain. Applying local heat can be helpful.

Rest
More rest may be helpful if dysmenorrhea

Nutrition
Many women need iron supplementation
cause dysmenorrhea.

Beginning at age 16, most adolescents wa
jobs to earn money. In addition, such jobs t
persons how to work with others, accept re
and spend money wisely.

When families were larger, each older c
sponsibility for a younger sibling and baby ca
ural activity. With small nuclear families, m
cents have never had the responsibility o
anyone younger than themselves. For their o
that of the children they care for, adolescen
to babysit should learn some basic rules of ch
safety. Many schools or Red Cross organiz
courses in babysitting just for the teenager.

Many adolescents engage in charitable en
ing middle to late adolescence. They learn t
strong and capable enough not only to take c
selves but also to help less fortunate people i
munity. Adolescents do well organizing and
swimming or gym programs for disabled chi
ing and delivering food to older shut-ins, or ra
to purchase equipment for a hospital. High s
may be organized to send money to childre
These activities fulfill the adolescent's need f
interaction with others and are indications
and willingness to accept adult roles.

Emotional Development

Developmental Task: Identity Versus Role Confusion

According to Erikson (1986), the developme
youngsters in early and midadolescence is to f
of **identity**, that is, to decide who they are an

All during adolescence, androgen stimulates sebaceous glands to extreme activity, sometimes resulting in acne, a common adolescent skin problem. The formation of apocrine sweat glands (glands present in the axillae and genital area) occurs shortly after puberty. Apocrine sweat glands produce a strong odor in response to emotional stimulation. Therefore, adolescents begin to notice they must shower or bathe more frequently than they once did in order to be free of body odor.

Teeth

Adolescents gain their second molars at about 13 years of age and their third molars (wisdom teeth) between 18 and 21 years of age. Third molars may erupt as early as 14 to 15 years of age; however, the jaw reaches adult size only toward the end of adolescence. As a result, adolescents whose third molars erupt before the lengthening of the jaw is complete may experience pain and may need these molars extracted because they do not fit their jawline.

CHECKPOINT QUESTIONS

1. Why does growth stop at 16 to 17 years of age?
2. What glands are responsible for adolescent body odor?

Sexual Development

Development of the reproductive organs begins during intrauterine life; full function is initiated at puberty when the hypothalamus synthesizes and releases gonadotropin-releasing factor stimulator (GnRf), which, in turn, triggers the anterior pituitary to form and begin to release follicle-stimulating hormone (FSH) and luteinizing hormone (LH). FSH and LH initiate the production of androgen and estrogen, which, in turn, initiate visible signs of maturity or secondary sex characteristics.

Pubertal Development

Adolescence is the physiologic period between the beginning of puberty and the cessation of bodily growth. **Puberty** is the stage of life at which secondary sex changes begin (Miller, 1997). Girls begin dramatic development and maturation of reproductive organs at approximately age 10 to 13 years; for boys, 12 to 14 years. Although the mechanism that initiates this dramatic change in appearance is not well understood, the hypothalamus under the direction of the central nervous system may serve as a gonadostat or regulation mechanism set to "turn on" gonad functioning at this age. Although not proven, theory is that a girl must reach a critical weight of approximately 95 lb (43 kg) or a critical mass of fat before the hypothalamus is "triggered" to send initial stimulation to the anterior pituitary gland to begin gonadotropic hormone formation. Studies of female athletes and dancers reveal that a lack of fat can delay or halt menstruation (Rice, 1997). The phenomenon of why puberty occurs is even less understood in boys.

The Role of Androgen. Androgenic hormones are the hormones responsible for muscular development, physical growth, and an increase in sebaceous gland secretions that causes typical acne in both boys and girls. In males, androgenic hormones are produced by the adrenal cortex and the testes; in the female, by the adrenal cortex and the ovaries.

The primary androgenic hormone, *testosterone,* is low in males until puberty (approximately age 12 to 14 years). At that time, it rises to influence the development of testes, scrotum, penis, prostate, and seminal vesicles; the appearance of male pubic, axillary, and facial hair; laryngeal enlargement and its accompanying voice change; maturation of spermatozoa; and closure of growth in long bones.

In girls, testosterone influences enlargement of the labia majora and clitoris and formation of axillary and pubic hair. This development of pubic and axillary hair due to androgen stimulation is termed **adrenarche.**

The Role of Estrogen. When triggered at puberty, ovarian follicles in females begin to secrete a high level of the hormone estrogen. This hormone is actually not one substance but three compounds (estrone [E1], estradiol [E2], and estriol [E3]). It can be considered a single substance, however, in terms of action.

The increase in estrogen level in the female at puberty influences the development of the uterus, fallopian tubes, and vagina; typical female fat distribution and hair patterns; breast development, and an end to growth as it closes epiphyseal lines of long bones. The beginning of breast development is termed **thelarche.**

Secondary Sex Characteristics. Secondary sex characteristics, for example, body hair configuration and breast growth, distinguish the sexes from each other but play no direct part in reproduction. The secondary sex characteristics that begin in the late school-age period (see Chapter 11) continue to develop during adolescence. The typical stages of sexual maturation are shown in Table 12-1.

Sexual maturity in males and females is classified according to Tanner stages, named after the original researcher on sexual maturity (Tanner, 1955). Stages of female sexual development are shown in Figure 12-1. Stages of male genital growth are shown in Figure 12-2.

There is wide variation in the times that adolescents move through these developmental stages; however, the sequential order is fairly constant. In girls, pubertal changes typically occur in the order of

1. Growth spurt
2. Increase in the transverse diameter of the pelvis
3. Breast development
4. Growth of pubic hair
5. Onset of menstruation
6. Growth of axillary hair
7. Vaginal secretions

The average age at which **menarche** (the first menstrual period) occurs is 12.5 years (Rice, 1997). It may occur as early as age 9 or as late as age 17, however, and still be within a normal age range. Irregular menstrual periods are the rule rather than the exception for the first year. Menstrual periods do not become regular until ovulation consistently occurs with them (menstruation is not dependent on ovulation), and this does not tend to happen until 1 to 2 years after menarche.

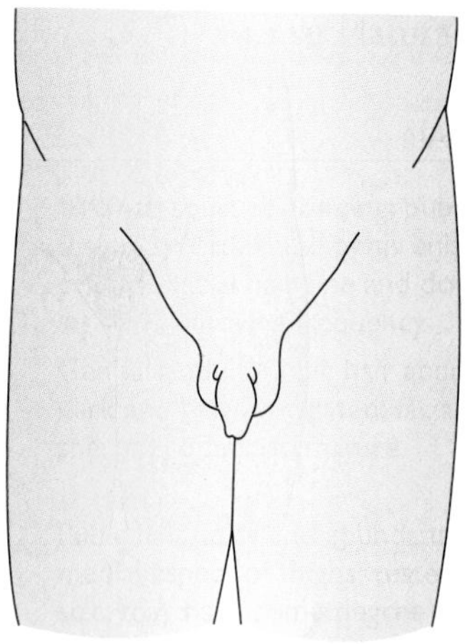

1

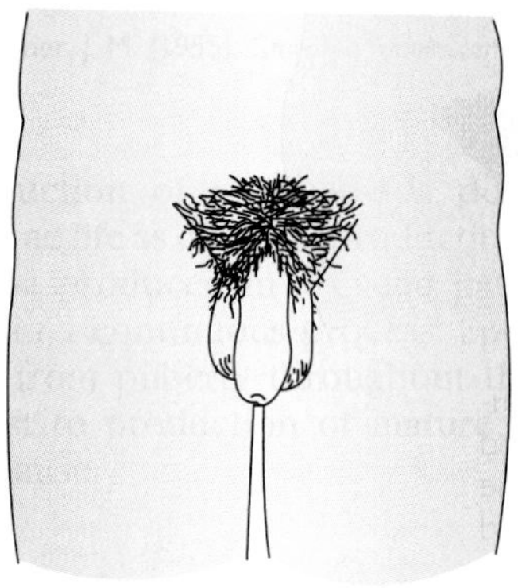

4

FIGURE 12.2 Male genital and pubic ha
development can differ in a typical boy at any giver
ily develop at the same rate. *Sex maturity rating 1:*
early childhood. *Sex maturity rating 2;* light, downy l
and testes may be slightly larger; scrotum becomin
extended across the pubis, testes and scrotum are
Sex maturity rating 4: more abundant pubic hair wi
has become larger and broader, scrotum is darker
pubic hair, with hair present along inner borders of
from Tanner, J. M. [1962]. *Growth at adolescence* [2

dysmenorrhea (painful menstruation) anc
syndrome are discussed in Chapter 26 wi
ductive tract disorders.

Developmental Milestones

Thirteen-year-old children are beyond the
ing time in any form of childhood play.
spend a great deal of time playing spo
school) loyalty is intense, and following
structions becomes mandatory. This attitu
the loyalty that 6-year-old children show to
grade teacher.

Young adolescents who do not have th
ity to compete successfully in sports may
tivities. Urge parents to encourage youn
sports for their own health and well-being
panionship involved, even though they d
not successful at sports, the young adole

portant for parents to keep the lines of communication open on the subject of sexuality (Woodson, 1997). Rates of teenage pregnancy and sexually transmitted diseases, including human immunodeficiency virus (HIV), are high and still rising. If parents suspect that their adolescent is sexually active, they must make sure their child is knowledgeable about safer sex practices. If they are going to have sexual relationships, adolescents should use condoms to try to prevent sexually transmitted diseases and pregnancy. (See discussion later in this chapter.)

Some adolescents may believe that intense sexual yearnings or peer pressure can only be alleviated by a sexual act. They can be reassured that they are pleasant people to be with because of the many fine qualities they possess and that sexual intercourse can be delayed until two persons have come to know these qualities in each other and have made a mutual commitment based on a deeper level than simply physical passion.

Intimacy involves this deeper level of relationships or developing a sense of compassion or concern for other persons. It means being able to discern when words will hurt, when a companion is unhappy and needs encouragement, or when a friend is floundering and needs support.

In our busy modern society in which adolescents can engage in such a variety of activities, they may need help learning how to project themselves into another person's situation and to ask themselves how the world looks from that position. This ability, *empathy*, is feeling for another in its finest form.

✓ CHECKPOINT QUESTIONS

5. What are the four tasks adolescents must achieve to gain a sense of identity?
6. Why do early adolescents often dress and act alike?
7. What should parents do if they suspect their adolescent is sexually active?

Socialization

Early teenagers may be full of self-doubt rather than self-confidence. They feel they should look grown up but, instead, they still look like children. The voices of most boys have not yet dependably deepened; thus, they cannot trust their voices to carry the serious tone they wish to convey. Most girls' bodies have not yet fully developed; they may look at themselves in a mirror and compare their profiles with those of girls in popular magazines and feel inadequate.

Both male and female 13-year-old children tend to be loud and boisterous, particularly when peers of the opposite sex, whose attention they would like to attract, are nearby. They are impulsive and very much like 2-year-old children in that they want what they want immediately, not when it is convenient for others.

Many 13-year-old children fall "in love," which at this early stage can be a painful kind of love. At this age, however, they spend more time longing for someone of the opposite sex than they do instituting an in-depth and rewarding relationship. They have too little experience with life, too limited a frame of reference to know how to offer a deep commitment to another or accept one from that person.

Fourteen-year-old children are often quieter and more introspective than 13-year-old children. They are becoming used to their changing bodies, have more confidence in themselves, and feel more self-esteem.

Adolescents watch adults carefully, searching for good role models with whom they can identify. They usually have a hero—a film star, writer, scientist, teacher, or athlete—whom they want to grow up to be like. Fourteen-year-old children often form a friendship with an older adolescent of the same sex, trying to imitate that person in everything from thoughts to clothing. If the older adolescent has dropped out of school, the younger person may express a wish to drop out, too.

Idolization of famous people or older adolescents fades as adolescents become more interested in forming reciprocal friendships. Attachments to older adolescents are often severed abruptly and painfully as the older teenagers make it clear they are more interested in being with persons their own age. Rejection by an older member of a pair forces the younger member to turn to friends of his or her own age and ends the intense hero worship so typical of early adolescence.

Most 15-year-old children fall in love five or six times a year. Many are sexually attracted to the opposite sex, however, because of physical appearance, not because of inner qualities or characteristics that are necessarily compatible with their own. Such infatuation can lead to extremely intense but brief attachments that fade once the two young people discover that they really have little in common. However, falling in love this often does not mean their feelings are any less strong or that they feel any less pain when the relationship ends (Figure 12-4).

By age 16, boys are becoming sexually mature (although they continue to grow taller until 18 years of age). Both sexes are better able to trust their bodies than they were the year before. By age 17, they tend to be quieter and thoughtful about interactions. They have left behind the childish behaviors they used in early adolescence—shoving and punching—to get the attention of the opposite sex.

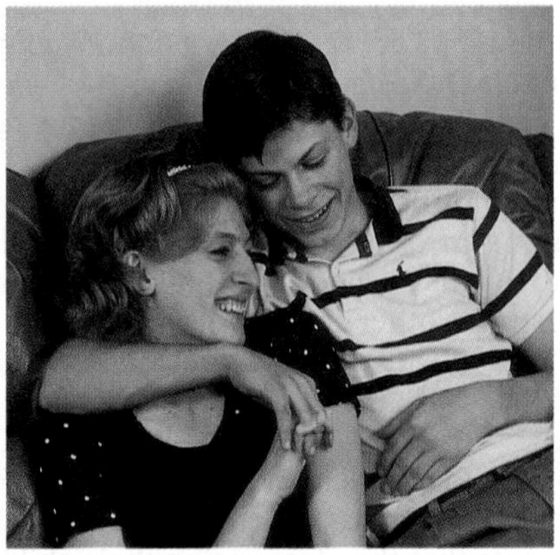

FIGURE 12.4 Although love can be fleeting, adolescents may feel intensely for each another.

Cognitive Development

The final stage of cognitive development, the state of **formal operations**, begins at age 12 or 13 years and grows in depth over the adolescent years (Piaget, 1969). This step involves the ability to think in abstract terms and use the scientific method to arrive at conclusions. The problems that adolescents are asked to solve in school depend on this type of thought (e.g., a boy rowing upstream at 5 miles per hour against a current of 2 miles per hour will go how far in 1 hour?). Problem solving in any situation depends on the ability to think abstractly and logically.

With the ability to use scientific thought, adolescents can plan their future. They can create a hypothesis (What if I go to college? What if I don't go to college?) and think through the probable consequences. Thinking abstractly is what allows adolescents to project themselves into the minds of others and imagine how others view them or their actions.

Moral and Spiritual Development

Because adolescents enlarge their thought processes to include formal reasoning, they are able to respond to the question, "Why is it wrong to steal from your neighbor's house?" with "It would hurt my neighbor by requiring him to spend money to replace what I stole," rather than with the immature response of the school-age child, "The police will punish me." Some adolescents, however, may have difficulty envisioning a department store or a large corporation as capable of suffering economic loss from stealing, which may contribute to the frequent practice of shoplifting at this age.

Almost all adolescents question the existence of God and any religious practices they have been taught (Kohlberg, 1981). This questioning is a part of forming a sense of identity and establishing a value system at a time in life when they draw away from their families.

✔ CHECKPOINT QUESTIONS

8. What is the final stage of cognitive development?
9. Why doesn't formal reasoning protect adolescents from shoplifting?

PLANNING AND IMPLEMENTATION FOR HEALTH PROMOTION OF THE ADOLESCENT AND FAMILY

Promoting Adolescent Safety

Accidents, most commonly those involving motor vehicles, are the leading cause of death among adolescents. Although adolescents are at the peak of physical and sensorimotor functioning, their need to rebel against authority or to gain attention leads them to take foolish chances while driving, such as speeding or driving while intoxicated.

In the interest of the adolescent's safety and that of others, parents should have the courage to insist on emotional maturity rather than age as the qualification for obtaining a driver's license. Encourage adolescents to take driver education courses to learn not only the techniques of driving but also a sense of responsibility toward others. The use of seat belts should also be demanded. Adolescents tend to dismiss seat belts as childish, and they need convincing that it is only sensible to use every precaution available when in a motor vehicle.

Equally dangerous for adolescents are motorcycles, motorbikes, and motor scooters, which are appealing because of their low cost and convenience in parking. Both drivers and riders should wear safety helmets to prevent head injury, long pants to prevent leg burns from exhaust pipes, and full body covering to prevent abrasions in case of an accident. Adolescents who choose these forms of transportation should be as familiar with safety rules as automobile drivers. They should be prevented from driving motorcycles or scooters until they are emotionally mature enough to use sound driving judgment.

Drowning is one of the chief accidents of adolescence, even though it is largely preventable. Teaching all children to swim is not the only preventive measure, because some drownings occur when good swimmers go beyond their capabilities on dares or in hopes of impressing friends. Teaching water safety, such as not attempting to swim alone or swimming when tired, is as important as teaching the mechanics of swimming.

Gunshots are another source of injury or accidental death in adolescents. The second most common cause of death in adolescents is homicide, related to the easy accessibility of guns to teenagers. Teenagers may carry guns in the streets or to school. Gang violence adds to this problem. Accidental gunshot injuries increase in early adolescence, often for the same reason that drowning increases: youngsters want to impress friends. Some teenagers play gunshot Russian roulette to prove to their friends that they are courageous. Both water and firearm safety must be taught creatively to adolescents by encouraging problem solving rather than lecturing, because they tend to rebel against such lectures or claim that they have heard it all before.

Athletic injuries tend to occur during adolescence because of the vigorous level of competition that occurs. In early adolescence, overuse injuries result from poor conditioning. Athletic injuries are discussed in Chapter 30. Health teaching measures to prevent accidents and athletic injuries are summarized in Empowering the Family.

Promoting Nutritional Health for the Adolescent

Adolescents experience so much growth that they may always feel hungry (Figure 12-5). If an adolescent's eating habits are unsupervised, however, he or she will tend to eat faddish or quick snack foods rather than more nutritionally sound ones. Some adolescents may turn away from the five pyramid food groups to eat great quantities of sweets, soft drinks, or empty-calorie snacks, which leaves them poorly nourished despite the large intake. One form of rebellion is to refuse to eat foods parents believe are good for them. Parents who stock their kitchens

EMPOWERING THE FAMILY: Measures to Prevent Accidents in Adolescents

Accident	*Health Teaching Measure*
Motor vehicle	Use seat belts whether as driver or passenger.
	Do not drink alcohol while driving, and refuse to ride with anyone who has been drinking.
	Wear helmet and long trousers as driver or passenger on a motorcycle.
	Accepting dares has no place in safe driving.
	Take driver education courses to learn safe driving habits for both two-wheel and four-wheel vehicles.
Firearms	Always consider all guns loaded and potentially lethal.
	Learn safe gun handling before attempting to clean a gun or hunt.
Drowning	Adolescents should learn safe water rules, such as never swimming alone, no diving into shallow end of swimming pools, no hyperventilating before swimming under water, no swimming beyond own limit.
	Taking dares has no place in water safety.
	All adolescents should learn how to swim.
Sports	Use protective equipment, such as face masks for hockey, pads for football.
	Do not attempt participation beyond physical limits.
	Careful preparation for sports through training is essential to safety.
	Recognize and set own limit for sports participation.

with more nutritious foods, always keeping plenty of milk, juice, and healthy snacks such as fruit and vegetables on hand, and who are willing to meet their adolescents halfway in terms of food preferences (e.g., serving pizza once a week) will be more certain their child is eating nutritious foods during the day. Giving the adolescent some responsibility for food planning or meals (e.g., making dinner every Wednesday night) may teach some important lessons about nutrition without conflict.

Adolescents who are slightly obese because of prepubertal changes may begin low-calorie or starvation diets to lose excess weight. Some develop eating disorders such as bulimia or anorexia nervosa (see Chapter 33). A weight-loss diet may be appropriate during adolescence, but it must be supervised to ensure that the adolescent consumes sufficient calories and nutrients for growth. For example, many adolescents omit breads and cereals entirely to lose weight rather than just reducing the amounts they consume. Diets such as these may be deficient in thiamine and riboflavin.

Recommended Daily Dietary Allowances

An adolescent needs an increased number of calories to maintain a rapid period of growth. Males continue to need more calories than females during this period. One of the most important things adolescents can learn is that just filling their stomachs will not provide adequate nutrition. Foods that supply the necessary carbohydrates, vitamins, protein, and minerals are essential.

The nutrients that are most apt to be deficient in both male and female adolescent diets are iron, calcium, and zinc. Large amounts of iron are necessary to meet expanding blood volume requirements. Females require a high iron intake not only because of increasing blood volume needs but also because iron begins to be lost with menstruation. Girls with a heavy menstrual flow (menorrhagia) may need to take an additional iron supplement to prevent iron-deficiency anemia (see Chapter 23). Increased calcium is necessary for rapid skeletal growth. Good intake during adolescence is important to "stockpile" calcium to prevent osteoporosis later in life (Rousseau, 1997). Zinc is necessary for sexual maturation and final body growth. Good sources of iron are meat and green vegetables; calcium is abundant in milk and milk products; meat and milk are also high in zinc.

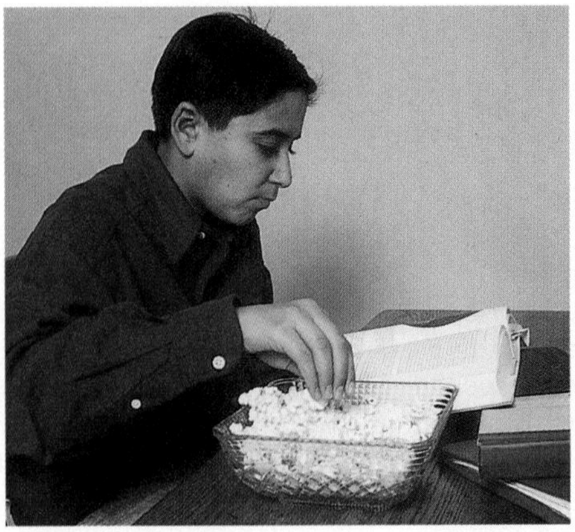

FIGURE 12.5 Adolescents experience rapid physical growth; typically, they are always hungry.

Promoting Nutritional Health With a Varied Diet

Vegetarian Diets. Because vegetables generally contain fewer calories than meat, adolescents need to consume large amounts to achieve an adequate caloric intake with a vegetarian diet. Textured vegetable protein can be purchased and added to meals to increase the amount of protein supplied and help meet adolescent growth needs. Some adolescents may find it difficult to follow a vegetarian diet because it makes them different from their peers and limits foods they can eat at parties or at school, such as pizza, meat tortillas, or hot dogs. Whether to continue to follow this type of diet is a decision the adolescent must make as part of achieving a sense of identity. Be certain that adolescent vegetarians are following a sound diet and not only eating fruits and vegetables as a way to lose weight (Neumark-Sztainer et al, 1997).

Glycogen Loading. Athletes need more carbohydrate or energy than do people who do not engage in strenuous activity, and the source of carbohydrate that best sustains athletes comes from the breakdown of glycogen because this supplies slow steady release of glucose. **Glycogen loading** is a procedure used to ensure there is adequate glycogen to sustain energy through an athletic event. Several days before a sports event, athletes lower their carbohydrate intake and exercise heavily to deplete muscle glycogen stores. They then switch to a diet high in carbohydrate. With the renewed carbohydrate intake, muscle glycogen is stored at approximately twice the usual level ready to supply twice the glucose for sustained energy. The effects of frequent glycogen loading are unknown, and it is not particularly recommended for adolescents. As a rule, the goals of nutrition that are best for everyone, such as eating a well-balanced diet, are also the best rules for athletes, rather than diets that interfere with carbohydrate, fluid, or fat intake (Lambert et al, 1997).

Promoting Development of the Adolescent in Daily Activities

Maintaining adequate nutrition to support rapid adolescent growth is essential to continued healthy development, as discussed above. Maintaining adequate sleep, hygiene, and exercise are also important and should become the adolescent's responsibility rather than the parents'. Parents can, however, encourage adolescents to engage in healthy patterns of living—primarily through role modeling.

Dress and Hygiene

Adolescents are capable of total self-care, and because of their body awareness, they may even be overly conscientious about personal hygiene and appearance. They often wash their hair every day, then grow dissatisfied because their hair has lost so much natural oil that it is dull and stringy. Both sexes try many types of shampoo, deodorant, breath fresheners, and toothpaste. They may take seriously (without admitting it) the content of ads showing toothpastes or deodorants helping to win an attractive person of the opposite sex or instant success. Remember this when caring for hospitalized adolescents. Providing time for self-care, such as shampooing hair, is important to include in an adolescent's nursing care plan.

Adolescents are acutely aware of what their peers are wearing. When adolescents cannot trust or are disappointed in their bodies, it is very reassuring to be dressed exactly like everyone else. When they first begin to work, many adolescents spend their first paychecks entirely on clothing. This seems inappropriate to many parents; they want their child to learn to spend money on more lasting items or to show an interest in saving. Adolescents may have to mature fully, however, before they discover that the real person shows through the clothing.

Remembering how important clothing is for adolescents also helps you plan care for them during a hospitalization. Most teenagers seem to improve markedly when allowed to wear their own clothing rather than a hospital gown.

Care of Teeth

Adolescents are generally very conscientious about tooth brushing because of a fear of developing bad breath. They should continue to use a fluoride paste rather than a brand advertised as providing white teeth. They tend to snack a great deal, so their teeth are always exposed to bacterial erosion. Some may develop cavities for the first time during this period. Those individuals with braces must be extremely conscientious in tooth brushing to prevent plaque buildup on tooth surfaces.

Sleep

Although it is widely believed that adults need 8 hours of sleep a night, some need more and others can adjust to considerably less. Protein synthesis occurs most readily during sleep. Because of this, adolescents need proportionately more sleep than school-age children to support the growth spurt during this time which demands the formation of so many new cells. In addition, because this is a stress period similar to first grade, adolescents may sleep restlessly as their mind reworks the day's tensions; sleep may not leave them feeling refreshed.

Many adolescents attempt to get by with too little sleep, because they are constantly busy and because staying up late is a symbol of the adult status they long for. Frequent lack of sleep can lead to chronic fatigue. Adolescents admitted to a hospital for even a minor illness may sleep as if exhausted for the day to make up for what they have lost at home.

✔ CHECKPOINT QUESTIONS

10. What is the leading cause of death among adolescents?
11. What three minerals are most apt to be deficient in an adolescent diet?

Exercise

Adolescents need exercise every day to maintain muscle tone and to provide an outlet for tension. Although they are constantly on the go, they often receive little real exercise. They ride a bus to school, sit for classes, sit at a mall after school and talk to friends, sit and watch a basketball game in the evening. They have put in a full day from 7:00 in the morning until 11:00 at night, yet they have had little exercise compared with the amount they used to get when they came home from school and played tag or hide-and-seek for several hours before dinner. Adolescents who have had an injury and must learn an activity such as crutch walking should do muscle-strengthening exercises at first, just as adults must.

Adolescents who are involved in structured athletic activities do receive daily exercise. If they have not participated in competitive sports before, they may need advice on increasing exercise gradually so they do not overdo and consequently develop muscle sprains or other injuries.

WHAT IF? What if an adolescent who previously maintained a daily exercise program is hospitalized? In what ways could such a program be continued?

THE NURSING ROLE IN HEALTH PROMOTION OF THE ADOLESCENT AND FAMILY

Promoting Healthy Family Functioning

During early adolescence, children may have many disagreements with parents that stem partly from wanting more independence and partly from being so disappointed in their bodies. It is frustrating for children to be told by parents that they are too old to behave in a certain manner when they still don't feel or look older. At other times, just when they begin to accept their maturing appearance, parents tell them they are too young to do something. It may be helpful to counsel parents to appreciate that, although it is not easy to live with a teenager, it is equally difficult to be the teenager.

At about age 15, parent–child friction tends to reach a peak. By 15, adolescents have discovered from careful observation that most adults are far from perfect. The teachers they previously thought of as all-knowing may be revealed to have very human shortcomings: they may not be able to answer every question; some may make it clear they do not have time for questions. Even a favorite coach may be discovered to be imperfect. School marks may slump as a reflection of this "fallen angel" syndrome.

Adolescents find even more fault in their parents and wonder how they can exist with their outdated ideas. They have trouble respecting parents who are so obviously imperfect. These adolescents may follow health advice poorly because they view health care personnel in the same light.

By the time they are 16 years old, adolescents generally become more willing to listen and to talk about problems. As a result, they may learn that adults are not as inadequate as they previously thought. Their parents, for example, may not be exactly the kind of persons these adolescents might wish they were, but generally, 16-year-old children can understand that adults are this way because they are, after all, only human. This changed perception does not mean that the adolescent of 16 is calm and quiet, free of parent–child discord. Adolescents may comprehend how hard it was for parents to get where they are, but they may not understand, for example, why they themselves are not allowed to stay out beyond midnight on weekends.

Seventeen-year-old children who have stayed in school are usually seniors, and for most this year is likely to be stormy. Looking ahead to leaving a school system with which they have been involved since they were very young may give some 17-year-old children a feeling of losing security. Even if going away to college or beginning a full-time job seems exciting, it may also be an unwelcome change from the people and routines that they feel so comfortable with to new contacts and new regulations that appear strange and even hostile.

The ambivalence that such feelings create makes 17-year-old children difficult to understand. They like to see parents perpetuating family traditions: a vacation in an old familiar place, the house decorated for a holiday in the same way, or the traditional birthday meal. Parents should appreciate that clinging to security this way is not the step backward it may seem. Instead, this behavior may be the preliminary working through to a time of separation that will be a major milestone in growing up.

To prove that they are old enough to leave high school and to enter into a more mature college or work world, adolescents may experiment with drugs or alcohol, sometimes interpreting their use as the mark of being an adult.

Common Health Problems of the Adolescent

A health maintenance schedule for the adolescent period and the assessments to be included at visits are shown in Table 12-2 (AAP, 1997).

Hypertension

Hypertension is present if blood pressure is above the 95th percentile, or 127/81 mm Hg for 16-year-old girls; 131/81 for 16-year-old boys for two consecutive readings (Wilson, 1997). Adolescents who are obese, African American, eat a diet high in salt, or have a family history of hypertension are most susceptible to developing the disease. Prevention and management of hypertension are discussed in Chapter 20. All children over 3 years of age should have their blood pressure taken routinely at health assessments to detect this. This is particularly true for adolescents.

Poor Posture

Many adolescents demonstrate poor posture, a tendency to round shoulders and a shambling, slouchy walk. This is due in part to the imbalance of growth, the skeletal system growing a little more rapidly than the muscles attached to it. Poor posture particularly seems to develop in adolescents who reach adult height before their peers. They slouch to appear no taller than anyone around them. Girls, especially, may slouch so as not to appear taller than boys in the belief that males will only date females shorter than themselves. Girls may also slouch to diminish the appearance of their breast size if they are developing more rapidly than their friends.

TABLE 12.2 Health Maintenance Schedule, Adolescent Period

AREA OF FOCUS	METHODS	FREQUENCY
Assessment		
Developmental milestones	History, observation	Every visit
Growth milestones	Height, weight plotted on standard growth chart; physical examination	Every visit
Hypertension	Blood pressure	Every visit
Nutrition	History, observation; height/weight information	Every visit
Hypercholesterolemia	Cholesterol level	During adolescence for children with family members with the disorder
Parent–child relationship	History, observation	Every visit
Behavior or school problems	History, observation	Every visit
Vision and hearing disorders	History, observation	Every visit
	Formal Snellen or Titmus testing	At 16 yr
	Audiometer testing	At 16 yr
Dental health	History, physical examination	Every visit
Scoliosis	Physical examination	Every visit to 16 yr
Thyroid	Physical examination, history	Every visit
Tuberculosis	Tine test	Depending on prevalence of tuberculosis in community
Bacteriuria	Clean-catch urine	At 16 yr
Anemia	Hematocrit	At 14–16 yr
Cervical or vaginal cancer	Pap test, pelvic examination	Every year for sexually active females or those whose mothers received diethylstilbestrol while in utero
Immunizations		
Tetanus & diphtheria (Td)	Check history and past records; inform caregiver about any risks and side effects; administer vaccine in accordance with health care agency policies	At 14–16 yr or 10 yr since last booster
Hepatitis		If not previously immunized
Anticipatory Guidance		
Adolescent care	Active listening and health teaching	Every visit
Expected growth and developmental milestones before next visit	Active listening and health teaching	Every visit
Accident prevention	Counseling about street and personal safety	Every visit
Problem Solving		
Any problems expressed by caregiver during visit	Active listening and health teaching regarding cigarette smoking, drug abuse, school adjustment	Every visit

Both sexes should be urged to use good posture during the rapid-growth years. Tall adolescents of both sexes are generally picked out by basketball or track coaches and thus may have the incentive, if properly guided, to maintain good posture. Assess posture at all adolescent health appraisals to detect the difference between normal posture and the beginning of scoliosis (lateral curvature of the spine; see Chapters 13 and 30).

Body Piercing and Tattoos

Body piercing and tattoos are becoming a mark of adolescence. Both sexes have ears, lips, chins, navels and breasts pierced and filled with earrings or tattoos applied to arms, legs, or their central body. These acts have become a way for adolescents to make a statement (I am different from you). Be certain they know the symptoms of infection at a piercing or tattoo site (redness, warmness, drainage, swelling, mild pain) and to report these to a health care provider if they occur. Caution them that sharing needles for piercing or tattooing carries the same risk as sharing needles for intravenous drug therapy.

Fatigue

So many adolescents complain of fatigue to some degree that it can be considered normal for the age group. Because fatigue may be a beginning symptom of disease, however, it is important that it be investigated as a legitimate concern and not underestimated. The adolescent's diet, sleep patterns, and activity schedules should be assessed, because all can contribute greatly to fatigue. Take a careful history, noting when the fatigue began. A short period of extreme tiredness is more likely to suggest disease than a long, ill-defined report of always feeling tired.

If an adolescent's sleep and diet appear to be adequate, the activity schedule is reasonable (in an attempt to be popular, some adolescents take on a schedule that would exhaust three people) and physical assessment suggests no illness, then the fatigue may be of emotional origin. It can be a means of avoiding school, avoiding conflict with parents (when children appear ill, parents are more sympathetic), or avoiding social situations. Those who are under stimulated by school may develop fatigue as a sign of boredom.

Blood tests may be indicated to rule out anemia and the infection that is so common in adolescents, infectious mononucleosis (see Chapter 22). After this, they can be assured that they are healthy and offered guidance to solve the problem with better diet, more sleep, fewer activities, and development of better problem-solving techniques to relieve tensions.

Menstrual Irregularities

Menstrual irregularities can be a major health concern of adolescent girls as they learn to adjust to their individual body cycles. Chapter 26 discusses these problems in detail.

Acne

Acne is a self-limiting inflammatory disease that involves the sebaceous glands that empty into hair shafts (the pilosebaceous unit) mainly of the face and shoulders. It is the most common skin disorder of adolescence, occurring slightly more frequently in boys than girls. The peak age for the lesions to occur in girls is 14 to 17 years; for boys, 16 to 19 years. Although not proven, genetic factors may play a part in their development. Cigarette smoking may also increase the number of inflammatory lesions.

Before the rapid increase in androgen secretion with puberty, the sebaceous glands that enter into hair follicles are small and relatively inactive, so acne is nonexistent. Changes associated with puberty cause acne through the following process:

- As androgen levels rise in both sexes, sebaceous glands become active.
- Abnormal keratinization (cell growth) of the lining of the ducts occurs; this overgrowth obstructs the ducts.
- The output of sebum increases. Sebum is largely composed of lipids, mainly triglycerides.
- If all of the material formed cannot be eliminated to the skin surface due to the narrow gland ducts, the glands enlarge, and trapped sebum causes whiteheads, or closed **comedones**.
- As trapped sebum darkens from accumulation of melanin and oxidation of the fatty acid component on exposure to air, blackheads, or open comedones, form.
- Bacteria (generally, *Propionibacterium acnes*) lodge and thrive in the retained secretions, forming papules.
- Leakage of free fatty acid from triglycerides causes a dermal inflammatory reaction.
- If glands rupture, sebum is extruded into adjacent skin, which produces reddened inflammatory cysts.

Acne is categorized as mild (comedones are present), moderate (papules and pustules are also present), or severe (cysts are present). The most common locations of acne lesions are the face, neck, back, upper arms, and chest (Figure 12-6). Flare-ups are associated with emotional stress, menstrual periods, or the use of greasy hair creams or makeup that can further plug gland ducts. Lesions are less noticeable in summer months, probably because of increased exposure to the sun, which increases epidermic peeling, and the reduction of stress, possibly as a result of being out of school (Tunnessen, 1997).

Assessment. Always ask adolescents at health assessments if they are troubled with acne and to what extent it interferes with their self-image. Inspect for facial, chest, and back lesions on physical examination.

Therapeutic Management. The goal of therapy is threefold:

1. To decrease sebum formation
2. To prevent comedones
3. To control bacterial proliferation

External Medication. Medications that are applied externally peel away the superficial skin layer to prevent sebum plugs from forming and are sufficient if only comedones are present. The most frequently used over-the-counter medications contain benzoyl peroxide. A common prescription medication is tretinoin (Retin-A cream). This reduces keratin formation and plugging of ducts. When using a vitamin A cream, adolescents should be cautioned to avoid prolonged sun exposure or use a sunblock of SPF 15 or higher, because the preparation makes their skin more susceptible to ultraviolet rays. Caution adolescents that, for the first week or two of therapy, peeling or oxidizing may make the complexion actually appear worse rather than better. Topical antibiotic creams such as erythromycin and clindamycin may be prescribed to reduce the bacterial level on skin, but usually only after oxidizing agents have not succeeded; these creams may sensitize adolescents unnecessarily to antibiotics.

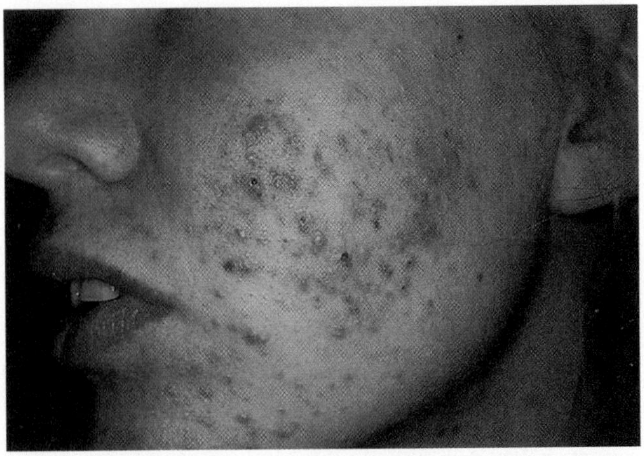

FIGURE 12.6 Facial acne in an adolescent.

Systemic Medication. In pustular and cystic acne, systemic (oral) antibiotics are helpful. Tetracycline (500 mg twice daily the first week, then tapered to 250 mg daily for maintenance) is effective against the anaerobic bacteria that break down sebum to form irritating acids. Improvement is not generally seen for 2 weeks, so adolescents must be supported to continue to take the medication during the waiting period. Without noticeable improvement, adolescents have a tendency to continue taking the higher dose or even increase the dose, hoping to initiate an effect. Tetracycline is not prescribed for children under age 12, because it can cause permanent staining of teeth. Because tetracycline may interfere with oral contraceptives, adolescent girls should use another method of birth control while on the antibiotic. Tetracycline should not be given to females who may be pregnant, because it causes faulty bone growth in a fetus.

Because food impairs the absorption of tetracycline, the drug should be taken on an empty stomach (2 hours before or after eating). Adolescents must be certain of the date of expiration of the drug; outdated tetracycline breaks down into an extremely toxic composition. Females taking systemic antibiotics for long periods become susceptible to developing candidal vaginitis and must be instructed about the symptoms of this: a white, pruritic vaginal discharge. Alternative antibiotics prescribed are erythromycin, minocycline, or clindamycin.

Isotretinoin (Accutane), a form of vitamin A, is an extremely effective oral drug for reducing sebum production and abnormal keratinization of gland ducts; it has become the drug of choice for cystic acne, although it is extremely teratogenic (Koren & Pastuszak, 1997).

Other Treatment Methods. If inflammatory reactions from acne are extreme, a corticosteroid such as prednisone or a nonsteroidal anti-inflammatory drug may be prescribed. Steroids must be used with caution in growing adolescents, because they can lead to stunted growth. Cortisone may be injected directly into cystic lesions to reduce them rapidly. This type of injection may reduce keloid formation, which is why it is usually reserved for adolescents who are prone to this permanent form of scarring.

Estrogen, alone or in combination with progesterone, suppresses sebaceous gland activity and is therefore useful therapy in some girls. However, Isotretinoin is more often prescribed instead of estrogen for two reasons: (1) high estrogen levels tend to close epiphyseal centers of long bones causing bone growth to stop; (2) long-term therapy does have dangerous side effects, including embolism and thrombophlebitis.

Although acne may be treated, some degree of scarring may result. Laser therapy is a follow-up possibility to reduce the effect of scarring (LeRoy, 1997).

NURSING DIAGNOSES AND RELATED INTERVENTIONS

Nursing Diagnosis: Risk for self-esteem disturbance related to development of acne during adolescence and lack of knowledge regarding treatment possibilities

Outcome Identification: Adolescent will express positive self-evaluation by next health maintenance visit.

Outcome Evaluation: Adolescent verbalizes positive aspects of self; states that acne does not affect his or her positive self-image; or if client admits to feelings of negative self-esteem, is able to discuss feelings and concerns about condition with nurse; describes way to prevent or reduce acne outbreaks and states realistic short- and long-term goals of treatment.

It is important to respect what acne means to the adolescent. The actual extent of the condition often is not as important as an adolescent's feelings about it. When one's face is constantly covered by red marks, it is extremely difficult for an individual to feel good about oneself (see the Nursing Care Plan).

When carrying out interventions, remember that acne is a potentially destructive disease that, if left untreated, can cause irreparable physical and emotional scarring. Parents and adolescents should therefore be advised to seek medical treatment rather than self-medicate if the condition is severe. At the same time, overconcern may lead to undue self-consciousness that affects performance in school and establishment of social relationships. Health teaching measures for the prevention and treatment of acne are summarized in Empowering the Family.

Obesity

Most overweight adolescents have obese parents, suggesting that both inheritance and environment may play a part in the development of obesity; the majority of such adolescents continue to be obese as adults. It can be difficult for adolescents to learn to like themselves (achieve a sense of identity) if they do not like their reflection in a mirror. It is equally difficult if they are always excluded from groups because of their weight. Some adolescents may be unaware that their food intake is excessive, because they have been told that they need excess nutrients for healthy adolescent growth and everyone in their family eats large portions.

A reducing diet of fewer than 1400 to 1600 calories per day can rarely be tolerated by adolescents. Such a diet would provide insufficient protein and be deficient in vitamins. If adolescents eat a diet that is too low in protein for any length of time, they can develop an inadequate nitrogen balance, which can seriously impair their growth. They generally can adhere to a diet of 1800 calories per day.

NURSING DIAGNOSES AND RELATED INTERVENTIONS

Nursing Diagnosis: Ineffective individual coping by overeating related to stresses of adolescent period that have led to obesity

Outcome Identification: Adolescent will determine cause of stress and demonstrate healthy ways of dealing with it by 1 month.

Outcome Evaluation: Adolescent identifies stressful situations in his or her life that lead to overeating; describes ways he or she might avoid those situations or other methods for coping with them.

Nursing Care Plan

THE ADOLESCENT WITH ACNE

A 15-year-old male comes to the clinic for his yearly health maintenance visit. He states, "Look at my skin. It's horrible!"

Assessment: 15-year-old male with history of acne for the last 6 months. Reports washing his face approximately 5 to 6 times a day with abrasive soap and covering lesions with cocoa butter cream twice a day. "I don't eat chocolate. And even with all this, my skin is getting worse instead of better. I dread going to school, and forget about getting my picture taken. My mom says to just wait it out." Physical examination reveals scattered pustules and comedones on forehead and face, very prominent on nose and both cheeks. Two lesions on right cheek with large erythematous base and tender to touch. Remainder of physical examination unremarkable.

Nursing Diagnosis: Knowledge deficit related to cause and treatment for acne

Outcome Identification: Adolescent verbalizes accurate information about acne.

Outcome Evaluation: Adolescent states causes of acne; identifies measures for prevention and treatment; demonstrates appropriate skin care measures.

Interventions	Rationale
1. Assess adolescent's understanding of acne and its causes.	1. Obtaining a baseline knowledge assessment provides a foundation on which to build future teaching strategies.
2. Review the structure and function of the skin and sebaceous glands and development of acne. Clarify any misconceptions.	2. Reviewing and clarifying aids in learning and strengthening understanding.
3. Discuss treatment options available. Refer to dermatologic health care provider for evaluation and treatment.	3. Discussion provides the adolescent with information about the numerous treatment options available for acne, providing him with the opportunity for making informed decisions, thereby enhancing control over the situation.
4. Instruct adolescent in measures to prevent and control acne, including twice daily washing with mild soap and water; a healthy, well-balanced diet; avoidance of picking or squeezing lesions; and avoidance of greasy or oily skin preparations.	4. Daily washing removes irritating fatty acids; excessive washing can rupture glands and exacerbate acne. A healthy, well-balanced diet is essential for overall good health. Picking or squeezing lesions ruptures glands and spreads sebum. Greasy or oily skin preparations can plug gland ducts, increasing comedone formation.
5. Review treatment program prescribed. Assist adolescent with setting up a schedule for prescribed therapy. Caution adolescent that results of therapy are not immediate.	5. Reviewing the program aids in the adolescent's understanding, thus helping to promote compliance, which is essential for successful treatment.
6. Arrange for a follow-up visit in 2 weeks.	6. A follow-up visit allows time for evaluation, feedback, review of compliance, and further teaching.

Nursing Diagnosis: Self-esteem disturbance related to appearance from acne

Outcome Identification: Adolescent will verbalize positive feelings about himself.

Outcome Evaluation: Adolescent states impact of acne on appearance and feelings of self-esteem; actively discusses feelings and concerns; participates actively in care and treatment; reports some degree of control over the situation.

(continued)

Interventions	Rationale
1. Attempt to identify the meaning of his appearance and acne to the adolescent.	1. Identifying the meaning assists in determining the degree of its possible effect on the client.
2. Encourage the adolescent to express feelings and thoughts about self, appearance, and acne.	2. Sharing of feelings and concerns permits a safe outlet for emotions and also aids in highlighting client's awareness of possible impact on self-esteem.
3. Review and reinforce with the adolescent positive attributes about self.	3. Positive attributes provide a foundation for rebuilding self-esteem.
4. Clarify any misconceptions he may have about acne.	4. Misconceptions can negatively impact self-esteem.
5. Assist with measures to prevent and control acne, encouraging independent role functioning and active participation in decision making.	5. Independence and ability to perform one's role promotes self-esteem; active participation enhances the feeling of control over situations.
6. Provide ample time for questions and concerns.	6. Providing time for questions and concerns helps clarify information, individualize information, and promote a feeling of control and trust.

Adolescents who are overweight because of stress need support until their pleasure in eating diminishes and their satisfaction with themselves as a "new" person or their friends' satisfaction with them can sustain them. They may have to visit a health care facility once or twice a week for encouragement and praise for their efforts. Weight control organizations are good if other adolescents also attend the meetings. They are ineffective if all the other members are adults because adolescents generally cannot relate to adult problems. It is important that the adolescent's self-esteem is maintained or he or she can switch to binge eating or such severe dieting that the opposite—extreme weight loss—occurs (Deramo-Melkus, 1997).

In addition, encourage activities that use up calories, such as swimming and participation in gym classes and other school activities. Adolescents could perhaps walk

EMPOWERING THE FAMILY: Guidelines for the Prevention and Treatment of Acne

1. Diet does not influence the development of acne lesions. Eat a healthy, well-balanced diet for good general health.
2. Do not pick or squeeze acne lesions, which ruptures glands and spreads sebum into the skin, thus increasing symptoms. The times you are most likely to do this are during periods of stress, such as when you are taking a test. When you find your hand on your face, distract yourself with some other motion, such as interlocking your fingers.
3. Makeup, greasy hair preparations, or tight sweatbands can plug ducts of glands and increase comedone formation. Avoid these, if possible. Using medicated makeup both covers and helps lesions heal.
4. Topical acne preparations work by unplugging glands. You must use them consistently to make them effective. Plan enough time in the morning before school and a time in the evening to apply these. Post a chart by your bathroom mirror to remind yourself.
5. Washing daily to remove irritating fatty acids is helpful. Excessive washing is not necessary to prevent lesion formation. Excessive washing can actually harm healing by rupturing glands.
6. Oral medications work by reducing sebum secretions or preventing bacterial invasion. These only work if you take them conscientiously. Make a chart to post in your bathroom or kitchen to remind yourself to take these, also. Remember that tetracycline must be taken on an empty stomach or it is not effective.
7. If you are taking oral vitamin A (Accutane), do not take another source of vitamin A in a tablet. Accutane is very harmful to fetal growth. Take measures to prevent pregnancy while taking the drug and for 1 month afterward. If you should become pregnant while taking the drug, stop taking it immediately and notify your physician.
8. Both topical and oral vitamin A make your skin very sensitive to sunlight. Avoid long exposures to sunlight, or you will sunburn readily.
9. No acne medication works immediately. While you are waiting for lesions to heal, keep yourself occupied with a new activity (join a school club, try dancing lessons). When your skin is clear once more, these experiences will help make you an interesting person as well as one with clear skin.

to school rather than ride, or walk the dog for three blocks rather than one. These activities are generally preferable to formal exercises, such as sit-ups and push-ups, which can be viewed as punishment.

Adolescents who continually cope with stress by overeating rarely succeed in losing weight. They may require psychological counseling rather than diet counseling if they are to develop a more mature emotional response. Behavior modification is sometimes successful with adolescents as a means of helping them lose weight, but it is rarely recommended for obesity alone. If the obesity is causing serious body image problems, lowered self-esteem, and depression, behavior modification might be suggested.

Measures to help an adolescent decrease overeating include:

- Making a detailed log of the amount they eat, the time, and the circumstances (including how they felt while they were eating) and then changing those circumstances
- Always eating in one place (the kitchen table) instead of while walking home from school or watching television
- Slowing the process of eating by counting mouthfuls, putting the fork down beside the plate between bites, and being served food on small plates so helpings look larger

These measures may be of little use, however, unless they are combined with a suitable diet and adequate activities. Despite all these interventions, weight reduction may not always be effective with adolescents. For some, a more realistic goal might be to prevent additional weight gain (O'Meara & Glenny, 1997).

✔ CHECKPOINT QUESTIONS

12. What type of infection are girls who take tetracycline for acne apt to develop?
13. What is the danger of a very low caloric diet for obese adolescents?

Sexuality and Sexual Identity

Sexuality is a multidimensional phenomenon that includes feelings, attitudes, and actions with both biologic and cultural components. It encompasses and gives direction to a person's physical, emotional, social, and intellectual responses throughout life. Born a sexual being, a child's gender identity and gender role behavior evolve from and usually conform to the societal expectations within that child's culture (Baldwin & Baldwin, 1997). Nurses can play a major role in promoting sexual health through education and discussion.

Biologic gender is the term used to denote chromosomal sexual development: male (XY) or female (XX). *Gender* or *sexual identity* is the inner sense a person has of being male or female, which may be the same as or different from biologic gender. *Gender role* is the behavior a person conveys about being male or female, which, again, may or may not be the same as biologic gender or gender identity.

Development of Gender Identity

Whether gender identity arises from primarily a biologic or psychosocial focus is controversial. The amount of testosterone secreted in utero (a process termed *sex typing*) may affect this characteristic. How appealing parents or other adult role models portray their gender roles may also influence how a child envisions himself or herself. For example, both sons and daughters often relate better to whichever parent is kinder and more caring. This may result in a son assuming characteristics often regarded as feminine or daughters developing interests typically regarded as masculine.

Gender role is also culturally influenced. In Western society, women have in the past been viewed as kind and nurturing, with sole responsibility for childrearing and homemaking. Men were viewed as financial providers for the family. Fortunately, gender roles today are more interchangeable than they once were: women pursue all kinds of jobs and careers without loss of femininity; men participate (some as primary homemakers) with childrearing and household duties without loss of masculinity.

An individual's sense of gender identity develops throughout an entire lifespan, and the stage is set by expectations even before a child is born. Although parents usually respond to the question, "Do you want a boy or a girl?" with the answer, "It doesn't matter as long as it's healthy," many parents actually have strong preferences for a male or female child. Although some parents may be disappointed if the child is not the gender they hoped for, most adapt quickly and will say later that they always wanted that sex child. Children who suspect their parents wanted a child of the opposite sex are more likely to adopt roles of the opposite sex than if they are confident parents are pleased with them as they are.

From the day of birth, female and male babies are treated differently by their parents. People generally bring girls dainty rattles and dresses with ruffles; on the whole, they are treated more gently by parents and held and rocked more than male babies. People tend to buy boys bigger rattles and sports-related jogging suits. Admonitions given babies can be different. A girl might be told, "Don't cry. You don't look pretty when you cry." A boy might be told, "You've got to learn to be tougher than that if you're ever going to make it in this world."

As early as the age of 2 years, children can distinguish between males and females. By age 3 or 4 years, they know what sex they are, having absorbed cultural expectations of that sex role.

Sex role modeling is reinforced through behavior toward and expectations of the child as well as from watching television, the color and decor of the child's room, and the child's clothing. Social contacts between the child and significant adults contribute to sexual identification and should be encouraged in this developmental period. A positive self-concept grows from parental love, effective relationships with others, success in play activities, and gaining skills and self-control.

Early school-age children typically spend play time imitating adult roles as a way of learning gender roles. They start to form strong impressions of what a feminine or male role should be (Mallet et al, 1997).

At puberty, as the adolescent begins the process of establishing a sense of identity, the problem of final gender role identification surfaces again. Most early adolescents maintain strong ties to their gender group; boys with boys, girls with girls. The advent of menstruation may provide a common bond for girls at this stage. Some adolescents choose a child of their own gender a few years older than themselves to use as their model of gender role behavior. This is a way that adolescents can be certain that they understand and feel comfortable with their own sex before they are ready to reach out and interact with members of the opposite sex.

Concerns Regarding Sexual Activity

Because of increasing exposure to and acceptance of premarital sexual relations in society today, more adolescents than ever before engage in sexual intercourse. Because of this, as part of routine health assessment of adolescents and preadolescents, you should ask about their sexual activity.

Interviewing adolescents for a sexual history needs to be done tactfully and with confidentiality, because this is a new and sensitive area for them. As many as 50% of ninth grade boys and 30% of ninth grade girls are already sexually active. As many as 75% of college sophomores are sexually active (NCHS, 1997; see the Focus on Nursing Research box).

Adolescents usually want to discuss this matter with a health care provider because they are concerned that they are exposing themselves to HIV infection or other sexually transmitted diseases and to pregnancy. At the same time, it is a difficult topic to discuss. Some adolescents may feel trapped into engaging in sex even though they are unwilling, because they perceive it as a way of having friends.

Counseling can help them improve their perspective and learn how to say no. In contrast, some would like to be sexually active but are not, because they believe myths: early sexual relations will drain their strength and make them poor athletes; having sex too early in life will stretch the vagina and make sexual relations later on unenjoyable. Unless these falsehoods are explored through discussion, the adolescents who believe them may never be comfortable with sexual relationships.

Sometimes adolescents use a mild cold or a mild acne condition as a reason to come to a health care facility, where they hope that someone will stumble onto their real concern of sexual activity. After asking adolescents at health maintenance visits if they are sexually active, ask if they have any questions or problems they want to discuss with you about this. Ask if they are interested in learning more about contraception. Be certain they are practicing safer sex measures. Overall guidelines on counseling the adolescent with respect to sexual activity are summarized in Box 12-1. Guidelines for safer sex practices are highighted in the Empowering the Family box.

Including such instructions in sexual counseling should help to reduce the incidence of sexually transmitted diseases as well as empower clients with better self-care skills. When discussing safer sex practices, be certain that adolescents not only understand when but how they will incorporate them into their lifestyle.

BOX 12.1

HEALTH TEACHING GUIDELINES FOR ADOLESCENTS REGARDING SEXUALITY

1. It is your choice whether or not to participate in sexual relations. Do not be influenced by friends who may be exaggerating stories to impress you or who ask you for involvement you do not want. When you say no, be firm and clear about your wishes.
2. Pregnancy can occur with *any* sexual encounter unless you use some prevention to avoid it. Be direct with a sexual partner in discussing abstinence or birth control measures.
3. Sexual relations neither add to nor detract from your physical strength or general wellness.
4. The mark of an adult sexual relation is that the activity is pleasurable to both partners. If a sexual partner is not interested in your enjoyment as well as his or her own, you should reconsider the relationship.
5. There is no "normal" mode of sexual expression. Any activity that is pleasurable to both partners is normal.
6. Learn about safer sex techniques and practice them (see Empowering the Family).

FOCUS ON NURSING RESEARCH

Why Do Adolescents Delay or Begin Coitus?

For this study, 218 adolescents aged 13 to 18 years were asked questions about their sexual decisions and the role of peer influence on those decisions. Reasons adolescents stated for delaying first intercourse were fear of pregnancy and sexually transmitted diseases, social sanctions, lack of developmental readiness and lack of opportunity. Morality was cited infrequently as a reason for postponing becoming sexually active. Many saw the beginning of sexual behavior in their peers as the trigger for them to become sexually active also.

The researchers suggest that valuable tools in helping teenagers delay becoming sexually active would be to help them learn to resist peer pressure and help them define how and when they know they are ready to become sexually active. This study has implications for nursing because nurses are often the people adolescents choose to first ask about questions of sexuality so are in front-line positions to give this help.

From Alexander, E., & Hickner, J. (1997). First coitus for adolescents: understanding why and when. *Journal of the American Board of Family Practice, 10* (2), 96.

EMPOWERING THE FAMILY: Guidelines for Safer Sex Practices

1. Be selective in choosing sexual partners. When you have sex, you are exposing yourself to the infections of everyone with whom your partner has ever had sex. The more partners you have relations with, the greater your danger of contracting a sexually transmitted disease.
2. Don't be reluctant to ask a sexual partner about his or her sexual lifestyle before engaging in sexual relations. If a partner has a history of casual contacts, bisexual or unprotected sex, there is a greater hazard of infection for you than if your partner is also choosy about partners.
3. Avoid sexual relations with IV drug users or prostitutes (male or female) or sexual partners who have had sexual relations with such people, because such people have a greater than usual chance of carrying HIV and hepatitis B infections.
4. Inspect your sexual partner for any lesions or abnormal drainage in the genital area. Do not engage in sexual relations with anyone who exhibits these signs.
5. Use a condom, the best protection against infection. Condoms should be latex; the chance of the condom tearing is less if it is a prelubricated brand. Those coated with the spermicide nonoxynol-9 appear to be effective in destroying HIV, herpes, gonorrhea, and chlamydia. Use water-based lubricants such as KY Jelly on condoms, because oil-based lubricants can weaken the rubber. Spermicidal cream or jelly impregnated with nonoxynol-9 not only provide lubrication but also some additional protection against infectious agents.
6. Protect condoms from excessive heat to avoid rubber deterioration and inspect them to be certain they are intact before use. Do not inflate condoms before use to test for intactness because this weakens the rubber.
7. Apply condoms over the erect penis with a small space left at the end to accept semen. The condom should be held against the sides of the penis while the penis is withdrawn to prevent spillage of semen.
8. Void immediately after sexual relations to aid in washing away contaminants on the vulva or in the urinary tract.
9. Be aware that anal intercourse carries a high risk for HIV and hepatitis B infection as well as infection from intestinal organisms. Use lubricants for anal penetration to keep bleeding and condom resistance to a minimum.
10. Do not engage in oral–penile sex unless the male wears a condom, because even preejaculatory fluid may contain viruses and bacteria. For safer oral–vaginal sex, a condom split in two or a plastic dental dam like that used for pediatric dentistry and covering the mouth should be used to protect against the exchange of body fluids.
11. Remember that hand-to-genital contact may be hazardous if open cuts are present on hands. Use a latex glove or finger cots for protection.
12. To decrease the possibility of transferring germs, do not share sexual aids such as vibrators.
13. If you think you have contracted a sexually transmitted disease, do not engage in sexual relations until you have contacted a health care provider and are again disease free. Alert any recent sexual partners that you might have an infection so they also can receive treatment.

Be certain to provide information on date rape and rape prevention as well, because adolescents are in a high-risk age group for date rape (Box 12-2; see also Chapter 34). Adolescent girls need to be cautioned about the dangers of flunitrazepam (Rohypnol), which is readily available to adolescent males (Anglin et al, 1997). Rohypnol, a benzodiazepine, has been implicated in date rape. Colorless, odorless, and tasteless, it can be dropped into a drink and remain undetected. The effect is drowsiness, impaired motor skills, and amnesia. Because of the amnesic effect, the adolescent who was raped has difficulty giving a history of the rape. Patients with a complaint of sexual assault who appear intoxicated or have amnesia for the event should be suspected of unknowingly ingesting flunitrazepam. In these instances, a urine specimen should be analyzed for the drug's metabolites.

CHECKPOINT QUESTIONS

14. What is meant by the term, sexual identity?
15. What are the effects of Rohypnol?

Reproductive Life Planning

Reproductive life planning includes all the decisions an individual makes about having children. These decisions usually include if and when to have children, how many children are desirable, and how they are spaced. Not so long ago, **contraceptive** products (products to prevent pregnancy) were not all that reliable or could not be easily purchased. Today, however, numerous contra-

BOX 12.2

HEALTH TEACHING GUIDELINES FOR THE PREVENTION OF RAPE IN ADOLESCENTS

Home

1. Do not advertise that you stay alone while a parent works or is on vacation.
2. Ask for identification from meter readers or repairmen before admitting them into the home.
3. Insist on adequate lighting for hallways in an apartment building or around your own home.
4. Have your house key in your hand when you approach your door; do not stand fumbling for it by the doorway.
5. Keep your doors and windows locked when you are alone at home.

Car

1. Avoid isolated parking places; park near a building or in a lot with a parking attendant.
2. Lock your car when waiting in it and after parking it.
3. Look in the back seat before unlocking and entering your car.
4. Have your car key ready when you approach your car; do not stand fumbling for it.

Work or School

1. Do not enter an elevator with a stranger.
2. Lock the outside door, and do not admit people you do not know when working alone at night.
3. Ask for security protection to walk out to your car.
4. When going to and from school or work after dark, walk in the street rather than next to shrubs or dark buildings.

Dates

1. Be clear with your date that when you say no, you mean no.
2. Limit alcohol use because this can lead to risk-taking behavior.
3. Make it clear that you consider date rape the same as any rape and you would press charges.
4. Rohypnol is a sedative, known as a "date rape" drug. Do not date any individual who brags that he knows how to obtain it or use it.

Personal Actions

1. Do not wear chains around your neck that could be used to strangle you.
2. Learn self-defense; scratch the attacker to obtain skin and blood specimens under fingernails.
3. Be aware that an attacker could take any weapon away and use it on you; use caution carrying a weapon or Mace.
4. Fight or stuggle cautiously to prevent harm to you beyond the rape itself. Actions such as kicking or gouging eyes may not be effective and may cause more violence.
5. If an attack occurs, observe the attacker's appearance as carefully as possible. Note identifying characteristics, such as a birthmark, scar, tattoo, words, or manner of speech, to be able to identify the individual later.
6. Press charges in court to make rape a crime of extreme magnitude and as an opportunity to fight back.
7. Work to provide rape prevention information and a united front against rape in your community.

ceptive choices, which range in reliability and accessability are available.

An individual's choice of contraceptive method should be made carefully with complete knowledge about the advantages, disadvantages, and side effects of the various options. This is a choice based on:

- Personal values
- Knowledge of each method
- How the method will affect sexual enjoyment
- Financial factors
- Status of an individual's relationship
- Prior experiences
- Future plans

Understanding how various methods of contraception work and how they compare in terms of benefits and disadvantages is necessary for successful counseling. It is also important to be able to answer questions about elective termination of pregnancy with accurate, up-to-date knowledge and objectivity for those whose contraceptive method failed. Legal and ethical issues (eg, client's age) must also be considered when counseling clients on the use of contraceptives. With information and the ability to discuss specific concerns, adolescents may be better prepared to make the decisions that are right for them (Slupik, 1998).

Education is an important nursing role. Most adolescents are uninformed or misinformed about the available options. An organization helpful for referral for reproductive life planning is Planned Parenthood, 810 7th Avenue, New York, NY 10019. When counseling, be certain to emphasize "safer sex" measures as well as contraceptive ones. For example, although many contraceptive options offer reliable pregnancy prevention, only condoms provide protection against STDs, an important concern if the relationship is not a monogamous one.

Interview Setting

An interview is best conducted in a private room with all parties seated comfortably; if not seated, a health care provider appears rushed and can't interact at eye level (Figure 13-1). Let parents know that their input and opinions about how their child is developing are valued by calling them by their names during the interview. A question such as "Does John sit up yet, Mr. Wiser?" is far more personal and a better form than "Does baby sit up yet?" As children grow they are able to answer questions and speak directly with the nurse.

Types of Questions Asked

The phrasing of questions varies, depending on the type of answer desired. Closed-ended and open-ended questions are two types of effective questions; compound, expansive, and leading questions, on the other hand, are three types to avoid.

Closed-Ended Question. This simplest form of question asks directly for a fact: "Does John walk yet?" "Did you take John's temperature?" This is an effective type of question if a particular point is being sought. It is limited in scope, however, because the response usually will be only a yes or no, with no further elaboration.

Open-Ended Question. An open-ended question allows the parent to elaborate. In contrast to "Did you take John's temperature?" the question "What did you do for John?" is open ended. The parent answers with a listing of all the things he or she did: the parent took John's temperature, had him lie on the couch, gave him extra fluid, and so on. It is important to ask open-ended questions with school-age children and adolescents so they are encouraged to fully describe a problem.

Compound Question. Compound questions are confusing and should be avoided because the information they elicit is often inaccurate and must be followed by a clarifying question. An example is, "Did John have nausea and vomiting?" The parent answers yes, but it still is not known whether John had vomiting and nausea, just vomiting, or just nausea.

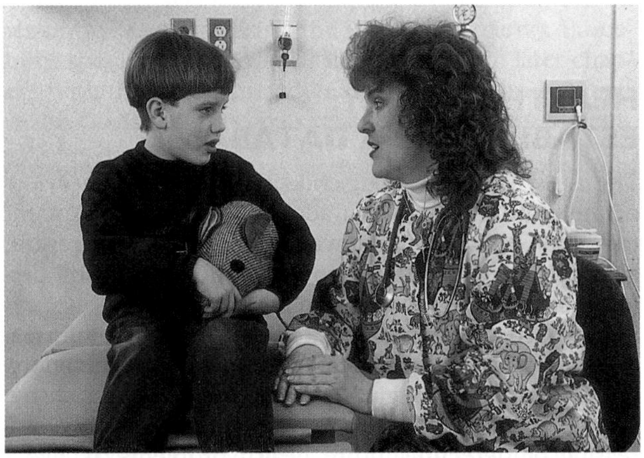

FIGURE 13.1 It is especially important to maintain good eye contact and allow children as active a part as possible in the assessment process.

Expansive Question. This is an open-ended question gone wrong because it is too broad to answer. "What can you tell me about John?" leaves a parent wondering where to start. "How has John been since his last visit?" limits the question and makes it answerable.

Leading Question. A leading question supplies its own answer, and thus should be avoided. "John has had all his immunizations, hasn't he?" implies that John should have had them and that the parent is somehow a poor caregiver if he or she answers that question any way but yes. The penalty for such an exchange could be a child left vulnerable to disease.

Conducting a Health Interview

Data gathering for an initial health assessment can be divided into nine categories:

1. Introduction and explanation
2. Demographic data
3. Chief concern
4. Present health status
5. Health and family profile
6. Day history
7. Past health history, including the pregnancy history
8. Family health history
9. Review of systems

At return visits, the categories that would be used are generally introduction and explanation, chief concern, health and family profile, interval history, and day history.

While conducting a health interview, be certain to make a transition statement before shifting from one part of an interview to another. Without a transition, the parent could be wondering what importance the questions have and may misinterpret their significance. For instance, if a parent has been providing information on the family's hospital insurance policy and, without a transition statement, is asked whether the child has been vomiting, a parent may think that the child needs hospitalization when that is not the intent at all. "Before we talk about Jane's current symptoms, let me ask you some general questions about your family as a whole" is an example of a good transition statement.

Introduction and Explanation

Parents and the child should be told as a matter of courtesy to whom they are talking and what they will be talking about. A short explanation and introduction such as "Hello, Ms. Wiser, I'm Janet Dickson, a nurse here in the One Day Surgery Department. I'd like to talk to you about John this morning" is an example of a suitable introduction. Because some families have never had the benefit of in-depth health care, it is helpful to include, as well, a statement about the subjects that will be discussed during the interview, for example, "So that I can get a picture of John's overall health, I'll be asking you questions about why you've brought him here today, your pregnancy with him, concerns you've had in the past, and questions about your typical day with John." The parent begins to concentrate on those areas because he or she realizes that health care providers in this setting are interested not just in John's health that particular day, but in his total health (see Focus on Cultural Competence).

FOCUS ON CULTURAL COMPETENCE

Health assessment of children is a skill that is learned with practice. Successful interviewing depends on respecting cultural variations. Whether people establish eye contact with an interviewer, for example, is a characteristic that is culturally determined. In Vietnam, touching the head of a child during physical assessment is thought to be harmful because the head is considered to be the seat of the soul.

Findings and techniques in children also differ depending on racial and ethnic characteristics. Assessing for cyanosis, for example, is more difficult in dark-skinned than in fair-skinned children (mucous membrane is the best place to detect this). Because height and weight charts are standardized on middle-class Caucasian children, measurements of children who do not fit this description may not plot well on these charts.

Recognizing that people hold differing cultural expectations and characteristics can help in establishing rapport with children and their families and help make health assessment more meaningful.

Demographic Data

To begin collecting demographic data, it is important to identify the client. Information such as the client's name, address, gender, and person who provided information should be included. To provide cultural competent care and make provisions for special needs, the child's culture, ethnicity, place of birth, religious or spiritual practices and primary and secondary language should also be identified. Ask if older children have a Social Security number.

In addition, it is important to identify the child's primary caregiver. If the parents are divorced or deceased, it is especially important to identify who has custody of the child (Barness, 1997).

Chief Concern

After gathering demographic data, begin data collection with the reason the parents have brought the child to the health care agency: the **chief concern.** This is what parents are most concerned about, and it is important that they get this immediate concern off their mind early in the interview (Boyle & Hoekelman, 1997). An effective way to elicit this information is to ask an open-ended question such as, "Why did you bring John to the clinic today, Ms. Wiser?" Such an opening allows the parent freedom to answer in a number of areas of concern: physical, emotional, nutritional, and developmental. If asked, "How is John feeling today?" or "Is John ill?" the parent is left to think about only physical aspects and may not voice his or her biggest concern—John's teething difficulty or his frequent temper tantrums. (See Enhancing Communication for more details on eliciting information about the client's chief concern.)

ENHANCING COMMUNICATION

Keoto Weigel is a 13-year-old girl you see at an ambulatory clinic. She has frequency and burning on urination. Her mother accompanies her.

Less Effective Communication

Nurse: Hello, Keoto. What's the reason you've come into the clinic today?
Mrs. Weigel: It hurts when she urinates.
Nurse: How long ago did that start, Keoto?
Mrs. Weigel: She started complaining about it yesterday.
Nurse: Has she had any blood in her urine?
Mrs. Weigel: She hasn't said anything about that. The important thing is the pain.
Nurse: Okay. I'm sure we need a urine specimen for culture. Let's get that to get started here.

More Effective Communication

Nurse: Hello, Keoto. What's the reason you've come into the clinic today?
Mrs. Weigel: It hurts when she urinates.
Nurse: Let's let Keoto answer for herself, Mrs. Weigel. Tell me what you think is the problem, Keoto.
Keoto: It hurts when I go to the bathroom.
Nurse: How long ago did that start, Keoto?
Mrs. Weigel: She started complaining about it last night.
Nurse: Keoto? When do *you* think it started?
Keoto: About an hour after I came in from my date last night.
Nurse: Have you had any blood in your urine?
Mrs. Weigel: She hasn't said anything about that.
Nurse: Keoto? Have you noticed your urine is red or dark brown?
Keoto: I had bright blood last night.
Nurse: Let me take you down to the lavatory and explain about a urine specimen. While we're there, I'd like to ask you some more questions about your date last night.

At about 10 years of age, children are able to supply much of a health history by themselves. As children become teenagers, it is increasingly important for them to do this because they may not have shared a total history with a parent. In the above scenario, for example, when the child is asked directly for information, she supplied more than when her history was given by the mother. Some urinary tract infections occur in girls after their first sexual relations. It would be important to ask Keoto if she is sexually active (what her date last night included), not only to document the probable cause of the urinary tract infection, but also to be certain she is knowledgeable about pregnancy prevention and safer sex practices.

Present Health Status

Once the parent has voiced this chief concern, ask him or her to describe at least six aspects of the problem:

1. Duration
2. Intensity

3. Frequency
4. Description
5. Associated symptoms
6. Actions taken

In discussing duration, it is important to know when the child was last well to determine when he or she became ill. For example, on Saturday morning, John began having long crying periods. On Monday night, he developed a fever. On Tuesday afternoon, he was brought into the clinic for a checkup. The parent states that John vomited three times Monday morning and thinks this was caused by teething. Unless the parent is asked when John was last well, he or she may pinpoint Monday as the beginning of the illness (the vomiting) when actually it was Saturday (the crying).

The intensity of the illness refers in this instance to the kind of vomiting the child is having. Is it drooling, spitting up, or actual vomiting? The description is the amount (a cupful? a mouthful?) and color (whether it contains blood, bile, or mucus). Associated symptoms might include fever, abdominal pain, difficulty eating, or signs of respiratory illness. A good question to obtain this information is "Is John ill in any other way?"

It is important to know the parent's actions for a number of reasons. First, it is important to know whether anything a parent has been doing has been making the illness worse (e.g., offering a great deal of fluid to replace that vomited and, by doing so, causing more vomiting; using a home remedy or alternative therapy). It also reveals what the parent has previously tried but found ineffective. There is no use telling a parent to give the child 2 tablets of acetaminophen (Tylenol) every 4 hours for fever if the parent has already done that and the fever has not improved. This information also reveals the parent's response to caring for an ill child. A parent who says "I tucked him into bed and gave him a little tea to drink" is different from one who replies, "Nothing. I fall all apart when my child is ill." If the child is going to be returned home for the parent to care for, the second parent will need more instructions and support before he or she leaves the health care setting than the first parent.

Obtaining this information about the chief concern puts the parent's observations in proper perspective. In the previous example, the parent is probably not describing teething difficulty (teething does not cause vomiting). More likely, the child has a viral gastroenteritis. Unless the problem is investigated, it is easy to accept the parent's statement at face value as a teething problem and not appreciate its full significance.

During this phase of the interview, it is also important to gather information about related or other health concerns. After the chief concern is documented, ask another open-ended question to elicit additional ones: "Is there anything else that worries you about John?" Now the parents might want to talk about John's temper tantrums. Unless asked about a second problem, the parents will go home with the first problem cared for but the second one still not addressed. When the parents arrive home and John begins stomping his feet in the car, unwilling to go into the house, they will begin to feel the health care John received was less than adequate because they did not receive help with this concern.

Do not assume that parents will always reveal their worst fears in the initial minute of an interview: it can be frightening to put these fears into words. As long as a concern is hanging as a nebulous thought in the mind, it is easy to tell oneself that it may not be true. Only when a parent voices the thought ("Do you think that John is retarded?" "Do you think this is leukemia?" "Could this be inherited?") does the fear become real. Before parents dare to speak openly this way, they must trust health care providers not to treat their statement lightly. For this reason, it is helpful to repeat the question about a second concern at the very end of the interview.

✔ CHECKPOINT QUESTIONS

1. What type of interview question supplies its own answer?
2. What are six areas to explore regarding a chief concern?

Health and Family Profile

Before pursuing the past history or development of a child, it is important to understand something about the circumstances in which the child lives (Kodadek, 1996). A good introduction to a health and family profile is a sentence such as, "Before we talk about any past illnesses or happenings with John, let me ask you some questions about John's health and your family as a whole."

Important information concerning the child's current health status includes:

- Who is the child's primary health care provider?
- How often is the child seen for routine health examinations?
- Can you describe the child's general state of health? How does this compare to the child's health 1 and 5 years ago (if appropriate)?
- Does the child have any known allergies?
- Does the child have a chronic illness or disability?
- Is the child taking any prescription medications? Over-the-counter medications? Home or folk remedies?
- How are medications administered (crushed in water, in a syringe, on a spoon)?
- Is the child undergoing any treatments?

Important information concerning the family includes:

- Is the parent married, single or divorced?
- Is the family nuclear or extended?
- How many children are in the family?
- What are the parents' occupations? This helps establish the family's socioeconomic level and means of family support.
- If parents both work, how do they manage child care?

Obtaining a health and family profile is sometimes delayed by medical interviewers until the end of the interview, when, theoretically, a parent or child is more comfortable and will answer these personal questions more readily. However, by following a nursing model and obtaining the information earlier in the interview, the healthcare practitioner can better assess the child and evaluate data.

Day History

The child's current skills, sleep patterns, hygiene practices, eating habits and interactions with the family can all be elicited by asking the parent to describe a typical day. Day histories are fun to obtain because most parents are eager to describe their day with their child. Information gained this way is surprisingly rich and pertinent, much more so than if parents are just asked how the baby sleeps, eats, or plays.

Begin by asking "Was yesterday a fairly typical day for John?" (The parent says, yes, it was.) "Would you describe for me all that John did yesterday, beginning with his awakening?" Some parents do this with a great deal of detail; with others, it is necessary to backtrack for particular details: "What did he eat for breakfast? Does he use a fork and spoon? Does he sit in a high chair or on your lap?"

Play. Play, the work of children, reveals a great deal about the child's development and overall well-being. Important questions regarding play include:

- Is John kept in a playpen or allowed room to run?
- Can the parent name his favorite toy?
- Does he play active, chasing games or quiet, pretending kinds?
- Does the parent spend time reading to the child?
- Does the parent play with him or let him play by himself? (This allows for an estimation of the quality of interaction during the day.)

Sleep. Every child needs adequate rest for healthy growth and development. Poor sleep patterns can often reveal a psychosocial or physical health problem. Important questions regarding sleep include:

- When the child sleeps, how long does he sleep?
- Is falling asleep a problem?
- Where does he sleep? Does he have night terrors?
- Does he sleep-walk?
- Does he wet his bed (depending on whether the child is toilet trained)?

Hygiene. Good hygiene practices promote healthy teeth, gums and skin; prevent infections; and improve self-esteem. Poor hygiene may reflect neglect, depression, drug abuse or low socioeconomic status. Important questions regarding hygiene include:

- How much self-care does the child do?
- Does he take baths or showers?
- Does he brush his teeth? How often? Does he floss regularly? (Responses depend on the age of the child.)
- Does he wash his hands before snacks and meals?
- Has there been a recent change in hygiene practices?

Eating Habits. Nutritional assessment is an important portion of a health assessment because it influences health so strongly (Byrnes, 1996). Characteristics of a nutritionally healthy child that can be revealed by assessment are summarized in Table 13-1. Food and nutrient intake risk factors are summarized in Box 13-1.

Taking a history of a child's food intake can help determine whether there are any foods missing in a typical meal plan or whether any quantities seem excessive. Be certain to assess not only the quantity of food taken but

BOX 13.1

FOOD AND NUTRIENT INTAKE RISK FACTORS

History or evidence of any of the following may be a potential risk:

Intake less or greater than standard for age and for calories, protein, and activity

Intake less or greater than standard for nutrients (i.e., vitamins and minerals)

Unusual food habits, such as pica, faddism, and meal skipping

Inappropriate use of supplements (vitamins, minerals, fortified food products)

A physician's order for NPO or a clear liquid diet for more than 3 days without enteral or parenteral nutrition

Inadequate transitional feeding, enteral support, or parenteral support

Minimal or no intake from a major food group

Fluid intake less than output

Eating or feeding disorders

Food allergies

Restricted diet

Council on Practice Quality Management Committee (1994). Identifying patients at risk: ADA's definition for nutrition screening and nutrition assessment. *J Am Diet Assoc, 94*(8), 838.

TABLE 13.1 Physical Signs of Adequate Nutrition

ASSESSMENT	FINDING
Overall impression	Alert, with good energy level; positive mood
Hair	Shiny, strong, with good body
Eyes	Good eyesight, particularly at night; conjunctiva moist and pink
Mouth	No cavities in teeth; no swollen or inflamed gingivae; no cracks or fissures at corners of mouth; mucous membrane moist and pink; tongue smooth and nontender
Neck	Normal contour of thyroid gland
Skin	Smooth; normal color and turgor; no ecchymotic or petechial areas present
Extremities	Normal muscle mass and circumference; normal strength and mobility; no edema present; no tender joints; normal reflexes; legs not bowed
Gastrointestinal	No diarrhea or constipation is present
Finger and toenails	Smooth, pink; not cracked or broken
Height and weight	Within normal limits on growth chart
Blood pressure	Normal for age

the quality as well (e.g., for the infant, cereal should be iron fortified).

To do this, ask parents to describe a typical day (24-hour recall), listing what the child ate for each meal and between meals as well. With an older child, the 24-hour recall can be a joint parent–child venture. Providing this history can be difficult, however, when the child consumes some meals at home and others at day care or school. It may be necessary to ask for a weekend history to get a complete picture.

When assessing the adolescent, take a 24-hour recall nutritional history without a parent present, if possible. In front of a parent, adolescents may add nutritional foods to a food intake history or leave out foods they have eaten (e.g., milkshakes, potato chips, or pizza) to avoid a lecture later; on the other hand, they may leave out healthy items or add less desirable ones because they may enjoy the obvious parental disapproval—a game that can appeal to them as part of their rebellion against adult authority.

After taking a history of the child's food intake, determine whether the child is receiving foods from the five pyramid groups. If whole food groups are absent or grossly inadequate, the follow-up evaluation should include a food frequency record as a double check to see if 24-hour recall was truly representative of a usual day. Remember that children do not have to eat food from all groups every meal, as long as they eat from them every day. If parents think in terms of days rather than meals, they may exert less pressure on a child at each meal.

WHAT IF? What if an adolescent tells you he eats a hamburger with lettuce, onion, and tomatoes on a bun, french fries, and a chocolate milkshake every night for dinner? Does this include the five pyramid food groups?

It is important to consider the role of food preferences and cultural, lifestyle and financial variations when assessing food intake. The number of meals eaten at home versus outside the home, form and content of traditional meals cooked at home, and the pattern of meals should all be considered. Any religious dietary restrictions should also be determined (see Focus on Cultural Competence).

FOCUS ON CULTURAL COMPETENCE

In addition to personal likes and dislikes, nutritional practices are culturally determined. Children whose religions prevent them from eating meat, for example, will be vegetarians. Some families prepare food with many spices, some blandly. Some families use corn as a dietary stable, some rice, and some potatoes or wheat. Lactose intolerance prohibits many Asian children from drinking milk. The main meal of the day is also culturally determined; for some families this is the noon meal; for others it is the evening meal. Assessment is always necessary to understand the meaning of food to a particular family.

Do not appear critical of a child's diet. If you convey dismay at erratic eating habits, parents or older children (especially adolescents) may begin to fabricate the food history to make it seem more acceptable.

Past Health History

For a past health history, ask whether the child ever had any serious illnesses. Parents do not generally think of childhood diseases such as measles, chickenpox, and mumps as serious illnesses; inquire about these separately. Has the child had any accidents? Any surgery? Parents may not think of a tonsillectomy as surgery because there were no stitches; ask about that separately. Did the child ever ingest anything that was inedible or harmful? Has the child been hospitalized for any reason? How many times has the child been seen in an emergency room?

The outcome of past illnesses is as important to obtain as the illnesses themselves. If the child had otitis media (middle ear infection) at age 2 years and received an antibiotic and recovered without complications, the parent has every reason to be confident that the child will get better from a present illness also. The parent has confidence in health care personnel. If the child had an allergic reaction to the antibiotic or was left with a hearing difficulty from the previous illness, the parent may distrust the care being given to the child now; he or she may not follow instructions well, thinking that nothing works anyway, or they may need extra support to follow instructions. This is important information for planning care.

When parents report a past health concern or outcome, be sure to ask for details and record the responses. This can help to minimize inaccurate data and ensure that the present and future care of the child is appropriate. For example, some parents believe that their child is allergic to an antibiotic because while the child was taking the drug he or she developed some diarrhea. There is a strong possibility that the diarrhea was associated with the reason for taking the antibiotic, not with the drug itself. In this example, you would want to ask about specific symptoms and record what the parent says about allergies so the person who prescribes medication for the child can decide whether a true allergy exists (Burns, 1996).

Pregnancy History. The health of children is affected by their mother's health during pregnancy. For children under age 5 years, therefore, a pregnancy history is usually obtained. Document which pregnancy this was for the mother. Were there complications in any past pregnancies? Abortions or miscarriages? Stillbirths? Children born prematurely? A history of the pregnancy of the child being assessed can begin with a question such as "How was your pregnancy with John?" This allows the mother to answer in physical and emotional areas. After exploring details she mentions, ask about specific events that are known to occur with pregnancy, such as:

- Did the mother have any complications such as bleeding, falls, swelling of hands and feet, high blood pressure, or unusual weight gain?
- Did she take any medication?
- Were any x-ray films taken?

- Did she smoke cigarettes or drink alcohol or use recreational drugs?
- Did the pregnancy end early or late?

Because life contingencies such as loss of finances or illness in the family during a pregnancy may affect a parent's ability to form a bond with a child, the emotional experiences of a woman during pregnancy are also important to obtain. Ask if the parents planned the pregnancy. A question such as "A lot of pregnancies come as a sort of surprise. Is that how it was with John?" or "Some unmarried women want to have children and some don't. How was it with you?" lets parents know you accept any answer they give.

Next, review labor and delivery. Questions to ask may include:

- Were they what the woman expected them to be?
- How long was labor?
- Were there any complications? Was the birth vaginal or cesarean?
- Was anesthesia used for delivery?
- Was the baby born vertex (head first) or breech?

Ask about the health of the child at birth as well. Questions to ask may include:

- Did the baby cry right away?
- Did he or she need special procedures or equipment either at birth or in the nursery?
- Was there cyanosis or jaundice?
- Did the infant go to a regular nursery?
- Was he or she discharged from the hospital with the mother?
- How did the parents feel about having a boy or girl?
- How did it feel for them to be new parents?

Family Health History

Because some diseases are inherited or familial, it is important to know which ones occur in a family. Ask if any family member has heart disease (childhood or adult type); kidney disease; a congenital anomaly; seizures; mental retardation; mental illness; diabetes (type 1 or 2); tuberculosis; a sexually transmitted disease (STD); or allergies. Keep in mind that events may have been misinterpreted and reports may be inaccurate so it is important to ask for details and record what is said about specific familial health problems and outcomes.

Review of Systems

The last step in a health interview is a summary of body symptoms or a **review of systems.** Once more, make certain to introduce this part of the history with a transition statement, otherwise a parent may think that the local problem (vomiting) he or she has been describing suggests other problems. To finish, "I'd like to ask about different parts of John's body, from his head down to his toes, just to be certain I don't miss anything" is such a transition statement.

Although the important items to be covered in a review of systems differ according to the age of the child, a basic list is shown in Box 13-2.

BOX 13.2

REVIEW OF SYSTEMS

Neuropsychiatric symptoms: Has the child ever had seizures? Head injury? Attention problems? Depression? Aggressive behavior? Has the parent ever had such difficulty rousing the child that the parent believed the child was unconscious? Have there been any problems with suspected substance abuse?

Eyes: Has the child had difficulty with eyes not focusing? Eye infection? Does the parent have any reason to believe that the child does not see well? *Does the child wear eye glasses? Contacts?*

Ears: Ear infections? Drainage from the ears? Earaches? *Tubes in ears?* Any infection from piercing? Reason to believe the child does not hear well?

Nose: Frequent drainage or cold symptoms? Difficulty breathing? Nosebleeds?

Mouth: Difficulty with teeth or teething? Mouth infections? Has the child seen a dentist (if older than age 2 years)? Does the child chew tobacco?

Throat: Throat infections? Difficulty swallowing?

Neck: Masses or swelling? Stiffness? Does the child hold his or her head straight? (Torticollis or wry neck will make the child hold his or her head crookedly; children with poor vision also may cock their heads to the side to try to see better.)

Chest: Is breast development in girls appropriate for age? For adolescent girls over 14 years and Tanner Stage V, ask about breast self-examination.

Lungs: Breathing problems? Infections? Pneumonia? *Asthma?* Does the child smoke any substance?

Heart: Has a physician ever said there was difficulty? What exactly was said?

Gastrointestinal system: Has there been an eating problem? Frequent nausea? Vomiting? Ask separately from nausea. (Children with *pyloric stenosis*—obstruction of the pyloric opening of the stomach—have vomiting but no nausea; children with a brain tumor may also have vomiting but no nausea; pregnant teenagers may have nausea but not vomiting.) Diarrhea? Any constipation? Is the child toilet trained? Any difficulty with this?

Genitourinary system: Pain or burning on urination? Blood in urine? Does the child have a good urine stream? If a girl is age 10 years or older, has she started menstruation? Any problems with menstruation? If an adolescent male, has he begun testicular self-examination? If an adolescent, is the child sexually active? Using contraception? Want more information on contraception? Ever had an STD? (*To protect privacy, it is essential to ask the adolescent, not the parents, questions regarding sexuality.*)

Extremities: Painful or swollen joints? Broken bones? Muscle sprains? Is the parent pleased with the child's coordination?

Skin: Rashes? Lesions such as warts?

Immunizations: What immunizations has the child received to date?

A review of systems covers a lot of ground, but it generally takes no more than 5 minutes. Do not think of it as just a mop-up operation and ask questions so quickly ("Has John ever had nausea-vomiting-diarrhea-painful joints-broken bones?") that the parent does not have time to answer or begins to believe this part of the interview is only an exercise and is unimportant. All the questions are important. If the child shows any of the symptoms described, an entirely new area needs to be explored.

Conclusion

A health history should close with one last open-ended question: "Is there anything more about John that we should know?" or "Is there anything I didn't mention that you want to ask about?" A parent may have been reluctant to bring up something earlier. Asking this final question gives the parent a final opportunity to do this.

CHECKPOINT QUESTIONS

3. What are the important areas to consider when obtaining a day history?
4. Why is it important to ask for a family health history?
5. What question should be asked at the end of every interview?

PHYSICAL ASSESSMENT

Physical assessment is one of the most frequently practiced skills of a nurse. The scope and extent of pediatric physical assessment vary, like health interviewing, depending on the circumstances of each health visit. Sometimes only a single segment is required to obtain the information needed. For example, if a child has a gastrointestinal disorder, assessment might be only a brief, multisystem examination concentrating on the gastrointestinal system (i.e., mouth, abdomen, and rectum) and fluid status (i.e., skin turgor, lips, and mucous membranes). At a first health care encounter, however, children usually receive a complete physical examination. Mastery of physical examination techniques is essential to incorporating physical assessment data into the assessment step of the nursing process.

Purpose and Techniques

The actual process of physical examination involves four separate techniques:

1. Inspection
2. Palpation
3. Percussion
4. Auscultation

These techniques are usually carried out in the above order in each area of the body except the abdomen (auscultation should follow inspection and precede palpation of the abdomen, because handling the abdomen may obliterate bowel sounds). **Inspection** is used to determine whether there is redness or swelling or any break in the skin. **Palpation** yields information on warmth and edema; **percussion** helps determine the consistency of tissue beneath the surface area (Figure 13-2) and **auscultation** reveals the presence of sound (Box 13-3). The findings from these techniques strengthen or validate history findings and help determine whether a problem requires immediate action.

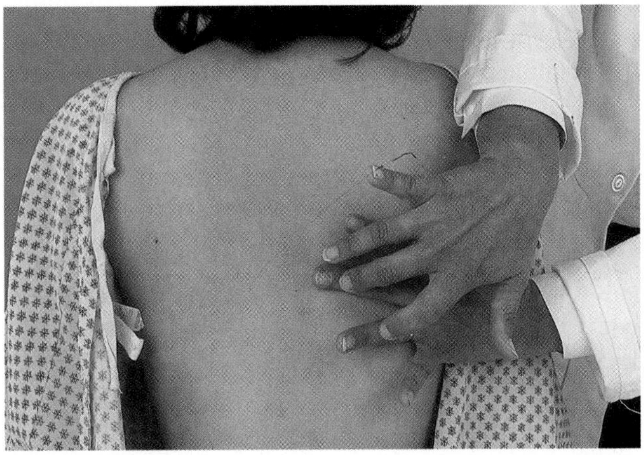

FIGURE 13.2 Percussion. The sound is made by one finger striking a second one.

BOX 13.3

TECHNIQUES OF PHYSICAL EXAMINATION

Inspection is examining a child or adolescent initially with your eyes or nose, being alert to visual indications or odors that may point to a health problem.

Palpation is examining by touch and can be either light or deep touch. Use light palpation before deep palpation so the child or adolescent does not tense muscles and make light palpation difficult. The tips of your fingers are most sensitive to texture, vibration, consistency, and contour; the back of your hand is most sensitive to warmth. If a child has a sensitive or painful body part, palpate that area last. Otherwise, the child may be unwilling to allow you to touch other parts for fear he or she will experience additional pain.

Percussion is the assessment of a body structure by determining the sound you hear in response to striking the part with an examining finger (Figure 13-2), and then interpreting the sound. Dense body areas such as bone have a dull, flat sound; those filled with air, such as lungs, are resonant. If an organ is stretched (a distended bladder), it has a hyperresonant or low and hollow sound. An organ stretched to an even greater point of distention has a tympanic or extremely hollow, ringing sound.

Auscultation is listening to sounds that are either discernible to the ear (wheezing or heavy breathing) or, as in most cases, made louder by means of a stethoscope. Always listen for four qualities of sound: duration, frequency, intensity (loudness), and pitch (high or low).

Use physical examination to complement the questions asked when a parent describes some symptom a child is experiencing. If a parent says he or she thinks the child has pain, for example, ask about the duration, intensity, frequency, associated symptoms, and any action or activity that precipitates the pain. Then examine the area for signs of inflammation and palpate for tenderness.

Effective use of physical assessment skills takes practice. Palpating an abdomen, for example, is a simple procedure; recognizing abdominal pathology through palpation is a second, more complicated step. It is difficult to distinguish between normal liver tissue and a distended liver, for example, until both these conditions have been felt many times.

Equipment, Setting, and Approach

A number of items are necessary for complete physical assessment: a thermometer, a stethoscope, a tongue depressor, an ophthalmoscope, an otoscope, a sphygmomanometer, a tape measure, a tuning fork, a reflex (percussion) hammer, rubber gloves, and perhaps a client drape or drawsheet. Nurses who work in community settings or clients' homes must be sure to carry any equipment that may be needed with them.

Examining body parts such as the mouth or an open lesion exposes the hands to body fluids. As part of infection prevention precautions, wear rubber gloves to examine such body parts. During a complete physical examination, every part of the child's body should be exposed for inspection. To protect against chilling and to provide for modesty, do this by exposing body parts individually and only for the amount of time necessary for the examination. Use a client gown or a drawsheet as a drape as necessary.

Be certain the temperature in an examining room is comfortable. Be certain to provide privacy. Paper table covers should be changed between children to avoid possible spread of illness.

People have the right not to have another person touch their body unless they permit them to do so. It is essential, therefore, to inform children that it is necessary to touch them for a physical examination and tell them what is happening at each step during a physical examination so they know when they will be touched (e.g., "Next, I will look at your throat"). If some action will cause discomfort, such as deep palpation of the abdomen, offer fair warning: "You'll feel pressure for a minute." Such explanations are also psychologically reassuring because they prevent surprises.

It can be assumed that adolescents will cooperate in placing themselves in whatever position is required to inspect body parts unless they are short of breath or in some other way unable to comply. Small children may not cooperate and so need to be restrained during an examination of body parts such as nose, throat, and ears. This is done not only to enable an examiner to see well but also to ensure that the instrument used will not accidentally injure the child. As a rule, do not ask parents to restrain with any procedure in which the child will be hurt—parents are best used as protectors and comforters. This is not usually a problem with physical examination, which rarely hurts, so parental participation is helpful. Some procedures, such as ear examination, do require a strong restraining hand, and this can be frightening to children. Urge parents to do this with a positive approach such as "I'll help you keep your hand still."

Variations for Age and Developmental Stage

Techniques of physical examination must be tailored to the age and developmental stage of the individual being assessed (Table 13-2). Expected findings also depend on the child's age and developmental stage.

Newborn

All newborns receive a physical examination immediately after birth and again after the first 24 hours of life. When examining newborns, remember that maintaining body temperature is one of the newborn's most difficult tasks. Cover body areas that are not being directly examined. Take axillary or tympanic temperatures to prevent rupture of rectal mucosa. Take the heart rate apically because peripheral pulses are too faint to be counted accurately. Be certain to take femoral pulses in newborns to rule out coarctation of the aorta. Include newborn reflexes, head circumference, and an assessment of gestational age (see Chapter 5) as routine parts of the examination. Do not take blood pressure because this value is unreliable in the newborn.

Infant

Infants are usually examined most effectively if a parent holds them during most of the examination. Use an "isn't this fun?" or "this is a game" approach. As a rule, assess heart and lung function first; intrusive procedures such as ear and throat assessment should be done last so the infant does not cry and complicate the remainder of the examination. Blood pressure is still not taken routinely. Include newborn reflexes until age 6 months; continue to take heart rate apically and temperature axillary or by tympanic membrane. Include head circumference for a full year.

Toward the end of the first year, children become fearful of strangers. Taking an extra minute to become well acquainted with the infant at the beginning of the examination helps to counteract this problem.

Toddler and Preschooler

Both toddlers and preschoolers may be afraid of examining equipment. To alleviate their fears, let them handle items such as stethoscopes, otoscopes, and blood pressure cuffs (Figure 13-3). Leave intrusive procedures such as assessment of the genitalia, ears, and throat until last. Give generous praise for cooperation (anything short of hysterical screaming or kicking is good cooperation for intrusive procedures in this age group). Empowering the Family describes ways parents can prepare young children for assessment.

Begin to include blood pressure as part of routine assessment at age 3 years; oral temperature by an electronic thermometer can also begin at this age. Before beginning an examination, establish a good rapport with the child's parents, because children this age sense parental trust or suspicion.

TABLE 13.2 Techniques of Physical Examination Based on Child's Age

AGE	TECHNIQUES
Newborn	Undress only the body part being examined or use radiant heat warmer to conserve heat (be certain all body parts are exposed during examination).
	Examine heart and respiratory systems first before infant cries, then follow head-to-toe procedure, performing all manipulative procedures such as throat and eyes last. Examine newborn with parents present, using this assessment time to teach them about normal appearance and development.
Infant	As with newborns, begin examination with heart and respiratory assessment, then follow head-to-toe procedure, performing all manipulative procedures such as throat and ears last.
	Begin examination while parent holds infant in arms or lap to calm the child. Talk to the infant as you proceed; infants calm to sound of your voice or the feeling tone that you radiate as much as they do to what you actually say. Positive feeling tone ("This is like a game") therefore often brings better cooperation than strict, businesslike approach. Infants older than 3 mo like to handle tongue blades. They can be distracted by brightly colored toys while you listen to their heart or lungs. They cooperate best if parent holds them for major portion of examination. Offering a bottle of water or pacifier may be necessary during heart assessment.
Toddler	Allow toddler to handle equipment; include games, such as blowing out otoscope light, to relax child.
	Ask parent to remove clothing or allow child to do it independently.
	Use head-to-toe procedure; leave uncomfortable procedures such as throat and ear examination for last.
Preschooler	Use games such as "Simon Says" to ease child's fright. Ask child to undress; do not remove underpants.
	Preschoolers are extremely threatened by intrusive procedures. Thus, they are frightened of examining instruments. Allow them to handle instruments before use. Assure them that instruments do not hurt. Children up to school age often need to be restrained for ear and throat examination because they grow fearful about procedures performed on a part of the body they cannot see (ears) or about a throat examination that may be uncomfortable.
School-age child	Ask whether child wants parent present or not.
	Proceed with head-to-toe assessment; leave genitalia for last.
	Allow child to undress except for underpants; supply gown.
	Explain equipment and reasons for procedures. Teach whys and hows of procedures.
Adolescent	Ask if the adolescent wants parent present or not.
	Teach adolescent about good health care during examination. Comment on body parts as you examine them: "Your heart sounds good," "Ears look fine." Sometimes an adolescent is so concerned with a part of his or her body (a supernumerary nipple, for example) that he or she is unable to voice this concern. A comment such as, "This is a supernumerary (extra) nipple. Does it ever worry you that you have that?" may help the adolescent to talk about what has indeed been worrying her for years.
	Use head-to-toe procedure; leave genitalia for last.
	Include health teaching on breast and testicular self-examination.

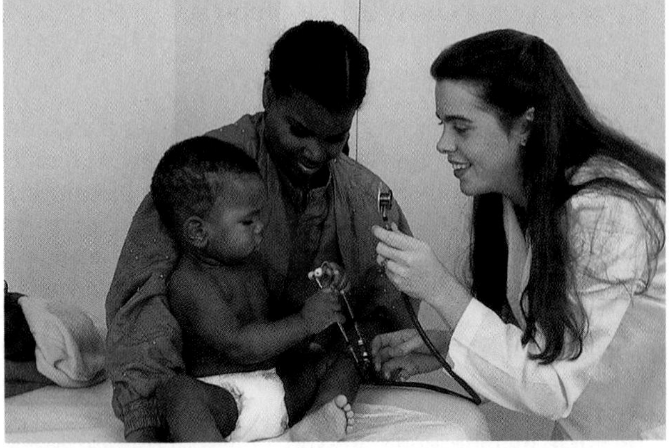

FIGURE 13.3 Children need the opportunity to play with examining equipment so they become more familiar with and less frightened by it.

School-Age Child and Adolescent

Some children of this age may still be unaware of what a physical examination includes and whether it will cause discomfort. Offer good explanations so they are not frightened by the unknown. Older children may enjoy having a parent with them while they are being examined or they may resent their presence; give them a choice. Adolescents are often worried about some normal physical finding such as a mole or supernumerary (extra) nipple. Make a habit of commenting on such findings—"This is a mole on your hand; that's normal"—as both a means of reassurance and health teaching.

Remember that school-age children and adolescents are particularly modest. Respect this by careful use of gowns or drapes. Begin to include teaching for breast and testicular self-examination when appropriate (usually age 14 and Tanner V stage for girls; age 13 for boys).

EMPOWERING THE FAMILY: Suggestions for Preparing a Child for a Health Assessment

- Promote the attitude that a health visit will be a positive experience for the child.
- Bring a comfort item from home (favorite doll or toy).
- Never threaten a child that if he is not good, a doctor or nurse will punish him.
- Review with the child what he can expect during an assessment (a nurse will ask some questions of his parent; she or he will then look at the child's head, hands, etc.)
- If a child has been taught not to let strangers touch his body (as he should have been taught), a child may need reassurance from a parent that it is all right for a nurse to examine him.
- Dress the child in easy to remove and replace clothing so you can quickly dress the child after an examination as a way of assuring him that the examination is over.

CHECKPOINT QUESTIONS

6. What four techniques are used in physical assessment?
7. At what age is blood pressure included as a routine procedure?

COMPONENTS OF PHYSICAL EXAMINATION

A physical examination may be done in any order, but traditionally the order proceeds from head to toe; examining each body part thoroughly before moving on to the next. With infants and young children, however, it is easiest to begin with the heart and lungs; this is because, if the infant cries, findings in these areas become difficult to assess over the sound of crying.

Presented here are the components of a routine or general physical assessment. If abnormalities were discovered during an examination, further assessment would be undertaken. A complete neurologic examination, for example, is not routine so is not included here (see Chapter 28 for details on neurologic examination). It is important to recognize what a "general" physical examination of this nature entails so you can interpret the extent of assessment that a child has received when the parent states, "He had a routine physical."

Vital Sign Assessment

Vital signs refer to temperature, pulse, respiration, blood pressure or the state of *vital* bodily functions (e.g., heart and lung function or metabolic rate). Because of the important information they provide, measurements of these signs are recorded not only with complete physical examinations but in many other instances of care (see Managing and Delegating Unlicensed Assistive Personnel). Techniques of these measurements and the nursing responsibilities that accompany them are discussed in Chapter 16.

General Appearance

Physical examination begins with inspection of **general appearance** to form a general impression of the child's health and well-being and to pinpoint specific body areas that will need detailed assessment (Figure 13-4). Assess such areas as:

- Does the child appear overall well or ill?
- Is the child's height and weight proportional?
- Does the child appear well nourished?
- What is the child's color? Pale? Yellow (jaundiced)? Cyanotic (blue)?
- Is posture normal? (Children who are in pain often assume an abnormal posture for relief.)
- What is the child's hygiene level?
- Are lesions or symptoms of a specific illness present?
- Are there any significant body odors? (Table 13-3)
- Does the child appear relaxed or distressed? Lethargic or active?
- Is breathing easy or distressed?

Mental Status Assessment

A mental status assessment is also made early in an examination as a complement to general appearance information.

MANAGING AND DELEGATING UNLICENSED ASSISTIVE PERSONNEL

Be certain unlicensed assistive personnel are aware of the need to clean examining equipment such as otoscope tips. If they are responsible for taking vital signs, be certain they understand that any conversation they have with the child or parents during this time should be reported because this can be interpreted by the parents as history taking. If parents interpret it this way, they may not repeat any of this information, assuming that it has been recorded and is now known by all health care personnel.

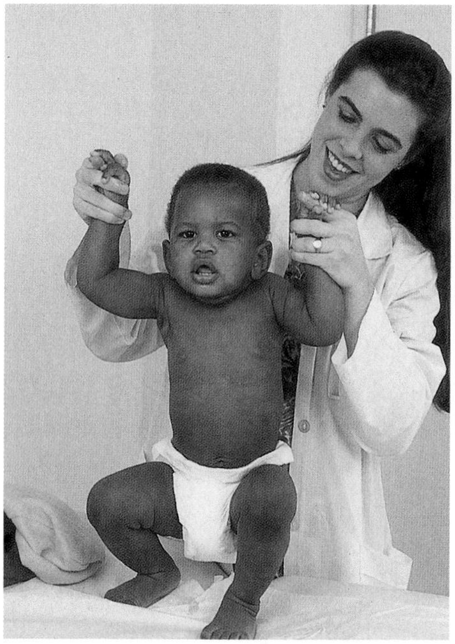

FIGURE 13.4 General appearance assessment reveals that this child is well proportioned and active.

As with general appearance, additional information is gained on mental status throughout the entire examination.

Begin by assessing the child's level of consciousness: Is the child alert? Able to respond to questions easily? Assess *orientation,* or awareness of person, place, and time (awareness of who they are, where they are, and the date). Assess the appropriateness of behavior and mood: hostile, frightened, or relaxed? At some point in the examination of children above preschool age, ask questions that test recent memory and distant memory.

Body Measurements

Body measurements are important determinants of health in children because with chronic illness the body expends so many nutrients combating the destructive process of the disease that normal height and weight cannot be maintained. Conversely, overweight (obesity) may be the cause of illnesses such as heart and lung disease later in life (Keller & Stevens, 1996).

Height

In children, height is as good a determinant of health and normal nutrition as weight. To accurately measure the height of infants and older children, see Nursing Procedure 13-1: Measuring the Child's Height.

Plot height measurements for children on a standard graph the same as for weight. Height and weight should follow the same percentiles. Remember that height-weight charts have been standardized for "typical" American children, so there will be variations among children of different cultural backgrounds. The important thing to look for is a consistency of measurements over time (always at the same percentile).

Weight

Until they can stand well, infants are weighed on a sitting or infant scale. Because diapers can be heavy in proportion to total body weight, infants are weighed nude. Always keep a sheltering hand over an infant on an infant scale (hovering but not touching), because infants squirm readily and there is danger of them falling (Figure 13-5A). Cover both infant scales and adult scales with scale paper before weighing to prevent spread of infection from one child to another.

TABLE 13.3 Significant Body Odors

SOURCE OF ODOR	POSSIBLE CAUSE
Breath	
Alcohol	Implies recent ingestion (important if coma or neurologic symptoms are present as cause of abnormal functioning)
Camphor	Mothball ingestion
Halitosis (bad breath)	Poor dental hygiene, lung infection; foreign body in respiratory tract
Burnt rope	Marijuana use
Sweet	Acidosis (seen in a child in diabetic coma)
Body	
Stale urine	Incontinence; poor kidney functioning leading to uremia; infrequently changed diapers; neglect
Sweat	May imply unusual fatigue recently, or that child has not maintained usual hygiene regimen
"Spoiled fruit"	Wound infection
Sweet	*Pseudomonas* infection
Urine	
Maple syrup	Protein metabolic condition
Musty or mousy	Phenylketonuria or a protein metabolism disorder
Ammonia	Urinary tract infection or poor hydration leading to concentrated urine
Stool	
Putrid	Fat in stool from inadequate absorption

NURSING PROCEDURE 13.1: MEASURING THE CHILD'S HEIGHT

Plan	Principle
INFANT	
1. Until they can stand securely (at approximately age 2 years), infants are measured lying down on a measuring frame or an examining table.	1. Promote accuracy.
2. Align the infant's head snugly against the top bar of the frame and ask an assistant to secure it there. Parents can help you restrain infants for height measurements because it is a painless procedure.	2. Provide a starting point for measurement.
3. Straighten the infant's body (Figure A).	3. Knees are difficult to straighten in infants because they always keep them flexed.

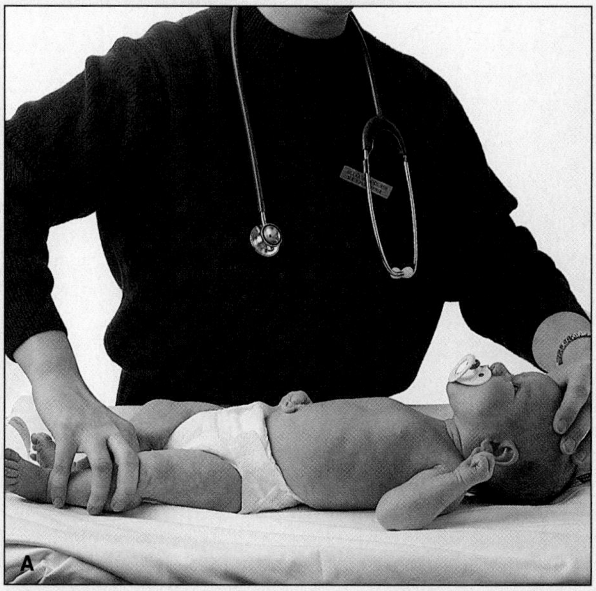

Plan	Principle
4. Hold the infant's feet in a vertical position. Bring the foot board up snugly against the bottom of the foot.	4. Complete measurement.
5. If an examining table is used, mark the spots at the top of the child's head and bottom of feet and then measure between the marks.	5. Alternative approach.
6. Plot height measurements on a standard graph.	6. Interpret findings.
OLDER CHILD	
1. Have the child remove his or her shoes.	1. Promote accuracy.
2. Have the child stand straight with his or her head held level.	2. Position child.
3. Align the measuring bar of a standing scale with the top of the head.	3. Perform measurement.

(continued)

Plan	Principle
4. If a scale with a measuring bar is not available, place a flat object such as a clipboard on the child's head in a horizontal position and read the height at the point at which the object touches a measuring tape on the back of the scale or a flat wall surface (Figure B).	4. Alternative approach.

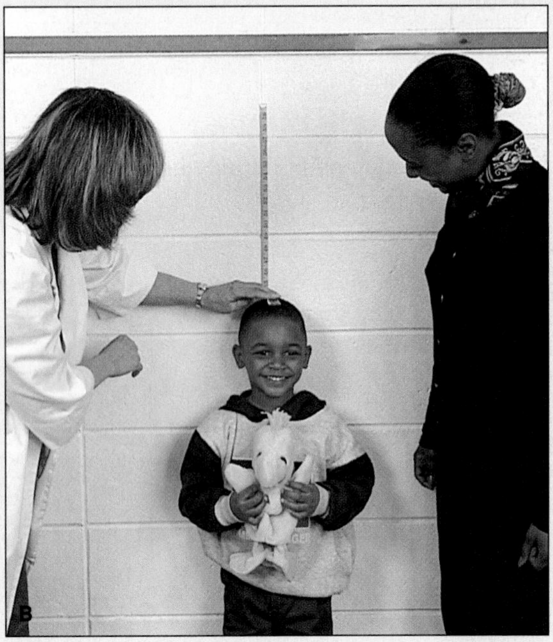

Plan	Principle
5. Plot height measurements on a standard graph.	5. Interpret findings.

Children older than age 2 years are weighed on standing scales, in street clothes (no shoes), or, if in a hospital, in a gown or robe (see Figure 13-5*B*). If children are going to have serial weights (weighed every day or several times a day), it is important that they wear the same clothing every time they are weighed so any discrepancy in weight is truly a difference in body weight and not a weight change due to more or less clothing. Take the weight at the same time each day (preferably before breakfast) on the same scale for greatest accuracy.

Most children and their parents want to know their weight. To convert from kilograms to pounds, multiply the kilogram amount by 2.2 (50 kg × 2.2 = 110 lb).

To assess whether weight is average for height, compare the child's weight with a standardized height-weight graph. Child and infant values of these are shown in Appendix E for easy reference. In the standardized scale for children, all weights between the 10th and 90th percentiles are considered normal (statistically, a range of weights that includes two standard deviations from the mean or the 50th percentile). As important as the fact that a child's weight falls between the 10th and 90th percentile on a growth chart is that over time the weight follows one of the percentile curves—that they are not at the 80th percentile the first time they are weighed and a month later at the 40th percentile, for example. Although both readings are within the normal range, they reflect a weight loss that needs investigation. Gaining weight in the same way could be equally serious. A child is defined as having a "failure to thrive" syndrome (medical diagnosis) if height or weight drops below the 3rd percentile on a standardized growth chart. Any height or weight in this category definitely needs to be reported so its cause can be investigated.

> WHAT IF? What if a 14-year-old girl weighs 93 lb? Is this reason for concern? What if 6 months earlier she weighed 110 lb and a year earlier she weighed 105 lb?

Head Circumference

Head circumference is measured at birth and routinely on physical assessment until age 1 year (many health care agencies measure routinely until age 2 years). Head growth occurs because the brain is growing, so head circumference is an important determinant of brain growth and potential neurologic function. The measurement is made by placing a tape measure around the head just above the eyebrows and around the most prominent portion of the back of the head, the occipital prominence (Figure 13-6). Babies generally push any object away from their head, so it may be difficult to carry out this otherwise simple procedure. Plot measurements on a standardized graph (Appendix E). Head

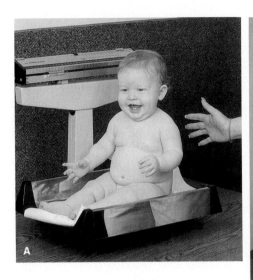

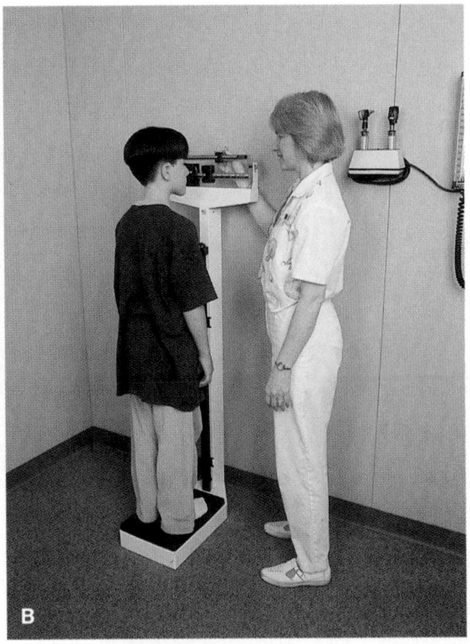

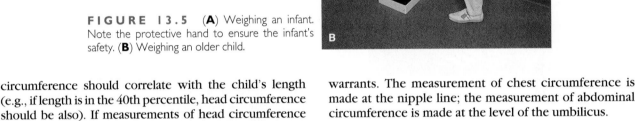

FIGURE 13.5 (**A**) Weighing an infant. Note the protective hand to ensure the infant's safety. (**B**) Weighing an older child.

circumference should correlate with the child's length (e.g., if length is in the 40th percentile, head circumference should be also). If measurements of head circumference plot at different percentiles over time, this should be reported because it implies that brain or skull growth is in some way abnormal and needs investigation.

Chest and Abdominal Circumference

Measurements of chest and abdominal circumference are not done routinely, but only when specific pathology warrants. The measurement of chest circumference is made at the nipple line; the measurement of abdominal circumference is made at the level of the umbilicus.

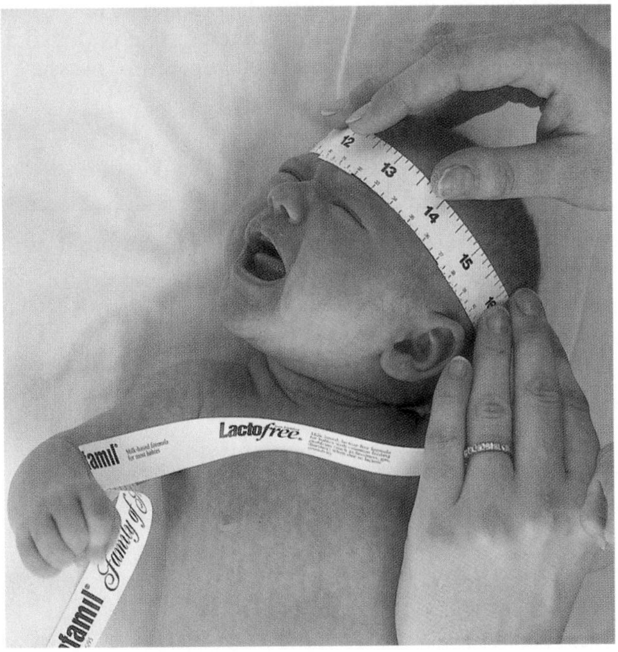

FIGURE 13.6 Measuring head circumference. The measuring tape passes just above the eyebrows and around the prominent posterior aspect of the head.

Skin

Skin is assessed along with the examination of each body region. Assess the following:

- Temperature
- Color
- Texture
- **Turgor,** which is the amount of fluid in body tissue (Figure 13-7)
- Presence of any lesions

Table 13-4 summarizes various other findings that may be detected. Be certain to examine the child's total skin surface at some time during an examination. Remove and replace as necessary adhesive bandages and other dressings that could hide important findings. Good lighting is imperative for accurate assessment of the skin, especially when assessing dark-skinned children.

Newborn and Infant

Newborns may appear ruddy because their layer of subcutaneous fat is thin and the intense redness of their blood circulation is visible. Erythema toxicum may be present. Birthmarks (hemangiomas, mongolian spots, or nevi) may be present. After the first few days of life, a diaper rash may be present.

Toddler, Preschooler and School-Age Child

Many children this age have minor lesions from mosquito bites or from flea bites if they own a pet. They also typically have a number of ecchymotic spots on their lower extremities from bumping into objects during active play. Ecchymotic spots on upper extremities suggest a blood

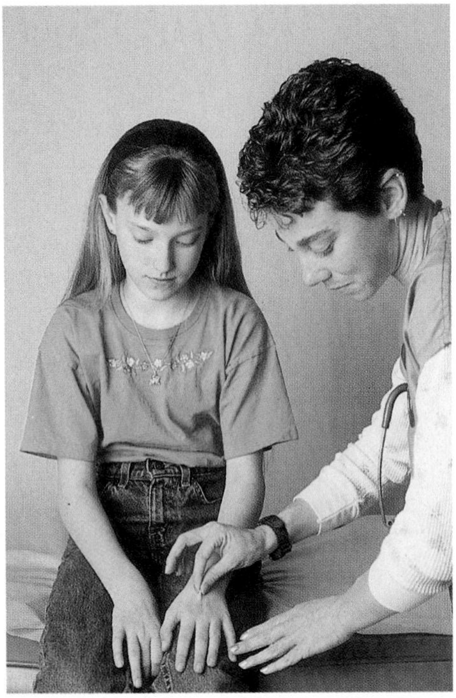

FIGURE 13.7 Assessing skin turgor. If the ridge of tissue does not immediately return to place, the child is poorly hydrated.

coagulation problem. Be certain in evaluating ecchymotic spots on all age children that the possibility of child abuse is considered.

Adolescent

Acne lesions on the face or back are usually present in the adolescent. Lesions or rashes caused by allergies to cosmetics may be apparent. If the child has a tattoo or body piercing, assess the site for inflammation to reveal beginning infection.

Head

To examine the head, slide a hand over the skull, assessing for irregular configurations or tenderness. Most children have a prominent occipital outgrowth; do not mistake this natural head contour as an abnormality. Assess the texture and cleanliness of the hair. Children who are well nourished usually have hair of good texture; poorly nourished children tend to have dry, brittle or limp hair. If hair is exceptionally oily, it may mean that a parent or the child has been too fatigued or depressed lately to wash it. If a serious protein deficiency is present such as **kwashiorkor,** the hair becomes striped with dark and light color because dark hair forms during periods of good protein intake and the light color forms during periods of protein deficit. Patches of hair loss (*alopecia*) suggest a fungal infection (*tinea capitis*), child abuse, or a possible drug reaction (chemotherapy will cause total hair loss, not patches).

Newborn and Infant

In the newborn, the head usually shows *molding* (an elongated shape due to pressure against the cervix before delivery). A caput succedaneum or cephalhematoma from the pressure of birth may be present (see Chapter 23). Skull suture lines may be palpable. In both newborns and infants, sit the child upright and palpate the skull for the presence of *fontanelles*—the places where the skull bones fuse. The anterior fontanelle is at the junction of the two parietal bones and the two fused frontal bones. It is diamond shaped and measures 2 cm to 3 cm (0.8 in to 1.2 in) in width and 3 cm to 4 cm (1.2 in to 1.6 in) in length. The posterior fontanelle is at the junction of the parietal bones and the occipital bone. It is triangular and measures approximately 1 cm (0.5 in) in length.

With the infant sitting, fontanelles should be felt as soft spots but should not appear indented (a sign of dehydration) or bulging (a sign of increased intracranial pressure).

TABLE 13.4 Skin Findings in Children That Suggest Illness

FINDING	INDICATION
Central bluish color	Cyanosis from decreased respiratory function or cyanotic heart disease. Acrocyanosis (blue hands and feet) are normal in newborn for first 48 hours.
White color	Edema (accumulated subcutaneous fluid is stretching the skin)
Pale color	Anemia or decreased circulation to a body part
Reddened area	Local inflammation or increased systemic temperature
Linear abrasion	Scratch marks from local irritation from an insect bite, or allergic reaction
Ecchymoses (black and blue marks)	Recent injury to skin
Petechiae (pinpoint blood marks)	Blood dyscrasia (poor clotting ability)
Yellow color	Jaundice from increased bilirubin in subcutaneous tissue; carotenemia (excess carotene in skin)
Moistness	Excess perspiration from elevated temperature
Localized cold temperature	Decreased circulation to particular body part
Warm temperature	Local irritation or elevated systemic temperature
Poor turgor	Dehydration
Rash	Infectious childhood illness, excessive heat, allergy

When an infant cries, cerebral pressure increases. Thus, with crying, fontanelles will feel tense, and sometimes even the fluctuation of a pulse is present. The anterior fontanelle normally closes at age 12 to 18 months and the posterior fontanelle by the end of age 2 months, so are not palpable after these times. The closing of fontanelles too early or too late may be an indication of decreased or increased brain or ventricle growth.

A scalp problem commonly encountered in infants is *seborrhea* (scaling, greasy-appearing, salmon-colored patches). This is referred to by parents as "cradle cap." Increasing the frequency of hair washing to once a day will effectively reduce this problem.

Toddler, Preschooler and School-Age Child

Examine the hair of children who attend school or day care carefully for small white-yellow, sand-sized particles attached to hair strands—the eggs (nits) of *pediculi* (head lice). Nits cling and cannot be readily removed from hair by running fingers the length of the hair. The child may have recent scratch marks on the scalp and generally states that the scalp feels "itchy." Pediculi spread easily in school-age children due to the sharing of combs and towels in school.

Examine the scalp carefully for round circular areas (perhaps weeping in the center, crusting and scaling on the edges) that would suggest **tinea capitis** (ringworm, a fungal infection). Like pediculi, fungal infections are spread readily among school-age children; a prescription medication is necessary to cure the condition (see Chapter 22).

Adolescent

Adolescents may streak their hair with dye or arrange it in a way that requires glue or use of a curling iron. Inspect to see that their scalp and hair are healthy underneath the styling.

Eyes

Observe the eyes for symmetry and signs of frequent blinking, crusting, squinting, or the child's rubbing the eyes. Observe lids and lashes for redness (erythema), which suggests infection. Common infections include **conjunctivitis** (called "pink eye" by parents; an infection of the thin conjunctiva that covers the eye) or a **hordeolum** or sty (an infection of the gland that lubricates an eyelash). Both conditions require an antibiotic for therapy (see Chapter 29).

Assess the location of eyes in relation to the nose (not unusually wide or narrow spaced) and the relationship of the globe to the socket (neither sunken nor protruding from the socket [exophthalmos]). Abnormalities in these areas occur in chromosomal or metabolic illnesses such as hyperthyroidism. Inspect the sclera of the eye for spots of hemorrhage (called *subconjunctival hemorrhage*) or yellowing. African-American children often have a slight yellowing of the sclera and small black spots on the sclera; do not mistake these for abnormal findings. Assess that no sclera shows above the pupil (if it does, this is termed a *sunset sign,* an indication of increased intracranial pressure).

Palpate the eye globe with eyelid closed to assess for tenseness, although the usual cause of this (glaucoma) is rare in children. Determine whether the eyelids completely close (edema or neurologic illnesses may make eyelids too short to do this), when the child shuts the eyes. Also determine whether the lids retract far enough so they do not obscure vision, when the child opens the eyes. When a lid obscures vision, a condition termed **ptosis,** it generally denotes neurologic involvement. Be certain not to mistake the normal absence of Eastern palpebral folds for abnormal findings. The difference in Western and Eastern eye creases is shown in Figure 13-8.

Examine the inner lining of the lower eyelid (the conjunctiva) by pulling the lid down slightly with a fingertip. The mucous membrane of this space should appear pink and moist. In children with anemia, it often appears pale; with allergy or infection, it may appear unusually red and irritated. Do not initiate a blink reflex by touching the cornea with a wisp of cotton, as can be done in adults; this is momentarily painful and frightening to children.

In addition, observe whether the eyes appear to be in good alignment. **Strabismus** refers to eyes that are not evenly aligned. If an eye is always turning in, the condition is called **esotropia**; if it always turns out, **exotropia.** Two screening procedures for straight eye alignment include a Hirschberg's test and a cover test. During a Hirschberg's test, the light of an otoscope should reflect evenly off both pupils if they are in equal alignment (Figure 13-9).

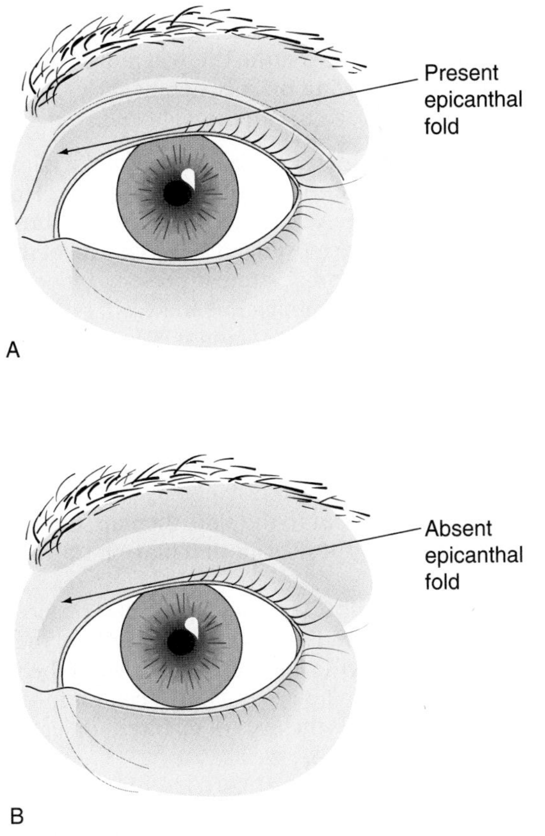

FIGURE 13.8 Differences in eye formation. (**A**) Western. (**B**) Eastern. The extra inner fold of tissue is an epicanthal fold.

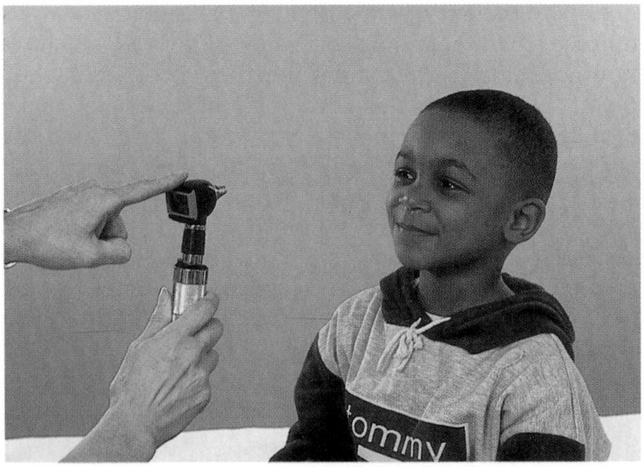

FIGURE 13.9 Testing of good eye alignment by Hirschberg's test. The child is asked to look directly at the light of the otoscope. The light reflex on the pupils of both eyes will be equal if the eyes are in straight alignment.

To perform a cover test (Figure 13-10), follow these steps:

- Have the child fix his or her vision on an attractive object, approximately 4 ft in front of the child.
- Hold a 3 × 5-in card over the left eye for a count of five. If any degree of strabismus is present, the eye will wander to its misaligned position while covered.
- Remove the card and observe the eye for movement.
- As the child again fixes his or her vision on the specified object in front, the eye will move back into line, thus revealing the misalignment.
- Repeat the process with the right eye.

Some children, particularly preschoolers who have wide epicanthic folds, may appear, at a quick glance, to show misalignment. A cover test is helpful in these children. There is no eye movement after removal of the card because there is no misalignment present, only the temporary appearance of misalignment. Reasons for true misalignment are discussed in Chapter 29.

Test the eyes for their ability to focus in all fields of vision. The steps of this procedure follow:

- Ask the child to follow a moving light (or catch the attention of an infant with a moving light) while holding the child's chin stationary.
- Move the light out to the side, then up, then down.
- Cross to the opposite side and move it up and down.
- Bring the light back to the midline and observe whether the child's eyes converge (follow the light to the nose) as the light moves in toward the nose. *Note:* Infants under age 3 months cannot follow past the midline; the eyes of children under school age do not converge well.

Observe if the pupil constricts (reduces in size) in response to a light, an indication that the third cranial nerve is intact. It is best to approach the child's eye from the forehead so the light suddenly appears on the pupil rather than advancing toward the child slowly. This makes the pupil constrict more dramatically. This should occur in response to a light shining directly on a pupil (direct constriction); when one pupil constricts, this will also occur in the opposite eye (consensual constriction). Record that pupils are equal in size and react to light as "PERL" (pupils equivalent, react to light). If the pupil converges (moves to follow a light in toward the nose), this is charted as "PEARL" or "PERLA" (pupils equal, react to light, accommodate).

For a final step, shine a flashlight or ophthalmoscope light into the pupil. A red reflex should appear. This is evidence that the retina is intact and the lens and cornea are clear (no tumor, cataract, scarring, or infection is present).

Newborn and Infant

Newborns often have a small, bright, red spot on the sclera (a subconjunctival hemorrhage) because the pressure of birth has ruptured a small conjunctival blood vessel. This is normal and will fade in 7 days to 10 days as the blood is absorbed.

Infants can easily be tested for a red reflex, but until they are age 3 months, they cannot follow an object or light across the midline or follow a light into all six positions of gaze. Even a newborn, however, can follow a bright light to the midline. Assessing for a red reflex is important because a congenital cataract can lead to loss of central vision if not discovered.

Toddler and Preschooler

Most young children are reluctant to let someone look into their eyes. Explaining what will happen during an eye examination is effective in reducing the child's anxiety about this part of the assessment.

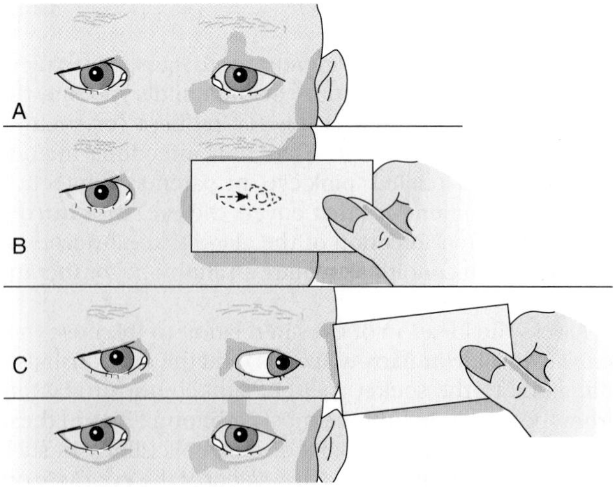

FIGURE 13.10 Cover test. (**A**) The child's eyes appear to be in good alignment. (**B**) The left eye is covered for 5 seconds. (**C**) When the card is removed, the left eye is seen to move perceptibly back to good alignment. This movement indicates that it "drifted" into a deviant position while covered, that is, that an exophoria (misalignment) is present.

School-Age Child and Adolescent

Many older children wear contact lenses (a red reflex is visible with a contact lens in place); some may be nervous about having their eyes examined because they know they should be wearing prescribed eyeglasses but have omitted wearing them because they do not like their appearance. Observe carefully for pupillary appearance and ability to constrict in adolescents as a sign of drug abuse. Many adolescent girls are anemic and so have pale conjunctiva.

CHECKPOINT QUESTIONS

8. On a standardized scale, what range of weight is considered normal for children?
9. What factors should be assessed during an examination of the skin?
10. How is a red reflex elicited?

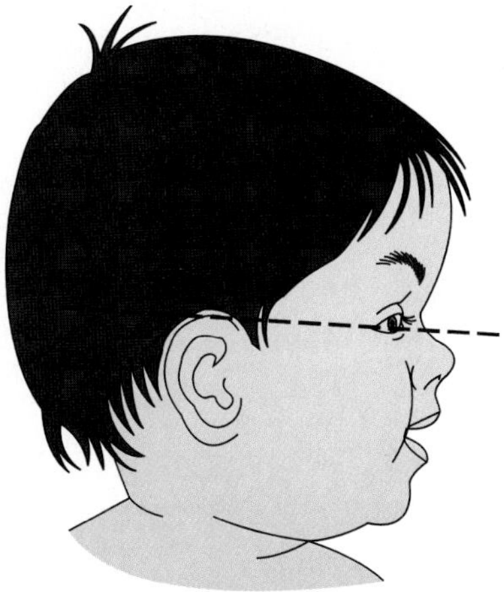

FIGURE 13.11 Normal ear alignment. When a line is drawn from the inner canthus through the outer canthus to the ear, the top of the ear pinna should meet the line. Abnormal ear alignment is associated with certain chromosomal abnormalities.

Nose

Observe the nose for flaring of the nostrils (a sign of need for oxygen). Using an otoscope light, observe the mucous membrane of the nose for color (it should be pink; pale suggests allergies, redness suggests infection). Note and describe any discharge. Document that the septum is in the midline (displaced septa such as those that occur after facial injuries can interfere with respiration and make nasal intubation in emergencies difficult). Press one nostril closed with gentle pressure and ask the child to inhale; repeat on the opposite side to ensure that both sides of the nose are patent (i.e., that no choanal atresia or no membrane obstructing the posterior nares exists). Sinuses do not fully develop until about age 6 years. For children 6 years or older, palpate the areas over the frontal and maxillary sinuses for tenderness, a symptom of sinus infection. Sense of smell can be assessed in school-age children and adolescents by asking them to identify a familiar odor such as chocolate or an orange.

Newborn and Infant

Infants are obligate nose breathers. They cannot coordinate mouth breathing, so become disturbed when the nose is temporarily blocked to check for patency; do this only momentarily to avoid discomfort. Most newborns have milia (small white papules) on the surface of the nose.

Older Children

Many children, preschool age and older, have upper respiratory infections that cause nasal mucous membranes to be reddened and also cause a purulent discharge. Allergies may cause a clear discharge. Children who have dry mucosa due to dry air (which leads to cracking and nosebleed) may be reluctant to allow inspection of their nose. Adolescents who sniff cocaine lose nasal hair and may have excoriations or abscesses in the mucous membrane. If the child has a nasal ring, inspect the site for redness or drainage.

Ears

Observe ears for proper alignment. In the average child, a line from the inner canthus of the eye to the outer canthus and then to the ear will touch the top of the pinna of the ear (Figure 13-11). Ears set lower than this are associated with chromosomal disorders such as trisomy 13. Observe the opening to the ear canal for any discharge. Touch the pinna and watch for evidence of pain (a sign of external canal infections). Observe immediately in

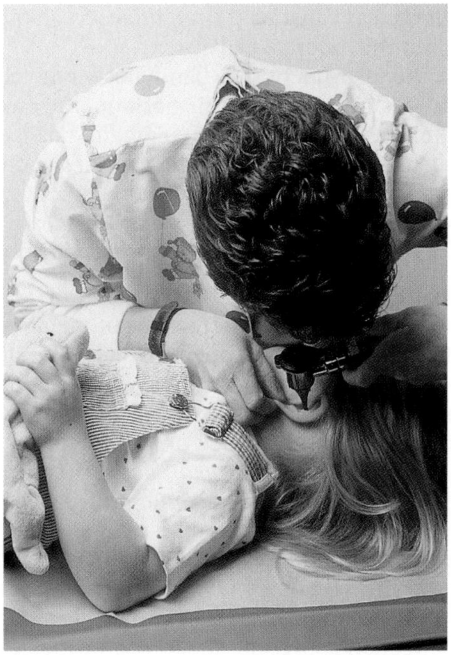

FIGURE 13.12 Otoscopic examination. Note how the nurse's hand rests between the otoscope and the child's head. Should the child move suddenly, no injury to the tympanic membrane will be sustained with this technique because the otoscope will move along with the child's head.

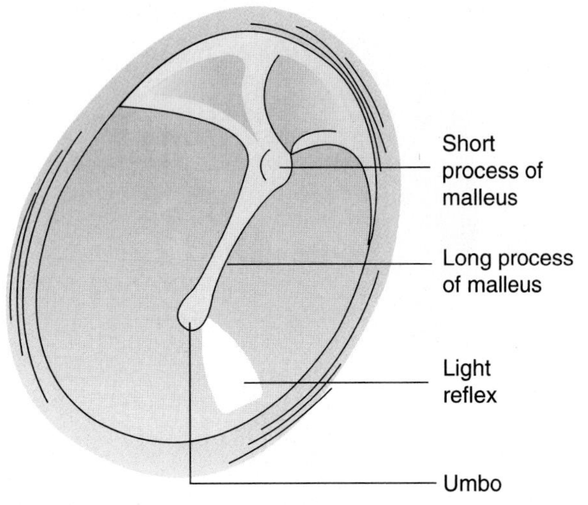

FIGURE 13.13 A tympanic membrane as viewed with an otoscope.

front of the ear for a dermal sinus or a skin tag (a finding that is usually innocent but may be associated with kidney abnormalities). Observe the ear lobes for redness or drainage from infected pierced earring sites.

To examine the ear canal, follow these steps:

- Straighten the ear canal by pulling the pinna gently down and back in the child under age 2 years and up and back in the older child.
- Select an otoscope tip. Otoscope tip sizes vary; use the smallest size possible that still gives adequate visibility.
- With the ear canal held straight, insert an otoscope tip into the external canal.
- Rest the instrument on a hand, not on the child's head (Figure 13-12). In this position, the otoscope will move with the child, avoiding the danger that the plastic tip will scratch the canal if the child should move his or her head suddenly.
- Inspect the sides of the ear canal and locate landmarks on the surface of the tympanic membrane.

Landmarks present should be the outline of the malleus of the inner ear through the translucent membrane (Figure 13-13). The color of the membrane is pinkish gray; if the tension of the membrane is normal, a cone of light—the light reflex—should be present in one of the lower corners (at either the 5 o'clock or 7 o'clock position).

Many children have wax (*cerumen*) in their ear canals, appearing as a dark-brown, glistening substance, but it is almost always possible to see the tympanic membrane past the wax. If a middle ear infection is suspected, it will be necessary to visualize the entire eardrum. If ear wax occludes visualization, it will need to be cleaned away.

If ear infection is present, the tympanic membrane appears reddened and often bulges forward so the malleus is no longer able to be discerned, and the cone of light is absent; if there is fluid in the middle ear, it may be possible to see bubbles of air through the membrane. With chronic middle ear disease (serous otitis media), the tympanic membrane may be retracted, the malleus is extremely prominent, and the cone of light is again missing. If the membrane has been torn from trauma or rupture, the jagged edge and opening to the middle ear are discernible. Inspect also for any ulcerated areas that could be a cholesteatoma or an ingrowing tumor (see Chapter 29).

The mobility of the eardrum can be tested by injecting a column of air into the ear canal against the drum by a pneumatic attachment on the otoscope that looks like the bulb of a blood pressure cuff (Figure 13-14). A normal drum is freely mobile and can be seen to move with pressure on the bulb; one with fluid behind it has decreased mobility. Warn children that this "tickles" before introducing air.

Finally, appraise hearing. Appraisal can be done grossly in older children by assessing their response to questions. Distract an infant with a toy; then make a sound behind the infant's back, out of peripheral vision, and watch for the response. Hearing infants will show some noticeable reaction, although they have difficulty looking directly toward or locating the sound until 4 months of age.

Newborn and Infant

Many newborns still have amniotic fluid or vernix caseosa in their ear canal, so inspecting the ear canal is ineffective. Be certain to assess for ear level and normal pinna contour. Assess for hearing by a gross check such as watching the infant startle to a sudden sound or quiet to the calming effect of quiet talking.

Older Children

Middle ear infection (*otitis media*) is a common childhood illness. This causes the ear to be painful when ex-

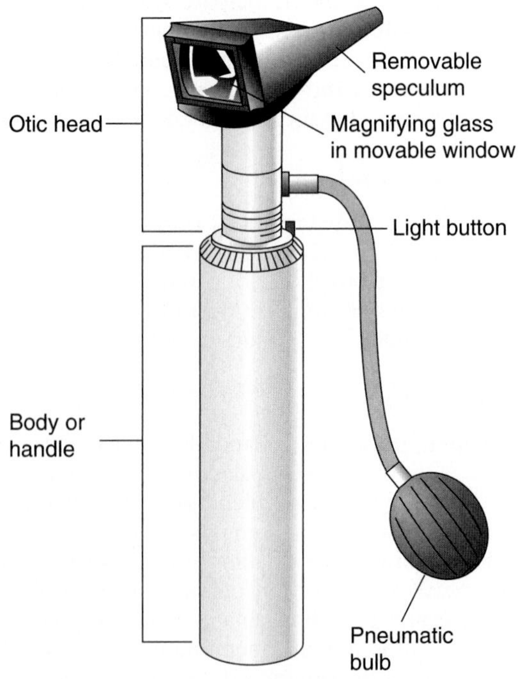

FIGURE 13.14 Otoscope with pneumatic attachment.

amined. An external ear infection (often called swimmer's ear) causes any movement of the pinna to be painful. For these reasons and because children are told many times never to put anything into their ears, they usually resist ear examinations. Explaining what is happening helps to allay fear. Beginning with preschool age, children may have myringotomy tubes (small circular plastic tubes in place on the tympanic membrane) to relieve chronic fluid collected in the middle ear. Inspect that the area surrounding the tube is not inflamed and the tube is not merely lying in the external canal and no longer inserted into the membrane (see Chapter 29).

Mouth

Assess the external appearance of the lips; look for symmetry and color. Ask the child to smile and to frown to evaluate the mobility of facial muscles. Count the number of teeth present and assess their condition (number missing or cavities present). Inspect the gum line (**gingivae**) for redness, tenderness, and edema, symptoms of periodontal disease. Inspect the buccal membrane and palate for color (pink) and the presence of any lesions. Ask the child to stick out his or her tongue and assess for midline position and no **fasciculations** (trembling). Inspect the area under the tongue for lesions in school-age children and adolescents who smoke or chew tobacco because this is the most common first site for oral cancer. A child's tongue is normally smooth and moist. With dehydration present, it often appears roughened and dry. **Geographic tongue** is a term for the rough-appearing tongue surface that often accompanies general symptoms of illness such as fever; it may also occur normally. If the child has had the tongue pierced, inspect for redness at the site. Assess that the object is secure so there is little chance of aspiration or that it is not striking tooth enamel and unnecessarily wearing this away.

Inspect the uvula to be certain it is in the midline. Use a tongue blade to press down and forward on the back of the tongue (Figure 13-15). The epiglottis can usually be observed with the tongue depressed. Observe for abnormal enlargement, palatine redness, or drainage of tonsils. Tonsillar tissue differs a great deal in size but should not be reddened or have pus in the crypts (indentations). After gagging an infant to view the back of the throat, always turn the infant's head to the side so he or she does not choke on any saliva that accumulated in the mouth during the throat examination, because an infant is less able to manage this than an adult.

It is important that the tongue of any child who is suspected to have epiglottitis or whose glottis is inflamed not be depressed. If a swollen, inflamed epiglottis rises with the pressure of a tongue blade, it can obstruct the respiratory tract so completely that the child is immediately unable to breathe. Symptoms of this condition are a sore throat, drooling, fever, difficulty with respiration, dysphagia, and a barking cough.

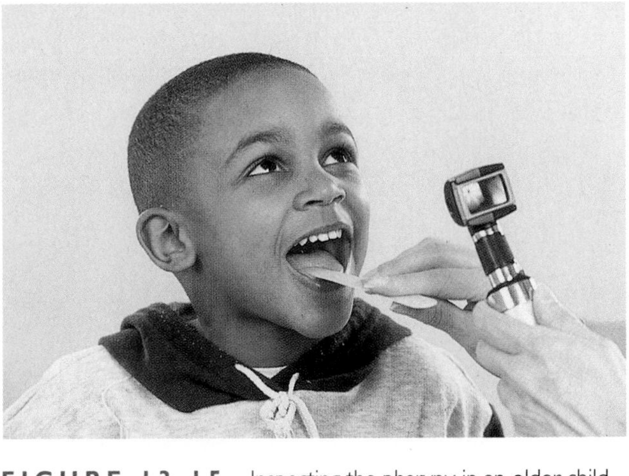

FIGURE 13.15 Inspecting the pharynx in an older child.

Newborn and Infant

Many newborns have considerable mucus in their mouths due to less ability to handle swallowing. If a newborn has teeth, evaluate them carefully for stability; if loose, they need to be removed to prevent aspiration. Assess carefully for white patches that do not scrape away from the buccal membrane or tongue (thrush), a frequent finding in infants.

Older Children

Tonsillar tissue in children reaches its maximum growth at early school age, making many preschool children appear to be "all tonsils." As long as the tissue does not appear reddened or tender, it can be assumed to be normal for the age. Many children have irregular, pale pink, elevated projections on the posterior pharynx as a normal finding. A stream of mucopurulent discharge in the posterior pharynx is not unusual if an upper respiratory infection and a "postnasal" flow of secretions are present. Assess carefully for pinpoint ulcers in the child with teeth braces to be certain the wires are not causing undue discomfort or infection. Cavities appear as dark brown areas on the tooth enamel. The average school-age child or adolescent may have at least one present.

Neck

Assess the neck for symmetry (the trachea should be in the midline; any deviation suggests lung pathology). Observe the outline of the thyroid gland (barely noticeable below puberty because it is obscured by the sternocleidomastoid muscle) on the anterior neck. Palpate the area in front of the ear (location of the parotid gland) and smooth a hand over the location of lymph nodes at the sides of the neck and under the chin to palpate for swelling. Figure 13-16 shows the location of lymph node chains of the head and neck. Because children have so many upper respiratory infections, a few shotty nodes (nodes that are freely movable, about the size of peas) are often present. Preauricular and postauricular nodes are palpable after ear infections, and postoccipital nodes after a scalp infection. Submental nodes generally denote a tooth abscess. Palpable submaxillary, anterior, and posterior cervical nodes follow throat infections.

Ask the child to move his or her head (or move it for the child) through flexion (touch chin to chest) and ex-

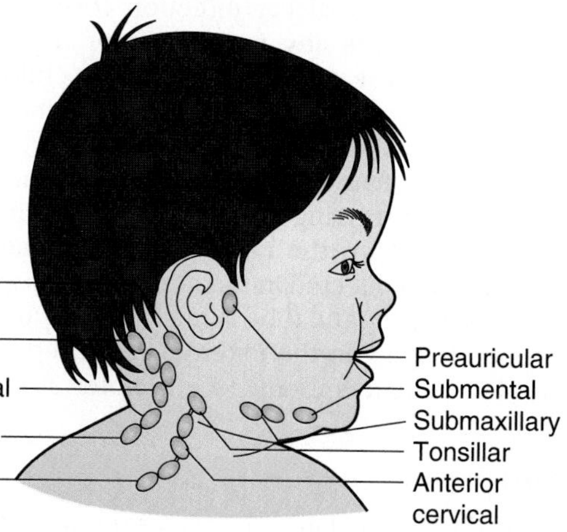

FIGURE 13.16 Location of lymph node chains in the head and neck.

tension (raise chin as high as possible), and turn it right and left (rotation) to see that the child does this easily. Pain on forward flexion is an important sign of neurologic (meningeal) irritation.

Newborn and Infant

With infants, the ability to control the head should be assessed. Lay the infant supine and pull child to a sitting position. Babies younger than age 4 months will let their heads lag backward as they are pulled up; they right their heads only as they reach a sitting position. After age 4 months, infants should bring their head up with them (no head lag) if their neuromuscular coordination is adequate for their age. This is a simple but important test in terms of the information it yields about overall neuromuscular control.

Adolescent

In adolescents, palpate the thyroid gland for symmetry and possible nodes. To do this, press on the right side of the gland to cause it to be more prominent on the left side; palpate the left half to discern any irregularities (areas of hardness). Repeat on the right side. A finding of a thyroid node needs to be investigated. It may be only an innocent transient cyst; alternatively, it may be the first indication of thyroid malignancy. Many adolescents have some increase in the size of the thyroid at puberty; this hypertrophy should not be accompanied by any nodes.

Chest

For ease in specifying the location of chest pathology, the chest is divided into sections by imaginary lines drawn through the midclavicle, midmammary, and midsternum points on the front; the midaxilla on the side; and the midscapula on the back. Pathology is described in terms of these lines (e.g., abnormal lung sound heard at left midaxillary line, and so forth). Other helpful means of locating pathology is by the suprasternal notch, the ribs, and the spaces between them (**intercostal spaces**). Intercostal spaces are numbered according to the ribs immediately above them (Figure 13-17). Inspect both front and back surfaces of the chest for symmetry of appearance and motion. An infant with a diaphragmatic hernia (intestine herniated into the chest cavity) may have a chest enlarged on

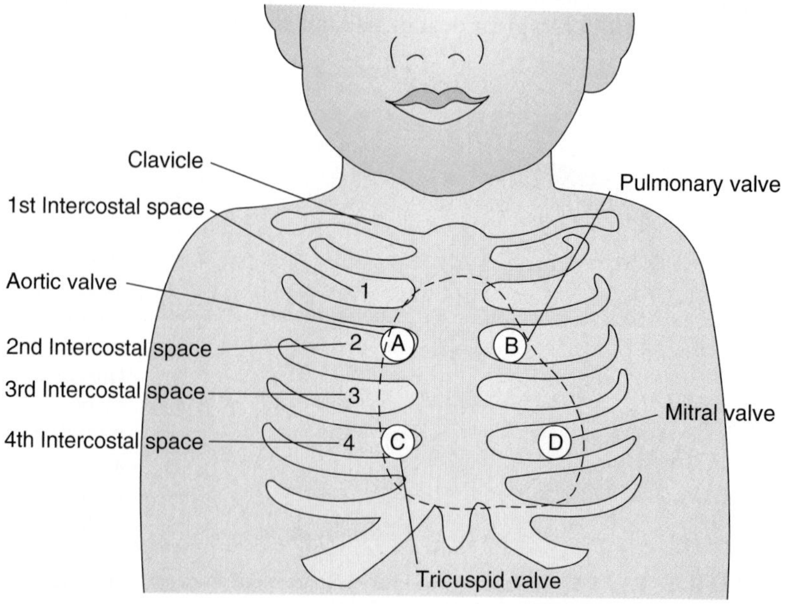

FIGURE 13.17 Intercostal (between rib) spaces are numbered according to the ribs immediately above them. The points (A, B, C, and D) to which the sounds of the heart valves radiate or where the sounds can be heard best are the listening posts of the heart.

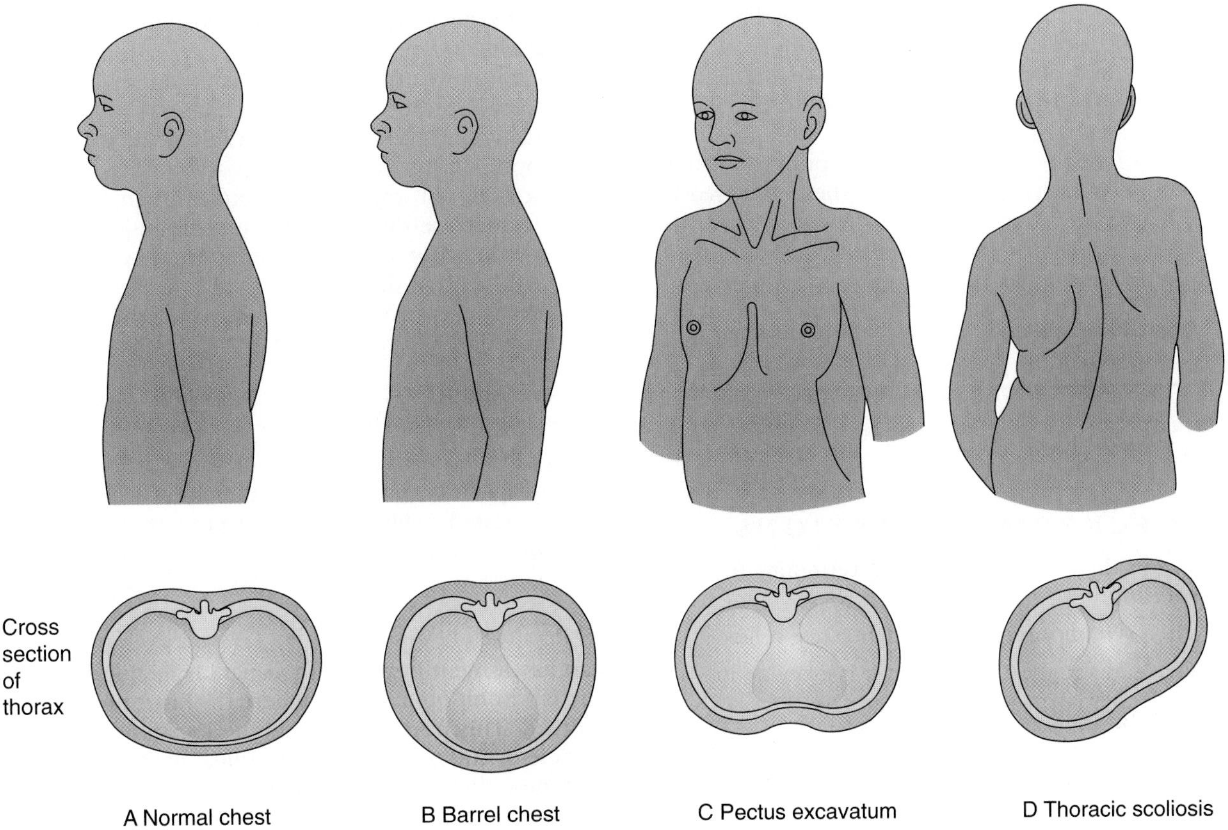

FIGURE 13.18 Chest contours that can be assessed by inspection. (**A**) Normal chest. (**B**) Barrel chest. (**C**) Funnel chest (pectus excavatum). (**D**) Thoracic kyphoscoliosis.

that side. An infant with an *atelectasis* (collapsed lung) may have a chest that is smaller on that side. If a child has an enlarged heart, the left side of the chest may appear large. Inspect for **retractions** or indentation of intercostal spaces or the suprasternal and substernal areas that reflect difficult respirations. Assess the proportion of anteroposterior to lateral diameter (normally 1:2). Children with chronic lung disease develop a broad (barrel) chest or one more rounded than normal. This and other chest abnormalities are shown in Figure 13-18.

Breasts

The degree of breast assessment depends on the child's age and development. As part of a normal breast assessment, inspect and palpate the breasts of all children to see if there are any deformities or abnormalities.

Newborn

Both male and female newborns may have breast edema from the influence of maternal hormones. A few drops of clear fluid may even be present from the nipples. This is normal. Document if a supernumerary nipple is present for baseline data.

School-Age Child and Adolescent

Breast examination should be done routinely on all children past puberty. This is also the time when girls should begin breast self-examination. If a girl younger than 8 years is beginning breast development, precocious puberty (see Chapter 26) should be suspected. Many preadolescent boys develop hypertrophy of breast tissue due to increased hormonal influences (termed *gynecomastia*); they are generally concerned and need reassurance that this is normal for their age and will fade as soon as androgen becomes their dominant hormone. Adolescent girls may be concerned their breast tissue is inadequate or that breast growth is uneven. They need assurance that not all women have completely symmetric breasts.

Inspection of breast tissue is easiest if the child sits on the examining table, arms at the sides, with both breasts exposed. Inspect for symmetry, although it is not unusual (and normal) for a girl to have breasts of slightly unequal size.

Inspect breasts for edema, erythema, wrinkling, retraction, or dimpling of the skin; all suggest that a tumor is growing in deeper layers of the tissue. Erythema occurs from inflammation due to abnormal, rapidly growing tissue; edema, from the blockage of lymph channels due to tumor pressure. Breast edema makes the skin appear not only swollen but pitted (an orange-peel effect). Note any nipple discharge or "pulled" nipple placement as another way to detect edema.

With the girl's arms at her sides to take pressure off breast tissue, palpate well into each axilla (because breast tissue extends this far), and also palpate to assess axillary lymph nodes. Normally, no nodes should be felt. Ask the girl to lie down; place a folded towel under her near shoulder. Palpate the near breast with her lying down with her arm raised and placed under her head because this spreads out breast tissue; begin at the nipple and palpate outward in a circular motion. The lower edge of each breast feels hard; do not mistake this or rib prominences underneath for a tumor.

Girls age 14 years or older (or at the point that they have developed breasts) should inspect their own breasts monthly on the day after the end of their menstrual period. This time not only serves as a marking point but is a time when hormonal influences on breast tissue are at a low ebb so breast tissue is not swollen or tender. The American Cancer Society's technique of breast self-examination is shown in Empowering the Family. A health examination is a good time to have the adolescent perform a breast-self examination so she can be provided feedback on the technique.

> **CHECKPOINT QUESTIONS**
>
> 11. What is the rule of thumb for determining normal ear level?
> 12. When is it important not to elicit a gag reflex?
> 13. What signs suggest that a tumor is growing in the deeper layers of breast tissue?

Lungs

Assess the rate of respirations and whether respirations are easy and relaxed or if accessory muscles are necessary for effective ventilation. Palpate over lung areas for vibrations caused by difficult respirations.

On the anterior chest, lung tissue extends from above the clavicles to the 6th or 8th rib. On the posterior chest, lung tissue is as low as the 10th to 12th thoracic vertebra. The right lung has three lobes; the left, only two. It is important when assessing lung tissue to attempt to evaluate all five lobes because lung disease can be specific for a lobe or involve the entire lung.

Next, percuss over lung tissue. Normal lung sounds in older children are resonant; normal lung sounds in infants and younger children are hyperresonant due to the thinness of the chest walls; overexpanded lungs sound hyperresonant in older children; and lungs filled with fluid sound dull in older children and less resonant in younger children (Burns, 1996). The lower anterior lobe of the right lung will sound dull, because liver covers it on the anterior surface below the fourth or fifth intercostal space. The space over the heart will also sound dull.

Diaphragmatic expanse (the distance the diaphragm descends with inhalation) is an estimate of lung volume. To establish this:

- Ask the child to take in a deep breath and hold it.
- Percuss downward to locate the bottom of the lungs (the percussion note changes from resonant to flat at this point).
- Ask the child to expire fully and momentarily hold that position.
- Percuss upward to locate the expired or empty lung position (the percussion note changes from flat to resonant).

The difference between these two points is the **diaphragmatic excursion.**

Auscultate breath sounds by listening with the diaphragm of a stethoscope over each lung lobe while the child inhales and exhales (preferably with his or her mouth open). Listen both anteriorly and posteriorly; compare left side with right side for equal findings. Normal breath sounds are slightly longer on inspiration than expiration. Consider whether there are any abnormal sounds. Table 13-5 describes normal breath sounds and transmitted airway sounds as well as adventitious sounds that, if heard, might reflect illness.

Newborn and Infant

Infants cannot breathe in and out on request. Try to listen to breath sounds early in an examination, because the breath sounds are difficult to hear clearly over the sound of crying.

Heart

Heart assessment begins with visual inspection to see if there is a point on the chest where the heart beat can be observed. This point represents the location of the left ventricle or the point where the apical heartbeat can be heard best. In children younger than age 7 years, this point is generally lateral to the nipple line and at the fourth intercostal space. In children older than age 4 years, it is at the nipple line or just medial to it and at the fifth intercostal space. This point is termed the **point of maximum impulse (PMI)** and is observable in approximately 50% of children.

Percuss the left side of the chest to discern the left side of the heart. Percussing in from the axillary, the sound will become dull as the heart is identified. If the heart is farther to the left than usual, it suggests an enlarged heart. Normally, the percussion note changes from resonant (percussing over lung) to flat (percussing over heart) midway between the midaxillary and midmammary line.

Heart Sounds

To hear heart sounds, auscultate at four main points. Although these are not the anatomic locations of heart valves, they are the listening points to which the sounds of the valves radiate and can be heard best (see Figure 13-17):

- The mitral valve is heard best at the fourth or fifth left intercostal space at the nipple line.
- The tricuspid is heard best near the base of the sternum (fourth or fifth right intercostal space).
- The pulmonary valve is heard best at the second left intercostal space.
- The aortic valve is heard best at the second right intercostal space.

Table 13-6 describes normal and abnormal heart sounds that may be heard on auscultation. Abnormal sounds are heard best if first the diaphragm and then the bell of the stethoscope is used.

To understand heart sounds, recall heart physiology. The first sound heard (S_1) is that of the mitral and tricus-

EMPOWERING THE FAMILY:
Breast Self-Examination

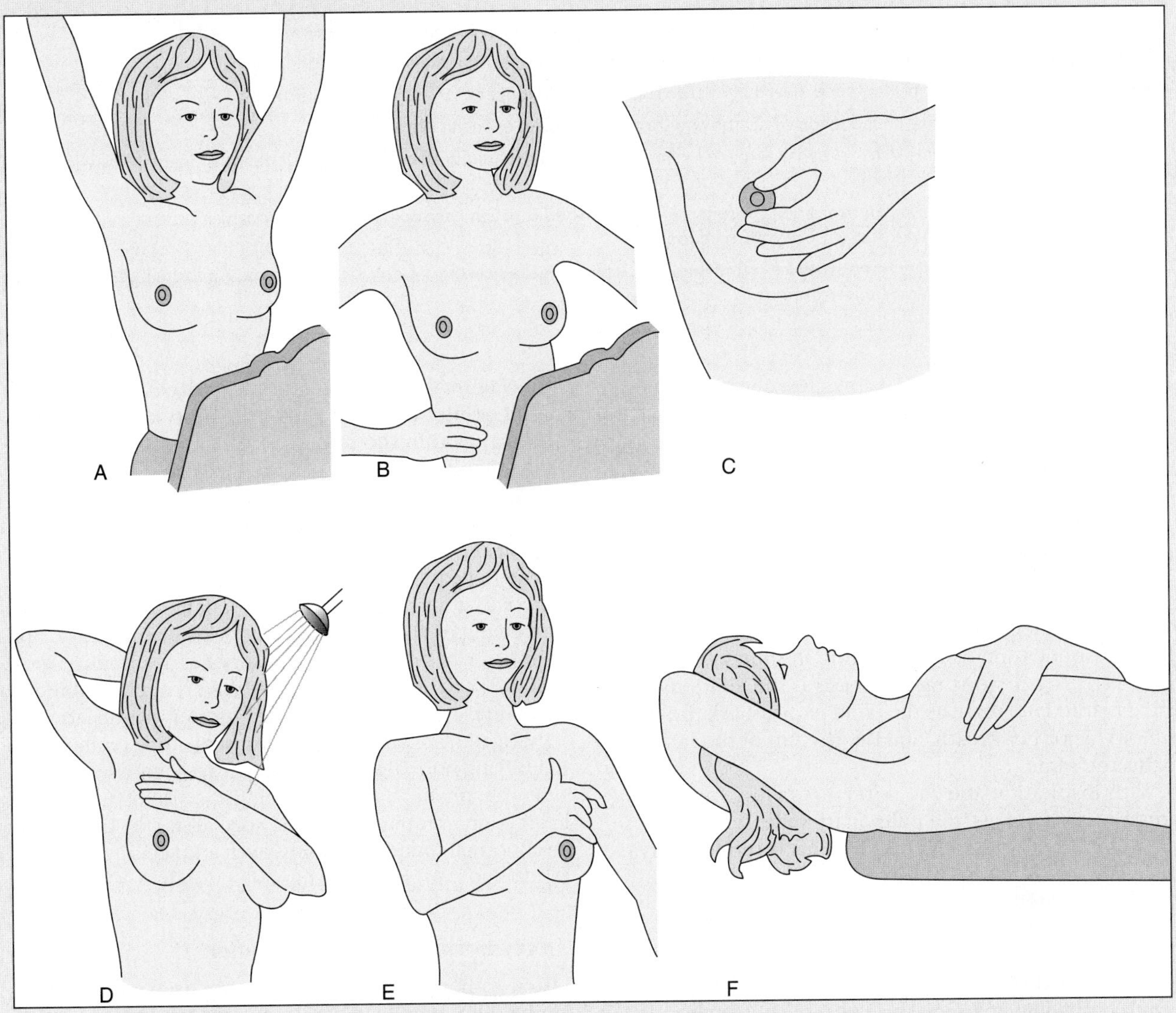

Step 1. Inspection

(A) In front of a mirror, look for any change in the size or shape of the breast, puckering or dimpling of the skin, or changes in the nipple.
(B) Inspect in three positions: (1) with arms relaxed at sides, (2) with arms held overhead, and (3) with hands on hips, pressing in to contract the chest muscles. Turn from side to side to view all areas.
(C) Nipple examination. Gently squeeze the nipple of each breast between thumb and index finger to check for discharge.

Step 2. Palpation or feeling

(D) In shower or bath, fingers will glide over wet, soapy skin, making it easier to feel changes in the breast. Check the breast for a lump, knot, tenderness, or change in the consistency of normal tissue. To examine your right breast, put your right hand behind your head. With the pads of your fingers of your left hand held flat and together, gently press on the breast tissue using small circular motions. Imagine the breast as the face of a clock. Beginning at the top (12 o'clock position), make a circle around the outer area of the breast. Move in one finger width; continue in smaller and smaller circles until you have reached the nipple. Cover all areas including the breast tissue leading to the axilla. Reverse the procedure for the left breast. At the lower border of each breast, a ridge of firm tissue may be felt. This is normal.
(E) Underarm examination. Examine the left underarm area with your arm held loosely at your side. Cup the fingers of the opposite hand and insert them high into the underarm area. Draw fingers down slowly, pressing in a circular pattern, covering all areas. Reverse the procedure for the right underarm.
(F) Lying down. While lying flat, place a small pillow or folded towel under the right shoulder. Examine the right breast using the same circular motion as was used in the shower. Cover all areas. Repeat this procedure for the left breast. Press firmly but gently while examining your breast, rolling the tissue between your fingers and the chest wall. (Courtesy of the American Cancer Society, New York State Division, Inc. East Syracuse, New York.)

TABLE 13.5 Breath Sounds Heard on Auscultation

SOUND	CHARACTERISTICS
Vesicular	Soft, low-pitched, heard over periphery of lungs, inspiration longer than expiration. Normal.
Bronchovesicular	Soft, medium-pitched, heard over major bronchi; inspiration equals expiration. Normal.
Bronchial	Loud, high-pitched, heard over trachea; expiration longer than inspiration. Normal.
Rhonchi	Snoring sound made by air moving through mucus in bronchi. Normal.
Rales	Crackle (like cellophane) made by air moving through fluid in alveoli. Abnormal; denotes pneumonia, which is fluid in alveoli.
Wheezing	Whistling on expiration made by air being pushed through narrowed bronchi. Abnormal; seen in children with asthma or foreign-body obstruction.
Stridor	Crowing or roosterlike sound made by air being pulled through a constricted larynx. Abnormal; seen in children with upper respiratory obstruction.

pid valves closing and the ventricles contracting (described as a "lub" sound). The second sound (described as a "dub" and termed S_2) is made by the closure of the aortic and pulmonary valves and atrial contraction. The first sound is generally longer and lower pitched than the second sound. It is louder than the second sound over the heart ventricles; otherwise, it is slightly quieter.

Listen for the rhythm of the heart sounds. Rhythm should be regular. **Sinus arrhythmia** is a phenomenon that most school-age and adolescent children demonstrate; it sounds abnormal but is not. In sinus arrhythmia, there is a marked heart rate increase as the child inspires and a marked decrease as the child expires; ask the child to hold his or her breath, and the rhythm of the heart remains the same.

With inspiration and the normal resulting increase of pressure in the lungs, the pulmonary valve tends to close slightly later than the aortic valve. This is termed **physiologic splitting** and is heard as "lub d-dub." As long as this is associated with inspiration, it is a normal finding. Fixed splitting implies that there is always difficulty with the pulmonary valve closing and suggests pathology.

At times, a distinct third heart sound (S_3) may be heard due to rapid filling of the ventricles. This sound should be investigated but it is not necessarily a serious finding. The presence of a fourth heart sound (S_4) generally signifies heart pathology because this sound (a gallop rhythm) is caused by abnormal filling of the ventricles.

Listen to the heart rate in all areas; assess rate and compare this to the child's age to determine if it is a normal rate (Figure 13-19). A *heart murmur* is caused by the sound of blood flowing with difficulty or in a different pathway within the heart (sounds like a swishing sound more than a murmur) and can be either innocent (functional) or pathogenic (organic). If a heart is pumping with abnormal force, there may be a palpable vibration termed a *thrill* on the chest wall. Palpate the precordium (area over the heart) for evidence of this (feels like the sensation of a cat purring) or a *heave* (a definite outward chest movement), which also denotes a struggling heart. Upon hearing or palpating any accessory heart sounds or movements, try to describe them with reference to Table 13-7.

All unusual heart sounds need further identification and investigation of their cause. The skills of listening to and identifying normal and abnormal heart sounds require considerable practice. Determining the cause of an abnormal heart sound requires a cardiac specialist. Determining that an abnormal sound exists, however, and securing proper referral is an important nursing role (Moody, 1997).

TABLE 13.6 Heart Sounds Heard on Auscultation

SOUND	CAUSE
S_1 (first heart sound)	Closure of tricuspid and mitral valves with beginning of ventricular contraction (systole)
S_2 (second heart sound)	Closure of pulmonary and aortic valves with beginning of atrial contraction (diastole)
S_3 (third heart sound)	Rapid ventricular filling
S_4 (fourth heart sound)	Abnormal filling of ventricles

Newborn, Infant and Toddler

Listen to heart sounds in young children early in an examination, before the child begins to cry, because it is almost impossible to evaluate heart sounds over the sound of crying. Allowing a parent to hold a child while doing this helps reduce fear.

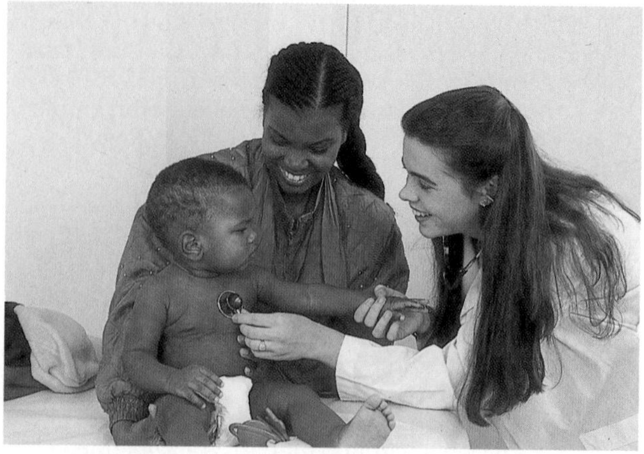

FIGURE 13.19 Auscultating heart sounds.

TABLE 13.7 Description of Accessory Heart Sounds

ASSESSMENT	INFORMATION TO BE GATHERED
Location	At which listening post is the sound most distinct?
Quality	Can sound be described as blowing, rubbing, rasping, musical?
Intensity	*Murmurs* are graded according to the following criteria:
	Grade 6: So loud it can be heard with stethoscope not touching the chest wall; has a thrill (palpable vibration).
	Grade 5: Very loud but must touch stethoscope to chest to hear; has a thrill.
	Grade 4: Loud; may or may not have a thrill.
	Grade 3: Moderately loud; no thrill.
	Grade 2: Quiet but easily discernible.
	Grade 1: Very quiet; difficult to hear.
Timing	When in relation to S_1 and S_2 did you hear it? A sound superimposed between S_1 and S_2 is a *systolic murmur*; one between S_2 and the next S_1 is a *diastolic murmur*. Innocent murmurs (functional, denoting no pathology) are usually systolic, although there are exceptions to this; pathologic murmurs are more likely to be diastolic.
Pitch	Can the sound be described as high- or low-pitched?
Radiation and thrills	Is there an accompanying thrill? Does sound radiate so it can be heard at another location, such as back of chest?

School-Age Child and Adolescent

Listen carefully for sounds of murmurs in children of school age and older. Refer them to a physician for further evaluation if any abnormalities are detected. Parents are always frightened by an unusual heart sound; unless the child has other symptoms, they can be assured that most murmurs are generally innocent (functional) and caused only by the normal flow of blood across valves.

Abdomen

The abdomen is divided anatomically into four quadrants. The quadrants and the organs that lie within them are shown in Figure 13-20. To assess the abdomen, first inspect the surface for symmetry and contour. It will be slightly protuberant in infants and scaphoid in older children. Note any skin lesions or scars.

Auscultate the abdomen for bowel sounds before palpating, because palpating may alter bowel movement (peristalsis) and therefore disturb bowel sounds. Bowel sounds can normally be heard in all quadrants of the abdomen. They are high "pinging" sounds that occur normally at time intervals of approximately 5 to 10 seconds and are heard best through the bell of a stethoscope. If a bowel is distended, the sounds occur more frequently; if the bowel is blocked so that there is no movement of contents, the sounds will be absent below the obstruction. Listen for 3 to 5 minutes before concluding that no bowel sounds are present (O'Hanlon-Nichols, 1998).

Listen along the middle of the abdomen over the aorta for irregular sounds. A **bruit** is a swishing or blowing sound that occurs if there is an outpouching of the aorta (an aneurysm), a condition that can be congenital, although it usually occurs with aging.

Palpate the abdomen in a systematic order to include all four quadrants. Palpate first lightly, then deeply (Figure 13-21). If the child has indicated that any portion of his or her abdomen is tender, begin assessment at the farthest point and work toward the tender area. If no tenderness is present, the order of palpation is unimportant as long as it is thorough. Ascertain whether any area is tender by watching the child's face while palpating; observe for "guarding" or the child tensing the abdominal muscles to keep anyone from pressing deeply at that point. Note any hard areas or masses. If a tender area is detected, "rebound tenderness" is a technique to determine its cause. To do this, press in on

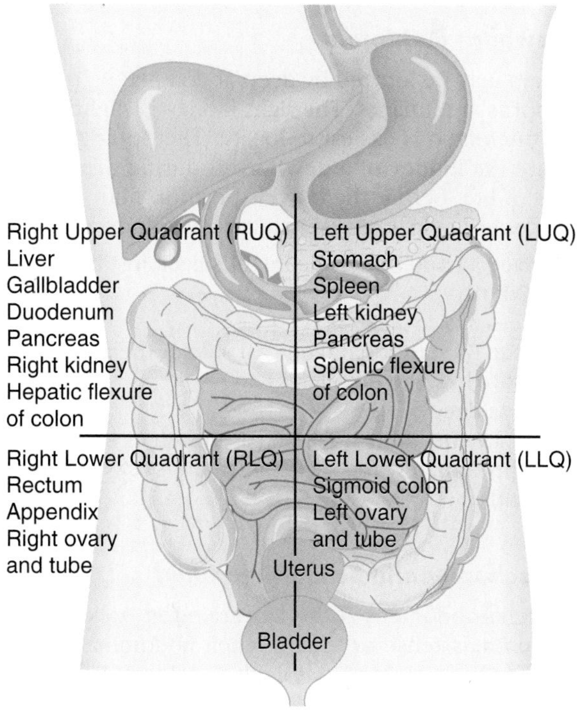

FIGURE 13.20 Quadrants of the abdomen and underlying structures.

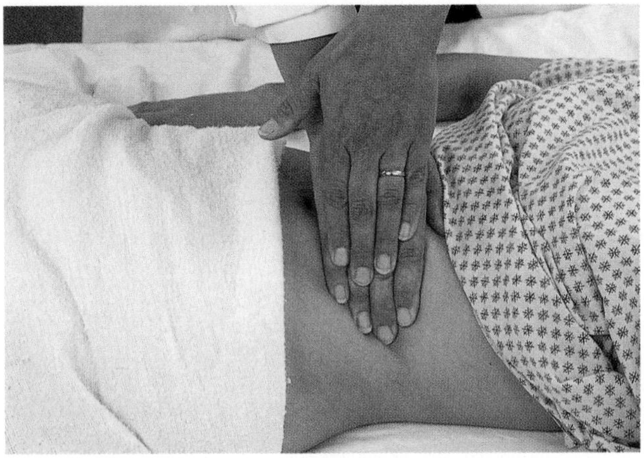

FIGURE 13.21 Deep palpation of the abdomen.

the abdomen, then lift your hand suddenly. This causes internal organs to vibrate. More pain with the vibration than with the original pressure is diagnostic of appendicitis.

By palpating from the right lower quadrant to the right upper quadrant, the hand will "bump" against the lower edge of the liver 1 cm to 2 cm below the right ribs. On the left side, the lower edge of the spleen may be discernible in the same way. A liver or spleen larger than this is suggestive of disease. Palpate the umbilicus to try to identify the presence of an umbilical hernia. A fascial ring at the umbilicus of more than 2 cm in diameter in an infant denotes a ring of fascia larger than will normally close spontaneously; when this is present, the child will generally need surgery to prevent an umbilical hernia. Liver, spleen, and bladder size can all be documented further by percussion.

Newborn and Infant

Kidneys may be located by deep abdominal palpation in newborns and infants. The right kidney is slightly lower than the left so is easiest to locate. The optimal time to palpate the kidney of a newborn is during the first few hours of life, before the bowels begin to fill up with air and obscure palpation. To palpate the kidneys:

- Place a hand under the infant's back just below the 12th rib.
- Press upward.
- Place the other hand on that side of the abdomen just below the umbilicus.
- Press deeply.
- Locate the kidney, which can be felt as a firm mass approximately the size of a walnut between the hands.

Preschooler and School-Age Child

Children's abdomens at this age are often "ticklish," and children may tense or "guard" their abdominal muscles when touched, making it difficult to palpate. Distract the child by asking him or her a question about home or school or let the child put his or her hand under the examiner's to help relax (Figure 13-22).

Genitorectal Area

In both sexes, the rectum should be inspected for any protruding hemorrhoidal tissue (rare in children) or fissures. Fissures may signify chronic constipation, intra-abdominal pressure or sexual abuse.

Female Genitalia

Inspection of external female genitalia and assessment of femoral nodes are included in every complete health assessment. An external examination consists of inspecting for Tanner stage of hair growth and configuration (an inverted triangle) and inspection of external genitalia (i.e., clitoris, labia majora, and labia minora) for normal contours. Look for signs of discharge or irritation. A vaginal discharge or fourchette tear in a young child may be another indication of sexual abuse.

Male Genitalia

Inspection of male genitalia consists of observing:

- The distribution and Tanner stage of hair, which has a diamond-shape pattern
- The penis for lesions
- Appearance and placement of the urethral opening, which should be slitlike and centered at the penis tip. Children with repeated urinary tract infections develop scarring of the meatal opening, making it small and round.
- The ability of the foreskin to retract if the boy is uncircumcised. *Phimosis* exists when the foreskin of a child older than 6 to 12 months is too tight to retract.

Hypospadias is a term for a urethral opening located on the inferior or ventral (under) surface of the penis; **epispadias** denotes a urethral opening on the superior or dorsal (upper) surface. Both these conditions need to be identified. If more than a slight deviation is present, repair is usually initiated before school age because such a urethral placement may interfere with fertility and self-image if not corrected.

Inspect the scrotum for size and the presence of testes. In most boys, the left testis is slightly lower than the right,

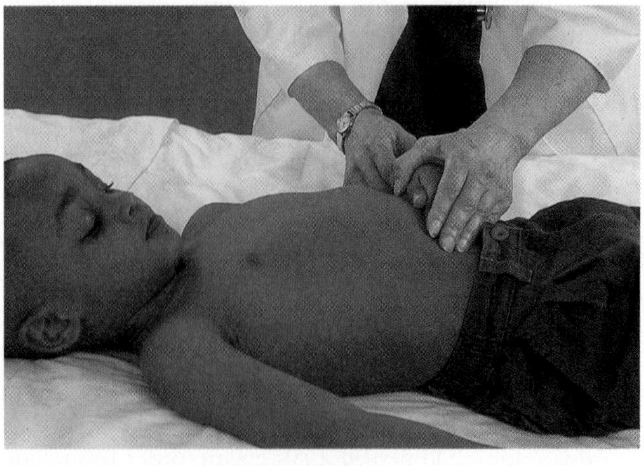

FIGURE 13.22 Decrease ticklishness during abdominal palpation by placing child's hand under yours.

EMPOWERING THE FAMILY: Testicular Self-Examination

Adolescent males should begin testicular self-examination with the same conscientiousness as girls do breast self-examination. Suggest that they select a certain day each month (first day, last day, and so forth) and do it in or immediately after a shower, because that is when scrotal skin is most relaxed. The adolescent should roll each testis gently between thumb and fingers to assess for hard lumps or nodules, change in consistency, or difference in size, any of which he should report. He should know that in most males one testis is slightly larger than the other and hangs a little lower in the scrotal sac, so he does not think these findings are abnormal. The epididymis, at the rear of the testes, feels like a strong cord; he should be familiar with its feel and recognize it as normal.

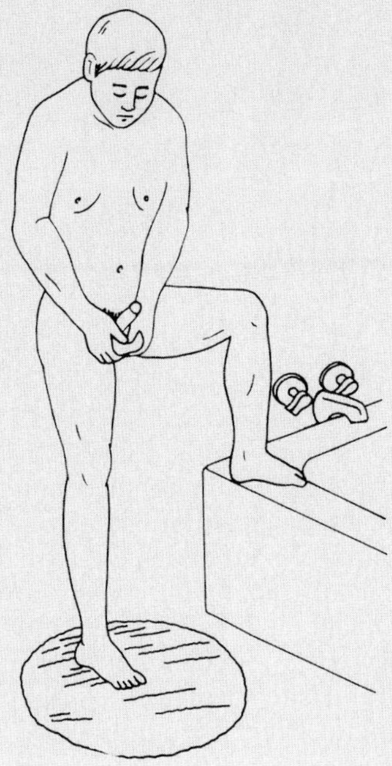

so the scrotum does not appear truly symmetric. Palpate to check that testes are both present by placing one hand over the top of the scrotum at the inguinal ring and then palpating the testis on that side (see Figure 23-18). This hand position prevents the testis from slipping up into the inguinal ring and appearing to be absent on palpation. Any swelling or mass in the scrotum needs to be identified. The most likely cause of such a condition is a **hydrocele,** or a fluid-filled sac; it could represent a serious finding such as testicular cancer in adolescents. Hydroceles can be transilluminated: when a flashlight is held in back of the scrotum, the fluid-filled cyst "glows." A **varicocele** (enlarged veins of the epididymis) may be palpated. These are not important findings in young boys; however, they may interfere with fertility in later life.

Assess the urethral meatus for any discharge that could reveal an STD such as gonorrhea or any lesions that would suggest herpes II infection or syphilis (see Chapter 26). Beginning at puberty, boys should be taught to do testicular palpation every month. The technique for this is shown in Empowering the Family: Testicular Self-Examination.

Inguinal Hernia

To assess for the presence of an inguinal hernia in an infant, simply observe the groin area for any bulging (especially while the infant is crying). In a school-age child or adolescent, with the child standing, place a fingertip against the inguinal ring in the groin area and ask the child to cough. If the tendency for a hernia is present, coughing tightens abdominal muscles and forces abdominal contents to bulge against the finger. Palpate femoral nodes (located in the groin and on the inner surface of the upper thigh) for any swelling, which suggests infection.

Extremities

Observe upper extremities for good color and warmth. Inspect fingernails for color, contour, and shape. Normally, nails are pink, smooth, and convex in shape. They should feel hard to touch and not brittle so they do not break readily. Signs of bitten fingernails in the school-age child may reflect a high level of stress. Darker-skinned children's nails are more deeply pigmented. A blue or purple tinge denotes cyanosis; a yellow tinge is jaundice. Children who have decreased respiratory function or cyanotic heart disease develop "clubbed" fingers (Figure 13-23); children with endocarditis often have characteristic linear hemorrhages under nails. Iron deficiency anemia may cause extremely concave surfaces (spoon shaped). Press against a fingernail, release the pressure, and time the refilling interval (should be under 5 seconds). Count the fingers,and check for webbing between fingers. Examine for the pattern of fingerprints. Distinctive dermatoglyphics are present on fingertips from the third month of intrauterine life; these are unique to every person but show patterns of circular grooves. Abnormal fingerprints may occur with chromosomal anomalies. Check for normal palmar creases. Children with chromosomal abnormalities often have one central palm crease

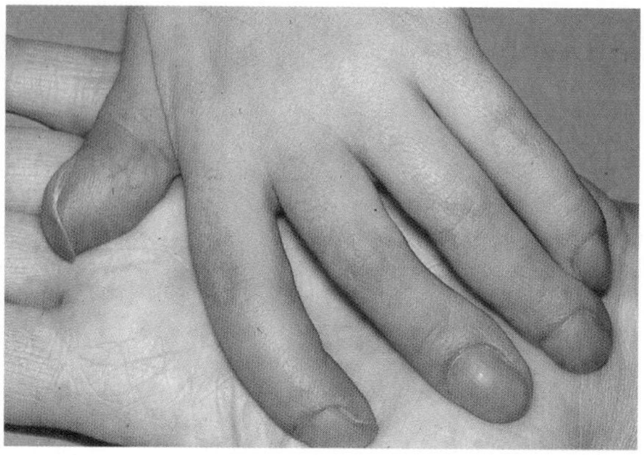

FIGURE 13.23 Clubbed fingers are a sign of cyanosis from heart or respiratory disease.

(a simian line) on each hand rather than the normal three. Check the wrist, elbow, and shoulder joints for movement and normal range of motion; palpate joints for swelling or warmth. Palpate to be certain that no lymph nodes are present in the antecubital space; palpate to check that the radial pulse is present.

Inspect the lower extremities for color and warmth. Count the toes, and check for webbing between toes. Check the ankle, knee, and hip joints for normal range of motion. Check for subluxated hip in infants by attempting to abduct fully the hip. Palpate to be certain that no lymph nodes are present in the groin or popliteal areas. Palpate to ensure that femoral pulses are present and equal bilaterally. Ask the older child to walk, and observe for ease of gait, limping, or any foot displacement such as toeing in or out. Toddlers typically walk with a wide-based gait; they walk best if allowed to walk toward their parent (a safe action) rather than away. Many adolescents are self-conscious and slouch or "amble" rather than presenting their true, natural gait.

Back

Inspect the back for symmetry and the spinal column for any deviation. Inspect the base of the spine for a *dermal sinus* (a pinpoint opening) or for a tuft of hair or a hemangioma that might reveal a *spina bifida occulta* (a defect of the bony structure of the canal). Inspect also for any dimpling that might denote a dermal cyst (*pilonidal cyst*). This is an innocent finding unless it becomes infected or connects to deeper tissue layers. Assess for tenderness along the spinal column by palpating each vertebra.

Routine assessment of the school-age child over 12 years and adolescent includes a scoliosis (sideways curvature of the spine) screening (Sponseller, 1997). Nursing Procedure 13-2: Scoliosis Screening details the steps to follow for a scoliosis checkup. (See Chapter 30 for more details on scoliosis.)

Neurologic Function

A full neurologic examination takes at least 20 minutes to complete. This is, therefore, not included in a routine physical examination. It is important, however, to assess for **deep tendon reflexes** (such as triceps, biceps, patellar, and Achilles reflexes) to test for motor and sensory function and balance and coordination. Techniques for eliciting deep tendon reflexes are shown in Figure 13-24. Grade reflexes according to the scale in Table 13-8. The biceps reflex tests 5th and 6th cervical nerves; the triceps reflex tests the 7th and 8th cervical nerves; the patellar reflex tests the 2nd, 3rd, and 4th lumbar; and the Achilles reflex tests the 1st and 2nd sacral. Test the sole of the foot for a *Babinski reflex*. This will demonstrate a fanning of the toes in an infant younger than age 3 months and a downward reflex of the toes beyond age 3 months. (Some normal infants demonstrate a flaring Babinski response until age 2 years; in the absence of other neurologic findings, this is not significant.)

Test for **superficial reflexes:** abdominal reflexes in both sexes, cremasteric reflex in males. An abdominal reflex is elicited by lightly stroking each quadrant of the abdomen. Normally, the umbilicus moves perceptibly toward the stroke. Presence of the reflex indicates integrity of the 10th thoracic nerve and the 1st lumbar nerve of the spinal cord. A *cremasteric reflex* is elicited by stroking the medial aspect of the thigh in boys. The testes move perceptibly upward in a normal male. The presence of this reflex indicates integrity of the 1st and 2nd lumbar nerves.

Motor and Sensory Function

Test general facial nerve function by asking the child to make a face. The child's ability to grasp with his or her hands and push against a surface with his or her feet establishes general motor ability. Recall whether gait was adequate when the child was observed walking to assess for balance and coordination.

To test sensory function, ask the child to close his or her eyes and identify the location where he is touched at six points (at least) on different body parts.

> ✔ **CHECKPOINT QUESTIONS**
>
> 14. At what point is the pulmonary heart valve heard best?
> 15. At what age should routine scoliosis screening begin?

VISION ASSESSMENT

Assessing vision is an important part of physical assessment because good vision is so important to development. The extent of testing depends on the age of the child (Stahlman, 1997).

Any child with congenital anomalies, low birth weight, or fetal alcohol syndrome is at risk for eye abnormalities, as is a child who received oxygen at birth. During an assessment, if you notice an unreported injury or infection or signs of neglected vision, make a special note. Because the average parent is careful of a child's eyes, these findings may be indicative of child neglect.

NURSING PROCEDURE 13.2: SCOLIOSIS SCREENING

Plan	Principle
1. Have the child remove clothing, except for the undergarments. Ask the child to stand up straight, with his or her feet together and arms at sides. Observe the child from a posterior view.	1. Promote optimal view of back.
2. Inspect for unequal shoulder or hip level, prominence of one scapula, or a curved spinal column (Figure A).	2. Signs of spinal curvature.

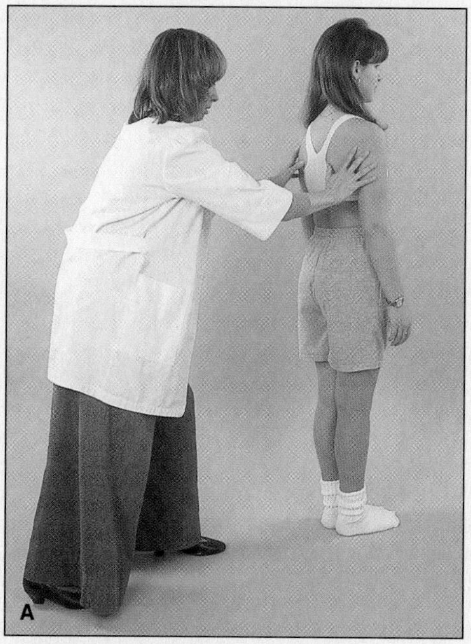
A

Ask yourself the following questions:
- Is one shoulder higher than the other?
- Is one shoulder blade more prominent than the other?
- Does one hip seem higher or more prominent than the other?
- Does the child seem to lean to one side?
- Does the spinal column appear curved?

Plan	Principle
3. Compare the level of the elbows in relation to the iliac crests. Be sure the arms are hanging down at the sides. Ask yourself the following questions: • Is the distance between one arm and body greater than on the other side? • Are the elbows uneven? • Do the elbows fall at the level of the crest or closer to the crest on the one side? (Normally the elbows fall above the iliac crest.)	3. Uneven posture will affect level of elbows.
4. Ask the child to bend over and touch his or her toes while you continue to observe the back (Figure B).	4. As the child bends, the rotation of the spine accompanying scoliosis becomes more prominent.

(continued)

Ask yourself the following questions:
- Is there a hump in the back?
- Does the spinal column appear to curve?
- Is one shoulder blade more prominent than the other?

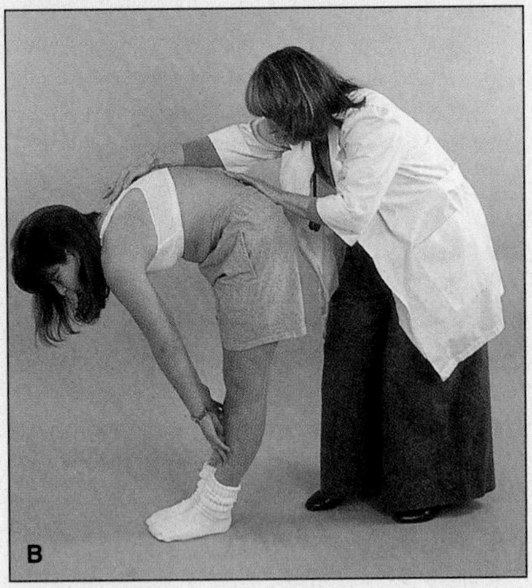
B

5. Refer the child to a physician for further examination if the answer to any of the above questions is yes. — 5. Provide proper referral.
6. Educate the child to inform parents or health care providers if signs of scoliosis, such as skirt hanging unevenly, bra straps need to be adjusted, begin to develop. — 6. Encourage health promotion.

Vision Screening

Routine vision screening is usually begun at 3 years of age. Common vision screening indicators and techniques for children of different ages are summarized in Table 13-9. Parents can provide important clues to possible problems: listen carefully any time a parent expresses concern about or questions a child's ability to see well.

Newborn and Infant

A parent's description of a child's activity may give clues to vision problems. Ask the parents if the infant's eyes follow them as they move around the room. Does the infant who is older than 6 weeks return their smile? Do the parents have any reason to think the child has difficulty seeing?

Newborns should be able to focus on a moving object such as a finger and follow it to the midline. Infants see black and white objects better than they do colored objects. They seem to see objects most clearly at a distance of 19 cm (8 in to 10 in).

Toddler and Preschooler

Ask the parents of an older infant, toddler, or preschooler if their child does any of the following:

- Rub his or her eyes, blink frequently, squint, or frown
- Cover one eye to look at objects
- Tilt the head to see things better
- Stumble over objects in the path
- Hold books and toys extremely close or extremely far away to look at them

Asking whether children sit close to a television set is meaningless because almost all children do that if allowed.

School-Age Child and Adolescent

Ask the parents if their child does any of the following:

- Complains of frequent headaches
- Does poorly with classwork
- Avoids sports that require long-distance vision, such as baseball or softball
- Avoids watching movies
- Skips over words when reading aloud
- Has blurriness or double vision
- Has reddened conjunctivae or drainage from the eyes
- Blinks at bright light

Techniques of Vision Testing

Vision is tested by asking the child to read an eye chart. All children need good orientation to such testing so they can appreciate that this is not a "test" in the usual sense of the word. Otherwise, they may be unusually anxious or try to pass it by cheating.

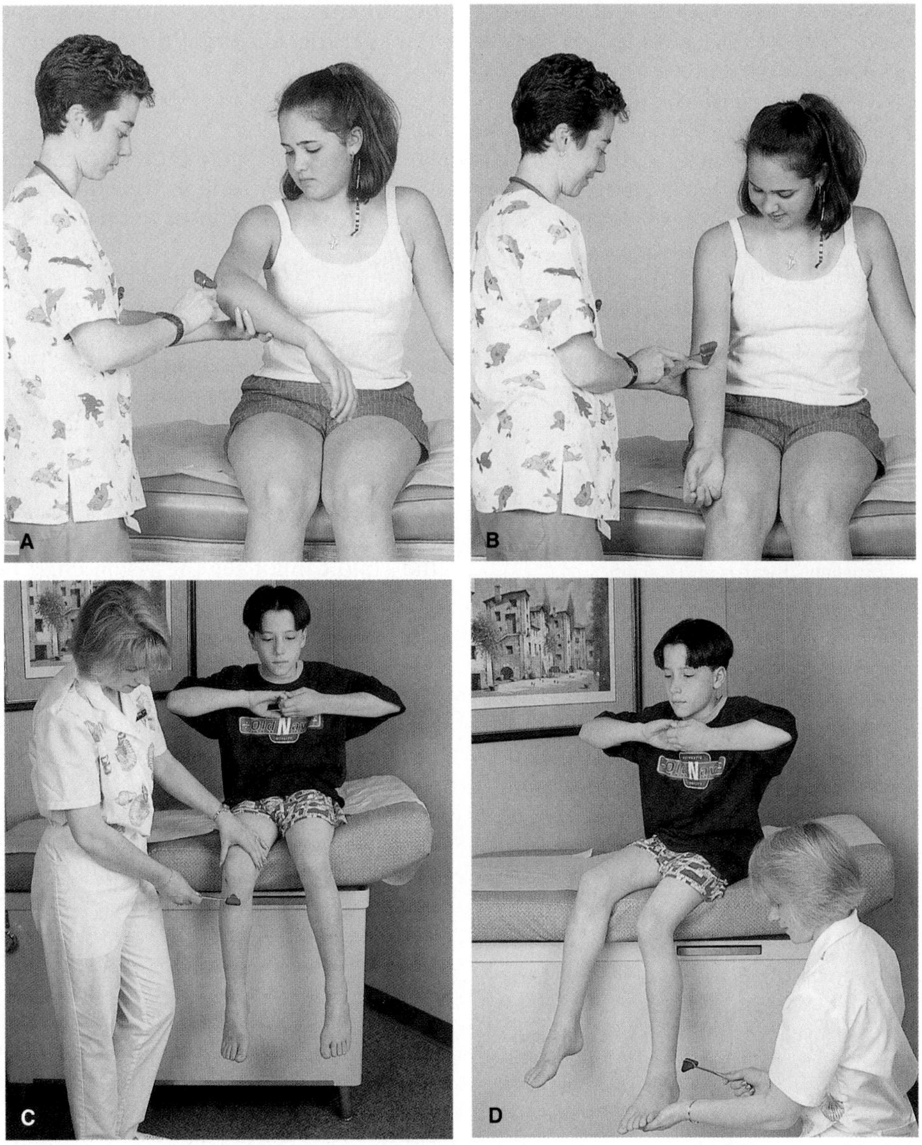

FIGURE 13.24 Deep tendon reflexes. (**A**) Triceps reflex. The triceps tendon is struck. The forearm will move perceptibly if the reflex is elicited. (**B**) Biceps reflex. The examiner's thumb is placed over the biceps tendon. The reflex hammer actually strikes the examiner's thumb. The examiner will feel the child's forearm move when the reflex is elicited. (**C**) Patellar reflex. (**D**) Achilles reflex. In both **C** and **D**, the child grasps his hands together and pulls as a means of distracting him away from what the nurse is testing. This helps to decrease muscle tension, facilitate the reflex arc, and elicit more accurate results.

TABLE 13.8 Grading of Deep Tendon Reflexes

GRADE	INTERPRETATION
4+	Hyperactive; extremely marked reaction; abnormal
3+	Stronger than average but within normal range
2+	Average response
1+	Less than average response but within normal range
0	No response; abnormal

Snellen Chart

As soon as children can identify letters of the alphabet (early school age), their vision can be tested at a health checkup by using a Snellen eye chart. This chart is standardized, so set procedures must be followed when using it to test vision (see Nursing Procedure 13-3: Snellen Eye Chart Assessment).

Preschool E Chart

Between age 3 years and the age they can read the alphabet, children can have vision tested by using a preschool E chart (Figure 13-25). This chart is also helpful in testing children who are cognitively challenged or those who

TABLE 13.9 Common Vision Screening Indicators and Procedures

AGE	COMMON TEST
Newborn	General appearance*
	Ability to follow moving object to midline; focus steadily on an object at 10–12 in.
Infant and toddler	General appearance*
	Ability to follow light past midline
3 yr–school age	General appearance*
	Random dot E for stereopsis (depth perception)
	Allen cards or preschool E chart for visual acuity
	Ishihara's plates for color awareness
School age–adult	General appearance*
	Snellen's test for visual acuity

* Note redness, blinking, squinting, crusting, and so forth.

speak a foreign language. The procedure is similar to that of the standard Snellen chart:

1. The child stands 20 ft from the chart. The child should read first with the right eye, then with the left, then both eyes, as with standard testing. Young children do not understand the importance of not pressing the card against their eye or of not peeking, so a second person is often needed to hold the occluder card for children of this age.
2. It is helpful to compare the *E* with a table with three legs and ask the child which way the legs of the table point. Children age 3 years are familiar with tables, but *E*s are strange symbols. Tell the child to point with the entire arm and hand in the direction the legs point so you do not confuse his or her motion.
3. Begin at the 40-ft line, as with the standard Snellen chart, and work downward until the child passes all lines or cannot read the majority of symbols on a line.

National Association for the Prevention of Blindness Home Test

A home eye test is available from the National Association for the Prevention of Blindness for parents to use to test children age 3 years to 6 years at home. It is similar to the preschool E chart except smaller; the child stands only 10 ft away. The test can help alert parents that a child needs a professional eye examination; it can be given or suggested to parents whose child is tired or for some other reason has not tested well in a health care facility.

Allen Cards

Preschool children may be tested with Allen cards on which are pictures of common objects such as a horse and rider, car, house, and birthday cake. These are shown to the child at a 15-ft distance, and the child is asked to identify the pictures (proof that the child sees them). Be certain the child has time to examine the cards before the test so he or she knows the names of the objects.

Stycar Cards

For this test, the child is given cards with nine letters: *H, C, O, L, U, T, X, V,* and *A*. The child holds up the card that matches the one pointed to on a chart.

Titmus Vision Tester

Another useful method for testing the vision of children is the Titmus Vision Tester. This is the same instrument used by many motor vehicle license offices. As the child looks into the eyepieces of the machine, alphabet letters or preschool *E*s are projected onto a well-lighted screen for the child to identify. Closed vision testers such as the Titmus have an advantage over wall charts in that the child is less easily distracted during testing. Also, because the child cannot see the vision chart beforehand, he or she cannot memorize letters to enable passing the test.

Color Vision Deficit Testing

Color vision deficit is a sex-linked recessive characteristic that tends to occur in males rather than in females, although females carry the gene for the disorder. All male children should be screened once for the disorder during their early school years.

This can be tested for by asking the child to identify the colored stripes at the top of a Snellen eye chart. This type of screening can also be done by showing the child a series of colored diagrams (Ishihara's plates) in which a person with color vision can see hidden figures, but people with red-green or yellow-blue color vision deficits cannot. Detecting color vision deficit in children is important because many educational materials depend on the ability to identify color, and certain occupations are closed to people who cannot identify colors. Even such a simple childhood pleasure as riding a bicycle safely on city streets depends on being able to distinguish colors, such as red from green on a traffic light.

Vision Referrals

Children should be screened twice before being referred to a physician for corrective eye care, because some children do not perform well on eye tests because they are easily distracted or do not know their alphabet as well as they pretend. For example, they may say that they do not see a letter when they really mean they do not know or remember its name. Testing twice helps eliminate or identify this type of misleading result.

After a second screening, general rules for when children should be referred are:

- Preschool children who have 20/50 vision in one or both eyes
- Children in kindergarten or later who have 20/40 vision or worse in one or both eyes
- Any child with a two-line difference between the eyes, which might be the beginning of amblyopia
- Any child who states or shows symptoms of visual disturbance

NURSING PROCEDURE 13.3: SNELLEN EYE CHART ASSESSMENT

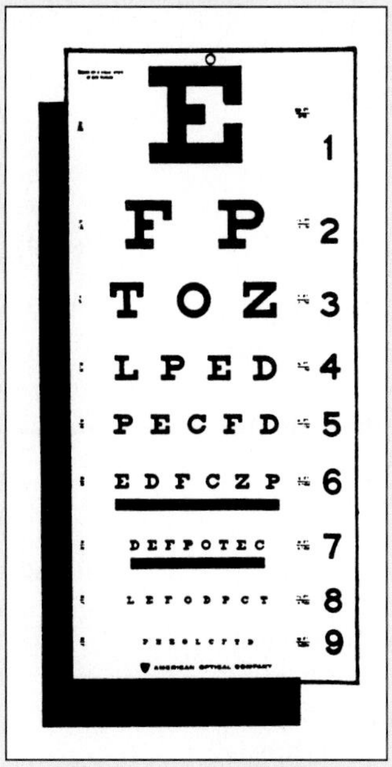

Plan	Principle
1. Hang the chart so the 20-ft line is at the child's eye level.	1. The child who has to look up or down must look farther than the child who is looking straight across at the chart. A possible solution to avoid moving the chart is to have smaller children stand and taller children sit. To accommodate children in wheelchairs, the chart needs to be lowered (or else have all children sit for the test).
2. Provide a good light for the chart and place it so there is no glare. A light intensity of 20 foot-candles is recommended.	2. Provide optimal test conditions.
3. Measure a distance of 20 ft from the chart. Mark the floor at this point with a piece of masking tape or other similar mark. For younger children, it is helpful to cut out paper footprints and paste them to the floor with the *heels* of the footprints touching the 20-ft line. If the child sits in a chair, the back legs of the chair should touch the 20-ft line.	3. Provide optimal distance from chart.
4. Provide an individual 3 × 5-in card (to cover the eye not being tested) for each child who is examined.	4. Allows one eye to be tested at a time.
5. If the child wears glasses, screen the child while he or she is wearing the glasses. If a child has forgotten his or her glasses, defer the screening until the child can bring the glasses. Do not screen the child first without glasses and then with them, because this forces the child to strain to read the chart.	5. Screen for corrected eyesight. After squinting, a child may have difficulty readjusting to reading with glasses and this makes the prescription appear too weak or too strong.
6. To begin testing, tell the child to stand with his or her shoes on the footprints (heels against the line); keep both eyes open; and cover the left eye with the occluding card. Be certain the child does not press the card against the eye (instead, the edge of the card should rest across the child's nose).	6. Provide optimal test conditions. Pressure will cause blurred vision when the child removes the card to test that eye.

(continued)

7. Begin at the 40-ft line of the chart and, using a pointer or pencil, point to each symbol on the line from left to right (the order in which children are taught to read). If the child reads a majority of symbols in a line, he or she sees the line satisfactorily.	7. Use standardized testing procedure.
8. If the child "passes" the 40-ft line, have the child read the 30- and 20-ft lines or the last line the child can read. Record the last line read. If the child fails to read the 40-ft line satisfactorily, then begin at the top of the chart and move downward to identify the last line the child can read. Record this reading. Because the 200-ft, 100-ft, and 70-ft lines have so few symbols, the child must read all the symbols on them to have read satisfactorily.	8. Use standardized testing procedure.
9. Visual acuity is always stated as a fraction. The top number is the distance in feet the child stands from the chart (always 20). The bottom of the fraction represents the last line the child read correctly. The adult with good (average) vision can read the 20-ft line from 20 ft away and thus is said to have 20/20 vision.	9. Use standardized reporting procedure.
10. It is important to test the eyes separately, then together. For example, Tony reads all the symbols on the 40-ft line with his right eye; he misses three out of four on the 30-ft line. His visual acuity for his right eye is 20 (the distance from the chart) over 40 (the last line he read correctly). With his left eye, Tony reads the 40-ft, 30-ft, and 20-ft lines correctly. His vision in that eye is 20/20. With both eyes, Tony reads the 40-ft, 30-ft, and 20-ft lines correctly. His visual acuity for both eyes is 20/20.	10. If only this last reading were taken, the right eye weakness (a symptom of *amblyopia* or "lazy eye") would be missed.
11. Observe the child for straining or squinting as he or she reads the chart.	11. By squinting and changing the shape of the eyeball, a child can improve his or her vision and will score higher. The child will appear to see better than he or she actually does in everyday situations.

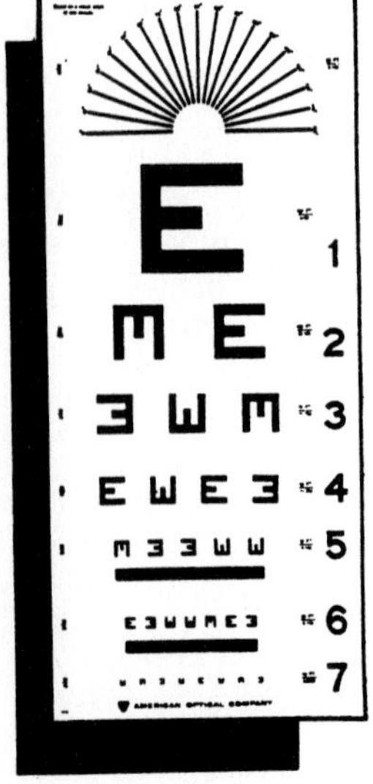

FIGURE 13.25 Astigmatic and preschool E chart. (From the American Optical Corporation, with permission.)

HEARING ASSESSMENT

A thorough health assessment should include an evaluation of hearing, including both history and observation, because good hearing is necessary for the development of age-appropriate skills. When taking an auditory history, be certain to ask the accompanying adult or parent an overall question such as, "Do you have any reason to believe Lucy doesn't hear as she should?" Parents and grandparents are usually attuned to hearing difficulty in children and may be suspicious of it in advance of its official detection.

Auditory Screening

Routine screening for adequate hearing levels is usually begun at 3 years of age. This requires knowledge of the technique and use of an audiometer. It requires a quiet, undistracting setting.

Newborn and Infant

Certain infants who are at risk should be screened at birth. These may include any of the following conditions:

- History of childhood hearing impairment in the family
- Perinatal infection, such as cytomegalovirus, rubella, herpes, toxoplasmosis, or syphilis
- Anatomic malformations involving the head or neck
- Birth weight less than 1500 g
- Hyperbilirubinemia at a level exceeding indication for exchange transfusion
- Bacterial meningitis, especially when caused by *Hemophilus influenzae*
- Severe birth asphyxia: infants with an Apgar score of 0 to 3, those who failed to breathe spontaneously within 10 minutes of birth, or those with hypotonia persisting to age 2 hours

If a newborn's hearing is assessed, it usually is done through simple response testing (observing whether an infant stirs or responds to a sound made or delivered to the child with a commercial device). It can also be done by brain-stem auditory-evoked response (BAER) testing (Figure 13-26). For this method, an earphone is placed on the infant and an electrode is attached to the scalp. When sound is transmitted to the child's ear through the earphone, the electrical potential created as the sound is processed by the brain stem is read by the scalp electrode, processed by a microcomputer, and plotted on a graph such as the one in Figure 13-26. This type of testing may be used at any age and is even successful for comatose or anesthetized persons. Smaller units using transient evoked otoacoustic emissions (TEOAE) are also available (Watkin, 1996). With these, a click stimulus delivered to a normal ear produces an echo from the cochlea. This can be detected by a miniature microphone to reveal even minor hearing loss.

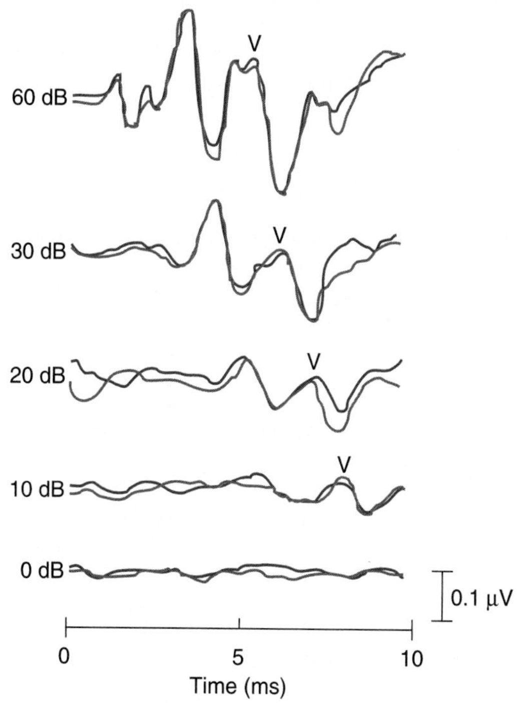

FIGURE 13.26 Wave pattern produced by brain stem auditory-evoked responses. (Stool, S. E. [1984]. Current methods of screening for hearing impairment. *Consultant, 24,* 131, with permission.)

Older Children

Older children who are at risk for hearing loss are those who have been exposed to loud noises, were of low birth weight, have congenital anomalies, have a repaired cleft palate, or have had repeated ear infections. During history taking, ask children if they ever worry that they have difficulty hearing. Ask them how they are doing in school. Some children with a minimum hearing impairment are considered to have behavioral problems in school because they do not follow directions or appear not to be following the teacher's discussion. In fact, they may be unable to hear what is being said. Be certain not to confuse difficulty hearing with shyness or recalcitrance in answering. Children with an ear infection (otitis media) or allergies should be tested after the fluids in their ears clear because their hearing may be temporarily affected by these conditions. Cerumen in the ear canal has not been documented to substantially decrease hearing.

Principles of Audiometric Assessment

Frequency

Sound is the result of vibration; frequency is the number of vibrations a sound creates per second. When frequency is increased, the pitch of the sound increases. For audiometric testing, frequency is measured in Hertz units. Normal speech sounds fall into a narrow range, 500 Hz to 2000 Hz. To function adequately and speak effectively, a child must be able to hear in this range. Children are tested for a wider frequency range than this, from 500 Hz to 6000 Hz, on a routine screening assessment.

Loudness

Decibels are an expression of the intensity of loudness of a sound (or vigor of the vibrations). A decibel level of 0 dB is the softest sound that can be heard. Normal conversation is approximately 50 dB to 60 dB. The sound level at which inner ear damage can occur is about 90 dB. Sound levels of 140 dB are so intense they actually cause pain. Screening audiometry is done at 25 dB.

Hearing Loss

Table 13-10 lists levels of hearing impairment. A hearing loss of 30 dB means the child has some difficulty hearing normal instructions and questions. A loss of 50 dB or more is severe: the child misses most normal conversation and cannot hope to achieve in a regular classroom environment. The child's speech will be impaired because he or she does not hear normal speech sounds.

If a child can hear all frequencies at the 25-dB level, he or she has passed an audiometric screening check. If the child fails to hear two or more frequencies at 25 dB, in either or both ears, the child has failed a screening audiometry test and should be referred to a physician or an otologist. An **audiogram** is a record of audiometric testing. Figure 13-27 shows an audiogram of a child with nor-

TABLE 13.10 Levels of Hearing Impairment

dB LEVEL	HEARING LEVEL PRESENT
Slight (less than 30)	Unable to hear whispered words or faint speech
	No speech impairment present
	May not be aware of hearing difficulty
	Achieves well in school and home, compensating by leaning forward, speaking loudly
Mild (30–50)	Beginning speech impairment may be present
	Difficulty hearing if not facing speaker; some difficulty with normal conversation
Moderate (55–70)	Speech impairment present. May require speech therapy.
	Difficulty with normal conversation
Severe (70–90)	Difficulty with any but nearby loud voice
	Hears vowels easier than consonants
	Requires speech therapy for clear speech. May still hear loud sounds such as jets or whistle of train.
Profound (more than 90)	Hears almost no sound

mal hearing in the right ear (the child heard all frequencies at the 20-dB level) but a loss of 45 dB in the left ear at frequencies of 1000 Hz, 2000 Hz, and 4000 Hz.

Acoustic Impedance Testing

Acoustic impedance testing is based on the principle that sound entering the ear canal meets resistance at the tympanic membrane. If the middle ear is functioning normally, there will be a symmetric pattern of resistance on a tympanogram printout. If the middle ear is functioning abnormally, the level of resistance will be greater or less than normal, so the pattern will be abnormal.

Acoustic impedance testing is performed by audiologists. For the assessment, the child's ear to be tested is plugged with a rubber disc. Sound is then administered to the ear through the center of the disc. The resistance met at the eardrum is registered and recorded as a graph. Tympanograms are inaccurate in children younger than age 7 months because the tympanic membrane is too compliant under that age to register normal impedance.

Conduction Loss Testing

Although not very accurate, both the Rinne and the Weber tests can be used to help determine the cause of hearing loss in older children.

Rinne Test

Strike a 500-Hz tuning fork and hold the stem of it against the child's mastoid bone. Ask the child to say when he or she no longer hears the tuning fork ringing. When the child says it is no longer audible, move the fork forward so it is at the auditory meatus. Because air conduction is normally better than bone conduction, the child should hear it when it is held in front of the meatus, although he or she no longer heard it when it was held against the bone (Figure 33-28). If the child does not hear it when it is brought forward, then the child's air conduction is probably reduced.

Weber's Test

Strike a 500-Hz tuning fork and hold the stem of it against the top of the child's head. The child with normal hearing in both ears will hear the sound equally well with both ears. If the child has an air conduction loss in one ear, the child will hear the sound better in that ear than in the good ear (Figure 13-29). The test must be used in conjunction with other evaluation tools because, if the sound is intensified in one ear, it may mean that there is no hearing perception (there is nerve loss) in the opposite ear.

✔ CHECKPOINT QUESTIONS

16. What is a good type of eye chart for cognitively impaired or non-English-speaking children?
17. What is the decibel level of normal conversation?

SPEECH ASSESSMENT

Speech problems are directly related to hearing problems: the child who does not hear will make preliminary babbling sounds but then will not develop intelligible speech because he or she is unable to hear and repeat sounds. Speech difficulties may also be related to:

- Motor development (e.g., the child cannot control tongue and facial muscles well enough to form proper words)
- Cognitive development (e.g., the cognitively challenged child does not grasp the concept of speech or word use until later than normal, or possibly not at all)
- Cultural influences (e.g., the parents speak two languages, making it difficult for the child to accurately learn and articulate either language)

Speech screening begins by asking the child a few simple questions to determine his or her language pattern. Parents are also asked if they have noticed any difficulties with their child's pronunciation or comprehension. Standardized tests, such as the Denver Articulation Screening Examination (DASE), may also be administered.

Denver Articulation Screening Examination

Assessing for language development is double assessment in that it assesses for both cognitive and hearing ability. The DASE is designed to detect significant developmental delays and normal variations in the acquisition of speech

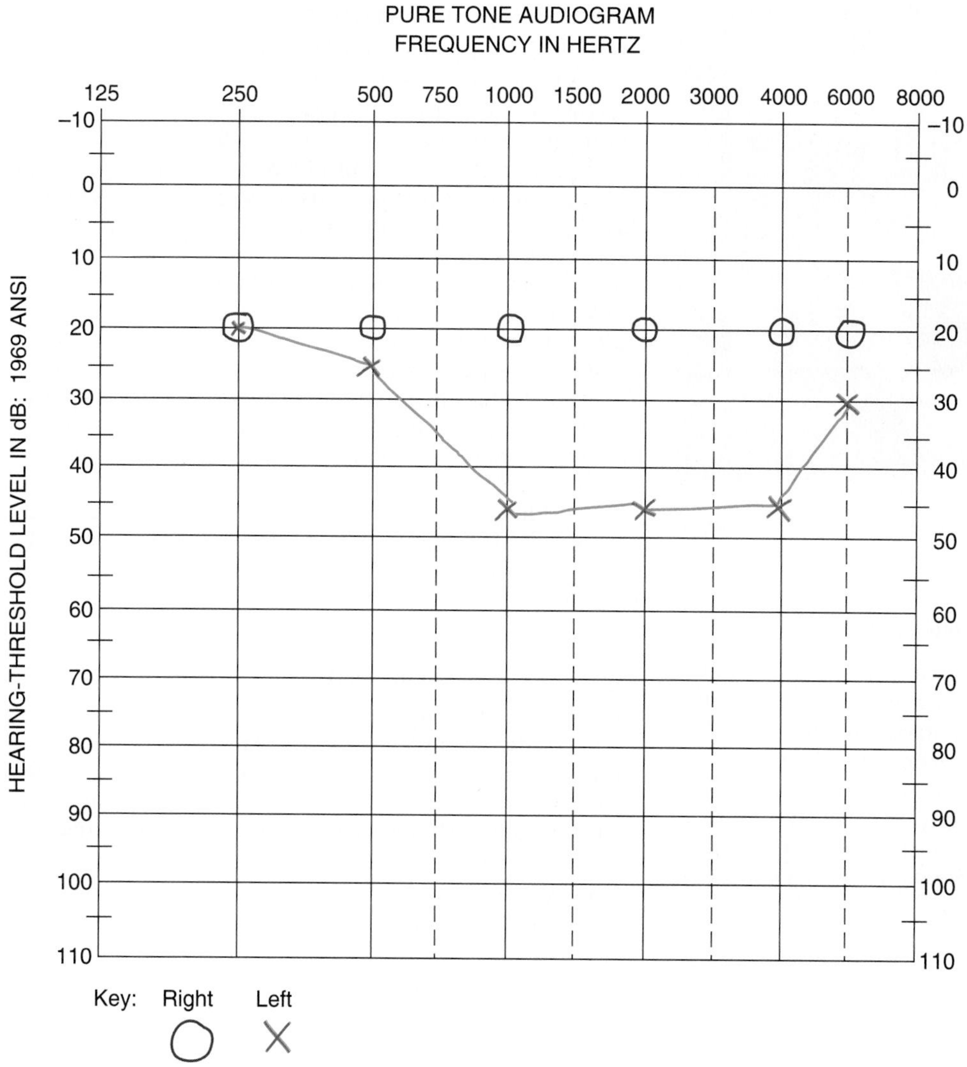

FIGURE 13.27 An audiogram done as a screening procedure. Notice that hearing is normal in the right ear (all frequencies are heard at the 20-dB level). In the left ear there is hearing loss (the frequencies 1000, 2000, and 4000 Hz are heard only at the 45-dB level). (Courtesy of Dr. H. Schill, Speech Pathology and Audiology Department, Boston University.)

sounds. Because it is a standardized test, its directions must be followed carefully. The test is only useful with English-speaking children.

Administration

For the test, explain that the child will need to repeat some words he or she hears. Give enough examples so the child will understand what he or she is to do: "When I say 'boat,' then you say 'boat.' " When certain that the child understands the directions, say each of the 22 words shown on the DASE form (Figure 13-30*A*). Convey the impression that there are no right or wrong answers. Give the child approval for responding and following directions correctly, no matter how inaccurately the child repeats the word.

Scoring

The DASE is designed for use with children between ages 2½ years and 6 years. In scoring, consider the child's age to be the closest previous age shown on the percentile rank chart (see Figure 13-30*B*). Score the child's pronunciation of the underlined sounds or blends in each word on the test form. A perfect raw score is 30 correctly articulated sounds.

Match this raw score on the percentile rank chart with the column representing the child's age. The number at which the raw score line and the age column meet is the percentile rank of the child (how the child compares with other children of that age). Percentiles shown above the heavy line are abnormal; those below the line are normal. For example, a 3-year-old who says only 12 sounds correctly ranks in the 9th percentile (abnormal ranking); the 3-year-old who scores 20 sounds correctly ranks in the 58th percentile (normal ranking).

In addition to determining the percentile ranking, rate the child's spontaneous speech in terms of intelligibility as 1, easy to understand; 2, understandable half the time; 3, not understandable; or 4, cannot evaluate (e.g., the child does not speak in sentences or phrases during the contact with the child). Score intelligibility according to the chart in Figure 13-30*B*. For a final score, rate the child's total test result (normal or abnormal on the DASE or intelligibility).

Children who score abnormally on this screening test should be retested in 2 weeks. If they still score abnormally, they should be referred for complete speech evaluation.

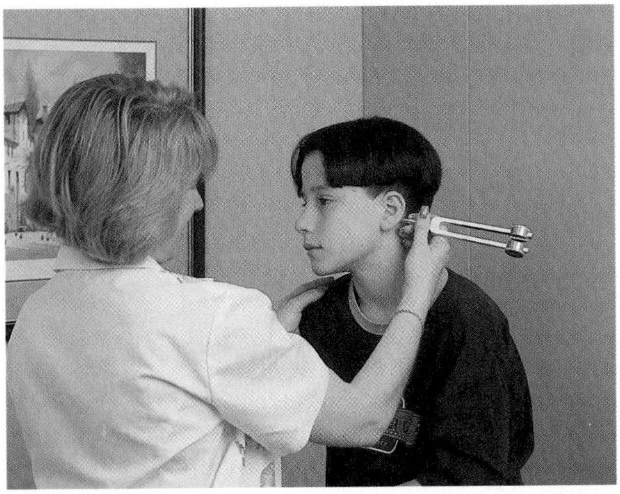

FIGURE 13.28 Rinne test to assess bone conduction.

DEVELOPMENTAL APPRAISAL

It would be ideal if children demonstrated all the developmental skills of which they are capable every time they are asked to demonstrate them. Rarely, however, do they accomplish this feat. Infants may become hungry, sleepy, or upset during testing. Older children may become shy. A portion of developmental information on almost all health assessments, therefore, must be elicited by history taking. All previous developmental milestones must be obtained this way.

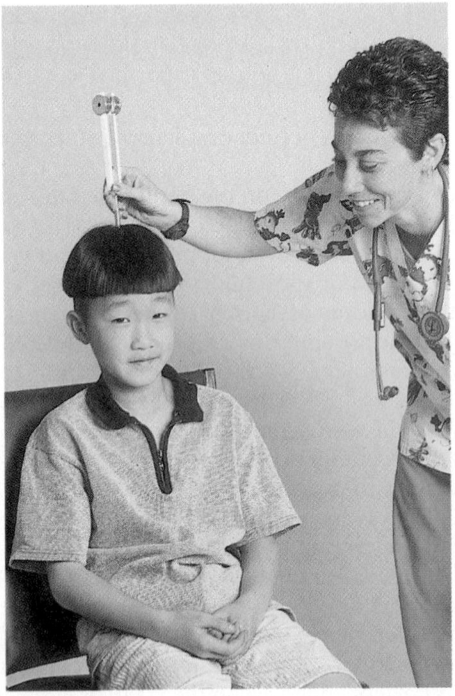

FIGURE 13.29 Weber's test. When the child has an air conduction hearing loss, he or she will hear the sound of the tuning fork better in the affected ear than in the normal ear.

Developmental History

Many parents keep careful records of their first child's development, a less careful record of their second, a scanty record of the third, and so on. Most of this information must, therefore, be obtained by recall.

Parents may not be able to recall the month during which a skill was first demonstrated. It is often helpful to ask them to try to remember in terms of holidays or seasons. For example, they may not know at which month the infant first used a *pincer grasp* (grasped cleanly with index finger and thumb) but do recall the way the child pinched the ear of the family dog at a summer picnic.

If parents seem to have no recall at all of developmental milestones that are important for the child's present evaluation, suggest that they ask other family members or look through family photographs to jog their memories and then call with as much information as they can gather.

In addition to getting the parents' description of the skills a child has mastered, it is often helpful to watch the child perform skills and rate him or her according to standard criteria.

Denver Developmental Screening Test

The Denver Developmental Screening Test (DDST; Denver II) is the most widely used tool to assess development and has been recently revised (Frankenburg, 1994; Figure 13-31). The DDST detects developmental delays during infancy and preschool years. Four main categories of development are rated:

1. Personal-social
2. Fine motor-adaptive
3. Language
4. Gross motor skills

Administration

The Denver II ideally should be presented when the child is approximately age 3 months or 4 months, again at age 10 months, and again at age 3 years. It is a supplement to the developmental evaluation by history that should be a part of every well-child assessment.

The materials to administer the test must be purchased as a kit. They include a skein of red wool, a box of raisins, a small bottle, a bell, a rattle with a narrow handle, a tennis ball, ten 1-in brightly colored blocks, a small plastic doll, a toy baby bottle, a plastic cup, and a pencil.*

Although administration of the Denver II is not difficult, it should not be attempted except by health care providers trained specifically in its procedures and interpretation. This precaution is necessary to ensure the validity of its developmental norms. Periodic retraining and proficiency testing are recommended to sustain a high degree of accuracy in administration.

* Denver II test and training materials may be purchased from Denver Developmental Materials, Inc., P.O. Box 6919, Denver, CO 80205-0919; phone: 303-355-4729.

(text continues on page 389)

A

DENVER ARTICULATION SCREENING EXAM
for children 2 1/2 to 6 years of age

Instructions: Have child repeat each word after you. Circle the underlined sounds that he pronounces correctly. Total correct sounds is the Raw Score. Use charts on reverse side to score results.

NAME

HOSP. NO.

ADDRESS ______________________

Date: __________ Child's Age: ________ Examiner: ____________________ Raw Score: ________
Percentile: ________ Intelligibility: ______________ Result: ____________________

1. table	6. zipper	11. sock	16. wagon	21. leaf
2. shirt	7. grapes	12. vacuum	17. gum	22. carrot
3. door	8. flag	13. yarn	18. house	
4. trunk	9. thumb	14. mother	19. pencil	
5. jumping	10. toothbrush	15. twinkle	20. fish	

Intelligibility: (circle one) 1. Easy to understand 2. Understandable 1/2 the time. 3. Not understandable 4. Can't evaluate

Comments:

Date: __________ Child's Age: ________ Examiner: ____________________ Raw Score ________
Percentile: ________ Intelligibility: ______________ Result: ____________________

1. table	6. zipper	11. sock	16. wagon	21. leaf
2. shirt	7. grapes	12. vacuum	17. gum	22. carrot
3. door	8. flag	13. yarn	18. house	
4. trunk	9. thumb	14. mother	19. pencil	
5. jumping	10. toothbrush	15. twinkle	20. fish	

Intelligibility: (circle one) 1. Easy to understand 2. Understandable 1/2 the time. 3. Not understandable 4. Can't evaluate

Comments:

Date: __________ Child's Age: ________ Examiner: ____________________ Raw Score ________
Percentile: ________ Intelligibility: ______________ Result: ____________________

1. table	6. zipper	11. sock	16. wagon	21. leaf
2. shirt	7. grapes	12. vacuum	17. gum	22. carrot
3. door	8. flag	13. yarn	18. house	
4. trunk	9. thumb	14. mother	19. pencil	
5. jumping	10. toothbrush	15. twinkle	20. fish	

Intelligibility: (circle one) 1. Easy to understand 2. Understandable 1/2 the time. 3. Not understandable 4. Can't evaluate

Comments:

B

To score DASE words: Note Raw Score for child's performance. Match raw score line (extreme left of chart) with column representing child's age (to the closest previous age group). Where raw score line and age column meet number in that square denotes percentile rank of child's performance when compared to other children that age. Percentiles above heavy line are ABNORMAL percentiles, below heavy line are NORMAL.

PERCENTILE RANK

Raw Score	2.5 yr.	3.0	3.5	4.0	4.5	5.0	5.5	6 years
2	1							
3	2							
4	5							
5	9							
6	16							
7	23							
8	31	2						
9	37	4	1					
10	42	6	2					
11	48	7	4					
12	54	9	6	1	1			
13	58	12	9	2	3	1	1	
14	62	17	11	5	4	2	2	
15	68	23	15	9	5	3	2	
16	75	31	19	12	5	4	3	
17	79	38	25	15	6	6	4	
18	83	46	31	19	8	7	4	
19	86	51	38	24	10	9	5	1
20	89	58	45	30	12	11	7	3
21	92	65	52	36	15	15	9	4
22	94	72	58	43	18	19	12	5
23	96	77	63	50	22	24	15	7
24	97	82	70	58	29	29	20	15
25	99	87	78	66	36	34	26	17
26	99	91	84	75	46	43	34	24
27		94	89	82	57	54	44	34
28		96	94	88	70	68	59	47
29		98	98	94	84	84	77	68
30		100	100	100	100	100	100	100

To Score intelligibility:

	NORMAL	ABNORMAL
2 1/2 years	Understandable 1/2 the time, or, "easy"	Not Understandable
3 years and older	Easy to understand	Understandable 1/2 time Not understandable

Test Result: 1. NORMAL on Dase and Intelligibility = NORMAL

2. ABNORMAL on Dase and/or Intelligibility = ABNORMAL

* If abnormal on initial screening rescreen within 2 weeks. If abnormal again child should be referred for complete speech evaluation.

FIGURE 13.30 Denver Articulation Screening Exam (DASE). (**A**) Test form. (**B**) Percentile rank form. (Reprinted by permission. Copyright 1971 by Amelia F. Drumwright, University of Colorado Medical Center, Denver, CO.)

ages by which 25%, 50%, 75%, and 90% of children normally have mastered that item. The left end of the bar is the 25% mark; the tick mark at the top of the bar, 50%; the left end of the colored (gray) area, 75%; and the right end of the bar, 90%. Looking at the form, notice, for example, the item "plays pat-a-cake" in the area of personal-social development. With this item, 25% of children show the trait at age 7 months, 50% between ages 9 months and 10 months, 75% between ages 10 months and 11 months, and 90% by ages 11 months to 12 months. Interpretation of performance is detailed in the manual.

Prescreening Test

A Denver Prescreening Developmental Questionnaire (R-PDQII) is available in addition to the Denver II. The PDQII is designed to identify the child who requires further testing with a full Denver II. It is a questionnaire, which the parent completes, of 10 developmental items. A child who scores 8 out of 10 or fewer should be retested in approximately 2 weeks. If the initial score is under 6 or the retest score is 8 or below, the child should have a full DDST.

INTELLIGENCE

Children must learn many important concepts or ideas such as near, far, here, there, number sequences, how to judge time intervals, how to reason and solve problems, and how to judge weight before they can function effectively in the world.

This type of learning—gaining concepts—is called **cognitive learning.** It is measured by intelligence tests. **Intelligence** can be defined as an ability to think abstractly, to adjust to new situations, and to profit from experience. Almost everyone has had his or her intelligence quotient (IQ) rated at some point in a school career. Although intelligence tests are not part of routine health appraisals, it is helpful to be familiar with those that are used for childhood measurements because these findings are helpful in evaluating children's development.

The *intelligence quotient* is the ratio of mental age as measured by an intelligence test to chronologic age. The formula is as follows:

$$\text{Mental age/Chronological age} \times 100 = \text{IQ}$$

A child aged 9 years old (chronologic age) who passes all the items on an intelligence test that an average 9-year-old child passes would be scored as follows:

$$9 \text{ (mental age)}/9 \text{ (chronological age)} \times 100 = 100 \text{ (the child's IQ)}$$

If a child passes no more items than the average 5-year-old child would, the IQ would be scored as:

$$5 \text{ (mental age)}/9 \text{ (chronological age)} \times 100 = 55$$

If a child passed all the items that a 12-year-old child normally passes, the IQ would be scored as:

$$12 \text{ (mental age)}/9 \text{ (chronological age)} \times 100 = 133$$

Children may score poorly on intelligence tests because of test anxiety. Cultural bias and past experience can also affect how they score. Therefore, labeling children by IQ and classifying them into divisions is often unfair and must be done with considerable thought and study.

It is difficult to test young children with any degree of accuracy because they lack the ability to complete tasks in the areas used for scoring intelligence tests: comprehension, imagination, reasoning, memory, and vocabulary. The most common tests used with infants are the Cattell Infant Intelligence Scale, the Bayley Mental Scale, and the Gesell Developmental Schedule. These tests rely heavily on perceptual and motor skills as rating devices.

The two most frequently used tests for older children are the Wechsler Intelligence Scale for Children and the Stanford-Binet test. All schoolchildren take one of these tests during the primary school grades. The results are made available to child health teams if they can demonstrate to school officials that such information is necessary for total health care or planning. If the information is unavailable, the child can be referred to a psychologist or a psychological testing clinic for assessment.

Goodenough-Harris Drawing Test

A child's drawing can reveal information on developmental or emotional problems. A Goodenough-Harris Drawing Test is a quick intelligence measurement that can be administered without special training (Goodenough, 1926). Give a child between ages 3 and 10 years a pencil and paper and ask the child to draw a person. Urge the child to draw it carefully in the best way he or she knows how and to take enough time to do it well (Box 13-4).

The child receives one point for each of the items in the drawing listed in Box 13-4. For each four points scored, 1 year is added to a base age of 3 years to get the child's mental age. The picture shown in Box 33-4 was drawn by a 4½-year-old child: it received eight points. The child's IQ level is

$$5.0/4.5 \times 100 = 111$$

Scores on the test are reasonably reliable, correlating well with a Stanford-Binet test, although results may not be as reliable with children who are mentally ill. A child who scores significantly lower than his or her chronologic age (after allowing for fatigue, illness, strange surroundings, nervousness, physical ability to use a pencil, and previous practice using a pencil and paper) should be referred for more refined testing.

TEMPERAMENT

Temperament refers to a child's innate behavioral characteristics such as activity level, rhythmicity, tendency to approach or withdraw, and adaptability to situations (see Chapter 7). A child with an "easy" temperament is generally adaptable and easy to care for; a child with a "difficult" temperament, in contrast, will almost automatically create childrearing concerns. Helping parents to assess their children's temperament helps them, in turn, to recognize their children's uniqueness and to anticipate and ideally prevent personality conflicts as a child grows older and expresses identified reactions to situations. If a be-

BOX 13.4

GOODENOUGH–HARRIS DRAWING TEST

Score one point for each characteristic listed below that is present on drawing. For every four points, 1 year is added to a base mental age of 3 years.

1. Head present
2. Legs present
3. Arms present
4a. Trunk present
 b. Length of trunk greater than breadth
 c. Shoulders indicated
5a. Both arms and legs attached to trunk
 b. Legs attached to trunk; arms attached to trunk at correct point
6a. Neck present
 b. Neck outline continuous with head, trunk, or both
7a. Eyes present
 b. Nose present
 c. Mouth present
 d. Nose and mouth in two dimensions, two lips shown
 e. Nostrils indicated
8a. Hair shown
 b. Hair nontransparent, over more than circumference
9a. Clothing present
 b. Two articles of clothing nontransparent
 c. No transparencies, both sleeves and trousers shown
 d. Four or more articles of clothing definitely indicated
 e. Costume complete, without incongruities.
10a. Fingers shown
 b. Correct number of fingers shown
 c. Fingers in two dimensions, length greater than breadth, angle less than 180 degrees
 d. Opposition of thumb shown
 e. Hand shown distinct from fingers or arms
11a. Arm joint shown, either elbow, shoulder, or both
 b. Leg joint shown, either knee, hip, or both
12a. Head in proportion
 b. Arms in proportion
 c. Legs in proportion
 d. Feet in proportion
 e. Both arms and legs in two dimensions
13. Heel shown
14a. Firm lines without overlapping at junctions
 b. Firm lines with correct joining
 c. Head outline more than circle
 d. Trunk outline more than circle
 e. Outline of arms and legs without narrowing at point of junction with body
 f. Features symmetric, correct position
15a. Ears present
 b. Ears in correct position and proportion
16a. Eye detail: brow and lashes shown
 b. Eye detail: pupil shown
 c. Eye detail: proportion correct
 d. Eye detail: glance directed to front in profile drawing
17a. Both chin and forehead present
 b. Projection of chin shown

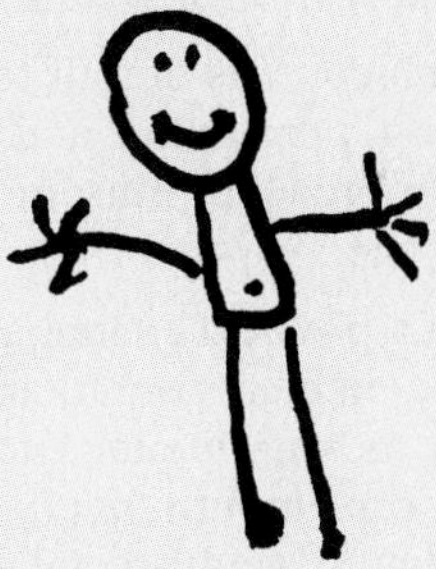

A person drawn by a 4½-year-old.

From Goodenough, F. L. (1926). *Measurement of intelligence by drawings.* New York: World Book Company, with permission.

havior or parent–child interaction problem is already present, a nursing assessment can be useful to determine whether temperament is a factor in the problem and assist parents with constructive solutions (Thomas & Chess, 1977).

One instrument that is helpful in evaluating temperament is the Carey-McDevitt Infant Temperament Questionnaire (Carey & McDevitt, 1978). This consists of 95 responses and can be answered by a parent in approximately 25 minutes. General categories center on the child's responses to feeding, sleeping, soiling and wetting, dressing, bathing, and diapering, as well as to people and new situations.

The questionnaire should be given to parents when their infant is between ages 4 and 8 months (before this, temperament is not developed enough to be evident). The parent reads each behavioral description and then selects the option that most accurately describes the child. If an item does not apply at all, the parent crosses it out. Finally, the parent is asked to describe general impressions of the child's temperament, activity level, positive and negative moods, and distractibility.

When scored, a child can be categorized into one of four groups:

1. Difficult—arrhythmic, withdrawing, low in adaptability, intense, and negative in mood
2. Slow to warm up—inactive, low in approach and adaptability, and negative in mood
3. Intermediate—some characteristics of both groups
4. Easy—rhythmic, approaching, adaptable, mild, and positive in mood

CONCLUDING A HEALTH ASSESSMENT

At every health maintenance visit, the parents and the child, if the child is old enough to understand, should be informed of any available results of screening procedures performed. After learning the results, some parents may require counseling to assist them with health or behavior concerns.

Parents should be asked whether questions remain. If some findings were positive and follow-up procedures are planned, the reason for the upcoming tests should be made clear. Suggest to parents that follow-up phone calls are welcome after they return home from a health assessment so additional questions can be answered. Provide parents with the best hours to call so someone may be available to answer questions for them.

KEY POINTS

A health history is an important part of a health assessment. The purpose is to gather information that will supplement physical or laboratory examinations to complete a more thorough health evaluation.

The parts of a complete health history consist of introduction, chief concern, present health, family profile, history of past illnesses, day history, family health history, and review of systems.

Physical examination consists of four techniques: inspection, palpation, percussion, and auscultation. Techniques and approaches must be varied according to the child's age.

The components of a physical examination are vital sign assessment; general appearance; mental status assessment; body measurements; and assessment of head, eyes, nose, ears, mouth, neck, chest, breasts, lungs, heart, abdomen, genitorectal area, extremities, back, and neurologic function.

Adolescent girls can be taught breast self-examination and boys testicular self-examination at the time of a health appraisal.

Vision assessment consists of asking children to read a standardized chart such as a Snellen Chart, cover testing, or color awareness assessment.

Hearing assessment consists of such assessments as audiometric testing and a Rinne and Weber test.

Development is an important part of total assessment. The Denver Developmental Screening Test (Denver II) and the Denver Articulation Screening Examination are specific development tests.

The Goodenough-Harris Drawing Test correlates well with intelligence quotient (IQ) and is an easy test to administer to children between the ages of 3 and 10 years.

Temperament refers to a child's innate behavioral characteristics such as activity level, rhythmicity, and tendency to approach or withdraw and adapt to situations. Assessing this can help parents to better understand behavior in their child.

Health assessment always causes some degree of apprehension for both parents and children because of worry that some illness will be detected. Giving reassurance of wellness during examinations helps to alleviate this worry.

Be certain to use examining instruments safely (supporting an otoscope base so if the child moves, the otoscope moves with the child). Be certain that young children are not left unsupervised on an examining table or a fall could result.

CRITICAL THINKING EXERCISES

1. Terry is the 5-year-old boy you met at the beginning of the chapter. His father has brought him to your ambulatory clinic for a preschool checkup because he is worried that he needs glasses because he sits so close to the television set. His mother was reluctant to bring him because she doesn't want him to be prescribed glasses. What questions on history would be important to ask the father or Terry? What type of eye chart would you use with Terry to assess his vision?
2. A 2-year-old child, who is seen in a health maintenance clinic for well-child care, is very resistant to being examined. What techniques would you use to help the toddler adjust better to a physical examination?
3. Children may cheat on vision and hearing tests because they do not understand the importance of them. What are techniques to use to keep children from doing this with these assessments?
4. Children should be completely undressed for physical examinations, and all body surfaces should be inspected. What would be your response if a parent said she did not want to undress a child? What if she did not want to remove a Band-Aid from a child's hand?

REFERENCES

Barness, L. A. (1997). The pediatric history and physical examination. In Johnson, K. B., & Oski, F. A. *Oski's essential pediatrics.* Philadelphia: Lippincott.

Boyle, W. E., Jr., & Hoekelman, R. A. (1997). The pediatric history. In Hoekelman, R. A., et al. *Primary pediatric care* (3rd ed.). St. Louis: Mosby.

Burns, C. E. (1996). Child assessment in pediatric primary care. In Burns, C. E., et al. *Pediatric primary care: a handbook for nurse practitioners.* Philadelphia: W. B. Saunders.

Byrnes, K. (1996). Conducting the pediatric health history: a guide. *Pediatric Nursing 22*(2), 135.

Carey, W. B., & McDevitt, S. C. (1978). Revision of the infant temperament questionnaire. *Pediatrics, 61*(4), 735.
Department of Health and Human Services. (1995). *Healthy people 2000: midcourse review*. Washington, DC: DHHS.
Frankenburg, W. K. (1994). Preventing developmental delays: is developmental screening sufficient? *Pediatrics, 93*(4), 586.
Goodenough, F. L. (1926). *Measurement of intelligence by drawings.* New York: World Book Co.
Keller, C., & Stevens, K. R. (1996). Assessment, etiology and intervention in obesity in children. *Nurse Practitioner, 21*(9), 31.
Kodadek, S. M. (1996). Family assessment in pediatric primary care. In Burns, C. E., et al. *Pediatric primary care: a handbook for nurse practitioners.* Philadelphia: W. B. Saunders.
Leff, S., & Bennett, J. (1996). Audit of school entry health assessments: to maximize efficient use of health personnel at school entry assessment at 5 years. *Public Health, 110*(5), 289.
Moody, L. Y. (1997). Pediatric cardiovascular assessment and referral in the primary care setting. *Nurse Practitioner, 22*(1), 120.
O'Hanlon-Nichols, T. (1998). Basic assessment series: Gastrointestinal system. *American Journal of Nursing, 98*(4), 48.
Sponseller, P. D. (1997). Bone, joint and muscle problems. In Johnson, K. B., & Oski, F. A. *Oski's essential pediatrics.* Philadelphia: Lippincott.
Stahlman, E. R. (1997). Vision screening. In Hoekelman, R. A., et al. *Primary pediatric care* (3rd ed.). St. Louis: Mosby.
Tesler, M. D. et al. (1998). Pain behaviors: postsurgical responses of children and adolescents. *Journal of Pediatric Nursing, 13*(1), 41.
Thomas, A., & Chess, S. (1977). *Temperament and development.* New York: Brunner/Mazel.
Ulione, M. S. (1997). Health promotion and injury prevention in a child development center. *Journal of Pediatric Nursing, 12*(3), 148.
Watkin, P. M. (1996). Outcomes of neonatal screening for hearing loss by otoacoustic emission. *Archives of Disease in Childhood, 75*(3), 158.

SUGGESTED READINGS

Canady, M. (1996). Headaches in children: sorting through the pain. *Journal of Pediatric Health Care, 10*(5), 223.
Coleman, W. L. (1995). The first interview with a family. *Pediatric Clinics of North America, 42*(1), 119.
Coody, D., et al. (1997). Eye trauma in children: epidemiology, management, and prevention. *Journal of Pediatric Health Care, 11*(4), 182.
Daya, M., et al. (1996). Otoacoustic emissions: assessment of hearing after tympanostomy tube insertion. *Clinical Otolaryngology, 21*(6), 492.
Garber, K. M. (1996). Enuresis: an update on diagnosis and management. *Journal of Pediatric Health Care, 10*(5), 202.
Jones, M. E., & Clark, D. (1997). Increasing access to health care: a study of pediatric nurse practitioner outcomes in a school-based clinic. *Journal of Nursing Care Quality, 11*(4), 53.
Kerr, C. (1998). Vision screening of primary school children. *Nursing Standard, 12*(13), 46.
Mitchell, M. A., & Jenista, J. A. (1997). Health care of the internationally adopted child. *Journal of Pediatric Health Care, 11*(3), 117.
Riportella-Muller, R., et al. (1996). Barriers to the use of preventive health care services for children. *Public Health Reports, 111*(1), 71.
Snowdon, S. & Stewart-Brown, S. (1998). The value of preschool vision screening. *Nursing Times, 94*(4), 53.
Thomas, R., & Taylor, K. (1997). Assessing head injuries in children. *MCN: American Journal of Maternal Child Nursing, 22*(4), 198.

Health and Wellness Teaching With Children and Families

14

CHAPTER

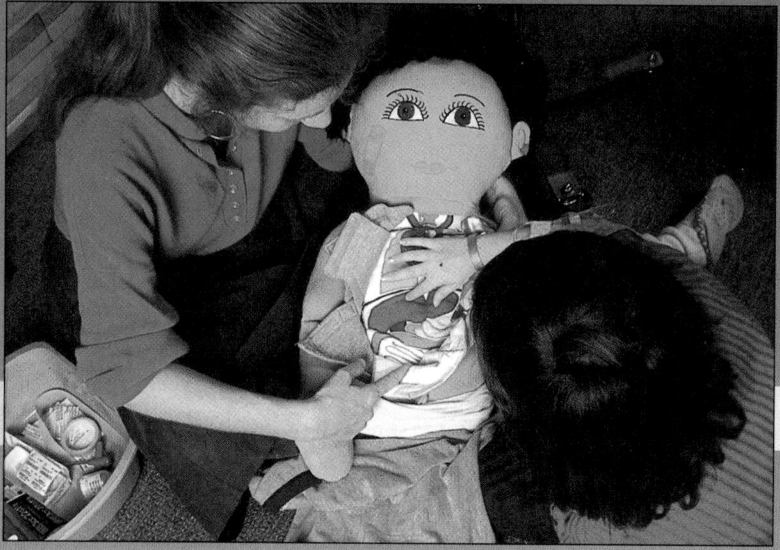

Key Terms

- affective learning
- behavior modification
- cognitive learning
- demonstration
- health fairs
- positive reinforcement
- psychomotor learning
- redemonstration
- teaching plan

Objectives

After mastering the contents of this chapter, you should be able to:

1. Describe principles of teaching and learning and their specific application to health teaching with children.
2. Assess children for their readiness to learn.
3. State nursing diagnoses related to health teaching and children.
4. Identify appropriate health teaching outcomes for a specific child based on the child's age, developmental maturity, emotional needs, and learning style.
5. Plan nursing care based on health teaching priorities.
6. Implement health teaching (e.g., devising a puppet show) using principles of teaching–learning.
7. Evaluate outcome criteria to be certain that nursing goals established for care have been achieved.
8. Identify National Health Goals related to teaching and children that nurses could be instrumental in helping the nation achieve.
9. Identify areas of care related to health teaching of children that could benefit from additional nursing research.
10. Use critical thinking to analyze ways that health teaching can be further incorporated into the nursing care of children and families.
11. Integrate knowledge of teaching–learning with the nursing process to achieve quality child health nursing care.

Bill is a 3-year-old boy who is scheduled for repair of syndactyly (webbed fingers) next week. One of his favorite activities is coloring. His mother is concerned that he will be hard to entertain after surgery because the large pressure bandage he will have afterward will prevent him coloring with that hand. "I don't even want to begin to talk to him about surgery," she tells you. How would you help her? What would be a good strategy for teaching about this type of surgery to a 3-year-old child?

In the previous chapters, you learned about normal growth and development and how children's understanding increases with age. In this chapter, you'll add information about techniques for health teaching with children. This is important information because it builds a base for disease prevention and health promotion for the age group.

After you've studied the chapter, turn to the Critical Thinking Exercises at the end of the chapter to sharpen your skills and test your knowledge.

Health teaching is an independent nursing action that accompanies all nursing care. It is probably the most frequently used intervention for nurses working with childbearing and childrearing families for whom health promotion is such a priority. Education is a prime method for empowering families to assume responsibility for their own health. It is as important as any intervention for families experiencing some type of illness or injury; it is especially important when preparing a child for surgery or some other medical procedure. New areas that require teaching are constantly arising as the health care environment continues to change (Engvall & McCarthy, 1996).

Health teaching may be offered to an individual or to a group of children with similar learning needs. It is offered both formally (e.g., teaching a group of preschoolers about hospitalization) and informally (e.g., when a nurse assures a parent that his or her child is getting enough nutrition, even though the child snacks rather than sits down to regular meals). The same principles of effective teaching and learning apply whether teaching is informal or formal, or offered to an individual or to a group. National Health Goals regarding health teaching and children are shown in Focus on National Health Goals.

FOCUS ON NATIONAL HEALTH GOALS

A number of National Health Goals address health teaching, because it is such an important mechanism of preventive health care. These include:

- Increase to at least 75% the proportion of the nation's elementary and secondary schools that provide planned and sequential quality school health education for kindergarten through 12th grade.
- Increase to at least 50% the proportion of counties that have established culturally and linguistically appropriate community health promotion programs for racial and ethnic minority populations.
- Increase to at least 90% the proportion of hospitals, health maintenance organizations, and large group practices that provide patient education programs, and to at least 90% the proportion of community hospitals that offer community health promotion programs addressing the priority health needs of their communities (DHHS, 1995).

Nurses can be instrumental in helping the nation achieve these goals by consulting with schools and health care organizations to develop health teaching programs and by teaching such programs. Areas that could benefit from nursing research include ways in which busy health care providers can better incorporate health teaching into care; what special techniques are needed to be certain that minority populations are addressed; and whether different teaching techniques are necessary for material with immediate application than for material for long-term care.

NURSING PROCESS OVERVIEW

for Health Teaching

Assessment

Health teaching cannot be effectively accomplished unless it is placed within the context of the nursing process. Learner needs and characteristics, teacher characteristics, available support people and level of content are all factors that will affect learning so must be assessed to formulate nursing diagnoses that clearly state the specific health needs that teaching will address (see Assessing the Child's Learning Capabilities).

Nursing Diagnosis

The following are examples of common nursing diagnoses related to health teaching:

- Knowledge deficit related to importance of taking medicine daily
- Health-seeking behaviors related to ways to improve the child's nutritional intake
- Anxiety related to perceived amount of material needed to be learned for home care of child

Outcome Identification and Planning

After formulation of a nursing diagnosis, an individualized teaching plan is constructed. A plan should detail not only what is to be learned but also methods that will be used for teaching and evaluation. The most effective way to ensure that the desired outcomes are achieved is to establish goals and develop the teaching plan in partnership with the child and family.

Implementation

The step of implementation involves the actual teaching of the plan. Teaching children is not always

Brown, A. L. (1997). Transforming schools into communities of thinking and learning about serious matters. *American Psychologist, 52*(4), 399.

Capen, C. L., et al. (1994). The team approach to pediatric asthma education. *Pediatric Nursing, 20*(3), 231.

Freda, M. C. (1998). Can patient education help mothers of sick children cope? *MCN: American Journal of Maternal Child Nursing, 23*(1), 52.

Lester, C., et al. (1996). Teaching schoolchildren cardiopulmonary resuscitation. *Resuscitation, 31*(1), 33.

Litman, R. S., Berger, A. A., & Chibber, A. (1996). An evaluation of preoperative anxiety in a population of parents of infants and children undergoing ambulatory surgery. *Paediatric Anaesthesia, 6*(6), 443.

Mooney, K. M. (1997). Perioperative management of the pediatric patient. *Plastic Surgical Nursing, 17*(2), 69.

Snowdon, A., & Dane, D. (1995). Parental needs following the discharge of the hospitalized child. *Pediatric Nursing, 21*(5), 425.

Wolraich, M. L. (1997). Addressing behavior problems among school-age children: traditional and controversial approaches. *Pediatrics in Review, 18*(8), 266.

Worthington, R. (1995). Family matters. Effective transitions for families: life beyond the hospital. *Pediatric Nursing, 21*(1), 86.

UNIT

3

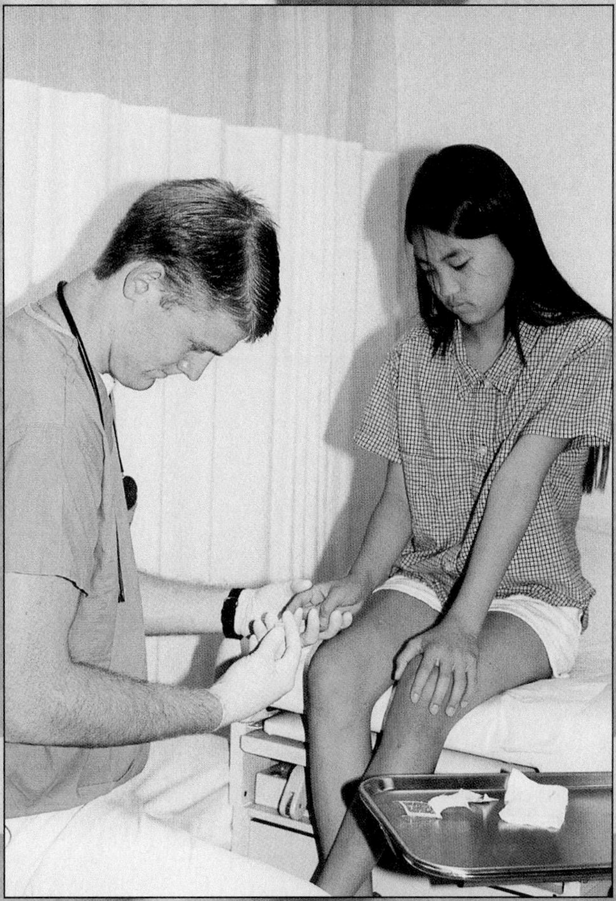

The Nursing Role in Supporting the Health of Ill Children and Their Families

Care of Ill Children and Their Families

15

CHAPTER

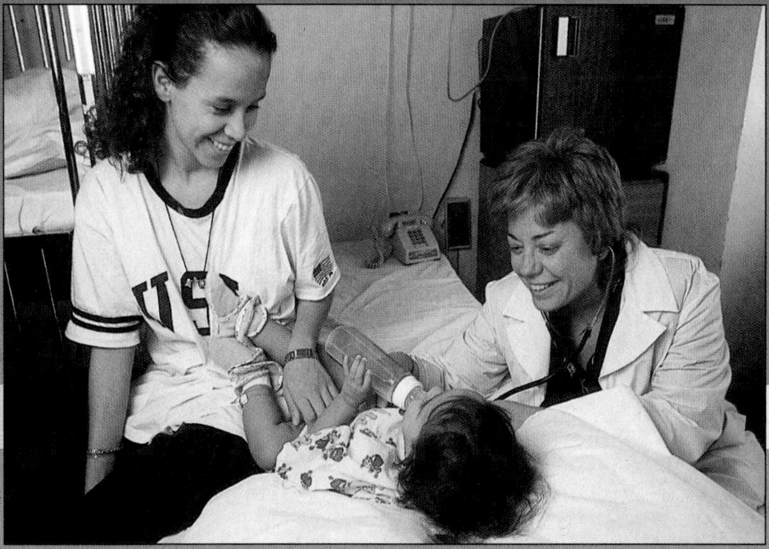

Key Terms

- case management nursing
- calorie counting
- direct care
- home care
- hospice care
- indirect care
- non–rapid-eye movement (NREM) sleep
- play therapy
- primary nursing
- rapid-eye movement (REM) sleep
- skilled home care
- sensory overload
- sleep deprivation
- therapeutic play

Objectives

After mastering the contents of this chapter, you should be able to:

1. Describe the meaning of illness and home care, ambulatory, and in-hospital experiences to children.
2. Assess the impact of an illness, especially that requiring hospital stay, on a child.
3. Formulate nursing diagnoses related to the stress of illness in children.
4. Establish appropriate outcomes for the ill child.
5. Plan nursing care to reduce the stress of illness, such as helping parents plan for hospitalization or home care.
6. Implement measures such as orientation, education, and therapeutic play to reduce the stress of illness.
7. Evaluate outcomes for achievement and effectiveness of care for the ill child.
8. Identify National Health Goals related to hospitalization or health care that nurses can be instrumental in helping the nation to achieve.
9. Identify areas related to illness in children that could benefit from additional nursing research.
10. Use critical thinking to analyze ways in which illness care can be made more family centered and less traumatic for children.
11. Integrate knowledge about the child's response to illness with the nursing process to achieve quality child health nursing care.

Becky is a 7-year-old who burned her foot in a campfire accident. She is going to be admitted to the hospital for 1-day surgery to have the wound debrided. Becky's parents tell you that Becky has not "been herself" since the injury. She has reverted to temper tantrums and sulking, more like a 4-year-old than one of early school age. Even though she's been told that eating meat is important because it provides protein for healing, she refuses to eat anything but Jello or soup. In the admission suite of the hospital, she picked up a doll and twisted its leg off. "What can I do with her?" her mother asks you. "How can we get our old daughter back again?"

Becky is obviously showing some effects of her accident. What type of additional explanation might be helpful to her? What advice would you give her mother to help her better prepare Becky for the upcoming debridement procedure?

In previous chapters, you learned about normal growth and development of children and their special needs at each stage of development. In this chapter, you'll add information about the additional needs of children when they become ill. This is important information because it builds a base for care and health teaching.

After you've studied the chapter, turn to the Critical Thinking Exercises at the end of the chapter to help sharpen your skills and test your knowledge.

Illnesses that require the attention of health care professionals are outside the usual occurrences of childhood, so most children have little knowledge about them. Helping a child and family prepare or adjust to such an experience is a fundamental nursing role. This role goes well beyond providing information on what to expect throughout an illness. Nurses can work to provide orientation programs before hospital admissions and advocate for more open parental visiting and overnight stay policies whenever these are not already in effect. Nurses can help families provide a therapeutic environment for care of the ill child in the home. For individual families, nurses can perform a number of interventions that promote comfort, safety, security, and continued growth and development. Play is one of the more powerful tools available to a nurse working toward this objective. National Health Goals related to children and illness are shown in the National Health Goals box.

NURSING PROCESS OVERVIEW

For the Ill Child

When children become ill, many of their needs, such as those for nutrition, play, and family support, change. If a child will need long-term home care or hospitalization, the entire family will find their priorities and needs changing. Unless these changing needs are examined, recognized, and met, a child may achieve physical wellness again but not mental or emotional health. The family may be left severely incapacitated. Identifying additional needs this way and putting in place necessary services or interventions is an important nursing role.

FOCUS ON NATIONAL HEALTH GOALS

Illness can be a major stress to children and thus a major threat to mental health. Two National Health Goals address the mental health of children:

- Reduce to less than 10% the prevalence of mental disorders among children and adolescents from a baseline of 12%.
- Increase to at least 75% the proportion of providers of primary care for children who include in their clinical practices assessment of cognitive, emotional, and parent–child functioning with appropriate counseling, referral, and follow-up (DHHS, 1995).

Helping with assessment of children's stress level and reducing the stress of hospitalization or health care are ways that nurses can help the nation achieve these goals. Areas where additional nursing research could aid understanding are: What measures do parents want taken to be able to feel most comfortable in a hospital setting; what are the deterrents to therapeutic play on hospital units and how could these be removed; and are there additional contributions nurses could make to shortening hospital stays for children?

Assessment

Assessment for the ill child begins with an interview of the child and parents to identify ways they think the illness will change their lives. This could include a wide range of situations such as increased expenses, changes in time schedules to visit or stay with a hospitalized child, necessity for one parent to take a leave from work to care for an ill child at home, necessity to schedule frequent ambulatory visits, consultation to handle body image changes, and the necessity to arrange for child care for other children. Because these needs change as the course of an illness changes, assessment must be ongoing. (See Assessing the Child for Effects of Illness.)

Nursing Diagnosis

Nursing diagnoses vary greatly depending on the extent of a child's illness, the care needed, and the age of the child. Those often used with families of children seen in ambulatory settings include:

- Health-seeking behaviors related to lack of knowledge regarding illness
- Anxiety related to pending hospital admission
- Risk for social isolation related to planned hospitalization

Nursing diagnoses established for children in the home are the same as those that would be established with the same findings in a health care facility. Often, however, because of the increased participation of the family necessary for home care, nursing diagnoses are more family oriented. Home care can

ASSESSING the Child for Effects of Illness

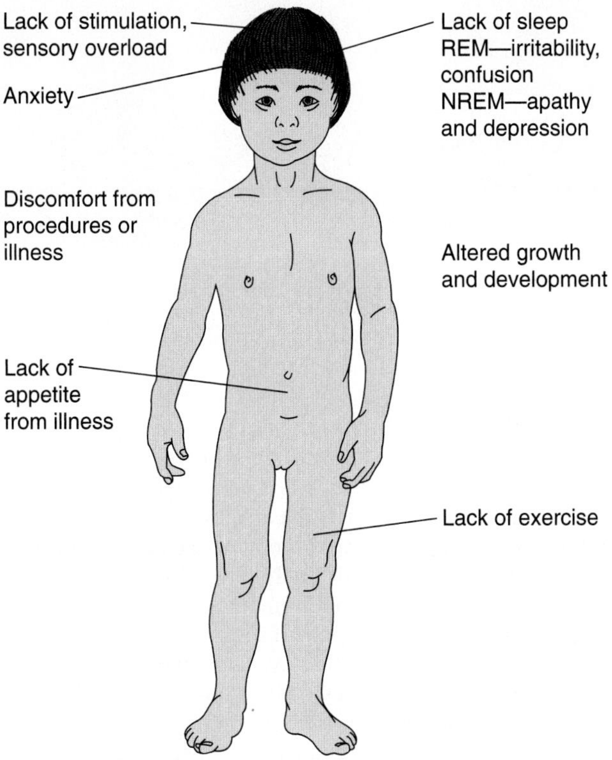

place a heavy burden on the family. The stress of being responsible for an ill child's daily health status can damage a parent's self-esteem or a couple's marital relationship or it can prevent parents from spending time with their other children. Examples are:

- Family coping, potential for growth, related to increased time together because of home care
- Health-seeking behaviors related to skills needed to continue home care
- Risk for altered growth and development related to lack of usual childhood activities
- Altered family processes related to dependence of ill child
- Coping: disabled, related to changes in family routine brought about by home care needs of ill child

Outcome Identification and Planning

Planning for the care of an ill child needs to consider all aspects of a child's and family's life: financial, social, and personal.

Implementation

Five hazards that may occur with all illnesses are (1) harm or injury, such as physical discomfort, pain, mutilation, and death; (2) separation from routines, parents, peers, and respected adults; (3) facing the unknown (new and strange sights and sounds and happenings); (4) facing uncertain limits (unclear definition of acceptable and expected behavior); and (5) loss of control (loss of competence or loss of the ability to make decisions).

It is important to be aware of these potential problems to guard against those that are preventable and to reduce the child's anxiety associated with those that cannot be prevented (such as facing new sights and sounds). Discussing these hazards with older children is important so that implementations to reduce their impact can be tailored to each individual child. Good preparation such as reading to the child, role playing, and puppetry are all useful techniques for easing the younger child's experience. Be certain that the techniques used are appropriate not only to the child's age but to his or her individual learning style.

Nursing interventions for home care often involve teaching family members how to give care. This may include encouraging members to voice the frustration they feel at being constantly confined at home or what they perceive to be a lack of progress in their child's condition. If the child has a terminal illness, parents need support to express their grief. They can also grow discouraged, because the work they are accomplishing is making the child comfortable but not preventing death.

Outcome Evaluation

Outcome criteria for evaluation of ill children should include specific measures such as whether discomfort was kept to a minimum during the experience. Long-term criteria should include whether the child was able to return to his or her usual behavior after the experience. The following are examples of outcome evaluation criteria regarding a hospital experience:

- Parents state that their level of anxiety regarding hospitalization of their infant is now at a tolerable level.
- Parents have effectively changed work schedules to be able to stay with child in hospital.
- Social isolation of toddler is reduced to a minimum through case manager nursing assignment.

Because a home setting is less structured than a health care facility setting, evaluation will show that some goals for care are more difficult to accomplish in the home; for the same reason, because there is more room for innovation at home, some goals will be more easily accomplished. Examples of outcomes might be:

- Parents state that they have been able to make adjustments to accommodate care of ill child at home.
- Child states he or she enjoys respite care in hospice setting 1 weekend a month.
- Parents state they believe they are supplying adequate growth experiences for siblings in light of home care of oldest child.

THE MEANING OF ILLNESS IN CHILDREN

The response of children to illness depends on their cognitive development, past experiences, and level of knowledge. From early school age, children generally know quite a bit about the workings of their major body parts. As general guidelines, early grade school children are usually able to name the function of the heart, lungs, and stomach. They may not be able to do that for kidneys or bladder. This lack of information may reflect the difficulty some parents have in discussing elimination with their children.

Younger children may think the cause of illness is magical (no one knows where it comes from) or that it occurs as a consequence of breaking a rule (e.g., walking in the rain or eating candy after school). With this perspective, they can think that getting well again is possible only if they follow another set of rules, such as staying in bed and taking medicine. By fourth grade, children are generally aware of the role of germs in illness but may be fooled by thinking that all illness is caused by germs. Because of this, they may see a passive role for themselves in getting well, because illness comes from outside influences. At about eighth grade, children are able to voice an understanding that illness can occur from several causes, such as being susceptible to germs from walking in the rain, and that they can take an active role in getting better. These concepts parallel cognitive development (see Chapter 7).

Knowing how children of each age view illness has implications for planning nursing care. In a classic study of children's reactions to illness, Perrin and Gerrity (1981) use the example "There's edema in your belly" being interpreted by a child as "There's a demon in your belly" to illustrate how confused children can be by technical explanations. Other examples are saying you are going to "stick" the child for blood work (interpreted as meaning you are actually going to put a stick in him or her), or saying that the child will receive a dye for a test (interpreted as the child will "die" during the procedure). Children who think illness comes as punishment for breaking rules can interpret nursing procedures (e.g., taking a rectal temperature or giving an injection) as punishment. They can be confused about explanations of procedures because some words sound alike or have double meanings (e.g., "drawing" as in making a picture versus drawing blood). Because of these distorted perceptions, explanations of procedures do not always successfully relieve children's stress level.

Differences in Responses of Children and Adults to Illness

Children are not just small adults. This is important to keep in mind when evaluating how children react to illness, perceive an illness, or react to health care (Figure 15-1). Their body images, as evidenced in their drawings, are different from those of adults. They can have difficulty telling which body parts are indispensable and which are not (this is why it is wise to talk to preschool and early school-age children about "fixing" body parts, such as tonsils, rather than "taking them out.").

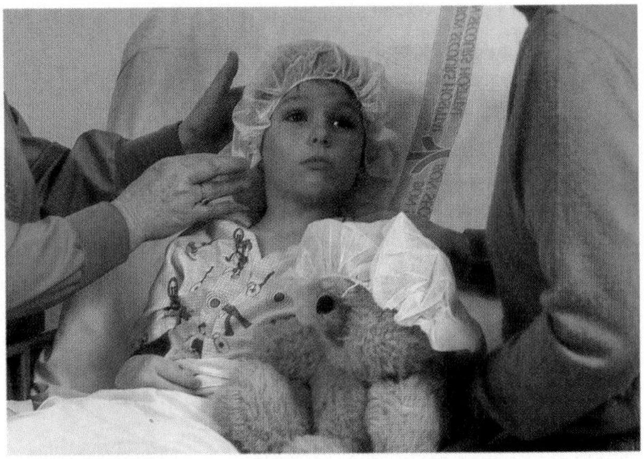

FIGURE 15.1 Illness is potentially traumatic because of the unknown and pain and discomfort that may be involved. Children need extra attention and reassurance to calm their fears.

Inability to Communicate

Very young children do not have the vocabulary to describe symptoms. Headache is an example of a symptom that children younger than 5 years have a great deal of difficulty describing. Dizziness and nausea can be equally bewildering because children this age do not know the words to express these phenomena.

By the time they reach school age, most children can describe symptoms with accuracy. They may intensify their concerns, however, if they believe that someone expects symptoms to be more serious. They may minimize symptoms if they are afraid illness will interfere with an activity.

Determine a child's symptoms as much by observation as by the child's report. The crying, whining preschooler who is "just not herself" probably has a symptom she cannot describe. The school-age child who guards her abdomen (keeps abdominal muscles rigid) is in pain just as clearly as the child who verbalizes the source of discomfort. Considerable observational ability is necessary to ascertain the extent of a child's illness at any given time.

Inability to Monitor Own Care and Manage Fear

Adults who are ill often ask about medication or procedures they are scheduled to undergo. For example, if a hospitalized man knows he is to receive a diuretic three times a day and by 10:00 AM has not been given it, he usually reminds someone of the oversight. School-age and younger children are unable to monitor their own care this way because they may not know which medicine or procedures they are to receive. If they do know, they may be confused about time. In addition, children have fears that adults do not. The infant, for example, fears separation above all else; the toddler and preschooler fear such things as separation, the dark, the unknown, intrusive procedures, and mutilation of body parts. The school-age child and adolescent are concerned about the loss of body parts, loss of life, and loss of friends. Adults have fears also, but most have learned to cope with them. Children in a strange environment (such as a hospital) require more support and active intervention to cope with their stress and fears.

Nutritional Needs

In addition to psychological differences, there are major physiologic differences in the way illness affects children compared with adults. This is because children have different physiologic needs and respond to imbalances in different ways.

Children need more nutrients (calories, protein, minerals, and vitamins) per pound of body weight than adults, for example, because their basic metabolic rate is faster, and they must take in not only enough to maintain body tissues but also enough to allow for growth. The infant requires 120 kcal per kilogram of body weight per day; the adult requires only 30 to 35 kcal/kg/day. An ill child who must limit food intake because of nausea or vomiting, therefore, may require hospitalization that would be unnecessary for an adult under the same circumstances.

Fluid and Electrolyte Balance

In the adult, extracellular water (in plasma and outside body cells) composes approximately 23% of total body water; in a newborn, extracellular water is closer to 40%. This means that an infant does not have as much water stored in the cells as an adult and thus is more likely to lose a devastating amount of body water with diarrhea or vomiting. Because of this, there is no such thing as "only diarrhea" or "simple diarrhea" in a child younger than 1 year. The full implications of both vomiting and diarrhea are discussed in Chapter 24.

Systemic Response to Illness

Because their bodies are immature, young children tend to respond to disease systemically rather than locally. The child with pneumonia, for example, may be brought to an emergency room not because of a cough (although the child has one) but because of accompanying systemic symptoms such as fever, vomiting, and diarrhea. Nausea and vomiting, in fact, occur so frequently in children with any type of illness that these symptoms do not have the diagnostic value they have in adults. Systemic reactions can delay diagnosis and therapy and cause increased fluid and nutrient loss, circumstances that compound an initial illness and can result in hospitalization.

Age-Specific Diseases

Because of their growth requirement and their immaturity, children are susceptible to some diseases that do not affect adults. For example, because infants are growing, a lack of vitamin D will cause rickets, but this same lack does not affect adults. Most adults have achieved immunity to common infectious diseases; children, however, are susceptible to childhood diseases such as measles, mumps, and chickenpox because of lack of immunity. Children younger than 5 years who have a high temperature may respond with generalized convulsions (febrile seizures), a phenomenon that rarely occurs after this age. Children younger than 1 year of age are subject to iron-deficiency anemia, because fetal red blood cells are destroyed after birth and are replaced by mature red blood cells very slowly.

✔ CHECKPOINT QUESTIONS

1. How well do school-age children understand the workings of major body parts?
2. Why are newborns more likely to lose a devastating amount of body fluid with diarrhea or vomiting?

CARE OF THE ILL CHILD AND FAMILY IN THE HOSPITAL

Based on the theory that hospitalization can be an unnecessary stress to children, only those who cannot successfully be managed on an ambulatory basis are now admitted to the hospital. This was not always true. For example, most children with head injuries automatically stayed overnight for observation. Currently, unless a child is unconscious or shows other signs of neurologic injury, he or she is sent home to be observed by parents for signs of increased intracranial pressure. This policy requires that time be spent in teaching parents skills such as how to take a pulse or evaluate consciousness. Teaching them requires patience because parents under stress can have difficulty comprehending instructions; however, because psychological trauma as well as excessive health care costs are prevented by allowing a child to return home, it is important teaching.

Instead of being admitted to the hospital, many children will have procedures such as tonsillectomy done on a 1-day basis. This prevents the major problem of separation anxiety; it does not necessarily reduce parents' or children's anxiety about the procedure (Freda, 1998). Some parents actually feel less confident and more anxious with 1-day procedures than they did with in-hospital admissions because they sense their responsibility for preparation and follow-up care will be significantly greater. They often comment that the system is not as good as when children were admitted and that this change is a result of cost containment by insurance companies. Although it is true that such short hospital stays reduce cost, it is helpful to inform parents that 1-day procedures are as safe as hospital admissions and are scheduled for other reasons than containing cost.

Preparing the Ill Child and Family for Hospitalization

Many childhood illnesses such as febrile convulsions, appendicitis, poisonings, and asthma attacks strike suddenly, making advance preparation for hospital admission impossible. However, when hospitalization is planned ahead of time, for orthopedic or second-stage surgeries, for example, preparation is possible. As a rule, parents eagerly seek guidance from nurses on what and how much to tell their children about an anticipated admission. The preparation a parent makes for a child obviously varies according to the child's age and individual experience. No matter what the child's age, however, parents should be encouraged to above all convey a positive attitude. Statements such as "They'll make you behave in the hospital" or "Wait until you have to stay in bed all day" should be avoided.

TABLE 15.9 Therapeutic Play Techniques for Children After Procedures

PROCEDURE	PLAY ACTIVITY
Radiograph	Provide a doll and table and box labeled "x-ray machine"; children sometimes worry that x-rays have injured them, just as laser rays in science fiction shows do.
Blood drawing	Provide a doll and syringe, alcohol wipes, tourniquet, or finger lancets; remember that finger pricks are as frightening for children as are needles.
Clean-catch urine	Provide a doll (anatomically correct), alcohol wipes, and a collection cup; children are often more embarrassed by urine collection than adults realize.
Intravenous therapy	Provide a doll with intravenous tubing, as well as restraints and armboard; some children are as angry about being restrained as having the needle inserted.
Bronchograms, cystograms, and so forth	Provide a doll and catheters or a penlight to simulate a scope.
Scans	Scans usually require the intravenous injection of isotopes; provide a doll and intravenous fluid and tubing.
Bone marrow	Provide a doll, alcohol wipes, syringe.
Electroencephalogram, electrocardiogram	Provide a doll and electrode leads that attach to a box; children might be afraid of these procedures because of their fear of electricity.
Surgery	Provide a doll, an anesthesia mask, and a blunt kitchen knife; watch and listen for where the child cuts and how he or she describes the experience.
Dental examination	Provide a doll, a suction catheter, a penlight to simulate a drill, and a 4 × 4 piece of plastic to simulate a dental dam; some children are angered by the use of plastic in their mouth.
Dressing changes	Provide a doll, gauze, and adhesive tape.
Cast application or removal	Provide plaster to soak and apply; simulate a cast cutter with an electric razor or hair dryer.
Nasogastric tube, enema, catheterization	Provide a doll and tubes.
Temperature taking	Provide a doll and thermometer.

such play sessions reveal fears, a child should be scheduled for other play sessions, perhaps one daily.

Furnish children with a wide range of equipment and then let them choose those items with which they wish to play. Children invariably choose a piece of equipment that has been used with them. They poke at a doll with a syringe or enjoy giving it a "shot." They wrap the doll in bandages or put tubes into its mouth or stomach, acting out things that were done to them or that they saw done to other children on a nursing unit or at a clinic visit or that they fear will be done to them. Play should be nondirective (let the child proceed at his or her own pace, choosing freely what equipment to play with and what he or she wants to do with the equipment). As a child works through an experience this way, the experience becomes less fearful and the child masters increased control of it.

Observe for children who may be using equipment in an unusual way, such as hitting dolls with stethoscopes or poking them in the eye with a thermometer (suggesting they are confused about the purpose of such equipment). Such behavior alerts health care providers to the importance of explaining the purpose of equipment to children. Listen to what children say as they play. A comment such as "I'm giving shots to all the bad dolls" suggests the child thinks injections are punishment. It would be important to stress the next time the child needs an injection that medicine is to make the child feel well again. A comment such as "This doll is going to surgery so you won't have her anymore" could suggest that the child thinks she will not return from surgery (she may have heard a family member describe someone who died after surgery and is asking for reassurance that such a thing is not going to happen to her). Do not be surprised about the force with which children insert nasogastric tubes into dolls. In part, this reflects how they perceive these procedures, but it also represents energy or anxiety release, in the way that pounding or hitting releases anger.

To better understand how the child feels, repeat what the child says verbally: "You're giving the bad dolls shots?" or ask the child to tell you more about what he or she said: "Do you think that's the only kind of children who get shots? Bad children?" Don't rush to reassure ("Don't worry—that isn't going to happen to you"). Quick reassurance rather than being reassuring tells the child that he or she should not ask any more questions or that the topic is not open for discussion.

Sometimes even children who seem well prepared may be taken by surprise during a procedure. For example, 7-year-old Tanya, seen in an ambulatory setting for a diagnostic workup after a urinary tract infection, showed little interest in dolls and syringes and tubing in the playroom. She had been prepared by her mother for the experience and seemed to understand what would happen during her x-ray procedure. After returning from the x-ray room where she had a voiding cystourethrogram, however, she was obviously upset. Her nurse brought her a rag doll, a doctor and a nurse figure, a play x-ray machine, and some tubing that could simulate a urinary catheter and encouraged Tanya to play with them. Tanya picked up the girl doll and put her under the x-ray machine. She imitated the doctor doll shouting, "Pee in front of everybody!" Tanya's mother had not realized that she would have to void during a cystourethrogram and so had not prepared her for that. Tanya felt betrayed by not being really prepared for this embarrassing situation. Her play brought her emotion out in the open where it could be talked about and handled. When Tanya was scheduled the next day for ureteral reflux surgery, her parent was alerted to make the preparation absolutely thorough.

Children older than 9 and 10 years find playing with dolls too childish to be of benefit. They enjoy handling syringes, however, and being able to see and handle such equipment as nasogastric tubes in advance of their being placed. Active handling helps to eliminate fear because it identifies exactly what the child has to face; it meets their concrete level learning needs.

Creative Play

Some children are too angry to be able to act out their feelings through dramatic play. However, they may be able to draw a picture that expresses their emotions or conveys the extent of their knowledge. To encourage this, give a child a blank paper and crayons or markers. If a child seems reluctant to draw something spontaneously, suggest a topic: "Why don't you draw a picture of yourself?"

Some children are so concerned with particular parts of their bodies that when asked to draw pictures of themselves, they draw only the body parts about which they are worried. Such a child generally is saying that he or she needs to talk about that part of the body, to be given reassurance that it is going to be all right. Figure 15-14*A* shows a picture drawn by a 9-year-old who was admitted to the hospital for 1-day surgery for debridement of a campfire burn on her left foot. She stated on admission that she was being admitted to have the burn on her foot "cleaned out." This sounds like a child who understands what debridement involves. Note, however, that the figure she drew has no left leg. One has to wonder whether she was concerned that she was going to surgery to have more than debridement. After the word *debridement* was explained to her, she drew the picture in Figure 15-14*B*. The child in the drawing now has a left and a right leg, the left leg covered by a bandage. Through a drawing, this child was able to say something she could not express without this help.

Many ill children draw pictures that reflect punitive images: a boy or girl tied to a bed or shut behind bars, or doctors and nurses frowning at them, obviously unhappy with them. Such children may need assurance that they are not being punished; they need to stay in bed or are being cared for by doctors and nurses to be made well (Figure 15-15). Other children draw pictures that are symbolic of death: airplanes crashing, boats sinking, buildings on fire, children in graveyards. They need assurance that they will not die.

Other concerns such as fear of abandonment and loss of independence may also be manifested in drawings. For example, preschoolers may draw a child in one corner of a picture and an adult in a far corner. They may comment that the parent cannot find the little child because she's gone to the hospital. They need to be reassured that their parents know where they will be and will visit them each day after work.

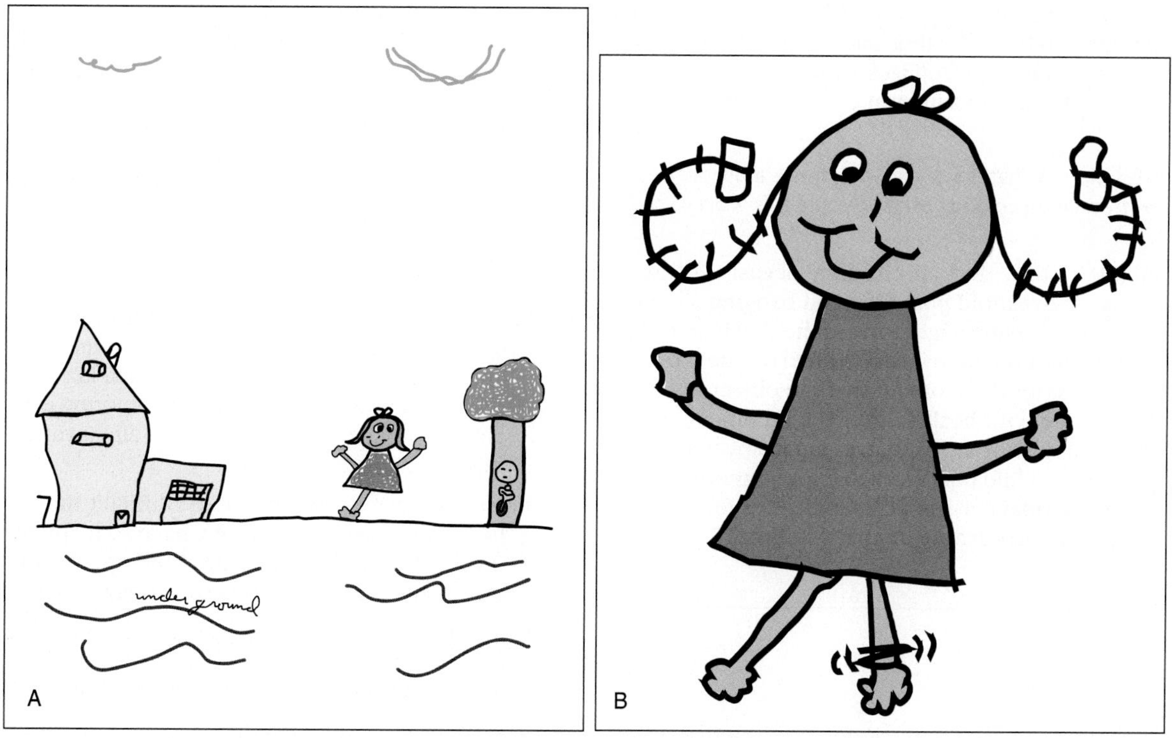

FIGURE 15.14 (**A**) Children who are concerned about body parts may draw pictures with that part missing or exaggerated. Note the missing left leg here. (**B**) After reassurance that her leg will be all right, the girl who did the drawing in **A** now draws a girl with two legs.

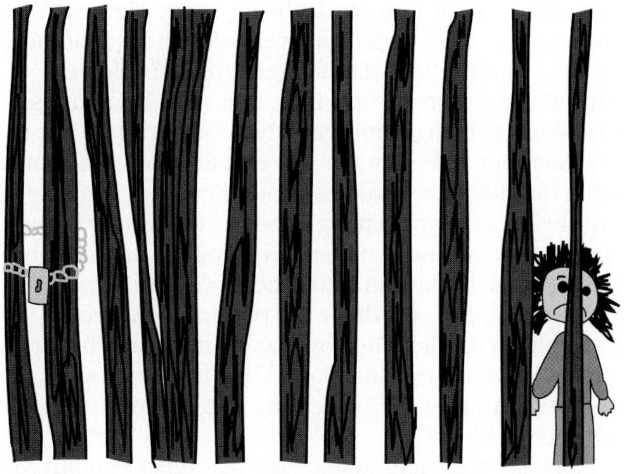

FIGURE 15.15 A picture drawn by a hospitalized child. Note the prison-like appearance of the crib. (Courtesy of Rita Crever.)

Older school-age children and adolescents may not be interested in drawing but can be interested in making a list of procedures or experiences they like and dislike. Examine the dislike list for procedures such as "shots" or "chemo." Mark the nursing care plan for nurses to take special time to explain these procedures and to offer special support when they must be done.

Guidelines for Conducting Therapeutic Play

It is important to use common sense when conducting therapeutic play. Be certain not to interpret a child's black and gloomy drawing as meaning the child is depressed when a black marker was the only one available. Many children 4 to 5 years of age draw a person lacking many body parts because that is the best human form they can draw.

WHAT IF? What if a 3-year-old draws a purple person with only three body parts? Would this worry you?

Remember, too, that all children occasionally treat dolls badly. A 2-year-old pounding and banging a rag doll may not be expressing anger toward the doll image at all, but may be intent on discovering the feel of a new texture and is unaware for the moment that the object is a doll.

A conference with health care team members, including a psychologist or a psychiatric nurse specialist, may be called for if a child continues to express mutilating behavior after normal reassurance. Guidelines for conducting therapeutic play are summarized in Box 15-4.

BOX 15.4

GUIDELINES FOR THERAPEUTIC PLAY

1. Allow a child to choose the articles with which he or she wants to play (something may be too frightening for a child to play with immediately; he or she needs time to work up to the activity).
2. Provide the materials specific to the child's experiences of which you, the nurse, are aware (e.g., nasogastric tube, syringe, or bandages), but do not supply only those things; a child may have misunderstandings and fears of situations you cannot know about.
3. Allow play to be unstructured or let the child use the materials however he or she wishes. If a child seems uninterested in materials, then begin to play with her (e.g., give a doll an injection) to see if this reduces her anxiety enough to be able to handle items.
4. If a child cannot manipulate materials himself (due to such things as a cast or traction), ask the child what he would like you to do with it.
5. Reflect only what the child expresses (verbal expression).
6. Do not criticize play; this inhibits further expression.
7. Use a therapeutic response, not "Don't worry, that won't happen," but "Are you worried that could happen?"
8. Ask children to describe paintings, not "That's a good picture of yourself," but "Tell me about your picture."
9. Do not be reluctant to use real equipment (e.g., real catheters and blood lancets). Handling real equipment best helps to reduce stress.
10. Supervise the therapeutic play, because some equipment could cause an accident (and therapeutically responding to the child's comments is necessary).

KEY POINTS

Illness may be more traumatic for children than for adults because of their inability to communicate and monitor their own care and because they have different nutrition, fluid, and electrolyte needs.

Separation from parents because of hospitalization can have permanent psychological effects on children. Methods to reduce this include keeping hospital stays as brief as possible, promoting open parent and sibling visiting, and providing primary or case management nursing.

Preschoolers may have the most difficult time during hospitalization because they have so many fears. Preparation and promotion of therapeutic play are essential to reduce trauma to a tolerable level.

Currently, many medical procedures can be done on an ambulatory basis. Advocating for care to be done in such settings is a nursing responsibility.

The presence of parents during health care can help reduce trauma to children. Making parents as welcome as possible makes it possible for them to room in. Include the parents in both the planning and the implementation of care. Parents reinfect children with fear if their own fear is not reduced.

Because hospitalizations currently are so brief, parents need good discharge instructions to continue to care for children safely at home. Providing clear instructions and danger signs for parents to watch for are nursing responsibilities.

Home care is increasing as a way of providing care to chronically ill children. It has the advantages of being cost-effective and providing meaningful comfort and support to the child. Disadvantages are that parents can become fatigued, the loss of a job for the primary caregiver can cause financial hardship, and social isolation and disruption of normal home life may occur.

Not all homes are ideal for home care. Assess that a primary care provider is present; the family is knowledgeable about the care necessary; necessary resources are available; and safety features such as a smoke detector, a safe area for oxygen storage, and a safe refrigerator for food or medicine are present.

Important elements to consider when planning home care are ways to provide a therapeutic environment; provide for adequate nutrition and mobility; meet care requirements for respiratory function and elimination; administer medication; and encourage self-care.

Home care can be exhausting for parents. Be certain that they devise a schedule of care that allows them enough rest. Advocate for medicine or treatment schedules that allow for administering medications during the day rather than a schedule that requires medication administration at night.

Parents may need respite care to continue to be effective care providers, just as professionals need time off. Help parents to relieve each other so each has some free time during a week.

CRITICAL THINKING QUESTIONS

1. Becky is the 7-year-old you met at the beginning of the chapter. Her foot was burned in a campfire accident. Since then she has refused to eat anything but Jello or soup. In the hospital playroom, she picked up a doll and tore off its leg. Her mother asked you why her daughter is acting this way. What suggestions would you make to her? The burn occurred because Becky was left momentarily unsupervised by a campfire. Is there a possibility her mother may not be acting her usual self because of guilt over the injury?
2. A 3-year-old has had emergency surgery while on vacation with her single mother. Her mother had to return home because of work responsibilities, so the 3-year-old will have no family with her for a week. What measures would you take to help make hospitalization and separation less traumatic for her?
3. A 14-year-old will be cared for at home after orthopedic surgery. She is concerned that because her home stay will be lengthy she will be cut off from her friends for a long time. What suggestions could you make to her to help her maintain contact with friends?
4. A 6-year-old is on home care for chronic respiratory disease. His parents state that they are exhausted because of the necessity for round-the-clock care. What suggestions could you make to them to make care easier?

REFERENCES

Burns, L.S. (1997). Advances in pediatric anesthesia. *Nursing Clinics of North America, 32*(1), 45-71.

Corser, N.C. (1996). Sleep of 1- and 2-year-old children in intensive care. *Issues in Comprehensive Pediatric Nursing, 19*(1), 17-31.

Department of Health and Human Services, (1995). *Healthy people 2000: midcourse review*. Washington, D.C.: DHHS.

Doman, M. (1998). Nursing children in a range of hospital settings. *Paediatric Nursing, 10*(1), 10.

Freda, M. C. (1998). Can patient education help mothers of sick children cope? MCN: *American Journal of Maternal Child Nursing, 23*(1), 52.

Krebel, M.S., Clayton, C. & Graham, C. (1996). Child life programs in the pediatric emergency department. *Pediatric Emergency Care, 12*(1), 13-15.

Kristensson-Hallstrom, I. & Elander, G. (1997). Parents' experience of hospitalization: different strategies for feeling secure. *Pediatric Nursing, 23*(4), 361-367.

Kuntz, N. et al. (1996). Therapeutic play and bone marrow transplantation. *Journal of Pediatric Nursing, 11*(6):359-367.

McConnochie, K.M. et al. (1997). Ensuring high-quality alternatives while ending pediatric inpatient care as we know it. *Archives of Pediatrics and Adolescent Medicine, 151*(4), 341-349.

Perrin, E.C. & Gerrity, P.S. (1981). There's a demon in your belly: children's understanding of illness. *Pediatrics, 67*(4), 841-847.

Pokorni, J.L. (1997). Promoting the overall development of infants and young children receiving home health services. *Pediatric Nursing, 23*(2), 187-190.

Robertson, J. (1958). *Young children in hospitals.* London: Tavistock.

Rossen, B.E. & McKeever, P.D. (1996). The behavior of preschoolers during and after brief surgical hospitalizations. *Issues in Comprehensive Pediatric Nursing, 19*(2), 121-133.

Rowe, J. (1996). Making oneself at home? Examining the nurse-parent relationship. *Contemporary Nurse, 5*(3), 101-106.

Spitz, R.A. (1945). Hospitalism: an inquiry into the genesis of psychiatric conditions in early childhood. *Psychoanalytic Study of the Child, 1*(3), 53-59.

Thorne, S.E., Radford, M.J. & Armstrong, E.A. (1997). Long-term gastrostomy in children: caregiver coping. *Gastroenterology Nursing, 20*(2), 46-53.

Tiedeman, M.E. (1997). Anxiety responses of parents during and after the hospitalization of their 5- to 11-year-old children. *Journal of Pediatric Nursing, 12*(2), 110-119.

SUGGESTED READINGS

Charron-Prochownik, D. et al. (1997). Outpatient versus inpatient care of children newly diagnosed with IDDM. *Diabetes Care, 20*(4), 657-660.

Dokken, D. L., & Sydnor-Greenberg, N. (1998). Helping families mobilize their personal resources. *Pediatric Nursing, 24*(1), 66.

Hatton, D.L. et al. (1995). Parents' perceptions of caring for an infant or toddler with diabetes. *Journal of Advanced Nursing, 22*(3), 569-577.

Liptak, G.S. (1997). Home care for children who have chronic conditions. *Pediatrics in Review, 18*(8), 271-273.

Lowes, L. & Davis, R. (1997). Minimizing hospitalization: children with newly diagnosed diabetes. *British Journal of Nursing, 6*(1), 28-33.

Melnyk, B.M., et al. (1997). Helping mothers cope with a critically ill child: a pilot test of the COPE intervention. *Research in Nursing and Health, 20*(1), 3-14.

Nelson, V.S. et al. (1996). Home mechanical ventilation of children. *Developmental Medicine and Child Neurology, 38*(8), 704-715.

Toder, D.S. & McBride, J.T. (1997). Home care of children dependent on respiratory technology. *Pediatrics in Review, 18*(8), 273-280.

Woodgate, R. & Kristjanson, L.J. (1996). "Getting better from my hurts": toward a model of the young child's pain experience. *Journal of Pediatric Nursing, 11*(4), 233-242.

Nursing Care of the Ill Child and Family: Diagnostic and Therapeutic Techniques

16

CHAPTER

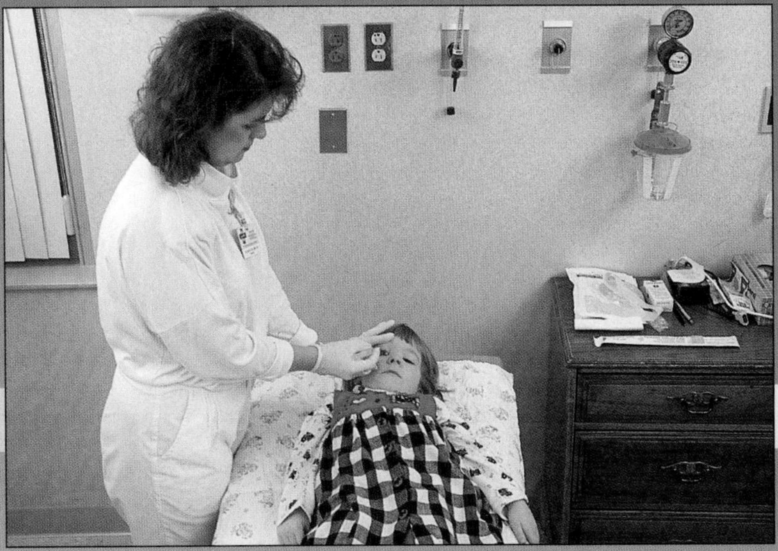

Key Terms

- aspiration studies
- barium contrast studies
- bronchoscopy
- central venous access devices
- clean-catch urine specimen
- computed tomography (CT)
- electrical impulse studies
- endoscopy
- gavage feedings
- intermittent infusion devices
- magnetic resonance imaging (MRI)
- positron emission tomography (PET)
- radiopharmaceutical
- single photon emission computerized tomography (SPECT)
- total parenteral nutrition (TPN)
- ultrasound
- venipuncture

Objectives

After mastering the contents of this chapter, you should be able to:

1. Describe common nursing interventions used in the health care of children to aid diagnosis and therapy.
2. Assess children as to developmental stage and knowledge level before beginning any diagnostic technique, therapeutic procedure, or other nursing intervention.
3. Formulate nursing diagnoses related to common diagnostic therapeutic techniques used with children.
4. Identify outcomes for the child undergoing a diagnostic or therapy technique.
5. Plan nursing interventions to aid in diagnosis or therapy for children.
6. Implement nursing procedures.
7. Evaluate outcome criteria to be certain that nursing goals related to diagnostic and therapeutic techniques were achieved.
8. Identify National Health Goals related to care of children that nurses could be instrumental in helping the nation achieve.
9. Identify areas related to nursing procedures with children that could benefit from additional nursing research.
10. Use critical thinking to analyze ways that procedures can be modified to meet the needs of children of all ages.
11. Integrate knowledge of common procedures with nursing process to achieve quality child health nursing.

Wally is a preschooler who is scheduled to have magnetic resonance imaging (MRI) study for a possible head injury. "How can I agree to this?" his mother asks you. "He's afraid of the dark. How can I allow him to be wheeled into a long dark machine that way?" How would you explain magnetic resonance imaging to Wally to make the procedure more acceptable to him?

In previous chapters, you learned about the growth and development of well children. In this chapter, you'll add information about how to care for children when they become ill. This is important information because it builds a base for care and health teaching.

After you've studied the chapter, turn to the Critical Thinking Exercises at the end of the chapter to help sharpen your skills and test your knowledge.

Illness can be particularly stressful if many diagnostic and therapeutic procedures are necessary for care. In today's health care climate, there is less time for teaching and preparation than once available, so good planning and follow-through are essential. Chapter 15 describes measures to make the experience of illness a more positive one. Health teaching, discussed in Chapter 14, is a cornerstone in this process. However, everything that nurses do with and for ill children will have a major influence on the child's progress toward health as well as on the child and family's perception of professional health care and the ability to carry out healthful practices in the future.

Many nursing actions offer an opportunity to accomplish several goals: Supporting the child and family during a diagnostic procedure, for instance, not only can aid in efficient diagnosis but also may help establish a trusting relationship between the family and health care providers that will make all future interactions more successful. This chapter describes the most common diagnostic and therapeutic techniques used in the care of ill children, including modifications needed to make these procedures safe and reduce associated stress, depending on the child's age and outlook. National Health Goals that address this area of child health practice are shown in the Focus on National Health Goals display.

FOCUS ON NATIONAL HEALTH GOALS

A basic part of carrying out procedures with children is keeping them safe during procedures. One National Health Goal concerns keeping patients safe from nosocomial infection:

- Reduce by at least 10% the incidence of surgical wound infections and nosocomial infections in intensive care patients.

A second concern for health care providers is to feel safe themselves from infection while carrying out procedures involving possible exposure to blood or body secretions. A National Health Goal also addresses this:

- Extend to all facilities where workers are at risk for occupational transmission of HIV, regulations to protect workers from exposure to bloodborne infections, including HIV infection (DHHS, 1995).

Nurses can be instrumental in helping to prevent nosocomial infection by enforcing measures such as frequent handwashing and being certain to use sterile technique for dressing changes. They can be instrumental in reducing the possibility of health care provider exposure to infection by being certain that they and their coworkers are following standard precautions, especially proper needle containment.

Areas related to these goals that could benefit from additional nursing research are whether the type or thickness of surgical dressings or length of hospital stay affect the incidence of incision infections; whether allowing parents or children to change dressings affect the incidence, and under what circumstances breaks in standard precautions are most apt to occur and how this could be prevented.

NURSING PROCESS OVERVIEW

for Care of the Ill Child and Family

Assessment

Before performing procedures such as assisting with a diagnostic test, collecting laboratory specimens, or administering medication, it is important to first carefully evaluate the child's age and developmental stage, as well as any special needs the child may have. Even the most common and painless procedures produce a certain amount of stress for the child and parents. During complex diagnostic procedures, this stress level is almost certain to increase. Unfamiliar doctors and nurses, high-tech supplies and equipment, and strange surroundings all add up to a frightening experience for most adults; imagine how frightening they can seem to children.

Assess the child's level of anxiety associated with unfamiliar equipment, circumstances, and surroundings as well as the child's knowledge concerning a technique before initiating a procedure or beginning health teaching. It may be possible to increase cooperation by acknowledging and respecting the child's past experience with the procedure.

Nursing Diagnosis

Common nursing diagnoses related to diagnostic procedures are as varied as the procedures and environment but include:

- Fear related to new and strange surroundings of the procedure room
- Pain related to lumbar puncture
- Knowledge deficit related to technique for 24-hour urine collection
- Diversionary activity deficit related to lack of appropriate toys in required setting
- Sleep pattern disturbance related to timing of medication administration

- Altered nutrition, less than body requirements related to lack of familiar foods
- Risk for injury related to a biopsy procedure

Outcome Identification and Planning

Illness in itself creates anxiety in the child; unless the child is helped to feel comfortable and safe, every procedure can result in even more stress. An important nursing goal is to perform interventions with the least degree of anxiety possible. To achieve this goal, plan specific ways to prepare children in advance. Planning should include the best way to explain the procedure to a particular child and also how to ensure that the child is not overwhelmed by the number of diagnostic or therapeutic procedures performed in any one day. With small children, it may make more sense to stagger ambulatory diagnostic tests over a number of days to preserve the child's coping ability. Conversely, some older children (and parents) do better if they can complete all necessary tests in 1 day, so that they do not have to anticipate more testing over a long period. Use nursing judgment and data from periodic assessment to help primary care providers determine what sort of schedule is in the child's and family's best interest.

Implementation

Whether assisting with a procedure or performing a therapeutic intervention, it is necessary to function in several roles at the same time: performing (or assisting with) the procedure, providing active support to the child and parents, and observing and then documenting the child's reactions. Providing support is a major role, and there are many ways to do this, such as holding a child's hand or placing a hand on the parent's shoulder. Playing a distracting game with an older child can also be helpful. Important observations to be made are signs of discomfort, changes in vital signs, or other signals of distress such as pallor or dizziness. Maintain a flowsheet of observations during a procedure. After a procedure, the procedure, the child's reaction, and specimens obtained can then be documented accurately and efficiently in the child's record.

As a final follow-through step, think of therapeutic play techniques to introduce that would be helpful in relieving stress caused by the procedure.

Outcome Evaluation

Evaluating goals related to procedures not only helps in determining the effect of the procedure but also helps in planning, should other procedures be required. Recording that a particular child who did not appear nervous during a procedure later admitted to being "more scared than he'd ever been before," for example, can help another nurse provide reassurance to this child, even when the child is successfully masking his emotions the next time. Examples of outcome criteria might be:

- Child voices she is able to cope with further bone marrow aspiration.
- Child voices steps to take to collect 24-hour urine at home.
- Child participates in 1 hour of active play daily.
- Child sleeps a minimum of 4 uninterrupted hours at night.
- Child eats a minimum of 1000 calories per day.
- Child experiences minimal loss of blood (less than 10 mL) during diagnostic procedures.

NURSING RESPONSIBILITIES WITH DIAGNOSTIC AND THERAPEUTIC TECHNIQUES

Responsibilities of the nurse in assisting with procedures performed on children include the following:

- Helping to obtain consent as needed
- Explaining the procedure to the child and his or her parents to prepare them psychologically
- Scheduling the procedure
- Preparing the child physically
- Obtaining equipment for the procedure and ensuring that standard precautions are followed
- Accompanying the child to the treatment room or hospital department where the procedure will be performed
- Providing support during the procedure
- Assessing the child's response to the procedure
- Providing care to the child and specimens obtained once the procedure is completed.
- Overseeing unlicensed assistive personnel to ensure the safety and efficacy of all procedures (see Managing and Delegating Unlicensed Assistive Personnel)

Obtaining Consent

Consent to perform a procedure must be obtained if the procedure carries any risk that would not be present if it were not performed (Williams et al, 1997). For a parent to sign a consent form, he or she must be informed about the content of the procedure and the risks of having or not having it performed. Although actually obtaining this is the physician's responsibility, seeing that it is obtained is a nursing responsibility. Acting as an advocate for the family if they do not understand the consent, procedure, or risk is also an important nursing role. Be certain that

MANAGING AND DELEGATING UNLICENSED ASSISTIVE PERSONNEL

Unlicensed assistive personnel may be asked to assist with diagnostic or therapeutic procedures, especially ones such as urine collection or vital sign measurement. Be certain that they do not become so used to taking these measurements that they grow careless with them. Help them also to develop sufficient patience to explain procedures to children as many times as needed to gain children's cooperation. Remind them that children cannot relax until their parents are also relaxed, so spending time to help parents understand a procedure is also important.

FOCUS ON NURSING RESEARCH

What Factors Influence Parents' Decisions to Consent to Their Child's Participation in Anesthesia Research?

To answer this question, 246 parents were approached in an outpatient waiting room and asked for permission to allow their child to participate in a clinical anesthesia study. They were then asked to complete a questionnaire detailing the reason for their decision to consent or decline to consent. One hundred and sixty-eight parents agreed to consent; 78 declined. Perceived low risk and the importance of the study were the primary factors in the parents' decision to consent to the study. Only 2.8% considered a lack of privacy as a deciding factor in their decision; 15.3% stated they had insufficient time to make a decision; none reported having felt pressured.

This study is important for nurses because it documents the important information that parents need to agree to allow their child to participate in a research study. It stresses the importance of preventing parents from feeling rushed while they read and sign a consent form.

Tait, A. R., Voepel-Lewis, T., Siewert, M., & Malviya, S. (1998). Factors that influence parents' decisions to consent to their child's participation in clinical anesthesia research. *Anesthesia & Analgesia, 86*(1), 50–53.

the rights of emancipated minors are respected and that in single-parent families the custodial parent has given the permission (see Focus on Nursing Research.)

Explaining Procedures

To be able to explain procedures clearly and answer questions about them appropriately, it is important to see as many procedures performed as possible. Asking a child after any procedure what sensations he or she experienced not only helps the child work through a possibly frightening situation (often called "debriefing") but also increases your knowledge of common procedures.

As a general guide, a child needs a detailed description of the procedure, such as "I'll clean your finger. You will feel a small pinprick . . .", and an explanation of the following:

- Why the procedure is performed—e.g., "The doctor needs to look at your blood to see why you're so sick."
- Where the procedure will be done—e.g., the x-ray department or a treatment room
- Any unusual sensations to be expected during the procedure—e.g., alcohol for cleaning skin will feel cold
- Any pain involved—e.g., "The needle will sting, although I'll put some cream on first to dull the feeling."
- Any strange equipment used—e.g., a large x-ray machine
- The approximate length of time the procedure will take
- Any special care after the procedure—"You will need to lie quietly for 15 minutes afterward."

It is important to use age-appropriate language when explaining procedures (Bar-Mor, 1997). Be careful not to use words that might be confusing during an explanation, such as "transducer" or "electrode," without defining them. Try to associate the procedure with something with which the child is already familiar and comfortable (e.g., an x-ray machine is a "big camera"). Try not to use the word "test" in explanations. School-age children associate the word "test" with a "pass/fail" situation. This can make them unduly worried after a procedure about whether they have "passed" it.

If unfamiliar with what a procedure entails, do not guess: nothing is more confusing to a child or parents than being told two different versions of something. Most technical personnel will take the time to describe over the telephone to you important information that a child should know about a study or procedure, because having a well-informed patient makes their job easier. Be certain that parents also receive an explanation of the procedure. A child has difficulty relaxing if parents are still anxious because they do not understand what is going to happen. Encourage parents to stay with the child during most procedures, because they can be extremely helpful in reducing a procedure's threatening aspects.

Scheduling

Most diagnostic procedures are scheduled on an ambulatory basis. Try to arrange for the child to have time for meals and some free play time between procedures. If food or fluid must be restricted for procedures, monitor the child's degree of discomfort and physiologic needs related to this; advocate as necessary for a time lapse between examinations or improved coordination in scheduling to decrease the time spent without food or fluid.

Physical Preparation

Physical preparation varies depending on what procedure is to be performed. In many instances, preparing a child for an examination (e.g., barium enema) involves another procedure (a saline enema), so physical preparation becomes education for the real examination. In all instances, be certain to explain both the preparative and actual procedures.

Accompanying the Child

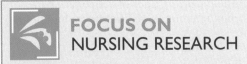

If a procedure will be done at another site rather than the primary care clinic or hospital unit with which a child is comfortable, ideally a nurse who the child knows should accompany the child to the other department and remain with the child for the procedure, or at least until the child has met a primary person who will be with him or her during the assessment. Older children do well without being accompanied as long as they have been introduced in advance to the new person who will give them care. A parent who can accompany a child is of invaluable help.

Before leaving the patient unit or clinic, have the child void for comfort unless this is a contraindication to the procedure. Check for any medication or a specific assessment procedure such as a blood pressure recording that should be given or done before leaving the unit for another department, in case the child is away from the primary unit for an extended time. If the child is an inpatient, check also that the identification band is securely in place and readily visible despite any intravenous equipment. If there will be a considerable wait in another department, ask the child if he or she would like some activity during a wait, such as a game or book. Hallways can be cool. Provide adequate blankets for comfort, especially for infants. Always use cart straps and side rails for safety.

Providing Support

Children do well with diagnostic and evaluative procedures as long as they have adequate support from a concerned provider or parent. Provide this both verbally (explain what is going to happen; assure a child that he or she is sitting still effectively) and nonverbally (a hand on the arm or a nearby presence).

Modifying Procedures According to the Child's Age and Developmental Stage

A child's age and potential understanding of procedures must be considered when planning the number and order of tests as well as the way they are performed.

The Infant

The number of painful or uncomfortable procedures done on infants should be kept to a minimum to avoid interfering with the infant's developing a sense of trust. Parents should be allowed to accompany their child to hospital departments and remain during procedures to offer support. Some parents may ask to hold their child during a procedure that causes pain, but do not ask parents to restrain the child during such a procedure. Their role should be a supportive and comforting, not a pain-causing, one.

Infants need to be picked up and comforted after procedures (a child of any age likes a hug or honest compliment for cooperation). Be aware that blood drawing (which can deplete blood stores) and x-rays (which are possibly harmful to bone marrow) should both be kept to a minimum in infants. Help parents understand why these procedures are being limited, so they do not think that their infant's care is being compromised by few diagnostic procedures.

The Toddler and Preschooler

Toddlers and preschoolers resist any diagnostic testing that involves any degree of discomfort or pain or that is unfamiliar. Give children this age short explanations of what to expect. Such explanations should be given close to the time of the procedure so that little time can be spent worrying over it.

The School-Age Child and Adolescent

School-age children are interested in the theory and reason for procedures; they often can be persuaded to cooperate for a procedure by being promised a look at their x-ray or laboratory report afterward. Be careful when promising children that they can see these results that this is actually possible. Otherwise, it can be difficult to obtain any further cooperation. Adolescents may project an air of maturity or sophistication beyond their years to remain in control of themselves in the face of frightening procedures. Do not be misled into thinking a child this age would not appreciate an explanation or a comforting hand on a shoulder during a procedure.

> WHAT IF? What if an adolescent who was scheduled for a series of diagnostic tests said, "I'm not a kid, you know," and refused to listen when you started to explain a procedure? Later, he acted angry because he had been "tricked" into having the procedure. How could you give explanations to him without offending him? Why do you think he acts this way?

Promoting Safety During Procedures

Safety is an important component of all patient care. When your patient is a child, there is an even greater concern for safety. Children's immaturity, which makes them unable to form mature judgments, leaves them vulnerable to harm unless their caretakers give special consideration to promoting safety (Huffman & Sandelowski, 1997).

NURSING DIAGNOSES AND RELATED INTERVENTIONS

Nursing Diagnosis: Risk for injury related to diagnostic procedures

Outcome Identification: The child will not sustain any injury during series of diagnostic procedures.

Outcome Evaluation: Child does not sustain injury from diagnostic equipment.

Children need special precautions taken so they remain safe during procedures. As a basic safety measure, before giving any medication or food or before performing any procedure, look at the identification band. If an armband must be removed because it interferes with an intravenous infusion site, cut it away but immediately anchor it to another extremity with adhesive tape. Ask the admissions department to provide a new armband as soon as possible. Do not leave the old one off while waiting for a replacement band. This leaves the child susceptible to the danger of mistaken identity during the waiting period.

Children tend to fuss with equipment to see what will happen if they turn a knob or spin a dial. They need close

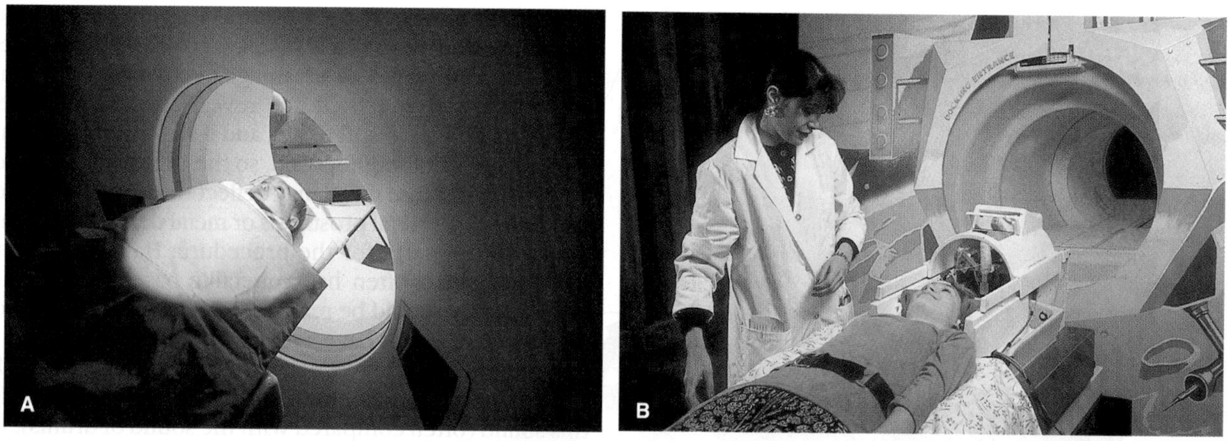

FIGURE 16.4 Some procedures are potentially frightening because of the size of the machinery used. (**A**) A CT scanner. (**B**) An MRI scanner.

ization include **endoscopy,** in which an endoscope is passed through the mouth to examine the gastrointestinal tract; **bronchoscopy,** in which a bronchoscope is passed through the nose or mouth to observe the larynx, trachea, bronchi, and alveoli; and colonoscopy, in which a colonoscope is passed through the anus to examine the rectum or colon.

Endoscopy. Endoscopy has become a common method of diagnosis for gastrointestinal disorders in children. When first developed, endoscopes were straight, stiff, metal instruments, which limited their use. Currently, endoscopes are *fiber optic* (a flexible, easily maneuvered, brightly lit tube), so these examinations are more common and not as uncomfortable as before.

The procedure is often frightening, however. A child can easily understand an explanation of the procedure (the physician will extend the child's head and pass a tube down into the child's stomach for direct observation), but the child is uncomfortable at the thought of someone doing it. A child may need a sedative or conscious sedation so he or she can lie quietly for the time needed (Landrum, 1997). Good support during the procedure is also important (Figure 16-6). Ask whether the child can have a Polaroid photo taken during the procedure to keep as a souvenir. Endoscopy is also used as an emergency measure to remove objects such as quarters or safety pins swallowed by children.

After an endoscopy study, edema may occur from pressure of the scope on the esophagus and pharynx. Aftercare consists of close assessment to see that edema is not interfering with a vital function such as respiration or causing discomfort.

Virtual endoscopy is computer-simulated endoscopy. By simulating the endoscopic examination this way, the child is spared the discomfort and possible complications of an actual examination (Blezek & Robb, 1997).

Bronchoscopy. Bronchoscopy is the direct visualization of the larynx, trachea, and bronchi through a lit, flexible, fiber-optic tube (a bronchofiberscope). The procedure is used with children who have aspirated a foreign object such as a peanut or to take culture and biopsy specimens (Martinot et al, 1997). Before the procedure, the child may be administered atropine by injection to reduce bronchial secretions and encourage bronchial relaxation. A sedative or conscious sedation may be administered because the pro-

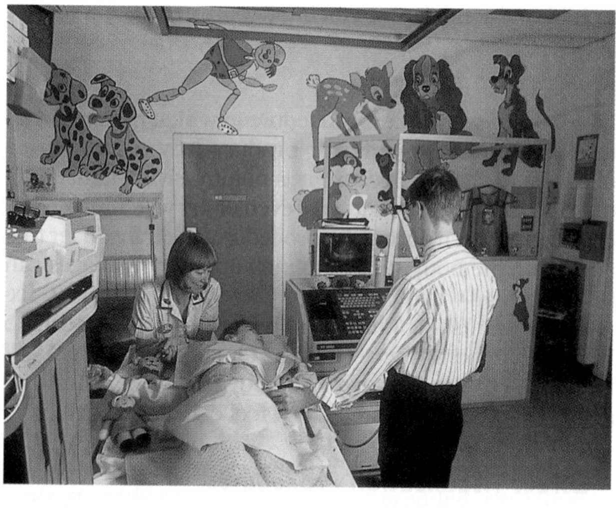

FIGURE 16.5 Sonography can be potentially frightening for children. Seeing the image on the television screen helps to relieve their fright.

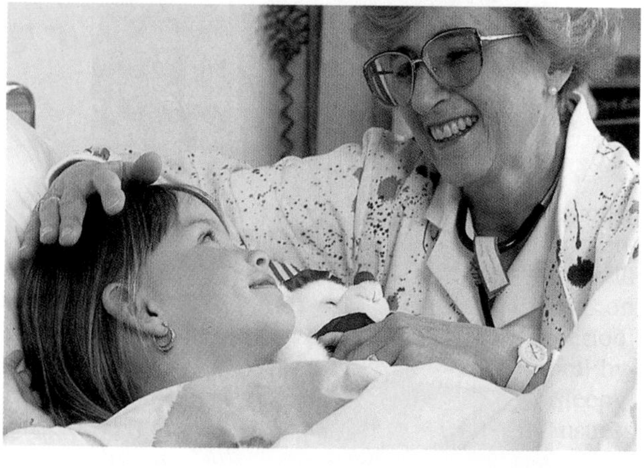

FIGURE 16.6 Examination with a flexible fiberoptic endoscope.

cedure is so frightening it is difficult for the child to cooperate. Because any manipulation of the airway has the potential to cause increased bronchial secretions and edema leading to narrowing of the airway, children need to be observed closely for respiratory function for at least 4 hours after the procedure. An ice bag applied to the neck often helps reduce the possibility of edema and relieve throat discomfort. Observe children carefully the first time they drink after the procedure to be certain their gag reflex is intact despite edema.

Aspiration Studies

Aspiration studies (removal of body fluids by such techniques as lumbar puncture or bone marrow aspiration) are always frightening procedures; often just looking at the size of the needle is frightening. A child may need a sedative or conscious sedation so that he or she can lie quietly. Support and restrain the child by talking and touching as appropriate. Assess for bleeding at the puncture site after the procedure and apply pressure as needed to completely halt bleeding. Remind children to lie quietly after lumbar puncture to help prevent spinal headache (see Chapter 28).

> **✓ CHECKPOINT QUESTIONS**
>
> 3. Why do most children have a blocking agent administered before a procedure with radioactive iodine?
> 4. What is the difference between endoscopy and bronchoscopy?

Measurement of Vital Sign

Vital signs and their measurements differ according to the size and age of children. Appendix G shows the average pulse rates, respiration rates, and blood pressures, respectively, for children of different ages.

Pulse Rate

As children grow older, the heart rate slows, and the range of normal values narrows. If possible, pulse rate should be measured with children at rest. An apical pulse (listening at the heart apex through a stethoscope) is taken in children younger than 1 year because their radial (wrist) pulse is too faint to palpate accurately. In an infant, the point of maximum intensity, or the point on the chest wall where the heart beat can be heard most distinctly, is just above and outside the left nipple (just lateral to the midclavicular line at the third or fourth interspace). This point gradually becomes more medial and slightly lower until by 7 years of age it is at the fourth or fifth interspace at the midclavicular line. For greatest accuracy, pulse rate should be counted for 1 full minute.

Respiration Rate

Respirations also should be measured before an infant is disturbed because respiration rate increases with crying. Take this while the child is sitting in the parent's lap or lying quietly in a crib before lowering the side rail. Infants tend to breathe with their abdominal muscles; therefore, it is as accurate to take respirations by counting movements of the abdomen as it is to count chest movements. Again, for greatest accuracy, respirations should be counted for 1 full minute.

Temperature

Temperature values in children are the same as in adults: axillary, 97.6°F (36.5°C); oral or tympanic, 98.6°F (37.0°C); and rectal, 99.6°F (37.6°C). Thermometers that assess tympanic membrane temperature are ideal for assessment in children because they register within 2 seconds and therefore cause less fear in the child because he or she does not have to be restrained for long (Figure 16-7*A*).

Newborns should always have their temperature taken in the axilla or by tympanic membrane because of the danger of damaging their rectal mucosa with a rectal thermometer (Figure 16-7*B*). Because preschoolers generally fear intrusive procedures, consider taking axillary or tympanic temperatures in children until 4 years of age.

For a tympanic temperature recording, insert the tip of the tympanic thermometer gently into the child's ear canal. Straighten the ear canal by pulling down on the ear lobe in a child younger than age 3; up on the child older

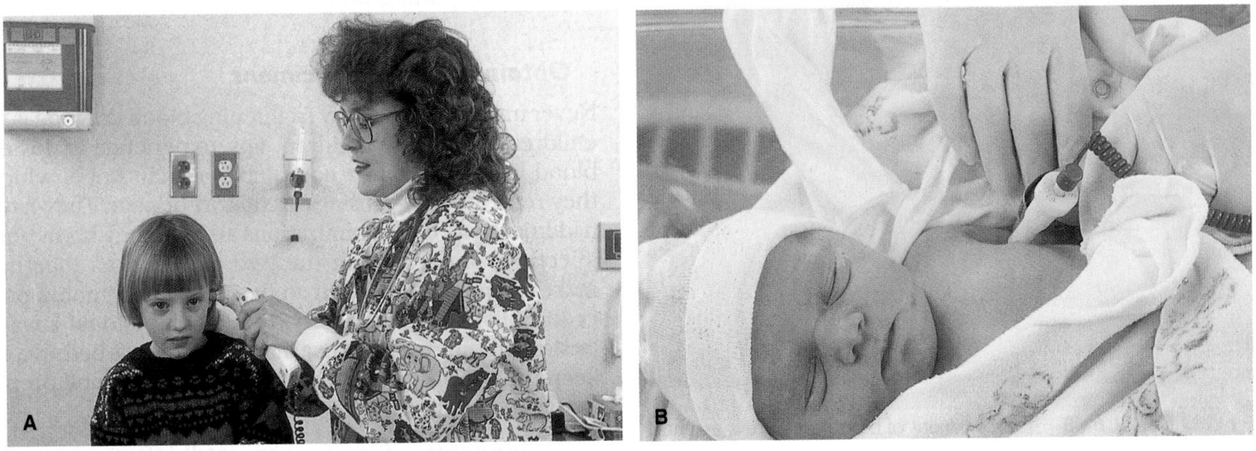

FIGURE 16.7 Temperature taking. (**A**) Tympanic membrane temperature. (**B**) Axillary temperature.

NURSING PROCEDURE 16.1: TECHNIQUE FOR FINGERTIP OR HEEL CAPILLARY PUNCTURE

Plan	Principle
1. Wash your hands; identify child; explain procedure to child.	1. Prevents spread of microorganisms from you to child. Promotes safety and well-being.
2. Assess status of puncture site.	2. Site must be warm and free of lesions.
3. Analyze appropriateness of procedure; adjust plan to individual circumstances.	3. Nursing care is always individualized based on professional judgment of client need.
4. Plan and give health teaching and preparation information as necessary.	4. Health teaching and preparation is an independent nursing action always included in care.
5. Implement care by assembling equipment: gloves, alcohol swab, lancet, collecting capillary blood tube, dry compress or cotton ball, adhesive bandage.	5. Conserve energy through organization and preparation.
6. Fingertips and heels must be warm. Warm by holding finger or heel in your hand for a moment or two. Warming heels or fingers by immersing them in warm water or covering with a warm compress is not advised.	6. Help blood flow freely. Warm water methods increase the flow of blood so much that values become comparable with arterial, not venous, values.
7. Select puncture site: sides of tip of finger; right or left of medial artery of heel (see figure below). Allow child to choose finger if appropriate.	7. Use child's nondominant hand to avoid child having to use tender finger on dominant hand afterward. Allowing choices adds to child's feelings of control and self-esteem.

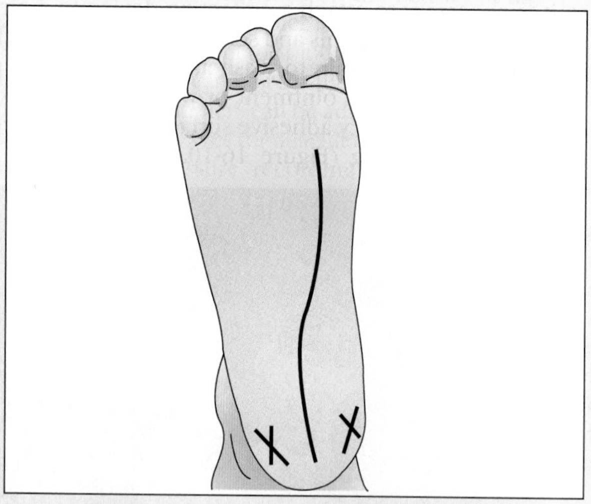

8. Apply gloves. Swab site with alcohol; puncture with a quick thrusting movement; wipe away first drop of blood with dry cotton ball.	8. Wipe away first drop so alcohol does not contaminate or dilute specimen.
9. Hold heel or finger lower than proximal extremity; touch capillary tube to blood drop and tip to encourage flow. Do not squeeze tissue around site.	9. Capillary action will quickly fill the collecting tube; squeezing causes tissue injury.
10. After filling required number of blood tubes, apply dry compress to site; apply adhesive bandage.	10. Applying dry compress to site halts bleeding.
11. Label specimen appropriately and send to proper laboratory for analysis.	11. Ensures continuity of care.
12. Evaluate effectiveness, efficiency, cost, safety, and comfort aspects of procedure; record procedure and child's reaction.	12. Documents nursing care and client status.

tempts to loosen the collector, cover the device with a diaper to keep it out of reach. Otherwise, leave it visible so that it can be observed for voiding. Offer the child something to drink. Most infants void shortly after a feeding, so if the collector is put in place just before a regular feeding, voiding will probably result. Remove the collector as soon as the infant voids and transfer the specimen to a specimen cup by clipping a bottom corner of the bag.

Urine may be aspirated from diapers for tests such as specific gravity, dipstick protein, pH, or glucose. This does not pull enough lint into the specimen to change its specific gravity (Figure 16-10*B*). With disposable diapers, urine tends to be pulled into the diaper and is best available for testing if the diaper is torn apart. Placing cotton balls inside the diaper can be a help because they can be squeezed for additional urine. Urine extracted from a disposable diaper can be analyzed for bacteria for urinary tract infections (Cohen et al, 1997).

The Preschooler or School-Age Child. It may be difficult to obtain routine urine specimens from preschoolers or toilet-trained toddlers because they can only void when they feel a definite urge to do so, not on command. Another problem is language. It is not unprofessional to use words such as "pee-pee" if this is what the child will understand. Provide a potty chair if one is available; if not, put a dutch cap collector on a toilet. A generally successful approach with a child this age is to act as if voiding is not a difficult procedure. Offer the child a glass of water or other fluid, and ask a parent to reinforce the request to void so that the child knows a parent approves. Do not encourage children to drink more than one glass of fluid to induce voiding, however, or else their urine production may be so diluted that the specific gravity, protein, and glucose levels will be inaccurate. A school-age child is usually able to void when asked, although the child may find it more difficult than the adult.

The Adolescent. Adolescents are usually knowledgeable and cooperative about providing urine specimens. As with adults, give them a clean specimen container and tell them what is needed. Unless they have voided recently, they are able to void "on command." Remember, however, that adolescents are concerned and self-conscious about body functions and therefore are often reluctant to carry a urine specimen through a crowded waiting room or desk area. They may be too self-conscious to void if they know someone is nearby—just outside a curtain, for example. Send them to a nearby bathroom with a closed door, or leave the area to give them privacy.

Some adolescents are suspicious that a urine specimen is being requested for drug testing; providing a good explanation of its actual purpose relieves this fear. Adolescent girls may be embarrassed to mention that they are menstruating; ask them about this so that the presence of any red blood cells in a urine specimen can be explained.

To avoid having a urine specimen contaminated by menstrual blood (which changes the specific gravity, protein, and red blood cell analysis), ask the girl who is menstruating to wash her perineum well with soap and water and rinse and dry it to remove menstrual blood. Next, supply a sterile cotton ball for her to insert gently into her vagina just before voiding (and remove again following voiding). Mark the specimen "possibly contaminated by menstrual blood" even though it does not appear discolored, because red blood cells may be present microscopically.

Twenty-Four-Hour Urine Specimens. Although urinalysis of a single urine specimen will indicate the presence of such substances as protein or glucose, a *24-hour urine specimen* is necessary to determine the quantitative amount of many substances or how much of a substance is excreted during a day (quantitative analysis). To begin a 24-hour urine collection, ask the child to void (with an infant, attach a collecting bag and wait for the child to void). This specimen (the discard specimen) is then thrown away so that a specific time for the ensuing collection is known. If the urine collection was started early in the morning and this first specimen was counted as part of the collection, the urine collected during the next 24 hours would include urine that had been forming all night, resulting in an approximately 32-hour collection period that would distort the analysis.

Record the start of the collection period as the time of the discarded urine. Save all urine voided for the next 24 hours and place it in one collection bottle. Have the child void (or watch for an infant to void) at the end of the 24-hour period and add the final specimen to the collection bottle. Record the time of the collection as being from the time of the discarded urine to the final specimen added to the collection.

The Infant and Toddler. For an infant, use a 24-hour urine collector. A collector will adhere for this length of time only if the child's perineum is thoroughly dry at the time of application. Applying tincture of benzoin to toughen the perineal skin and make removal of the collector easier is helpful; tincture of benzoin also makes the perineum slightly sticky and aids in firm contact. Commercial sprays that encourage adhesiveness are also available. Place an infant in a semi-Fowler's position, if possible, to encourage urine to flow freely into the collector. Make certain that the tubing from the collector is pinned out of the infant's reach or the infant may pull the collector free. It may be necessary to place a diaper on the infant to keep the apparatus out of sight. Provide activities; make sure the parents understand that they can pick up the infant and hold him or her during this time, as long as they take care not to kink or pull the tubing.

To keep bacterial count to a minimum, 24-hour collections are generally kept on ice or poured into a container that is then refrigerated during the 24-hour period and until they are transported to the laboratory for analysis.

With active infants, fitting them with a colostomy bag applied to cover the urinary meatus may be more effective than using a collector with tubing (Figure 16-11). Puncture a small hole in the corner of the top of the bag. Insert a small feeding tube through this into the bottom of the bag. When the child voids, attach a syringe to the feeding tube and aspirate the urine. Transfer the specimen to the collection bottle. This type of urine collector has an advantage in that it allows the child to be ambulatory. For the active toddler, this collector may be the only type that is acceptable to the child.

is filled with a dilute solution of heparin or normal saline through the rubber stopper and flushed again with solution every 2 to 8 hours (depending on hospital policy) to keep it patent. Intravenous medication can be added as needed. The tubing and stopper must be firmly secured to the wrist and an armboard taped in place to remind the child to protect the site from careless trauma.

Children who are hospitalized or on home care for a long time and who need only intravenous medication, not additional fluid, are good candidates for such devices. Heparin locks also can be used with children when frequent venous blood samples are required. If blood is drawn from the already inserted tubing, the child is pricked only once (when the device is originally placed) no matter how many samples are drawn. Similar devices may be inserted into arteries when arterial blood is required—for example, for the child who is having blood gases monitored frequently.

Venous Access Catheters and Devices

Venous access for long-term intravenous therapy can be gained by insertion of a catheter into the vena cava just outside the right atrium; the catheter exits the chest just under the clavicle (Figure 16-21*A–D*). Typical catheters

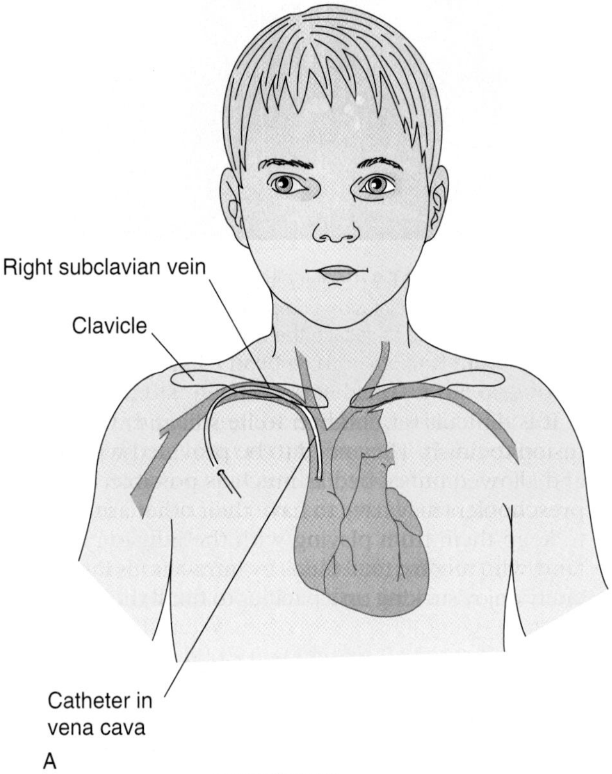

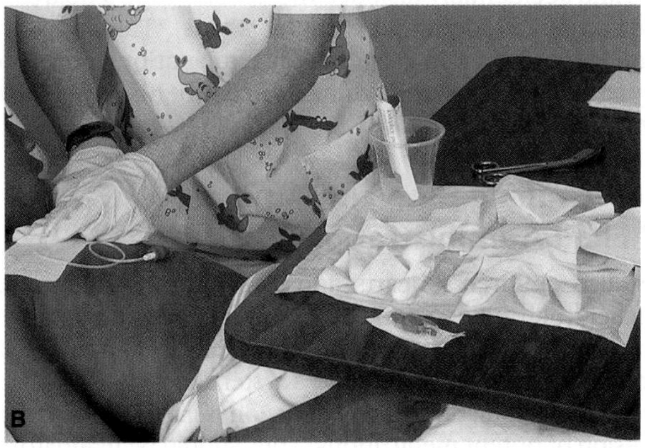

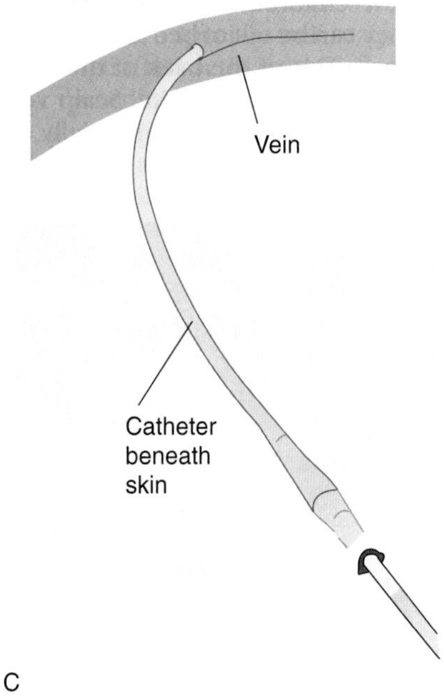

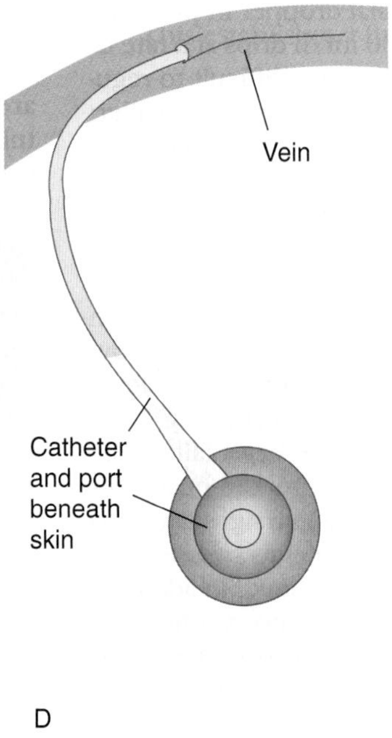

FIGURE 16.21 (**A**) Insertion site for placement of a subclavian fluid line for intravenous infusion. (**B**) Changing a dressing for a subclavian catheter. (**C**) Subclavian catheter beneath the skin. (**D**) A central venous access device beneath the skin.

used in this way are Broviacs, Hickmans, or Groshongs. Such catheters have a wrinkle-resistant fabric (Dacron) cuff that adheres to subcutaneous tissue and helps to seal the catheter in place and keep infection out. Care of the catheters (depending on agency policy) consists of daily or weekly changes of dressings over the exit site and periodic irrigation with heparin or saline to ensure patency.

Such catheters have the advantage of not involving any further skin punctures, so they cause no further discomfort. One disadvantage is that the catheter could be snagged on something and accidentally pulled out. It is an emergency if this happens because the child could lose an appreciable amount of blood from the point of entrance into a vein as major as the vena cava. Children with a catheter in place are usually not allowed to swim or take showers, to avoid infection.

Central venous access devices (infusion ports that can be implanted) are small plastic devices that are implanted under the skin, usually on the anterior chest just under the clavicle (Figure 16-21*D*). A small catheter threads from the port internally into a central vein. Common brands are Port-A-Cath, Infus-A-Port, and Groshong Venous Port. Blood samples can be removed or medication can be injected by a puncture through the chest skin into the port. Although this device requires a skin puncture (causes pain), it may be well accepted by children because it is not as visible as a central venous catheter, no dressing is required, and it allows a full range of activities such as showering and swimming. Be certain when accessing these ports to use only the needle supplied by the manufacturer. A regular needle has the tendency to "core" or remove a small circle of the membrane over the port and destroy the integrity of the device. Use EMLA cream to decrease discomfort.

Children also may have peripherally inserted central catheters (PICC lines) for therapy. These are inserted into an arm vein (usually at the antecubital space into the median, cephalic, or basilic vein) and advanced until the tip rests in the superior vena cava. If a shorter catheter is used, the tip of it will rest closer to the head of the clavicle (a "midline" insertion). Many parents seem more comfortable with this type of insertion than with a central line because it appears so much more like a routine IV. Total parenteral nutrition (TPN) should not be administered through a midline insertion site because the hypertonic solution will be irritating to this peripheral a site. Newborns can have a catheter inserted into an umbilical vessel and fluid administered by that route (see Chapter 6).

Intraosseous Infusion

Intraosseous infusion (IO) is the infusion of fluid into the bone marrow cavity of a long bone, usually the distal or proximal tibia, the distal femur, or iliac crest. Because the bone marrow communicates directly with the circulatory system, the time at which fluid reaches the bloodstream when administered this way is the same as if it were administered intravenously. All fluids that can be administered intravenously, including whole blood or medicine, can also be administered by this route.

Intraosseous infusion is used in an emergency when it is difficult to establish usual IV access or in a child with such extensive burns that the usual sites for intravenous infusion are not available.

Intraosseous infusion is a temporary measure until a usual route of administration can be opened because of the danger of causing osteomyelitis, a devastating infection with long-term effects to bone marrow. It must be initiated with sterile technique, and if continued for an extended time, the infusion point is rotated about every 2 to 3 days to try to minimize infection.

Intraosseous infusion is painful as the needle enters the bone marrow cavity and again at the time of the bone marrow aspiration. Prepare the child for this and offer support.

The steps to initiate the infusion are as follows:

- The skin over the chosen site is cleaned with povidone-iodine and anesthetized with a local anesthetic.
- A small incision is made into the skin with a scalpel blade.
- A large hypodermic or bone marrow needle is inserted through the incision into the cavity of the bone.
- To ensure that the needle tip has reached the bone marrow cavity, a syringe is attached to the needle and aspirated for bone marrow.
- If bone marrow is obtained, the syringe is removed and intravenous tubing, including a filter and the fluid to be administered, is attached to the needle and opened to a gravity flow.
- A dressing with additional iodine is then applied over the needle site.
- A restraint is applied to the leg to help the child hold the leg still.

Tubing must be changed about every 48 hours and the dressing over the site about every 24 hours—again, to try to reduce the possibility of infection. Assess for a distal pulse and adequate temperature and color of the leg every hour during the length of the infusion to ensure that circulation to the leg is not becoming impaired. If the needle should become dislodged, symptoms of circulatory impairment or pain and taut skin over the site will occur.

Occasionally during the course of fluid administration, a bone chip or thick marrow will occlude an intraosseous needle and slow the infusion. If this occurs, a stilette passed through the needle clears it and allows for continued fluid administration.

Subcutaneous (Hypodermoclysis) Infusion

Before safe intravenous infusion was perfected with infants, fluid was given to them subcutaneously (perfusing fluid into subcutaneous skin layers by means of an intravenous infusion set). The technique is still appropriate for children with blood disorders who receive a medication to remove stored iron from their body by this route. Sites used for hypodermoclysis are generally the pectoral region, the back, or the anterolateral aspects of the thighs. The intravenous needle is inserted into the subcutaneous layer of the skin and the infusion apparatus opened. The rate is governed by the rate of absorption by the subcutaneous layer of skin; it is not a set rate.

✔ CHECKPOINT QUESTIONS

13. What are three safety devices for the administration of intravenous fluid in children?
14. When are intraosseous transfusions used?

HOT AND COLD THERAPY

Children who sustain muscle sprains or undergo procedures such as bronchoscopy or tonsillectomy may have cold applications prescribed to prevent inflammation and edema (Figure 16-22). If inflammation or edema is already present, application of heat may be prescribed to help it resolve. It is important to implement measures to prevent both burns and boredom in the child during treatments. Guidelines for hot and cold applications are shown in Box 16-2.

PROVIDING NUTRITIONAL CARE

Because almost all illnesses affect children's nutritional and fluid balance, assessment of these sheds a great deal of light on a child's general health. Nutritional assessment begins with asking a child or parent for a 24-hour recall of all the foods eaten during that time followed by more specific measures such as intake and output measurements. Common therapies for nutritional deficiencies include enteral, gastrostomy, and TPN.

NURSING DIAGNOSES AND RELATED INTERVENTIONS

Nursing Diagnosis: Risk for nutrition, less than body requirements, related to chronic illness

Outcome Identification: Child will ingest a diet adequate for nutritional needs during illness.

Outcome Evaluation: Skin turgor is good; no signs of dehydration are present; child gains a minimum of 1 pound weekly.

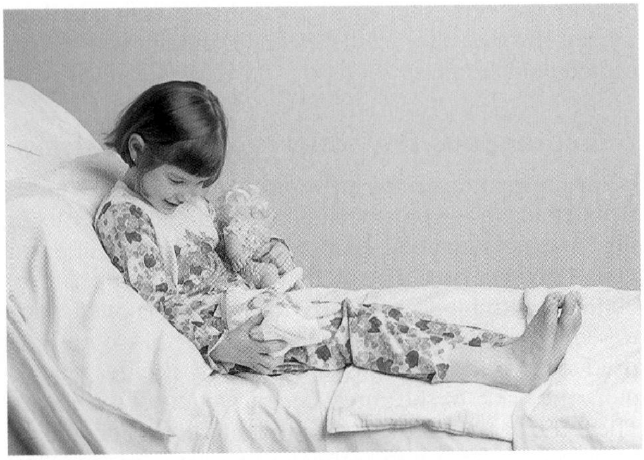

FIGURE 16.22 A rubber glove used as an ice pack. The face on it helps to make it seem friendlier.

BOX 16.2

GUIDELINES FOR HOT AND COLD APPLICATIONS WITH CHILDREN

1. Neither heat nor cold should be applied for longer than 20 minutes unless prescribed otherwise, because after this time, the vasoconstriction caused by cold and the vasodilatation caused by heat is reversed.
2. When using electrical sources of heat with toddlers and preschoolers, never make a game of plugging in and pulling out the apparatus that makes the light come on or a dial glow. Otherwise, the child may play with it after you leave.
3. Supply a special activity for a child to enjoy while a hot or cold application is in place (playing a board game or reading a story to the child) so that the procedure is not viewed as a chore but as a pleasant time to look forward to because of the accompanying enjoyable activity.
4. Put tape on the gauge of an electric appliance at the point where you want it so that a child cannot change the setting.
5. Always test the warmth of solutions or heat sources with your inner wrist or dorsal surface of your hand before applying them to the child, to be certain they are not too hot.
6. Do not apply ice packs or ice directly to the skin. Cover the pack or ice with a towel or other cover to prevent frostbite and cell damage from cold.
7. Be cautious about heat or cold applications with a child who is receiving an analgesic because the child's perception of heat or cold may be reduced, and he or she could easily be burned.

Measure Fluid Intake and Output

Fluid is an essential element of nutrition because of the water supplied and because it can also be a source of calories and vitamins. To document fluid balance, some children may have fluid intake and output measured and recorded. This is especially true for children with vomiting, diarrhea, burns, hemorrhage, dehydration, cardiac and kidney disease, draining wounds, gastrointestinal suction, edema, and diuretic or intravenous therapy.

Intake

Estimating the intake of infants who are formula-fed is simply a matter of estimating the kind and amount of fluids that were swallowed. Intake in breast-fed infants is merely recorded as "breast-fed." If it is necessary to estimate the amount more closely than this, the infant can be weighed before and after a feeding. The difference in weight in grams is the number of milliliters of breast milk ingested. This measurement is not very accurate, however, because if the child voided or had a bowel movement, weight would be affected by these losses.

With preschool children, be certain to record fluids ingested during snacks, because children this age usually have many during the day. At approximately 10 years of age, children can be depended on to record their own intake as long as they have a list of how many milliliters are contained in each glass or cup they use (an average cup is 150 mL; a glass, 180 mL). Be certain to check that they remember that soup, flavored frozen ice such as Popsicles, and sherbet are liquids and should be counted.

Output

Diapers can be readily used as a method of measuring urine output. Weigh the diaper before it is placed on the infant and record this weight conspicuously (mark it on the front of the plastic covering with a ballpoint pen). Reweigh the diaper after it is wet and subtract the difference to determine the amount of urine present. This difference will be in grams. Because 1 g = 1 mL, the amount can be recorded in milliliters. In infants who have liquid stools, it is difficult to separate stool from urine because these blend together in a diaper. Separate urine from stool by applying a urine collector; check it frequently for filling.

Girls often void along with bowel movements when they use a toilet, which means that a urine specimen is easily lost. To separate urine from bowel movements, teach older children to void first.

Provide Enteral Feedings

Enteral feedings (nasogastric tube feedings) are a common means of supplying adequate nutrition to an infant who is unable to suck or tires too easily when sucking, or to an older child who cannot eat. In infants, such feedings are traditionally called **gavage feedings.** To prepare for an enteral feeding, an infant may have to be loosely swaddled to be sure that the arms will be out of the way. Next, the space from the bridge of the infant's nose to the ear lobe to a point halfway between the xiphoid process and the umbilicus is measured against a no. 8 or no. 10 feeding tube (Figure 16-23). For children older than 1 year of age, measure from the bridge of the nose to the ear lobe to the xiphoid process. The tube is marked at this point by a small Kelly clamp or piece of tape. It is important that the tube be measured in this way to ensure that it enters the stomach after it is passed. A tube passed too far will curl and end up in the esophagus; a tube not passed far enough will also be in the esophagus. Both situations could cause the feeding to be aspirated into the lungs. The tip of the catheter is next lubricated with water.

An oil lubricant should never be used. Although the tube is going to be passed into the stomach, it is occasionally passed into the trachea accidentally; oil left in the trachea could lead to lipoid pneumonia, a complication that a child already burdened with a disease may be unable to tolerate.

Whether enteral catheters should be passed through the nares or the mouth is controversial. Because newborns are nose breathers, it seems reasonable that passing the catheter through the mouth will lead to less distress than passing it through the nose. This can also decrease the possibility of striking the vagal nerve and causing bradycardia. If the tube is to be left in place, however, it may be passed through a nostril. Insertion through a nostril is easier for the older child.

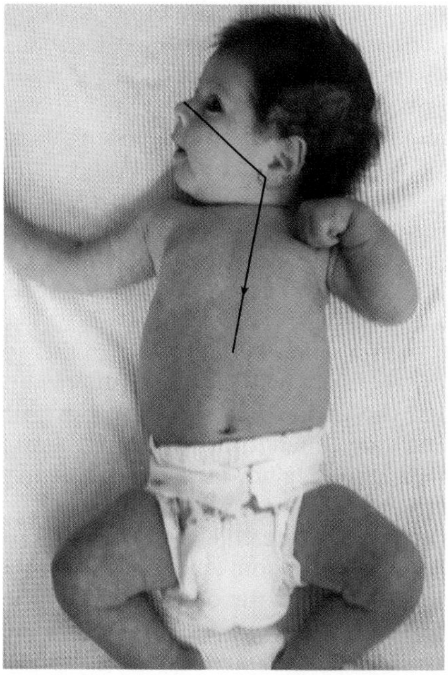

FIGURE 16.23 A nasogastric tube in an infant is measured from the bridge of the nose to the earlobe to a point halfway between the umbilicus and the xyphoid process.

The catheter is passed with gentle pressure to the point of the clamp or tape. If the catheter is inadvertently passed into the trachea rather than the esophagus, the child usually has some dyspnea; the catheter should be withdrawn and replaced. The catheter must be checked for position (that it is not in the trachea) before any feeding is given. Checking may be done in either of the two ways described in Table 16-3. With some infants, it is im-

TABLE 16.3 Methods to Determine Proper Gavage Tube Placement

METHOD	CONSIDERATIONS
Attach syringe to the tube and aspirate stomach contents.	In most instances, stomach contents aspirated this way are returned to the stomach before the feeding; in small infants, the amount of stomach contents is subtracted from the prescribed amount of feeding; because stomach contents are highly acid, discarding them at each feeding can lead to alkalosis.
Inject 5 mL air into the gavage tube and listen over the stomach with a stethoscope to the sound of injected air.	The injected air is heard as a whistling or growling sound; do not use an adult size stethoscope on small infants to listen for it; the diaphragm of the stethoscope will be partially over lung, and where one is hearing the air injection is unknown.

portant to evaluate whether the entire previous feeding has been absorbed. Testing for tube placement by aspiration allows you to both test placement and evaluate stomach contents in one step. If the amount aspirated is only a small amount (a few milliliters), it is merely replaced at the beginning of the feeding. If it is a large amount (large is determined by a physician's order), it will be replaced through the tubing, and the amount of the feeding is then reduced by that amount. Replacing stomach secretions rather than discarding them is important to prevent electrolyte loss.

Once it is certain that the catheter is in the stomach, attach a syringe or special feeding funnel to the tube. Be certain that the child's head and chest are slightly elevated to encourage fluid to flow downward into the stomach. Then add the specific kind and amount of feeding ordered to the syringe or funnel and allow it to flow by gravity drainage into the child's stomach (Figure 16-24). The fluid should be at room temperature to prevent chilling. The syringe end of the tube should not be elevated more than 12 inches above the child's abdomen so that the gravity flow is not too fast. Feedings should never be hurried by using the plunger of the syringe or a bulb attachment for more pressure. The result could be stomach overflow and aspiration.

Offering a pacifier (non-nutrient sucking) during the feeding may make the feeding experience more normal for the infant and supply the normal sucking time the infant would otherwise be missing by being gavage-fed. When the total feeding has passed through the tube, the tube is reclamped securely and then gently and rapidly withdrawn. Clamping the tube before it is withdrawn is important, because this prevents any milk remaining in the tube from flowing out as the tube is removed and, again, reduces the risk of aspiration. If the tube is to remain in place, it should be flushed with 1 to 5 mL clear water and capped to seal out air. If it is to remain in place, tape it below the nose and to the cheek. Do not tape it to the forehead or pressure can be put on the anterior naris and cause ulceration there. Children with long-term neurologic disabilities may have enteral tubes left in place and continual feedings administered by an entero feeding pump.

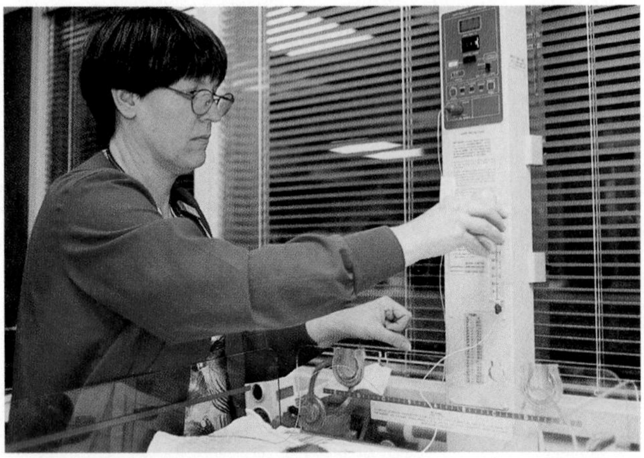

FIGURE 16.24 A gavage feeding. Formula enters the gavage tube by the force of gravity only.

A baby should be bubbled after an enteral feeding, just as after a bottle feeding or breastfeeding. This extra handling not only prevents regurgitation of formula along with bubbles after the infant is laid down but gives the close contact so essential to the baby's development. Both infants and older children should be unswaddled and placed on the right side with the head slightly elevated after a feeding or held and rocked in this position. Older children fed by nasogastric tube require mouth care at least twice a day, or their mouths become dry and ulcers may form.

Provide Gastrostomy Tube Feedings

Children who may have gastrostomy tubes placed as a method of feeding include, for example, those who cannot swallow and those with esophageal atresia, severe gastroesophageal reflux, or esophageal stricture. With the use of regional or general anesthesia, the tube is inserted through a puncture wound in the abdominal wall into the stomach (Figure 16-25). The tube used in children is usually a Foley catheter rather than a true gastrostomy tube. This is because a Foley catheter can be removed easily and changed if it should become plugged, and the balloon is small enough not to obscure and fill the small stomach space.

As with nasogastric feedings, gastrostomy feedings should be at room temperature to prevent chilling. Before a feeding, elevate the child's upper trunk 30 to 40 degrees so the food will remain in the stomach and not flow upward into the esophagus and possibly cause aspiration. Do this by holding an infant in the lap or placing him or her in an infant seat; for an older child, use pillows or elevate the head of the bed. Use a syringe to aspirate the tube for any stomach residual. After noting the amount, replace this fluid. To administer the feeding, attach a syringe to the tube; allow the specified amount to flow by gravity drainage only (again, to prevent reflux and possible aspiration).

After the feeding, flush the tube with a specified amount of clear water and either clamp or suspend the tube in an elevated position. Leaving the tube unclamped and elevated ensures that if the child should vomit, vomitus will be evacuated by the stomach from the tube rather than the esophagus. If a tube is left elevated and unclamped, cover it with a clean piece of porous gauze to prevent bacteria from settling into it. Leave the child in a head-elevated position for at least 1 hour after a feeding.

Infants who are fed by gastrostomy tube miss the pleasure of sucking. Offer a pacifier to suck on during the procedure. Talk or sing to the child as if the feeding were being given orally.

The biggest problem with gastrostomy tubes is that often they do not fit snugly, and formula or gastric secretions can leak around the tube onto the abdominal skin. These secretions are irritating because of their high hydrochloric acid content. Consult an enterostomal therapy nurse for wound care. Placing stomadhesive around the tube can protect the skin. One method of helping to provide a snug fit for the tube is to place a soft nipple used with premature infants (enlarge the nipple opening slightly) over the catheter (nipple tip up) so the base of the nipple fits against the stomadhesive on the skin. Tape the tube to the nipple at the tip, which brings the balloon of the tube up against the stomach wall and prevents leakage.

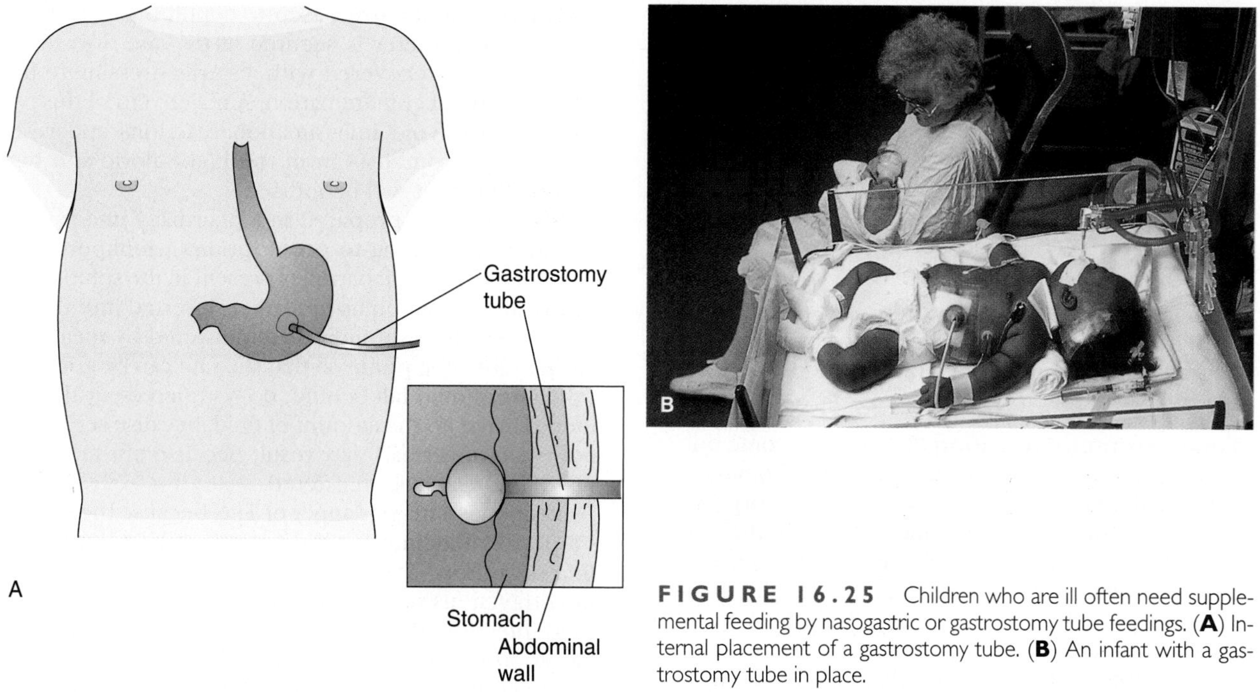

FIGURE 16.25 Children who are ill often need supplemental feeding by nasogastric or gastrostomy tube feedings. (**A**) Internal placement of a gastrostomy tube. (**B**) An infant with a gastrostomy tube in place.

Tape the nipple to the skin and stomadhesive securely using nonadhesive tape. Clean the skin around the nipple daily with half-strength hydrogen peroxide; change the stomadhesive every 2 to 3 days. At the time of the change, expose the skin to air for approximately 1 hour.

The most important complication of a gastrostomy tube is that it can move into the duodenum through the pyloric sphincter and cause obstruction. Observe and report any vomiting, abdominal distention, or brown or green tube drainage (duodenal secretions that would suggest the tube has moved). Testing residual aspiration fluid to see that it is acid is a guarantee that the tube is in the stomach (stomach secretions are acid; duodenal secretions are alkaline). Putting a mark on the tube with a ballpoint pen just above the nipple lets you check that the tube has not migrated into the stomach but is remaining securely in place.

Tubes are replaced approximately every 6 weeks. To replace a tube, deflate the Foley balloon by withdrawing the water in it and gently pull the tube free. Insert a clean Foley catheter into the stomach opening approximately 1 inch beyond the balloon; inflate the balloon with 2 to 4 mL water. Attach a nipple and tape in place.

Most children who have gastrostomy feedings will have the tube in place for an extended time. Teach the parents how to feed their child this way, how to remove and to replace a tube, and the danger signs to watch for (e.g., vomiting, abdominal discomfort, or skin excoriation). Help parents to see this as an alternative way of feeding, not a totally different one. Be certain that they are comfortable with the procedure before the child is discharged from the hospital, so that they can feed the child by this method. Be certain they understand that it does not hurt the child to have the tube replaced or to have pressure put against the tube, so that they need not worry about holding the child snugly. Many children on long-term gastrostomy feedings have gastrostomy buttons implanted for easier stomach access (Figure 16-26). For feeding, a catheter is inserted through the device; it is removed following the feeding. With this in place, only a small access device is visible, not a large bulky tube.

> WHAT IF? What if a parent wants to take her child with a gastrostomy tube in place to a restaurant so the child learns about "eating out"? Would you agree with her that this is a good idea?

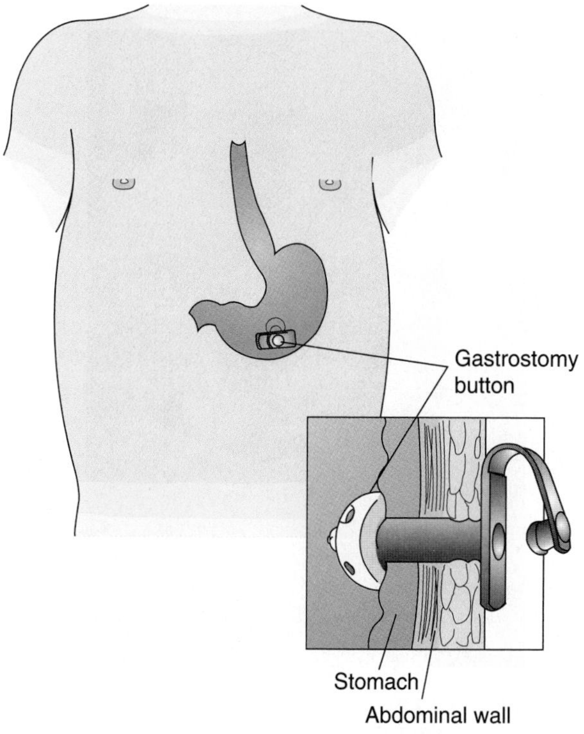

FIGURE 16.26 Placement of a gastrostomy button.

Provide Total Parenteral Nutrition

NURSING DIAGNOSES AND RELATED INTERVENTIONS

Nursing Diagnosis: Altered nutrition, less than body requirements related to malabsorption of nutrients

Outcome Identification: Child will receive adequate nutrients for physiologic needs during course of illness.

Outcome Evaluation: Skin turgor is good; no signs of dehydration are present; child loses no weight during therapy; intestinal cramps and distention lessen.

Total parenteral nutrition (TPN) has become one of the most important therapies for children who have gastrointestinal illnesses that prevent proper absorption of basic caloric or fluid requirements. Traditional intravenous therapy contains fluid, electrolytes, and sugars but not protein and fat, which are essential for the maintenance and growth of body tissues. With TPN, all of a child's nutritional needs can be met by a concentrated hypertonic solution of intravenous therapy containing glucose, vitamins, electrolytes, trace minerals, and protein. An intralipid solution (emulsified fat able to be administered intravenously) given once or twice per week supplies needed fatty acids. Children with chronic diarrhea or vomiting, bowel obstruction, anorexia, or extreme immaturity are examples of children who benefit greatly from TPN (Figure 16-27).

Solutions may be administered into central intravenous or peripheral intravenous sites. If a central line is chosen, a catheter is inserted through the right external jugular vein into the superior vena cava or directly into the subclavian vein under strict aseptic conditions (see Figure 16-21). The catheter is secured at the site of insertion with sutures and covered with a sterile dressing to help reduce bacterial contamination. A major vein of this type is chosen to avoid inflammation reactions and resulting venous thrombosis from the high-caloric and high-osmotic fluid that will be infused.

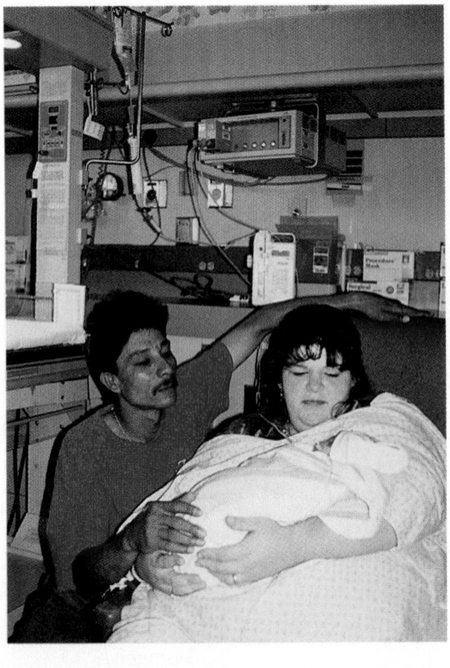

FIGURE 16.27 An infant receiving total parenteral nutrition. One pump controls the flow of a hyperalimentation solution, the other a lipid solution.

TPN solution is prepared in a pharmacy under sterile conditions according to prescription. A millipore filter, which removes small particles present in the solution that might cause an embolus to form, is inserted into the tubing. The solution should be administered by means of a constant infusion pump so that the rate can be governed. If the rate should fall behind, do not increase it the next hour to make up the amount of fluid, because serious cardiovascular overload may result because of the concentrated fluid being administered.

Infection is a major danger of TPN because the solution is a perfect medium for the growth of bacteria or *Candida* organisms. The dressing over the insertion site and the intravenous tubing are changed every 1 to 2 days to avoid infection; the tubing should not be used for drawing blood or for adding medications (unless a double-barreled tube is used), because either process may introduce infection. Sterile technique is required in changing bottles of solution so that the tubing is not contaminated. Some health care facilities require nurses to wear both masks and gloves while doing this to avoid airborne and direct contamination. Fewer restrictions are necessary for home care. The insertion site should be inspected at the time of the dressing change for indication of local infection: redness, tenderness, or discharge.

A second major problem that can occur with TPN is dehydration. A TPN solution contains approximately twice the amount of glucose normally administered in an intravenous solution to ensure that the amino acids in the solution will be used not for energy but for protein synthesis. Dehydration may occur as the body tries to reduce the amount of glucose recognized by the kidneys as excessive by excreting it (the same phenomenon that leads to high urine output in persons with diabetes mellitus). When TPN is first begun, urine should be tested for glucose and for specific gravity with each voiding. If two or more consecutive samples indicate a 3^+ or 4^+ glucose level, either the rate of the infusion or the amount of glucose in the solution should be decreased or insulin added to the solution to counteract the excess glucose. Generally, decreasing the concentration of glucose and then gradually increasing it again allows the child's body to adjust to the glucose overload.

After the first few days of TPN, a rebound effect (the child's body produces increased insulin) may cause hypoglycemia. A urine sample that suddenly is negative for glucose after a series that has been highly positive is therefore not necessarily an encouraging sign, but it may be a warning that the child's glucose level is dangerously low. The TPN solution should not be discontinued abruptly but gradually tapered or a glucose rebound effect will occur. If a TPN catheter should be accidentally pulled out by a child, the child must be immediately assessed for hemorrhage from the insertion site and closely observed in the next few hours for signs of hypoglycemia (i.e., lethargy, incoordination, fidgetiness, or seizures). Parents need to be alerted to these concerns for safe home care.

Remember that, to a child, eating is more than a means of receiving nourishment. It is a means of receiving love. Even though children are able to voice the reason they must have TPN and appear to understand that they are receiving all the needed nutrients, they still may miss eating food and the natural social interaction that comes with it. While in the hospital, they may be upset by the smell of food from a hospital unit kitchen or by the fact that playmates have to leave to eat a meal. Finding an activity for the child while other children eat (e.g., helping to check supplies on the emergency cart or stamping laboratory slips) may be helpful in supplying the interaction the child misses. Ask whether the child can be allowed chewing gum or occasional hard candy for chewing and taste sensations. Tooth brushing twice a day is necessary to keep the oral mucous membrane healthy because the child is not chewing. An infant needs sucking pleasure from a pacifier.

Many children on long-term TPN are cared for by parents at home. Careful coordination with the home care agency is necessary to ensure that parents are familiar with the system and know how to obtain TPN fluid so the child's care continues safely. Parents need to arrange for special time each day with the child to make up for the time normally spent at meal interaction time.

CHECKPOINT QUESTIONS

15. How do you measure the correct length for a feeding tube in an infant?
16. Why might dehydration occur with TPN therapy?

AIDING ELIMINATION

Two aspects of intestinal elimination that require special care are administration of enemas and ostomy care.

Administering Enemas

Enemas are rarely used with children unless they are therapy for Hirshsprung's disease or a part of preoperative preparation or a radiologic study. If an enema is necessary, offer a careful explanation of what the child can expect to experience. The usual amounts of enema solutions used are as follows:

Infant: Less than 250 mL (exact amount should be stipulated by physician's order)
Preschooler: 250–350 mL
School-age child: 300–500 mL
Adolescent: 500 mL

For an infant, use a small, soft catheter (no. 10 to 12 French) in place of an enema tip to prevent rectal trauma. Infants and children up to ages 3 or 4 years are unable to retain enema solutions, so they must rest on a bedpan during the procedure. Pad the edge of the pan so that it is not cold or sharp. Place a pillow under the infant's or young child's upper body for positioning and comfort. Lubricate the catheter generously with a water-soluble jelly and insert it only 2 to 3 inches (5 to 7 cm) in children and only 1 inch (2.5 cm) in infants. Be certain to hold the solution container no more than 1 foot above the level of the sigmoid colon (12 to 15 inches above the bed surface) so the solution flows at a controlled rate. If the child experiences intestinal cramping, clamp the tubing to halt the flow temporarily and wait until the cramping passes before instilling any more fluid. An older child can be asked to take a deep breath to help the cramping sensation pass. The amount of solution used in infants is so small that this is not usually a problem. If the enema solution is to be retained, such as an oil solution, hold the child's buttocks together for about a count of 10 after administration.

Until late school age, children cannot retain an enema as adults can (rarely more than 5 to 10 minutes). For this reason, be certain the bathroom the child will use is available before administering the enema.

Fleet enemas are not routinely administered to children younger than 2 years because of the harsh action of the sodium biphosphate and sodium phosphate they contain. Tap water is not used because it is not isotonic and causes rapid fluid shifts of water in body compartments, leading to possible water intoxication. Normal saline (0.9% sodium chloride) is the usual solution. It can be made by parents at home by adding 1 teaspoonful of salt to 1 pint (500 mL) of water.

After enema administration, praise the child for cooperating. Allow a preschooler an opportunity for therapeutic play, because this is a frightening procedure for a child of this age.

Providing Ostomy Care

An *ostomy* is an opening of the bowel on the surface of the abdomen. Ostomies in newborns are created to relieve bowel obstruction caused by conditions such as ileal atresia, necrotizing enterocolitis, and imperforate anus. In older children they are constructed for such conditions as inflammatory bowel syndrome. If an ostomy is created in the ileum (an *ileostomy*), the stoma is located on the right side of the abdomen and drains liquid stool, which is extremely irritating to the skin because of the digestive enzymes it contains. If an ostomy is created in the sigmoid portion of the bowel (*colostomy*), the stoma is on the left lower abdomen and passes normally formed stool (Figure 16-28).

An ileostomy requires the use of a collecting ostomy appliance to contain acid stool and prevent excoriation of the abdominal skin; older children also may use an appliance with a colostomy. For an infant colostomy, parents may choose (with support and advice) whether to use an appliance.

There are two basic problems to using an ostomy appliance with an infant: it may be difficult to locate one small enough to contain liquid drainage without leaking, and the skin under the appliance may become extremely irritated. Consulting with an enterostomal therapy nurse can be helpful. Clear plastic colostomy bags without a ring can often be cut more easily to fit the size of the stoma and the contour and size of an infant's abdomen than a ring type. A commercial skin sealant is helpful to

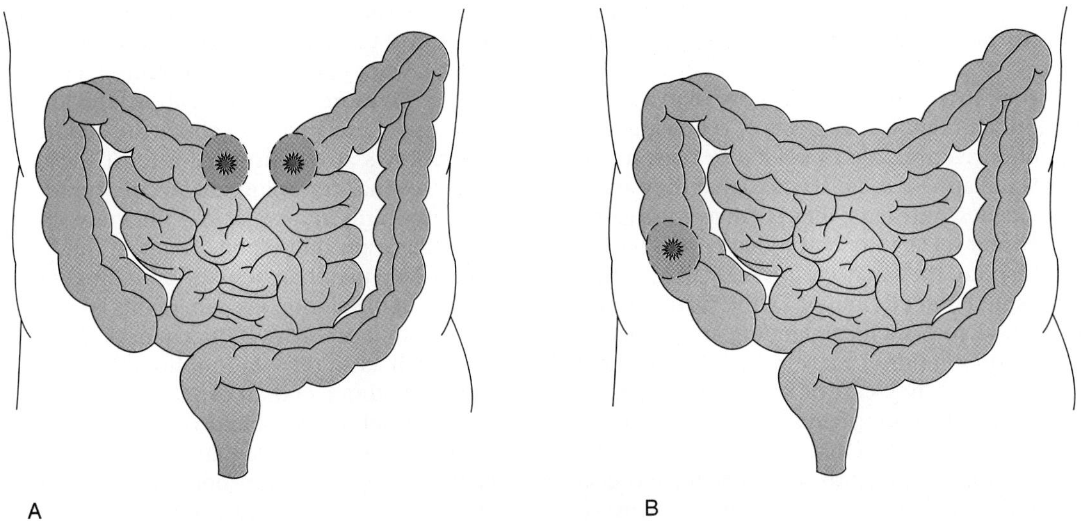

FIGURE 16.28 Different sites for ostomies. (**A**) A double-barrel colostomy. (**B**) A single-barrel colostomy.

harden the skin surrounding the stoma. Apply according to the brand directions and fan to dry. If a spray is used, protect the infant's face so that he or she does not inhale the solution. Apply the chosen stoma collection appliance. Tuck it inside the diaper to help keep the infant from pulling it loose.

Check the appliance or bag for collecting stool at least every 4 hours. To protect the underlying skin, do not remove a self-adhering bag if it is full, but drain collected stool from the bottom of the appliance into a basin or paper cup for disposal. To reduce odor, flush the appliance bag with a warm water and soap solution, using an asepto syringe, and rinse with clear water. Change the bag no more frequently than the point at which leakage occurs (perhaps as long as 1 week) to reduce skin irritation. To remove a bag that was placed with a sealant, be certain to use the designated solvent to prevent pulling or harming underlying skin. The solvent must then be washed away with soap and water or it will become an irritant itself. Because most infants enjoy tub bathing, a long, soaking bath is also an excellent way to loosen an appliance.

If an appliance or bag is not used, stool will be discharged onto the abdomen three or four times a day (no different than a usual newborn or infant stool pattern). To care for a colostomy without using an appliance, wash and dry the stoma and surrounding skin area well; apply karaya powder, an ointment such as Desitin, or a stomadhesive to protect the skin. Apply ample absorbent gauze (fluffed) and an absorbent pad. Secure in place with nonadhesive tape or a binder. Check the dressing approximately every 4 hours. Remove and replace it when soiled, washing the skin well and applying new powder or ointment as necessary. Without an appliance in place, stool is kept from touching the skin only by the protection of the ointment and frequent changing of the dressing. Turning an infant from side to side after every feeding keeps stool from always flowing to one side and may be helpful. Leaving the abdominal skin exposed to air for at least 1 hour per day also helps healing.

Stress to parents that caring for an infant with an ostomy is little different from usual. All parents must change their infant's diapers frequently and clean the diaper area. Stress that the stoma has no nerves so a parent can feel free to wash it without hurting the child and that compression against the stoma will not hurt so the parents feel comfortable laying the infant on his or her abdomen or holding the infant closely against their body for comfort.

Colostomies are rarely irrigated in children. On occasion, to prepare a child for second-stage abdominal surgery, irrigation of the *"blind-end" bowel* (bowel between the rectum and colostomy) of a double-barreled colostomy may be ordered irrigated daily to keep it lubricated and to maintain bowel tone. The exact amount of fluid to be used should be specified by the physician, but it is only a small amount (40 to 100 mL in infants). Normal saline (0.9% sodium chloride) should be used in place of tap water, which could lead to water intoxication because it is not isotonic.

Children who have had a colostomy since infancy adapt well to it, because they have never known another method of defecation. Parents should begin toilet training for urine control at the usual time. In contrast, school-age children often have a great deal of difficulty adjusting to a colostomy. Encourage children to perform self-care as fully and as soon as possible so they can be independent. Preschool children usually benefit from therapeutic play that helps them work through their feelings. Provide some time for older children to discuss concerns about being accepted by others and how to answer questions about a colostomy for other children. Adolescents with a colostomy may have questions regarding sexuality and need reassurance that this should not interfere with intimate relationships. They may appreciate open discussion of how they see this affecting their life (Zoucha & Zamarripa, 1997).

PREPARING A CHILD FOR SURGERY

Preparing a child for surgery is a major responsibility for the child health nurse, because surgery is a potentially very frightening procedure (Algren & Algren, 1997). Such preparation differs according to the type of surgery being performed, but certain activities apply to all surgery and all children. Psychological preparation of both child and parents is aimed at reducing the child's fears about the procedure and consists primarily of providing health teaching and opportunities for therapeutic play. Physical preparation includes providing for restrictions on food and fluid intake before surgery, preparing the incision site on the child's skin, and arranging for transportation of the child to surgery. Because many children's surgical procedures are done on an ambulatory basis, preparation must also include informing the parents about the details of the preparation techniques, the surgery, and the postoperative period and the steps they must take toward preparation.

Emotional Preparation

Preparing a child emotionally for surgery requires the prevention of fears common to all children (e.g., fear of separation, fear of mutilation, or fear of death). This can be accomplished by telling the child about the procedure and describing any specific equipment and techniques that will be used, such as anesthesia, eye bandages, nasogastric tubes, sutures, or special aftercare. A teaching plan is essential for explaining all of these features of surgery to the child (see Chapter 14). Be certain that preparation is appropriate to age. Most children undergoing surgery will receive a general anesthetic, rather than a local or regional anesthetic as might be used with adults, because this minimizes their fears of intrusive or mutilating procedures, and because children who are not yet adolescent are not mature enough to cooperate adequately during surgery.

Physical Preparation

Most children will be on nothing by mouth (NPO) status for surgery. The length of the time the child will remain NPO depends on the child's age. Adolescents and school-age children may be restricted from food or fluid from midnight until the time of surgery the following morning; if infants younger than 6 months were held NPO for as long a time as this, they would be taken to surgery in dehydration. Therefore, infants younger than 6 months may be kept NPO for as little as 4 hours. At the end of the 4 hours, as the infant becomes hungry, he or she will begin to cry and fuss for fluid. Parents need an explanation that infants who vomit during surgery because of recent feedings may aspirate, and therefore, even though they are becoming hungry, they must be restricted from fluid. Infants who are used to pacifiers can be offered them, although a hungry child will usually not suck on one for long.

Preparing the Incision Area

Preparation of surgical sites varies. In most instances, shaving of the area and final cleansing are done in a holding room adjacent to the operating room after the child is anesthetized. A povidone-iodine wash may be ordered before transport to the operating room for some types of surgery. Washing a particular body part in this manner can be interpreted as an intrusive procedure by a preschooler. He or she needs a great deal of assurance that the solution being used will not sting.

Transportation

Children should have their identification band checked to see that it is legible and secure. If not, it must be replaced or secured before surgery.

Immediately before transport, remove barrettes and bobby pins from the child's hair and check the mouth for loose teeth (particularly in children ages 6, 7, and 8 years, who are losing their central and lateral incisors) or for dental appliances. It is rare to find a child with full dentures but not uncommon to find a "post" or screw-in tooth that may have to be removed before surgery or a "retainer" used to maintain an orthodontic correction after brace removal. Teeth braces do not need to be removed. Make certain the anesthesiologist knows about any loose teeth before an airway for surgery is inserted (a loose tooth could be knocked totally free and aspirated during the procedure).

For some children, having to give up their own pajamas or their bedroom slippers or outside shoes to change to a hospital gown is a terrifying moment. Giving up underpants is a step that many preschool and early school-age children cannot tolerate, so many children are allowed to wear their own pajamas or clothes until they are under an anesthetic.

In ambulatory settings, children may walk to surgery. If they will ride in a cart, this should have been introduced during preparation. The child should have a restraining strap fastened for safety (presented with "Here's your seat belt; it's just like going in a car."). Preschoolers may need to take a favorite toy or blanket to surgery with them. Ideally, they should be allowed to keep this with them until they are under an anesthetic. Parents should be allowed to accompany their children to the operating suite. Some parents can accompany their child into an anesthesiologist's induction room; for others, this is asking more than they are capable of doing. A nurse whom the child knows should accompany the child to the operating room and remain there until the child is under the anesthetic. The bravest child can feel his or her courage fail at the moment everyone says goodbye at the door of surgery and turns the child over to a green-dressed, firmly capped stranger (even if the child has been well prepared for the exchange of personnel).

Although it may not be cost-effective to have a staff nurse wait with a child until he or she is under an anesthetic, the nurse's wait will probably not be long if the child has been called for surgery when the surgical suite is almost ready. The psychological benefit of a familiar nurse's comforting presence is well worth the wait.

PROVIDING WOUND CARE AFTER SURGERY

Children frequently have a dressing or bandage in place to cover a surgical incision or sutured laceration. Such dressings differ from adult dressings in terms of material, size, and methods used to secure them. Keeping a dressing dry to avoid introducing infection to the wound in infants and toddlers who are not toilet trained can be a major problem. In many instances after surgery, collodion (a clear substance similar to nail polish) is applied to a suture line to serve as the dressing. This keeps the suture line from being contacted by urine or feces and, because it is clear, allows good visualization of the healing surface. Parents need to be assured that such a covering is adequate and actually preferable if the incision is in the groin, such as a hernia repair.

If a gauze dressing is used, it can be covered with plastic, securely held in place with nonadhesive, waterproof tape. Be certain when cutting plastic to cover a dressing not to leave an extra piece behind in the crib; the child could pull it over his or her head and suffocate.

Occlusive dressings (hydrogel sheets, hydrocolloids, or polyurethane films) are dressings especially designed to provide a healing surface over a wound. These need to be applied and removed according to each product's directions (Strickland, 1997).

Infants and young children usually have skin that is too sensitive for adhesive tape to be used to secure dressings. Use nonadhesive tape (silk or paper) instead or secure a dressing with a nonadhering bandage (Kling) or roller gauze. Young children, as a rule, find bandages comforting and accept them as a "badge of courage," displaying them proudly. Apply adhesive bandages (Band-Aids) generously after venipuncture or finger punctures for this reason. Preschool children have little concept of how long it takes healing to occur. They are often surprised that their incision or wound has not yet healed the day after surgery. Preschoolers are often worried that a part of their body under a dressing is missing and find it reassuring to see that the body part is still there (they may pull a dressing away to do this). It is better to know what something is like than to worry about the unknown. Therefore, do not discourage children from looking at their incision during dressing changes. Even if the area looks raw and unhealed, it may look better than what the child has envisioned was under the dressing.

REDUCING ELEVATED TEMPERATURE IN CHILDREN

NURSING DIAGNOSES AND RELATED INTERVENTIONS

Nursing Diagnosis: Risk for hyperthermia related to illness affecting temperature regulation, medications, or surgery

Outcome Identification: Child's temperature will return to normal with appropriate interventions within 2 hours.

Outcome Evaluation: Child's temperature is at 98.6°F (37°C) orally.

Many illnesses cause elevated temperatures. Because children's temperature-regulating mechanism is immature, fever tends to be more marked in them than in adults and may even be out of proportion to the seriousness or extent of the disease. An increased temperature occurs because the child's temperature-regulating point (*set point*) has been elevated. The temperature cannot be reduced until the set point returns (or is returned) to normal. An important nursing intervention with infants and young children is helping to reduce high temperatures, or giving a parent instructions on how to reduce the temperature at home. Any infant younger than age 3 months with a fever should be seen by a primary care provider as soon as possible because of the high incidence of febrile convulsions in infants.

Acetaminophen (Tylenol) is an excellent *antipyretic* (i.e., it acts to reduce temperature set point), and it is the drug most often prescribed to reduce fever in children. Children's ibuprofen is also effective (Simon, 1996). Parents often do not give enough of an antipyretic such as acetaminophen to be effective because they are afraid the child will have a bad reaction to it. They must be encouraged to give the full dose every 4 hours up to five doses a day until their child's temperature is reduced. Conversely, they must be careful not to give too much or a severe overdose with liver or kidney toxicity can occur (Heubi, et al, 1998). An antipyretic is generally ordered for any child whose oral or tympanic temperature is more than 101°F (38.4°C) or whose rectal temperature is more than 102°F (39.0°C) (see the Drug Highlights). Caution parents not to give acetylsalicylic acid (aspirin) to children with fever because aspirin is associated with Reye's syndrome.

Teach parents that fever is actually a body protection measure, and unless it is exceptionally high (more than 41.1°C [106°F]) it does no specific harm. In fact, there is some evidence that fever may be of value in helping to combat infection, because it aids in destroying microorganisms. In addition to antipyretic administration, children with fever should be dressed in lightweight clothing, such as summer pajamas. All clothing but the diaper can be removed from an infant. Many parents dress febrile children warmly in flannel nightgowns to "keep them from getting a

DRUG HIGHLIGHT

Acetaminophen (Tylenol)

Action: Used for moderate temperature elevation or pain; does not have anti-inflammatory properties

Pregnancy risk category: B

Dosage: Oral: 10–15 mg/kg every 4–6 hours as needed; may repeat 4–5 times per day; do not exceed 5 doses in 24 hours

Possible adverse effects: Elevated liver enzymes, jaundice, rash

Nursing Implications:

- Caution parents that drug can cause severe liver toxicity with overdose.
- Educate parents to not administer a larger dose or more frequently than prescribed.

DRUG HIGHLIGHT

Ibuprofen (Advil, Pediaprofen)

Action: Used to reduce inflammation and mild to moderate pain

Pregnancy risk category: B; D if used in last trimester

Dosage: (for fever or pain) 5–10 mg/kg every 6–8 hours; do not exceed 40 mg in 24 hours

Possible adverse effects: Gastric upset, headache, dizziness, nausea, occult blood loss, prolonged bleeding, peptic ulceration

Nursing Implications:
- Use with caution in children with gastrointestinal irritation.
- Drug can cause renal failure if child becomes dehydrated.
- Administer with food or drink to minimize gastrointestinal irritation.

chill." This increases the child's temperature and does not prevent the shaking, trembling reaction that comes with high fever. Placing a cool cloth (not ice) on the child's forehead feels comforting. Sponging children to lower the temperature is no longer recommended because it can lead to extreme chilling and shock to an immature nervous system.

CHECKPOINT QUESTIONS

17. How far should an enema catheter be inserted in an infant?
18. Would you recommend a parent give aspirin (ASA) or acetaminophen for a child's fever?

KEY POINTS

Preparing children for procedures reduces anxiety. Prepare a child and parents by trying to relate a procedure to something the child is already familiar with, such as comparing an x-ray machine to a camera.

Include parents in both the planning and implementation of care. Parents reinfect children with fear if their own fear is uncontrolled. Give explanations on two levels: "I'm going to change the dressing on her suture line" for a parent; "I'm going to put a clean bandage on your tummy" for the child.

Reduce painful procedures to the minimum possible (combine blood sampling procedures, if possible).

Perform any procedures that will cause pain in a treatment room or away from the child's bedside so the bed remains a "safe place."

Perform treatments without chilling or exposure. Be aware that even small children expect modesty to be respected.

Allow the child to voice anger or fear of a procedure. Provide therapeutic play after a procedure to help reduce these reactions.

Identify a child well before a procedure; children do not monitor their own care as do adults.

Children enjoy adults who are secure in their actions. Practice as necessary the steps of a procedure before you begin so you radiate confidence in your manner.

Once you have announced that a procedure needs to be done, proceed to do it; waiting for something to happen is often as stressful as actually having it done.

Involve children in procedures because this gives them a sense of control. Allow a child to examine electrodes or apply lubricant for electrode contact. Give the child a portion of an ECG strip as a badge of courage after the procedure, or let the child apply his or her own adhesive bandage.

Praise children for cooperation even if none was visibly obvious. For painful procedures, any behavior short of hysterical screaming counts as cooperation.

CRITICAL THINKING EXERCISES

1. Wally is the 4-year-old you met at the beginning of the chapter who is frightened of dark places. He is scheduled to have an MRI of his head done, which means he will be wheeled into a huge, dark, hollow tube. How would you prepare him for this?
2. An infant who has had three seizures is scheduled to have a CT scan done with dye injected. The mother asks you to assure her that her son will not have a reaction to the dye. How will you answer her?
3. An infant who had bowel surgery at birth and now has a temporary colostomy is ready for hospital discharge. His grandmother will be caring for him two mornings a week while his mother attends school. The grandmother tells you that she cannot imagine how she will care for an infant with a colostomy. What could you do to try to make her feel more comfortable with the baby's care? Will his care really be much different from that for other newborns?

REFERENCES

Algren, C.L. & Algren, J.T. (1997). Pediatric sedation: essentials for the perioperative nurse. *Nursing Clinics of North America, 32*(1), 17.

Bar-Mor, B. (1997). Preparation of children for surgery and invasive procedures: milestones on the way to success. *Journal of Pediatric Nursing, 12*(4), 252.

Bartlett, E.M. (1996). Temperature measurement: why and how in intensive care. *Intensive and Critical Care Nursing, 12*(1), 50.

Blezek, D.J. & Robb, R.A. (1997). Evaluating virtual endoscopy for clinical use. *Journal of Digital Imaging, 10*(3.1), 51.

Brouhard, B.H. (1997). Fluid and electrolyte therapy. *Clinical Pediatrics, 36*(7), 401.

Cohen, H.A. et al. (1997). Urine samples from disposable diapers: an accurate method for urine cultures. *Journal of Family Practice, 44*(3), 290.

Cusumano, A. (1998). Three-dimensional ultrasound imaging: clinical applications. *Ophthalmology, 105*(2), 300.

Department of Health and Human Services. (1995). *Healthy people 2000: Midcourse review*. Washington, D.C.: DHHS.

Heubi, J.E. et al. (1998). Therapeutic misadventures with acetaminophen hepatoxicity after multiple doses in children. *Journal of Pediatrics, 132*(1), 22.

Huffman, C. & Sandelowski, M. (1997). The nurse-technology relationship: the case of ultrasonography. *Journal of Obstetric, Gynecologic and Neonatal Nursing, 26*(6), 673.

Landrum, L. (1997). Conscious sedation in the endoscopy setting. *Critical Care Nursing Clinics of North America, 9*(3), 355.

Martinot, A. et al. (1997). Indications for flexible versus rigid bronchoscopy in children with suspected foreign-body aspiration. *American Journal of Respiratory and Critical Care Medicine, 155*(5), 1676.

Niederhauser, V.P. (1997). Prescribing for children: issues in pediatric pharmacology. *Nurse Practitioner, 22*(3), 16.

Selekman, J. & Snyder, B. (1997). Institutional policies on the use of physical restraints on children. *Pediatric Nursing, 23*(5), 531.

Sherazi, Z. & Gordon, I. (1996). Quality of care: identification and quantification of the process of care among children undergoing nuclear medicine studies. *Nuclear Medicine Communications, 17*(5), 363.

Simon, R.E. (1996). Ibuprofen suspension: pediatric antipyretic. *Pediatric Nursing, 22*(2), 118.

Strickland, M.E. (1997). Evaluation of bacterial growth with occlusive dressing use on excoriated skin in the premature infant. *Neonatal Network, 16*(2), 29.

Tait, A.R. et al. (1998). Factors that influence parents' decisions to consent to their child's participation in clinical anesthesia research. *Anesthesia and Analgesia, 86*(1), 50.

Williams, L. et al. (1997). Consent to treatment by minors attending accident and emergency department guidelines. *Journal of Accident and Emergency Medicine, 14*(5), 286.

Zoucha, R. & Zamarripa, C. (1997). The significance of culture in the care of the client with an ostomy. *Journal of Wound, Ostomy and Continence Nursing, 24*(5), 270.

SUGGESTED READINGS

Berlin, C.M. (1997). Advances in pediatric pharmacology and toxicology. *Advances in Pediatrics, 44*(3), 545.

Beyea, S.C. & Nicoll, L.H. (1996). Back to basics: administering IM injections the right way. *American Journal of Nursing, 96*(1), 35.

Lesar, T. S. (1998). Errors in the use of medication dosage equations. *Archives of Pediatrics and Adolescent Medicine, 152*(4), 340.

MacKenzie, J.R. (1997). The role of nuclear medicine in children. *British Journal of Hospital Medicine, 57*(6), 248.

Matsui, D.M. (1997). Drug compliance in pediatrics: clinical and research issues. *Pediatric Clinics of North America, 44*(1), 1.

Mee, C.L. & Possanza, C.P. (1997). How to record an accurate 12-lead ECG. *Nursing, 27*(3), 60.

Molnar, J. (1997). Consent in the 90's. *Medicine and Law, 16*(3), 567.

Perez, A. (1996). Cardiac monitoring: mastering the essentials. *RN, 59*(8), 32.

Selekman, J. & Snyder, B. (1996). Uses of and alternatives to restraints in pediatric settings. *AACN Clinical Issues, 7*(4), 603.

Thigpen, J. (1995). Minimizing medication errors. *Neonatal Network, 14*(2), 85.

Pain Management in Children

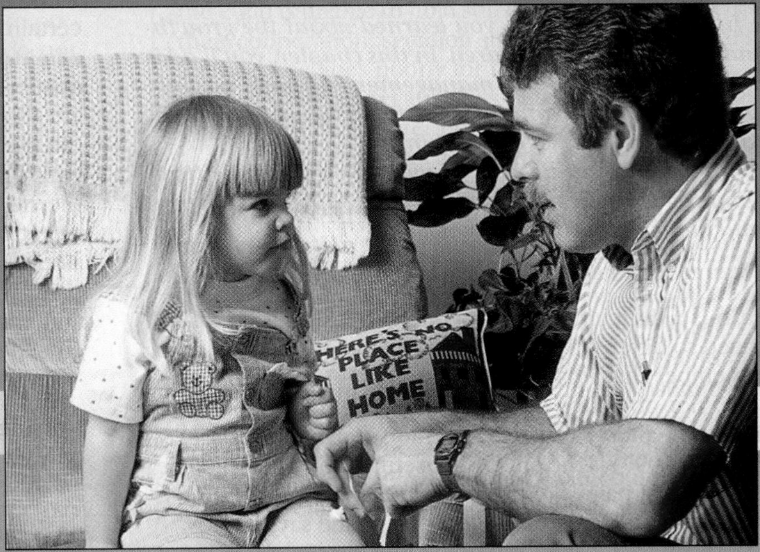

17

CHAPTER

Key Terms

- conscious sedation
- distraction
- epidural analgesia
- gate control theory
- imagery
- pain
- patient-controlled anesthesia
- substitution of meaning
- thought stopping
- transcutaneous electrical nerve stimulation

Objectives

After mastering the contents of this chapter, you should be able to:

1. Describe the major methods of pain management in children.
2. Assess the child for needed pain management.
3. Formulate nursing diagnoses for the child with pain.
4. Identify appropriate outcomes for the child with pain.
5. Plan nursing care for the child with pain.
6. Implement nursing care related to the child with pain.
7. Evaluate outcomes for achievement and effectiveness of care.
8. Identify National Health Goals related to children with pain that nurses could be instrumental in helping the nation achieve.
9. Identify areas related to care of children with pain that could benefit from additional nursing research.
10. Use critical thinking to analyze ways that nursing care for a child with pain could be more family centered.
11. Integrate knowledge of pain in children with nursing process to achieve quality child health nursing care.

- Child describes ways to reduce pain when it returns.
- Child resumes age-appropriate behaviors.

PHYSIOLOGY OF PAIN

As in adults, pain in children occurs for one of four reasons: (1) reduced oxygen in tissues from impaired circulation, (2) pressure on tissue, (3) external injury, or (4) overstretching of body cavities with fluid or air. The stimuli causing pain is not always visible or measurable. In addition, anxiety can lead to increased pain regardless of the physical stimuli.

ASSESSING TYPE AND DEGREE OF PAIN

Pain assessment is difficult with children because some will suffer with pain rather than report it, often because of fear. Using only subjective measures such as observation can be misleading because some children do not appear to be in pain. They may distract themselves by such methods as concentrating on play. Some children may sleep, not from comfort but from the exhaustion caused by pain. Cultural differences also influence how pain is expressed (see Focus on Cultural Competence).

Parents also may have difficulty evaluating their child's pain. Sutters & Miaskowski (1997) studied children after tonsillectomy to see if their parents were able to successfully rate their degree of pain. In this study, although children displayed symptoms of nausea, anxiety, restless sleep and difficulty taking oral fluids, parents rated their children's worst pain as only 0 to 3 on a ten-point scale. The study revealed that because parents expected their children to have pain, they did not rate their pain as being very intense. Better pain assessment would have helped them meet their children's needs.

FOCUS ON CULTURAL COMPETENCE

Because pain is an individual sensation, it can be experienced totally differently by different children. In South American countries, for example, pain may be expressed very openly and freely. In Asian or northern European countries, children are expected to be more stoic about pain. In China, children may not accept something offered for pain relief until it has been offered twice. Because the expression of pain is culturally determined this way, two children having the same degree of pain may express it very differently.

Additionally, perception of the situation influences the response to a situation independent of the intensity of the stimuli. Therefore, a child experiencing a procedure less intrusive than another child's may still describe the degree of pain as more intense based on their perception. Assessment for pain must be individualized.

Developmental Considerations

Pain assessment techniques vary widely from assessment of the nonverbal infant to the adolescent. Keep in mind the child's developmental level when assessing for pain.

The Infant

In the past, it was believed that infants do not feel pain because of incomplete myelinization of peripheral nerves. This is no longer believed because myelinization is not necessary for pain perception.

A second argument against needing to provide pain relief to infants is that they have no memory. It can be shown, however, that physiologic changes do occur with pain. So even with a lack of memory, it is clear that pain is experienced. In all age populations, including premature infants, pain has been shown to have the potential for serious physical harm. Because they are preverbal, assessing pain in infants is especially difficult. Observing for cues such as diffuse body movement; tears; a high-pitched, sharp, harsh cry; stiff posture; lack of play; and fisting can all be helpful (Seymour et al, 1997). Even newborns instinctively guard a body part by holding an extremity still or tensing the abdomen. Perhaps the chief mark of pain in infants is that when pain is present, they cannot be comforted completely. Preterm neonates may not be able to organize a distress response to cue a health care provider to the presence of pain (Rutledge & Donaldson, 1997). When working with infants of this age, be sensitive to situations that could cause pain. Be alert for subtle alterations in facial expression, such as eyes squeezed shut or quivering chin that might signal pain.

The Toddler and Preschooler

Determining when pain is present and its extent continues to be difficult with toddlers and preschoolers because they may not have a word in their limited vocabularies to describe it. They may have difficulty comparing it to past pain (is it better or worse) because they have had little experience with past pain. Words such as "sharp," "nagging," or "aching" have no meaning in relation to pain until the child has experienced each type. Parents may have encouraged children this age to refer to pain as "my boo-boo" or some other word instead of the word "pain." To assess such a child's pain accurately, use the child's term (or teach the child pain is the same as boo-boo). For some toddlers, pain is such a strange sensation that, aside from crying in response to it, they may react aggressively (pounding and rocking) as if to fight it off. They also may avoid being touched or held.

Preschool children can describe that they have pain but continue to have difficulty describing the intensity. They are able to begin to use comforting mechanisms, such as gritting teeth, pressing a hand against a forehead, pulling on their ear, holding their throat, rubbing an arm, or grimacing, to control or express pain. Some preschoolers do not think to mention they have pain because they believe no one wants to help them. They may think the pain is punishment for some act so this is what they deserve. They also can believe that, if they admit to pain, they will receive a "shot," a circumstance seen as worse than the original pain. It is sometimes difficult to comfort children this age during painful procedures because they do not yet have a perception of time. Soothing statements such as "It's only for a minute" are not comforting to the preschooler who does not know how long that is. The preschool child, due to their egocentric thinking, may expect that adults are aware of the child's pain.

For all young children who are unable to fully verbalize their pain state, behavior must be carefully examined. In addition to behaviors already discussed, young children may regress when in pain or become very withdrawn. The health professional should ask the question: "What would this child normally be doing (for example, playing, eating, sleeping)?" Deviations from usual behavior may, in the absence of any other verbal description, be signs that the child is in pain. Input from parents on how their child usually behaves is very valuable. Any procedure or condition that would normally cause pain in an adult will cause pain in a child. In a nonverbal child, a trial dose of analgesia may be used. The nurse can evaluate behavior changes after the dose is given. The child who resumes usual behavior after analgesia was probably in pain before it.

The School-Age Child and Adolescent

Children who think concretely (preadolescents) can have difficulty envisioning that a word like "sharp" applies both to knives and to the feeling in their abdomen. They may continue to have difficulty describing pain. They may assume that because the nurse is an authority figure, the nurse knows they have pain. They may be in middle school before they are able to understand how to use a pain rating scale or that the scale intensifies from left to right. Doing some preassessment work with them, such as giving them ten different size triangles and asking them to arrange them from smallest to largest, is a good way to evaluate if they understand incremental measurements. The child who can arrange triangles this way understands the concept of less to most. Once children have grasped this concept, they are able to describe pain intensity in a very measurable way. A scale of 1 to 5 can be used in younger children.

Adolescents commonly use adult mechanisms for controlling pain. Some are more stoic in the face of pain than adults, trying to avoid the stereotypes of "cry-baby" or "chicken." This makes assessing for body motions such as clenched hands, clenched teeth, rapid breathing, and guarding of body parts that might indicate pain not as helpful as they may be in adults. Some children of school age will regress with pain (e.g., talking "baby-talk" or lying in a fetal position). Children this age can understand that if pain will last only an instant, such as with an injection, it can be controlled through nonpharmacologic activities such as distraction techniques.

✔ CHECKPOINT QUESTIONS

1. What are frequent physiologic findings that indicate pain in infants?
2. What if a toddler uses the word "oowie" for pain? Should you use his word or insist he learn the word "pain"?

PAIN ASSESSMENT

The techniques of pain assessment vary depending on the age of the child and the type and extent of pain. Although monitoring for physiologic findings such as a change in pulse or blood pressure may give some indication that the child is under stress, these are not the most dependable indicators of pain. Common fallacies about pain in children are shown in Table 17-1. Because pain is a subjective finding, once children can speak, asking them to tell you about their pain (self-reporting on a pain rating scale) is the most accurate method for assessment.

Pain Rating Scales

A variety of pain rating scales have been devised for use with children. Despite the large amount of research in this area, one study revealed that only 36% of pediatric surgical nurses had ever used a pain assessment scale specifically adapted for children (Colwell, Clark &

TABLE 17.1 Common Fallacies About Pain in Children

FALLACY	FACT
1. Nurses can accurately estimate children's pain from physical appearance or activity.	1. Nurses commonly underestimate children's pain when they do not rely on children's self reports.
2. Young children, particularly newborns, do not feel pain.	2. Newborns and children do feel pain.
3. A child who resumes usual activity or sleeps cannot be in pain.	3. Some children distract themselves with play or music while in pain. They may sleep from exhaustion from the pain.
4. Because of the possible adverse effects, narcotic analgesics are too dangerous for young children.	4. Narcotics can be used safely with children, including low-birth-weight infants.
5. Experiencing pain will not harm an infant or young child.	5. Newborns with pain can become cyanotic and bradycardic; no one knows the psychological stress of pain at this age.
6. If a child denies he or she is feeling pain, you should believe him or her.	6. Children may deliberately deny pain to avoid another possible painful procedure, such as an injection, which they view as more painful. They may be afraid, fearing that they are being punished or believe others know how they feel.

Perkins, 1996). Part of this lack of application to practice has resulted because of a controversy over which scale is best to use. At present, all of them can be used because none has been proven to be consistently better than the others, mainly because both children and the type of pain they can be experiencing vary so much. As a rule, pick one scale to use with a child and then use that scale consistently for the child rather than asking the child to adapt to different assessment techniques. Be sure to follow the individual instructions for that scale (Rutledge & Donaldson, 1997; see Enhancing Communication).

Pain Experience Inventory

The Pain Experience Inventory is a set of eight questions for children and eight separate questions for the child's parents to elicit the terms the child uses to denote pain and what actions the child thinks will best alleviate the pain. Such a form can be used when a child is admitted to an acute care facility or on an initial home care visit (Box 17-1). If possible, it should be used before the child has pain.

CRIES Neonatal Postoperative Pain Measurement Scale

The CRIES inventory is a 10-point scale on which five physiologic and behavioral variables frequently associated with neonatal pain can be assessed and rated. These include:

- Amount and type of crying
- Need for oxygen administration
- Increased vital signs
- Facial expression
- Sleeplessness (Krechel & Bildner, 1995)

Each area is scored from 0 to 2, and then a total score is obtained (Table 17-2). On the scale, infants with a score of 4 or more are most likely to be in pain and need pain management interventions to reduce discomfort. The scale cannot be used with infants who are intubated or paralyzed for ventilatory assistance because they would have no score for cry and perhaps none for facial expression.

FLACC Pain Assessment Tool

The FLACC Pain Assessment Tool (Merkel et al, 1997) is a scale intended to be rated by health care providers without the need for self-report input by the child. It incorporates five types of behaviors usually seen with pain: facial expression; leg movement; activity; cry; and consolability. Preliminary data indicate that the scale is reliable and valid. It has the advantage of rating pain level in children who are not able to verbalize pain or self-report.

Poker Chip Tool

The Poker Chip Tool (Hester & Barcus, 1986) uses four red poker chips placed in a horizontal line in front of the child. It can be used with children as young as 4 years of age, provided the child can count or has some concept of numbers. To use the tool, tell the child, "These are pieces of hurt." Beginning at the chip nearest the child's left side and ending at the one nearest child's right side, point to chips and say, "This is a little bit of hurt, this is a little more hurt, this is more hurt, and this (the fourth chip) is the most hurt you could ever have." Then ask the child, "How many pieces of hurt do you have right now?" Children without pain will reply that they do not have any so do not give children an option for zero hurt. Clarify the child's answer by a follow-up question such as, "Oh, you have a little hurt? Tell me about the hurt." This is an effective tool for young children because the poker chips are concrete items (Figure 17-1).

FACES Pain Rating Scale

This scale consists of six cartoonlike faces ranging from smiling to tearful. Explain to the child that each face is for a person who has no hurt to a lot of hurt. Use the words

ENHANCING COMMUNICATION

Faye Harvey is a 4-year-old girl who has just returned from tonsillectomy surgery. You know this type of surgery is painful so you want to assess her level of pain.

Less Effective Communication

Nurse: Faye? How are you feeling?
Mrs. Harvey: Her throat is too sore to talk.
Nurse: I'm going to show you some faces, Faye. Just point to the one that looks the way you feel. If you point to a sad one, I'll get you a shot to take away your pain.
Faye: (Points to the first face—the "no pain" face.)
Nurse: No pain? Good. That's probably because your anesthetic is still working.

More Effective Communication

Nurse: Faye? How are you feeling?
Mrs. Harvey: Her throat is too sore to talk.
Nurse: Faye? Remember the faces we looked at this morning before surgery? I want you to use them to tell me how you feel. This one means "no hurt." This one means "the most hurt you could have." Point to the one that shows how much hurt you have.
Faye: (Points to the middle face—the "moderate pain" face.)

It is important when using pain rating scales that they are introduced to children before surgery or before they will have pain from procedures so both the pain and the rating tool are not new to the child at once. It is important also to give the correct instructions for standardized assessment tools or the results will not be accurate. Mentioning bringing a "shot for pain" can cause children not to report pain because they imagine the injection causing even more pain rather than relieving pain.

BOX 17.1

PAIN EXPERIENCE INVENTORY

Questions for Child

Tell me what pain is.
Tell me about the hurt you have had before.
What do you do when you hurt?
Do you tell others when you hurt?
What do you want others to do for you when you hurt?
What don't you want others to do for you when you hurt?
What helps the most to take away your hurt?
Is there anything special that you would like me to know about you when you hurt? (If yes, have child describe.)

Questions for Parents

Describe any pain your child has had before.
How does your child usually react to pain?
Does your child tell you or others when he/she is hurting?
How do you know when your child is in pain?
What do you do for your child when he/she is hurting?
What does your child do for himself/herself when he/she is hurting?
Which of these actions work best to decrease or take away your child's pain?
Is there anything special that you would like me to know about your child and pain? (If yes, have parents describe.)

Hester, N. O., & Barcus, C. S. (1986). Assessment and management of pain in children. *Pediatrics: Nursing Update, 1*(14), 2. Princeton, N.J.

under each face to describe the amount of pain. Ask the child to choose the face that best describes his or her own pain (Wong & Baker, 1996). Record the number under the face the child chooses. Children as young as 3 years can use this scale. This scale appeals to health care providers because it is cute. However, it is not as concrete a measure as the Poker Chip tool and, therefore, may not be as effective with all children (Figure 17-2).

Oucher Pain Rating Scale

The Oucher (Reyer, Denyes & Villarruel, 1992; Jordan-Marsh et al, 1994) scale consists of six photographs of children's faces representing "no hurt" to "biggest hurt you could ever have." Also included is a vertical scale with numbers from 0 to 100. To use the photograph portion, point to each photograph and explain what each means: first photograph from the bottom (0) is "no hurt"; the next (photograph 1) means "a little hurt"; the next (photograph 2) means "a little more hurt"; the next (photograph 3) means "even more hurt"; the next (photograph 4) is "pretty much or a lot of hurt"; and the top photograph (photograph 5) is the "biggest hurt you could ever have."

To use the scale portion, point to each section of the scale and explain what it means: 0 means "no hurt"; 1 to 29 means "little hurt"; 30 to 69 means "middle hurt"; 70 to 99 means "big hurt"; and 100 means "the biggest hurt you could ever have." Ask the child to point to the section of the scale that represents his or her level of hurt. Children as young as 3 can use the tool by pointing to the photograph that best describes their level of pain. If the child can count to 100 by ones and understands the concept of increasing value, the numbered scale can be used. The Oucher scale has African-American and Hispanic-American

TABLE 17.2 CRIES Neonatal Postoperative Pain Measurement Scale

	Infant's Score		
Assessment	*0*	*1*	*2*
Crying	No	High-pitched	Inconsolable
Requires oxygen for saturation above 95%	No	<30%	>30%
Increased vital signs	Heart rate and blood pressure within 10% of preoperative values	Heart rate or blood pressure 11%–20% higher than preoperative value	Heart rate or blood pressure 21% or more above preoperative value
Expression	None	Grimace	Grimace/grunt
Sleepless	No	Wakes at frequent intervals	Constantly awake
TOTAL INFANT SCORE			

Krechel, S. W., & Bildner, J. (1995). CRIES: a new neonatal postoperative pain management score. *Pediatric Anesthesia, 5*(1), 53.

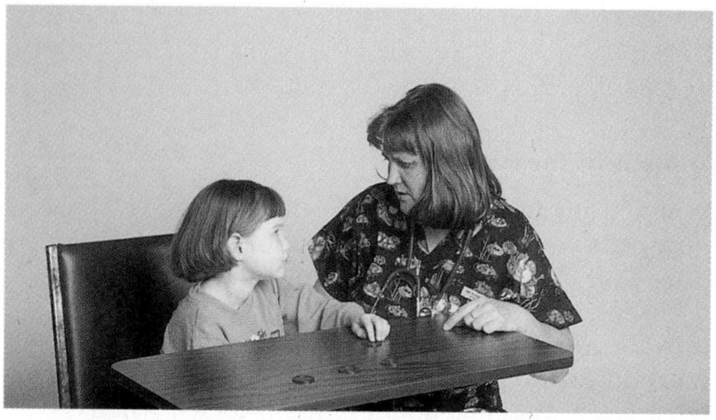

FIGURE 17.1 The child points to the poker chip indicating the degree of pain she is experiencing.

versions. Allow children to select the version they want to use or present the version that most closely matches the cultural characteristics of the child.

Numerical or Visual Analog Scale

A numerical or visual analog scale uses a straight line with end points marked "0 = no pain" on the left and "10 = worst pain" on the right. Divisions along the line are marked in units from 1 to 9. Explain to children that the left end of the line (the 0) means a person feels no pain. At the other end is a 10, which means a person feels the worst pain possible. The numbers 1 to 9 in the middle are for "a little pain" to "a lot of pain." Ask children to choose a number that best describes their pain. As soon as they can count and have a concept of numbers, children can use a numerical scale. Be certain to actually show school-age children the scale; don't just say score your pain from 0 to 10. Until children reach late adolescence, they use concrete thought processes and may need the help of seeing the line to accurately rate their pain.

Adolescent Pediatric Pain Tool

The Adolescent Pediatric Pain Tool (APPT) combines a visual activity and a numerical scale (Savedra et al, 1992). On one half of the form (Figure 17-3) is an outline figure showing the anterior and posterior view of a child. The child is asked to color in the areas as big or as small as the place where the pain is on the figures to show where he or she has pain. On the right side of the form, the child rates the pain in reference to "no pain," "little pain," "medium pain," "large pain" and "worst possible pain." For a third activity, children are asked to point to or circle as many words as possible on the form that describe their pain (words such as horrible, pounding, cutting and stinging).

Many school-age children need help reading and interpreting the multitude of words that describe pain. This is a useful tool for involving parents to talk with the child about his or her pain. Reading the words together helps the child examine the type, location, and level of pain he is experiencing. It also helps parents to better understand what their child is experiencing. The scale is suggested for children 8 through 17 years of age.

Logs and Diaries

Keeping a log or diary of when pain occurs and to self-rate pain each time it occurs is useful for assessing children with chronic but intermittent pain. Examining such a diary can provide direction for pain management. For example, if it shows that the child always awakens with pain in the morning, the child needs longer acting analgesia at bedtime. Or if the pain is worse during weekends spent at her grandparent's house, then something different is happening in that setting than at home.

> WHAT IF? What if a child completely colored in the figures on the Adolescent Pediatric Pain Tool? Would you assess that the child has pain all over? Explain why or why not. If not, then what might account for this?

PAIN MANAGEMENT

Pain management techniques vary greatly depending on the age of a child and the degree and type of pain present. Many health care agencies are employing nurses specially prepared in pain management to serve on an interdisciplinary team of health care providers including physicians, anesthesiologists, patient advocates, and wound therapy nurses to individually plan pain management programs for children. In the past, children frequently were not prescribed potent analgesics because of the fear that common drugs used, such as morphine, would decrease their respiratory rate to an unsafe level. Those children who had adequate analgesia prescribed may not have received it because a nurse was overly concerned about causing respiratory distress. Today, it is recognized that if the dose of an opiate such as morphine is regulated to the child's size, there is no more danger of respiratory depression in children than in adults. The risk of respiratory depression is not very great if the drug is administered correctly. When administered by IV bolus injection, opiates should be given slowly. After checking that the correct dose has been prescribed, opiates can be given with confidence to decrease pain without untoward effects. A good rule for determining whether children need pain relief for a procedure is to remember that if a procedure would cause pain in an adult, it will also cause pain in a child. Often a combination of nonpharmacologic

FIGURE 17.2 The FACES pain rating scale. *(Whaley and Wong's essentials of pediatric nursing,* ed. 5. 1997, p. 1216. Copyright by Mosby-Year Book, Inc. Reprinted by permission.)

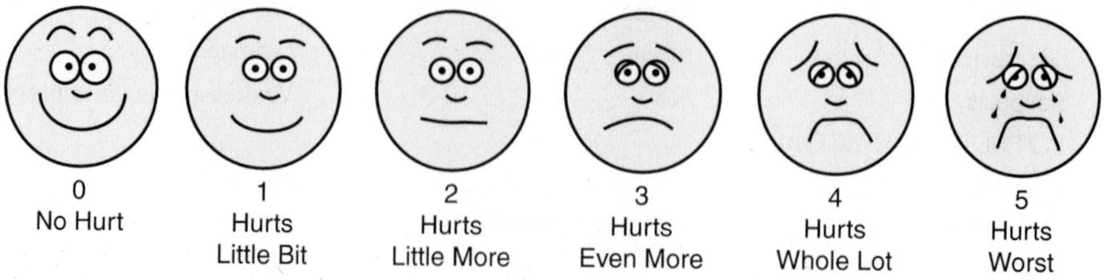
0
No Hurt
1
Hurts
Little Bit
2
Hurts
Little More
3
Hurts
Even More
4
Hurts
Whole Lot
5
Hurts
Worst

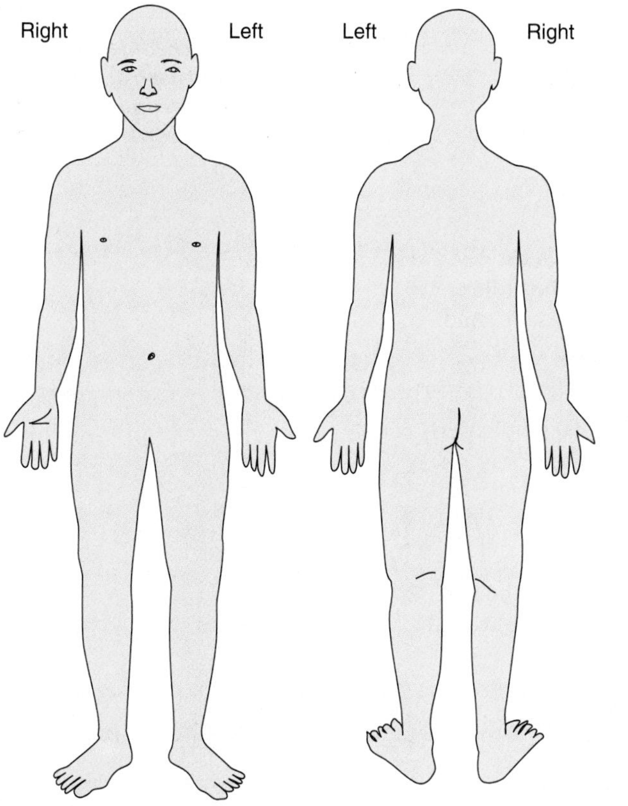

FIGURE 17.3 Adolescent Pediatric Pain Tool (APPT). (Savedra, M. C., Tesler, M. D., Holzemer, W. L. and Ward, J. A. [1992]. *Adolescent pediatric pain tool: User's manual.* San Francisco: University of California-San Francisco)

and pharmacologic methods is most effective (see Nursing Care Plan). Children with chronic pain or pain not relieved with standard approaches may benefit from a referral to pain management specialists. Relief of frequent pain episodes or prolonged pain may require intense, consistent assessment and intervention, which is difficult to achieve in an acute care setting or during infrequent office visits. Whatever tools are used for assessment, the staff should become very familiar and comfortable with their use. It is important that pain be assessed in an organized and consistent manner so relief and interventions do not vary based on the health care provider (Hamers et al, 1998). Pederson and coworkers (1997) surveyed nurses in critical care units to discover that, even in the light of this, there are gaps in effective pain management (see Focus on Nursing Research). General measures to alleviate pain that are helpful to parents as well as health care providers are summarized in Empowering the Family. These guidelines are based primarily on the gate control theory described below.

Gate Control Theory

The **gate control theory** of pain (Melzack & Wall, 1965) attempts to explain how pain impulses travel between a site of injury and the brain where the impulse is actually registered as pain. This theory envisions that gating mechanisms in the substantia gelatinosa of the dorsal horn of the spinal cord, when activated, are capable of halting an impulse at that level of the cord. This prevents the pain impulse from being received at the brain level and interpreted as pain. Gating mechanisms can be stimulated by three techniques: (1): cutaneous stimulation, (2) distraction, and (3) anxiety reduction.

Pain impulses are carried by small peripheral nerve fibers. If large peripheral nerves next to an injury site are stimulated, the ability of the small nerve fibers at the injury site to transmit pain impulses appears to decrease. Rubbing an injured part such as a stubbed toe or applying heat or cold to the site is an effective maneuver to suppress pain because it activates large fibers. This technique is especially effective with children because the rubbing is not only comforting from a physical standpoint but also conveys psychological warmth.

Distraction allows the cells of the brain stem that register an impulse as pain to be preoccupied with other stimuli so the pain impulse cannot register. Having a child focus on an action or a thought is a common form of distraction (Figure 17-4). Telling a child to say "ouch" while an injection is administered is the simplest use of this technique.

Pain impulses are perceived more quickly if anxiety is also present. Therefore, attempt to reduce the child's anxiety as much as possible. Teaching a school-age child about what to expect with a procedure is one method. As well as knowing when something is going to happen, children also should know when nothing is going to happen. Being told that a clinic visit will not involve painful procedures allows a child to relax and feel less anxiety.

Gate Control Theory Techniques

The effectiveness of gate control theory techniques varies with the child's age, ability to cooperate, degree of pain, and time allowed for learning and applying the techniques. Because memory may influence the sensation of pain (expecting to have pain produces anxiety, which increases pain), these techniques are best taught to children before they begin to have pain. In all instances, teach children to use them just before or at the moment they first feel the pain. If they wait until the pain is intense, the pain may be so distracting that they cannot concentrate on using the technique. Children who were able to effectively use a distraction technique in the past but are no longer able to do so need to be evaluated for what is changing. Is it their ability to cope with the pain or is the pain increasing in intensity? Contrary to common belief, familiarity with procedures does not necessarily lessen the fear nor the pain experienced.

Substitution of Meaning or Imagery. **Substitution of meaning** or **guided imagery** is a distraction technique to help the child place another meaning (a nonpainful one) on a painful procedure. Children are often more adept at this than adults because their imagination is less inhibited. Success with this technique requires practice, so has limited application in an acute care setting. A venipuncture, for example, could be viewed as a silver rocket probing the moon to transport specimens back to earth or a submarine diving under the water to escape torpedoes just in time. Be certain a child thinks of a *specific* image. Help him or her elaborate on the image to make it more concrete each time

A 5-year-old is scheduled for a bone marrow aspiration to rule out the possibility of a hematologic disorder.

Nursing Care Plan

THE CHILD REQUIRING PAIN MANAGEMENT

Assessment: 5-year-old female with a history of frequent nosebleeds, petechiae, and bruising is admitted for diagnostic testing. This is the child's first experience with hospitalization. Parents at bedside talking with child. Bone marrow aspiration scheduled in 3 hours. Child upset and crying, "Why must I have this test? It's gonna hurt so much."

Nursing Diagnosis: Anxiety related to fear of the unknown, lack of experience with previous testing, and anticipation of painful procedure

Outcome Identification: Child will express feelings and concerns verbally and through play.

Outcome Evaluation: Child talks openly about the test; identifies the reason for the test; exhibits age-appropriate coping behaviors; relates options for minimizing pain.

Interventions	Rationale
1. Assess the child's understanding about the reason for the bone marrow aspiration. Explore with the child her thoughts and feelings about it.	1. Assessment and exploration reveal information about the child, her knowledge base, and possible clues to her anxiety, providing a foundation on which to build future strategies and teaching.
2. Talk with the child about what she thinks the test will be like, acknowledging her anxieties and providing feedback to clarify misconceptions.	2. Talking with the child allows her to share her feelings and concerns openly and safely. Acknowledging her anxieties validates her feelings. Feedback helps correct misinformation.
3. Explain the procedure to the child at the appropriate age level. Incorporate the use of play materials and role play.	3. Explanations that also include play aid in the child's learning and understanding. Role playing can be an effective technique for preparing children for new and unfamiliar experiences.
4. Inform the child about various techniques, both nonpharmacologic and pharmacologic, for pain control. Allow the child to practice nonpharmacologic methods. Include the parents in these practice sessions.	4. Information about pain-relief measures may help to alleviate some of the child's anxiety about the hurt. Practice helps the child become proficient with the technique, thereby enhancing its effectiveness.
5. Introduce the child to the pain assessment tool to be used, such as the poker chip tool or Oucher pain scale.	5. Introducing the child to the tool prior to the onset of pain minimizes the anxiety associated with a new experience and increases the tool's usefulness and accuracy in determining the child's pain level.

Nursing Diagnosis: Pain related to invasive procedure of bone marrow aspiration

Outcome Identification: Child will verbalize that pain is within tolerable limits.

Outcome Evaluation: Child states pain is controlled; identifies pain as no higher than one with poker chip tool or Oucher pain scale; exhibits few to no nonverbal indicators of pain.

(continued)

Interventions	Rationale
1. Apply EMLA cream to intended aspiration site and cover with an occlusive dressing at least 2 to 3 hours before scheduled procedure.	1. EMLA cream is a topical analgesic cream that acts to anesthetize the skin. An occlusive dressing enhances absorption and tissue penetration.
2. Anticipate the need for possible conscious sedation. If ordered, prepare the child for its use. Administer analgesic as ordered. Anticipate the use of intravenous route if child will receive conscious sedation.	2. A bone marrow aspiration is painful. If the child experiences pain, analgesia is necessary for relief. Conscious sedation results in a pain-free, sedated state that leaves the child's protective reflexes intact. Preparation for this technique helps to minimize the child's anxiety and fears.
3. Assess the child's pain immediately prior to the procedure using the appropriate tool.	3. Pain assessment prior to the procedure provides a baseline for evaluation.
4. Just prior to the procedure, remove the occlusive dressing and wipe away the EMLA cream. Look for reddened or blanched skin.	4. Removal prior to the procedure is necessary to prevent injury. Reddened or blanched skin indicates that the drug has been effective.
5. Warn the child of the possible feeling of pressure with needle insertion and of sharp pain with aspiration. Encourage the child to use guided imagery.	5. Anticipatory knowledge of events and feelings helps to prepare the child and aids in coping.
6. After the procedure, assess the child's pain and compare to baseline.	6. Assessment and comparison to baseline identifies the child's level of pain postprocedure.
7. Engage the child in quiet activities for the first hour after the procedure.	7. The child is at risk for bleeding from the puncture site. Quiet activities reduce the risk for bleeding and also provide distraction.
8. Provide opportunities for therapeutic play with a doll and syringe.	8. Therapeutic play helps the child express her feelings now that the procedure is completed.

they use the image so the child's mind stays on the image (what color is the rocket ship? Are there stripes on the sides? What does the pilot look like?).

When helping parents teach a distraction technique to their child, be certain they don't interpret distraction as just talking to the child or suggesting a video game to divert attention. Although this is distraction, simple distraction like this will allow pain to break through.

Thought Stopping. Thought stopping is a technique whereby children are taught to stop anxious thoughts by substituting a positive or relaxing thought. As with imagery, this technique also requires a great deal of practice before using it in the actual situation. Anticipatory anxiety is a negative force because it increases the pain experience during a procedure and makes the time before it full of anxiety also. For this technique, help the child to think of a set of positive factors about the approaching feared procedure. For a bone marrow aspiration, for example, this might include, "It doesn't take long; the doctor and nurse who do it are helping me; it's important to help me get better." Next, tell the child that when he or she starts to think about the impending procedure, to stop whatever he or she is doing and recite the list of positive thoughts to himself or herself if others are present or out loud if the child is alone or important support people are present. The child can then return to the activity. Every time the anxious thoughts appear, however, the child should stop and recite the exercise.

Thought stopping is an effective technique because it allows children to feel in control of their thoughts, which is different from merely saying, "Don't think about it." This technique does not suppress thoughts. Rather, it changes them into positive ones. The secret is for the child to use the technique every time the disturbing, anxious thought appears even if, at first, such thoughts crowd in as frequently as every few minutes.

FOCUS ON NURSING RESEARCH

Are Pediatric Critical Care Nurses as Knowledgeable as They Could Be About Children's Pain Management?

To measure pediatric critical care nurses' knowledge of pain management, a descriptive exploratory study was conducted by three nurse researchers. For the study, a pain management knowledge test developed by the researchers was distributed to 50 pediatric ICU nurses. Disappointingly, only 38% of the nurses returned the questionnaire. Findings from this group, however, revealed that some nurses were not knowledgeable about specific medication interactions. Only 63% indicated that when a child states that the child has pain, pain exists. The researchers concluded that gaps in nurses' pain management knowledge do exist.

Pederson, C., Matthies, D., & McDonald, S. (1997). A survey of pediatric critical care nurses' knowledge of pain management. *American Journal of Critical Care, 6*(4), 289.

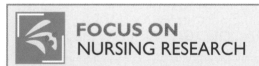

EMPOWERING THE FAMILY: Offering Additional Pain Relief Measures

- Administer pain medication before pain becomes intense to help prevent pain rather than just relieve it. If the child is hospitalized, inform the staff if one approach works or doesn't work.
- Let the child know it is important to try to take the pain away and that you will work with the child to relieve it. Use a positive approach: "This medicine will take away the pain," not "Let's see if this works or not."
- Never just give an analgesic. Make the child comfortable, such as straightening the sheets or offering a backrub.
- Ask your child about measures she or he thinks will be helpful such as an additional pillow, the television turned on, a favorite toy nearby.
- Help your child talk about and describe the pain. This can help to make it more concrete and not as psychologically frightening.
- Relieve anxiety about other phases of life, if possible. Relaxation reduces muscle strain and tension that add to pain.
- Offer support to your child. Pain never seems as bad when a support person is present. Reassuring your child that he or she is loved and you will be there for him or her can be very comforting.

Hypnosis. Hypnosis is not a common pain management technique with children but, when a child is properly trained in the technique, can be very effective. For best results, the child needs to train with a therapist before anticipated pain, so at the time of the pain, the child can use a trancelike state to avoid sensing pain.

Transcutaneous Electrical Nerve Stimulation. Transcutaneous electrical nerve stimulation (TENS) involves applying small electrodes to the dermatones that supply the body portion where pain is experienced. When children sense pain, they push a button on a control box, which then delivers a small electrical current to their skin. The principle underlying this technique is the same as rubbing an injured part. The current interferes with the transmission of the pain impulse across small nerve fibers.

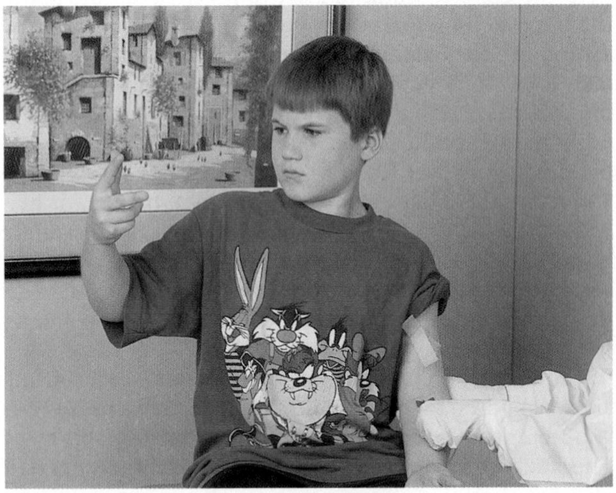

FIGURE 17.4 A child using distraction as a pain management technique.

TENS can be used to manage either acute or chronic pain. Some children (and parents) dislike TENS therapy because they are afraid or nervous about the electric current. Assure them that the current is a very mild one and will not harm the child. TENS is not recommended if the child is incontinent or has a wound with a high probability of causing the electrodes to grow wet.

CHECKPOINT QUESTIONS

3. Why does a technique such as imagery work better for children to reduce the sensation of pain?
4. How do the techniques of thought stopping and substitution of meaning differ?

PHARMACOLOGIC PAIN RELIEF

Pharmacologic pain relief refers to the administration of a wide variety of analgesic medications. Many children need analgesic agents in addition to nonpharmacologic techniques for pain relief, especially for acute pain. Medications can be applied topically, or given orally, intramuscularly, intravenously, or by epidural injection. As a rule, intramuscularly administered analgesia should be avoided if possible.

Topical Anesthetic Cream

To reduce the pain of procedures such as venipuncture, lumbar puncture and bone marrow aspiration, two local anesthetic creams (EMLA, consisting of lidocaine and prilocaine, and TAC, consisting of tetracaine, adrenaline, and cocaine) are available (Zempsky & Karasic, 1997). EMLA can be easily obtained from local pharmacies. TAC is most frequently used in the emergency department. These are applied to the skin and covered with an occlusive dressing, such as Tegaderm or plastic wrap. EMLA must be applied at least 1 hour before an expected procedure (see Drug Highlight). Parents can apply EMLA cream at home before bringing a child to a clinic visit for a procedure such as bone marrow aspiration (Figure 17-5). Caution them not to allow the child to remove the dressing and eat the cream (it could anesthetize the gag reflex). It also is potentially dangerous if rubbed into the eyes. EMLA, the more frequently used cream, has changed procedures such as blood drawing from painful procedures to procedures to which children can submit without experiencing pain. A disadvantage of EMLA cream is that a procedure must be anticipated by at least 1 hour for the medication to be effective. However, it can be applied up to 3 hours before a procedure and still be effective. A number of research studies have been conducted to evaluate its efficiency in reducing the pain of circumcision at birth. It has been shown to be efficient and safe for this use (Taddio et al, 1997).

DRUG HIGHLIGHT

EMLA Cream

Action: EMLA is a topical analgesic cream containing lidocaine and prilocaine, which acts to anesthetize skin before potentially painful procedures.

Pregnancy risk category: B

Dosage: Dollop of cream to intended skin site for at least 1 hour before procedure (2 to 3 hours before deeper procedures such as lumbar puncture or bone marrow aspiration)

Possible adverse reactions: Possible hypersensitivity

Nursing Implications:

- Explain to the child that the cream will help take the hurt away.
- Apply a dollop of cream to the intended site and cover with a transparent occlusive dressing at least 1 hour before the procedure. Do not spread cream or rub it in.
- If the cream is to be applied at home, instruct the parents how to apply the cream and the occlusive dressing. Suggest that the parents use plastic wrap, such as Saran wrap for the occlusive dressing.
- Instruct the child not to touch the dressing while it is in place. If necessary, cover the occlusive dressing with an opaque material to prevent the child from touching or playing with the dressing.
- Just before the procedure, remove the dressing and then wipe the skin to remove cream.
- Observe the skin. Look for reddened or blanched skin, which indicates that the drug has penetrated the skin.
- Do not use the drug for a child with a known history of sensitivity or allergy to local anesthetics such as lidocaine.
- Know that the drug is not approved for use in infants under 1 month of age.

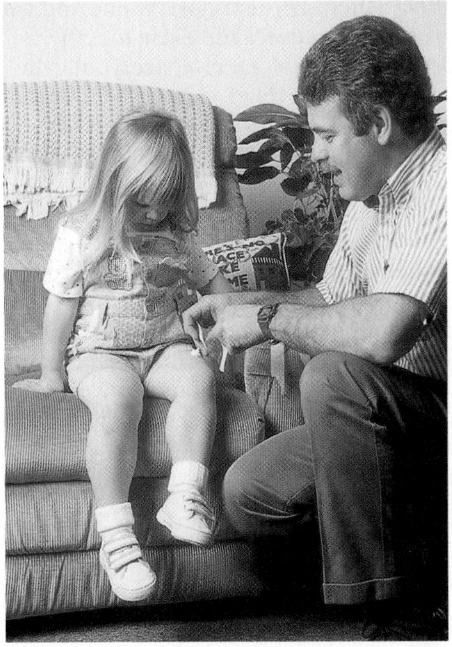

FIGURE 17.5 A father applies EMLA cream at home prior to a painful procedure.

WHAT IF? What if a child is scheduled to have a bone marrow aspiration at 10:00 and, to prepare for this, you apply EMLA cream at 9:00, but the surgeon who is going to do the aspiration arrives early? Would you ask the surgeon to wait for the hour, or explain to the child that the cream isn't going to work?

Oral Analgesia

Oral analgesia is advantageous because it is cost-effective and relatively easy to administer. Analgesia can be adequately achieved if correct dosing is given. Many analgesics can be prepared as elixirs or suppositories for children unable to swallow pills.

Over-the-counter analgesics, such as acetaminophen (Tylenol) are flavored deliberately to make them taste good. Caution parents about this. Reinforce with them the need for proper storage (locked or out of the child's reach). Otherwise, children may help themselves to more when the parent leaves the room. Toxicity from too frequent or too large doses of acetaminophen can lead to severe liver damage in children. The rule of safe medicine administration never to refer to medicine as "candy" applies here.

Nonsteroidal anti-inflammatory drugs (NSAIDs) are excellent for reducing the pain that accompanies inflammation in injuries such as sprained ankles or rheumatic conditions. They also are effective in reducing bone pain. Drug examples include ibuprofen and naproxen. Long-term administration of any NSAID can lead to severe gastric irritation. Help parents giving any analgesia around the clock for a number of days to make out a medication sheet to hang on their refrigerator door. This both reminds them when the next dose is due and alerts them not to give the drug doses too close together.

Children should not receive acetylsalicylic acid (aspirin) for routine pain relief, especially in the presence of flulike symptoms. There is an association between aspirin administration and the development of Reye's syndrome (see Chapter 28).

For managing severe or acute pain, such as postoperatively or with sickle-cell crises, opioids, such as morphine, codeine, and hydromorphone (Dilaudid), are the drugs of choice. Codeine is often given in combination with acetaminophen. Because this class of drugs is also referred to as narcotics, parents may be reluctant to give their children these medications, concerned that their child will become addicted. Acknowledge their concern and reassure them that the risk for addiction is remote. Reinforce that the main concern is supplying adequate pain relief for their child.

Intramuscular Injection

Few analgesics for children are given by intramuscular injection. This route is associated with pain on administration and also produces great fear in children. It is associated with a number of risks including uneven absorption, unpredictable onset of action and nerve and tissue damage. Other routes should be used whenever possible.

✔ CHECKPOINT QUESTIONS

5. Can a child's pain management program include both nonpharmacologic and pharmacologic methods of pain management?
6. Why is the intramuscular route infrequently used to administer analgesia to children?

Intravenous Administration

Intravenous administration is the method of choice for administering an analgesic in emergency situations, in the child with acute pain because it is the most rapid-acting route, and in children requiring frequent doses of analgesia but who are unable to use the gastrointestinal tract. Common opioids given by this route include morphine, fentanyl and hydromorphone (Dilaudid). They can be given by bolus injection or by continuous infusion. If doses will be added periodically to an IV line, advocate the use of an intermittent infusion device (a heparin lock) to avoid repeated venipunctures with each new dose.

If a child's pain is frequent or constant, continuous IV administration may be used. When the child is able to take medications by mouth, oral forms of analgesics should be administered. It is important that, when changing from IV to oral medications, equianalgesic doses be used. As needed (prn) dosing should be avoided because it leads to inconsistent administration.

All opioids have the potential to decrease respiratory rate. Other side effects include nausea, pruritus, vasodilatation, cough suppression and constipation. If toxicity with opioids should occur, naloxone (Narcan) can be administered to counteract the effects of the toxicity.

Hydromorphone is eight to ten times stronger than morphine but very similar to morphine in action. Fentanyl has a shorter duration of action than morphine. Side effects of pruritus and vasodilatation are less. These features make it an ideal drug to use for short painful procedures such as debriding a burn or inserting a chest tube to relieve a pneumothorax.

Patient-Controlled Analgesia

Patient-controlled analgesia (PCA) is a form of administration that allows a child to self-administer IV opiate boluses with a medication pump. Children as young as 5 or 6 years may be able to assess when they need a bolus of medicine and press the button on the pump that will deliver the new dose to an established IV line. Parents or a nurse can administer a new dose to children younger than this. Morphine is a common analgesic used for PCA administration (McNeely & Trentadue, 1997). The pump is set so that after each dose the pump will not release further medication even if the button is pushed again (a lockout time). Thus a child cannot overmedicate himself. If the pain is constant, a continuous infusion should be used so pain relief is not lost while the child is sleeping. The pump can still be programmed for bolus dosing to cover episodes of increased pain.

Conscious Sedation

Conscious sedation refers to a state of depressed consciousness obtained by IV analgesia therapy (Figure 17-6). The technique allows the child to be both pain free and sedated for a procedure. Unlike the child under general anesthesia, protective reflexes are left intact, and the child is able to respond to instructions during the procedure. The technique is used for procedures such as extensive wound care; bone marrow aspiration, which is potentially very painful; procedures such as magnetic res-

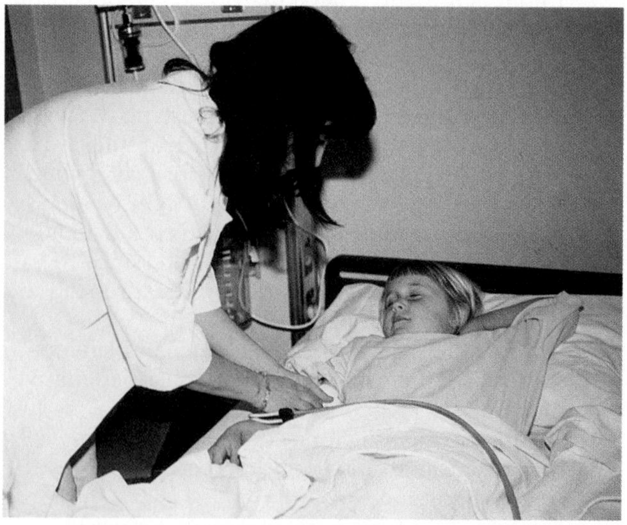

FIGURE 17.6 The nurse monitors the vital signs of a child who has received conscious sedation.

onance imaging that require a child to lie still for a long period of time; and endoscopy, which is both potentially frightening and requires the child to lie still for a period of time (Landrum, 1997). In many health care settings, conscious sedation is administered and monitored by nurses, specially prepared in the technique. Drugs commonly used for conscious sedation include a combination of pentobarbital sodium (Nembutal), which produces sedation, and midazolam and fentanyl, which provide relief of both anxiety and pain.

Intranasal Administration

Midazolam (Versed) is a short-acting adjuvant sedative that can be administered intranasally by nasal drops or nasal spray (Ljung & Andreasson, 1996). (It may also be administered intravenously.) It may be used for sedation before surgery and procedures such as nuclear medicine scanning. It has a very short duration of action and may require readministration. Because midazolam has no analgesic action, analgesia, such as with morphine, should be added if the procedure is painful.

Local Anesthesia

Children can receive local anesthetic injections (lidocaine) before procedures such as bone marrow aspiration and peritoneal dialysis. For many children, the sight of the anesthetic needle is so frightening that they are unable to listen to the assurance that the momentary needle stick of the anesthetic will prevent further pain. The use of EMLA cream before the injection relieves the needle stick pain and allows the anesthetic to numb the deeper tissues.

Epidural Analgesia

Epidural analgesia, injection of an analgesic agent into the epidural space just outside the spinal canal, can be used to provide analgesia to the lower body for 12 to 24 hours. An opioid often combined with a long-acting anesthetic is instilled continuously or administered intermittently. When used, opiate receptors in the spinal cord are affected directly, providing analgesia without the undesirable effects that would occur when opiate receptors in the brain would be affected. Children who have spinal fusion, for example, may have an epidural catheter inserted in the operating room and may receive analgesia by this method (Kester, 1997). This can be a very effective route of analgesia in the postoperative child in the first few days.

Some parents may be reluctant to allow this type of analgesia because they equate it to spinal anesthesia, which can be followed by severe headaches. They can be assured that an epidural needle does not enter the cerebral spinal fluid so this will not occur.

ONGOING PAIN RELIEF

Be certain children who begin a pain management program in a health care setting are provided with support and follow-up pain management. Otherwise, lack of pain relief at home can be overwhelming.

Oral analgesia in the home setting may be needed. Parents need instruciton on dosing, administration, frequency, and expected outcomes and level of relief. Provide them with the name and number of a health care professional that they can call about pain management. Earlier discharge and the increased use of outpatient surgery necessitate adequate pain management in the home setting.

✓ CHECKPOINT QUESTIONS

7. Does conscious sedation provide analgesia or just sedation?
8. Does epidural analgesia lead to spinal headaches?

KEY POINTS

Many children and infants are undermedicated for pain relief because of common misperceptions by health care personnel, such as infants do not feel or remember pain. Inviting parents and the child, if preschool age or older, to participate in assessment and pain management is an important aspect of pain therapy.

Pain in children is best assessed by means of a standardized self-report tool such as the Poker Chip or FACES tool. Without self-report forms, both nurses and parents may underestimate children's pain. Nurses should choose tools and become very familiar with their use.

Many children benefit from a combination of nonpharmacologic and pharmacologic methods of pain management.

Many nonpharmacologic pain relief measures such as imagery, distraction, and TENS are based on the theory of gate control.

Few analgesics are administered intramuscularly to children. IV administration is the method of choice for the child with acute pain. Patient-controlled analgesia, commonly used to administer morphine, can be used effectively with children.

Conscious sedation is useful for short procedures. Protective reflexes are left intact, and the child is able to respond to instructions during the procedure.

CRITICAL THINKING EXERCISES

1. Robin is the 3-year-old girl you met at the beginning of the chapter. She was given IV morphine in the emergency room an hour ago for a burn on her

hand. Her mother asks you now if Robin can have some more, not because her pain has returned, but because the mother wants to give it before the pain comes back. Is this mother's assessment of her child's pain apt to be accurate? Would this be the best intervention for Robin?
2. A 6-year-old girl is scheduled for daily debridement of a pressure ulcer, a very painful procedure. She screams before the procedure begins. What type of analgesic management should be used? How should the child's anxiety be addressed?
3. A fellow nurse tells you that she does not use self-report tools with children; she feels they take the place of her nursing judgment. You like to use rating scales. How would you justify your view? What types of approaches could be used to change staff behavior about pain management?

REFERENCES

Agency for Health Care Policy and Research. (1992). *Acute pain management in infants, children, and adolescents: operative and medical procedures*. Washington, DC: DHHS.

Beyer, J., Denyes, M., & Villarruel, A. (1992). The creation, validation, and continuing development of the Oucher: a measure of pain intensity in children. *Journal of Pediatric Nursing, 7*(5), 335.

Colwell, C., Clark, L., & Perkins, R. (1996). Postoperative use of pediatric pain scales: children's self report vs nurse assessment of pain intensity and affect. *Journal of Pediatric Nursing, 11,* 375.

Department of Health and Human Services. (1995). *Healthy people 2000: midcourse review.* Washington, DC: DHHS.

Hamers, J. P. et al. (1998). Are children given insufficient pain-relieving medication postoperatively? *Journal of Advanced Nursing, 27*(1), 37.

Hester, N. O., & Barcus, C. S. (1986). Assessment and management of pain in children. *Pediatrics: Nursing Update, 1*(14), 2.

Jordan-Marsh, M. et al. (1994). Alternate Oucher form testing: gender, ethnicity, and age variations. *Research in Nursing and Health, 17*(2), 111.

Kester, K. (1997). Epidural pain management for the pediatric spinal fusion patient. *Orthopaedic Nursing, 16*(6), 55.

Krechel, S. W. & Bildner, J. (1995). CRIES: a new neonatal postoperative pain measurement score. *Paediatric Anesthesia, 5*(1), 53.

Landrum, L. (1997). Conscious sedation in the endoscopy setting. *Critical Care Nursing Clinics of North America, 9*(3), 355.

Ljung, B., & Andreasson, S. (1996). Comparison of midazolam nasal spray to nasal drops for the sedation of children. *Journal of Nuclear Medicine Technology, 24*(1), 32.

McCaffery, M. & Pasero, C. L. (1997). Pain ratings: the fifth vital sign. *American Journal of Nursing, 97*(2), 15.

McNeely, J. K., & Trentadue, N. C. (1997). Comparison of patient-controlled analgesia with and without nighttime morphine infusion following lower extremity surgery in children. *Journal of Pain and Symptom Management, 13*(5), 268.

Melzack, R., & Wall, P. (1965). Pain mechanisms: a new theory. *Science, 150,* 971.

Merkel, S. I., et al. (1997). Practice applications of research: the FLACC: a behavioral scale for scoring postoperative pain in young children. *Pediatric Nursing, 23*(3), 293.

Pederson, C., Matthies, D., & McDonald, S. (1997). A survey of pediatric critical care nurses' knowledge of pain management. *American Journal of Critical Care, 6*(4), 289.

Rutledge, D. N., & Donaldson, N. E. (1997). *Pain assessment and documentation, part III.* Glendale, CA: CINAHL Information Systems.

Savedra, M. C., Tesler, M. D., Holzemer, W. L., & Ward, J. (1992). *Adolescent pediatric pain tool: user's manual.* San Francisco: University of California-San Francisco.

Seymour, E. et al. (1997). Modes of thought, feeling and action in infant pain assessment by pediatric nurses. *Journal of Pediatric Nursing, 12*(1), 32.

Sutters, K. A., & Miaskowski, C. (1997). Inadequate pain management and associated morbidity in children at home after tonsillectomy. *Journal of Pediatric Nursing, 12*(3), 178.

Taddio, A., et al. (1997). Efficacy and safety of lidocaine-prilocaine cream for pain during circumcision. *New England Journal of Medicine, 336*(17), 1197.

Wong, D., & Baker, C. (1996). *Reference manual for the Wong-Baker FACES Pain Rating Scale.* Duarte, CA: CHNMC.

Zempsky, W. T., & Karasic, R. B. (1997). EMLA versus TAC for topical anesthesia of extremity wounds in children. *Annals of Emergency Medicine, 30*(2), 163.

SUGGESTED READINGS

Caty, S., et al. (1995). Assessment and management of children's pain in community hospitals. *Journal of Advanced Nursing, 22*(4), 638.

Corbett, J. V. (1995). Pharmacopoeia: EMLA cream for local anesthesia. *MCN: American Journal of Maternal Child Nursing, 20*(3), 178.

Deady, A., & Gorman, D. (1997). Intravenous conscious sedation in children. *Journal of Intravenous Nursing, 20*(5), 245.

Hodgins, M. J., & Lander, J. (1997). Children's coping with venipuncture. *Journal of Pain & Symptom Management, 13*(5), 274.

Jonas, D., & Day, A. (1997). Assessing pain in children. *Community Nurse, 3*(10), 23.

Pasek, T. (1997). Controlling pain: assessing pediatric pain. *Nursing, 27*(8), 18.

Phillips, P. (1995). Neonatal pain management: a call to action. *Pediatric Nursing, 21*(2), 195.

Twycross, A. (1997). Nurses' perceptions of pain in children. *Paediatric Nursing, 9*(1), 16.

Warnock, F. F. & Lander, J. (1998). Pain progression, intensity and outcomes following tonsillectomy. *Pain, 75*(1), 37.

Zeigler, V. L., & Brown, L. E. (1997). Conscious sedation in the pediatric population: special considerations. *Critical Care Nursing Clinics of North America, 9*(3), 381.

UNIT

4

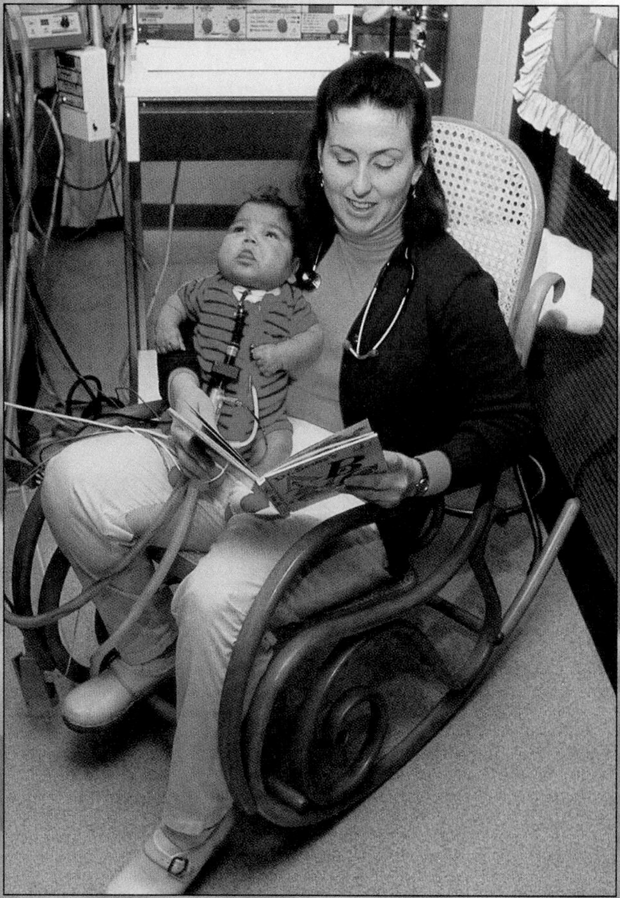

The Nursing Role in Restoring and Maintaining the Health of Children and Families With Physiologic Disorders

Nursing Care of the Child Born With a Physical Developmental Disorder

18

CHAPTER

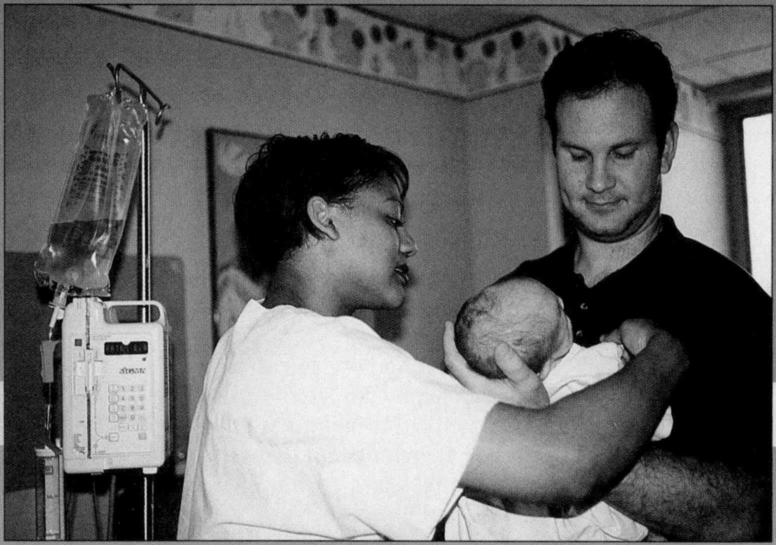

Key Terms

- ankyloglossia
- atresia
- cleft lip
- cleft palate
- developmental hip dysplasia
- fistula
- frenulum
- hydrocephalus
- meconium plug
- omphalocele
- polydactyly
- spina bifida
- stenosis
- syndactyly
- transillumination
- volvulus

Objectives

After mastering the contents of this chapter, you should be able to:

1. Describe common physical birth disorders.
2. Assess a newborn who is born physically challenged.
3. Develop nursing diagnoses for the child born with a physical developmental disorder.
4. Establish outcomes to meet the needs of the child with a physical developmental disorder.
5. Plan nursing care to meet the established outcomes of care for the child born with a physical developmental disorder.
6. Carry out nursing interventions in the care of children born with physical developmental disorders, such as preventing infection in the child with spina bifida.
7. Evaluate outcome criteria to determine achievement and effectiveness of care.
8. Identify National Health Goals related to children born with physical disabilities that nurses could be instrumental in helping the nation achieve.
9. Identify areas related to developmentally challenged infants that could benefit by additional nursing research.
10. Use critical thinking to analyze the impact of a developmentally challenged child on the family and propose ways to make care more family centered.
11. Integrate knowledge of congenital physical anomalies with the nursing process to achieve quality child health nursing care.

Mrs. Sparrow is a 29-year-old woman whose baby was admitted to the intensive care unit because of a diaphragmatic hernia. Mrs. Sparrow is obviously upset over the diagnosis. She asks you why the intestine would have herniated into the chest. If the diaphragm is incomplete, does it mean the baby has other incomplete parts as well? Most important, could this have happened from the cough medicine she took during pregnancy? How would you answer Mrs. Sparrow? What type of advice would be most helpful to her?

In previous chapters, you learned how important it is to assess all infants at birth. In this chapter, you'll add information about common congenital anomalies, structural disturbances and genetic disorders that may be assessed in children. This information is important both as the basis for newborn assessment and also as the basis for health teaching for parents.

After you've studied the chapter, turn to the Critical Thinking Exercises at the end of the chapter to sharpen your skills and test your knowledge.

Few things, other than maternal hemorrhage during delivery, can change the usually expectant, joyous tone of a birthing room faster than the birth of a baby with a developmental defect. Physicians or nurse-midwives, who are used to saying "perfect boy" or "beautiful girl" and holding up the infant for the parents' first glance, are suddenly without words. The nurse is in the same predicament. Words of congratulations hang, unsaid, in the air.

When a child is born with an apparent physical developmental defect, nurses play an even bigger role in supporting and educating the parents. Some disorders are easily repaired; others require surgery but the prognosis is good; some disorders, however, represent serious, even life-threatening problems for the infant, possibly resulting in long-term care needs. This chapter covers the physical congenital disorders that are apparent at birth or soon after. Such disorders primarily involve the gastrointestinal, neurologic, and skeletal systems. Congenital disorders of the cardiovascular system, which also represent life-threatening problems for the infant, are addressed in Chapter 20. National Health Goals related to children with congenital anomalies are shown in the Focus on National Health Goals box.

FOCUS ON NATIONAL HEALTH GOALS

Many congenital anomalies such as omphalocele and spinal cord defects can be detected during intrauterine life. The following National Health Goal addresses the importance of prenatal care and counseling:

- Increase to at least 90% the proportion of women enrolled in prenatal care who are offered screening and counseling on prenatal detection of fetal abnormalities.

Another National Health Goal emphasizes the importance of the coordination of services for complex disorders such as cleft lip and palate:

- Increase to at least 40 from a baseline of 25 states that have an effective system for recording infants with cleft lip and palate and referring them to craniofacial anomaly teams (DHHS, 1995).

Nurses can be instrumental in helping the nation achieve these goals by ensuring that appointments for follow-up care or further diagnosis made at prenatal visits or in the newborn period are arranged at times convenient for parents so that such visits are kept.

Additional nursing research in this area is needed concerning what factors determine which women will continue their pregnancy after a congenital anomaly is discovered in their fetus; how far is reasonable to ask parents to travel for follow-up care for a newborn; and what measures do parents feel were most helpful to them at the time of a fetal or newborn anomaly diagnosis.

NURSING PROCESS OVERVIEW

for Care of the Physically Challenged Child

Assessment

Nursing assessment of the physically challenged child, a child born with a physical defect, focuses on determining the child's immediate physiologic needs required to sustain life and the parents' immediate emotional needs to promote bonding between child and parents. Evaluate how the anomaly affects the infant's eight primary needs:

- Establishment and maintenance of adequate respiration
- Establishment of extrauterine circulation
- Establishment of body temperature control
- Ability to take in adequate nourishment
- Establishment of waste elimination
- Prevention of infection
- Development of an infant–parent bond
- Exposure to adequate stimulation

The parents' response to the diagnosis of a congenital defect must also be assessed. Anomalies that affect the child's appearance may have the most immediate effect on the parents' ability to establish a positive feeling about their child. It is important, however, not to jump to conclusions about parents' responses. Assessment of the family's verbal and nonverbal responses must be as thorough and objective as assessment of the infant's health status.

Nursing Diagnosis

Many nursing diagnoses established for children born with congenital anomalies address their effect on body function, including the child's primary needs and also on family interaction. The following diagnoses are examples:

- Altered nutrition, less than body requirements, related to inability to take in adequate nutrition secondary to physical defect
- Impaired physical mobility related to congenital anomaly

FOCUS ON CULTURAL COMPETENCE

The cause of most congenital anomalies is unknown, although they probably arise from a combination of environmental and genetic factors. Still, many people persist in believing that infants with congenital anomalies are born to people less deserving than others or who have sinned or have been looked on by someone with envy during pregnancy. Eating raisins during pregnancy causes brown spots and strawberries cause hemangiomas are beliefs that still proliferate. New parents need a chance to talk about why they believe their child's disorder occurred, to relieve their guilt that they were the cause and allow them to regain sufficient self-esteem to be able to parent a child with a congenital disorder.

The way that parents carry infants may contribute to the formation of hip dysplasia. Infants who are carried straddled on their parents' hips the way Latino American mothers carry their infants may have less hip dysplasia than those carried with their legs consistently brought together such as Native American infants carried by swaddling boards.

- Risk for altered parenting related to birth of child with anomaly
- Anticipatory grieving (parental) related to loss of "perfect" child

Outcome Identification and Planning

When establishing outcomes and planning care, be certain to consider both the short- and long-term needs of the newborn and how these needs may affect the family. Also, consider the family's resources—both emotional and financial and devise a plan of care with these in mind. A parent or parents with supportive family members nearby may be able to accept the limits of a child's disorder and turn their attention to the planned treatment regimen or care priorities sooner than those without close friends or relatives to whom they can turn for comfort and support. For the latter, you may need to act not only as a source of information and support but also as a sounding board and advocate until the parents can begin to develop positive coping mechanisms that will help them come to terms with this unexpected turn of events. Referrals for support groups may also be beneficial, allowing parents to learn that they are not alone in this situation.

Implementation

Nursing interventions for the newborn with a physical anomaly include immediate life-sustaining measures such as providing for adequate intake of nutrients when a defect prevents the infant from sucking. Educating the parents regarding pre- and posttreatment procedures and encouraging them to hold, touch, and talk with their babies are especially important to the future emotional well-being of the child and family.

Parents may have difficulty caring for a child with a congenital anomaly because they suffer a loss of self-esteem at the child's birth. They feel as if the baby is proof that something in the combination of their genes or the prenatal environment they provided was inadequate (see Focus on Cultural Competence). They need to hear positive comments about themselves and be given support until they can realize that by caring for the child they are accomplishing more—not less—than other couples.

Parents can be expected to move through the same stages of grief as those whose child has died at birth.

Parents are acutely aware of what people think of their children. They watch closely how the nurse or unlicensed assistive personnel handle their baby to see if he or she is giving as much attention to their baby as to other babies (see Managing and Delegating Unlicensed Assistive Personnel). It is important for the baby with an anomaly, and for the parents' acceptance of their child, to treat the child with an anomaly in the same manner as any other child, for example, rocking the baby after feeding and cooing and talking to the baby as much as with the other babies in the nursery. Otherwise, parents may think that if a professional finds their child distasteful, how will they dare show the child to their family and friends? If a nurse is able to look past the anomaly to the whole child, however, they begin to do so, too. Through positive role modeling, a nurse is setting the stage for healthy parent–child interaction every time he or she handles an infant born with a congenital anomaly.

Parents may also need the assistance of support groups and community organizations. The following

MANAGING AND DELEGATING UNLICENSED ASSISTIVE PERSONNEL

Unlicensed assistive personnel may be assigned to care for newborns and infants with congenital physical anomalies because they are able to manage the routine care of these children, such as bathing and feeding. Be certain they are aware how important it is to handle these infants the same as other infants. Reinforce the need for rocking, cooing, and gentle talking with the infants as much as possible. In addition, ensure that they are aware of the need for close monitoring of the child, even with routine care, such as measuring an infant's head circumference accurately. They also need to recognize the danger signs in the newborn and infant such as failure to pass meconium, bile-colored vomitus, and abdominal distention because these are frequently associated with some of the most common anomalies that occur.

organizations may be helpful sources of support for parents:

National Easter Seal Society
70 East Lake Street
Chicago, IL 60601

Spina Bifida Association of America
4590 MacArthur Boulevard
Suite 250
Washington, DC 20007

American Cleft Palate-Craniofacial Association
1218 Grandview Avenue
Pittsburgh, PA 15211

Outcome Evaluation

Evaluation should focus on outcomes established for the child's physical health and developmental needs, as well as the family's ability to cope with whatever special care and growth needs the child may have in the future. Be sure parents have numbers to call for questions, follow-up care, and support.

Outcome criteria may include:

- Child is ambulatory with walker in 3 months.
- Parent voices positive features of child by 2 weeks.
- Parents voice they accept talipes anomaly as a correctable condition by 1 month.

RESPONSIBILITIES OF THE NURSE AT THE BIRTH OF AN INFANT WITH A PHYSICAL ANOMALY

Most physicians and nurse-midwives believe that relating the news of congenital physical anomalies to parents is their responsibility. However, because the physician or nurse-midwife must deliver the placenta and suture the perineum if an episiotomy was used for birth, if a neonatal specialist is not immediately available, many minutes may pass before this person is ready to make a second inspection of the baby, assess the extent of the anomaly from the physical symptoms present, and tell the parents about the defect and the baby's prognosis. This delay affects the parents in two ways: It leaves them believing for that time either that they delivered a perfect child among people who do not share their enthusiasm or they have just given birth to a child so deformed that all the professionals in the room find it too horrible to even talk about. Because parents are aware of the atmosphere in a birthing room, the second response is by far more likely. In terms of parent–child interaction, this response is unhealthy. Parents begin anticipatory grieving for a deformed child. Even when they are told later that the defect is not extensive, is easily correctable, and that as soon as the correction is made the child will be perfect, the anticipatory grief reaction may be hard to stop. They may continue to cut themselves off emotionally from the child.

Nurses should be familiar enough with the most frequently encountered physical anomalies that they can make truthful statements and explain the problem to parents. This transfer does not represent "passing the buck" by physicians. Rather, the responsibility then falls to the person who at that moment in the delivery process is free to assume it. If a physician does not feel comfortable in allowing a nurse to take on this role, the nurse must be ready to serve as a back-up informant, to answer the parents' questions after being told that their child has been born less than perfect. It is probably best to explain to parents what the defect is and what the prognosis for the defect is before showing the baby to them. Parents may find it hard to look at an infant with a cleft lip or palate or exposed abdominal contents and also listen. Their minds are so consumed with the visual image their eyes are sending them, so unlike the child of their imagination, that they cannot hear. Provide, for example, the following explanation:

"Your baby's upper lip isn't completely formed. That's called a cleft lip. Your doctor will call one of the plastic surgeons here to look at your baby. This is a problem that can be repaired so well surgically that you'll barely be able to tell your baby had this problem. I'll bring the baby over so you can see her. Remember when you look at her that this can be repaired. She seems perfect in every other way."

These statements define and limit the problem for the parents. They also give them direction about where and how they should proceed in beginning to seek help for their child.

ANOMALIES OF THE GASTROINTESTINAL SYSTEM

Many of the most common congenital anomalies involve the gastrointestinal system. The gastrointestinal tract forms first as a solid tube, then undergoes canalization. If this subsequent canalization does not occur, a blockage or obstruction will occur. Other defects of the tract, such as cleft lip and cleft palate, are the results of midline closure failure extremely early in intrauterine life.

Ankyloglossia (Tongue-Tie)

Ankyloglossia is an abnormal restriction of the tongue caused by a tight **frenulum,** the membrane attached to the lower anterior tip of the tongue. Most children adapt well to this condition, but if it causes speech problems later on or if the condition places destructive pressure on gingival tissue, surgical release may be performed. Because parents may be concerned, even if surgery is not indicated, they need a thorough explanation of the normal appearances of newborns' tongues. Normally the frenulum is short and near the tip of the tongue, but as the anterior portion of the tongue grows, the frenulum becomes located farther back. Showing them other newborns or photographs of normal tongues is helpful in convincing them that a short frenulum is normal. Explore with them why they are concerned. Is there a child in the family with a speech defect or a cleft lip and palate? Do the parents need assurance in any other way that their child is all right?

Thyroglossal Cyst

A *thyroglossal cyst* arises from an *embryogenic fault* (a persistent opening to the anterior surface of the neck that did not close normally). It may be a dominantly inherited trait.

A cyst may form at the base of the tongue, possibly involving the *hyoid bone* (the bone at the anterior surface of the neck at the root of the tongue), or containing aberrant thyroid gland tissue. As the cyst becomes filled with fluid, the obstruction can cause respiratory difficulty. If infected, the cyst becomes swollen, appears reddened, and drains mucus or pus from the anterior neck (Kuint et al, 1997).

Treatment is surgical removal of the cyst to avoid future infection of the space or, if thyroid tissue is present, the possibility of carcinoma. Observe infants closely in the immediate postoperative period for respiratory distress, because the operative area will have some nearby edema. Position such children on their sides so secretions drain freely from their mouths. Intravenous fluid therapy is given after surgery until the edema at the incision recedes somewhat and swallowing is safe once more (approximately 24 hours). If the mother is breastfeeding, encourage her to express her milk manually to preserve her milk supply. Observe infants closely the first few times they take fluid orally to be certain they do not aspirate. Be certain parents feed them before they are discharged from the hospital to make sure they can see the infant swallowing safely. This is important to their development of confidence in themselves as parents and their ability to feed the infant at home in a relaxed and comfortable way.

Cleft Lip and Palate

The fusion of the maxillary and median nasal processes normally occurs between weeks 5 and 8 of intrauterine life. In infants with **cleft lip,** the fusion fails in varying degrees, with the defect ranging from a small notch in the upper lip to a total separation of the lip and facial structure up into the floor of the nose. Upper teeth and gingiva may be absent. The nose is generally flattened because the incomplete fusion of the upper lip has allowed it to expand in a horizontal dimension. The deviation may be unilateral or bilateral. Cleft lip is more prevalent among males than females. It occurs at a rate of approximately 1 in every 1000 live births (Smith, 1996).

Cleft lip demonstrates a familial tendency or most likely occurs from the transmission of multiple genes. It is twice as prevalent in the Japanese population. It occurs rarely in African Americans. Formation may be aided by teratogenic factors present during weeks 5 to 8 of intrauterine life such as avitaminosis or viral infection. Parents of a child with a cleft lip should be referred for genetic counseling to ensure they understand that future children are at a greater risk than usual for this problem.

The palatal process closes at approximately weeks 9 to 12 of intrauterine life. A **cleft palate,** an opening of the palate, is usually on the midline and may involve just the anterior hard palate, or the posterior soft palate, or both (Figure 18-1). It may be a separate anomaly but as a rule occurs in conjunction with a cleft lip. As a single entity, it tends to occur more frequently in females than males. Like cleft lip, it appears to be the result of polygenic inheritance or environmental influences such as maternal smoking (Kallen, 1997). In connection with cleft lip, the incidence is approximately 1 in every 1000 births. As a single entity, it occurs in approximately 1 in every 2500 births.

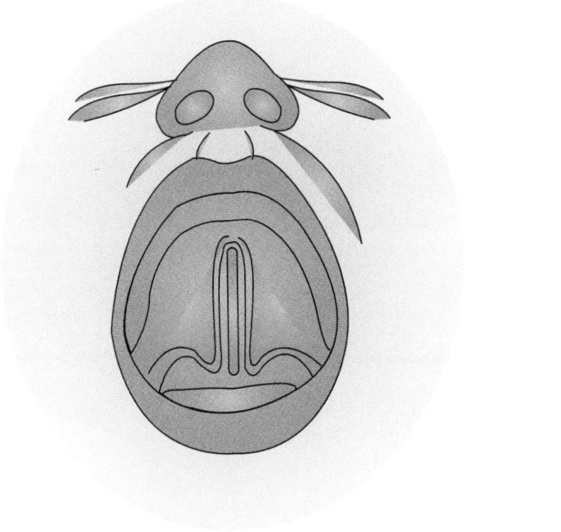

FIGURE 18.1 Appearance of a cleft palate. Both the hard and soft palate are involved.

Assessment

Cleft lip is readily apparent on inspection at birth. Cleft palate can be determined by depressing the tongue with a tongue blade. This reveals the total palate and the extent of a cleft palate. Be sure to have good lighting to visualize the palate clearly. Because cleft palate is a component of many syndromes, a child with a cleft palate must be assessed for other congenital anomalies that would suggest it is only one of a combination of problems.

Therapeutic Management

Cleft lip may be detected by sonogram while the infant is in utero. The condition can even be repaired by fetal surgery at this early time. In most children, it is not discovered until birth. A cleft lip is repaired surgically shortly after birth, sometimes at the time of the initial hospital stay and sometimes between 2 and 10 weeks. Because the deviation of the lip interferes with nutrition, infants may be a better surgical risk at birth than they are after a month or more of poor nourishment. Early repair also helps infants experience the pleasure of sucking as soon as possible. It is equally important from a psychological standpoint that these disorders be repaired early. Parents may find it extremely difficult to bond with an infant whose face is deformed in this way. This is not a sign of a "bad" parent. It is reality and a problem that should be dealt with as realistically as the actual oral construction.

The repair of cleft palate is usually postponed until the child is 18 to 24 months old. It is postponed until the anatomic change in the palate contour that occurs during the first year of life has taken place (Gorlin, 1997). Repairs made before this change (the palate arch increases) may be ineffective and have to be repeated.

Currently, the results of surgical repair of cleft lip and cleft palate are excellent (Figure 18-2). It is helpful to show parents photographs of babies with good repairs to assure them that their child's outcome can also be good. The older term for this condition, "harelip," should not be used when talking with parents about the problem. Be-

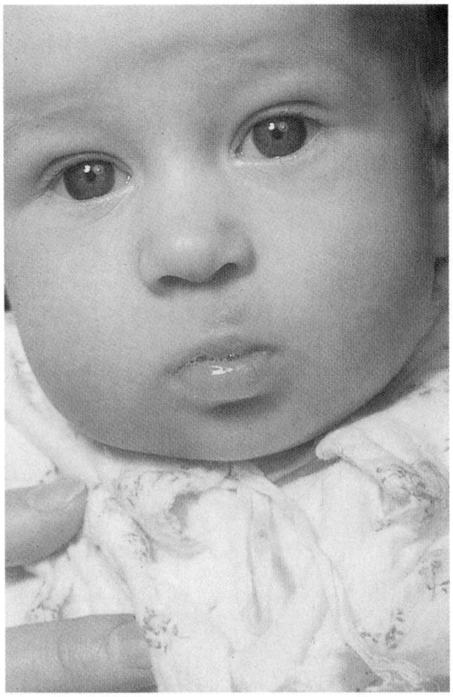

FIGURE 18.2 Infant showing surgical repair of cleft lip. Parents can be encouraged that the results of cleft lip repair are generally excellent.

fore modern surgical techniques were available, children were left with large lip scars, gross speech impediments, and a poor appearance after surgery. Harelip tends to be associated with these negative outcomes rather than with the current positive outlook.

Some infants with a cleft lip have an accompanying deviated nasal septum, which may need to be repaired in later years for good air exchange. Because palate repair narrows the upper dental arch or because the original cleft may have involved the dental arch, there may be less space in the upper jaw for the eruption of teeth, causing a defect in teeth alignment. These children need follow-up treatment by a pedodontist or a dentist skilled in children's dental problems so that, as the children grow, extractions or realignment of teeth can be done as indicated.

NURSING DIAGNOSES AND RELATED INTERVENTIONS

Nursing Diagnosis: Risk for altered nutrition, less than body requirements, related to feeding problems caused by cleft lip or palate

Outcome Identification: Child will demonstrate adequate nutritional intake until anomalies are fully repaired.

Outcome Evaluation: Child will ingest a diet of 50 kcal/lb in 24 hours; weight is maintained within 10% of birth weight.

Preoperative Period. Before a cleft lip or palate is repaired, feeding the infant is a problem because the infant has difficulty maintaining suction. Despite this, the child must take in an adequate amount of food and also be prevented from aspirating.

It may be possible for an infant with a cleft lip to breastfeed, because the bulk of the breast tends to form a seal against the injured upper lip. Although the baby needs the enjoyment of sucking, some surgeons do not want the baby to breastfeed or suck on a nipple before surgical correction of the defect to avoid any local bruising of tissue. The best feeding method for the child with cleft lip may be to support the baby in an upright position and feed the child gently by a commercial cleft lip nipple. Be careful when feeding these infants. A hurried approach can easily cause the infant to aspirate. A Breck feeder, an apparatus similar to a bulb syringe, may also be used. Newer devices, such as the Haberman feeder, may be used as well (Figure 18-3). If the surgical repair will be done immediately, the mother will be able to breastfeed as early as 7 to 10 days after surgery. Teach her how to pump or manually express breast milk to maintain a milk supply for this time. If surgery will be delayed for 1 month, she will need to decide whether she wants to continue to express milk for this period of time; if she chooses to do so, she may need continuing support and encouragement from the nursing staff.

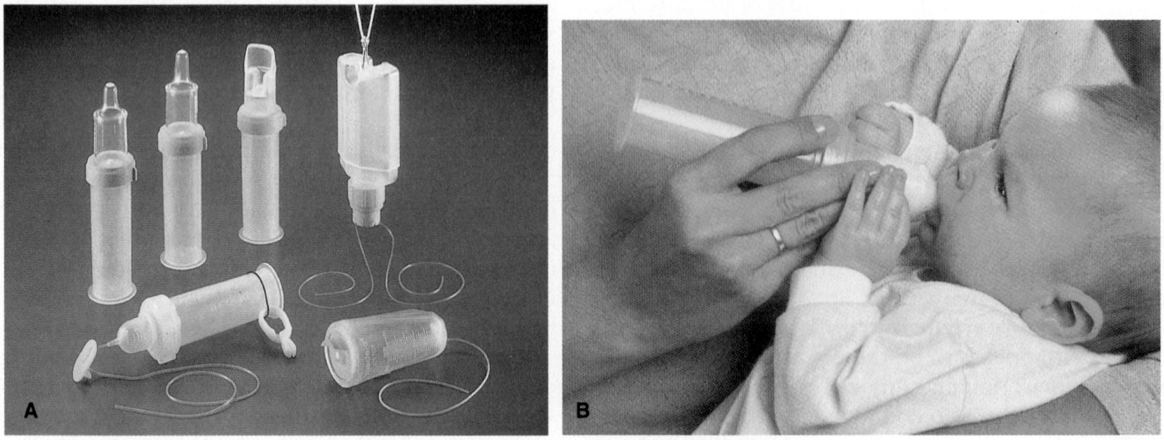

FIGURE 18.3 (**A**) Specialty feeding devices used for infants with cleft lip and cleft palate. (**B**) An infant uses a Haberman Feeder™.

The infant with a cleft lip needs to be held and bubbled well after feeding because of the tendency to swallow air caused by the inability to grasp a nipple or syringe edge securely with the mouth. If the cleft extends to the nares, the infant will breathe through the mouth; the mucous membrane becomes dry and the infant's lips may become dry, too. Small sips of fluid between feedings may keep the mucous membrane moist and prevent cracks and fissures that could lead to infection.

Infants with cleft palate cannot suck effectively either, because pressing their tongue or a nipple against the roof of their mouth would force milk up into their pharynx and cause aspiration. The most successful method for feeding this infant, then, like the child with cleft lip, is to use a commercial cleft palate nipple with an extra flange of rubber to close the roof of the mouth. The nipple can be used with a plastic bottle that can be squeezed gently to increase the flow of the feeding to the infant's mouth to compensate for poor sucking. A Breck feeder may also be used.

If surgery is delayed beyond age 6 months or the time solid food is introduced, teach parents to be certain food offered is soft. Particles of coarse food could invade the nasopharynx and cause aspiration. Infants whose surgery is delayed to this point can be fitted with plastic palate guards to form a synthetic palate and help prevent this.

Postoperative Period. After surgery for both cleft lip and palate, the infant is kept on nothing-by-mouth (NPO) status for at least 4 hours. The infant is introduced to liquids (plain water) at the end of this time; begin the process gradually to prevent vomiting.

No tension should be placed on a lip suture line to keep sutures from pulling apart and leaving a large scar. Bottle- or breastfeeding is contraindicated during this immediate postoperative period. The infant is usually fed using a Breck feeder.

After palate surgery, liquids are generally continued for the first 3 or 4 days, then a soft diet is given until healing is complete. Learn from parents what fluids the child prefers so they will be available postoperatively.

After a cleft palate repair, when the child begins eating soft food, he or she should not use a spoon, because the child will invariably put it against the roof of the mouth and possibly disrupt sutures. If being fed evokes an intense reaction, it is better to leave the child on a liquid diet, including milkshakes or concentrated formulas, until the sutures are removed. Be certain milk is not included in the first fluids offered because milk curds tend to adhere to the suture line. After a feeding, offer the child clear water to rinse the suture line and keep it as clean as possible.

Nursing Diagnosis: Risk for ineffective airway clearance related to oral surgery

Outcome Identification: Child's airway will remain patent.

Outcome Evaluation: Child's respiratory rate is between 20 and 30 respirations per minute without retractions or obvious distress.

Because of the local edema that occurs after cleft lip or palate surgery, observe children closely in the immediate postoperative period for respiratory distress. Before surgery, the infant with a cleft lip breathed through the mouth. After surgery, the infant now has to breathe through the nose, possibly adding to respiratory difficulty. Generally, however, this is not a problem because newborns normally are strict nose-breathers.

Infants may need suction to remove mucus, blood, and unswallowed saliva. Be gentle and do not touch the suture line with the catheter. After cleft lip surgery, *do not* lie infants on their abdomen. Doing so puts pressure on the suture line, possibly tearing it. Position them on their side or, as soon as awake, in an infant chair.

Nursing Diagnosis: Impaired tissue integrity at incision line related to cleft lip/cleft palate surgery

Outcome Identification: Child's incision will heal without signs or symptoms of infection or trauma.

Outcome Evaluation: Incision line is clean and intact, free of erythema or drainage during postoperative period.

The suture line is held in close approximation by a *Logan bar* (a wire bow taped to both cheeks; Figure 18-4) or an adhesive bandage such as a Band-Aid simulating a bar that approximates the incision line but does not cover the incision. The Logan bar or Band-Aid-simulated bar must be checked after each feeding or cleaning of the suture line to be certain it is secure and protecting the suture line. The infant should not be allowed to cry, because crying increases tension on the sutures. This means having to anticipate the infant's needs. Have formula ready to feed the infant on demand—do not wait until after the infant is awake and crying. Use whatever measures, such as rocking, carrying, or holding, are necessary to make the child feel secure and comfortable. He or she also will need to be bubbled well after a feeding because there is a tendency to swallow more air than the average infant. This tendency is due to the non-sucking method of feeding used.

Nothing hard or sharp must come in contact with the cleft suture line. Observe infants after palate repair carefully to be certain they do not put toys with sharp edges into their mouths. Use elbow restraints as necessary to reduce the risk. They should not use a straw to drink nor should they brush their own teeth—they will certainly brush the suture line accidentally. Keep elbow restraints

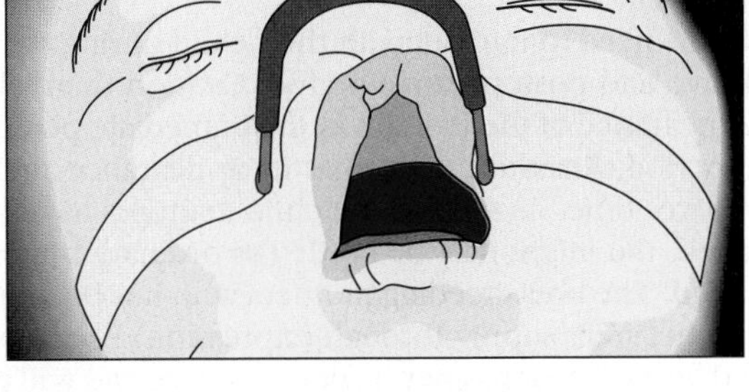

FIGURE 18.4 A Logan bar is an apparatus that may be used to protect the surgical incision for a cleft lip repair.

in place so they do not put their fingers in their mouth and poke or pull at the sutures. Most children run their tongues over their sutures because of the odd feeling in the roofs of their mouths, and most children this age do not respond to a caution not to do this. Because this often occurs when children have nothing to think about, provide diversional activities such as reading, singing to them, and showing them things out the window.

Acetaminophen (Tylenol) may be given to keep children comfortable. Keeping infants content after cleft palate repair is much more difficult than keeping a newborn quiet after cleft lip repair, because the older child is more aware of the strange hospital surroundings. They need a great deal of attention, holding, and active play. Encourage parents to stay in the hospital with them if at all possible. If the procedure is performed as 1-day surgery, be certain parents are aware of their responsibility to protect suture lines at home until healing is complete.

Nursing Diagnosis: Risk for infection related to surgical incision

Outcome Identification: Infant will remain free of infection during postoperative period.

Outcome Evaluation: Infant's temperature is below 37°C axillary; incision site is clean, dry, and intact without erythema or foul drainage.

Infection, and subsequent severe scarring, may result if crusts are allowed to form on a cleft lip suture line. Clean the suture line with a sterile solution such as sterile water, sterile saline, or 50% hydrogen peroxide in sterile water and sterile cotton-tipped applicators after every feeding and whenever the normal serum that forms on suture lines accumulates. Apply the solution in a smooth, gentle rolling motion. Do not rub because this can loosen sutures. If hydrogen peroxide is used (usually half strength), it will foam as it reacts with the protein particles at the suture line. Rinse the area with sterile water afterward. Dry the suture line with a dry cotton-tipped applicator. Remember that the infant has sutures on the inside of the lip that need the same meticulous care as those visible on the outside.

Nursing Diagnosis: Risk for altered parenting related to infant's congenital anomaly

Outcome Identification: Parents will demonstrate acceptance of infant by 48 hours postoperatively.

Outcome Evaluation: Parents voice a belief in a positive outcome for child; they demonstrate positive coping behaviors, evidenced by holding and helping with infant care.

Parents need to interact with their child during the preoperative and postoperative period. Caution them about the appearance of the incision in the immediate postoperative period. Reassure them that its appearance will improve over time. As soon as the child's sutures have been removed, the infant may be bottle (an ordinary bottle) or breastfed. The breastfeeding mother (who has been maintaining her milk supply through expression) needs assurance that the infant has never sucked before and will need time to learn, just as a newborn does. The infant may have an equally difficult time learning to suck from a bottle.

Notice whether the parents look at their baby's face while feeding the baby. Help them to understand that any negative feelings directed toward the child or themselves, such as sadness or anger that their baby was born this way, are normal. This does not instantly make them feel better about the child, but the knowledge that what they are experiencing is normal will help them begin to deal with such emotions. Many communities have support groups for parents of children born with a cleft lip or palate. Referral to these groups can be helpful.

Nursing Diagnosis: Risk for self-esteem disturbance related to facial surgery

Outcome Identification: Child will demonstrate age-appropriate self-esteem.

Outcome Evaluation: Child participates in normal childhood activities that involve contact with other people; states activities he or she enjoys at health care visits; demonstrates age-appropriate developmental milestones.

If a scar remains after cleft lip surgery, the child may need some help with adjusting to it. Explaining that what is inside people is more important than what shows on the surface may be helpful to strengthen self-esteem. As children reach adolescence, the inheritance pattern of cleft lip may need reviewing so adolescents are informed of the possible risk of transmission to their own children.

Nursing Diagnosis: Risk for infection (ear) related to altered slope of eustachian tube with cleft palate surgery

Outcome Identification: Child experiences few to no middle ear infections during childhood.

Outcome Evaluation: Parents state possible signs and symptoms of ear infection; state importance of early treatment; parents list signs of hearing loss.

Changing the contour of the palate also changes the slope of the eustachian tube to the middle ear. This can lead to a high incidence of middle ear infection (otitis media). Parents of children with a cleft palate must be alert to the signs of infection (e.g., fever, pain, pulling on the ear, or discharge from the ear). They need to report pharyngeal infection to their primary care provider so it can be treated promptly before spread to the middle ear can occur. Because the eustachian tube may remain partially closed owing to its changed position, serous otitis media, or accumulation of fluid in the middle ear, also tends to occur more frequently in these children than in others. The child needs routine screening for hearing loss during childhood, because this is a sign of serous otitis media. Parents should be cautioned to watch for signs of hearing loss (after being made aware that all children seem deaf when they are watching television or involved in play).

Nursing Diagnosis: Risk for altered pattern of communication related to cleft palate

Outcome Identification: Child will communicate clearly enough to make needs known by 2 years.

Outcome Evaluation: Family members voice satisfaction with child's speech; developmental milestone of two-word sentences by age 2 years is met.

Infants with a cleft palate will begin to make speech sounds at the normal time (age 2 months); their speech may be guttural and harsh; at age 9 months, when other children begin to say meaningful words ("bye-bye," "mama," "dada"), assuming the cleft palate is still unrepaired, their sounds will be unclear. Some parents try to discourage their baby from talking, thinking that if he or she does not talk until after the cleft palate repair is made, a speech impediment will not develop. Speech occurs at a specified developmental time, however, and, despite the unfused palate, should be encouraged at these age-appropriate times. The child with a cleft palate can enunciate vowel sounds with the most clarity, so these are the sounds a parent should encourage the child to voice. Words such as "me," "they," "no," "mama," "home," "moon," "rain," "yell," and "row" are words consisting largely of vowel sounds and thus can be enunciated by the child before the cleft palate repair.

Almost all children with cleft palates continue to have accompanying speech problems after the repair. The soft palate must function for the child to pronounce *p* and *b* sounds. If cleft palate surgery is going to be delayed much past age 2 years (as might happen if the child has other congenital anomalies, such as heart disease), a plastic prosthesis to cover the palate defect may be prescribed. This allows children to articulate more normally.

If children learned to speak in a defective manner before the repair, they generally continue to speak this way after repair. Speech training by a speech therapist is usually necessary. Children may be asked to perform blowing games, such as blowing a feather or a table tennis ball (a blowing motion is what is required to pronounce *p* and *b*). Children do not spontaneously outgrow bad speech patterns. Without therapy, they continue to speak into adulthood as if the cleft were still present. Speech therapy is an important follow-up measure, therefore, not a luxury. No repair can be considered successful if a child speaks incoherently afterward.

Pierre Robin Syndrome

The Pierre Robin syndrome is a triad of *micrognathia* (small mandible); cleft palate; and *glossoptosis* (a tongue malpositioned downward). It is an example of cleft palate occurring as only one of a syndrome of defects. Children with Pierre Robin syndrome may have associated disorders of congenital glaucoma, cataract, or cardiac disorders. They need thorough physical and genetic assessment to be certain that none of these associated disorders is present.

All infants with Pierre Robin syndrome need to be observed carefully to be certain they are free of airway obstruction (Perkins et al, 1997). They may need frequent nasopharyngeal suction to remove unswallowed saliva. Beginning with birth, children with this syndrome are apt to have episodes in which they have difficulty breathing because, due to the small jaw, their tongue is too large for their mouth. This causes it to drop backward and obstruct the airway. This is most noticeable when they are lying in a supine position. No infant with this syndrome, therefore, should be placed in a supine position; they are in grave danger of anoxia if left in this position and should be positioned on the side. Occasionally, infants have extensive airway obstruction; attaching a suture to the anterior aspect of the tongue and pulling it forward is used to give relief. This position can be maintained if the suture is attached to the mucous membrane of the lower lip (creating an artificial tongue-tied condition).

Feed these infants with the same care and concern given all children with cleft palate. A gastrostomy tube may be inserted to relieve feeding difficulty (see Chapter 16). As the child grows older, the jaw grows somewhat, although the mandible will always be small. Growth, coupled with a repair of the cleft palate, will decrease the respiratory problems.

Parents of the child with Pierre Robin syndrome take on a great deal of responsibility when first assuming the infant's care. They need a health care provider to call when they have questions about care. Many of these parents grow exhausted during the first few weeks of the child's life, afraid they may fall soundly asleep at night and miss their child having respiratory difficulty. As their confidence grows in their ability to provide care, this problem lessens, but it may be months or even years before a high level of confidence is achieved.

✔ CHECKPOINT QUESTIONS

1. In which sex is cleft lip more prevalent?
2. Would it be good technique to allow a child to drink fluid with a straw after a cleft palate repair?
3. Before surgery, why is feeding the infant with cleft lip a problem?

Tracheoesophageal Atresia and Fistula

Between weeks 4 and 8 of intrauterine life, the laryngotracheal groove develops into the larynx, trachea, and beginning lung tissue. The esophageal lumen also is formed. A number of anomalies may be found in infants if the trachea and esophagus are affected by some teratogen that does not allow the esophagus and trachea to separate normally.

The five usual types of esophageal atresia and **fistula** (opening) that occur (Figure 18-5) are:

1. The esophagus ends in a blind pouch; there is a tracheoesophageal fistula between the distal part of the esophagus and the trachea (Figure 18-5*A*).
2. The esophagus ends in a blind pouch. There is no connection to the trachea (Figure 18-5*B*).
3. A fistula is present between an otherwise normal esophagus and trachea (Figure 18-5*C*).
4. The esophagus ends in a blind pouch. A fistula connects the blind pouch of the proximal esophagus to the trachea (Figure 18-5*D*).
5. There is a blind end portion of the esophagus. Fistulas are present between both widely spaced segments of the esophagus and the trachea (Figure 18-5*E*).

These are serious disorders because, during a feeding, milk can fill the blind esophagus and overflow into the trachea or a fistula can allow milk to enter the trachea, re-

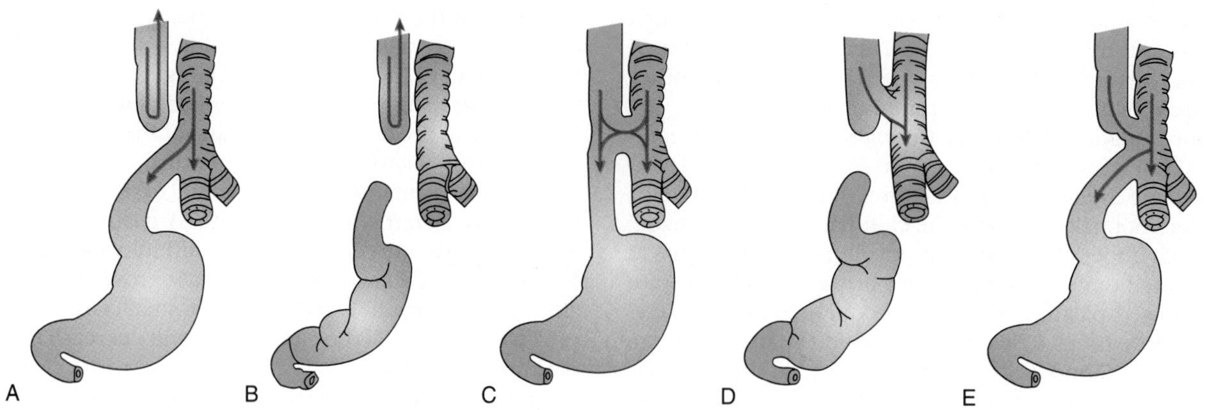

FIGURE 18.5 Esophageal atresia and tracheoesophageal fistula. (**A**) In the most frequent type of esophageal atresia, the esophagus ends in a blind pouch. The trachea communicates by a fistula with the lower esophagus and stomach (approximately 90% of infants with the defect have this type). (**B**) Both upper and lower segments end in blind pouches (5% to 8% of infants with the defect have this type). (**C**) Both upper and lower segments communicate with the trachea (2% to 3% of infants with the defect have this type). (**D**) Very rarely the upper segment ends in a blind pouch and communicates by a fistula to the trachea, or (**E**) a fistula connects to both upper and lower segments of the esophagus.

sulting in aspiration (Newman & Bender, 1997). The incidence of tracheoesophageal fistula is approximately 1 in 3000 live births.

Assessment

Tracheoesophageal atresia must be ruled out in any infant born to a woman with hydramnios (excessive amniotic fluid). A normal fetus swallows amniotic fluid during intrauterine life. The infant with a tracheoesophageal atresia cannot swallow, so the amount of amniotic fluid may thus become abnormally large. Many infants are born preterm because of the accompanying hydramnios, compounding the problem with immaturity. The infant needs to be examined carefully for other congenital anomalies that could have occurred from the teratogenic effect at the same week in gestation that caused the tracheoesophageal fistula, such as vertebral, anorectal, and renal disorders (VATER syndrome; Botto et al, 1997).

An infant who has so much mucus in the mouth that he or she appears to be blowing bubbles should be suspected of having tracheoesophageal fistula. The condition can be diagnosed with certainty if a catheter cannot be passed through the infant's esophagus to the stomach and stomach contents cannot be aspirated. Be certain to use a firm catheter because a soft one will curl in a blind-end esophagus and appear to have passed. If a radiopaque catheter is used, it can be demonstrated coiled in the blind end of the esophagus on x-ray. A flat plate x-ray of the abdomen may reveal a stomach distended with the air, which is passing from the trachea into the esophagus and stomach. Either a barium swallow or a bronchial endoscopy examination will reveal the blind-end esophagus and fistula. It is important that the condition be diagnosed before the infant is fed or, at this time, the infant will cough, become cyanotic, and have obvious difficulty in breathing as fluid is aspirated.

Therapeutic Management

Emergency surgery for the infant with tracheoesophageal fistula is essential to prevent pneumonia from leakage of stomach secretions into the lungs, dehydration, or electrolyte imbalance from lack of oral intake. A gastrostomy may be performed (under local anesthesia) and the tube allowed to drain by gravity to keep the stomach empty of secretions and prevent reflux into the lungs. Upper right lobe pneumonia from aspiration is one of the major complications of this disorder. Thus, antibiotics also may be started to prevent this complication.

Surgery consists of closing the fistula and anastomosing the esophageal segments. It may be necessary to complete the surgery in different stages and to use a portion of the colon to complete the anastomosis if the esophageal segments are far apart from each other. Leaks occurring at anastomosis sites are a common complication, most frequently at postoperative days 7 to 10 when sutures dissolve. Fluid and air leak out into the chest cavity, and *pneumothorax* (collapse of the lung) may occur.

In some infants, some stenosis or stricture at the anastomosis site occurs and necessitates esophageal dilatation at periodic intervals to keep the repaired esophagus fully patent. Gastroesophageal reflux may also occur. This can lead to recurrent fistula formation from the presence of stomach acid in the esophagus.

The ultimate prognosis for the child will depend on the extent of the repair necessary, the condition of the child at the time of surgery, and whether other congenital anomalies were present. If surgery can be performed on the child before pneumonia develops and the defect is amenable to surgical correction, the prognosis is good. However, the mortality rate for the condition remains high because of the presence of other congenital defects or low birth weight that often accompanies the tracheal defect.

NURSING DIAGNOSES AND RELATED INTERVENTIONS

Outcomes established for the child with tracheoesophageal fistula must be realistic in terms of the extent of the defect, the timing of anticipated surgery, and stage of grief or readiness for decision making and planning that the parents have reached.

Nursing Diagnosis: Risk for altered nutrition, less than body requirements, related to inability for oral intake

Outcome Identification: Child will ingest adequate nutrition during course of therapy.

Outcome Evaluation: Child will maintain weight within 10% of birth weight; will maintain weight in same percentile on growth curve.

Before surgery, because oral fluid cannot be given until the esophagus is repaired, intravenous therapy infusion supplies fluid and calories to the infant. This is continued for a time after surgery until the possibility of vomiting from the anesthetic is decreased. Then the infant is started on gastrostomy feedings. The glucose water or formula ordered for a feeding should be introduced into the tube slowly and allowed to run by gravity, never by pressure, to prevent it from entering the esophagus and putting pressure on the suture line. After the feeding, the end of the tube should be elevated, covered by sterile gauze, and kept in that position. It should not be clamped. In this way, air introduced during the feeding will bubble from the tube and not enter the esophagus and pass the fresh suture line. This also helps to ensure that, if the infant vomits the feeding, the vomitus will be projected into the gastrostomy tube and not contaminate the fresh sutures. Most newborns enjoy sucking a pacifier during gastrostomy feedings for sucking pleasure. If the mother wishes to breastfeed, she can manually express breast milk for the infant's gastrostomy feedings.

The infant may be given sips of clear fluid by mouth as early as the day after surgery, although some infants are kept NPO for 7 to 10 days until the suture line is healed. Early introduction of fluid may help to ensure patency of the esophagus, because it helps to decrease adhesions from the anastomosis and allows the infant the enjoyment and practice of sucking. The infant is introduced to a full oral fluid diet as soon as he or she begins to tolerate it and the suture line is healed. When the child is taking oral feedings satisfactorily, the gastrostomy tube is removed. If the child is to return home to await a second-stage operation, the gastrostomy tube will be left in place and the parents must be shown how to do gastrostomy feedings. If the gastrostomy tube is only a temporary measure for surgery, the parents do not need to learn the procedure. The parents' time with the child is better spent in holding him or her, gently stroking or talking to the child, and getting to know the child better.

Nursing Diagnosis: Risk for infection related to aspiration or seepage of stomach secretions into lungs

Outcome Identification: Child will remain free of infection during course of therapy.

Outcome Evaluation: Child's temperature remains below 37°C axillary; absence of rales on auscultation.

Preoperative Care. Before surgery, the infant should be kept in an upright position and on the right side to prevent gastric juice from entering the lungs from the fistula. Because the infant cannot swallow mucus, frequent oropharyngeal suctioning to prevent aspiration of collected mucus is necessary. A catheter may be passed into the blind-end esophagus and attached to low continuous or intermittent suction to keep this segment of the esophagus from filling with fluid and causing aspiration. Irrigation of the catheter may be necessary to keep it patent, because mucus tends to dry and plug it.

If surgery will be delayed, the infant may have a *cervical esophagostomy* (the distal end of the blind esophagus is brought to the surface just over the sternum so that mucus can drain). Use absorbent gauze around the opening to absorb moisture and prevent excoriation of the skin. Apply a protective ointment liberally to protect skin. A consult by a enterostomal therapy nurse may be needed.

Keeping the infant under a radiant heat warmer with a high-humidity oxygen source will both maintain body heat and liquefy bronchial secretions. The infant should be kept from crying to prevent air from entering the stomach from the trachea, distending the stomach, and thus causing vomiting into the lungs. A pacifier may help relax the baby and also satisfy the sucking need.

Postoperative Care. After surgery, because the chest cavity was entered for the repair, the infant will have one or two chest tubes in place. The posterior tube drains collecting fluid; the anterior tube allows air to leave the chest space, reexpanding the lung. Care of the child with chest tubes is discussed in Chapter 19.

Observe the infant closely for respiratory distress in the first few days after surgery. Continue to suction the child frequently because mucus tends to accumulate in the pharynx from surgery trauma. Suctioning must be done only shallowly, however, to prevent the suction catheter from touching the suture line in the esophagus. Oxygen and high humidity are needed to keep respiratory secretions moist. Turn the child frequently to discourage fluid from accumulating in the lungs. This turning and handling generally makes the child cry. Postoperatively, *crying helps expand lung tissue* (an older child or adult can be told to take deep breaths; the newborn cannot). An infant laryngoscope and endotracheal tube should be available at the bedside in case extreme edema develops and the infant's airway is obstructed.

Nursing Diagnosis: Risk for altered skin integrity related to gastrostomy tube insertion site

Outcome Identification: Child's skin will remain intact during course of therapy.

Outcome Evaluation: Child's skin remains clean and dry without erythema.

There is a possibility that gastric secretions may leak onto the skin from the gastrostomy site, irritating it because of the acid content of stomach secretions. Protect the skin by using a cream or commercial skin protector system. Consulting with an enterostomal therapy nurse can be helpful in reducing the possibility of skin irritation and breakdown.

Omphalocele

An **omphalocele** is a protrusion of abdominal contents through the abdominal wall at the point of the junction of the umbilical cord and abdomen. The herniated organs are usually the intestines, but they may include stomach and liver. They are usually covered and contained by a thin transparent layer of peritoneum. The deviation is evident on sonogram during pregnancy or at birth and reflects an arrest of development of the abdominal cavity at weeks 7 to 10 of intrauterine life. At approximately weeks 6 to 8 of intrauterine life, the abdominal contents are extruded from the abdomen into the base of the umbilical cord. Omphalocele occurs when there is failure of the abdominal contents to return to the abdomen (Figure 18-6).

Assessment

The incidence of omphalocele is as rare as 1 in 5000 live births. The child may have accompanying defects that also were caused by the teratogen insult that prevented normal intestinal growth. Most omphaloceles are diagnosed by prenatal sonogram (Dykes, 1996). If not, the presence of omphalocele is obvious on inspection at birth. Record its general appearance and its size in centimeters.

Therapeutic Management

Elastic bandaging to replace the omphalocele may be performed as conservative therapy (Belloli et al, 1996). Most infants will have immediate surgery to replace the bowel. If the defect is large, infants may be managed by topical application of a solution such as silver sulfadiazine to prevent infection of the sac, followed by delayed surgical closure. It is often difficult to replace the entire bowel immediately owing to the unusually small abdomen, which did not need to grow to accommodate the abdominal contents. If the total bowel were replaced, respiratory distress might result from the pressure of the visceral bulk on the diaphragm and lungs. For this reason, the bowel may be contained by a Silastic pouch that is suspended over the infant's bed and gradually over 5 to 10 days decreased in size as more bowel is gradually returned to the abdomen. During this time, the infant can be fed by total parenteral nutrition.

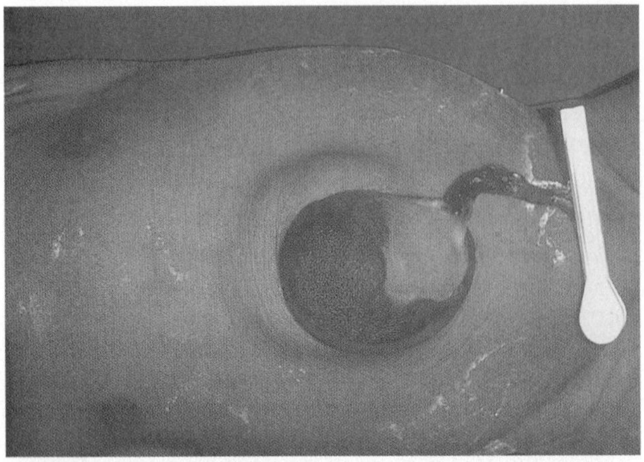

FIGURE 18.6 Omphalocele. This large example seen at birth contains intestine and liver.

NURSING DIAGNOSES AND RELATED INTERVENTIONS

Outcomes established must be realistic in terms of the extent of the defect, the timing of anticipated surgery, and stage of grief or readiness for decision making and planning that the parents have reached. Omphalocele is a shock to parents, being an anomaly that is obviously severe and yet one that is generally unknown.

Nursing Diagnosis: Risk for infection related to exposed abdominal contents

Outcome Identification: Child remains free of infection until repair is complete.

Outcome Evaluation: Child's temperature is below 37°C axillary; skin surrounding omphalocele is clean, dry and intact without erythema or foul drainage.

It is important that the lining of peritoneum covering the defect not be ruptured or allowed to dry out and crack. Otherwise, infection and malrotation of the uncontained intestine will complicate the surgical repair. Exposure of intestine to air causes a rapid loss of body heat. Immediately, place the baby in a warmed isolette. Do not leave infants under a radiant heat source because this will quickly dry the exposed bowel. To keep the sac moist, cover it with either sterile saline-soaked gauze or a sterile plastic bowel bag until surgery. The saline used must be at body temperature. Applying cold saline will lead to a decreased body temperature because so much intestinal surface is involved. Prepare to insert a nasogastric tube to prevent intestinal distention.

The prognosis for a final successful surgical repair is good. After this, the child with an omphalocele will be the child his or her parents once envisioned, with the exception of a rather large abdominal scar. Even then, if the scar is a problem for the child in later life, plastic surgery can reduce the scar's appearance.

Nursing Diagnosis: Risk for altered nutrition, less than body requirements, related to exposed abdominal contents

Outcome Identification: Child's nutritional intake will be adequate for needs during course of treatment.

Outcome Evaluation: Child's weight remains within 10% of birth weight; skin turgor is good; specific gravity of urine is between 1.003 and 1.030.

The child must not be fed orally or suck on a pacifier until the repair is complete. Doing so would distend the exposed bowel with food or air and make the return to the abdomen more difficult. Some infants have an accompanying **volvulus,** a twisting of the bowel causing obstruction, which is another reason to omit oral feedings. After surgery, the infant is maintained on total parenteral nutrition. Once the final stage of bowel repair is completed, a normal infant diet can be introduced gradually. Observe infants carefully for signs of obstruction (e.g., abdominal distention, constipation or diarrhea, or vomiting) when they begin eating.

Infants with omphalocele will be hospitalized or receive home care for a long time (a minimum of 1 or 2 months) waiting for a second-stage or even a third-stage operation. If the infant is hospitalized, parents need to be encouraged to visit frequently. The infant needs to be furnished age-appropriate toys for stimulation.

Many parents believe that surgeons can do anything and are distressed that their child's operation is being done in such small stages. They need support to accept that this treatment method is the best way to manage this type of intestinal disorder.

Gastroschisis

Gastroschisis is a condition similar to omphalocele, except that the abdominal wall defect is a distance from the umbilicus and abdominal organs are not contained by peritoneal membrane but rather spill from the abdomen freely (Langer, 1996). It occurs at a higher than usual rate in infants of teenagers (Nichols et al, 1997). A greater amount of intestinal content tends to herniate, which increases the potential for volvulus and obstruction. The surgical procedure is the same as for omphalocele. Children with gastroschisis often have decreased bowel mobility and, even after surgical correction, they may have difficulty with absorption of nutrients and passage of stool.

✔ CHECKPOINT QUESTIONS

4. What is the chief danger of a tracheoesopheal fistula?
5. What is the most important consideration in the care of the child with an omphalocele at birth?

Intestinal Obstruction

If canalization of intestine does not occur in utero at some point in the bowel, an **atresia** (complete closure) or **stenosis** (narrowing) of the bowel can occur. The most common site for this is the duodenal bowel portion.

Obstruction may occur because of a twisting (rotation or volvulus) of the mesentery of the bowel as the bowel reenters the abdomen after being contained in the base of the umbilical cord early in intrauterine life, or because of severe twisting of the mesentery due to the looseness of the intestine in the abdomen of the neonate (this continues to be a problem for the first 6 months of life). Obstruction can also occur because of thicker than usual meconium formation.

Assessment

Intestinal obstruction may be anticipated if the mother had hydramnios during pregnancy (amniotic fluid could not be digested effectively) or if more than 30 mL of stomach contents can be aspirated from the newborn stomach by catheter and syringe at birth. If the obstruction is not revealed by either of these findings, then symptoms of intestinal obstruction in the neonate are the same as at any other time in life: the infant passes no meconium or may pass one stool (meconium that formed below the obstruction) and then halt; the abdomen becomes distended. As the effect of the obstruction progresses, the infant will vomit. Obstructions are rare above the ampulla of Vater, the junction of the bile duct with the duodenum, so vomitus will be bile stained (greenish). Because meconium is black, vomitus may also be dark. Bowel sounds increase with obstruction owing to the increased peristaltic action as the intestine attempts to pass stool through the point of obstruction. Waves of peristalsis may be apparent across the abdomen. The infant may evidence pain by crying—hard, forceful, indignant crying—and by pulling the legs up against the abdomen. The child's respiratory rate will increase as the diaphragm is pushed up against the lungs and lung capacity decreases. An abdominal flat plate x-ray will reveal no air below the level of obstruction in the intestines. A barium swallow or barium enema x-ray film may be used to reveal the position of the obstruction.

WHAT IF? What if a nursing assistant tells you that a baby born with meconium staining 2 days ago is spitting up green mucus? Would it be safe to assume the nursing assistant is reporting meconium-stained mucus? Is there a possibility she is reporting a baby vomiting bile-stained emesis?

Therapeutic Management

If bowel obstruction is established, an orogastric or nasogastric tube is inserted and then attached to low suction or left open to the air to prevent further gastrointestinal distention from swallowed air (see Chapter 36). Always use low intermittent suction with decompression tubes in neonates. Pressure greater than this can break down the stomach lining.

The infant should be started on intravenous therapy to restore fluid, and immediate surgery is scheduled because bowel obstruction is an emergency that must be treated before dehydration, electrolyte imbalance, or aspiration of vomitus occurs.

Repair of the defect (with the exception of meconium plug syndrome) is done through an abdominal incision. The area of stenosis or atresia is removed, and the bowel is anastomosed. If the repair is anatomically difficult or the infant has other anomalies that interfere with overall health, a temporary colostomy may be constructed and the infant discharged to home care, with surgery rescheduled for age 3 to 6 months. Care of the child with a colostomy is discussed in Chapter 16. The final surgical procedure will restore the child to full health unless a large portion of the bowel had to be removed.

NURSING DIAGNOSES AND RELATED INTERVENTIONS

Nursing Diagnosis: Risk for fluid volume deficit related to vomiting

ENHANCING COMMUNICATION

Mr. Marlow's son was born with hydrocephalus. The infant is scheduled to have a ventriculoperitoneal shunt inserted this afternoon. You talk with Mr. Marlow before surgery.

Less Effective Communication

Nurse: Is there anything I can explain to you about your son's surgery, Mr. Marlow?
Mr. Marlow: No. I just want to see him back here with a smaller head.
Nurse: The shunt won't actually make his head smaller. Its purpose is to keep his head from growing any larger.
Mr. Marlow: What is the chance that he'll die in surgery?
Nurse: All surgery has a risk, certainly, but he should do well.
Mr. Marlow: But there is a chance he'll die in surgery?
Nurse: You're worrying over nothing. Why don't you relax and go for coffee until he gets back?

More Effective Communication

Nurse: Is there anything I can explain to you about your son's surgery, Mr. Marlow?
Mr. Marlow: No. I just want to see him back here with a smaller head.
Nurse: The shunt won't actually make his head smaller. Its purpose is to keep his head from growing any larger.
Mr. Marlow: What is the chance that he'll die in surgery?
Nurse: All surgery has a risk, certainly, but he should do well.
Mr. Marlow: But there is a chance he'll die in surgery?
Nurse: You sound more worried than I'd expect. Is there something specific you're worried about?
Mr. Marlow: I'd like him to die in surgery. How are we going to take care of a child with such a deformed head?
Nurse: I can't give you a simple answer for that. Let's sit down and talk about this some more.

Because surgical procedures are so safe today and the results of surgery for newborns are so successful, it is easy to begin to think of these anomalies as more inconvenient than serious. The infant, after all, will grow up with only a few minor problems. To a parent, however, the difference between a child born with one of these anomalies and the "perfect" child the parent envisioned can be great. Careful listening is necessary to appreciate the extent of a parent's understanding of the problem. Handling a problem by giving quick reassurance, as in the first scenario above, can lead to missing a parent's concern. Better listening, as in the second scenario, reveals the true problem.

Nursing Diagnosis: Risk for altered cerebral tissue perfusion related to increased intracranial pressure

Outcome Identification: Child will remain free of signs of increased intracranial pressure during childhood.

Outcome Evaluation: Child shows no increased temperature and blood pressure, or decreased pulse rate, decreased respiratory rate, or decreased level of consciousness, PERLA; muscle strength equal and strong bilaterally, head circumference is maintained at age-appropriate level.

After a shunting or laser surgery, the infant's bed is usually left flat or only slightly raised (approximately 30 degrees) so the head remains level with the body. If the child's head is raised excessively, CSF may flow too rapidly and decompression may occur too rapidly with possible tearing of cerebral arteries.

A valve in the shunt is inserted to open when cerebrospinal pressure fluid has increased owing to an accumulating bulk of fluid. It closes when enough fluid has drained to reduce the pressure. The surgeon who performed the shunting procedure will write specific orders about how often the infant is to be turned and to what side after surgery. Often infants are not turned to lie on the side with the shunt to prevent putting pressure on the valve, which might cause it to open and rapidly decompress.

It is important to assess for signs of increased intracranial pressure after surgery: tense fontanelles; increasing head circumference; irritability or lethargy; decreased level of consciousness; poor sucking; vomiting; an increase in blood pressure (difficult to measure accurately in infants unless Doppler instrumentation is used); increasing temperature; and a decrease in pulse and respiratory rates (see Chapter 28 for a neurologic assessment). Symptoms of infection (i.e., increased temperature, increased pulse rate, general malaise, and signs of meningitis such as a stiff neck and marked irritability) must also be assessed (see Empowering the Family). Be certain the child receives adequate pain management to decrease crying because crying elevates cerebral fluid pressure.

Nursing Diagnosis: Risk for altered nutrition, less than body requirements, related to increased intracranial pressure

Outcome Identification: Child will ingest an adequate nutritional intake after shunt placement.

Outcome Evaluation: Child's weight remains within 5th to 95th percentile on height/weight chart; no vomiting occurs.

Because an abdominal incision is involved to thread the catheter into the peritoneum, most children have a nasogastric tube placed during surgery. They are kept NPO until bowel sounds return postoperatively and the tube can then be removed. Introduce fluid gradually in small quantities after removal of the tube. Vomiting that results from the introduction of fluid too soon after any surgery causes increased intracranial pressure.

If possible, infants with hydrocephalus should be held when fed. Be certain to support infants' heads well when

Nursing Care Plan

THE CHILD WITH HYDROCEPHALUS

A 3-month-old infant with hydrocephalus is admitted to the acute care facility for insertion of a ventriculo-peritoneal shunt.

Assessment: 3-month-old infant whose head circumference has continued to increase since birth. Head circumference at birth was normal (40th percentile); increased to 60th percentile at 6 weeks of age and now increased to 80th percentile. Mother reports being placed on bedrest late in pregnancy for elevated blood pressure. Delivered vaginally without problems at 39 weeks. Newborn's Apgar score 9/10. Mother noted increasing irritability and lethargy over the last few weeks.

On examination, infant's head is enlarged, with widened and tense anterior fontanel. Scalp veins prominent. Eyes appear sunset. Parents report two episodes of forceful vomiting yesterday. "His cry is so high pitched and shrill and he hasn't been feeding well lately." Mother is breastfeeding. Afebrile. Blood pressure 100/40; pulse 100 beats per minute; respirations 16. Parents asking many questions about the surgery. "The doctor said he has to put in a shunt. That'll fix everything, right?"

Nursing Diagnosis: Altered cerebral tissue perfusion related to increased intracranial pressure from hydrocephalus

Outcome Identification: Infant will exhibit signs of adequate cerebral tissue perfusion prior to surgery.

Outcome Evaluation: Infant's vital signs within age-appropriate parameters; head circumference measurements are maintained at current level and begin to decrease; infant responds to auditory stimuli.

Interventions	Rationale
1. Assess infant's neurologic status closely, including response to sound, behavior, pupillary response, and motor and sensory function. Watch for increasing irritability or lethargy.	1. Assessment of infant's neurologic status provides a baseline for evaluating changes, allowing for early identification and prompt intervention. Irritability and lethargy are signs of increasing intracranial pressure.
2. Measure and record head circumference every 4 hours. Assess anterior fontanel for tenseness and bulging.	2. Head circumference, if increasing, or a tense, bulging fontanel indicates accumulating cerebrospinal fluid and increased intracranial pressure.
3. Position the infant with the head of the bed elevated 15 to 30 degrees and prevent hyperextension, flexion, or rotation of the head. Maintain head in a neutral position.	3. Elevating the head of the bed facilitates venous return, helping to reduce intracranial pressure.
4. Monitor vital signs frequently, every 1 to 2 hours.	4. Changes in vital signs, such as increased blood pressure, increased temperature, decreased respiratory rate, and decreased pulse rate, are clues to increasing intracranial pressure.
5. Administer oxygen as ordered. Have emergency equipment readily available.	5. Increased intracranial pressure can cause brain stem compression, which could result in respiratory or cardiac failure.
6. Monitor intake and output closely. Administer osmotic diuretic and corticosteroids as ordered.	6. Adequate hydration is necessary to ensure renal function. Overhydration may increase intracranial pressure. Osmotic diuretics act to pull water from the edematous tissue, decreasing intracranial pressure. Corticosteroids aid in reducing cerebral edema and thus, intracranial pressure.
7. Anticipate the need for a ventricular tap should the infant's condition begin to deteriorate.	7. A ventricular tap removes excess cerebrospinal fluid, thus decreasing intracranial pressure.

(continued)

Nursing Diagnosis: Risk for altered nutrition, less than body requirements, related to vomiting episodes and difficulty feeding secondary to increased intracranial pressure

Outcome Identification: Infant will exhibit signs of adequate nutrition.

Outcome Evaluation: Infant's weight remains within age-acceptable parameters; skin turgor is good; intake and output within normal limits; episodes of vomiting decrease; infant ingests adequate calories from breastfeeding.

Interventions	Rationale
1. Encourage mother to breastfeed infant if possible.	1. Breast milk is considered the optimal nutrition for an infant.
2. Assist mother with positioning the infant properly, supporting the head without flexion or hyperextension during feeding.	2. Breastfeeding promotes parent–child interaction and bonding. Proper positioning is important for latching on and also preventing neck vein compression, which could increase intracranial pressure.
3. Administer intravenous fluids as ordered. Assess intake and output closely. Check skin turgor and urine specific gravity every 4 hours.	3. Intake and output, skin turgor, and urine specific gravity provide valuable clues about the infant's hydration status and aid in identifying possible problems with fluid excess or overload.
4. Obtain daily weights.	4. Weight is a reliable indicator of overall fluid status.
5. If vomiting occurs, have the mother attempt to refeed the infant.	5. Refeeding helps maintain adequate fluid and nutritional intake.
6. If vomiting continues, anticipate the need for enteral or total parenteral nutrition.	6. Alternative methods may be necessary to ensure optimal nutrient intake if the infant is unable to tolerate oral feedings.

Nursing Diagnosis: Parental knowledge deficit related to hydrocephalus and shunt insertion

Outcome Identification: Parents will express accurate information about their infant's condition and scheduled procedure.

Outcome Evaluation: Parents describe hydrocephalus and how it affects their infant; identify measures used to treat the condition; state realistic expectations about their infant following shunt insertion.

Interventions	Rationale
1. Assess the parents' understanding of hydrocephalus and treatment measures.	1. Obtaining a baseline knowledge assessment provides a foundation on which to build future teaching strategies.
2. Review the structure and function of the brain and how hydrocephalus develops. Clarify any misconceptions.	2. Reviewing and clarifying aid in learning and strengthening understanding.
3. Provide ample time for questions and concerns.	3. Providing time for questions and concerns helps to clarify information, individualize teaching, and promote a feeling of trust and control.
4. Review with the parents what the physician has told them about the shunt insertion procedure, including why it is necessary, and what parents might expect to see after the surgery.	4. Review and reinforcement help to prepare the parents for events both before and after the surgery, thereby helping to minimize their anxiety.
5. Instruct parents about the appearance and care of their infant postoperatively, including the need for follow-up visits, monitoring for infection, and providing stimulation.	5. Instruction helps to prepare the parents for what will be required of them.
6. Assist parents with caring for the child as much as possible; offer positive reinforcement frequently.	6. Caring for the child promotes active participation and parent–infant bonding. Positive reinforcement enhances self-esteem and aids in coping.
7. Refer parents to support group of other parents of children with hydrocephalus. Anticipate the need for home care following discharge.	7. Support groups of other parents in similar situations promote sharing, decrease feelings of isolation and loneliness, and provide opportunities for further learning. Follow-up home care provides continuing support, guidance, and education.

EMPOWERING THE FAMILY: Caring for a Child With a Ventriculoperitoneal Shunt

- Observe for signs of increased intracranial pressure, such as drowsiness, vomiting, headache, irritability, and anorexia.
- Observe the pump site daily for any sign of swelling or redness.
- Have your child sleep with his head slightly elevated at night to help ensure fluid flow through the tube. Do not allow your child to fall asleep with his head hanging over the side of a couch or bed.
- Do not allow your child to become constipated, because hard stool might press against and obstruct the shunt. Encourage fruit, vegetables, cereal, and a generous amount of fluid in his diet.
- Do not call attention to the pump behind your child's ear; teach him not to touch the pump when he's nervous or as an attention-getting action.
- Be certain your child wears a helmet for tricycle and bicycle riding (as should all children) to avoid injury to the shunt. Otherwise, there are no special precautions that need to be taken for normal play.
- If your child develops signs of infection such as an increased temperature, telephone your primary care provider. This is probably a simple infection of childhood but could indicate an infected shunt.
- Be certain to keep your regularly scheduled health assessment visits. As your child grows taller, the shunt will eventually need to be replaced for proper functioning.

moving them. Hold their head with the whole palm, not just the fingertips, because the skull is thinned to some degree and could actually puncture with a stiff, forceful touch. Use a rocking chair with an armrest to provide support for your arm. Otherwise, the infant's head will be so heavy that you may not want to spend as much time holding the infant after the feeding as you might spend with other infants the same age. There is no reason why mothers cannot breastfeed the infant with hydrocephalus. Encourage them as you would any other mother.

Note how the child sucks. Increased intracranial pressure may be noted first because of poor or ineffective sucking. Vomiting after feeding, without nausea (difficult to detect in a small infant), is also a sign of increased intracranial pressure.

Observe for constipation, because straining at passing stool causes increased intracranial pressure. This is not usually a problem of infants who are totally breast- or formula-fed. It can be a problem when children return for shunt replacement at an older age. Urge parents to increase fluid and roughage in the diet to prevent this.

Nursing Diagnosis: Risk for altered skin integrity related to weight and immobility of head

Outcome Identification: Child's skin will remain intact during course of illness.

Outcome Evaluation: Child's skin remains clean, dry and intact without signs of erythema or ulceration.

The head of the infant with hydrocephalus is so heavy it cannot be moved freely. The skin of the head is stretched thin, and skin breakdown tends to occur on the pressure points. Wash the child's head daily. Change position of the head approximately every 2 hours so no portion of the head rests against the mattress for a long period. A foam rubber or synthetic sheepskin pad, an air, water or alternating air mattress may help to relieve pressure points. If a Kling or stockinette bandage is used to hold the head dressing from surgery in place, place a piece of gauze or cotton behind the child's ear before the bandage is applied to prevent skin surfaces from touching and becoming excoriated. Observe that the bandage does not become wet from oral secretions draining backward or shunt leakage.

Nursing Diagnosis: Knowledge deficit related to home care needs of child with hydrocephalus

Outcome Identification: Parents will demonstrate understanding of shunt placement and voice confidence in their ability to care for child by hospital discharge.

Outcome Evaluation: Parents state fears regarding ability to provide care; state signs of increased cranial pressure for which to watch; demonstrate competence in shunt care.

Caring for a child with a shunt in place is a continuing responsibility for parents. If parents do not seem to be asking many questions about the child's care after surgery, do not assume this is because they are taking the child's care in stride. They may be too frightened or too bewildered to ask questions. An opening such as "Most parents are a little frightened when they think about taking a child home with a shunt in place; do you feel that way?" gives them an opportunity to admit how they feel. For many people, being able to talk about a problem suddenly brings it down to manageable size. Talking about how frightened they feel about the responsibility will not immediately make them more comfortable with the child's care. However, it may make them more comfortable with their emotions. Assure them that health care providers caring for their child are interested in helping and supporting them.

If a valve is inserted in the shunt, it can be palpated below the skin just behind the ear. Parents must be certain that their child understands that this strange object is not to be felt continually. A child nervously fidgeting with a pressure pump can inadvertently evacuate CSF from the ventricles at a dangerously rapid rate.

Before an infant is discharged, be certain the parents have ample opportunity to feed and care for the child, so they can be comfortable and feel that they "know" him or her. Because irritability, lethargy, vomiting, and a change in the baby's cry are signs of increased intracranial pressure, the parents must report these symptoms immediately to their primary care provider. Before parents can report a change in the infant's disposition in this way, they must know the infant well. A referral for home care follow-up is often appropriate.

Nursing Diagnosis: Risk for altered growth and development related to potential neurologic impairment

Outcome Identification: Child will achieve developmental growth to the maximum of his or her potential.

Outcome Evaluation: Child demonstrates regular observable growth and achieves age-appropriate developmental milestones.

Remember that the mental functioning of a child with hydrocephalus may remain intact despite extreme thinning of the brain cortex. After a shunting procedure, the head may remain larger than normal but intelligence may be normal. Like all children, children with hydrocephalus need stimulation—to be talked to, smiled at, played with. If the child's head is enlarged, turning it to look at things around him or her is difficult. It may be necessary to reposition mobiles or pictures so the child receives adequate visual stimuli. Role-model talking and singing to the child to help parents more quickly include these actions in their care.

On the child's discharge from the hospital, be certain parents have a telephone number of the person they should call if they have a question or concern about the child's condition or care, and a referral for home care follow-up. They also need an appointment for the child's first checkup. This helps to assure them, again, that they are not being left alone just because they are leaving the hospital. Infection of the shunt is a possibility and a severe complication because it can lead to meningitis. If this should occur, parents should look for signs of increased intracranial pressure as well as those of infection, such as increased temperature. The child will be admitted to the hospital and administered intravenous antibiotics. An extraventricular shunt to promote drainage will be inserted. This allows antibiotics to be administered directly to the cerebral fluid and ensures that infected CSF is not draining to the peritoneal cavity where it could cause peritonitis.

As the child reaches preschool and school age, conference with the school nurse may be necessary to make him or her aware that the child has a shunt in place and that the child may need special head protection, if necessary, for sports activities.

✔ CHECKPOINT QUESTIONS

11. What changes in vital signs occur with increased intracranial pressure?
12. After a shunting procedure, how should the infant's bed be positioned?

Neural Tube Disorders

Because the neural tube forms in utero first as a flat plate and then molds to form the brain and spinal cord, it is susceptible to malformation. The term **spina bifida** (Latin for "divided spine") is most often used as a collective term for all spinal cord disorders, but there are well-defined degrees of spina bifida involvement, and not all neural tube disorders involve the spinal cord. All these disorders, however, occur because of lack of fusion of the posterior surface of the embryo in early intrauterine life. They can be compared with cleft palate or cleft lip—these are also closure defects.

The incidence has fallen dramatically in recent years from 3/1000 to 0.6/1000. No specific cause for many such disorders can be isolated, but poor nutrition, especially a diet deficient in folic acid, appears to be a major contributing factor. Pregnant women are advised to ingest 0.4 mg of folic acid daily to help prevent these disorders (CDC, 1995). Such disorders may occur as a polygenic inheritance pattern. The risk of bearing a second child with a neural tube defect once one child is born with such a defect increases to as much as 1 in 20. For this reason, women who have had one child born with a spinal cord defect are advised to have a maternal serum assay or amniocentesis of alpha-fetoprotein (AFP) levels to determine if such a defect is present in a second pregnancy (levels will be abnormally increased if there is an open spinal lesion). Serum assessment is done at week 15 of pregnancy when AFP reaches its peak concentration and is a routine test in many prenatal settings. If the result is elevated, an amniocentesis will be done to assess the level of AFP in amniotic fluid. A sonogram is also helpful to determine the presence of the defect.

Types of Defects

Anencephaly. *Anencephaly* is absence of the cerebral hemispheres. It occurs when the upper end of the neural tube fails to close in early intrauterine life. It is revealed by an elevated level of AFP in maternal serum or on amniocentesis.

Infants with anencephaly may have difficulty in labor, because the malformed head does not engage the cervix well. Many such infants present in a breech delivery position. On visual inspection at birth, the disorder is obvious (Figure 18-11). Children cannot survive with this disorder, because they have no cerebral function. Because the respiratory and cardiac centers are located in the intact medulla, however, they may survive for a number of days after birth.

When the condition is discovered prenatally, parents are offered the option of abortion. An ethical problem has arisen in a number of instances when parents, aware that the child cannot survive, elect to carry the infant to term so the organs can be used for transplant. Nurses need to think through their feelings about caring for such infants, because it can be difficult to give care to a child who will most likely die slowly or who has been born only to help others live.

Microcephaly. *Microcephaly* is a disorder involving brain growth so slow that it falls more than three standard

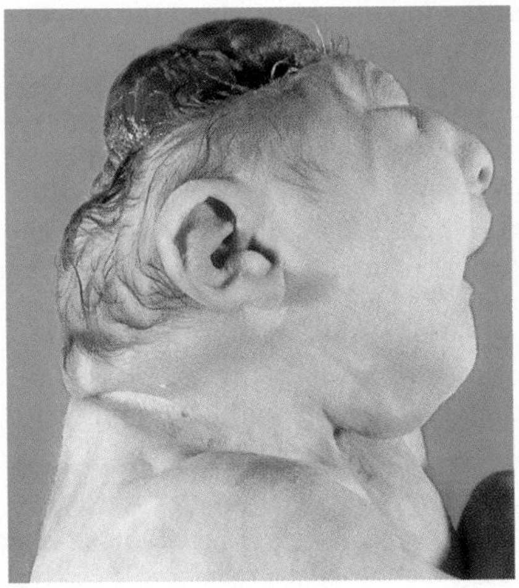

FIGURE 18.11 An infant with anencephaly.

deviations below normal on growth charts. The cause might be a defect in brain development associated with maternal phenylketonuria or an intrauterine infection such as rubella, cytomegalovirus, or toxoplasmosis. It is apparent at birth in these instances. Microcephaly may also result from severe malnutrition or anoxia in early infancy.

Microcephaly generally results in mental retardation because of the lack of functioning brain tissue. True microcephaly must be differentiated from *craniosynostosis* (normal brain growth but premature fusion of the cranial sutures), which also causes decreased head circumference. Infants with craniosynostosis have abnormally closed fontanelles and often show bulging (bossing of the forehead and signs of increased intracranial pressure). Such children must be identified, because with surgery, craniosynostosis can be relieved and brain growth will be normal.

The prognosis for a normal life is guarded in children with microcephaly and depends on the extent of restriction of brain growth and on the cause.

Spina Bifida Occulta. *Spina bifida occulta* occurs when the posterior laminae of the vertebrae fail to fuse. This occurs most commonly at the fifth lumbar or first sacral level but may occur at any point along the spinal canal. The normal spinal cord is shown in Figure 18-12*A*. The defect may be noticeable as a dimpling at the point of poor fusion; abnormal tufts of hair may be present (Figure 18-12*B*). Simple spina bifida occulta is a benign defect; it occurs as frequently as in one of every four children.

The term *spina bifida* is often used wrongly to denote all spinal cord anomalies. Because of this wrong usage, parents, when told that their child has a spina bifida occulta, may interpret this as meaning that the child has an extremely serious defect. Health professionals should use the terms correctly to reduce confusion.

Meningocele. If the meninges covering the spinal cord herniate through unformed vertebrae, a *meningocele* occurs. The anomaly appears as a protruding mass, usually approximately the size of an orange, at the center of the back (Figure 18-12*C*). It generally occurs in the lumbar region, although it might be present anywhere along the spinal canal. The protrusion may be covered by a layer of skin or only the clear dura mater.

Myelomeningocele. In a *myelomeningocele,* the spinal cord and the meninges protrude through the vertebrae defect the same as with a meningocele. The difference is that the spinal cord often ends at the point of the defect, so motor and sensory function is absent beyond this point (Figure 18-12*D*). Because this results in lower motor neuron damage, the child will have flaccidity and lack of sensation of the lower extremities and loss of bowel and bladder control. The infant's legs are lax, and he or she does not move them; urine and stools continually dribble because of lack of sphincter control. Children often have accompanying *talipes* (clubfoot) defects and subluxated hip. Hydrocephalus may accompany myelomeningocele in as many as 80% of infants; the higher the myelomeningocele occurs on the cord, the more likely hydrocephalus will accompany it. It is generally difficult to tell from the gross appearance whether it is myelomeningocele or the simpler meningocele (Figure 18-13).

Encephalocele. An *encephalocele* is a cranial meningocele or myelomeningocele. The defect occurs most often in the occipital area of the skull but may occur as a nasal or nasopharyngeal defect. Encephaloceles generally

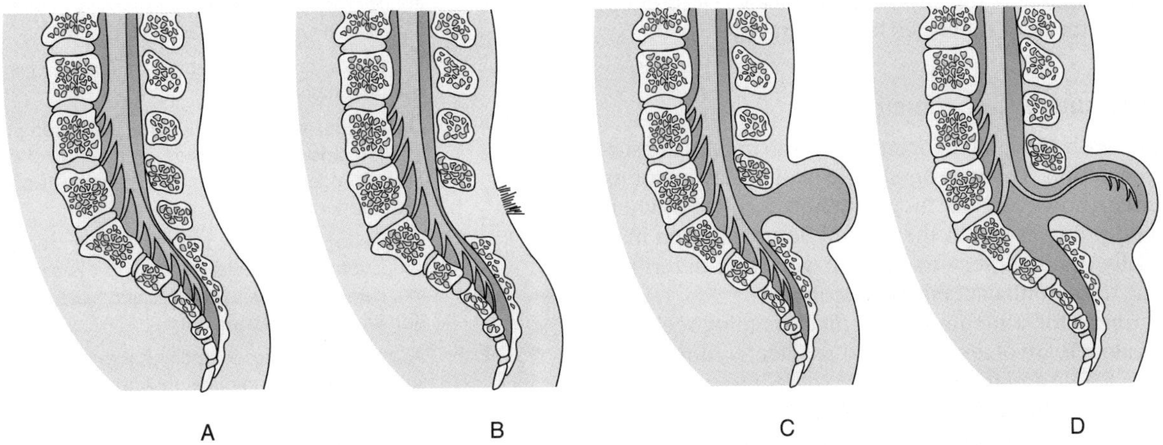

FIGURE 18.12 Degrees of spinal cord anomalies. (**A**) Normal spinal cord. (**B**) Spina bifida occulta. (**C**) Meningocele. (**D**) Myelomeningocele.

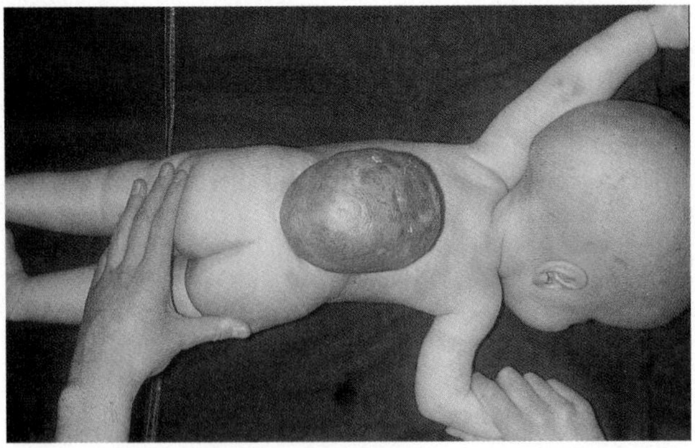

FIGURE 18.13 A myelomeningocele. The infant also has hydrocephaly and a subluxated hip.

are covered fully by skin, but they may be open so that infection will occur. It is difficult to tell from the size of the encephalocele how much brain tissue is trapped in the defect. Transillumination of the sac will reveal solid substance or fluid in the sac. X-ray or sonography will reveal the size of the skull defect.

Assessment

All types of neural defects except spina bifida occulta are readily visible at birth (Sarwark, 1996). They may be discovered during intrauterine life by sonography, fetoscopy, amniocentesis (discovery of AFP in amniotic fluid), or analysis of AFP in maternal serum. When infants are detected as having meningocele or myelomeningocele, they may be delivered by cesarean birth to avoid pressure and injury to the spinal cord. Observe and record whether an infant born with a myelomeningocele has spontaneous movement of lower extremities. Also assess the nature and pattern of voiding and defecation. A normal infant appears to be "always wet" from voiding but actually voids in amounts of approximately 30 mL and then is dry for 2 or 3 hours before voiding again. An infant without sphincter control voids continually. This pattern is the same for defecating. Observing these features aids in differentiating between meningocele and myelomeningocele. Differentiation can be further established by sonography.

Therapeutic Management

Children with spina bifida occulta need no immediate surgical correction. The parents should be made aware of its existence, however, so they are not surprised when someone points it out to them later. Some children may eventually need surgery to prevent vertebral deterioration due to the unbalanced spinal column.

Treatment for a meningocele, myelomeningocele, or encephalocele involves surgery to replace contents that are replaceable and to close the skin defect to prevent infection. The child with myelomeningocele will continue to have paralysis of lower extremities and loss of bowel and bladder function. Table 18-1 provides a classification of motor function disability. In the past, this surgery was done after the infant had survived the newborn period. Currently, it is done as soon after birth as possible (usually within 24 hours) so infection does not occur. Parents need to be cautioned that the surgery is not without risk and that brain defects accompanying an encephalocele may limit the child's potential.

The future prognosis will depend on the extent of the defect. The loss of meninges by surgery may limit the rate of absorption of CSF. It may build up in amount, resulting in subsequent hydrocephalus. Parents need a great deal of support to care for a child with a myelomeningocele because their child has a multiple disability. Referral to a community support group can be helpful.

WHAT IF? What if a parent tells you he wants to let his newborn die rather than undergo palliative surgery to close the defect? Whose rights should be honored, the parents' or the child's, and how should these rights be determined? What would be your role?

NURSING DIAGNOSES AND RELATED INTERVENTIONS: IMMEDIATE CONCERNS

Although parents were told before surgery that their child's spinal deformity is a type that means motor and sensory function are absent in the child's lower extremities, parents do not necessarily hear this information. Only after surgery do they begin to comprehend the extent of their child's disability. When the child is discharged from the hospital, they need to be certain of the next step in follow-up care. This

TABLE 18.1 Motor Function Disability in Myelomeningocele

SPINAL CORD LESION	DYSFUNCTION
T6–12	Complete flaccid paralysis of the lower extremities; weakened abdominal and trunk musculature in higher lesions; kyphosis and scoliosis common; ambulation with maximal support
L1–2	Hip flexion present; paraplegia, ambulation with maximal support
L3–4	Hip flexion, adduction, and knee extension present; hip dislocation common; some control of hip and knee movement possible; ambulation with moderate support
L5	Hip flexion, adduction, and varying degrees of abduction; knee extension and weak knee flexion; paralysis of the lower legs and feet; ambulation with moderate support
S1–2	As above, with preservation of some foot and ankle movement; ambulation with minimal support
S3	Mild loss of intrinsic foot muscular function possible; ambulation without support

prevents them from feeling deserted when they most need support—the time when they begin to appreciate what this problem will mean to them in the coming years, and what it will mean to the child throughout life.

Nursing Diagnosis: Risk for infection related to rupture of neural tube sac

Outcome Identification: Child will not develop an infection before surgery.

Outcome Evaluation: The neural tube sac remains intact; the child's temperature remains below 37°C.

If the sac should be allowed to dry, it might crack and allow CSF to drain and microorganisms to enter. Pressure on the protruding mass might cause rupture of the sac, leading to quick decompression of the CSF (which can lead to herniation of the brain stem into the spinal cord and interference with respiratory and cardiac centers) and possibly to infection (meningitis). Such pressure may also force CSF from the sac into the spinal column and, therefore, increase intracranial pressure.

Preoperative Positioning. Before surgery, infants should be positioned carefully so pressure on the spinal defect does not occur. They can be placed in a prone position or supported on their side. When they are on their side, use a rolled blanket or diaper placed behind their upper backs (above the defect) and a separate one behind their lower back (below the defect). This way, no pressure will be exerted on the lesion, and the infant will be protected from rolling backward onto it. Placing infants on their abdomen has the added advantage of keeping the flow of feces and urine away from the defect as well as keeping the lesion free from pressure. This is important because in many instances the skin covering of the defect is incomplete. A folded towel under the abdomen helps to flex the hip, reduce pressure on the sac, and ensure good leg position. If an infant is on his or her side, putting a folded diaper between the legs prevents skin surfaces from touching and rubbing (and also helps to keep the hips from internally rotating). Notice the position of the infant's legs. If they are paralyzed because of lack of motor control, the infant cannot move and straighten them.

Placing a piece of plastic or sturdy plastic wrap below the meningocele on the child's back like an apron and taping it in place is another method of preventing feces from touching the open lesion. A sterile wet compress of saline, antiseptic, or antibiotic gauze over the lesion may be used to keep the sac moist. Rather than remove this to wet it again and risk rupturing the sac, merely add additional fluid.

Although no pressure should be exerted on the open lesion by a top sheet, make certain that the child is warm enough. The presence of the sac adds to the amount of body surface area exposed, thus increasing heat loss. He or she may need to be kept in an Isolette to maintain body heat if a large area of the back cannot be covered. Use caution when placing the infant under a radiant heat source for warmth. Radiant heat can dry the lesion and cause cracking. Any seepage of clear fluid from the defect should be reported promptly, because this is probably escaping CSF. Checking any leakage with a test tape and reading it for glucose will confirm the fluid is CSF fluid (urine or mucus will not test positive for glucose).

Postoperative Care. After surgery, a child is again placed on the abdomen until the skin incision has healed (7 to 14 days). The same careful precautions against allowing urine or feces to touch the incision area must be taken.

Nursing Diagnosis: Risk for altered nutrition, less than body requirements, related to difficulty assuming normal feeding position

Outcome Identification: Infant will take in adequate nutrition during period of healing.

Outcome Evaluation: Infant's skin turgor is good; weight maintained within 10% of birth weight; specific gravity of urine remains between 1.030 and 1.003.

To maintain nutrition, the infant should be held in as normal a feeding position as possible. Make certain that a supporting arm does not press against the lesion. When bubbling the infant, remember not to pat the back over the defect. If the defect is large and the risk in picking up the infant is too great, the infant may be fed while lying on his or her side in bed or prone on a Bradford frame. Raise the infant's head slightly by slipping a folded diaper under it. Stroke the head, arms, or upper back while the infant sucks to give the child the same comfort and assurance at feeding time as a baby receives while being held. Talk to the infant and let him know that someone loves and cares for him. The infant may enjoy a pacifier after feeding, because he does not experience the enjoyment of sucking while feeding that would be experienced if he could be held and cuddled. If a mother planned on breastfeeding and the infant can be held, urge her to do this. Caution her not to allow the sac or postoperative incision line to press against her arm. Every new mother has some difficulty getting comfortable with feeding an infant. The mother who must feed her child in an unusual position or with the infant on a support frame will have even more difficulty. She needs to observe a warm, comforting role model so she can begin a positive mother–child interaction.

Children with increased intracranial pressure tend to suck poorly. If this complication develops after the surgery, nursing may be difficult. Parents need a realistic explanation of treatment planned for the child so they can decide whether to continue to plan on breastfeeding. If it is necessary to forgo breastfeeding for this child, assure parents that the child will thrive on commercial formula.

Nursing Diagnosis: Risk for altered cerebral tissue perfusion related to increased intracranial pressure

Outcome Identification: Infant remains free of symptoms of compression from increased intracranial pressure or an increase in skull circumference during childhood.

Outcome Evaluation: Infant's head circumference remains within present percentile on growth chart; absence of signs and symptoms of increased intracranial pressure.

Preoperative Care. Increasing head size from poor absorption of CSF (hydrocephalus) is a complication of neural tube disorders. To detect increased head size (development of hydrocephalus), measure head circumference once daily (or more frequently if ordered) in the preoperative period. Head circumference measurements are only accurate if the tape measure is placed on the same points of the child's head each time. Placing an indelible or ballpoint pen mark on the forehead just above the eyebrows and at the most prominent point of the occiput allows different people to measure the head during the day and yet be sure that they all measure at the same point.

Postoperative Care. Children may develop hydrocephalus after surgery, probably because of interference with subarachnoid absorption of CSF. The shortening of the meninges creates an Arnold Chiari disorder (see below) or traction of the hind brain into the spinal cord. The child must be observed frequently for signs of increased intracranial pressure, such as changes in vital signs, neurologic signs such as pupillary changes, or an increase in head circumference or bulging fontanelles, as well as behavioral changes such as irritability or lethargy. Keep the infant prone or on the side to prevent pressure on the incision.

Nursing Diagnosis: Risk for altered skin integrity related to required prone positioning

Outcome Identification: Infant will not experience disruption in skin integrity during preoperative or postoperative period.

Outcome Evaluation: Infant's skin remains intact without erythema or ulceration.

Preserving skin integrity is a major problem because of frequent dressing changes and because the constant prone position puts pressure on the infant's knees and elbows. Laying the infant on a synthetic sheepskin helps reduce friction; use paper tape or stockinette for dressing changes or place Stomahesive on the skin under the area where the tape will touch. Change diapers frequently to prevent excessive contact of acid urine with skin. If hydrocephalus has developed, the head will be heavy and pressure areas at the temples can occur if the head is not turned every 2 hours.

NURSING DIAGNOSES AND RELATED INTERVENTIONS: LONG-TERM CONCERNS

Nursing Diagnosis: Impaired physical mobility related to neural tube disorder

Outcome Identification: Child will be mobile within the limits of nerve involvement after surgery.

Outcome Evaluation: Child ambulates with the least amount of accessory equipment possible.

Parents must provide normal stimulation and activities for the child because his or her mobility is limited. They need to be encouraged to take the infant to the places a child would normally accompany parents—relatives' homes, shopping, the zoo, and so forth. They need to encourage the child to be as independent as possible so he or she can lead as normal a life as possible (Figure 18-14).

If a child has impaired lower-extremity motor control, parents will need to perform passive exercises to prevent muscle atrophy and formation of contractures. The child

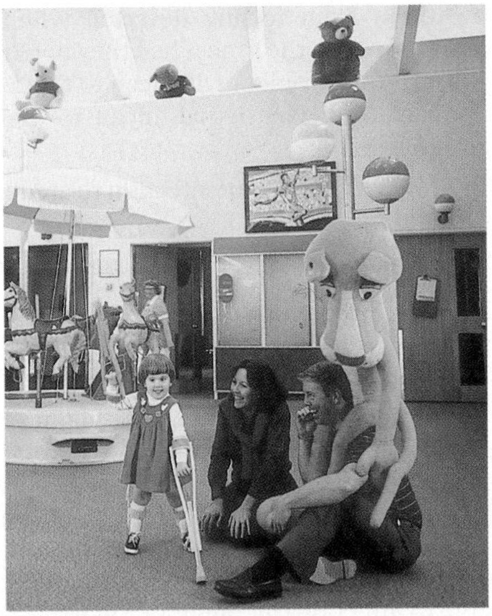

FIGURE 18.14 A child born with a neural tube impairment demonstrates her ability to walk using braces and a crutch.

may need braces to help maintain good alignment and make walking with crutches possible in childhood. Parents are generally anxious to do something for their child and follow routines of passive exercises well if they are given sufficient support for their accomplishments at health care visits. As the child grows older, tendon transplants and osteotomy may be necessary to prevent contractures and poor bone alignment. Because these children have no sensation in their lower extremities, parents must make a routine of inspecting the child's lower extremities and buttocks daily for any area of irritation or possible infection. Teach children as they grow older to do this themselves. When children are using a wheelchair, be certain to teach them to press with their arms on the armrests to raise their buttocks off the wheelchair seat at least once every hour. This will help provide adequate circulation to lower extremities.

Nursing Diagnosis: Risk for altered elimination related to neural tube disorder

Outcome Identification: Child will achieve a satisfactory method of elimination by school age.

Outcome Evaluation: Child demonstrates ability to independently manage bowel and bladder elimination.

To ensure bladder emptying, intermittent clean urinary catheterization is taught to parents. As the child reaches school age, he or she can be taught clean self-catheterization (inserting a clean catheter every 4 hours to drain urine from the bladder; Box 18-1). A potential danger is that, because catheters are latex, the child may develop a latex sensitivity. It is possible for artificial bladder sphincters to be placed to help establish continence. Prescription of a drug such as oxybutynin chloride (Ditropan) may improve bladder capacity (see Drug Highlight). In some children, a continent urinary reservoir or ureterosigmoidostomy (see Chapter 25) is constructed to bypass the nonfunctioning bladder. However, children who are begun on intermittent clean catheterization from birth require less bladder aug-

BOX 18.1

INSTRUCTIONS FOR SELF-CATHETERIZATION

1. The purpose of self-catheterization is to keep the bladder empty through using clean technique and frequent emptying so microorganisms do not have time to grow in urine in the bladder. It is important that you always use clean equipment and that you self-catheterize at least every 4 hours to accomplish this.
2. Always carry your self-catheterization equipment with you (a plastic bag containing a clean catheter and water-soluble lubricant). This enables you to stay longer away from home if you wish. If you will be using a public lavatory, you might want to include a presoaped washcloth rather than have to use rough paper towels.
3. To begin self-catheterization, wash your hands in warm, soapy water. This reduces the chance that you will introduce germs from your hands into the bladder.
4. Next wash your perineum or penis with a clean washcloth and warm, soapy water. Rinse the washcloth and wash again with clear water. This reduces the chance that germs on your skin will be pushed into the bladder.
5. Coat a clean catheter with a water-soluble lubricant. This reduces friction and makes the catheter slide into the bladder easily.
6. Females use one hand to spread the lips of the perineum so the bladder entrance is exposed. Locate the urinary meatus and gently but quickly insert the catheter approximately 1 inch (males insert the catheter approximately 4 inches). Urine should begin to flow immediately through the catheter. Let this drain into the toilet.
7. When urine stops flowing, gently remove the catheter. Clean the catheter with soap and water, rinse with clear water, and replace in the plastic bag with the lubricant.
8. Examine your schedule at the beginning of each day and plan ways that you will be able to use a bathroom or school lavatory every 4 hours.
9. Be certain that on special days (e.g., school trips or vacation) that you do not forget the importance of self-catheterization.
10. Ask your parents to telephone your health care provider if urine is ever blood tinged, smells foul, or is cloudy rather than clear; if you have pain in your abdomen or lower back; or if you have an elevated temperature, because these may be symptoms of a urinary tract infection.

DRUG HIGHLIGHT

Oxybutynin Chloride (Ditropan)

Action: Oxybutynin is a urinary antispasmodic that relaxes smooth muscle to relieve symptoms of bladder instability associated with patients with neurogenic bladders.

Pregnancy risk category: C

Dosage: 5 mg orally, b.i.d.

Possible adverse effects: Drowsiness, dizziness, blurred vision, decreased sweating

Nursing Implications:
- Advise the parents to give or the child to take the medication exactly as prescribed.
- Alert the parents about the need for frequent bladder examinations required during treatment to document the drug's effect.
- Ask the child to report complaints of drowsiness or blurred vision. Caution the child not to attempt activities that require balance while taking the drug.
- Caution the child and parents that with decreased sweating, high temperatures will not be tolerated. Encourage the parents to keep the child's environment cool and avoid high temperatures.

mentation procedures than those who are not (see Focus on Nursing Research).

Arnold-Chiari Deformity (Chiari II Malformation)

The Arnold-Chiari deformity is caused by overgrowth of the neural tube in weeks 16 to 20 of fetal life. The specific anomaly is a projection of the cerebellum, medulla oblongata, and fourth ventricle into the cervical canal. This causes the upper cervical spinal cord to jackknife backward, obstructing CSF flow and causing hydrocephalus. A lumbosacral myelomeningocele is also present in approximately 50% of children with this anomaly (Fishman, 1997).

The prognosis for the child with an Arnold-Chiari malformation depends on the extent of the defect and the surgical procedure possible. Because of the upper motor neuron involvement, gagging and swallowing reflexes may be absent, increasing the risk for tracheal aspiration.

CHECKPOINT QUESTIONS

13. Why should a meningocele sac be kept moist?
14. When is surgery performed to repair a neural tube defect?

FOCUS ON NURSING RESEARCH

Does Intermittent Clean Catheterization Have a Positive Long-Term Effect in Children With a Neurogenic Bladder Such as Those With Myelomeningocele?

To answer this question, 46 patients started on intermittent clean catheterization before 1 year of age, and 52 patients who were not begun on the procedure until after 1 year of life were compared. The results of the comparison showed that persistent hydronephrosis was the same in both groups. Significantly fewer bladder augmentation procedures were required in the patients in the earlier group. The researchers concluded that intermittent clean catheterization may help prevent irreversible bladder dysfunction.

This is important research for nurses because teaching intermittent clean catheterization is a nursing responsibility. Helping parents appreciate how important it is can increase their motivation to learn the procedure and carry it out conscientiously.

Wu, H. Y., et al. (1997). Neurogenic bladder dysfunction due to myelomeningocele: Neonatal versus childhood treatment. *Journal of Urology, 157*(6), 2295.

SKELETAL ANOMALIES

A number of physical developmental defects result in skeletal deformities in the newborn.

Absent or Malfomed Extremities

Congenital bone defects may result from unknown reasons, drug ingestion, virus invasion during pregnancy, or amniotic band formation in utero. If a child is born with a bone deformity, record a careful pregnancy history. In most instances, however, the cause of the anomaly cannot be established. Children born without an extremity or with a malformed extremity can be fitted with a prosthesis early in life. In most instances, children will have better function if the malformed portion of an extremity is amputated before a prosthesis is fitted. This is a difficult decision for parents to make as it is one that they cannot undo later. They need assurance that arms that appear like seal flippers, for example, will not later grow to become normal. A well-fitted prosthesis that a child learns to use at an early age will provide more function and allow a more normal childhood and adult life than if the original deformity is left unchanged (Figure 18-15). Lower-extremity prostheses are fitted as early as age 6 months (so an infant will learn to stand at the normal time). Upper-extremity prostheses are fitted this early also, so an infant will handle and explore objects readily.

Introducing a prosthesis early also prevents a child from adjusting to a missing extremity, such as writing with the feet or sliding across a floor rather than walking. Children can become so proficient at these adjustments that later in life they do not see the advantage of a prosthesis and refuse to use one. Although these self-adjustments may be cute in infants, in the long run they greatly limit the child's potential.

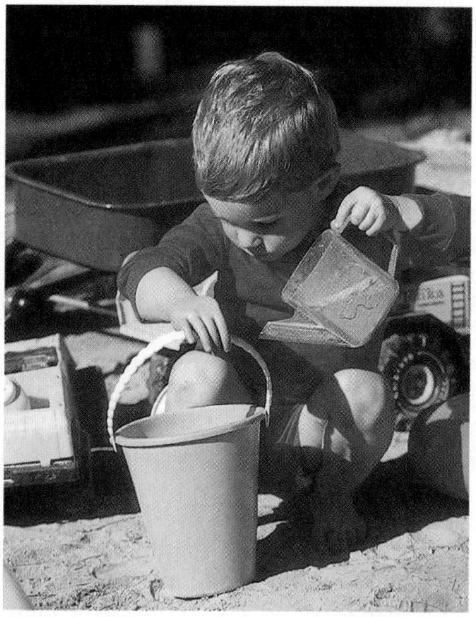

FIGURE 18.15 A young child learns to use a hand prosthesis during play.

Learning to use a hand prosthesis takes weeks to months; help parents think of interesting activities to introduce so a child uses a prosthesis to accomplish something rather than feeling he or she is only undergoing a ritual. Gait training for use of lower-extremity prostheses begins by use of parallel bars and proceeds to independent walking and mastery of steps. Children who are born with an absent extremity need help not only in mastering the use of a prosthesis but also in mastering a positive body image of themselves as whole.

Parents often feel devastated at the child's birth and search to discover the cause of the defect. They should be introduced to a rehabilitation team in the newborn period if possible. Further steps then will be outlined for them to help them move past the helplessness they feel to more positive action. Visiting with a child who uses a prosthesis well can be a great help in convincing them that their child can lead a normal life. Children with a congenital extremity loss do not grieve over the lost extremity as do adults or older children, which means they are often better prepared to quickly move on to rehabilitation.

Finger Conditions

Polydactyly is the presence of one or more additional fingers. When this occurs, the supernumerary finger is usually amputated in infancy or early childhood. These extra fingers are often just cartilage or skin tags, and removal is simple and cosmetically sound. In **syndactyly** (two fingers are fused) the fusion is usually caused by a simple webbing (Figure 18-16); separation of the fingers into two sound and cosmetically appealing ones is usually successful. In other instances, the bones of the fingers are also fused, and the cosmetic appearance and function of fingers will always be impaired.

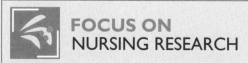

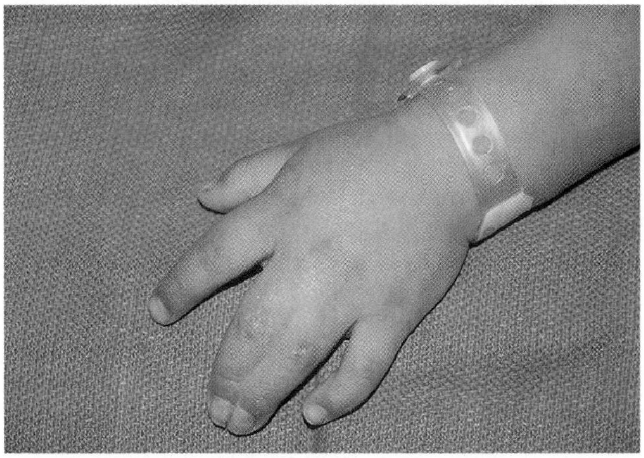

FIGURE 18.16 Syndactyly.

These hand anomalies are always upsetting to parents (one of the first things that new parents do is count the fingers and toes of newborns). Parents need time to air their feelings and concerns. They need reassurance at health maintenance visits throughout the child's development that he or she is normal in other ways so they can accept and love the child. Children need this same type of assurance so they can think of themselves as well people.

Pectus Deviations

Pectus excavatum is an indentation of the lower portion of the sternum. This usually occurs congenitally. It may also occur after chronic obstructive lung disease or rickets. The defect results in decreased lung volume and displacement of the heart to the left. Surgery can be done for cosmetic reasons or to expand lung volume. With *pectus carinatum,* the sternum is displaced anteriorly, increasing the anterior posterior diameter of the chest.

Torticollis (Wry Neck)

Torticollis is a term derived from *tortus* (twisted) and *collum* (neck). Torticollis (wry neck) occurs as a congenital anomaly when the sternocleidomastoid muscle is injured and bleeds during birth. This tends to occur in newborns with wide shoulders when pressure is exerted on the head to deliver the shoulder. The infant holds the head tilted to the side of the muscle involved; the head rotates to the opposite side. The injury may not be noticeable in the neck of the newborn and may become evident only as the original hemorrhage recedes and fibrous contraction occurs at age 1 to 2 months. A palpable mass over the muscle will be present.

Treatment consists of passive stretching exercises and encouraging the infant to look in the direction of the affected muscle. A mother could encourage this by holding the child to feed in such a position that the child must look in the desired direction. A mobile on the child's crib should be placed to encourage the child to look toward the affected side. The parents should speak to and hand the child objects always from the affected side to make the child look that way.

If the parents do this consistently, further treatment usually is not necessary. It is important that parents understand that this is important therapy. It seems so simple that they otherwise may not take it seriously and may not carry it out. In the few instances in which simple exercises are not effective and the condition still exists at a year, surgical correction followed by a neck immobilizer will be necessary (Sponseller, 1997). Torticollis can lead to the one shoulder continuing to be elevated. This has the potential to lead to scoliosis later in life.

Craniosynostosis

Craniosynostosis is premature closure of the sutures of the skull. This may occur in utero or early in infancy because of rickets or irregularities of calcium or phosphate metabolism; it also may occur without any known cause. It occurs more often in males than females (Gorlin, 1997).

It is important that craniosynostosis be detected early, because premature closure of the suture line will compromise brain growth. When the sagittal suture line closes prematurely, the child's head tends to grow anteriorly and posteriorly. If the coronal suture line fuses early, the child's face becomes deformed. The orbits of the eyes become misshapen, and the increased intracranial pressure may lead to exophthalmos, nystagmus, papilledema, strabismus, and atrophy of the optic nerve with consequent loss of vision. Premature closure of the coronal suture line is associated with syndactyly, so all infants with syndactyly should be observed closely for head circumference. Cardiac anomalies, choanal atresias, or defects of elbows and knee joints are also associated with craniosynostosis.

Head circumference should be measured on all children age 2 years or younger at all health maintenance visits and compared with normal head circumference charts. The posterior fontanelle closes normally at age 2 months, the anterior fontanelle at age 12 to 18 months. All children with premature closure of fontanelles must be observed closely for craniosynostosis.

Craniosynostosis can be established by x-ray film, which reveals the fused suture line. If the suture line is the sagittal one, treatment may involve only careful observation; if the coronal suture line is involved, it will need to be surgically opened.

Measuring head circumference at health maintenance visits is a nursing responsibility. Thoughtful comparison of an infant's head circumference with past measurements and with standard growth measurements can be important in detecting craniosynostosis and preventing brain compression.

Achondroplasia

Achondroplasia (chondrodystrophia) is a form of dwarfism inherited as a dominant trait (Tunnessen, 1997). It involves a defect in cartilage production in utero. The epiphyseal plate of long bones cannot produce adequate cartilage for longitudinal bone growth, which results in both arms and legs being stunted.

Because the bones of the cranium are of membranous origin, they continue to grow normally. Children's heads will therefore appear unusually large in contrast to extremities. The forehead is prominent and the bridge of the nose is flattened. Because it is a cartilage—not a brain—problem, intelligence generally is normal. Children's trunks are of near-normal size, but a *thoracic kyphosis* (outward curve) and *lumbar lordosis* (inward curve) of the spine may be present.

Achondroplasia dwarfism can be diagnosed in utero or at birth by comparing the length of extremities to the normal length (in the average child, the arms can be extended to the distance of the midthigh) or by x-ray film, which will reveal characteristic abnormal flaring epiphyseal lines. People with achondroplasia dwarfism rarely reach a height of more than 4½ ft (140 cm). Women with this condition will have difficulty with childbearing because of the small pelvis and generally have their children by cesarean birth.

Children with achondroplasia become aware of their unusual appearance as early as during the preschool years. They are apt to become acutely aware of it during school age, when they realize they do not "fit in" with the neighborhood children. Ideally, such children have parents who have adjusted well to short stature in themselves and therefore have developed good self-esteem and are able to implant these qualities in a child. The child nearing reproductive age must be informed that, as with all dominantly inherited disorders, there is a high probability that any children will inherit the disorder. Adolescence may be a particularly difficult time for these children, and continued guidance or counseling can help them to emerge from this period feeling good about themselves as adults.

Talipes Deformities

Talipes is a Latin word formed from the words *talus* and *pes*, meaning "foot" and "ankle," respectively. The talipes deformities are ankle-foot deformities, popularly called *clubfoot*. The term *clubfoot* implies permanent crippling to many people and should not be used when discussing talipes deformities with parents. With good orthopedic correction techniques currently available, correction should leave the child with no permanent deformity of the foot (Craig, 1995).

Approximately 1 in every 1000 live-born children has a talipes deformity, occurring more often in males than females. It probably is inherited as a polygenic pattern. It usually occurs only as a unilateral problem.

Some newborns have a pseudo talipes deformity from their intrauterine position. In these infants, the foot looks to be turned in but can be brought into a good position by manipulation. In a true defect, the foot cannot be properly aligned without further intervention. Be certain to demonstrate to parents that, if a pseudodeformity is present, the foot can easily be brought into line or is not deformed. Otherwise, the first time parents fit booties or shoes on the infant, they will notice this and worry that the foot is misshapen.

A true talipes deformity can be one of four separate deformities: (1) *plantar flexion* (an equinus, or "horsefoot" position with the foot lower than the heel); (2) *dorsiflexion* (the heel is held lower than the foot or the anterior foot is flexed toward the anterior leg); (3) *varus deviation* (the foot turns in); or (4) *valgus deviation* (the foot turns out). Most children with talipes deformities have a combination of these conditions, or have an equinovarus (Figure 18-17) or a *calcaneovalgus* deformity (a child walks on the heel with the foot everted).

Assessment

The earlier a true deformity is recognized, the better the correction. Make a habit of straightening all newborn feet to the midline as part of initial assessment to detect this defect.

Therapeutic Management

Correction is achieved best if it is begun in the newborn. This is accomplished by the foot being placed in a cast in an overcorrected position. Although the deformity involves the ankle, the cast extends above the infant's knee to ensure firm correction (Figure 18-17*B*). (Care of the child in a cast is discussed in Chapter 30.) Because talipes casts are high

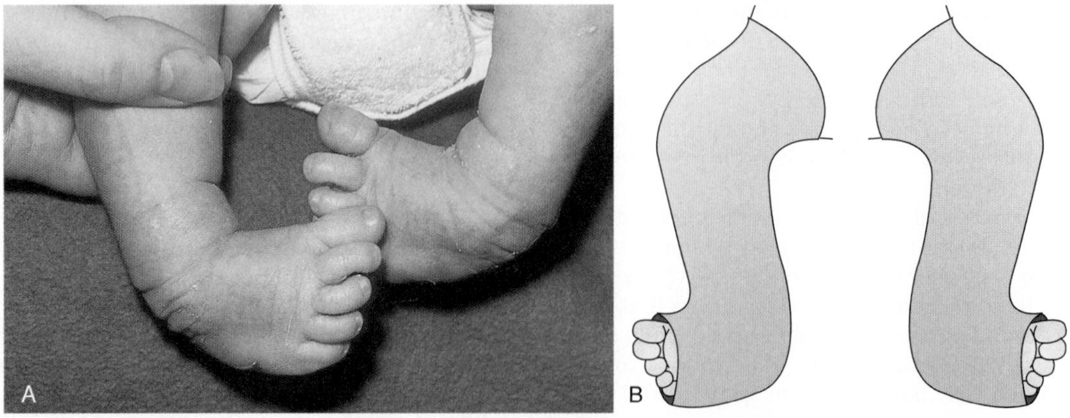

FIGURE 18.17 (**A**) Talipes equinovarus. (**B**) Casts for bilateral equinovarus.

on the leg, diapers should be changed frequently to prevent a wet diaper from touching the cast and causing it to become soaked with urine or meconium. Review with parents how to check the infant's toes for coldness or blueness and how to blanch a toenail bed and watch it turn pink to assess for good circulation. Because a newborn is unable to report pain except by generalized crying, crying episodes in the infant must be evaluated carefully. Such crying may be due to colic, hunger, or wet diapers; it might also be due to the tingling feeling of circulatory compression (as when a foot is "asleep" from too tight a cast).

Infants grow so rapidly in the neonatal period that casts for talipes deformities must be changed almost every 1 or 2 weeks. If a mother has a complication of childbirth or is exhausted from childbirth (depression due to the child having been born with a congenital defect may manifest itself as exhaustion), be certain she knows to make arrangements for another family member to bring the infant to the hospital for cast changes.

After approximately 6 weeks (the time varies depending on the extent of the problem), the final cast is removed. After this, parents may need to perform passive foot exercises such as putting the infant's foot and ankle through a full range of motion several times a day for several months. These seem like simple maneuvers, so their importance must be impressed on the parents; otherwise, they are easy exercises to omit when people's lives are busy. The infant may have to sleep in Denis Browne splints (shoes attached to a metal bar to maintain position) at night up to age 1 year. Although a successful correction cannot be guaranteed, the prognosis for a full correction is good. For those children who do not achieve correction by casting, surgery can be performed to achieve a final correction.

CHECKPOINT QUESTIONS

15. What is the name of the condition when two fingers are fused?
16. What is an important care measure to teach parents of the child with a torticollis?

Developmental Hip Dysplasia

Developmental hip dysplasia (often referred to as *congenital hip dysplasia*) is improper formation and function of the hip socket. It may be evident as subluxation or dislocation of the head of the femur (Figure 18-18).

A flattening of the acetabulum of the pelvis is present, which prevents the head of the femur from remaining in the acetabulum and rotating adequately. In *subluxated hip,* the femur "rides up" because of the flat acetabulum; in *dislocated hip,* the femur rides so far up that it actually leaves the acetabulum. Why the defect occurs is unknown, but it may be from a polygenic inheritance pattern. It may also occur from a uterine position that causes less than usual pressure of the femur head on the acetabulum (Sponseller, 1997).

Hip dysplasia is found in females six times more frequently than in males, possibly because the hips are normally more flaring in females and possibly because the hormone relaxin causes the pelvic ligaments to be more relaxed. Thus the femur does not press as effectively into the acetabulum during intrauterine life. It is usually, but not always, a unilateral involvement. It occurs most often in children of Mediterranean ancestry. Sociocultural methods of childrearing such as the way infants are carried may pro-

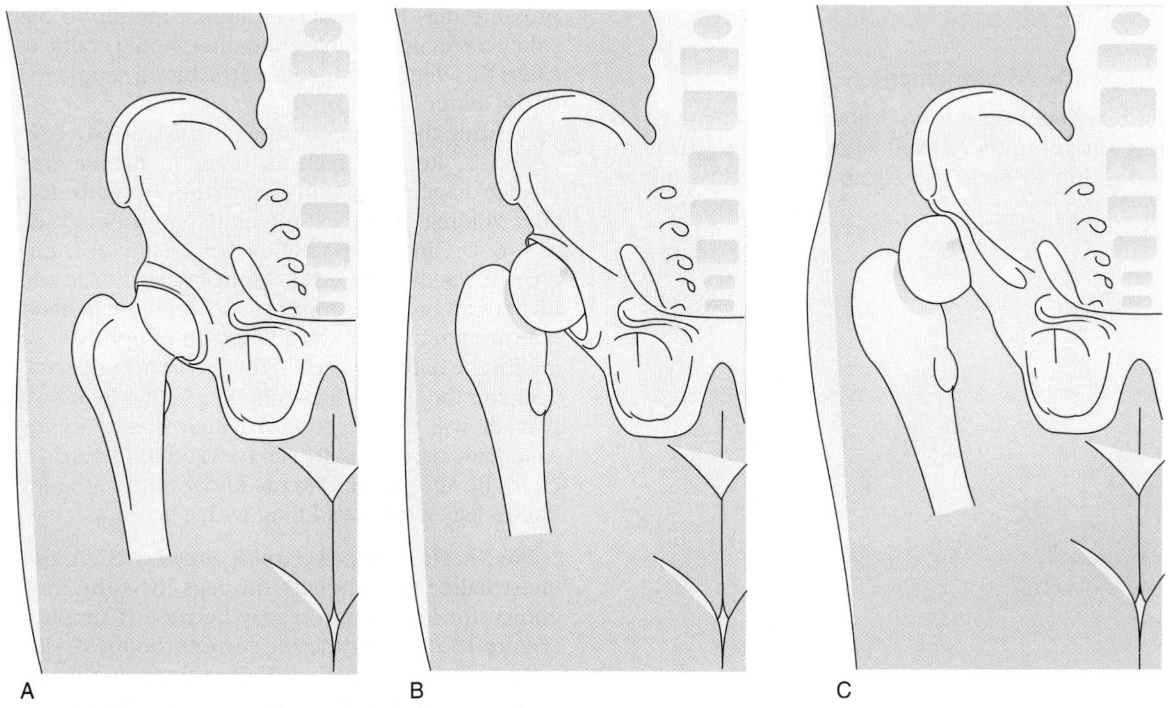

FIGURE 18.18 Hip dysplasia. (**A**) A normal femur head and acetabulum. (**B**) A subluxated hip. The femur head is "riding high" in the shallow acetabulum. (**C**) A dislocated hip. The femur head is not engaged in the shallow acetabulum.

mote or decrease the extent of the involvement (see Focus on Cultural Competence earlier in this chapter).

Assessment

It is important that developmental hip dysplasia be detected in the newborn because the longer it goes undetected, the more difficult it is to correct. Sometimes the affected leg may appear slightly shorter than the normal one because the femur head rides so high in the socket. This is most noticeable when the child is lying supine and the thighs are flexed to a 90-degree angle toward the abdomen. One knee will appear to be lower than the other (Figure 18-19*A*). An unequal number of skin folds may be present on the posterior thighs (Figure 18-19*B*). This finding is unreliable, however, because some infants with normal hips have an uneven number of posterior thigh skin folds. Diagnosis is confirmed by ultrasound or magnetic resonance imaging (Harding et al, 1997).

Subluxated or dislocated hip is best assessed by noting whether the hips abduct (see Nursing Procedure 18-1).

In some infants, the hip abducts properly at a newborn assessment, but at the time of the health maintenance visit at approximately age 4 to 6 weeks, a secondary shortening of the adductor muscles will have occurred, and the defect will be evident. Tight adductor muscles occur in children with cerebral palsy, so this disorder must be ruled out. An x-ray film or sonogram will reveal the shallow acetabulum and a more lateral placement of the femur head than is ordinarily seen.

Hip dysplasia is difficult to detect at birth in an infant who delivered from a footling or frank breech presentation, because the knees are stiff and do not flex readily. Always assess hip function in these infants at each health maintenance visit.

Therapeutic Management

Correction of subluxated and dislocated hip involves positioning the hip into a flexed, abducted (externally rotated) position to press the femur head against the acetabulum and deepen its contour by the pressure. Either splints, halters, or casts may be used. If the child is older, traction is used first to bring the femur head into good position with the acetabulum. The small number of children who do not achieve a correction by these methods will have surgery and a pin inserted to stabilize the hip.

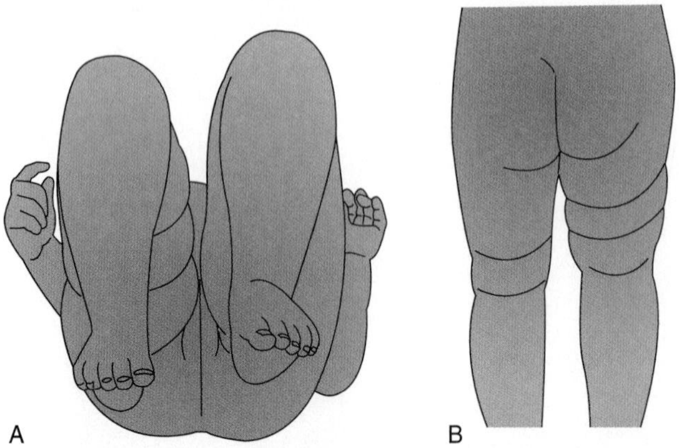

FIGURE 18.19 Signs of developmental dysplasia. (**A**) With child in a supine position, the right knee on the side of the subluxation appears lower than the left because of malposition of the femur head. (**B**) Asymmetry of skin folds and prominence of the trochanter on the right side.

NURSING DIAGNOSES AND RELATED INTERVENTIONS

Nursing Diagnosis: Parental knowledge deficit related to splint, halter, or cast correction for hip dysplasia

Outcome Identification: Parents will demonstrate increased knowledge of the care of the child in a splint, halter, or cast by discharge from the health care agency.

Outcome Evaluation: Parents correctly demonstrate application and removal of splint or halter device and care of device or cast.

Multiple Diapers or Splints. Often splint correction (to hold the legs in a frog-leg, or abducted, externally rotated position) is begun during the newborn's initial hospital stay by placing two or three diapers on the infant. The extra bulk of cloth between the child's legs effectively separates and spreads them. Many brands of disposable diapers are cut narrow between the legs; thus, they do not offer this much bulk and will not work as well as cloth diapers.

A Frejka splint is made of plastic and buckles onto the child as a huge confining diaper (Figure 18-20*A*). Parents need to keep the splint in place at all times, except when changing diapers or bathing the infant. Although firm pressure may be needed to abduct the hip to place the splint correctly, forcible abduction should not be used because this might compromise the blood supply to the leg or the femur head.

Wearing the splint continually can lead to a severe diaper rash. Remind parents of good diaper area care: change diapers frequently; wash the area with clear water after voiding or defecation, and apply an ointment such as A & D Ointment, Vaseline, or Desitin at each diaper change. Padding the edges of the brace with an additional diaper can increase comfort and decrease irritation. Parents are taught that swaddling babies tightly is comforting for the baby. Be certain these parents understand that bringing the child's legs together with a tight swaddling blanket will not be good for their infant. Some Native American parents still use a swaddling board for their child. Be sure these parents know not to straighten the child's legs while swaddling with a board.

Pavlik Harness. A *Pavlik harness* is an adjustable chest halter that abducts the legs. It is the method of choice for long-term therapy because it simplifies care (Figure 18-20*B*). Soft plastic stirrups (booties) with quick-fastening closures such as Velcro attach to the leg extension straps and hold the hips flexed, abducted, and externally rotated. To put it in place, the infant is laid supine, the thighs are grasped and abducted to place the femoral head into the acetabulum, and the harness is ap-

NURSING PROCEDURE 18.1: ASSESSING ORTOLANI'S AND BARLOW'S SIGNS

Purpose
To assist in detecting developmental hip dysplasia

Plan	Principle
1. Lay the infant supine and flex the knees to 90 degrees at the hips.	1. Proper positioning ensures accurate results.
2. Place your middle fingers over the greater trochanter of the femur and your thumb on the internal side of the thigh over the lesser trochanter.	2. Placing your fingers in this way allows for abduction of the hips.

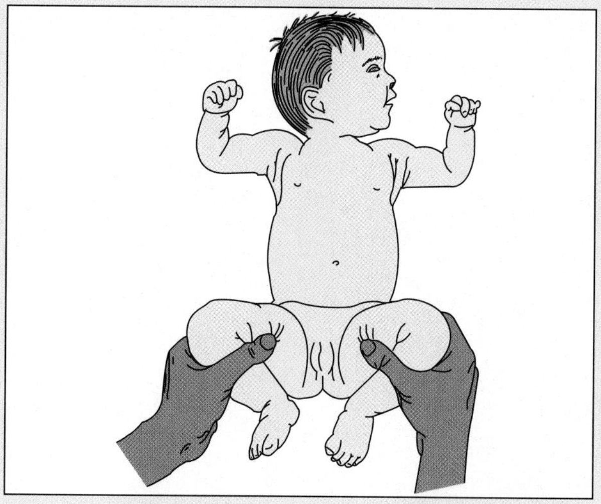

Plan	Principle
3. Abduct the hips while applying upward pressure over the greater trochanter and listen for a clicking sound.	3. Normally, no sound is heard. A clicking or clunking sound is a positive Ortolani's sign and occurs when the femoral head reenters the acetabulum.
4. Next, with your fingers in the same position, and holding the hips and knees at 90 degrees flexion, apply a backward pressure (down and laterally) and adduct the hips.	4. Normally, the hip joint is stable. A feeling of the femur head slipping out of the socket posterolaterally is a positive Barlow's sign indicative of hip instability associated with developmental hip dysplasia.

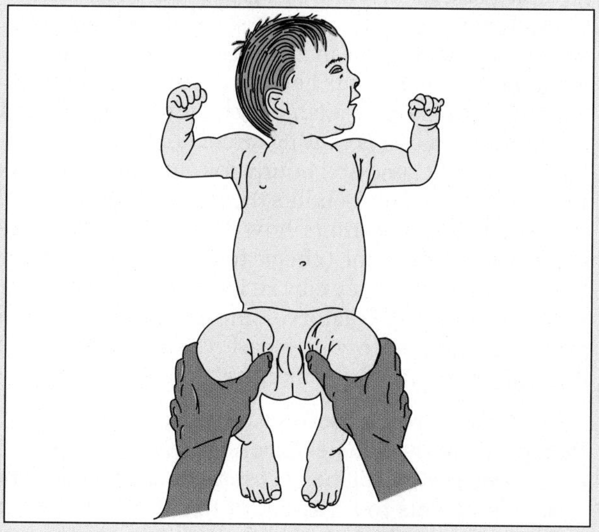

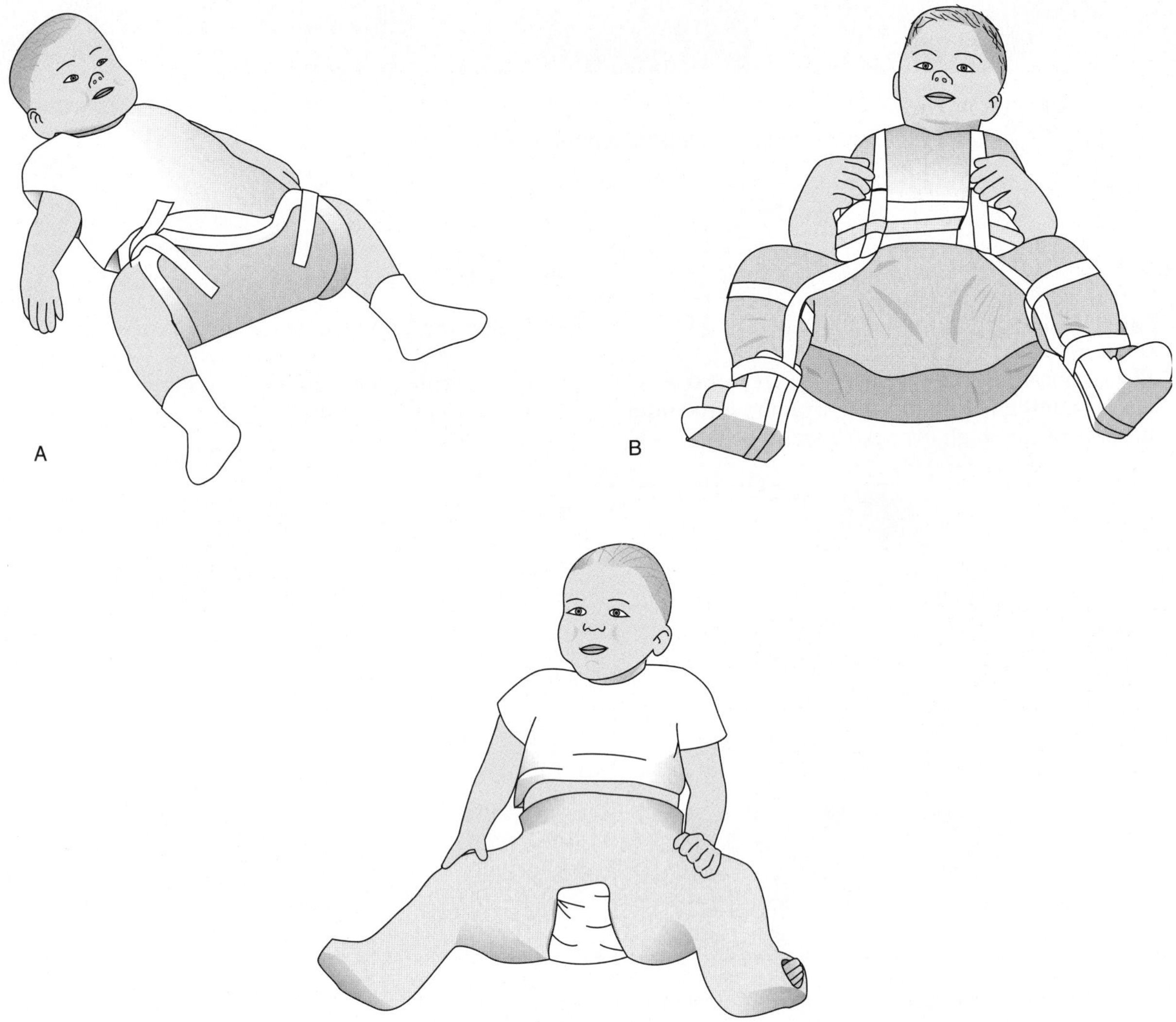

FIGURE 18.20 (**A**) Hip abduction splint (Frejka splint) holds the hips in an abduction position, forcing the femur head into the acetabulum. (**B**) A Pavlik harness. (**C**) A hip abduction cast for correction of subluxation of the hip.

plied. The harness is then worn continually (infants must be sponge bathed). With a few children whose hip is only mildly subluxated, parents may be taught to remove the harness for bathing and to reduce the hip again before it is replaced in the harness. Parents should assess the skin under the straps daily for irritation or redness. Because the harness does not show under a shirt and long trousers, many parents prefer a Pavlik harness as a means of correction.

An advantage of a Pavlik harness is that it promotes gentle reduction of the hip. A disadvantage may be that it is not firm enough if a hip is completely dislocated. It will be ineffective if parents remove it.

Spica Cast. If the hip is fully dislocated or the subluxation is severe, the infant may be placed immediately in a "frog-leg" cast or a spica cast to maintain an externally rotated hip position. The child may first be placed in Bryant's traction for a week to better position the hip. The hip is then placed in an abducted position and a large hip spica cast or an A-line cast is applied (Figure 18-20*C*). These casts are heavy and are so wide that dressing infants or sitting them in an infant car seat or bassinet is difficult. Be certain parents have a car seat that can be modified to accommodate a large cast. Newborns are unable to report that a cast is causing circulatory constriction, so they need to be assessed hourly for circulation to the extremities for the first 24 hours the cast is in place and daily thereafter. Teach parents how to do this type of neurovascular assessment (check temperature and circulation in toes) before they take an infant home from the hospital to prevent circulatory compression from a rapidly growing limb outgrowing a cast. Casts will be changed but maintained for 6 to 9 months.

General Care Guidelines. No matter what type of therapy is used—double-diapering, splint or harness or cast—surgery may still be necessary for a final correction. Teaching parents to be aware of this from the start prevents them from thinking that their child's condition is so serious that usual methods of treatment failed. It helps them from becoming discouraged or dissatisfied with health care. It also helps them to accept from the beginning that this condition is a long-term care concern. Some children will be 2 years old before the final cast is removed.

The child and parents will be visiting their orthopedist frequently during these early years. Assess that the parents also schedule general health maintenance visits for routine immunizations and overall growth and development assessment. Spend time during health maintenance visits talking with the parents about infant stimulation. Because the child is not fully mobile, this needs special thought. Teach parents to hold their child for feeding and to rock and cuddle the infant, even though a large cast or a brace may be bulky and awkward. Teach parents to bring experiences to the infant, because the child is unable to crawl and walk toward interesting objects in the environment. A child's wagon makes for convenient and fun transportation. The child may also be able to lie prone and move about on a large skate board. Many parents worry that the child who is still in a large cast at the normal age for walking (12 months) won't ever learn to walk. They can be assured that this is not a problem; when the cast is removed, the child will quickly catch up on this developmental step.

✔ CHECKPOINT QUESTIONS

17. How is developmental hip dysplasia best assessed?
18. How is the affected hip positioned to correct developmental hip dysplasia?

COMMON CHROMOSOMAL DISORDERS THAT RESULT IN PHYSICAL OR COGNITIVE DEVELOPMENTAL DISORDERS

A number of chromosomal disorders may be detected at birth on physical assessment. The most common chromosomal disorders revealed this way are nondisjunction syndromes. All have the potential for causing physical anomalies and mental retardation. (Care of the child with mental retardation is discussed in Chapter 33.)

Trisomy 13 Syndrome

Trisomy 13 syndrome (Patau's syndrome; 47XX13+ or 47Xy13+) is a condition in which children have an extra chromosome 13. Children with this disorder are severely cognitively impaired. The incidence is low, approximately 0.45 per 1000 live births. Midline body disorders are present, and common findings are microcephaly with abnormalities of the forebrain and forehead; eyes that are smaller than normal (microphthalmia) or absent; cleft lip and palate; low-set ears; heart defects, particularly ventricular septal defects; and abnormal genitalia. Most of these children do not survive past early childhood.

Trisomy 18 Syndrome

Children with trisomy 18 syndrome (47XX18+or 47Xy18+) have three number 18 chromosomes. They are severely cognitively impaired. The incidence is approximately 0.25 per 1000 live births. These children tend to be small for gestational age at birth. They have markedly low-set ears, a small jaw, congenital heart defects and misshapen fingers and toes (the index finger crosses over other fingers). The soles of the feet are often rounded instead of flat (rocker-bottom feet). These children do not survive beyond early infancy.

Cri du Chat Syndrome

Cri du chat syndrome (46XX5q−) is the result of a short arm on chromosome 5. In addition to an abnormal cry, which is much more like the sound of a cat's than a human infant's, children with the syndrome tend to have a small head, wide-set eyes, and a downward slant to the palpebral fissure of the eye. They have severe cognitive impairment.

Turner's Syndrome

The child with Turner's syndrome (gonadal dysgenesis; 45XO) has only one functional X chromosome. The child is short in stature. The hairline at the nape of the neck is low-set, and the neck may appear to be webbed and short (Williams, 1995). The newborn may have appreciable edema of the hands and feet and a number of congenital anomalies, most frequently coarctation (stricture) of the aorta and kidney disorders. The child has only *streak* (small and nonfunctional) gonads so that, with the exception of pubic hair, secondary sex characteristics do not develop at puberty. Lack of ovarian function results in sterility. The incidence of the syndrome is approximately 1 per 1000 live births.

Although children with Turner's syndrome may be cognitively challenged, more commonly, intelligence is normal. Some children may have learning disabilities that interfere with learning ability.

If treatment with estrogen is begun at approximately 13 years, secondary sex characteristics will appear. If females continue taking estrogen for 3 out of every 4 weeks, they will have withdrawal bleeding that results in a menstrual flow. This flow, however, does not correct the problem of sterility. The gonadal tissue is scant and inadequate for ovulation because of the basic chromosomal aberration. Growth hormone can be helpful to achieve additional height.

Klinefelter's Syndrome

Infants with Klinefelter's syndrome are males with an XXY chromosome pattern (47XXY) (Abramsky & Chapple, 1997). The incidence is about 1 in 1000 live births. Characteristics of the syndrome may not be noticeable at birth. At puberty, the child has poorly developed secondary sex characteristics and small testes that produce ineffective sperm. Boys with the disorder tend to develop gynecomastia (increased breast size). The syndrome may be associated with an increased risk of developing cancer, especially male breast cancer (Humphreys et al, 1997).

Fragile X Syndrome

Fragile X syndrome is an X-linked pattern of inheritance in which one long arm of a X chromosome is weakened.

The incidence is about 1 in 1000 live births. It is the commonest cause of cognitive impairment in boys.

Before puberty, boys with fragile X syndrome typically have maladaptive behaviors such as hyperactivity and autism. They have reduced intellectual functioning with marked deficits in speech and arithmetic. They may be identified by the presence of a large head, a long face with a high forehead, a prominent lower jaw, and large protruding ears. Hyperextensive joints and cardiac disorders may also be present. After puberty, enlarged testicles may become evident. Affected individuals are fertile and can produce.

Carrier females may show some evidence of the physical and cognitive characteristics. Although intellectual function of children with the syndrome cannot be improved, both folic acid and phenothiazide administration may improve symptoms of poor concentration and impulsivity.

Down Syndrome (Trisomy 21)

Trisomy 21 (47XX21+ or 47Xy21+), the most frequent chromosomal abnormality, occurs as frequently as 1 in 800 live births. The syndrome occurs most frequently in the pregnancies of women who are over 35 years of age (the incidence is as high as 1 in 100 live births for these women). Paternal age (over 55) may also contribute to the increased incidence (Shapiro, 1997).

The physical features of children with Down syndrome are so marked that fetal diagnosis is possible by sonogram in utero. The nose is broad and flat; the eyelids have an extra fold of tissue at the inner canthus (an epicanthal fold); and the palpebral fissure (opening between the eyelids) tends to slant laterally upward. The iris of the eye may have white specks in it called Brushfield's spots. Even in the newborn, the tongue may protrude from the mouth because the oral cavity is smaller than normal. The back of the head is flat; the neck is short, and an extra pad of fat at the base of the head causes the skin there to be so loose it can be lifted up (like a puppy's neck). The ears may be low-set. Muscle tone is poor, giving the baby a rag-doll appearance. This can be so lax that the child's toe can be touched against the nose (not possible in the average mature newborn). The fingers of many children with Down syndrome are short and thick, and the little finger is often curved inward. There may be a wide space between the first and second toes and the first and second fingers. The palm of the hand shows a peculiar crease (a simian line) or a horizontal palm crease rather than the normal three creases in the palm. Children with Down syndrome usually have some degree of cognitive impairment, but the impairment can range from that of an educable child (intelligence quotient [IQ] of 50 to 70) to one requiring institutionalization (IQ less than 20). The extent of cognitive impairment is not evident at birth. Educable children may represent mosaic chromosomal patterns. The fact that the brain is not developing well is shown by a head size that is generally under the 10th to 20th percentile.

These children appear to have altered immune function. They are prone to upper respiratory infections. Congenital heart diseases, especially atrioventricular defects, are common. Stenosis or atresia of the duodenum and strabismus and cataract disorders are also common. For unknown reasons, acute lymphyocytic leukemia occurs approximately 20 times more frequently in children with Down syndrome than in the healthy population. Even if children are born without an accompanying disorder such as heart disease, their lifespan generally is only 40 to 50 years as aging seems to occur faster than normally.

Children with Down syndrome need to be exposed to early educational and play opportunities (see Chapter 33). Because they are prone to infections, sensible precautions such as using good handwashing technique should always be taken when caring for them. The enlarged tongue may interfere with swallowing and cause choking unless the child is fed slowly.

As with all newborns, children with Down syndrome need physical examination at birth in order that the genetic disorder can be detected and counseling and support for parents can begin.

✓ CHECKPOINT QUESTIONS

19. What feature of Turner's syndrome results in sterility?
20. Are the muscles of children with Down syndrome unusually stiff or relaxed?

KEY POINTS

The earlier parents learn about a child's health problem, the easier it is for them to adjust to it. Advocate for parents by helping them obtain as much information as they need.

Cleft lip and palate result from the failure of the maxillary process to fuse in intrauterine life. Surgical repair is possible early in life with good prognosis for both these conditions.

Tracheoesophageal atresia and fistula occur from failure of the trachea and esophagus to divide appropriately in intrauterine life. Surgical intervention often needs to be completed in several procedures.

Omphalocele is the protrusion of abdominal contents through the abdominal wall at birth, protected only by a peritoneal membrane. When the membrane is not present, this is gastroschisis. Although several stages of repair are often necessary, surgical correction has a good outcome.

Intestinal obstruction can result from atresia (complete closure) or stenosis (narrowing) of a part of the bowel. Correction is surgical removal of the narrowed bowel portion.

A meconium plug occurs when an extremely hard portion of meconium blocks the lumen of the intestine. Infants with meconium plug syndrome need to be observed for continued bowel function and may have a sweat test done for cystic fibrosis, because meconium plug is often a symptom of this.

Diaphragmatic hernia occurs when the abdominal organs protrude through a defect in the diaphragm into the chest cavity. This prevents the lungs from fully expanding at birth. These infants are critically ill at birth and need extensive surgical correction.

Imperforate anus is stricture of the anus resulting in inability to pass stool. The infant may have a temporary colostomy done before a final surgical correction.

Physical anomalies of the nervous system include hydrocephalus (excess CSF in the ventricles) and spina bifida (incomplete closure of the spinal cord). Infants with hydrocephalus have a shunt implanted from their ventricles to the peritoneal cavity to remove excess CSF. Children with myelomeningocele, the most severe form of spinal cord defect, face permanent loss of lower neuron function that requires continued habilitation.

Absent or malformed extremities that may occur range from absence of a finger to absence of an entire limb. Children may need physical therapy and teaching on how to use a prosthesis to have full function.

Developmental hip dysplasia is the improper formation and function of the hip socket; talipes deformities are foot and ankle deformities. Children may need extensive bracing and casting to correct these disorders.

Common nondisjunction genetic disorders that cause physical developmental concerns include Down syndrome (trisomy 21), trisomy 13 syndrome, trisomy 18 syndrome, Turner's syndrome, and Klinefelter's syndrome. Most of these syndromes involve cognitive impairment.

Parent–infant bonding is often difficult to establish when the child is hospitalized at birth. Assess family relationships at health maintenance visits to see that bonding has occurred.

CRITICAL THINKING EXERCISES

1. Mrs. Sparrow is the mother of the child with diaphragmatic hernia you met at the beginning of the chapter. She asked you what caused the condition. Now she asks you why everyone is telling her diaphragmatic hernia is an emergency. She thought a simple hernia repair could be done later when the child is older. How would you explain this to her?
2. You are in the birthing room when a child with various anomalies including an omphalocele and a cleft palate is born. The neonatal nurse practitioner who examines the baby tells you she thinks the baby has trisomy 18 syndrome. The mother becomes upset when she is told the omphalocele repair will result in an abdominal scar because she wants her daughter to be a model when she grows up. How would you respond to the mother? Will her daughter be able to be this?
3. A newborn who has been diagnosed with a tracheoesophageal fistula is waiting transport to an intensive care nursery. What assessments would be important? How would you explain this disorder to his parents? What position would you place the child in while awaiting transport?
4. You notice that the 16-year-old mother of a child born with a cleft lip is obviously upset at the child's appearance. She doesn't want to feed the baby and voices the thought of placing her for adoption. The child's father, a 22-year-old man, in contrast, handles the baby warmly and asks questions about surgery. No grandparents visit. What interventions would you want to begin with this family?
5. Children with developmental hip dysplasia may be in casts for a full year or more. What suggestions could you make to a parent to help her instill a strong sense of trust in her child? A sense of autonomy?

REFERENCES

Abramsky, L., & Chapple, J. (1997). 47,XXY (Klinefelter syndrome) and 47,XYY: estimated rates of an indication for postnatal diagnosis with implications for prenatal counseling. *Prenatal Diagnosis, 17*(4), 363.

Agrons, G. A., et al. (1996). Gastrointestinal manifestations of cystic fibrosis: radiologic-pathologic correlation. *Radiographics, 16*(4), 871.

Belloli, G., et al. (1996). Management of giant omphalocele by progressive external compression: case report. *Journal of Pediatric Surgery, 31*(12), 1719.

Botto, L. D., et al. (1997). The spectrum of congenital anomalies of the VATER association: an international study. *American Journal for Medical Genetics, 71*(1), 8.

Centers for Disease Control. (1995). Knowledge and use of folic acid by women of childbearing age—United States, 1995. *MMWR, 44*(38), 716.

Craig, C. (1995). Congenital talipes equinovarus. *Professional Nurse, 11*(1), 30.

Currarino, G. (1996). The various types of anorectal fistula in male imperforate anus. *Pediatric Radiology, 26*(8), 512.

Department of Health and Human Services. (1995). *Healthy people 2000: midcourse review.* Washington, DC: DHHS.

Dykes, E. H. (1996). Prenatal diagnosis and management of abdominal wall defects. *Seminars in Pediatric Surgery, 5*(2), 90.

Fishman, M. A. (1997). Developmental defects. In Johnson, K. P., & Oski, F. A. *Principles and practice of pediatrics* (2nd ed.). Philadelphia: J. B. Lippincott.

Frenckner, B., et al. (1997). Improved results in patients who have congenital diaphragmatic hernia using preoperative stabilization, extracorporeal membrane oxygenation and delayed surgery. *Journal of Pediatric Surgery, 32*(8), 1185.

Gorlin, R. J. (1997). Craniofacial defects. In Johnson, K. P., & Oski, F. A. *Principles and practice of pediatrics* (2nd ed.). Philadelphia: J. B. Lippincott.

Grant, A. (1996). Varicella infection and toxoplasmosis in pregnancy. *Journal of Perinatal and Neonatal Nursing, 10*(2), 17.

Harding, M. G., et al. (1997). Management of dislocated hips with Pavlik harness treatment and ultrasound monitoring. *Journal of Pediatric Orthopedics, 17*(2), 189.

Humphreys, M., et al. (1997). Klinefelter syndrome and non-Hodgkin lymphoma. *Cancer Genetics and Cytogenetics, 97*(2), 111.

Kallen, K. (1997). Maternal smoking and orofacial clefts. *Cleft Palate-Craniofacial Journal, 34*(1), 11.

Kuint, J., et al. (1997). Laryngeal obstruction caused by lingual thyroglossal duct cyst presenting at birth. *American Journal of Perinatology, 14*(6), 353.

Langer, J. C. (1996). Gastroschisis and omphalocele. *Seminars in Pediatric Surgery, 5*(2), 124.

Laubscher, B., et al. (1997). Response to nitric oxide in term and preterm infants. *European Journal of Pediatrics, 156*(8), 639.

Newman, B., & Bender, T. M. (1997). Esophageal atresia/tracheoesophageal fistula and associated congenital esophageal stenosis. *Pediatric Radiology, 27*(6), 530.

Nichols, C. R., et al. (1997). Rising incidence of gastroschisis in teenage pregnancies. *Journal of Maternal and Fetal Medicine, 6*(4), 225.

Perkins, J. A., et al. (1997). Airway management in children with craniofacial anomalies. *Cleft Palate-Craniofacial Journal, 34*(2), 135.

Pokorny, W. J. (1997). Anorectal malformations. In Johnson, K. P., & Oski, F. A. *Principles and practice of pediatrics* (2nd ed.). Philadelphia: J. B. Lippincott.

Sarwark, J. F. (1996). Spina bifida. *Pediatric Clinics of North America, 43*(5), 1151.

Shapiro, L. J. (1997). Signs and symptoms of inborn errors of metabolism. In Johnson, K. P., & Oski, F. A. *Principles and practice of pediatrics* (2nd ed.). Philadelphia: J. B. Lippincott.

Smith, M. (1996). Cleft lip and palate. *Modern Midwife, 6*(6), 30.

Sponseller, P. D. (1997). Bone, joint and muscle problems. In Johnson, K. P., & Oski, F. A. *Principles and practice of pediatrics* (2nd ed.). Philadelphia: J. B. Lippincott.

Teo, C., & Jones, R. (1996). Management of hydrocephalus by endoscopic third ventriculostomy in patients with myelomeningocele. *Pediatric Neurosurgery, 25*(2), 57.

Thibeault, D. W., & Sigalet, D. L. (1998). Congenital diaphragmatic hernia from the womb to childhood. *Current Problems in Pediatrics, 28*(1), 1.

Tunnessen, W. W., Jr. (1997). Common syndromes with morphologic abnormalities. In Johnson, K. P., & Oski, F. A. *Principles and practice of pediatrics* (2nd ed.). Philadelphia: J. B. Lippincott.

Williams, J. K. (1995). Parenting a daughter with precocious puberty or Turner syndrome. *Journal of Pediatric Health Care, 9*(3), 109.

Wu, H. Y., et al. (1997). Neurogenic bladder dysfunction due to myelomeningocele: neonatal versus childhood treatment. *Journal of Urology, 157*(6), 2295.

SUGGESTED READINGS

Alexander-Doelle, A. (1997). Breastfeeding and cleft palates. *AWHONN Lifelines, 1*(4), 27.

Dagostino, J. A. (1997). Congenital diaphragmatic hernia: what happens after discharge? *MCN: American Journal of Maternal Child Nursing, 22*(5), 263.

Davies, B. W., & Stringer, M. D. (1997). The survivors of gastroschisis. *Archives of Disease in Childhood, 77*(2), 158.

Dunn, J. C., & Fonkalsrud, E. W. (1997). Improved survival of infants with omphalocele. *American Journal of Surgery, 173*(4), 284.

Fraser, R. (1996). Imperforate anus: nutritional care. *Paediatric Nursing, 8*(3), 16.

Javid, P. J. et al. (1998). Immediate and long-term results of surgical management of low imperforate anus in girls. *Journal of Pediatric Surgery, 33*(2), 198.

Lasswell, B. (1996). Myths and facts . . . about Down syndrome. *Nursing, 26*(3), 65.

Neal, M. R., et al. (1997). Neonatal ultrasonography to distinguish between meconium ileus and ileal atresia. *Journal of Ultrasound in Medicine, 16*(4), 263.

Stephens, P., et al. (1997). Neonatal cleft lip repair; a retrospective review of anaesthetic complications. *Paediatric Anaesthesia, 7*(1), 33.

Sullivan, G. (1996). Parental bonding in cleft lip and palate repair. *Paediatric Nursing, 8*(1), 21.

Tsai, J. T., et al. (1997). Esophageal atresia and tracheoesophageal fistula: surgical experience over two decades. *Annals of Thoracic Surgery, 64*(3), 778.

Urao, M., et al. (1996). Lingual thyroglossal duct cyst: a unique surgical approach. *Journal of Pediatric Surgery, 31*(11), 1574.

Zaleski, C. G., et al. (1997). Pediatric case of the day: small bowel (ileal) volvulus and ileal atresia. *Radiographics, 17*(2), 537.

Nursing Care of the Child With a Respiratory Disorder

19

CHAPTER

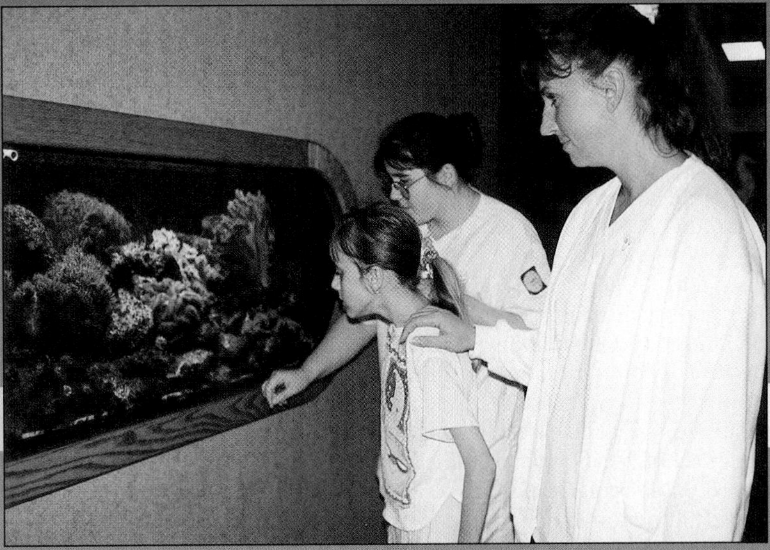

Key Terms

- adventitious sounds
- aspiration
- atelectasis
- clubbing
- cupping
- cyanosis
- expiration
- hypoxemia
- hypoxia
- inspiration
- paroxysmal coughing
- percussion
- pneumothorax
- postural drainage
- rales
- retraction
- steatorrhea
- stridor
- tachypnea
- tracheostomy
- tracheotomy
- vibration
- wheezing

Objectives

After mastering the contents of this chapter, you should be able to:

1. Describe common respiratory illnesses in children.
2. Assess the child with a respiratory illness.
3. Formulate a nursing diagnosis related to respiratory illness in children.
4. Establish outcomes that address the priority needs of the child with a respiratory illness
5. Plan the nursing care of the child with a respiratory illness.
6. Implement nursing care for the child with a respiratory illness.
7. Evaluate outcomes for achievement and effectiveness of care.
8. Identify National Health Goals related to children with respiratory disorders that nurses could be instrumental in helping the nation achieve.
9. Identify areas related to care of children with respiratory disorders that could benefit from additional nursing research.
10. Use critical thinking to analyze ways that nursing care for a child with a respiratory illness could be more family centered.
11. Integrate knowledge of respiratory illness in children with nursing process to achieve quality child health nursing care.

Michael is a 5-year-old who is seen in the emergency department. He was brought in by his nanny because he was coughing and obviously short of breath. He has such loud wheezing you can hear it without a stethoscope. "Get me oxygen!" Michael shouts at you. "Hurry!" the nanny shouts. "If he dies, everyone will say it's my fault!" What emergency care does Michael need? What about Michael's action would lead you to believe his airway is not yet completely obstructed?

In previous chapters, you learned about the growth and development of well children. In this chapter, you'll add information about the dramatic changes, both physical and psychosocial, that occur when children develop respiratory disorders. This is important information because it builds a base for care and health teaching.

After you've studied the chapter, turn to the Critical Thinking Exercises at the end of the chapter to help sharpen your skills and test your knowledge.

Respiratory disorders are among the most frequent causes of illness and hospitalization in children. Because the diseases range from minor illnesses such as a simple upper respiratory tract infection to life-threatening lower-respiratory tract diseases, such as pneumonia, and because the level of acuity changes quickly, respiratory disorders are often difficult for parents to evaluate. Overall, respiratory dysfunction in children tends to be more serious than in adults because the lumens in the child's respiratory tract are smaller and therefore more likely to become obstructed with disease. Both the child and parents need a great deal of nursing support when disease interferes with the function of breathing, because even very young children can panic when breathing becomes labored. Early diagnosis and treatment are essential in preventing a minor problem from turning into a more serious one.

Because respiratory disorders are a frequent cause of childhood illness and hospitalization, National Health Goals have been established for children with respiratory illnesses. These are shown in the Focus on National Health Goals box.

FOCUS ON NATIONAL HEALTH GOALS

A number of National Health Goals focus on respiratory illness in children:

- Reduce the initiation of cigarette smoking by children and youth so that no more than 15% have become regular cigarette smokers by age 20 from a baseline of 30%.
- Reduce asthma morbidity as measured by a reduction in asthma hospitalizations to no more than 225 per 100,000 children under 14 years of age, from a baseline of 284 per 100,000.
- Reduce pneumonia-related days of restricted activity in children age 4 and younger to 24 days per 100 children, from a baseline of 27 days per 100 children.
- Reduce tuberculosis to an incidence of no more than 3.5 cases per 100,000 people from a baseline of 9.1 per 100,000 (DHHS, 1995).

Nurses can be instrumental in helping the nation achieve these goals by teaching children to avoid beginning cigarette smoking, teaching programs to help children with asthma learn ways of increasing activity and steps to take to reduce the severity of an attack and reminding parents to come for child health maintenance visits so that children receive screening for tuberculosis.

Additional nursing research is needed on the accuracy of parents in reading and interpreting tine tests; what motivates children to keep participating in asthma exercise programs; and what new parents need to know to better manage respiratory illness in infants and young children.

NURSING PROCESS OVERVIEW

for Care of the Child With a Respiratory Disorder

Assessment

Respiratory illness can begin at birth when the newborn has difficulty initiating the first breath or establishing regular respirations. Knowing the newborn's Apgar score will help to quickly identify the newborn who may be experiencing respiratory difficulty at this early stage.

As a nurse in a well-child clinic or health maintenance organization, you are often the first health care provider to talk to a parent about a child's respiratory illness. It is important to establish both onset and duration of the problem so that its seriousness can be determined. Infants who cannot finish a bottle feeding because of exhaustion or rapid breathing or children who cannot run with other children because they do not have enough breath, for example, should be suspected of having a respiratory disorder. An episode of acute coughing is suggestive of an acute respiratory disorder.

The child admitted to the hospital with a respiratory disorder is usually in an acute stage of the illness. The child's condition may worsen rapidly in the first few hours until a prescribed medication, such as an antibiotic or bronchodilator, begins to take effect. Assessment that a child is developing tachypnea or retractions may be the first indication of a child's worsening condition.

Nursing Diagnosis

Nursing diagnoses established for the child with a respiratory disorder focus both on the alteration in mechanisms of breathing and on the emotional distress such problems can create. "Ineffective airway clearance" is a common diagnostic category used in this area. The problem may be related to any one of a variety of factors, such as ineffective cough, fatigue, weakness, viscous secretions, pain, aspiration of foreign body, or lack of knowledge about the importance of coughing.

The diagnostic categories "Impaired gas exchange" and "Ineffective breathing pattern" also may be used, although because the nurse does not generally prescribe definitive treatment for these problems (except when caused by hyperventilation), it may be appropriate for a nursing diagnosis to focus on the effects of impaired gas exchange or ineffective breathing on daily activities and psychosocial health (Carpenito, 1997). Additional nursing diagnoses include the following:

- Activity intolerance related to insufficient oxygenation
- Fatigue related to impaired gas exchange
- Fear related to inability to breathe without effort
- Impaired social interaction related to difficulty in keeping up with physical activities of peers
- Knowledge deficit related to need for continued treatment

Outcome Identification and Planning

If the child is experiencing an acute respiratory problem, the outcomes and plan of care will focus on supporting the child and family through prescribed therapy and keeping parents informed about their child's health status and response to treatment. Often the treatment period for respiratory illness may be prolonged, and parents of children with chronic conditions need to learn how to continue therapy at home. Helping parents to plan programs of exercise, chest physiotherapy, and continuing medication is an important nursing activity. Parents also need to understand that their approach to these programs must change as their children grow older. With an infant, they simply need to perform the prescribed procedures. Toddlers may be ready to learn how to do some things for themselves, and preschoolers should be ready. A game might be a good way to get across the necessary information ("Simon says cough. Simon says take five deep breaths"). Exercise programs for school-age children must be planned around the school day. If a home program, such as an exercise program or medication therapy, is not well designed or adapted to the child and family, parents may have difficulty carrying out the program or may only carry it out sporadically or not at all. Including other family members, such as older siblings (within reason) or grandparents, in this program may help to diffuse the burden of care and also to unite the family in working toward a common goal.

Implementation

Collaborative nursing interventions in the care of the child with respiratory dysfunction include suctioning to remove respiratory secretions, administering oxygen, and providing humidification and expectorant therapy to help the child maintain a clear airway. Some of the most important nursing interventions in this area are independent nursing functions: placing the child in an upright position to help her cough more effectively; providing an interesting game to teach him the importance of strengthening chest muscles; supporting the child and family through the anxiety created when the child is not breathing normally; and teaching parents of the child with chronic respiratory dysfunction the basics of percussion or chest physiotherapy techniques. All of these interventions require sound nursing judgment and skill.

Referral to community resources and organizations for support is also a key nursing function. Some organizations to recommend as support to parents of the child with a respiratory disorder include the following:

American Lung Association
1740 Broadway
New York, NY 10019-4374

National Easter Seal Society
70 E. Lake Street
Chicago, IL 60601

National Asthma Education Program
4733 Bethesda Avenue, Suite 530
Bethesda, MD 20814

Asthma & Allergy Foundation of America
1125 15th Street, NW, Suite 502
Washington, DC 20005

Cystic Fibrosis Foundation
6931 Arlington Road
Bethesda, MD 20814

Outcome Evaluation

An acute respiratory illness such as pneumonia is extremely frightening for parents. After the child has recovered, talk with the parents to determine whether they have come to terms with their fear and are able to treat the child as a well child again. Overprotection of children by their parents may result in well but dependent children. This pattern is one that nursing evaluation can help to prevent.

Outcomes for the child with chronic respiratory disease will change as the child grows and develops. No matter what the specific concerns are, however, evaluation should always include examination of how well the child individually and the family as a whole have adapted to manage the limitations imposed by the disorder while maintaining a lifestyle that fosters growth and development for all family members.

Expected outcomes may include the following:

- Infant maintains respiratory rate of at least 20 breaths/min.
- Child voices a reduced program of school activities he will maintain to reduce fatigue.
- Child's PaO_2 is maintained at 80 to 100 mm Hg in room air.
- Child lists steps she will take if breathing becomes impaired while at school.
- Parents demonstrate correct techniques for performing respiratory treatments at home.

ANATOMY AND PHYSIOLOGY OF THE RESPIRATORY SYSTEM

The respiratory system is usually separated into two divisions for discussion: the upper respiratory tract, composed of the nose, paranasal sinuses, pharynx, larynx, and epiglottis; and the lower tract, composed of the bronchi, bronchioles, and lungs. Through **inspiration**, the respiratory system delivers warmed and moistened air to the alveoli; transports oxygen across the alveolar membrane to hemoglobin-laden red blood cells; and allows carbon dioxide to diffuse from red blood cells back into the alveoli. Through **expiration**, carbon dioxide–filled air is discharged to the outside. Levels of oxygen and carbon dioxide in the lungs, blood, and body cells are shown in Figure 19-1.

The respiratory center is located in the medulla of the brain. Changes in body acidity, percentages of carbon dioxide and oxygen, temperature, and blood pressure all stimulate the respiratory center to slow or increase respiratory activity. In the pons, an inhibitory center halts inspiratory impulses before the lungs become overextended. Depth of respiration is influenced by proprioceptors located in the lung periphery that register lung fullness and in the oxygen concentration and pH of arterial blood. Often children with chronic lung disease have adapted so well to a chronically high $PaCO_2$ level that receptor sites in the blood vessels no longer register this as abnormal. In these instances, the main stimulus for respiration is a low oxygen level. In such children, administering high levels of oxygen may be dangerous, because it alleviates oxygen want and respiratory stimulus.

Respiratory Tract Differences in Children

The ethmoidal and maxillary sinuses are present at birth; the frontal sinuses (those sinuses most frequently involved in sinus infection) and the sphenoidal sinuses do not develop until 6 to 8 years of age. Tonsillar tissue is normally enlarged in early school-age children.

Respiratory mucus generally functions as a cleaning agent. However, newborns produce little respiratory mucus, which makes them more susceptible to respiratory infection than older children. Excessive production of mucus in children up to 2 years of age can readily lead to obstruction because the lumen is smaller in a child of this age.

After 2 years of age, the right bronchus becomes shorter, wider, and more vertical than the left. For this reason, inhaled foreign bodies more often lodge in the right bronchus. Infants use their abdominal muscles to inhale. The change to thoracic breathing begins at 2 to 3 years of age and is complete at 7 years. Because accessory muscles are used more in children than adults, weakness of these muscles from disease may result in respiratory failure.

In infants, the walls of the airways have less cartilage than in older children and adults and are more likely to collapse after expiration. A lessened amount of smooth muscle in the airway means that an infant does not develop bronchospasm as readily as an older child or adult. Wheezing, the sound of air being pushed through constricted bronchioles, therefore, may not be a prominent finding in infants even when the lumen of the airway is severely compromised.

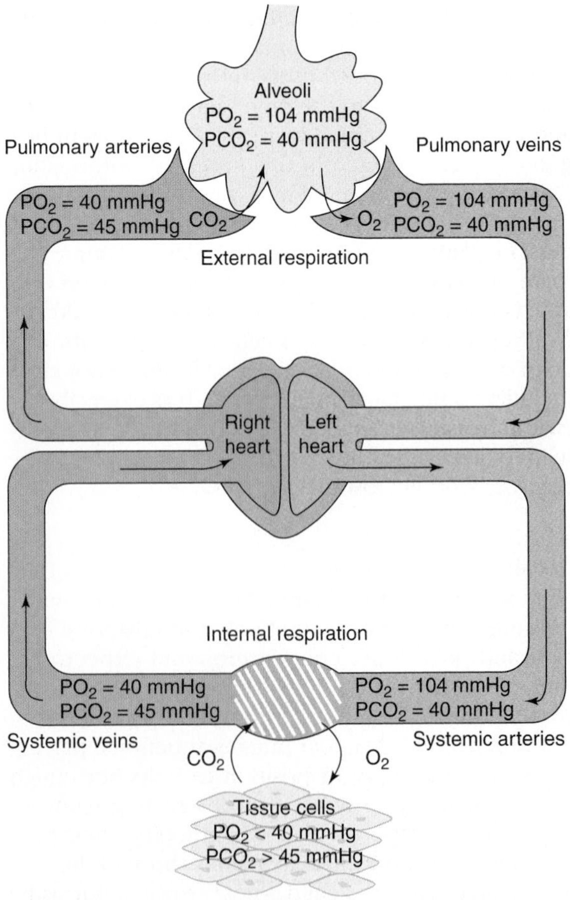

FIGURE 19.1 Partial pressure of gas (mm Hg) as measured in peripheral and systemic circulation. Because of the differences in partial pressure of the gases in the different areas, O_2 moves from alveoli to pulmonary capillaries (i.e., the gas moves from the area of greater concentration to one of a lesser concentration). When it reaches the tissue capillaries, O_2 partial pressure is less, so O_2 goes into the tissues and CO_2 moves out.

✓ CHECKPOINT QUESTIONS

1. Which sinuses do not develop until approximately age 6 years?
2. Where would you anticipate that an inhaled foreign body would lodge in a 4-year-old?

ASSESSING RESPIRATORY ILLNESS IN CHILDREN

Assessment of respiratory illness in children includes an interview, physical examination, and laboratory testing. If the child is in acute distress, the interview and health history may cover only the most important details: when the child first became ill and what symptoms are present. It is important, however, to get as accurate a picture as possible, because the problem could be the result of a variety of causes (see Assessing the Child for Signs and Symptoms of Respiratory Dysfunction.)

It is important to take a thorough history because the symptoms of **hypoxemia** (deficient oxygenation of the blood) are often insidious. Peripheral vasoconstriction (a mechanism to save the available oxygen for central life-sustaining body organs) leads to a pale appearance. Tachypnea and tachycardia (efforts to oxygenate better), anxiety, and confusion (caused by limited brain perfusion) may occur. A poor feeding pattern may be one of the first signs noted in the infant because an infant cannot suck and breathe rapidly at the same time. Cardiac arrhythmia may occur because of poor heart perfusion.

ASSESSING the Child for Signs and Symptoms of Respiratory Dysfunction

History

Chief concern: Cough, rapid respirations, noisy breathing, rhinitis, reddened sore throat, lethargy, cyanosis, difficulty sucking, fever.
Past medical history: Poor weight gain, difficulty with respirations at birth; prematurity.
Family history: History of family member with asthma; other family members with respiratory infection.

Physical examination

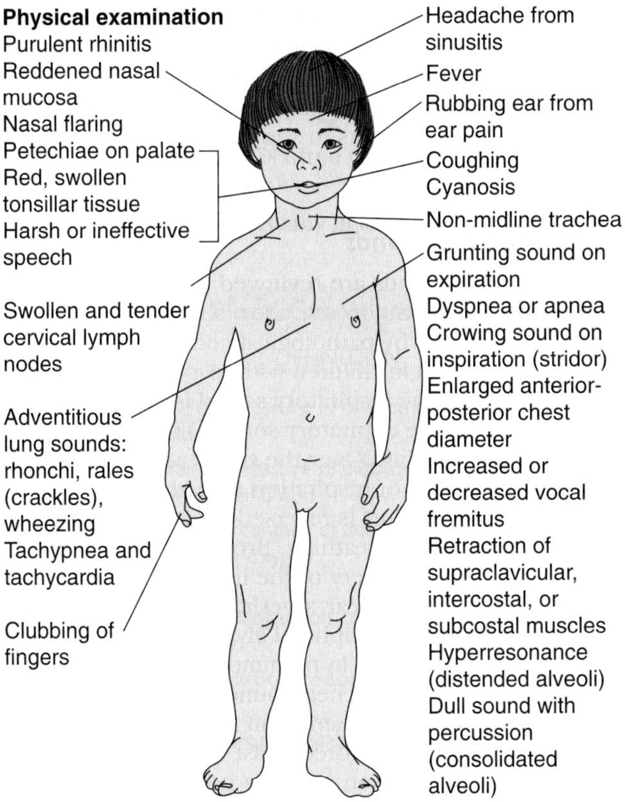

Physical Assessment

Physical assessment of the child with respiratory dysfunction includes observation of such presenting symptoms as cough, cyanosis, or pallor, as well as evaluation of respirations and lung sounds. While assessing the child, be alert for cultural factors such as home remedies that may have been used (see Focus on Cultural Competence). Lung sounds are heard best if an infant or child is not crying. Spending time comforting the child to stop crying is therefore time well spent.

Cough

A cough reflex is initiated by stimulation of the nerves of the respiratory tract mucosa by the presence of dust, chemicals, mucus, or inflammation. The sound of coughing is caused by rapid expiration past the glottis. Coughing is a useful procedure to clear excess mucus or foreign bodies from the respiratory tract. It becomes harmful and needs suppression only when there is no mucus or debris to be expelled. This might occur with respiratory tract inflammation. A series of expiratory coughs after a deep inspiration is **paroxysmal coughing.** Commonly, it occurs in children with pertussis (whooping cough). Coughing increases chest pressure and may decrease venous return to the heart. This lowers cardiac output and may lead to fainting (syncope). Paroxysmal coughing may increase the pressure in the central venous circulation to such an extent that there is bleeding into the central nervous system. Young

FOCUS ON CULTURAL COMPETENCE

Upper respiratory illnesses occur universally, making them a concern of parents the world over. Home remedies for such illnesses vary greatly, however. Hanging garlic around a child's neck is a frequent therapy in Mediterranean countries. Herbs may be used the same way by parents from the Far East or South America. It is important to respect these remedies and not remove them when they are discovered. Although the therapeutic value of these remedies may not be proven, it is important to the nurse-patient and nurse-family relationships to respect family traditions.

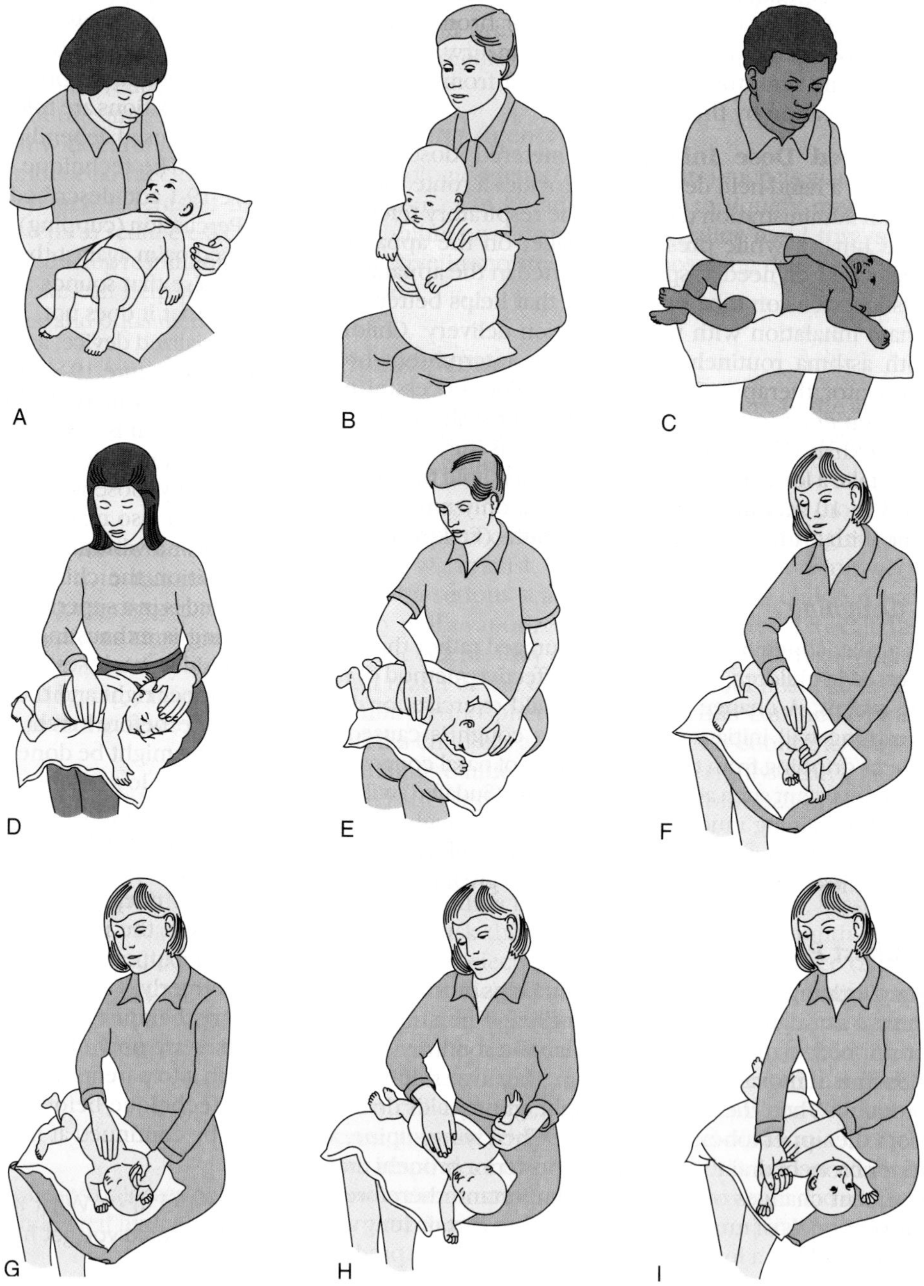

FIGURE 19.7 Positions for bronchial drainage for major segments of all lobes in infants. This procedure is most readily performed with the infant in the therapist's lap, with the therapist's hand on the chest indicating the area to be cupped or vibrated. (**A**) Apical segment of left upper lobe. (**B**) Posterior segment of left upper lobe. (**C**) Anterior segment of left upper lobe. (**D**) Superior segment of right lower lobe. (**E**) Posterior basal segment of right lower lobe. (**F**) Lateral basal segment of right lower lobe. (**G**) Anterior basal segment of right lower lobe. (**H**) Medial and lateral segments of right middle lobe. (**I**) Lingular segments (superior and inferior) of left upper lobe.

tory tract. Oxygen may be delivered to infants by flooding an Isolette or by using a plastic hood. This tight-fitting plastic enclosure can keep oxygen concentration at nearly 100% (Figure 19-10). The hood should fit snugly over the infant's head, making sure that it does not rub against the infant's neck, chin, or shoulders. Be sure that the gas does not blow directly into the infant's face. A nasal catheter or nasal prongs can be used for older children. These provide a concentration of approximately 50% with an oxygen flow of 4 L/min. Most children do not like nasal prongs because they are intrusive. Assess the nostrils carefully when using nasal prongs. The pressure of prongs can cause areas of necrosis, particularly on the nasal septum. A snug-fitting oxygen mask can supply nearly 100% oxygen (Figure 19-11). However, masks are often not well tolerated by children. If necessary, let children hold a mask rather than strapping it in place to allow them more control.

Oxygen tents also may be used. Although using an oxygen tent is the most comfortable form of administration to use with children, the oxygen concentration in a tent is difficult to control and maintain, and it rarely rises above 40%, a level inadequate to correct the oxygen need in many children. The moisture in oxygen tents also may harbor microorganisms and therefore be contraindicated.

Oxygen must be administered warmed and moistened, no matter what the route of delivery, because dry oxygen will dry mucous membranes and thicken secretions. It must be administered with the same careful observation and thoughtfulness as any drug. If concentrations are too low,

MANAGING AND DELEGATING UNLICENSED ASSISTIVE PERSONNEL

Unlicensed assistive personnel may be assigned to help with the care of children with respiratory disorders. When assigned, be certain they understand the importance of not allowing a child to grow fatigued during care. Instruct them in the need to maintain oxygen therapy as ordered, even with activity, and to watch oxygen saturation levels (if pulse oximetry is attached), reporting any changes in oxygen saturation levels below specified values. When oxygen is being used, review oxygen safety measures with them and reinforce the concept that oxygen supports combustion. Providing a birthday cake with lit candles, for example, might seem like a nice idea but could be very hazardous, even fatal, because of the risk for an explosion.

mucus membrane of the nose, reduce mucus production, and thereby enlarge the airway. These products also typically cause drowsiness. Bronchodilators such as albuterol, theophylline, and racemic epinephrine may be used to open the lower airway. Corticosteroids taken either orally or by inhalation enlarge the airway by reducing inflammation. Expectorants such as guaifenesin (Robitussin) help to raise mucus. Most of these agents also cause drowsiness, so the dose must be regulated, especially in adolescents who will be driving automobiles.

In children with asthma, a disorder that leads to inflammation, bronchoconstriction, and mucus production, a combination of drugs (an anti-inflammatory steroid and a beta-2 agonist bronchodilator) may be used. Antibiotics may be given intravenously, intramuscularly, orally, or inhaled through nebulization. These help enlarge the airflow by combating the infection that is the cause of unusual mucus production or inflammation.

Incentive Spirometry

Incentive spirometers, or devices to encourage children to inhale deeply to fully aerate lungs or move mucus, are manufactured in different configurations, but a common type consists of a hollow plastic tube containing a brightly colored ball that will rise in the tube when a child inhales on the attached mouthpiece and tubing. The deeper the inhalation, the higher the ball rises in the tube.

Children need instruction in how to use this type of device, because their first impression is that they should blow out against the mouthpiece rather than inhale (Figure 19-12*A*).

Breathing Techniques

Some children need exercises prescribed to help them better inflate alveoli or more fully empty alveoli. Blowing a cotton or plastic ball across a surface such as a table, blowing through a straw, or blowing out with the lips pursed all accomplish this (Figure 19-12*B*). Yet another method for increasing aeration includes asking the child to blow up a balloon, which requires the child to take a deep inhalation. For best results, make these activities a game or contest rather than an exercise.

CHECKPOINT QUESTIONS

7. Why do children find nebulizers uncomfortable?
8. What is the chief point to teach children about using incentive spirometers?

Tracheostomy

A **tracheostomy** involves an opening into the trachea to create an artificial airway to relieve respiratory obstruction that has occurred above that point. The procedure to create the airway is a **tracheotomy;** the resultant airway

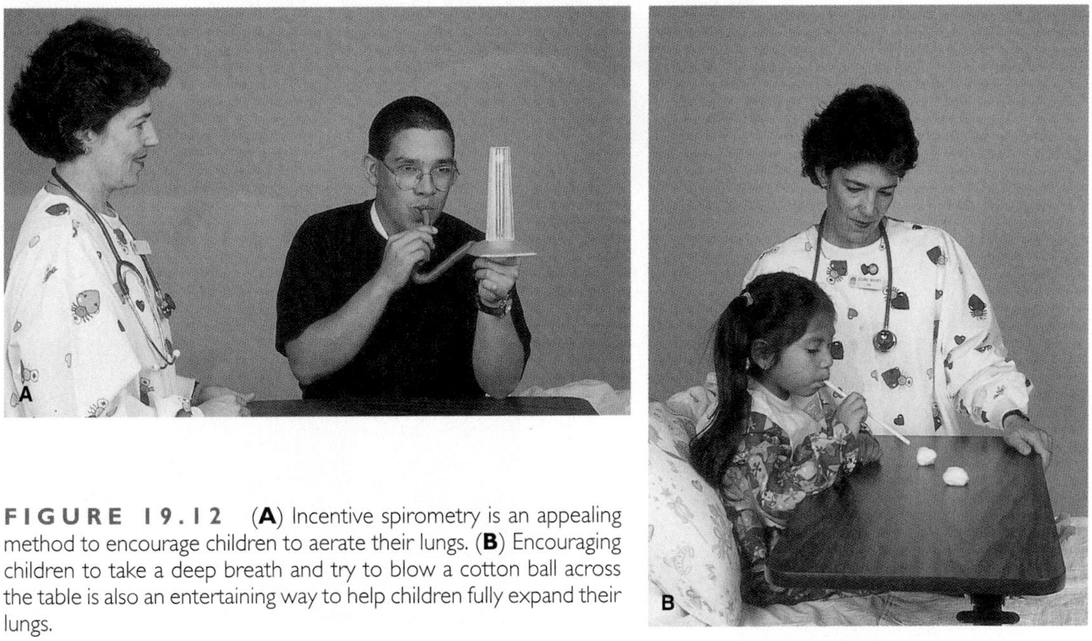

FIGURE 19.12 (**A**) Incentive spirometry is an appealing method to encourage children to aerate their lungs. (**B**) Encouraging children to take a deep breath and try to blow a cotton ball across the table is also an entertaining way to help children fully expand their lungs.

is the tracheostomy. Tracheostomies also may be used when accumulating mucus causes lower airway obstruction, because the accumulated fluid can be suctioned through the tracheostomy tube. Tracheostomy interferes with the cleansing action of the mucous membrane lining the airway. Children with tracheostomies will need frequent suctioning to eliminate mucus. Tracheostomy also eliminates the warming and filtering action of the nose and pharynx, making children more susceptible to infection. For these reasons, endotracheal intubation, not tracheostomy, has become the method of choice to relieve airway obstruction. The exception to this is obstruction in the pharynx, because it is often impossible to pass an endotracheal tube beyond obstruction at this point.

Emergency Intubation. Few medical emergencies are as frightening to a child or parents as an obstruction of a child's upper airway requiring a tracheotomy or endotracheal intubation. The child suddenly becomes limp and breathless with his color changing quickly from pink to pale, followed by systemic cyanosis. Tracheotomies are done more easily on a treatment room table than on a bed or crib, so it is generally best to carry the child immediately to the treatment room. If the child cannot be moved quickly, however, because of accessory equipment, no time should be lost in transport. For tracheotomy, the cricoid cartilage of the trachea is swabbed with an antiseptic; if readily available, a local anesthetic may be injected into the cartilage ring. (This is not necessary in the unconscious child.) An incision is made just under the ring of cartilage; a tracheostomy tube with its obturator in place is inserted into the opening (Figure 19-13*A*). When the obturator is removed, the child is able to breathe through the hollow tracheostomy tube. Suction equipment should be available for immediate use to clear any blood caused by the incision (this is minimal) and any obstructing mucus from the trachea.

A few sutures may be necessary at the tube insertion site to halt bleeding or to reduce the size of the incision so the tube fits snugly. The color change in children after tracheostomy is usually dramatic. They inhale deeply a number of times through the tube, and color returns to normal.

As children begin to breathe normally and, if unconscious, regain consciousness, they often thrash and push at people around them. Part of this reaction stems from oxygen deficit, part from fright. Children try to cry for a parent but make no sound, adding to their fright. Such a child needs to be assured that everything is all right. If preschool age or younger, the comforting sound of someone saying that it is all right that they cannot speak will have a calming effect (Figure 19-13*B*). A school-age child can understand a simple explanation, for example, "you cannot speak at the moment because of the tube in your throat." As soon as the child's respirations are even and no longer distressed, the child can be shown that by placing a finger over the tracheostomy tube, air will again flow past the larynx and allow the child to speak.

Explain to parents why the tube is in place. Assure them that it is a temporary measure (providing this is true). Let them see the child as soon as possible after the procedure to assure themselves that their child is again all

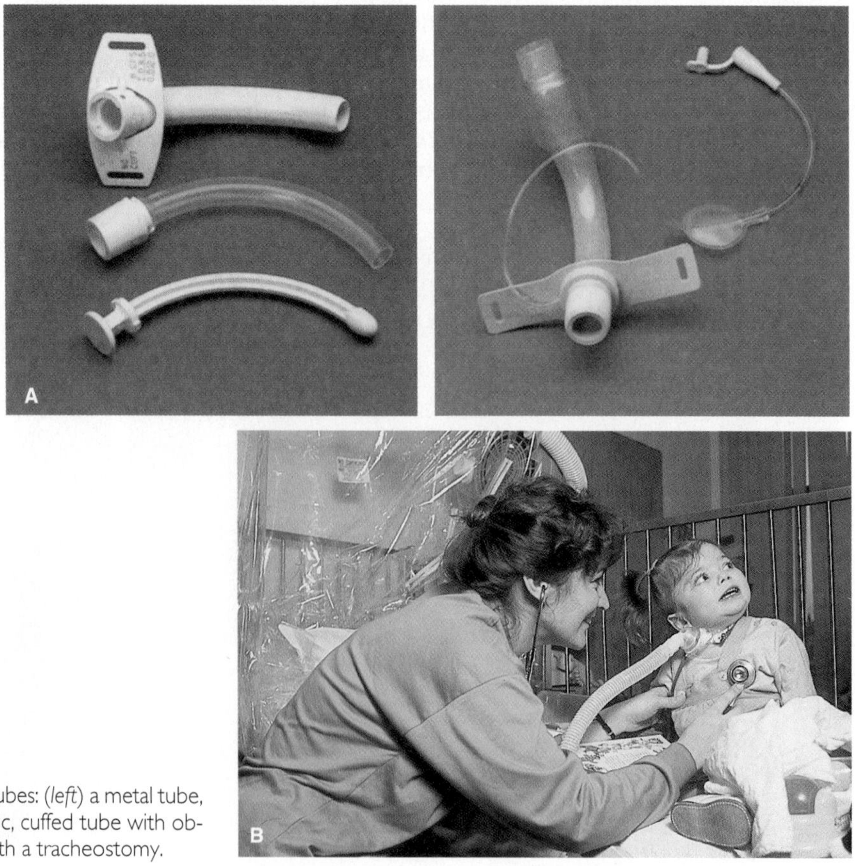

FIGURE 19.13 (**A**) Tracheostomy tubes: (*left*) a metal tube, inner cannula, and outer cannula; (*right*) a plastic, cuffed tube with obturator. (**B**) The nurse interacts with a child with a tracheostomy.

right. Explain well to parents why the tracheostomy was necessary. Children cannot relax and accept this strange new way of breathing until their parents can understand its need, relax and accept it. Some children hyperventilate, not because of respiratory difficulty, but because of their fear.

Suctioning Technique. Most tracheostomy tubes used with children today are plastic. They do not include an inner cannula that would require regular cleaning. Most children, however, do require frequent suctioning (perhaps as often as every 15 minutes) to keep the airway free of mucus. Suction gently and yet thoroughly. Ineffective suction does not remove obstructive mucus but, because of irritation, causes more mucus to form. Be certain you know how deeply to suction. Some children need only to be suctioned the length of the tracheostomy tube so that the catheter does not touch and irritate the tracheal mucosa. Others need to be deeply suctioned to reduce the possibility that mucus will become so copious or so thickened that it obstructs the trachea.

Tracheostomy suctioning technique is shown in Nursing Procedure 19-2. Because suctioning removes air as well as secretions from the trachea, children may become very short of oxygen during the procedure. Preoxygenating them by "bagging" or administering oxygen for 5 minutes before the procedure helps reduce this problem.

Dropping 1 or 2 mL sterile saline into the tracheostomy tube before suctioning may be helpful in loosening secretions. This is a controversial procedure, however, because it induces violent coughing, and possibly aspiration, and it may not actually aid the removal of secretions.

Young children may need to wear elbow restraints while being suctioned to keep their hands away from the catheter. In addition, restraints may be necessary at all times when they are alone to prevent them from fussing with the tracheostomy tube and accidentally removing it.

Frequently check on children with tracheostomies to assess for possible respiratory difficulty. Make certain that you spend time playing with them or just sitting and rocking them so that they come to think of you in ways other than as the person who comes to suction them. Be sure that parents are aware that you check on their child more frequently than what would be necessary for suctioning alone, to assure them that if the child should have another episode of acute obstruction, someone will be nearby. If the tracheostomy tube is to be left in place after discharge from the hospital, teach the parents how to care for it at home.

The tracheostomy tube is held in place by cloth ties that fasten at the back of the child's neck. These need to be changed when they become soiled or loose and checked frequently to be certain they remain tied. Children tend to fuss with such things, whereas adults may not. The ties should fit snugly but allow for one finger to be inserted underneath the ties. For preschoolers or younger children, it is a good idea to cover the tracheostomy opening with a gauze square tied to the child's neck like a bib while they are eating. This prevents crumbs or spilled liquids from entering. Do not give children small toys that could possibly fit into the lumen of the tube and cause obstruction (see Empowering the Family).

If the tracheostomy tube used has an inner cannula, remove and clean it as necessary, at least every 8 hours. Be certain that the school-age child who is old enough to understand this realizes that you are removing only the inner tube to clean it and that this action will not interfere with breathing in any way. Wear sterile gloves and use sterile solutions to clean an inner cannula to prevent introducing bacteria to the trachea. Always follow standard precautions. If secretions are moist and loose, a cotton-tipped applicator or tube brush dipped in sterile water may work well for cleaning the inner cannula. If secretions are tenacious, soaking the cannula in a solution such as half-strength hydrogen peroxide may be helpful to loosen the secretions. Dry an inner cannula well with a cotton-tipped applicator before you replace it in the outer tube, so that drops of water do not run from it into the trachea and add to the accumulating secretions.

Each child must be considered individually as to when it is time to remove a tracheostomy tube (Gray, Todd & Jacobs, 1998). Tracheostomy tubes are generally sealed off partially by adhesive tape for a day or two before removal. Then they are completely occluded (but not removed) for yet another day. In this way, suctioning is still possible if it is needed. Occasionally, children cough so forcefully that they dislodge a tracheostomy tube. You might be with a child when this occurs, or you might walk into the room and find the tube lying beside the child on the bedclothes. A new tube and obturator should always be kept at the bedside in case replacement is necessary. As long as a child is not in distress, this is not an emergency, because the incision site usually does not close completely to occlude the tracheal opening when a tube is dislodged. Slide the obturator into the tube and gently replace it in the tracheal opening. If you do this quickly yet calmly, children are less likely to become alarmed and protest. If, however, they sense your excitement or if you indicate that something is terribly wrong, they may begin to cry and turn away, thus making it difficult to replace the tube without assistance.

✔ CHECKPOINT QUESTIONS

9. Is it necessary to wear gloves when suctioning a tracheostomy?
10. What is a good method to keep crumbs out of a tracheostomy while a child eats?

Endotracheal Intubation

Endotracheal intubation (nasal or oral intubation) is another means of bypassing upper airway obstruction and allowing free entry of air to the trachea. Intubation tubes cause edema and local irritation and so cannot be left in place as a permanent solution. As with tracheostomies, children cannot speak while intubated. Those old enough to write should be supplied with a pencil and paper for effective communication. Preschoolers may want to draw pictures to indicate what they need. It is helpful to have simple drawings that a child can point to (a drink, a straw, a blanket, the television turned on, a urinal) to make needs known. Make sure that endotracheal tubes are care-

NURSING PROCEDURE 19.2: TRACHEOSTOMY SUCTION

Procedure	Principle
1. Wash hands, identify child, explain procedure to child.	1. Prevents spread of microorganisms; encourages cooperation.
2. Assess child, especially breath sounds; analyze appropriateness of procedure. Plan ways to modify care based on individual circumstances.	2. Assessment prior to procedure provides a baseline for future evaluation. Nursing care is always individualized based on client need.
3. Assemble supplies: suction source and tubing, sterile suction catheter (#12 or 14F), or sterile suction kit, sterile gloves, sterile bottle of normal saline, sterile medicine dropper or syringe, manual resuscitator. Plan method to keep child from touching sterile catheter (placing a restraint, distraction, or asking assistance from another nurse).	3. Organizing supplies will increase efficiency of procedure.
4. Open normal saline and suction catheter or kit. Pour a small amount of saline solution into disposable container included in kit. Prepare syringe or dropper with small amount of sterile normal saline; put on sterile gloves.	4. Sterile technique is important to prevent introducing microorganisms.
5. Hold suction catheter with one gloved hand, suction tubing with other gloved hand, and attach tubing to sterile catheter; dip tip of catheter into normal saline and suction a small amount through catheter.	5. Note that once sterile glove touches suction tubing, it is no longer sterile. Suctioning normal saline ensures that the tubing and catheter are patent.
6. If necessary, instruct assistant to hyperoxygenate child with manual resuscitator.	6. Hyperoxygenation prevents child from developing anoxia during suctioning.

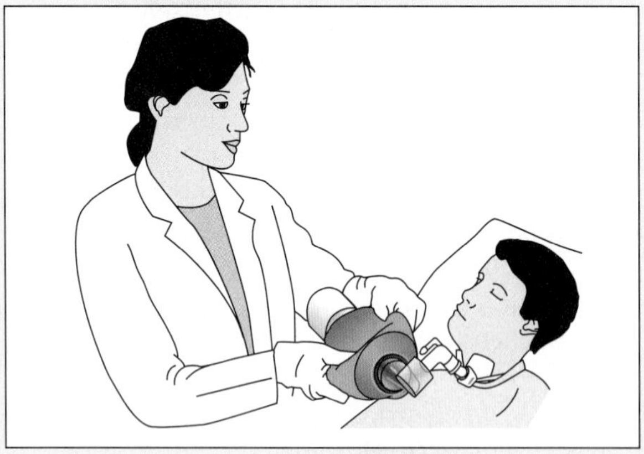

Procedure	Principle
7. If necessary, drop prescribed amount of normal saline into tracheostomy tube with dropper or syringe, and observe child closely for respiratory distress.	7. Normal saline helps to liquefy secretions enough to be suctioned readily.
8. Hold breath; introduce sterile catheter into tracheostomy tube to desired length. Apply suction for 5 to 10 sec and gently withdraw, rotating gently.	8. Holding breath helps you not to suction longer than is comfortable. Applying suction only on withdrawal allows catheter to pass freely without irritating the trachea and prevents oversuctioning. Prolonged suctioning longer than 10 seconds can cause hypoxia.

(continued)

Procedure	Principle
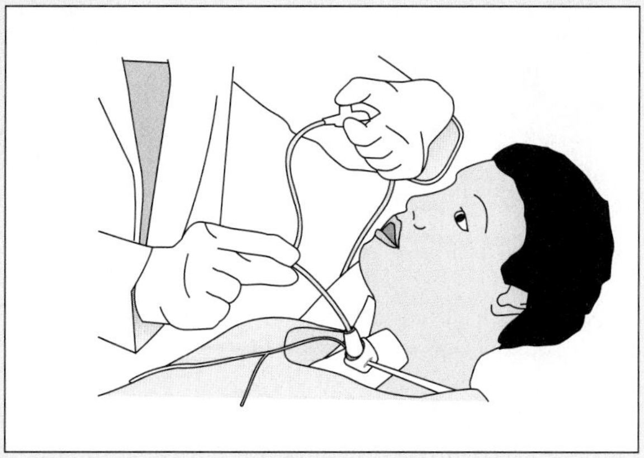	
9. Rinse catheter by dipping tip in normal saline and applying suction.	9. Rinsing catheter ensures that it remains patent.
10. Repeat procedure until airway sounds clear. Be careful not to suction longer than necessary.	10. Suctioning is fatiguing to children. Extended suctioning can lead to airway irritation and further mucus production.
11. Assess effectiveness and efficiency of procedure; plan teaching such as importance of procedure to parents; document procedure.	11. Comparing initial baseline assessments with post procedure status provides information about effectiveness of the procedure. Teaching is an independent nursing care measure always included as part of care.
12. Comfort child; remain with child for support. Provide opportunities for therapeutic play.	12. Suctioning is frightening; offer support and comfort after all such procedures to decrease fears and anxieties.

fully secured because children can easily dislodge them. Avoid frequent tape changes to protect the skin on the child's cheeks.

A capnometer is a device that measures the amount of CO_2 in inhaled or exhaled breaths. It uses infrared technology and is attached to the distal end of the endotracheal tube. By measuring the percentage of CO_2 in expired air, the arterial CO_2 ($PaCO_2$) can be estimated. A capnometer, used this way, can reduce the number of repeated arterial punctures that are needed for arterial blood gas analysis.

Assisted Ventilation

When it is not possible to improve oxygen saturation to sufficient levels by the methods described above, assisted ventilation may become necessary. Positive-pressure machines deliver moistened or nebulized air or oxygen to the lungs under enough pressure and with appropriate timing to produce artificial, periodical inflation of alveoli; they rely on the elastic recoil of the lungs to empty the alveoli.

Depending on the type of ventilator, the inspiration-expiration cycle is determined by a timed interval, a volume

EMPOWERING THE FAMILY: Preventing Aspiration in the Child With a Tracheostomy

- Use a bib tied loosely over the tracheostomy when your child is eating to prevent food from entering the tube.
- Avoid buying toys with small parts that could be removed and dropped into the tube.
- Inspect stuffed toys to be certain they don't shed (fur could enter the tube).
- Supervise play with other children to be certain they don't place anything in the tube.
- Stay with your child in a bathtub to be certain water doesn't splash into the tube.
- Keep sprays such as perfume or room fresheners to a minimum, because they can be irritating to the trachea.
- Avoid cold air because it can cause tracheal spasm (cover the child's throat with a loose cotton scarf when out in cold weather).

limit, or a pressure limit. Conventional mechanical ventilators supply high tidal volumes at a low frequency rate. High airway pressure is needed in this conventional system, which can, unfortunately, lead to bronchopulmonary disease. A newer method of ventilation depends on low tidal volumes delivered at high frequencies of 200 to 300 breaths/min. Hyperinflation of lungs can occur with high-frequency ventilation, because there is not enough time for expiration to occur. For this reason, some high-frequency ventilators are set so air is sucked out of the lungs rather than depending on the normal elastic recoil of the lungs.

Pancuronium (Pavulon) may be administered intravenously to a point of abolishing spontaneous respiratory action to allow mechanical ventilation to be accomplished at lower pressures (see Drug Highlight). Without normal respiratory action, there is no normal muscle resistance to overcome. Clearly, a child who has no spontaneous respiratory function needs critical observation and frequent arterial blood analysis, because he or she depends totally on caregivers at that point.

Mechanical ventilation for a prolonged period requires that children either have a tracheotomy performed or have an endotracheal tube passed (Figure 19-14). A cuffed tube must be used with a ventilator so the seal at the trachea is airtight. Infants need a nasogastric tube inserted to prevent stomach distension. Providing adequate nutrition may be difficult for the child on a ventilator. This can be provided by enteric (nasogastric) feedings or total parenteral nutrition. Providing a balance of rest and stimulation for the child can be a challenge for nursing personnel or parents.

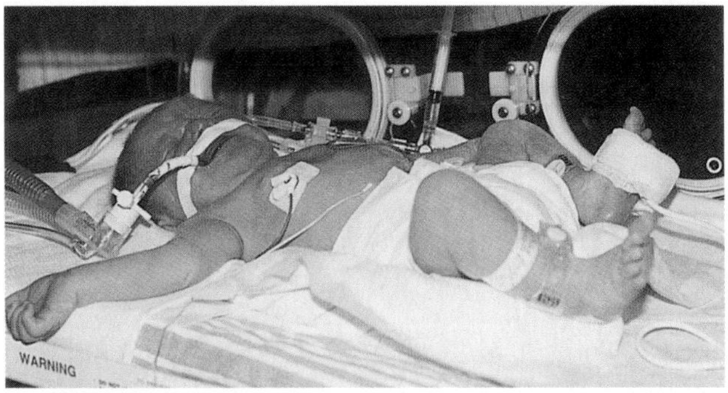

FIGURE 19.14 An infant with an endotracheal tube receiving assisted ventilation.

Children who need respiratory assistance are frightened. A great many fight ventilators or refuse to lie quietly and let the ventilator breathe for them. Their parents also are extremely anxious and fearful. A nurse who is comfortable with ventilator care automatically conveys assurance that the child will be safe during ventilation. Be certain that you are comfortable enough with the machinery being used that you can concentrate on providing total nursing care to the child (Table 19-4).

Once children become accustomed to ventilator care, it is sometimes difficult to discontinue a device, even when there is no longer a clinical indication for it. This is most pronounced in adolescents who are aware of the role of oxygen and proper ventilation in life function. Children may need a number of trial periods free of the ventilator with someone remaining close by them, so that they can be assured that if they do have difficulty breathing, someone is standing by to help. Many children are too afraid to fall asleep on the first night off a ventilator unless someone is with them and has assured them that he or she will be there through the night.

DRUG HIGHLIGHT

Pancuronium Bromide (Pavulon)

Action: Pancuronium is a neuromuscular blocking agent that relaxes skeletal muscles during assisted mechanical ventilation or endotracheal intubation.

Pregnancy risk category: C

Dosage: 0.03–0.04 mg/kg intravenously initially, then 0.03–0.1 mg/kg intravenously, repeated every 30 to 60 minutes as needed.

Possible adverse effects: Prolonged dose-related apnea; tachycardia, excessive salivation, and sweating.

Nursing Implications:

- Keep in mind that the child's respiratory muscles do not function after administration; maintain assisted ventilation.
- Know that the drug peaks in approximately 2 to 3 minutes and lasts approximately 1 hour (longer in children with poor renal perfusion).
- Remember that the drug does not alter state of consciousness. Anticipate the need for sedation or analgesia for procedures.
- Keep equipment for emergency resuscitation (Ambu bag) at bedside in case of a power or mechanical ventilator failure.
- Be sure to explain all events and procedures to the child; even though the respiratory muscles may be paralyzed, the child can still hear. Also encourage the parents to talk to the child when they visit.
- Be prepared to reverse the effects of the drug by administering atropine or neostigmine methylsulfate (prostigmin methylsulfate).
- Monitor all physiologic parameters, including vital signs, heart rate, and blood pressure. Obtain electrolyte levels as ordered, because electrolyte imbalances can potentiate neuromuscular effects.

Lung Transplantation

Lung transplantation is a possibility for children with a chronic respiratory illness such as cystic fibrosis. Lung transplantation may be done in conjunction with a heart transplantation if chronic respiratory disease has caused ventricular hypertrophy (Maurer & Chaparro, 1995).

✔ CHECKPOINT QUESTIONS

11. What device is used to measure the amount of carbon dioxide in exhaled air when the child is intubated?
12. What drug is sometimes used to abolish spontaneous respiratory activity to allow lower pressures for mechanical ventilation?

TABLE 19.4 Terms Commonly Used With Ventilator Therapy

TERM	DEFINITION	CLINICAL APPLICATION
IMV	Intermittent mandatory ventilation	Number of mandatory breaths the ventilator will deliver each hour. A child may breathe most of the time without assistance, but a set (mandatory) number of breaths per minute is delivered to ensure adequate lung expansion and oxygenation
PEEP	Positive end-expiratory pressure	Pressure delivered to lungs at the end of each expiration to keep alveoli from collapsing on expiration and to ensure adequate oxygenation
Sigh	A deep inhalation delivered by the ventilator	Used to fully inflate the lungs a number of times each minute
CPAP	Continuous positive airway pressure	A constant pressure exerted on the alveoli to keep them from collapsing on expiration
FIO_2	Concentration of oxygen the child is receiving (inspiring)	A child on oxygen therapy will have an FIO_2 from 22% to 100%

DISORDERS OF THE UPPER RESPIRATORY TRACT

The upper respiratory tract warms, humidifies, and filters the air that enters the body (Figure 19-15). As such, the structures of the upper respiratory tract constantly come into contact with a barrage of foreign organisms, including pathogens, which can sometimes lead to airway irritation and illness. Congenital malformation of respiratory structures also causes some upper respiratory tract disorders.

Choanal Atresia

Choanal atresia is congenital obstruction of the posterior nares by an obstructing membrane or bony growth, preventing a newborn from drawing air through the nose and down into the nasopharynx. It may be either unilateral or bilateral.

Newborns up to approximately 3 months of age are naturally nose breathers. Infants with choanal atresia, therefore, develop signs of respiratory distress at birth or immediately after they quiet for the first time and attempt to breathe through the nose. Passing a soft no. 8 or 10 catheter through the posterior nares to the stomach is in many hospitals a part of birthing room procedure. If such a catheter will not pass bilaterally, the diagnosis of choanal atresia is confirmed.

Choanal atresia can also be assessed by holding the newborn's mouth closed, then gently compressing first one nostril, then the other. If atresia is present, infants will struggle

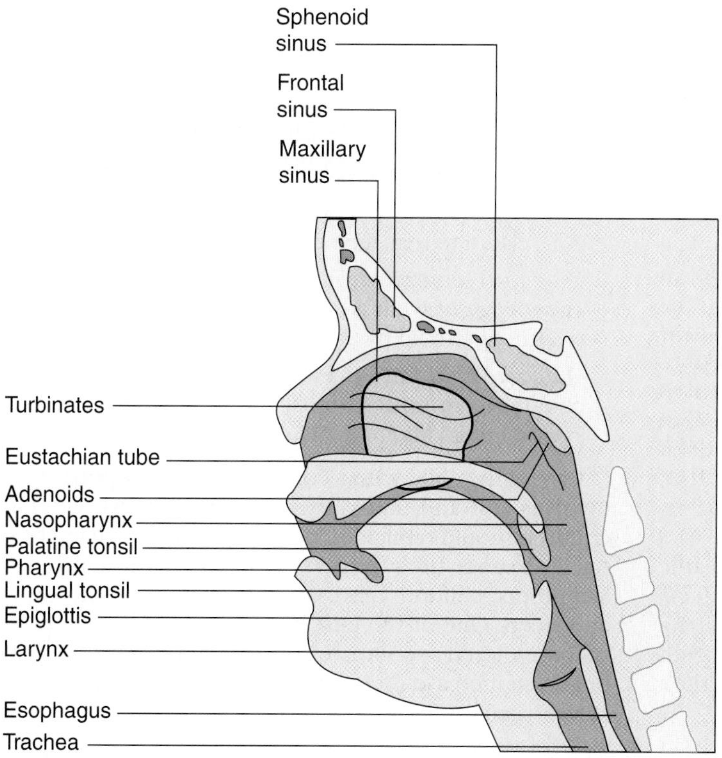

FIGURE 19.15 Structures of the upper respiratory tract.

as they experience air hunger when the mouth is closed. Their color improves when they open their mouth to cry. Atresia is also suggested if infants struggle and become cyanotic at feedings because they cannot suck and breathe through their mouth simultaneously.

Because infants with choanal atresia have such difficulty with feeding, they may receive intravenous fluid to maintain their glucose and fluid level until surgery can be performed. Some infants may need an oral airway inserted so they can continue to breathe through their mouths. The treatment for bilateral atresia is either local piercing of the obstructing membrane or surgical removal of the bony growth. The child then has no further difficulty or symptoms.

Acute Nasopharyngitis (Common Cold)

The common cold is the most frequent infectious disease in children. Toddlers have an average of 10 to 12 colds a year. School-age children and adolescents have as many as four to five yearly. The incubation period is typically 2-3 days. Most occur in the fall and winter (Coakley-Maller & Shea, 1997).

Acute nasopharyngitis (the common cold) is caused by one of several viruses, most predominantly by rhinovirus, coxsackie virus, respiratory syncytial virus, adenovirus, and parainfluenza and influenza viruses. Children are exposed to colds at school from other children. Those children who are in ill health from some other cause are more susceptible to the cold viruses than are well children if their immune system is compromised. Stress factors also appear to play a role. Although it is difficult to document phenomena such as drafts, cold feet, or chilling as causative factors, they probably play a role in susceptibility.

Assessment

Symptoms begin with nasal congestion, a watery rhinitis, and low-grade fever. The mucous membrane of the nose becomes edematous and inflamed. Children experience difficulty breathing because of the edema and congestion. Posterior rhinitis, plus local irritation, leads to pharyngitis. Draining pharyngeal secretions may lead to a cough. Cervical lymph nodes may be swollen and palpable. The process lasts about a week and then symptoms fade. In some children, a thick, purulent nasal discharge occurs because bacteria such as streptococci invade the irritated nasal mucous membrane and cause a secondary infection.

Infants can be critically ill and not develop an elevated temperature owing to their immature body systems. With the common cold, they often develop a fever elevated out of proportion to the symptoms, possibly as high as 102° to 104°F (38.8° to 40°C). Infants also may develop secondary symptoms, such as vomiting and diarrhea, as a general response. Because they cannot suck and breathe through their mouth at the same time, they refuse feedings. This can lead to dehydration. Older children will not develop as high a fever. Their temperature rarely exceeds 102°F (38.8°C). Because they can breathe through their mouth, the nasal congestion does not seem as acute.

Therapeutic Management

There is no specific treatment for a common cold. Antibiotics are not effective unless a secondary bacterial invasion has occurred. If children have a fever, it should be controlled by an antipyretic such as acetaminophen (Tylenol) or children's ibuprofen. It is important for parents to understand that these drugs are to control the fever symptoms. They do not reduce congestion or "cure" the cold. They should not be given unless children have fever, generally defined as an oral temperature over 101°F (38.4°C). You may need to remind parents that children younger than 18 years should not be given acetosalicylic acid (aspirin) because this is associated with the development of Reye's syndrome (see Chapter 28).

If infants have difficulty nursing because of nasal congestion, saline nose drops or nasal spray may be prescribed to liquefy nasal secretions and help them drain. A bulb syringe, used before feedings to clear away nasal mucus, will allow infants to suck more efficiently. Caution parents that when they use a bulb syringe, they must compress the bulb first, then insert it into their child's nostril. If they insert the bulb syringe first, then depress the bulb, they will actually push secretions further back into the nose, causing increased obstruction.

There is little proof that oral decongestants relieve congestion with the common cold. Most parents believe that these products give relief, however, and feel better if one is prescribed for the child. It is not good policy to suppress the cough of a common cold, because a cough raises secretions, thus preventing pooling of secretions and consequent infection. Guaifenesin is an example of a drug that loosens secretions but does not suppress a cough. Parents may use a cool mist vaporizer to help loosen nasal secretions. The efficiency of home vaporizers is questionable, however, and safe use of a vaporizer, including proper cleaning, must be stressed or it can serve as a reservoir for infection.

NURSING DIAGNOSES AND RELATED INTERVENTIONS

Nursing Diagnosis: Parental health-seeking behaviors related to management of child's cold

Outcome Identification: Parents will demonstrate knowledge of what is and what is not helpful in the treatment of cold by end of health visit.

Outcome Evaluation: Parents state intention to use cool mist vaporizer to loosen secretions, to encourage oral fluid, and to avoid cough medicine.

Care of the child with a cold is typically supportive and involves rest and fluids. Parents generally ask whether children should remain on bed rest. Children characteristically restrict their activity when ill. With acute cold symptoms, children may naturally curl up on the couch and sleep. One of the best ways that parents can judge when children are improving is to note that they have begun to increase their activity or are "acting like themselves" again.

Children with a cold often show a loss of appetite. They may prefer simple liquids to solid food for the first few days of a cold.

Parents can be assured that a cold is only a cold and nothing more. Because the symptoms in infants are so out of proportion to the seriousness of the disorder, it is easy to be fooled into thinking that this is a more serious disorder than it is. A complication of a cold in children can be otitis media (middle ear infection). Instruct parents about these symptoms such as sudden elevated temperature and ear pain. If this occurs, a child needs antibiotic administration and further evaluation to protect against hearing impairment.

Pharyngitis

Pharyngitis is infection and inflammation of the throat. It may be either bacterial or viral in origin. It may occur as a result of a chronic allergy in which there is constant postnasal discharge and resulting secondary irritation. Some pharyngitis often accompanies a common cold. The peak incidence of pharyngitis occurs between 4 and 7 years of age. The nursing diagnosis most often used with pharyngitis is pain.

Viral Pharyngitis

If the causative agent of the pharyngitis is a virus, the symptoms are generally mild: a sore throat, fever, and general malaise. On physical assessment, regional lymph nodes may be noticeably enlarged. Erythema will be present in the back of the pharynx and the palatine arch. Laboratory studies will indicate an increased white blood cell count.

If the inflammation is mild, children rarely need more than an analgesic such as acetaminophen or ibuprofen. By school age, children are capable of gargling (before this, they tend to swallow the solution unless the procedure is well explained and demonstrated to them). Gargling with warm water may be soothing; warm heat may be applied to the external neck using a warm towel or heating pad.

Because children's throats are sore, usually they do not eat well. They often prefer liquid to solid food. Infants, especially, must be observed closely until the inflammation and tenderness diminish to be certain that they take in sufficient fluid to prevent dehydration.

Streptococcal Pharyngitis

Group A beta hemolytic streptococcus is the organism most frequently involved in bacterial pharyngitis in children.

Assessment. Streptococcal infections are generally more severe than viral infections, although the fact that the symptoms are mild does not rule out streptococcal infection. With a streptococcal pharyngitis, the palatine tonsils are usually markedly erythematous (bright red) and enlarged. There may be a white exudate in the tonsillar crypts. Petechiae may be present on the palate. The pharynx is erythematous. There may be high fever, extreme sore throat, and lethargy. The child appears ill and reports difficulty swallowing. The temperature is usually elevated to 104°F (40°C). The child may complain of headache. Swollen abdominal lymph nodes may cause abdominal pain. A throat culture confirms presence of the *Streptococcus* bacteria. All streptococcal infections must be taken seriously because they can lead to cardiac and kidney damage. An extremely virulent form of streptococci that actually necroses tissue, causing extensive tissue damage, has also been identified. Identifying streptococci is a simple office procedure. However, these simple antigen tests may not yield more information than is gained from the appearance of a typical infection (Gerber, 1997).

Therapeutic Management. Treatment consists of a full 10-day course of an antibiotic such as penicillin. Cephalosporins or broad-spectrum macrolides may be prescribed if resistant organisms are known to be in the community (Watkins, et al, 1997). Parents should understand the importance of the full 10 days of therapy. The prolonged treatment is necessary to ensure that the streptococci are eradicated completely. If not, children may develop a hypersensitivity reaction to group A streptococci that results in rheumatic fever (although the chance of rheumatic fever occurring is probably as low as 1%) and glomerulonephritis. To ensure that the child receives the full antibiotic course, help parents make a reminder sheet to place on their refrigerator door. In addition, instruct parents about measures for rest, relief of throat pain, and maintaining hydration, the same actions as for a common cold.

Acute glomerulonephritis is also a possible complication. Symptoms of acute glomerulonephritis (blood and protein in urine) may appear in 1 to 2 weeks after the pharyngitis. There is no proof that antibiotic treatment prevents acute glomerulonephritis. If the strain of streptococci was nephrogenic, the chances are as high as 50% that kidney disease will develop.

Two weeks after treatment, children are asked to return to the health care facility with a urine specimen to be examined for protein so that developing acute glomerulonephritis can be detected. Because it is impossible for parents to discriminate between a pharyngitis caused by a virus (and needing no therapy other than comfort measures) and a streptococcal pharyngitis (needing definite therapy to prevent life-threatening illnesses), a child with pharyngitis always should be examined by health care personnel. "Simple" sore throats in children may not be simple at all.

Retropharyngeal Abscess

The lymph nodes that drain the nasopharynx are located behind the posterior pharynx wall. These nodes may become infected in an infant with an acute nasopharyngitis or pharyngitis. These nodes disappear by preschool age, so the problem is usually limited to young infants.

Assessment. Typically, children have an upper respiratory tract infection or sore throat for a few days. Suddenly, they refuse to eat. They may drool because they are unable to swallow saliva. They have a high fever. They "snore" with respirations because of the occlusion of the pharynx. To allow themselves more breathing space, they may hyperextend the head, a very unusual position for infants.

On physical assessment, regional lymph nodes will be enlarged. The mass itself may not be visible in the posterior pharynx if it is below the point of vision. An x-ray study using a swallowed contrast medium will reveal the bulging tissue in the pharynx. Laboratory studies will reveal leukocytosis.

Therapeutic Management. Because the most frequent cause of retropharyngeal abscess is group A beta-hemolytic streptococcus, amoxicillin or penicillin and rifampin are effective. Because they swallow poorly, infants' mouths may need to be suctioned to remove secretions. Be careful not to touch the suction catheter to the posterior pharynx, because this might rupture the abscess, possibly leading to aspiration of the abscess contents (producing respiratory obstruction or a pneumonia caused by the aspirated purulent material). Blood vessels invade some retropharyngeal abscesses, so that rupture of the structure also can lead to profuse bleeding (dangerous to the child because of the loss of blood from major arteries such as the carotid artery and because the blood can be aspirated).

Infants need to be placed in a prone or side-lying position to allow difficult-to-swallow mouth secretions to drain forward. Food is generally restricted, and intake may be limited to fluids. Make certain that parents understand this so they do not offer a hard food such as a toast crust (a substance good for teething). The sharp edges could rupture the abscess.

Postpharyngeal abscesses may be incised by a surgeon to promote drainage. This is done in surgery with the child in a Trendelenburg position, so that drainage from the abscess can be suctioned away to prevent aspiration. After surgery, maintain the child in a Trendelenburg or a prone position to encourage further drainage and prevent aspiration. Monitor vital signs closely. Observe drainage from children's mouths to detect fresh bleeding. Frequent swallowing is also a sign of postpharyngeal bleeding. Increased respiratory rate suggests airway obstruction.

Oral fluid is introduced as soon as the swallowing and gag reflexes are intact after surgery. Although the throat is undoubtedly still sore, most infants suck eagerly and need supplemental intravenous fluid administration for only a short time.

Parents need to handle infants and care for them while in the hospital so that they can regain their confidence in themselves as parents. On admission they may be thoroughly frightened by the extent of the child's symptoms (gurgling or snoring sound, high temperature, dyspnea). They need time and opportunity to work through their fear to restore their confidence with child care.

CHECKPOINT QUESTIONS

13. When would the child with choanal atresia typically develop signs of respiratory distress?
14. Why are infants not prescribed acetosalicylic acid (aspirin) for the pain of pharyngitis?

Tonsillitis

Tonsillitis is the term commonly used to refer to infection and inflammation of the palatine tonsils. *Adenitis* refers to infection and inflammation of the adenoid (pharyngeal) tonsils.

Tonsillar tissue is lymphoid tissue that acts to form antibodies and to filter pathogenic organisms from the head and neck area. The palatine tonsils are located on both sides of the pharynx; the adenoids are in the nasopharynx. Tubal tonsils are located at the entrance to the eustachian tubes. Lingual tonsils are located at the base of the tongue. All of the tonsils may be referred to collectively as *Waldeyer's ring*. They are easily infected because of the bacteria that pass through or are screened through them.

Assessment

Infection of the palatine tonsils gives all of the symptoms of a severe pharyngitis. Children drool because their throat is too sore for them to swallow saliva. They may describe swallowing as so painful that it feels as though they are swallowing bits of metal or glass. They usually have a high fever and are lethargic. On physical assessment, tonsillar tissue appears bright red and may be so enlarged that the two areas of palatine tonsillar tissue meet in the midline. Pus can be detected on or expelled from the crypts of the tonsils.

In addition to fever, lethargy, pharyngeal pain, and edema, the symptoms of adenoidal tissue infection are a nasal quality of speech, mouth breathing, difficulty hearing, and perhaps halitosis. The mouth breathing and change in speech come from the postpharyngeal obstruction by the enlarged tissue. The difficulty with hearing occurs because of eustachian tube obstruction. Eustachian tube blockage can contribute to both serous and acute otitis media (middle ear infection). Enlarged adenoidal tissue may be a cause of sleep apnea because of underaeration.

Tonsillitis is most common in the school-age child. The responsible organism is identified by a throat culture. In school-age children, the organism is generally a group A beta-hemolytic streptococcus. In children younger than 3 years of age, the cause is often viral.

Therapeutic Management

As therapy for bacterial tonsillitis, children need an antipyretic for fever, an analgesic for pain, and a full 10-day course of an antibiotic such as penicillin. If the cause is viral, no therapy other than comfort or fever reduction strategies are necessary. Although the pain of the infection will subside a day or two after the antibiotic administration is begun, remind parents that children need the full 10-day course of antibiotic to eradicate streptococci completely from the back of the throat. After a tonsillar infection, tonsillar tissue may remain hypertrophied or it may atrophy and appear smaller than normal.

Tonsillectomy. *Tonsillectomy* is removal of the palatine tonsils. *Adenoidectomy* is removal of the pharyngeal tonsils. In the past, tonsillectomy was a common therapy after tonsillitis. In current practice, however, tonsillectomy is not recommended unless all other measures prove ineffective. Tonsillar tissue is removed by ligating the tonsil or by laser surgery. Because sutures are not placed, the chance for hemorrhage after this type of surgery is higher than after surgery involving a closed incision. The danger of aspiration of blood at the time of surgery and the danger of a general anesthetic compound the risk.

Chronic tonsillitis is about the only reason for removal of palatine tonsils. Adenoids may be removed if they are so hypertrophied that they are causing obstruction. At one time, adenoids and palatine tonsils were always removed together; today, depending on the symptoms and the extent of hypertrophy and infection, children may have a tonsillectomy, an adenoidectomy, or both.

Tonsillectomy or adenoidectomy is never done while the organs are infected, because an operation at such a time might spread pathogenic organisms into the bloodstream, causing septicemia. Parents often ask why an operation to remove tonsils must be delayed. They think that as long as the tonsils are sore, they should be immediately removed. They need an explanation of why this is not possible and why it is safer to schedule surgery for a later date. Most parents report an improvement in their child's general health and performance after surgery (Conlon, et al, 1997).

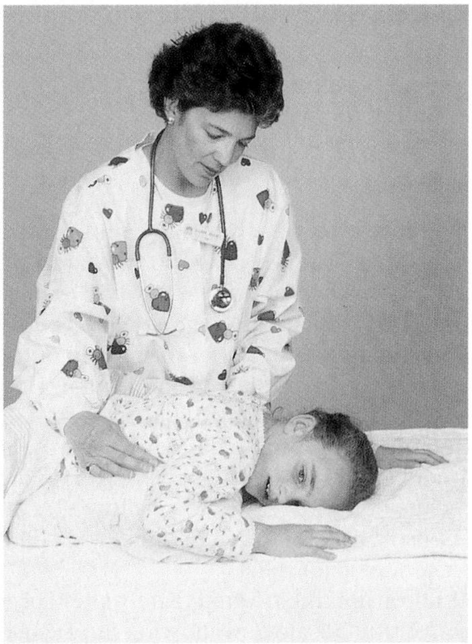

FIGURE 19.16 Positioning a child after tonsillectomy. The pillow under the chest helps secretions flow out of mouth.

NURSING DIAGNOSES AND RELATED INTERVENTIONS

Nursing Diagnosis: Risk for fluid volume deficit related to blood loss from surgery

Outcome Identification: Child will maintain adequate fluid volume balance postoperatively.

Outcome Evaluation: Child's pulse and blood pressure are normal for age-group; there is absence of extensive bleeding; intake and output are within acceptable parameters.

Tonsillectomies are done as ambulatory or 1-day surgery. Before surgery, a complete history and physical examination and laboratory tests, including bleeding and clotting times, complete blood count, and urinalysis, should be done. Another important aspect of assessment is to observe for loose teeth that could be dislodged during surgery and aspirated. If loose teeth are present, mark this fact on the front of the child's chart and report it to the anesthesiologist. Teach parents to use common sense in their child's care during the weeks before hospital admission, so that the child does not have a cold or recurrent tonsillitis at the time planned for surgery.

After surgery, observe vital signs carefully to make certain that the child is not bleeding from the denuded surgical area. Place the child on the side or abdomen with a pillow under the chest so that the head is lower than the chest. This allows blood and unswallowed saliva to drain from the child's mouth rather than back to the pharynx, where it might be aspirated (Figure 19-16).

Hemorrhage after tonsillectomy can be acute and intense. Because children will swallow any blood that is oozing from the surgical site, a child can be bleeding heavily and yet little blood is apparent. To detect bleeding, assess for subtle signs of hemorrhage, including an increasing pulse or respiratory rate; frequent swallowing; throat clearing, and a feeling of anxiety. A child's first line of defense against hemorrhage is a nurse who recognizes these subtle signs of bleeding before the bleeding is so intense that symptoms of shock occur.

If bleeding does occur, elevating the child's head and turning him or her on the side reduces vascular pressure on the operative site yet continues to prevent obstruction. Physicians who examine the child need a good light source and a dentist's mirror so that they will have a good view of the posterior throat. Secure these items so the examination can be thorough and effective. If extreme hemorrhage of the surgical area occurs, the child may need to be returned to surgery for a suture or two to halt bleeding.

The most dangerous periods after a tonsillectomy are the first 24 hours, when the clots covering the denuded surgical area are forming, and the fifth to seventh days, when the clots begin to lyse or dissolve. If new tissue is not yet present when the clots dissolve, hemorrhage from the denuded surface may result. If children have no complications from surgery, are able to swallow fluids, and have voided, they are generally discharged later the same day of surgery. Parents need careful instruction concerning the danger signs to watch for in children during their first day home (frequent swallowing, clearing the throat, increasing restlessness). They are usually advised to restrict their child's activity (no running, swimming) until after the seventh day, when firm healing should have taken place. The child needs a return appointment to a health care facility approximately 2 weeks after surgery for follow-up assessment that the surgical area has healed without complication.

Nursing Diagnosis: Pain related to surgical procedure

Outcome Identification: Child's level of discomfort will be limited to a tolerable level.

Outcome Evaluation: Child states that level of pain is tolerable.

Tonsillectomy is an uncomfortable and painful procedure for children. They need good preparation for the procedure and for the sensations they will experience afterward. Although tonsils are removed, it is better to talk about tonsils being "fixed" rather than taken out; children may be extremely frightened to know that a body part will be removed, however small it is.

Tonsillectomy leaves the child with a very painful posterior throat. Liquid analgesics are better than pills or tablets because they are easier to swallow. Rectal administration is also a possibility. Occasionally, a child may require intravenous pain relief.

Most children are thirsty immediately after surgery, and drinking is helpful because swallowing fluid causes active pharyngeal movement, increasing the blood supply to the area and reducing edema and pain. Frequent sips of clear liquid or ice chips can be offered as soon as children have completely awakened from the anesthesia. Choose fluids carefully. Acid juices sting the denuded tissue and so are uncomfortable. Carbonated beverages also can irritate the area unless they are allowed to stand for a time to become "flat." Avoiding red fluid such as Koolaid is a good idea, too, so, if vomited, it isn't mistaken for swallowed blood.

Children are generally promised by well-meaning people that they can have all the ice cream they want after a tonsillectomy. Because it forms tenacious secretions that are difficult to swallow, it is not a food of choice. A better treat is a Popsicle, which is a frozen clear liquid.

Children can be gradually advanced to a soft diet including foods such as gelatin, mashed potatoes, soups, and cooked fruits after 24 to 48 hours. They should continue to eat only soft foods for the first week. A selective diet can be given the second week (no toast crusts or other foods that could cause pharyngeal irritation if not chewed well). Be certain that parents know the telephone number they should call (clinic, hospital, or pediatrician) if they have a question or concern about a child's condition or care. Caution parents that some children develop a mild earache after tonsillectomy for the first week, probably caused by shifting pressure on the eustachian tube.

Epistaxis

Epistaxis (nosebleed) is extremely common in children. It usually occurs from trauma, such as picking at the nose or from being hit on the nose by another child. In older homes that lack humidification, the hot dry environment makes children's mucous membranes dry, uncomfortable, and susceptible to cracking and bleeding. In all children, epistaxis tends to occur during respiratory illnesses. It may occur after strenuous exercise. It is associated with a number of systemic diseases, such as rheumatic fever, scarlet fever, measles, or varicella infection (chickenpox). It can occur with nasal polyps, sinusitis, or allergic rhinitis. There apparently is a familial predisposition.

Nosebleeds are always frightening because of the visible bleeding and a choking sensation if blood should run down the back of the nasopharynx. The fear is generally out of proportion to the seriousness of the bleeding.

Keep children with nosebleeds in an upright position with their head tilted slightly forward to minimize the amount of blood pressure in nasal vessels and to keep blood moving forward, not back into the nasopharynx. Apply pressure to the sides of the nose with your fingers (Figure 19-17). Make every effort to quiet children and to help them stop crying, because crying increases pressure in the blood vessels of the head and prolongs bleeding. If these simple measures do not control the bleeding, epinephrine (1:1000) may be applied to the bleeding site to constrict blood vessels. A nasal pack may be necessary.

Every child has occasional nosebleeds. Chronic nasal bleeding, however, should be investigated to rule out a systemic disease or blood disorder.

> WHAT IF? What if a parent tells you his child has "nosebleeds that just will not stop"? How would you advise the parent to position the child?

Sinusitis

Sinusitis is rare in children younger than 6 years of age, because the frontal sinuses do not develop fully until age 6. It occurs as a secondary infection in older children when streptococcal, staphylococcal, or *Haemophilus influenzae* organisms spread from the nasal cavity. They will develop a fever, a purulent nasal discharge, headache, and tenderness over the affected sinus. Children should have a nose and throat culture taken to identify the infectious organism.

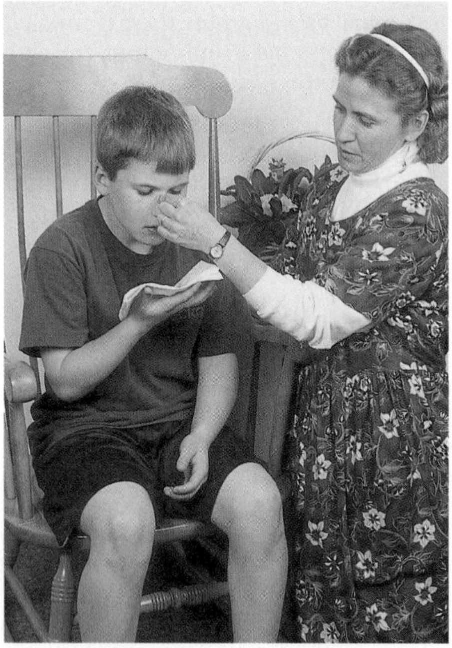

FIGURE 19.17 Emergency therapy for a nosebleed is to tilt the head slightly forward and apply pressure to the sides of the nose.

Treatment for acute sinusitis consists of an antipyretic for fever, an analgesic for pain, and an antibiotic for the specific organism involved. Saline nose drops or sprays keep nasal secretions moist but do not reach the sinuses. Nose drops such as oxymetazoline hydrochloride (Afrin) to shrink the nasal congestion will allow drainage from the sinuses. Teach parents not to use over-the-counter nasal sprays without their primary care provider's approval. Also caution them that the prolonged use of nasal drops or sprays can lead to nasal polyps. To avoid a rebound effect, they should be used for only 3 days at a time; otherwise, they actually cause more nasal congestion than was present originally. Some children need acetaminophen (Tylenol) for pain. Warm compresses to the sinus area may both encourage drainage and relieve pain.

Sinusitis is considered by many adults to be a minor illness. It needs to be treated, however, because it can have serious complications if the infection spreads from the sinuses to invade the bone (osteomyelitis) or the middle ear (otitis media). Chronic sinusitis can interfere with school and social performance because of the constant pain.

Laryngitis

Laryngitis is inflammation of the larynx. It results in brassy, hoarse voice sounds or inability to make audible voice sounds. It may occur as a spread of pharyngitis or from excessive use of the voice, as in cheerleading. Laryngitis is as annoying for children as it is for adults. Sips of fluid (either warm or cold, whichever feels best) offer relief from the annoying tickling sensation often present. The most effective measure, however, is for children to rest their voice for at least 24 hours, until inflammation subsides. Be certain to meet infants' needs before they have to cry for things. Older children simply need to be cautioned not to speak. Having children stay in bed is generally ineffective, because this requires them to shout to another room of the house to make their needs known; this merely adds to the irritation of the larynx.

Congenital Laryngeal Stridor

Congenital laryngeal stridor (laryngomalacia) results when the child's laryngeal structure is weaker than normal and collapses more than usual on inspiration. The stridor is generally present from birth, possibly intensified when the child is in a supine position.

Assessment

The infant's sternum may become retracted on inspiration because of the increased effort to pull air into the trachea past the collapsed structure. The stridor may become most noticeable when infants suck. Most infants with this condition must stop sucking frequently during a feeding to maintain adequate ventilation. They become exhausted easily, interrupting their feeding to rest.

Therapeutic Management

Stridor is a frightening sound. When parents wake at night and listen in a quiet house to the sound of stridor, it seems unbearably loud. They may need to be reassured at every health care visit that although the sound is raucous, it is safe for them to care for the infant at home. They may need to see a weight chart that shows them that their child is growing and thriving despite this problem. Many parents sleep at night with the child's crib brought next to their bed or with one hand resting on the infant's chest so they can be assured during the night that the child is continuing to breathe. At health care visits, assess whether the parents are receiving enough sleep at night and are not becoming too exhausted to be able to continue to work or give care.

Most children with congenital laryngeal stridor need no routine therapy other than to have parents feed them slowly, providing rest periods as needed. The condition improves as children mature, because cartilage in the larynx becomes stronger at about 1 year of age.

Parents must be certain to bring the child for early care if signs of an upper respiratory tract infection develop. If not, laryngeal collapse will be even more intense during these times, and complete obstruction of the trachea could occur. Any time stridor becomes more intense, advise parents to have the infant seen by their primary care provider, because generally this indicates beginning obstruction and probably the beginning of an upper respiratory tract infection. As parents become more used to the sound their infants make while breathing, they will become astute reporters of change in their infant's condition; listen to them carefully when they report a change so you do not miss this important information.

✓ CHECKPOINT QUESTIONS

15. Which tonsils are typically involved with tonsillitis?
16. What subtle sign best reveals post-tonsillectomy bleeding?
17. What is the most effective treatment for laryngitis?

Croup (Laryngotracheobronchitis)

Croup (inflammation of the larynx, trachea, and major bronchi) is one of the most frightening diseases of early childhood. In children between 6 months and 3 years of age, the cause of croup is usually a viral infection such as parainfluenza virus. In children between 3 and 6 years, it may occur from *H. influenzae* (Madden, 1997). Routine immunization of infants against *H. influenzae* should decrease the incidence.

Assessment

With croup, children typically have only a mild upper respiratory tract infection at bedtime with no fever or only a low-grade one. During the night, they develop a barking cough (croupy cough), inspiratory stridor, and marked retractions. They wake in extreme respiratory distress. The larynx, trachea, and major bronchi are all inflamed. Cyanosis is rarely present, but the danger of glottal obstruction from the larynx inflammation is very real. The severe symptoms typically last a number of hours and then, except for a rattling cough, subside by morning. Symptoms may recur the following night. Pulse oximetry and transcutaneous CO_2 monitors are helpful measures to document whether hypoxemia is occurring.

Therapeutic Management

One emergency method of relieving croup symptoms is for a parent to run the shower or hot water tap in a bathroom until the room fills with steam, then keep the child in this warm, moist environment. If this does not relieve symptoms, instruct the parents to bring the child to an emergency department for further evaluation and care. When a child is seen at the emergency room, cool moist air with budesonide, a steroid, or racemic epinephrine, given by nebulizer, results in reduced inflammation and effective bronchodilation to open the airway. Dexamethasone, a steroid given orally, also helps to reduce airway edema (Folland, 1997). Intravenous therapy may be prescribed to keep the child well hydrated.

NURSING DIAGNOSES AND RELATED INTERVENTIONS

Nursing Diagnosis: Ineffective airway clearance related to edema and constriction of airway

Outcome Identification: Child will demonstrate adequate airway clearance by 1 hour.

Outcome Evaluation: Respiratory rate is below 22 breaths/min; no cyanosis is present; PaO_2 is 80 to 100 mm Hg.

Remain constantly with a child, not only to observe closely but to reduce anxiety. Encourage a parent to remain for the same reason. Take vital signs as often as every 15 minutes, because extreme restlessness and thrashing, increased heart and respiratory rates, and cyanosis are symptoms of air hunger. A tracheostomy or endotracheal intubation may be necessary if these symptoms occur. (It is difficult to intubate children with croup because of the severe respiratory tract edema.) Increasing stridor is also a good indication of increasing inflammation. In some children, it is difficult to distinguish between fright from the newness of the experience (and their sense of their parents' fright) and the anxiousness that comes from oxygen want. Keep a continuous record of vital signs and activity as a way to demonstrate increasing respiratory rate and restlessness. Arterial blood gases may be taken to assess for sufficient oxygenation if pulse oximetry is not being used.

WHAT IF? What if a child who had loud stridor suddenly has no stridor present? Would you be relieved (his condition must be improving) or worried (his airway may be so blocked not enough air is entering to make the sound of stridor)?

Ensure that the child remains hydrated and secretions stay moist by offering frequent sips of oral fluid. If the child has such rapid respirations that drinking is not possible, intravenous fluid therapy will be necessary. Measure intake and output and urine specific gravity to evaluate hydration.

Laryngospasm with total occlusion of the airway is most apt to occur when a child's gag reflex is elicited or when the child is crying. Comfort to prevent crying. Do not elicit a gag reflex in any child with a croupy, barking cough.

Croup is a frightening disease for parents, because the symptoms of distress appear so suddenly. If the severe symptoms disappear by morning, parents may feel foolish that they rushed to a hospital with the child in the middle of the night. Assure them that their judgment was correct. When they brought the child in, he or she was seriously ill. Parents may be reluctant to see children discharged in the morning until they are convinced that they are now well enough to go home.

Epiglottitis

Epiglottitis is inflammation of the epiglottis (the flap of tissue that covers the opening to the larynx to keep out food and fluid during swallowing). Although it occurs rarely, inflammation of the epiglottis creates an emergency situation because the swollen epiglottis is unable to rise and allow the airway to open. This occurs most frequently in children from 3 to about 6 years of age (Mangione, 1997).

Epiglottitis can be either bacterial or viral in origin. *H. influenzae* type B is the most common bacterial cause of the disorder, but pneumococci, streptococci, or staphylococci may be responsible. Echovirus and respiratory syncytial virus also can cause the disorder.

Assessment

Children's symptoms begin as those of a mild upper respiratory tract infection. After 1 or 2 days, as inflammation spreads to the epiglottis, they suddenly develop severe inspiratory stridor, a high fever, hoarseness, and a very sore throat. They may have such difficulty swallowing that they drool saliva. They may protrude their tongues to increase free movement in the pharynx.

If the child's gag reflex is stimulated with a tongue blade, the swollen and inflamed epiglottis rises in the back of the throat as a cherry-red structure. It can be so edematous, however, that the gagging procedure causes complete obstruction of the glottis and respiratory failure. Therefore, *in children with symptoms of epiglottitis (dysphagia, inspiratory stridor, fever, and hoarseness), never attempt to visualize the epiglottis directly with a tongue blade or obtain a throat culture unless a means of providing an artificial airway, such as tracheostomy or endotracheal intubation, is readily available.* This is important for the nurse functioning in an expanded role, who performs physical assessments and routinely elicits gag reflexes.

Laboratory studies will show leukocytosis (20,000 to 30,000 mm^3) with the proportion of neutrophils increased. Blood cultures may be done to evaluate for septicemia. Arterial blood gases may be obtained to evaluate oxygen saturation. However, because excessive crying can precipitate entrapment of the epiglottis and obstruction, such tests may be delayed in preference to a lateral neck x-ray film or sonogram, which will show the enlarged epiglottis. Do not allow a child with possible epiglottitis to go to the x-ray department accompanied only by parents or a nursing aide, in case obstruction occurs while in the x-ray room.

Therapeutic Management

Children need moist air to reduce the epiglottal inflammation. If cyanosis is present, they need oxygen. An antibiotic, such as a second-generation cephalosporin, for example, cefuroxime, known to be effective against *H. influenzae,* may be prescribed until a throat culture indicates a specific antibiotic drug. Being unable to swallow, children need intravenous administration of fluid to maintain hydration. They may need a prophylactic tracheostomy or endotracheal intubation to prevent total obstruction. It is often difficult to intubate children with epiglottitis because the tube cannot be passed beyond the edematous epiglottis. After antibiotic therapy, the epiglottal inflammation recedes rapidly. By 12 to 24 hours, it has reduced in size enough that the airway may be removed. Antibiotic administration will continue for a full 7 to 10 days. Siblings of the ill child may be prescribed prophylactic antibiotic therapy to prevent them from developing the same symptoms.

The symptoms of epiglottitis are not unlike those of croup. Parents may not realize the extent of the occlusion in their child if the child has had croup on other occasions. They may question why a prophylactic tracheostomy was necessary this time when it was not used when the child had croup. Explain to them the difference between the two diseases (Table 19-5). Routine immunization for *H. influenzae* type B should decrease the incidence of epiglottitis in the future.

Some infants with epiglottitis die because obstruction occurs before a tracheotomy can be accomplished. If this should happen, parents need to be assured that they could not realize the seriousness of their child's symptoms. They may become overcautious, bringing other children to health care settings repeatedly for symptoms that are obviously not serious. It takes these parents time to regain confidence in themselves as parents and in their ability to judge a child's health again.

Aspiration

Aspiration is inhalation of a foreign object into the airway (Cataneo et al, 1997). Objects are most frequently aspirated by infants and toddlers. When a child aspirates a large foreign object, the immediate reaction is choking and hard, forceful coughing. Usually, this results in dislodging the object. However, if the cough becomes ineffective (no sound with cough, or if there are signs of increased respiratory difficulty accompanied by stridor), some intervention is essential. A series of Heimlich subdiaphragmatic abdominal thrusts are recommended for children (but not for infants; American Heart Association, 1992). Stand behind the child and place a fist just under the child's diaphragm (a point immediately below the anterior rib cage). Embrace the child, grip your fist with your other hand, and pull back and up with a rapid thrust. This action of pushing up on the diaphragm forces the aspirated material out of the trachea (Figure 19-18).

If a child is lying on his or her back at the time of the aspiration, stand at the head of the bed or table, place your hands in the same position as described above, and exert the same inward and upward thrust. A Heimlich maneuver may cause the child to vomit as well as expel an aspirated object. Turn the child's head to the side to prevent aspiration of vomitus.

Heimlich thrusts are not recommended for infants because of possible liver laceration (American Heart Association, 1992). A combination of back blows and chest thrusts is considered the most effective method for relieving complete foreign body airway obstruction in infants. Turn the infant prone over your arm and administer up to five quick back blows forcefully between the infant's shoulder blades, using the heel of the hand (Figure 19-19*A*). If the object is not expelled, turn the infant while carefully supporting the head and neck and holding the infant in a supine position draped over your thigh. Be sure to keep the infant's head lower than his chest. Pro-

TABLE 19.5 Comparison of Laryngotracheobronchitis (Croup) and Epiglottitis

ASSESSMENT	LARYNGOTRACHEOBRONCHITIS	EPIGLOTTITIS
Causative organism	Usually viral	Usually *Haemophilus influenzae*
Usual age of child	6 mo–3 yr	3–6 yr
Seasonal occurrence	Late fall and winter	No seasonal variation
Onset pattern	Preceded by upper respiratory infection; cough becomes worse at night	Preceded by upper respiratory infection; suddenly very ill
Presence of fever	Low grade	Elevated to about 103°F
Appearance	Retractions and stridor; prolonged inspiratory phase of respirations; not very ill appearing	Drooling; very ill appearing; neck is hyperextended to breathe. (Do not attempt to view enlarged epiglottis, or immediate airway obstruction can occur.)
Cough	Sharp, barking	Muffled cough
Radiographic findings	Lateral neck radiograph shows subglottal narrowing	Lateral neck radiograph shows enlarged epiglottis
Possible complications	Asphyxia due to subglottic obstruction	Asphyxia due to supraglottic obstruction

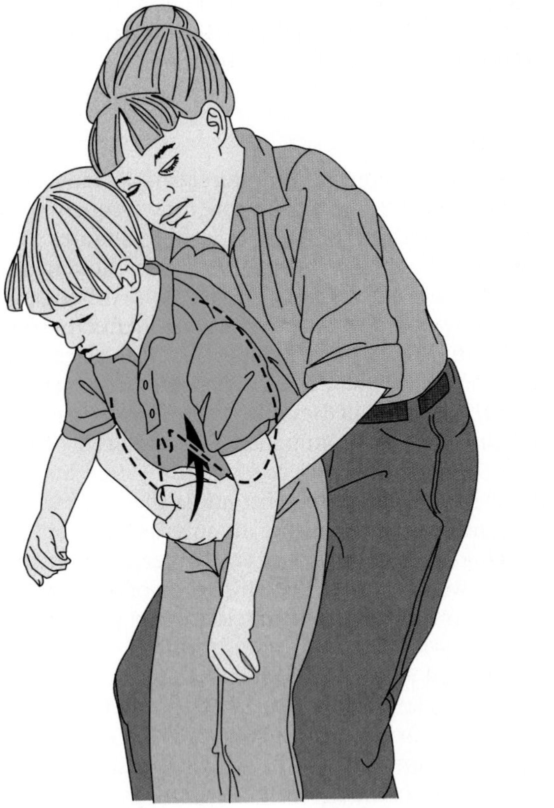

FIGURE 19.18 Heimlich maneuver on a school-age child.

vide up to five quick downward thrusts in the lower third of the sternum (Figure 19-19*B*; American Heart Association, 1992). This is generally enough to dislodge the foreign object. However, if this does not occur, rescue breathing may then be attempted.

Bronchial Obstruction

The right main bronchus is straighter and has a larger lumen than the left bronchus in children older than 2 years of age. For this reason, an aspirated foreign object that is not large enough to obstruct the trachea may lodge in the right bronchus, obstructing a portion or all of the right lung. The alveoli distal to the obstruction will collapse as the air remaining in them becomes absorbed (**atelectasis**), or hyperinflation and pneumothorax may occur if the foreign body serves as a ball valve, allowing air to enter but not leave the alveoli.

Assessment

After aspirating a small foreign body, the child generally begins to cough violently and may become dyspneic. Hemoptysis, fever, purulent sputum, and leukocytosis will result if the object scratches the airway or infection develops. Localized wheezing (a high whistling sound on expiration made by air passing through the narrow lumen) may occur. Because it is localized, it is different from the generalized wheezing of a child with asthma.

A chest x-ray film will reveal the presence of a radiopaque object. Objects most frequently aspirated are bones, nuts, coins, and safety pins. As a rule, nuts or popcorn should not be given to children younger than school age, because these objects are so frequently aspirated. These objects are coated with oil, and as they swell with moisture in the respiratory tract, they cause not only obstruction but lipid pneumonia, which is difficult to treat. Foreign bodies that are inhaled this deeply are rarely coughed up spontaneously, despite the severe coughing that ensues. Because objects such as bones and nuts cannot be visualized well on x-ray film, an x-ray study may be inconclusive. Most objects can be removed successfully by laryngoscopy or bronchoscopy.

Therapeutic Management

Children who are seen in emergency departments because of this type of aspirated foreign body are in distress from pain and are choking and coughing. Their parents

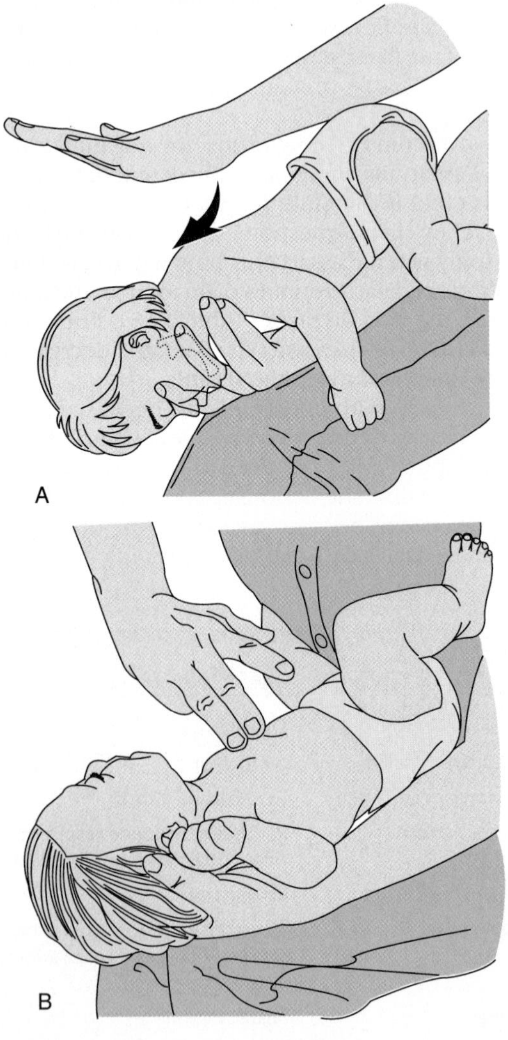

FIGURE 19.19 Back blows (**A**) and chest thrusts (**B**) to relieve complete foreign body airway obstruction in an infant. (From American Heart Association. [1992] Pediatric basic life support. *Journal of the American Medical Association, 268,* 2251-2261, with permission.)

are frightened by the degree of distress. They may have reason to feel badly about having offered a child (or allowing the child to reach) a food such as a peanut. Children need quick orientation to the treatment environment, because they often go from one department to another, such as the emergency department, x-ray, and then possibly to surgery or treatment room. If possible, allow their parents to go with them as appropriate. Throughout, be ever vigilant in observing the child for coughing up the foreign body or increasing respiratory distress.

A bronchoscopy may be performed to remove the foreign body. Children are often given conscious sedation for the procedure. For details of a bronchoscopy procedure, see Chapter 16. After bronchoscopy, assess the child closely for signs of bronchial edema and airway obstruction. Obtain frequent vital signs (increasing pulse and respiratory rate suggests increased edema and obstruction). The edema, which causes increased respirations, is in the airway and cannot be visualized. Thus, other indicators, such as vital signs, are important.

The child is kept on NPO status for at least an hour after the procedure. Check for return of the gag reflex. Once the gag reflex is present, give the first fluid cautiously to prevent possible aspiration. Cool fluid may be more soothing and also helps to reduce the soreness in the throat. Breathing cool, moist air or having an external ice collar applied may further reduce edema. Secretions that collect in the bronchus because of the irritation or manipulation can be kept moist and liquefied by encouraging the child to use a cool nebulizer.

Obviously, parents need to be cautioned about the danger of aspiration to keep it from happening again. Do not lecture, however. A parent whose child has just been through this experience recognizes the danger of aspiration and the need to be more careful in the future.

CHECKPOINT QUESTIONS

18. If a child has epiglottitis, what should you never attempt?
19. What two maneuvers are used to dislodge an aspirated foreign body in an infant?

DISORDERS OF THE LOWER RESPIRATORY TRACT

The structures of the lower respiratory tract are subject to infection by the same pathogens that attack the upper respiratory tract structures. Inflammation and infection of the lungs, or pneumonia, is particularly troublesome and is seen in many different forms in children. Other illnesses that occur in the lower respiratory tract, such as asthma and cystic fibrosis, can lead to secondary pneumonia infections.

Common disorders of the lower respiratory tract are discussed in the following sections.

Bronchitis

Bronchitis, or inflammation of the major bronchi and trachea, is one of the more common illnesses affecting preschool and school-age children. It is characterized by fever and cough, usually in conjunction with nasal congestion. Causative agents include the influenza viruses, adenovirus, and *Mycoplasma pneumoniae,* among others.

Assessment

On auscultation, rhonchi and coarse **rales** (the sound of crackles) can be heard. The child may have a mild upper respiratory tract infection for 1 or 2 days; the child then develops a fever and a dry, hacking cough that is hoarse and mildly productive in older children. The cough is serious enough to wake the child from sleep. These symptoms may last for a week, with full recovery sometimes taking as long as 2 weeks.

A chest x-ray film will reveal diffuse alveolar hyperinflation. There may be some markings at the hilus of the lung.

Therapeutic Management

Therapy is aimed at relieving the symptoms of illness, reducing fever, and maintaining adequate hydration. An antibiotic is prescribed for bacterial infections. If mucus is viscid, an expectorant may be helpful. It is important that children with bronchitis cough to raise accumulating sputum. Cough syrups to suppress the cough, therefore, are rarely indicated.

Bronchiolitis

Bronchiolitis is inflammation of the fine bronchioles and small bronchi. It occurs most often in children younger than age 2 years, peaking at 6 months of age. Incidence is highest in the winter and spring months. Many children who develop asthma later in life have numerous instances of bronchiolitis during their first year of life. Viruses, such as adenovirus, parainfluenza virus, and respiratory syncytial virus (RSV), in particular, appear to be the pathogens most responsible for this illness (Darville & Yamauchi, 1998).

Assessment

Typically, children have 1 or 2 days of an upper respiratory tract infection, then suddenly begin to have nasal flaring, intercostal and subcostal retractions on inspiration, and an increased respiratory rate. They may have a mild fever, leukocytosis, and an increased erythrocyte sedimentation rate. Mucus and inflammation block the small bronchioles, and air can no longer enter or leave alveoli freely. Most children develop alveolar hyperinflation because air enters more easily than it leaves inflamed, narrowed bronchioles. The expiratory phase of respiration is prolonged, and wheezing may be present. After initial hyperinflation, areas of atelectasis may occur as alveoli are blocked and the air they contain is absorbed. Infants develop tachycardia and cyanosis from hypoxia. Soon they become exhausted from the rapid respirations. A chest x-ray film may show pulmonary infiltrates caused by a secondary infection or collapse of alveoli (atelectasis). Pulse oximetry shows low oxygen saturation.

Therapeutic Management

For children with less severe symptoms, antipyretics, adequate hydration, and maintaining a watchful eye on progression to more serious illness is all that is necessary. Hospitalization is warranted for children in severe distress (e.g., if the child is tachypneic, has marked retractions, seems listless, or has a history of poor fluid intake). Oxygen, critical monitoring of vital signs and blood gas levels, and ventilatory support may be necessary.

Antibiotics are not commonly used in the treatment of bronchiolitis, because bacteria is rarely a causative factor. Children need humidified oxygen to counteract hypoxemia and adequate hydration to keep respiratory membranes moist. Nebulized bronchodilators and steroids may be used. A number of children may need assistance to achieve adequate ventilation. They all need to be carefully observed because, if RSV is the cause, apnea may occur. In some infants, extracorporeal membrane oxygenation (the same as that used for heart surgery) is necessary to maintain adequate oxygenation. Infants with prior cardiac disease may receive anti-RSV immunoglobulin (Jeng & Lemen, 1997).

Infants are usually positioned in a semi-Fowler's position to facilitate breathing, although some appear to be more comfortable on their abdomen. The prone position allows the weight of the body to help empty the chest more completely on expiration. Feeding is often a problem because the infants tire easily and therefore cannot finish a feeding. Intravenous fluids may be given for the first 1 or 2 days of illness to eliminate the need for oral feeding.

NURSING DIAGNOSES AND RELATED INTERVENTIONS

Nursing Diagnosis: Parental anxiety related to respiratory distress in child

Outcome Identification: Parents will demonstrate reduced anxiety regarding child's illness by 24 hours.

Outcome Evaluation: Parents state that anxiety level is tolerable as signs and symptoms of disease decrease.

Parents need a good explanation of the child's condition. Most parents are aware of bronchi but are unfamiliar with the word *bronchiole.* They may be unable to understand how a simple cold has become so severe. They wonder whether they should have sought medical attention sooner. Parents may lose confidence in themselves as parents when such a young infant becomes so severely ill. They can be assured that bronchiolitis begins first as only a cold. They could not have known at that point that this cold would take a more serious turn.

The acute phase of bronchiolitis lasts 2 or 3 days. After this time, the child's condition improves rapidly. Although mortality from bronchiolitis is less than 1%, it is a serious disorder of infancy; without treatment, a larger number of infants certainly would die.

Asthma

Asthma is an immediate hypersensitivity (type I) response (See Chapter 21). It is the most common chronic illness in children, accounting for many days of absenteeism from school and many hospital admissions each year. It tends to occur initially before age 5 years, although in these early years it may be diagnosed as frequent occurrences of bronchiolitis rather than asthma (Table 19-6). The condition may be intermittent, with periods of being symptom free, or chronic, with continuous symptoms.

Asthma results in diffuse obstructive and restrictive airway disease because of inflammation and bronchoconstriction. Severe bronchoconstriction can be induced by cold air or irritating odors, such as turpentine or smog, as well as inhalation of a known allergen. Air pollutants such as cigarette smoke may lower the threshold for hypersensitivity reactions and worsen the condition. Most children with asthma can be shown to have sensitization to inhalant antigens such as pollens, molds, or house dust. Food also may be involved. Although there may be a seasonal factor responsible for the child's symptoms, most of these children have multiple sensitivities and are affected all year long.

TABLE 19.6 Comparison of Bronchiolitis, Pneumonia, and Asthma

ASSESSMENT	BRONCHIOLITIS	PNEUMONIA	ASTHMA
Cause	Usually respiratory syncytial virus	May be bacterial (pneumococcal, or *H. influenzae*), viral, or mycoplasmal; can occur from aspiration	Hypersensitivity type I immune response
Age of child	Under 2 yr	All through childhood	Onset 1–5 yr
Onset pattern	Follows an upper respiratory infection	Follows an upper respiratory infection	Follows initiation by an allergen
Appearance	Fatigued, anxious, shallow respirations, increasing anteroposterior diameter of chest	Fatigued, anxious, shallow respirations	Wheezing, exhausted, frightened
Cough	Paroxysmal, dry	Productive, harsh cough	Paroxysmal, with thick mucus production
Fever	Low grade	Elevated	None
Auscultatory sounds	Barely audible breath sounds, rales, expiratory wheezing	Decreased breath sounds, rales	Wheezing

Mechanism of Disease

Asthma primarily affects the small airways and involves three separate processes: (1) bronchospasm, (2) inflammation of bronchial mucosa, and (3) increased bronchial secretions (mucus). All three processes act to reduce the size of the airway lumen, leading to acute respiratory distress. Bronchial constriction occurs because of stimulation of the parasympathetic nervous system (cholinergic mediated system), which initiates smooth muscle constriction. Inflammation occurs because of mast cell activation to release leukotrienes, histamine, and prostaglandins. These increase bronchospasm and mucus production. Once viewed as a long-term, poorly controlled disorder, newer therapy makes this a reversible disorder (Fehrenbach, 1997).

Assessment

The word *asthma* is derived from the Greek word for "panting." Typically, after exposure to an allergen, an episode begins with a dry cough, often at night as bronchospasm begin. Because bronchioles are normally larger in lumen on inspiration than expiration even with bronchospasm, children may inhale normally or have little difficulty. However, they have difficulty exhaling because they cannot force air through the narrowed lumen of the bronchioles filled with mucus. This causes the dyspnea and the wheezing (the sound caused by air being pushed forcibly through obstructed bronchioles). The child coughs up mucus, which is generally copious. The sputum produced after a severe attack may contain white casts bearing the shape of the bronchi from which they were dislodged. It is important to remember that wheezing is heard primarily on expiration. However, when severe, wheezing may be heard on inspiration as well.

History. Assessment should include a thorough history of the development of the child's symptoms, actions before the attack, and any other factors, such as triggers that would have been involved in initiating the current attack. When an acute attack has passed, ask the parent or child to describe the home environment, including any pets, the child's bedroom, outdoor play space, classroom environment, and type of heating in the house to see whether inhalants in the environment could be eliminated.

Physical Assessment. A physical assessment includes examining for the specific symptoms of asthma. On auscultation, wheezing will be present on expiration. The bronchospasm has led to CO_2 trapping and retention; thus, arterial O_2 saturation monitored by a pulse oximeter may be decreased because of the inability to fully aerate the lungs. The child may be cyanotic and is often frightened because of an acute feeling of suffocating. A peak flow meter will show decreased respiratory capacity.

In many children, the initial wheezing may be so loud that it can be heard without a stethoscope. In others, it will be evident only by auscultation. Asthma affects all lobes of the lungs, so, although the wheezing may be more prominent in one lobe than in another, it is generally audible in all lung fields. Audible wheezing in only one lobe suggests that only one bronchus is plugged, which may indicate that a foreign body such as a peanut is responsible, rather than asthma. This possibility should be investigated.

The lungs will be hyperresonant to percussion (i.e., they will make louder, hollower noise on percussion than usual) because of pockets of trapped air behind clogged bronchi. The length of expiration will be increased beyond normal limits. In normal respirations, the inspiration phase of breathing is longer than the expiration phase. During an attack of asthma, children must work so hard to exhale that the expiration phase becomes longer than the inspiration phase. Time the two phases to demonstrate this. To achieve full breaths, children use intercostal accessory muscles, producing retractions.

As constriction becomes acute, the sound of wheezing may decrease because so little air is able to leave the alveoli. Hypoxemia and possibly cyanosis will become severe. When blood gases show an increased CO_2 level and the sound of wheezing suddenly stops, respiratory failure is imminent.

During attacks, children with asthma are generally more comfortable in a sitting or standing position rather than lying down. If seated in a chair, they lean forward and raise their shoulders, to give themselves more breathing space. Do not urge children to "lie down and relax." This causes severe anxiety and increased difficulty in breathing. Children who do agree to lie down are either at the end of an attack and so beginning to feel less threatened by the dyspnea or are so exhausted by the paroxysms of coughing that they no longer have the strength to sit upright.

Over time, as the child has many bouts of asthma, the child may develop a shieldlike or barrel-shaped chest from constant overinflation of air in alveoli. Clubbing of the fingers from polycythemia in response to poor tissue oxygenation in distal parts may be noticeable. If the child has been treated for a long period with steroids, growth may be stunted. On laboratory examination, the eosinophil count will be elevated, and pulmonary function studies will be reduced.

Pulmonary Function Studies

Good pulmonary function depends on good ventilation (drawing adequate air into the lungs and expelling it again); adequate transfer of gases across the alveolar capillary membranes; and the volume and distribution of pulmonary capillary blood flow. In children with asthma, the vital capacity may be low or the capacity may be normal but, because of narrowed bronchioles as a result of bronchospasm, the expiratory rate may be abnormally long (more than 10 seconds rather than the normal 2 or 3 seconds). If the child has atelectasis, the vital capacity will be low because of air absorption behind bronchial plugging. When a vital capacity test is abnormal, the child may have it repeated after an inhalation treatment. A gross measure of vital capacity is to ask a child to blow out a match. A child with an average vital capacity should be able to do this when the match is held at 6 in.

Peak Expiratory Flow Rate (PEFR) Monitoring. Children often use a home peak flow meter daily to measure gross changes in peak expiratory flow over time. This can help in the planning of an appropriate therapeutic regimen (Figure 19-20). Children with asthma

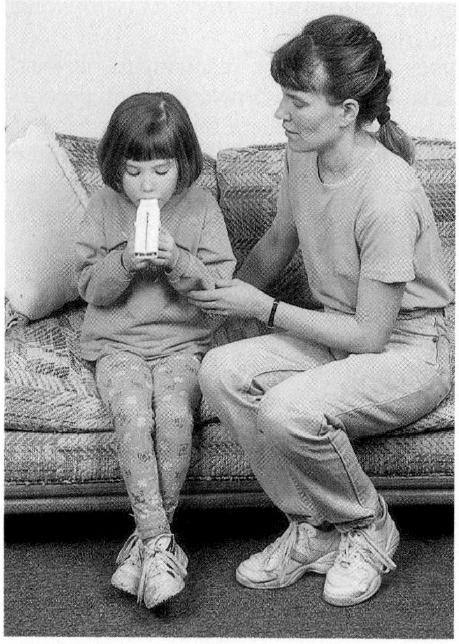

FIGURE 19.20 Children with any chronic illness require periodic evaluation and sometimes home monitoring. Children with asthma may use a home peak flow meter and track their peak expiratory flow readings on a daily or weekly basis.

should be able to tell you their usual reading and personal best score.

To effectively use a peak flow meter, a child places the indicator at the bottom of the numbered scale, and takes a deep breath. He or she places the meter in the mouth and then blows out as hard and fast as he can. He then repeats this two more times and records the highest number achieved as the peak flow meter result. During a 2-week period when the child feels well, he or she should do this daily. The highest number recorded during this time is recorded as the child's "personal best."

Children are assigned "zones" to rate their expiratory compliance.

- Green zone (80% to 100% of their personal best) means no asthma symptoms are present, and they should take their routine medications.
- Yellow zone (50% to 80% of personal best) signals caution. An episode of asthma may be beginning.
- Red zone (below 50% of personal best) indicates an asthma episode is beginning. The child should immediately take an inhaled beta 2-agonist and then repeat the peak flow assessment. If the second reading is not in the green zone, the parent should alert the child's primary care provider.

Therapeutic Management

Therapy for children with asthma involves planning for the three goals of all allergy disorders: (1) avoidance of the allergen by environmental control, (2) skin-testing and hyposensitization to identified allergens, and (3) relief of symptoms by the use of pharmacologic agents.

In the past, children with asthma were maintained on an oral preparation of a methylxanthine such as theophylline and administered epinephrine to relieve acute attacks. Asthma is managed today by the stepwise administration of medication. If the child has only mild intermittent symptoms, no daily medication is usually needed. When symptoms occur, the child should take a short-acting inhaled beta 2-agonist bronchodilator such as albuterol (see Drug Highlight). If the child needs to do this more than twice a week, long-term control therapy may be indicated.

The child with mild but persistent asthma will be prescribed an inhaled anti-inflammatory corticosteroid daily. If the child needs to supplement the primary therapy this way on a daily basis, additional long-term control therapy may be necessary.

For children who have moderate persistent symptoms, the child takes an inhaled anti-inflammatory corticosteroid daily and a long-acting bronchodilator at bedtime. Children who have severe persistent asthma symptoms take a high dose of an inhaled anti-inflammatory cortico-

DRUG HIGHLIGHT

Albuterol Sulfate (Proventil, Ventolin)

Action: Albuterol is a beta-2 adrenergic agonist that acts selectively to cause bronchodilation and vasodilation for relief of bronchospasm.

Pregnancy risk category: C

Dosage: Orally, 2 or 4 mg 3 or 4 times daily not to exceed 32 mg/day in children older than 14 years; 2 mg 3 or 4 times daily not to exceed 24 mg/day in children ages 6 to 14 years; 0.1 mg/kg 3 times daily not to exceed 2 mg, gradually increasing to 0.2 mg/kg 3 times daily not to exceed 4 mg in children ages 2 to 6 years. By inhalation, 2 puffs every 4 to 6 hours in children 12 years of age and older or 2.5 mg (0.5 mL of 0.5% solution diluted with 2.5 mL of 0.9% sodium chloride) or 3 mL of 0.083% solution 3 or 4 times daily.

Possible adverse effects: Restlessness, apprehension, anxiety, fear, nausea, cardiac arrhythmias, paradoxical airway resistance with repeated, excessive use of inhalation preparations, sweating, pallor, and flushing.

Nursing Implications:

- Instruct parents and child in method to administer drug. Teach child and parents about use and care of nebulized solution or metered dose inhaler and spacer devices if ordered.
- Warn child and parents not to exceed the number of ordered puffs to prevent possible tolerance to drug.
- If more than one inhalation is ordered, advise child to wait 1 to 2 minutes before taking the second puff.
- If the child is also receiving an inhaled corticosteroid, advise the child and parents to have the child use the albuterol first to open the airways and then wait approximately 5 minutes before using the corticosteroid, to maximize its effectiveness.

steroid daily, a long-acting bronchodilator at bedtime, and an oral corticosteroid (NAEAPP, 1997). Children who have such severe symptoms they are admitted to the hospital may receive theophylline, a methylxanthine. Theophylline needs to be titrated to a therapeutic blood level (peak and trough levels need to be drawn) to prevent toxicity (signs are vomiting, severe gastrointestinal distress, and dysrhythmias). Cromolyn sodium is a mast cell stabilizer given by a nebulizer or metered dose inhaler that can prevent bronchoconstriction and thereby prevent the symptoms of asthma (see Drug Highlight). It is not effective once symptoms have begun.

If children are to receive medication by nebulizer or inhaler, it is important that they learn to use these wisely. It is easy to take this type of medication lightly (because it is "not really medicine"), and so overdose from constant use of nebulizers or metered dose inhalers can occur. Metered dose inhalers require that the child trigger the inhaler at the same time he or she breathes in (Figure 19-21*A*). Because it is difficult for children younger than approximately 12 years to do this, placing a "spacer" tube between the inhaler and the mouthpiece eliminates this problem (Figure 19-21*B*).

Dehydration occurs rapidly in children during an asthma attack from decreased oral intake (children stop drinking because they are coughing, or coughing makes them vomit and parents stop offering fluid) and increased insensible loss from tachypnea. If theophylline is administered, its diuretic effect contributes to fluid loss. Dehydration leads to increased mucus plugging and further airway obstruction. Encourage children to continue to drink oral fluid (ask what are favorite beverages and offer small sips of them). Avoid milk or milk products because they cause thick mucus and difficulty swallowing. In an emergency setting, an intravenous line will be established to supply continuous fluid therapy.

DRUG HIGHLIGHT

Cromolyn Sodium (Intal)

Action: Cromolyn is a mast cell inhibitor that acts to inhibit the release of histamine and slow-releasing substance of anaphylaxis, and leukotriene, thus decreasing the overall allergic response. In asthma, it is used prophylactically to prevent severe bronchospasms.

Pregnancy risk category: B

Dosage: Initially, 20 mg inhaled (via inhaler or as nebulized solution) 4 times daily at regular intervals

Possible adverse effects: Dizziness, headache, nausea, dry and irritated throat, cough, nasal congestion, epistaxis, and sneezing.

Nursing Implications:

- Instruct parents and child that this drug is not effective in an acute attack.
- Caution child and parents to take the drug exactly as prescribed and to continue other agents, such as bronchodilators. Advise the parents as the cromolyn therapy is started that corticosteroids, if ordered, will be continued and then gradually tapered.
- Instruct child and parents in the use of metered dose inhaler or nebulizer for administration of cromolyn.
- Instruct parents and child to watch for a possible recurrence of asthmatic symptoms if dosage is decreased.
- Know that this drug is only given once the acute episode is over and the child's airway is clear and he can inhale on his own.
- Warn child and parents not to exceed the number of ordered puffs to prevent possible tolerance to drug.
- If more than one inhalation is ordered, advise child to wait 1 to 2 minutes before taking the second puff.
- If the child is also receiving an inhaled bronchodilator, advise the child and parents to have the child use the bronchodilator first to open the airways and then wait approximately 5 minutes before using the cromolyn, to maximize its effectiveness.

NURSING DIAGNOSES AND RELATED INTERVENTIONS

Nursing Diagnosis: Fear related to sudden onset of asthma attack

Outcome Identification: Parents and child will demonstrate ability to manage sudden attacks within 1 month.

Outcome Evaluation: Parents and child express confidence in their ability to prevent attacks and handle any that occur.

Asthma is a frightening disease. At the time it is diagnosed, parents may have already gone through a long period of wondering what was wrong (Horner, 1997). Parents may be afraid to allow children to attend school for fear that they will have an attack while in school. They may be afraid to leave them alone with baby sitters or even relatives so that they may have evenings to themselves or enjoy a vacation. Help parents to allow a child enough freedom for growth and development while still being certain that he or she is safe. Taking steps to slow breathing, better emptying alveoli through pursed lip breathing, and beginning medications to prevent symptoms from becoming severe are key measures to teach. Children can have long periods without attacks. When a new one occurs after a long absence, it is almost as frightening as the original attack because everything seems so new again.

Nursing Diagnosis: Health-seeking behaviors related to prevention of and treatment for asthma attacks

Outcome Identification: Parents and child within 1 month will demonstrate understanding of ways to prevent attacks and measures to manage attacks when they occur.

Outcome Evaluation: Parents and child accurately state triggers; child correctly demonstrates breathing exercises, use of inhaler, and PEFR meter.

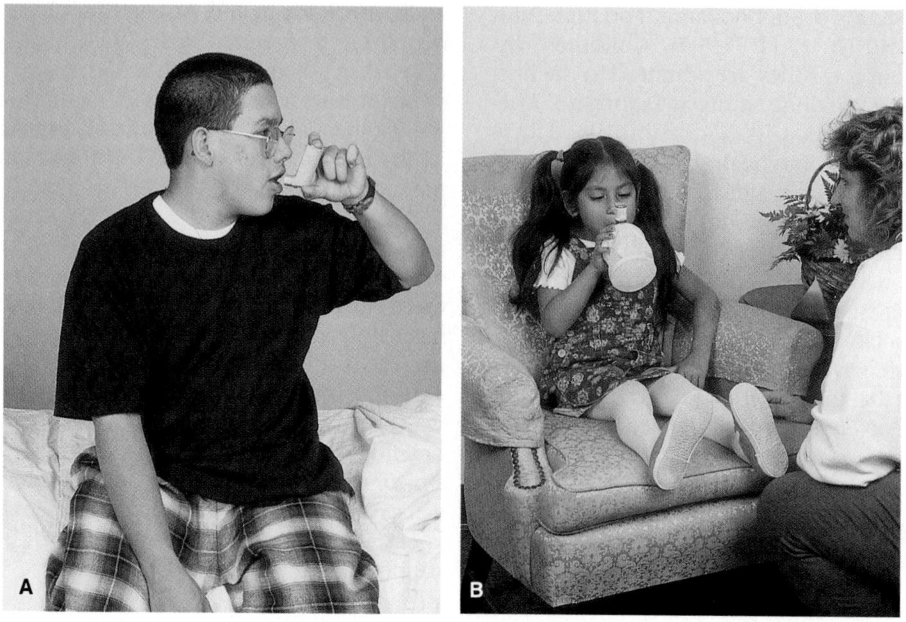

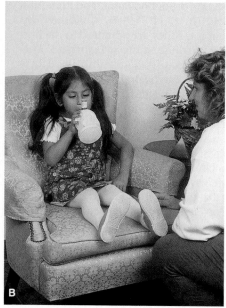

FIGURE 19.21 (**A**) Many children with asthma use a metered dose inhaler to administer a bronchodilator to themselves. Be certain children respect such medicine as medicine and thus use sensible precautions. (**B**) Younger children need a "spacer" with inhalers so they do not need to correlate administration with inhalation.

Children need to learn how to avoid possible triggers. (For more information about controlling triggers in the home, see Chapter 21). If foods are a trigger, children need to learn to be responsible for their own diets so they can avoid these foods. Children as young as age 6 years can learn the foods they cannot eat and to stay away from triggers such as cats or dogs. They must take responsibility to tell a friend's parent if at a birthday party or a schoolteacher that they must not eat certain foods. They must learn to use a metered dose inhaler or nebulizer if that is prescribed for them. At the same time, they must not become inhaler dependent or carry the inhaler with them constantly, afraid to go anywhere without it. This will invariably result in their using the inhaler much more often than is necessary.

To prevent children with asthma from losing chest mobility and to decrease their tendency to develop a "barrel chest," they frequently are taught a number of breathing or mobility exercises to do daily at home. Using an incentive spirometer also can be effective in helping the children "exercise their lungs."

Mobility exercises consist of such activities as bending side to side, bending forward and touching the left foot with the right hand, and swinging the arms rhythmically in front of the body like a windmill. These keep chest muscles supple.

Breathing exercises are aimed at increasing expiratory function (diaphragmatic or side-expansion breathing). These exercises can be incorporated into a bedtime or after-school routine. Parents (and nurses) who do the mobility exercises with the children find that the exercises help to reduce abdominal size, because they tighten abdominal muscles as well.

The prognosis in children who develop asthma is good if they adhere to their treatment regimen. Children do not "out-grow" asthma, although most of them may become symptom free as adults, probably because the lumens of major airways enlarge with adulthood.

In informing parents of these facts, be certain not to convey the impression that asthma is a disease that is outgrown. Although asthma may not always last into adulthood, the need for careful environmental control, conscientious administration of medication, and hyposensitization during childhood should not be diminished.

Status Asthmaticus

Under ordinary circumstances, an asthma attack responds readily to the aerosol administration of a bronchodilator such as albuterol and steroids. When children fail to respond and an attack continues, they are in status asthmaticus. This is an extreme emergency because if the attack cannot be relieved, the child may die of heart failure caused by exhaustion, atelectasis, or respiratory acidosis from bronchial plugging.

Assessment

Status asthmaticus is often caused by pulmonary infection, which acts as the triggering mechanism for the prolonged attack (Johnston, 1997). Cultures should be obtained from coughed sputum, and a broad-spectrum antibiotic will be ordered until the cultures are returned. Be sure the sputum obtained for culture is coughed from deep in the respiratory tract and not just from the back of the throat.

Therapeutic Management

By definition, the child in status asthmaticus has failed to respond to first-line therapy. Continuous nebulization with an inhaled beta 2-agonist, intravenous corticosteroids and methylxanthine therapy all may be necessary to reduce symptoms. Pulse oximetry will show that the child in status asthmaticus needs oxygen, which is best given by face mask or nasal prongs. These methods supply good oxygen concentrations and yet leave the child unobscured. To prevent drying of pulmonary secretions, oxygen must be given with humidification. Oxygen is best administered at a concentration of 30% to 40%, not 100%. If concentrations greater than 40% are needed, a Venturi mask may be used. Some children in severe status asthmaticus have such a carbon dioxide buildup (because they cannot exhale properly) that they develop carbon dioxide narcosis with no stimulation for inhalation. The child's respiratory stimulus, therefore, is hypoxia, or lack of oxygen. If 100% oxygen were administered, the oxygen lack would disappear, and respirations would cease. The idea "if a little is good, a lot is better" does not apply here. After it has been ascertained that the child is not in acidosis (from blood gas and pH studies), oxygen levels may be increased, but, for initial therapy, keep the level at 30% to 40%.

After an acute stage of status asthmaticus, children need increased fluid to keep airway secretions moist. Drinking tends to aggravate coughing, so they are unlikely to drink, and they are often dehydrated on admission to the hospital. An intravenous infusion of 5% glucose in 0.45 saline is started to supply fluid. If the child is able to drink, do not offer cold fluids because these tend to aggravate bronchospasm. Also, the child should not be given any cough suppressants. As long as they continue to cough up mucus, they are not in serious danger. When they stop coughing up mucus, it forms thick mucus plugs that may lead to pneumonia, atelectasis, and acidosis. Loss of cough and no wheezing is, therefore, an ominous sign. Monitor intake and output; measure the specific gravity of urine. Under stress, antidiuretic hormone is released so fluid retention and overhydration may occur.

The PaO_2 level usually is maintained at more than 90 mm Hg with oxygen administration. An increasing $PaCO_2$ level is a danger sign because it indicates the degree of hypoventilation. In severe attacks, endotracheal intubation and mechanical ventilation may be necessary to maintain effective respirations.

✓ CHECKPOINT QUESTIONS

20. When is bronchiolitis most commonly seen?
21. What is the major presenting symptom in a child with asthma?
22. What is the chief medication given for an acute asthma attack?

Bronchiectasis

Bronchiectasis is chronic dilatation of the bronchi. It may follow pneumonia, aspiration of a foreign body, pertussis, or asthma. It is often associated with cystic fibrosis.

Children develop a chronic cough that produces mucopurulent sputum. Young infants may have accompanying wheezing or stridor. If a large area of lung is obstructed, children may have cyanosis. As the disease becomes chronic, children may develop symptoms of chronic lung disease, such as clubbing of the fingers and easy fatigability. Their physical growth may become retarded. Their chest may become enlarged from overinflation of alveoli caused by the air trapped behind inflamed bronchi.

Chest physiotherapy may be necessary to raise tenacious sputum. An antibiotic will be necessary if infection is present. The cause of the bronchiectasis must be identified and relieved before the chronic process can be relieved. Surgery to remove the affected lung portion may be necessary (Larroquet et al, 1997).

Pneumonia

Pneumonia is inflammation of the alveoli, occurring at a rate of 2 to 4 children in 100 (Modlin, 1997). It may be of bacterial origin (pneumococcal, streptococcal, staphylococcal, or chlamydial) or viral origin such as respiratory syncytial virus (RSV). Aspiration of lipid or hydrocarbon substances also causes pneumonia. Pneumonia is the most common pulmonary cause of death in infants younger than 48 hours of age. It occurs most often in late winter and early spring. Newborns who are born more than 24 hours after rupture of the amniotic membranes and those who aspirated amniotic fluid during delivery are particularly prone to developing pneumonia in their first few days of life. When it is known that the membranes have been ruptured for more than 24 hours before birth, prophylactic broad-spectrum antibiotics may be given to prevent pneumonia. Differences between bronchiolitis, pneumonia, and asthma are summarized in Table 19-6. *Pneumocystis carinii* pneumonia, the type seen almost exclusively with human immunodeficiency syndrome, is discussed in Chapter 21.

Pneumococcal Pneumonia

The onset of pneumococcal pneumonia is generally abrupt and follows an upper respiratory tract infection. In infants, pneumonia tends to remain bronchopneumonia with poor consolidation (infiltration of exudate into the alveoli). In older children, pneumonia may localize in a single lobe, and consolidation may occur. With this, children may have blood-tinged sputum as exudative serum and red blood cells invade the alveoli. After 24 to 48 hours, the alveoli are no longer filled with red blood cells and serum but fibrin, leukocytes, and pneumococci. The child's cough no longer raises blood-tinged sputum but thick purulent material.

Assessment

Children develop a high fever, nasal flaring, retractions, chest pain, chills, and dyspnea. Some children report the pain as being abdominal. The fever with pneumococcal pneumonia may rise so fast that a child has a febrile convulsion (see Chapter 28).

Children with pneumococcal pneumonia appear acutely ill. Physical assessment will show tachypnea and tachycardia. Because lung space is filled with exudate, respiratory function is diminished. Breath sounds become bronchial (sound transmitted from the trachea) because air no longer or poorly enters fluid-filled alveoli. Adventitious breath sounds may be present. Rales (sound of crackles) may be present as a result of the fluid. Percussion will indicate dullness over a lobe in which consolidation has occurred. Chest radiographs will show lung consolidation in older children and patchy diffusion in young children. Laboratory studies will indicate leukocytosis.

Therapeutic Management

Before antibiotic therapy was available for pneumonia, it was almost always a fatal disease, especially in infants, so parents may be more worried about a child's condition than is warranted (see Enhancing Communication).

Therapy for pneumococcal pneumonia is antibiotics. Either ampicillin or amoxicillin are effective against pneumococci. Amoxicillin-clavulanate (Augmentin) also may be prescribed. Infants need rest to prevent exhaustion. Plan nursing care carefully to conserve a child's strength. At the same time, turn and reposition frequently to avoid pooling of secretions. Intravenous therapy may be necessary to supply fluid, especially in infants, because infants tire so readily with sucking that they cannot achieve a good oral intake. They may need an antipyretic such as acetaminophen to reduce fever (Modlin, 1997) (see the Nursing Care Plan).

Humidified oxygen may be necessary to alleviate labored breathing and prevent hypoxemia. Oxygen saturation levels need to be assessed frequently. Chest physiotherapy will encourage the movement of mucus and prevent obstruction. Older children may need to be encouraged to cough so that secretions do not pool and become further infected.

After pneumonia, children usually have a period of at least a week when they tire easily and need frequent, small feedings. Parents need to be cautioned that this is an expected outcome and not a complication in itself. Children with chronic illness, those who have had a splenectomy, or those who are immunocompromised should receive a pneumococcal vaccine to prevent pneumococcal pneumonia.

ENHANCING COMMUNICATION

B.J. is a 2-year-old who has been admitted to your hospital unit with pneumonia. His mother called home to tell the grandmother about the diagnosis. Since she returned from the telephone, she seems tearful and visibly upset.

Less Effective Communication

Nurse: Is something wrong, Mrs. Silver? You seem upset.
Mrs. Silver: I am. I didn't realize pneumonia was so serious until I talked to my mother.
Nurse: Because it's serious is why B.J.'s been admitted to the hospital.
Mrs. Silver: She told me my brother had pneumonia when he was a baby. Is this oxygen? My mother said to check B.J.'s getting oxygen.
Nurse: It sure is. He's also going to get an antibiotic. Why don't you stay with him while I get the equipment for that?

More Effective Communication

Nurse: Is something wrong, Mrs. Silver? You seem upset.
Mrs. Silver: I am. I didn't realize pneumonia was so serious until I talked to my mother.
Nurse: Because it's serious is why B.J.'s been admitted to the hospital.
Mrs. Silver: She told me my brother had pneumonia when he was a baby. Is this oxygen? My mother said to check B.J.'s getting oxygen.
Nurse: Let's talk about everything your mother told you about pneumonia. Because the treatment has changed so much, what happened years ago isn't the same as what happens now.

Before the advent of antibiotics, a diagnosis of pneumonia in a young child was almost automatically a fatal diagnosis. Ask enough questions of parents today to be certain they understand that their child's prognosis, although serious, is not the fatal diagnosis of years ago.

Chlamydial Pneumonia

Chlamydia trachomatis pneumonia is most often seen in newborns up to 12 weeks of age. Symptoms usually begin gradually with nasal congestion and a sharp cough; children fail to gain weight. Symptoms progress to tachypnea with wheezing and rales (the sound of crackles) audible on auscultation. Laboratory assessment will show an elevated level of immunoglobulin IgG and IgM antibodies, peripheral eosinophilia, and a specific antibody to *C. trachomatis.* Such an infection is treated with erythromycin with good results (Boyer, 1997).

Viral Pneumonia

Viral pneumonia is generally caused by the viruses of upper respiratory tract infection: the RSVs, myxoviruses, or adenoviruses. The symptoms begin as an upper respiratory tract infection. After a day or two, symptoms such as a low-grade fever, nonproductive cough, and tachypnea begin. There may be diminished breath sounds and fine rales on chest auscultation, although few symptoms of lung disease may be noticed. Chest radiographs will show diffuse infiltrated areas. Respiratory syncytial virus may cause apnea.

Because this is a viral infection, antibiotic therapy usually is not effective. The child needs rest and, possibly, an antipyretic for the fever; intravenous fluid may be necessary if the child becomes exhausted from feeding or is dehydrated and refusing fluids. After recovery from the acute phase of illness, the child will have a week or two of lethargy or lack of energy, as occurs with bacterial pneumonia. Parents may be confused because their child is not receiving an antibiotic, despite the diagnosis being pneumonia. They need an explanation of the difference between viral and bacterial infections, so that they can better understand their child's therapy and plan of care.

Nursing Care Plan

THE CHILD HOSPITALIZED WITH PNEUMONIA

A 3-year-old brought to the emergency department by his parents is admitted to the hospital with a diagnosis of pneumococcal pneumonia. His parents state, "He just had a cold but now he's coughing up some thick yellow mucus."

Assessment: 3-year-old male within age-acceptable parameters for height and weight. Child is diaphoretic and pale. Tympanic temperature—102.2°F (39.0°C); pulse—146; respirations—40. Nasal flaring and intercostal retractions noted. Lungs with decreased breath sounds. Scattered rales (crackles) auscultated and dullness to percussion noted in right upper and middle lobes. Productive cough with thick purulent sputum. Child complains of difficulty breathing. Mother states, "He hasn't been drinking much because of his coughing. And all he seems to want to do is lie on the couch."

Chest x-ray reveals patchy diffusion; white blood cell count reveals leukocytosis. Unable to obtain sputum specimen for culture.

Nursing Diagnosis: Ineffective breathing pattern related to physiologic effects of pneumonia

Outcome Identification: Child will exhibit signs and symptoms of adequate ventilation.

Outcome Evaluation: Respiratory rate, oxygen saturation, and arterial blood gas levels within age-acceptable parameters without the use of supplemental oxygen. Lungs clear to auscultation. Child states breathing is easier; demonstrates measures to improve ventilation and ease the work of breathing.

Interventions	Rationale
1. Administer supplemental, humidified oxygen via face mask at prescribed rate. Obtain arterial blood gases (ABGs) as ordered and monitor oxygen saturation levels via pulse oximetry.	1. Supplemental, humidified oxygen aids in improving ventilation without drying the mucous membranes and in minimizing the risk for hypoxemia. ABGs and pulse oximetry provide objective evidence of the child's tissue oxygenation.
2. Assess vital signs and respiratory status, including lung sounds, initially every 1 to 2 hours and then according to institution's policy.	2. Frequent assessment of vital signs and respiratory status provides information about any improvement or deterioration in the child's condition.
3. Administer antibiotic therapy, such as ampicillin or amoxicillin, as ordered.	3. Amoxicillin and ampicillin are effective against pneumococcus.
4. Place the child in a semi-Fowler's to high Fowler's position. Reposition the child frequently.	4. An upright position facilitates breathing and promotes optimal lung expansion by relieving diaphragmatic pressure. Frequent repositioning prevents pooling and stasis of secretions.
5. Perform chest physiotherapy as ordered.	5. Chest physiotherapy helps to mobilize secretions to prevent mucous plugging and aids in expectoration.
6. Use play to encourage the child to cough, deep breathe, and use incentive spirometry every 1 to 2 hours. Involve the parents in these activities.	6. Coughing, deep breathing, and incentive spirometry help to maximize ventilation. Play helps to enhance the child's participation. Involving the parents promotes active participation in the child's care.
7. Assist the child and parents with measures to relax.	7. Anxiety and stress increase the child's oxygen demands. Assisting the parents to relax also helps to minimize the effect of the parents' anxiety on the child.

(continued)

Nursing Diagnosis: Risk for fluid volume deficit related to diminished oral intake and increased insensible fluid losses secondary to tachypnea, diaphoresis, and fever

Outcome Identification: The child will exhibit signs and symptoms of adequate fluid balance.

Outcome Evaluation: Skin turgor good. Intake and output, urine specific gravity, laboratory studies, and weight remain within age-appropriate parameters.

Interventions	Rationale
1. Obtain baseline weight and monitor daily.	1. Weight is an accurate indicator of fluid balance.
2. Administer intravenous fluid therapy at prescribed rate, using an infusion pump or controller.	2. Intravenous fluid therapy assists in replacing fluid losses, especially when there is difficulty with ingesting appropriate amounts of oral fluid. Using a pump or controller ensures an accurate flow rate, minimizing the risk for fluid overload.
3. Offer the child sips of fluid frequently. Try different forms of fluid such as gelatin, popsicles, or fruit bars based on the child's likes. Incorporate the use of play to encourage the child to drink, such as taking a sip or spoonful of gelatin each time after his turn in a game. Involve the parents in these activities.	3. Oral fluid intake is necessary for replacement. Different forms of fluid may be more appealing to the child and enhance his intake. Using games and play are effective methods for encouraging fluid intake in a child. Involving the parents promotes active participation in the child's care.
4. Institute measures to control fever, such as administering acetaminophen as ordered and dressing child in summer clothing.	4. Reducing fever aids in reducing insensible fluid loss.
5. Monitor intake and output, urine specific gravity, urine and serum electrolytes, blood urea nitrogen, creatinine, and osmolality.	5. Intake and output and urine specific gravity are reliable indicators of fluid balance. Fluid loss can result in dehydration, leading to decreased renal function and ability to eliminate wastes.

Nursing Diagnosis: Activity intolerance related to effects of pneumonia and tachypnea

Outcome Identification: Child will exhibit a return to pre-illness activity level.

Outcome Evaluation: Child's oxygen saturation level and vital signs within age-acceptable parameters with activity. Child participates in self-care activities with minimal to no complaints of difficulty breathing.

Interventions	Rationale
1. Provide a balance of activity with rest periods. Cluster nursing care to prevent overexertion.	1. Activity increases myocardial oxygen demand, further compromising respiratory function.
2. Continue to administer supplemental oxygen and monitor vital signs, oxygen saturation levels, and breathing difficulties before and after any activity.	2. Oxygen is necessary for adequate tissue perfusion. A decrease in oxygen saturation levels or vital signs or increasing difficulty breathing in response to activity indicates an increase in oxygen demand that the child is not able to meet.
3. Provide small, frequent meals.	3. Eating requires energy expenditure. Small, frequent meals prevent overtiring, which could further compromise respiratory function and also interfere with nutrition.
4. As the pneumonia resolves, gradually allow an increase in activity, such as self-care activities, getting out of bed to a chair, and ambulation, using oxygen saturation levels as a guide.	4. Gradual increase in activity within acceptable oxygen saturation levels minimizes the risk for further respiratory compromise.
5. Provide frequent support and contact with the child and family.	5. Frequent contact and support helps to alleviate anxiety, which increases the child's oxygen demands.

Mycoplasmal Pneumonia

The *Mycoplasma* organisms are similar to, yet larger than, viruses. Mycoplasmal pneumonia occurs more frequently in older children (over 5 years) and more often during the winter months.

The symptoms of a mycoplasmal pneumonia make it difficult to differentiate from other pneumonias. The child has a fever and a cough and feels ill. Cervical lymph nodes will be enlarged. The child may have a persistent rhinitis.

Mycoplasmal organisms generally are sensitive to erythromycin or tetracycline. Erythromycin is the preferred drug for children younger than 8 years of age, because tetracycline tends to stain teeth brown and possibly stunt long bone growth.

Lipid Pneumonia

Lipid pneumonia is caused by the aspiration of oily or lipid substances. It is much less common than it once was, because children are not given castor oil or cod liver oil as they were in the past. Lipid pneumonia may be caused by aspirated oily foreign bodies such as peanuts. A proliferative inflammatory response occurs when lung lipases act on the aspirated oil. This may be followed by diffuse fibrosis of the bronchi or alveoli. The area may become secondarily infected.

A child may have an initial coughing spell at the time of aspiration. A period follows during which the child is symptomless. Then a chronic cough, dyspnea, and general respiratory distress will occur. A chest radiograph will show densities at the affected site.

Antibiotic therapy is ineffective unless a secondary bacterial infection occurs. Surgical resection of a lung portion may be done to remove a lobe or segment if the pneumonitis does not heal by itself.

Hydrocarbon Pneumonia

A number of common household products such as furniture polish, cleaning fluids, turpentine, kerosene, gasoline, lighter fluid, and insect sprays have hydrocarbon bases. These products are a common cause of childhood poisonings and can result in hydrocarbon pneumonia.

Assessment. The child who has swallowed a hydrocarbon-based product usually will exhibit gastrointestinal symptoms such as nausea and vomiting. The child may become drowsy because of inhalation of the vapors of the substance and may develop a cough as vapors from the stomach rise and are inhaled. As bronchial edema occurs from irritation and inflammation, the child's respirations become increased and dyspneic. Physical assessment will show an increased percussion sound caused by the presence of air trapped in the alveoli beyond the point of inflammation. There may be rales as air passes through collected mucus and diminished breath sounds because air does not reach and inflate the alveoli fully.

Therapeutic Management. Hydrocarbon aspiration may occur when children initially swallow the fluid. If they are given an emetic to induce vomiting, they may aspirate at the time of vomiting. This is why vomiting is never induced if a child has swallowed a hydrocarbon. Parents should telephone a poison control center to ask for advice before inducing vomiting if they do not know the substance ingested or are unsure whether it was a hydrocarbon. The poison control center may recommend that the parents administer an oily substance such as olive oil or mineral oil to delay gastric absorption of the substance. Gastric lavage may be done by health care personnel with great care to remove the substance from the stomach.

The child is usually admitted to the hospital for observation. Vital signs and general appearance must be watched carefully for symptoms of increased respiratory tract obstruction. Careful observation for signs of increasing drowsiness or other symptoms of central nervous system involvement is also necessary. Cool, moist air administered by a nebulizer with supplemental oxygen may decrease lung inflammation. If febrile, the child needs an antipyretic. Frequent changes of position will prevent pooling of secretions, which could lead to a secondary infection. Chest physiotherapy will help to move secretions and reduce areas of stasis.

The initial inflammation reaction may lead to such occlusion that emphysema (pocketing of air in alveoli) occurs, causing rupture of the alveoli into the pleural space, with consequent pneumothorax and atelectasis.

Children who swallow a household cleaner or other substance are often aware that they should not have been handling substances kept under the sink. Such children cannot help but interpret the hospitalization, blood drawing, and other uncomfortable procedures as punishments for their action. They may benefit from therapeutic play with puppets or dolls that will help alleviate their guilt and anger at being "punished" so severely; you may see them treating the dolls roughly or poking them with needles.

After the illness, parents should be cautioned to put poisons in a safe place. They need a listening ear so they can explain that they did not mean this to happen and were unaware of the dangers of these everyday household products.

Atelectasis

Atelectasis is the collapse of lung alveoli. It may occur in children as a primary or secondary condition.

Primary Atelectasis

Primary atelectasis occurs in newborns who do not breathe with enough respiratory strength to inflate lung tissue or whose alveoli are so immature or so lacking in surfactant that they cannot expand. This is seen most commonly in immature infants or in infants with central nervous system damage. It may occur if infants have mucus or meconium plugs in the trachea.

When atelectasis occurs, the newborn's respirations become irregular, with nasal flaring and apnea. After a few minutes, a respiratory grunt and cyanosis may occur. The sound of a respiratory grunt is caused by the newborn's glottis closing on expiration. With this, pressure in the respiratory tract becomes increased, forcing more air into the alveoli in an attempt to inflate them. As hypoxemia increases, the infant becomes hypotonic and flaccid. The Apgar score invariably will be low.

As infants cry or are administered oxygen, more alveoli become aerated, and cyanosis may decrease. The cause of the atelectasis must be established so that therapy directed to the specific cause can be initiated.

Secondary Atelectasis

Secondary atelectasis occurs in children when they have a respiratory tract obstruction that prevents air from entering a portion of the alveoli. As the residual air in the alveoli is absorbed, the alveoli will collapse. The causes of obstruction in children include mucus plugs that may occur with chronic respiratory disease and aspiration of foreign objects. In some children, atelectasis occurs because of pressure on lung tissue from outside forces, such as compression from a diaphragmatic hernia, scoliosis, or enlarged lymph nodes (Figure 19-22).

The signs of secondary atelectasis depend on the degree of collapse. Asymmetry of the chest may be noticed. Breath sounds on the affected side will be decreased. If the process is extensive, tachypnea and cyanosis will be present. A chest radiograph will show the collapsed lung (a "white-out").

Children with atelectasis are prone to secondary infection because mucus continues to be secreted. Stasis of body fluid provides a good culture medium for bacteria.

Therapeutic Management

Atelectasis caused by inspiration of a foreign object will not be relieved until the object is removed by bronchoscopy. Atelectasis caused by a mucus plug will resolve as the plug resolves or is moved or expectorated. Children may need assisted ventilation to maintain adequate respiratory function during this time.

Make certain that the chest of a child with atelectasis is kept free from pressure so that lung expansion is as full as possible (to allow as much breathing space as possible). If restraints are being used to keep an infant positioned, make certain that body restraints are not crossing the chest area and interfering with chest expansion. Check clothing to be certain that it is loose and nonbinding. Make certain that children's arms are not positioned across the chest, where their weight could interfere with deep inspiration.

A semi-Fowler's position generally allows for the best lung expansion, because it lowers abdominal contents. The humidity of the child's environment should be increased to prevent further bronchial plugging; suction and chest physiotherapy may be necessary to keep children's respiratory tracts clear and free of mucus. Children need close observation so that increased respirations or cyanosis can be detected. Atelectasis is a serious disorder in children of all ages. It must be considered as a possibility in all children with respiratory distress.

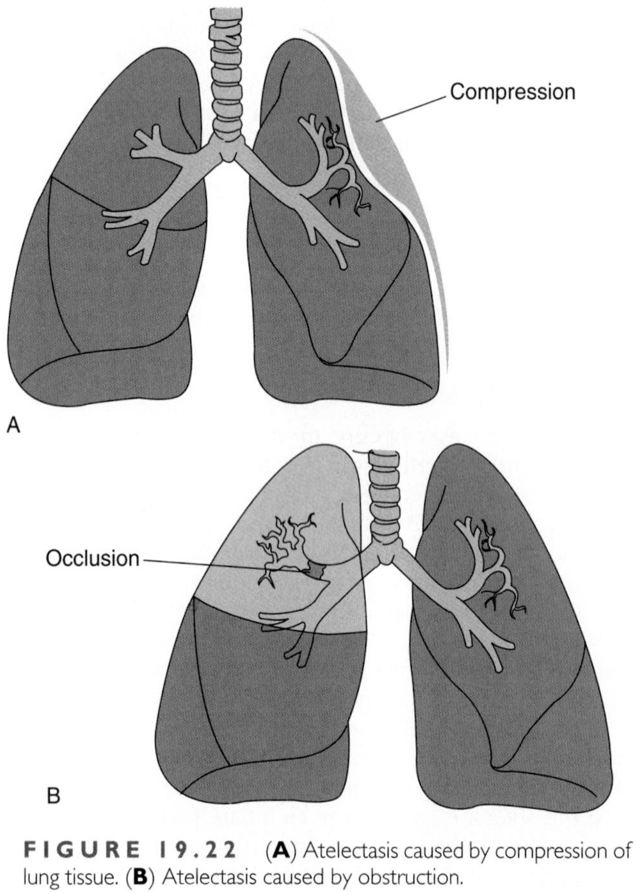

FIGURE 19.22 (**A**) Atelectasis caused by compression of lung tissue. (**B**) Atelectasis caused by obstruction.

Pneumothorax

Pneumothorax is the presence of atmospheric air in the pleural space; its presence causes the alveoli of the lungs to collapse (Alter, 1997; Figure 19-23). Pneumothorax in children usually occurs when air seeps from ruptured alveoli and collects in the pleural cavity. It also can occur when puncture wounds allow air to enter the chest from the outside.

Pneumothorax occurs in approximately 1% of newborns, probably from the extreme intrathoracic pressure needed to initiate the first inspiration. The infant develops tachypnea, grunting respirations, flaring of the nares, and cyanosis. Auscultation will indicate absent or decreased breath sounds on the affected side. Percussion may not be revealing, despite the hollow air space; the sound may be hyperresonant. A more revealing sign may be the shift of the apical pulse (mediastinal shift) away from the site of the pneumothorax and the resulting atelectasis. A chest film will show the darkened area of the air-filled pleural space.

Children need oxygen therapy if they are in respiratory distress. A thoracotomy catheter or needle may be placed in the pleural space and low-pressure suction with water-seal drainage applied to remove accumulated air. In most children with pneumothorax, symptoms are relieved within 24 hours after suction is begun. The use of water-seal drainage with children is discussed in Chapter 20.

If the air in the pleural space is from a puncture wound, the chest wound must be covered immediately by an impervious material, such as petrolatum gauze, to prevent further air from entering. In an emergency, the impervious object can be your gloved hand.

Pneumothorax is always a serious respiratory problem. The extent of the symptoms and the outcome will depend on the cause of entry of air into the pleural space.

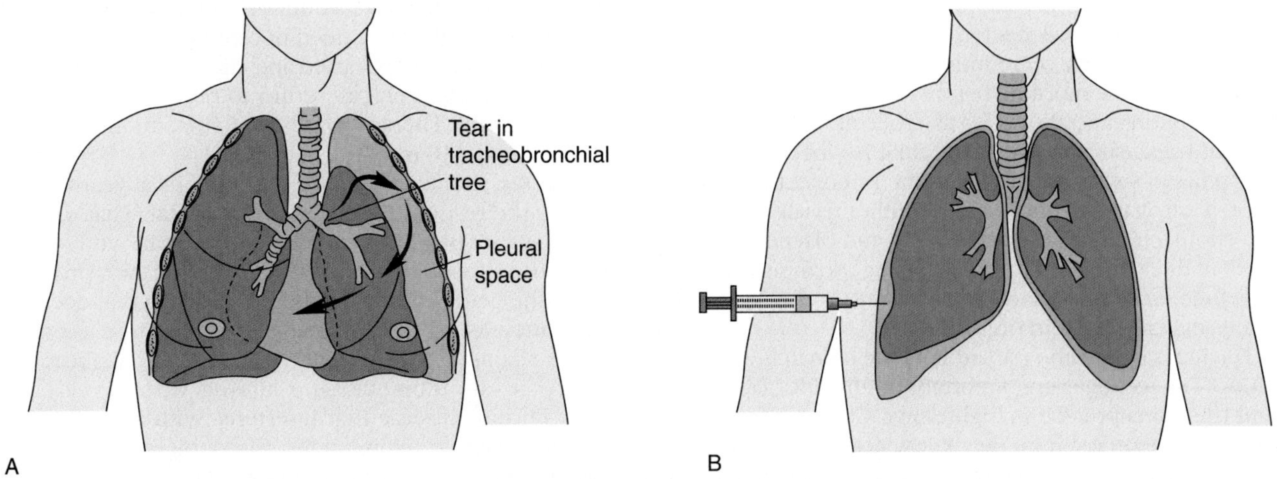

FIGURE 19.23 (**A**) Pneumothorax. A tear in the tracheobronchial tree has caused air to move into the pleural space; the lung collapses and the mediastinum shifts to the unaffected side. (**B**) Aspiration of air from the pleural space allows lung to reexpand after a pneumothorax.

CHECKPOINT QUESTIONS

23. Which children should receive a vaccine to prevent pneumococcal pneumonia?
24. What position is best to aid lung expansion?

Tuberculosis

Tuberculosis is a highly contagious pulmonary disease. The causative agent is *Mycobacterium tuberculosis* (tubercle bacillus). The mode of transmission is inhalation of infected droplets. The incubation period is from 2 to 10 weeks.

Children generally contract this disease from someone in the immediate family. When any member of a family contracts tuberculosis, all family members must be tested (tine or Mantoux) to screen for the disease. In some children, the contact is not known, and the disease is first detected when symptoms appear. Nonwhite children tend to be more susceptible than white children. Children with chronic illness or malnutrition are more susceptible than healthier children because of their overall susceptibility to infection.

When *M. tuberculosis* invades the child's lung, there is primary inflammation. The child develops a slight cough. Leukocytes invade the area and are joined by a formation of new cells, effectively walling off the primary infection. The area calcifies and confines the organism permanently. This development of a primary focus is the most usual form of tuberculosis in children. If a child is in poor health or does not have adequate calcium intake for the body to confine the infection, tuberculosis may spread to other lung areas or to other parts of the body (miliary tuberculosis). As miliary tuberculosis develops, a child develops signs of anorexia, loss of weight, night sweats, and low-grade fever. Other body sites that may be affected are bones and joints, lymph nodes, kidneys, and the subarachnoid space (tuberculosis meningitis).

Assessment

The diagnosis of tuberculosis is suggested by the history of a recent contact. All children should have a tuberculin test as part of basic preventive health care at 9 to 12 months of age, and yearly thereafter if they live in an area in which there is a high risk of tuberculosis. The test should not be done after measles immunization or the test will read false-negative (a child with tuberculosis will be considered free of the disease). Also, the measles vaccine can cause a primary tuberculosis focus to become miliary; thus, it is important to have a negative tuberculin result before administration.

For a tine test, a small, four-pronged applicator, dipped in purified protein derivative (PPD) vaccine, is pressed against the inner aspect of the child's arm so that the prongs break the skin after the skin has been cleansed with acetone or alcohol. A health care professional inspects the area in 72 hours and notes the reaction. A positive reaction (the formation of one or more papules, 2 mm or larger in diameter) indicates that the child has been exposed to tuberculosis (has developed a sensitivity to the foreign products of the tuberculosis organism). Children with positive reactions need follow-up care, such as a chest radiograph, to ascertain the importance of the reaction; that is, whether a current infection exists. Skin testing should not be done on children who are known to have had tuberculosis. Such a child will have such an intense reaction that the skin at the site of the test may slough off and necrose. A more definitive skin test is a Mantoux test, in which PPD vaccine is injected directly into the dermis layer of skin. The reaction is read in the same way as a tine test.

As a second diagnostic procedure, sputum may be analyzed. Make certain that children understand that you want them to expectorate mucus raised from the lungs, not just from the back of the throat. Have the child demonstrate a deep cough to you, so that you can be sure you are both talking about the same thing. Infants and young children do not raise sputum but swallow it. In children younger than 9 or 10 years of age, therefore, gastric lavage is necessary to obtain the sputum specimen (because tuberculosis bacteria are acid-fast they are not destroyed by gastric secretions). Gastric lavage should be done early in the morning before the child eats. This prevents vomiting and allows for the collection of large numbers of organisms, because the child has been coughing sputum and swallowing it all night. To collect the specimen, a nasogastric tube is passed either nasally or orally. The stomach contents are aspirated and placed in a sterile container for laboratory processing. Analysis is generally done for 3 consecutive days, because individual specimens may not contain organisms.

Having a large tube passed into the stomach is frightening. The feeling is uncomfortable—choking, gagging—and the concept itself is frightening. Children need support from people whom they know and trust. They need time to express their feelings about the procedure. They may enjoy playing with a plastic catheter and a doll into which a tube can be inserted. It is revealing to see the force and the anger they use to insert the tube into the doll. This indicates how they envision the procedure being done to them.

In the early course of the disease, because the initial focus of the tuberculosis is so small, it may not be evident on a chest radiograph. As local inflammation occurs, however, a cloudiness in the inflamed area will be noticeable on the film, as will calcification as it occurs.

Parents are concerned when their child is diagnosed as having tuberculosis. Before drug therapy was available, a diagnosis of tuberculosis meant a long-term hospital stay of approximately a year. Parents who believe that tuberculosis is still treated this way will need assurance that it is all right for their child to return home and for him or her to attend regular school.

Therapeutic Management

The treatment of tuberculosis is based on the administration of a combination of specific antituberculin drugs. More resistant strains of the disease are making these drugs less effective (Starke, 1997). Para-aminosalicylic acid (PAS) is bacteriostatic to *M. tuberculosis* and for a long time served as the mainstay of therapy. PAS administration may lead to such gastrointestinal disturbances in children that it is not used as much as in the past. If it is prescribed, it should be administered after meals and never on an empty stomach. Isoniazid (INH) is now the drug of choice for therapy. INH may lead to peripheral neurologic symptoms if pyridoxine (vitamin B_6) is not administered concurrently. Rifampin is often used in combination with INH.

Ethambutol is used with older children (Trebucq, 1997). It is used with caution with infants because one side effect is optic neuritis; inability to do adequate eye examinations in children under school age to discover this side effect can make ethambutol unsafe for long-term use. In addition to drug therapy, children should receive a diet high in protein, calcium, and pyridoxine, especially if INH is used as therapy, to effectively wall off organisms in lung tissue.

Children who have primary tuberculosis are not infectious, because they have a minimal pulmonary lesion and little or no cough. They need not be isolated. As soon as drug therapy has been started and clinical symptoms have disappeared, children can return to regular activities, including school. Therapy may have to be continued, however, for up to 18 months.

Children should have chest radiographs at yearly intervals for the rest of their life to make certain that the disease does not become active later. A woman who had tuberculosis as a child must tell her primary care provider when she becomes pregnant; lung changes that occur in pregnancy as a result of the pressure of the growing uterus against the lungs can break down calcifications and reactivate tuberculosis. Children who develop another chronic disease that interferes with appetite and, therefore, with calcium intake have a high risk of reactivation of calcium-contained tuberculosis.

Because children will be taking medicine for a long time, they need periodic health care facility visits to evaluate the extent of drug compliance. They must receive regular childhood immunizations so that they do not contract a second disease until they have fully recovered from tuberculosis. It is most important that pertussis (whooping cough) be prevented, because the paroxysmal cough caused by this illness could break and reactivate tuberculosis lesions.

The bacilli Calmette-Guérin (BCG) vaccine is available against tuberculosis, but it is not used routinely with children. A skin test will be strongly positive after effective BCG vaccination. For this reason, most people advocate placing children on prophylactic INH when there is known tuberculosis in the home rather than vaccinating them against tuberculosis. As long as a repeat tine test remains negative, you know that they are disease free. After BCG vaccine, the value of skin testing is lost.

Cystic Fibrosis

Cystic fibrosis (CF) is a disease in which there is generalized dysfunction of the exocrine glands. Mucus secretions of the body, particularly in the pancreas and the lungs, have difficulty flowing through gland ducts. There is also a marked electrolyte change in the secretions of the sweat glands (chloride concentration of sweat is two to five times above normal). The cause of the disorder is an abnormality of the long arm of chromosome 7. This results in the inability to transport small molecules across cell membranes; this leads to dehydration of epithelial cells in the airway and pancreas (Rosenstein, 1997).

The disorder is inherited as an autosomal recessive trait. It occurs in approximately 1 in 2500 live births. It occurs most commonly in whites, rarely in blacks and Asians. Although the disease is fatal in early life, as many as 50% of children now live to be past 28 years of age. With the availability of lung transplants, full life expectancy has increased. Because the gene that causes the disorder can be isolated, chorionic villi sampling or amniocentesis can be done early in pregnancy to detect fetuses who have the disease. In the future, gene therapy will reverse the effect of the involved gene (Bellon, 1997).

Boys with CF may not be able to reproduce, because they have tenacious plugging and blocking of the vas deferens from tenacious seminal fluid. Girls may have such thick cervical secretions that sperm penetration is limited. Artificial insemination or in vitro fertilization can be accomplished if they desire to become pregnant.

Pancreas Involvement

The acinar cells of the pancreas normally produce lipase, trypsin, and amylase, enzymes that flow into the duodenum to digest fat, protein, and carbohydrate. With CF, these enzyme secretions become so tenacious that they plug the ducts; eventually, there is such back pressure on the acinar cells that they become atrophied and are then no longer capable of producing the enzymes. The islets of Langerhans and insulin production are little influenced by this process until late in the disease because they have endocrine activity (they are ductless cells).

Without pancreatic enzymes in the duodenum, children are unable to digest fat, protein, and some sugars. The child's stools will be large, bulky, and greasy (**steatorrhea**). The intestinal flora increases because of the undigested food and, when combined with the fat in the stool, gives the stool an extremely foul odor often compared with that of a cat's stool. The bulk of feces in the intestine leads to a protuberant abdomen. Because children are benefiting from only about 50% of the food they ingest, they show signs of malnutrition—emaciated extremities and loose, flabby folds of skin on their buttocks. The fat-soluble vitamins, particularly A, D, and E, cannot be absorbed because fat is not absorbed, so children develop symptoms of low levels of these vitamins. These four symptoms—malnutrition, protuberant abdomen, steatorrhea, and fat-soluble vitamin deficiencies—are the same four symptoms that are part of celiac disease (malabsorption syndrome), so they are referred to as the *celiac syndrome* (see Chapter 24).

The meconium in a newborn is normally thick and tenacious. In approximately 10% of children with CF, it may be so thick, because pancreatic enzymes are lacking, that it obstructs the intestine (meconium ileus). The newborn will develop abdominal distention with no passage of stool. Meconium ileus should be suspected in any infant who does not pass a stool by 24 hours of life. Rectal prolapse from straining to evacuate hard stool is another common finding in infants.

Lung Involvement

Pockets of infection begin in pooled thick secretions of the bronchial tree, which obstruct the bronchioles. The organisms most frequently cultured from lung secretions in children with CF are *Staphylococcus aureus, Pseudomonas aeruginosa,* and *H. influenzae.* Secondary emphysema (overinflated alveoli) occurs because the air cannot be pushed past the thick mucus on expiration, when all bronchi are narrower than they are on inspiration. Bronchiectasis and pneumonia occur. Atelectasis occurs as a result of complete absorption of air from alveoli behind blocked bronchioles. Children's fingers become clubbed because of the inadequate peripheral tissue perfusion. Children's chests become distended in the anteroposterior diameter. Respiratory acidosis may develop because obstruction interferes with the ability to adequately exhale carbon dioxide.

Sweat Gland Involvement

Although the sweat glands themselves do not appear to change in structure, the electrolyte composition of perspiration does change. In children with CF, the level of chloride to sodium is increased two to five times above normal. Some parents report that they knew their newborn had the disease before they had laboratory tests done, because when they kissed their child they could taste such strong salt in the perspiration.

Assessment

CF is diagnosed by the history, the abnormal concentration of chloride in sweat, the absence of pancreatic enzymes in the duodenum, and pulmonary involvement.

The newborn with CF loses the normal amount of weight at birth (5% to 10% of birth weight), but then does not gain it back at the usual time of 7 to 10 days and perhaps not until 4 to 6 weeks of age. Failure to regain birth weight as a newborn is a significant sign, which nurses, who often weigh babies, may be the first to detect. As mentioned, at birth, meconium may be so tenacious that the baby has intestinal obstruction (meconium ileus) and so is unable to pass stool. All babies with meconium ileus should be tested for CF. This can be done by analysis of serum immunoreactive trypsin (IRT), which is elevated in newborns with the disease because of obstruction in the pancreas as early as during fetal life.

Children may be seen in a health care setting at about 1 month of age because of a feeding problem. Using only about 50% of their intake because of their poor digestive function, they are always hungry. This causes them to eat so ravenously that they tend to swallow air. This is manifested as colic or abdominal distention and vomiting. Stools are large, bulky, and greasy and may be loose and frequent. The appearance of the stools is an important finding because children with simple colic do not show changes in stool consistency this way.

Children may be seen by health care providers between 4 and 6 months of age because of frequent respiratory infections, a chronic cough, and failure to gain weight. On auscultation of the chest, wheezing and rhonchi may be heard.

By the time the child with CF is a preschooler, a cough is a prominent finding. On percussion, the chest will be hyperresonant, reflecting the emphysema present. Rales and rhonchi will be heard. Clubbing of the fingers may already be apparent. It is rare for a child to go undiagnosed beyond this time because the symptoms of the illness have become so persistent and evident.

Sweat Testing. A sweat test is a test for the chloride content of sweat. Infants may not be tested until 6 to 8 weeks of age because newborns do not sweat a great deal, and interpretation of the test may not be accurate. With newer testing procedures, however, sweat testing can be done even in newborns.

For a sweat test, pilocarpine (a cholinergic drug that stimulates sweat gland activity) is dropped onto a gauze square. This is placed on the child's forearm, and copper electrodes are connected to it. A small electrical current is then applied to carry the pilocarpine into the skin. Because the electrical current is of such low intensity, it should be painless. After the application of the electrical current, the area on the arm is washed with water and dried, and a filter paper is applied to collect the sweat that forms. The filter paper must be lifted by forceps rather than touched by the examiner's fingers, because the sweat from the examiner's skin could transfer to the paper and make the test analysis inaccurate.

A normal concentration of chloride in sweat is 20 mEq/L. A level of more than 60 mEq/L chloride in children is diagnostic of CF. Values between 50 and 60 mEq/L are suggestive of the disease and call for a repeat of the test.

Duodenal Analysis. Analysis of duodenal secretions for detection of pancreatic enzymes is done by passing a nasogastric tube into the duodenum and then aspirating secretions for analysis. This test may take a considerable amount of time because the tube is allowed to pass through the pylorus and into the duodenum by natural peristaltic action. You can tell a tube has passed from the stomach into the duodenum by aspirating secretions from the tube and testing them for pH. Stomach secretions are acid (less than 7.0); duodenal secretions are alkaline (more than 7.0). The initial insertion of the tube typically is frightening to children because they may choke and gag as it passes the pharynx. Children, however, are generally surprised that once the initial insertion is done, the tube usually is not too uncomfortable. They need a great deal of support during the procedure, however, because it is so unusual for them and initially so uncomfortable.

The secretions removed from the duodenum are sent to the laboratory for analysis of trypsin content, the easiest pancreatic enzyme to assay. Keep the secretions cold during transport. They should be analyzed immediately for accurate results.

Stool Analysis. Stool may be analyzed for fat content, although description of the large greasy appearance may be all that is necessary.

Pulmonary Testing. A chest radiograph will generally confirm the pulmonary involvement (pockets of emphysema and perhaps beginning pneumonia infiltration). Pulmonary function tests may be done to determine the extent of the lung involvement.

Therapeutic Management

Therapy for children with CF consists of measures to reduce the involvement of the pancreas, lungs, and sweat glands.

NURSING DIAGNOSES AND RELATED INTERVENTIONS

Nursing Diagnosis: Altered nutrition, less than body requirements, related to inability to digest fat

Outcome Identification: Child will absorb an adequate nutritional amount daily.

Outcome Evaluation: Child's height and weight follow percentile growth curves, quantity of stool decreases.

Children with CF are placed on a high-calorie, high-protein, moderate-fat diet. Water-miscible forms of vitamins A, D, and E are supplemented. During the hot months of the year, extra salt may be added to food to replace that which may be lost though perspiration. Medium-chain triglycerides are used with the diet because these are more readily digested than other oils.

Infants with CF are generally not totally breastfed because there is not enough protein in breast milk for them (they need large amounts because they cannot make use of all the protein they ingest). Breastfeeding with supplementary formula is required. Some of these children, unfortunately, are initially diagnosed as having a milk allergy and are treated by being placed on a soybean formula. This does not contain enough protein either, and their malnutrition increases greatly while they are taking this formula. A high-protein formula, such as Probana, is generally the formula that should be recommended.

Children with CF have a ravenous appetite and eat well. Before each meal or snack, they need to take a synthetic pancreatic enzyme, pancreatic lipase (Cotazym or Pancrease) to replace the enzyme they cannot produce (see Drug Highlight). These synthetic enzymes are supplied in large capsules that must be opened for young children because they cannot swallow such a big capsule, and infants, in particular, may not have enough gastric acids to dissolve the capsule. The powder from the capsule is then added to a small amount (no more than a teaspoonful) of food. It should not be added to hot food or a large portion of enzyme activity will be destroyed. Also, it must not be added to the infant's bottle of formula, because the infant may not drink the entire bottle and therefore will not receive the total benefit of the enzymes. When children are taking a synthetic source of pancreatic

DRUG HIGHLIGHT

Pancrelipase (Cotazym)

Action: Pancrelipase is an enzyme replacement used for children with cystic fibrosis

Pregnancy risk category: C

Dosage: 2000 U orally per meal (children 6 months to 1 year of age); 4000 to 8000 U orally with each meal and 4000 U with snacks (children 1 to 6 years of age); 4000 to 12,000 U orally with each meal and with snacks.

Possible adverse effects: Nausea, abdominal cramps, diarrhea, hypersensitivity

Nursing Implications:

- Administer the drug before or with meals and snacks. Instruct parents and child in the same.
- Caution child and parents to avoid inhaling powder or spilling it on the hands because it may irritate the skin or mucous membranes.
- Do not crush or let the child chew the enteric form of the drug.
- Instruct the child and parents about possible adverse effects and encourage them to contact the health care provider should any become severe.

enzymes this way, the size of stools and the accompanying foul odor decreases. Children begin to gain weight. In adolescence, children may have a great deal of difficulty eating enough to maintain weight even with enzyme therapy, because their growth spurt requires so many additional calories.

If a child with CF becomes overheated, the child will begin to lose excessive sodium and chloride through perspiration and become dehydrated. Caution parents to keep the room temperature at 72°F or below; and to offer water frequently. Supervise outside play to guard against overexertion or heat exposure.

Nursing Diagnosis: Ineffective airway clearance related to inability to clear mucus from tract

Outcome Identification: Child's airway will remain patent during course of illness.

Outcome Evaluation: Child's temperature is below 38.0°C; PaO_2 is 80 to 90 mm Hg; $PaCO_2$ is 40 mm Hg.

Unfortunately, the pulmonary effects of CF progress despite supplementation with pancreatic enzymes; infection from plugged airways is always a possibility. Therefore, it is important to try to keep bronchial secretions as moist as possible so they can drain from the bronchial tree. This is done by frequent nebulization or aerosol therapy followed by chest physiotherapy.

Moistened Oxygen. Oxygen is supplied to children by mask, prongs, ventilators, or nebulizers and rarely by tent. Mist can be supplied by an ultrasonic compressor and delivered through a nebulizer mask, which makes droplet size so small that the mist reaches the smallest bronchial spaces.

Provide Aerosol Therapy. Three or four times a day, children may be given aerosol therapy by means of a nebulizer to provide antibiotics or bronchodilators. Antibiotics are specifically determined by culture. A mucolytic, such as acetylcysteine (Mucomyst), can be added to the mist to aid in diluting and liquefying secretions. Children's coughs will become loose and productive after they have used aerosol therapy. Provide a box of tissues for them so they can cough up these loose secretions. Observe them to ensure that they are able to cough and keep their airway clear. Never give cough syrups to suppress their cough, because getting secretions out is essential to air exchange. Likewise, they should never receive codeine as an analgesic, because codeine suppresses the cough reflex.

Chest Physiotherapy. Because the bronchial secretions with CF are so tenacious, even with liquefaction by mist or aerosol therapy, children may be unable to raise them. To aid drainage of secretions, children need chest physiotherapy frequently, approximately three to four times a day.

Activity. Children with CF need frequent position changes if they are in bed so that, at various times of the day, all lobes of their lungs will be encouraged to drain by being in a superior position. Therefore, they should alternately lie on either side, on their abdomen, and on their back. They should sit up part of the day to drain the upper lobes. This change in position also helps to prevent skin breakdown over bony prominences, and it helps to aerate their lungs by furnishing some activity for them.

Frequent Observations. Children with CF require frequent observation because their condition can change rapidly. If a portion of a lung becomes obstructed from a plug of mucus, they may quickly be in respiratory difficulty. Also, the right side of the heart enlarges in children with chronic respiratory disease because the congestion in the lungs increases pressure in the pulmonary artery. After a period of stress or exercise, children may begin to show signs of cardiac failure.

Respiratory Hygiene. The sputum that a child coughs up may have a disagreeable taste or odor. The child needs frequent mouth care, toothbrushing, and a good-tasting mouthwash to make his or her mouth feel fresh.

Adequate Rest and Comfort. Any child who has compromised lung function has a degree of dyspnea that leads to exhaustion. Children need periods of rest during the day rather than being disturbed every few minutes. At the same time, they must not have too many procedures done all at once. Many procedures done one right after another will exhaust them. Allow for a rest period before meals so that they are not too tired to eat. They may need a long rest period before CPT so that they may be able to tolerate it better. Achieving a balance between allowing periods of rest and yet not doing all procedures at once is not an easy task.

Growth and Development. Children need to be exposed to as many normal life experiences as possible. It may be necessary to spend significant time with parents before they are able to do this if the child tires easily.

Nursing Diagnosis: Risk for altered skin integrity related to acid stools

Outcome Identification: Child's skin will remain intact during course of illness.

Outcome Evaluation: Child does not have areas of erythema or ulceration; rectal prolapse is not present.

Children who are not toilet-trained need to have their diapers changed immediately after they wet or pass stool so that they do not develop skin irritation and breakdown in the diaper area. Until children are regulated on pancreatic enzymes, the stool is particularly irritating because of its high fat content.

After a bowel movement, check the child's rectum for rectal prolapse. Because of weak musculature of the rectal area, this is a common complication. A prolapse of rectal mucosa appears as a bright red mass protruding from the anal sphincter. This mucosa must be replaced promptly before its blood supply is compromised. Place the child on the slant board used for chest physiotherapy in a position with the head lower than the buttocks; then, with a lubricated, gloved hand, gently replace the prolapsed rectal mass. Afterward, compress the buttocks together to maintain gentle pressure on the anus for a few minutes. This is much less of a problem in children who are receiving pancreatic enzymes than in those who are not, because the incidence of rectal prolapse decreases with better nutrition.

Nursing Diagnosis: Risk for ineffective family coping, compromised, related to chronic illness in a child

Outcome Identification: Family members demonstrate an adequate level of coping ability during course of illness.

Outcome Evaluation: Family members state they have adequate resources to cope with current circumstances.

The parents of these children are asked to assume a great deal of responsibility for care of their child. Discharge planning begins when a child is first admitted to a hospital in terms of what changes need to be made at home to accommodate the child's homecoming and to familiarize parents with the necessary care measures. For example, many children with this disorder sleep with oxygen by cannula at night when they are at home. Thus, parents will need to be taught the functions of oxygen and how to regulate the flow. The program is most effective if a little is taught every day (for example, "Could you turn the oxygen on for me, Mrs. Smith? I'm ready to tuck Brian in to sleep" rather than a sit-down, let-me-tell-you-how-oxygen-works lecture given close to the day of discharge). Teach parents how to do CPT the same way.

The family will have to think through how the care of this child will affect their home life (see Focus on Nursing Research). They are going to be spending a great deal of time caring for the child. The parents need to balance work, care of the child, and care of the rest of the family.

FOCUS ON NURSING RESEARCH

How Well Do the Parents of Children With Cystic Fibrosis Manage With the Stress of This Illness?

Fifty mothers and 44 well siblings of children or adolescents with cystic fibrosis participated in this study to identify how well mothers of children with cystic fibrosis felt about themselves and what factors led to well-being. Participants completed mailed questionnaires that assessed maternal well-being, problems experienced during the illness and treatment, and the nature of the sibling relationship. It was anticipated that mothers of children with cystic fibrosis would experience higher levels of stress and consequent poorer well-being than the normal population. Findings showed, however, that these mothers, as a group, did not rate themselves as experiencing more stress than those in the general population. This is an important study because it points out the enormous ability of parents to adjust to chronic stress. It stresses the importance of teaching them not only how to manage techniques of their child's illness, but also how to manage the long-term stress of chronic illness.

Foster, C. L., Byron, M. & Eiser, C. (1998). Correlates of well-being in mothers of children and adolescents with cystic fibrosis. *Child Care, Health & Development, 24*(1), 41–56.

Many parents become fatigued after the first week of having the child at home, because they are afraid to fall soundly asleep at night for fear of not hearing the child call if he or she should be in distress. As they grow more confident in their ability to evaluate the child's condition before bedtime, the apprehension will lessen, but real confidence may not come for months, even years. This may always be a problem for some parents.

Parents need the telephone number of the health care provider they should call when the pressure they are under is more than they can bear. Encourage parents to join a support group, so that there are other understanding people available to whom they can voice their concerns. At these times, one of the most important needs they have is to verbalize to someone what it feels like to be the parent of a child with CF.

Children need to attend regular school if at all possible. If not, a home tutor should be provided for them. They should participate to the extent that they can in physical fitness activities in school. Also, they must remember to take pancreatic enzyme with them if they are going to be eating lunch in the school cafeteria. Instruction for health maintenance and illness prevention measures, such as proper clothing and hygiene, need to be stressed with the child and parents and those involved with the child, such as teachers.

Children with CF need periodic health assessment the same as all children so that routine childhood immunizations can be given. It is not unusual for children with a chronic disease to fall behind in immunizations because they are hospitalized at the times these are routinely given. It is particularly important that these children be given pertussis and measles vaccine, because these two infections cause severe respiratory complications. Children also generally receive influenza, meningococcal, and pneumococcal vaccines to try to prevent them from contracting these illnesses. When death occurs, it is usually from a combination of infection and cor pulmonale. If there are other children in the family with CF (not an uncommon occurrence), parents need a great deal of support if the first child should die. Supporting parents after a child dies is discussed in Chapter 35. Family members may wish to have genetic testing done to see whether they are carriers of the disease.

✔ CHECKPOINT QUESTIONS

25. What term is used to describe tuberculosis that has spread to other parts of the body?
26. What result of a sweat test would be diagnostic for CF?

KEY POINTS

Respiratory tract disorders tend to occur more frequently in children than adults, because the lumens of bronchi are narrow and obstruction can occur more easily.

Infants with respiratory illness need extremely close observation, because they cannot describe oxygen hunger. Young children do not appreciate the fact that oxygen supports combustion. They need more observation than adults do to be certain that no flames, such as birthday candles, are brought within 10 ft of an oxygen source.

Acute nasopharyngitis (common cold) is the most frequently seen infectious disease in children. There is no specific therapy for a cold other than comfort measures.

Tonsillitis is infection and inflammation of the palatine tonsils. Adenitis is infection and inflammation of the adenoid tonsils. Children with recurring infections may have tonsils surgically removed.

Laryngotracheobronchitis (croup) is inflammation of the larynx, trachea, and major bronchi. Epiglottitis is inflammation of the epiglottis. Both of these conditions can cause severe impairment of the airway. Children with epiglottitis should never be gagged with a tongue blade or the elevated epiglottis can completely occlude the airway.

Bronchitis is inflammation of the major bronchi and trachea. Bronchiolitis is inflammation of the fine bronchioles.

Respiratory syncytial virus infection is an infection that accounts for the majority of lower respiratory infection in young children. Infants with RSV infections must be observed closely because they are prone to apnea.

Asthma, a type I hypersensitivity reaction, is a diffuse and obstructive airway disease. The major symptom is wheezing.

Pneumonia may occur from a variety of organisms (viral, pneumococcal, chlamydial, mycoplasmal, lipid, and hydrocarbon). Unless viral, children need specific antibiotics depending on the organism present.

Tuberculosis is a lung infection that is growing in incidence, with some strains becoming very resistant to the usual therapy.

Cystic fibrosis is a disease in which there is generalized dysfunction of the exocrine glands. This results in malabsorption and tenacious pulmonary secretions.

CRITICAL THINKING EXERCISES

1. Michael is the 5-year-old you met at the beginning of the chapter. His nanny brought him to the emergency room because his respirations were rapid and he was wheezing. He is diagnosed as having asthma. Both he and his nanny shouted instructions at you. What about Michael's actions would lead you to believe his airway is not yet extremely constricted? Would you encourage him to lie down and rest? What emergency care does Michael need?
2. A 3-year-old has a permanent tracheostomy tube in place. Her parents are going to enroll her in a preschool center. What precautions would you want to review with the parents to keep this experience safe?
3. A 10-year-old has just returned from tonsillectomy surgery. What observations would be most important to make? Why is the 7th day after tonsillectomy surgery a particularly important day?
4. The parents of a 16-year-old with CF want to take her on an extended vacation in the Caribbean next summer. What anticipatory guidance would you give the adolescent and her parents?

REFERENCES

Alter, S.J. (1997). Spontaneous pneumothorax in infants: A 10-year review. *Pediatric Emergency Care, 13*(6), 401.

American Heart Association. (1992). Pediatric basic life support. *Journal of the American Medical Association, 258*(11), 2251.

Bellon, G. (1997). Cystic fibrosis (CF) gene therapy. *Pediatric Pulmonology, 16*, 278.

Boyer, K.M. (1997). Nonbacterial pneumonia. In Johnston, K.B. & Oski, F.A. *Oski's essential pediatrics*. Philadelphia: Lippincott.

Carpenito, L. (1997). *Nursing diagnosis: application to clinical practice*. Philadelphia: J.B. Lippincott.

Cataneo, A.J. et al. (1997). Foreign body in the tracheobronchial tree. *Clinical Pediatrics, 36*(12), 701.

Coakley-Maller, C. & Shea, M. (1997). Respiratory infections in children: preparing for the fall and winter. *Advances for Nurse Practitioners, 5*(9), 2027.

Conlon, B.J. et al. (1997). Improvements in health and behavior following childhood tonsillectomy: a parental perspective at 1 year. *International Journal of Pediatric Otorhinolaryngology, 4*(2), 155.

Darville, T. & Yamauchi, T. (1998). Respiratory syncytial virus. *Pediatrics in Review, 19*(2), 55.

Department of Health and Human Services. (1995). *Healthy people 2000: midcourse review*. Washington, D.C.: DHHS.

Fehrenbach, C. (1997). New thinking on childhood asthma. *Community Nurse, 3*(3), 20.

Folland, D.S. (1997). Treatment of croup: sending home an improved child and relieved parents. *Postgraduate Medicine, 101*(3), 271.

Foster, C.L., Bryon, M., & Eiser, C. (1998). Correlates of well-being in mothers of children and adolescents with cystic fibrosis. *Child Care, Health and Development, 24*(1), 41.

Frakes, M.A. (1997). Asthma in the emergency department. *Journal of Emergency Nursing, 23*(5), 429.

Gazarian, P.K. (1997). Teaching your patient to use a metered-dose inhaler: the direct route for asthma therapy. *Nursing 27*(10), 52.

Gerber, M.A. (1997). Use of antigen detection tests in the diagnosis and management of patients with group A streptococcal pharyngitis. *Pediatric Infectious Disease Journal, 16*(12), 1187.

Gray, R.F., Todd, N.W., & Jacobs, I.N. (1998). Tracheostomy decannulation in children: approaches and techniques. *Laryngoscope, 108*(1.1), 8.

Horner, S.D. (1997). Uncertainty in mother's care for their ill children. *Journal of Advanced Nursing, 26*(4), 658.

Jeng, M.J. & Lemen, R.J. (1997). Respiratory syncytial virus bronchiolitis. *American Family Physician, 55*(4), 1139.

Johnston, S.L. (1997). Influence of viral and bacterial respiratory infections on exacerbations and symptom severity in childhood asthma. *Pediatric Pulmonology, 16*, 88.

Larroquet, M. et al. (1997). Video-assisted thoracoscopic surgery for bronchiectasis. *Pediatric Pulmonology, 16*, 180.

Madden, V. (1997). Croup. *Professional Care of Mother and Child, 7*(4), 93.

Mangione, R.A. (1997). Selected pediatric emergencies in community practice. *Journal of the American Pharmaceutical Association, 37*(1), 22.

Maurer, J.R. & Chaparro, C. (1995). Lung transplantation in cystic fibrosis. *Current Opinion in Pulmonary Medicine, 1*(6), 465.

Modlin, J.F. (1997). Bacterial pneumonia. In Johnston, K.B. & Oski, F.A. *Oski's essential pediatrics*. Philadelphia: J.B. Lippincott.

National Asthma Education and Prevention Program. (1997). *Expert panel report II: guidelines for the diagnosis and management of asthma*. Washington, DC: DHHS.

Rencken, I., Patton, W.L., & Brasch, R.C. (1998). Airway obstruction in pediatric patients. *Radiologic Clinics of North America, 36*(1), 175.

Rosenstein, B.J. (1997). Cystic fibrosis. In Johnston, K.B. & Oski, F.A. *Oski's Essential Pediatrics*. Philadelphia: J.B. Lippincott.

Starke, J.R. (1997). Drug-resistance in tuberculosis: mechanisms and prevention. *Pediatric Pulmonology, 16*, 154.

Trebucq, A. (1997). Should ethambutol be recommended for routine treatment of tuberculosis in children? *International Journal of Tuberculosis Lung Disease, 1*(1), 12.

Watkins, V.S. et al. (1997). Comparison of dirithromycin and penicillin for treatment of streptococcal pharyngitis. *Antimicrobial Agents and Chemotherapy, 41*(1), 72.

SUGGESTED READINGS

Agasthian, T. et al. (1996). Surgical management of bronchiectasis. *Annals of Thoracic Surgery, 62*(4), 976.

Bone, R. (1996). Goals of asthma management: a step care approach. *Chest 109*(6), 1056.

Chiocca, E.M. (1996). Actionstat: epiglottitis. *Nursing, 26*(9), 25.

Geelhoed, G.C. (1997). Croup. *Pediatric Pulmonology, 23*(5), 370.

Lask, B. (1997). Understanding and managing poor adherence in cystic fibrosis. *Pediatric Pulmonology, 16*, 260.

Marrie, T. J. (1998). Epidemiology of mild pneumonia. *Seminars in Respiratory Infections, 13*(1), 3.

Meyer, S.B. et al. (1996). Postoperative care of the lung transplant recipient. *Critical Care Nursing Clinics of North America, 8*(3), 239.

Pichichero, M.E. (1997). Sore throat after sore throat after sore throat: Are you asking the critical questions? *Postgraduate Medicine, 101*(1), 205.

Toder, D.S. & McBride, J.T. (1997). Home care of children dependent on respiratory technology. *Pediatrics in Review, 18*(8), 273.

Uba, A. (1996). Infraglottic and bronchial infections. *Primary Care, 23*(4), 759.

Wright, C. (1997). Improving asthma care. *Community Nurse, 3*(3), 6.

Nursing Care of the Child With a Cardiovascular Disorder

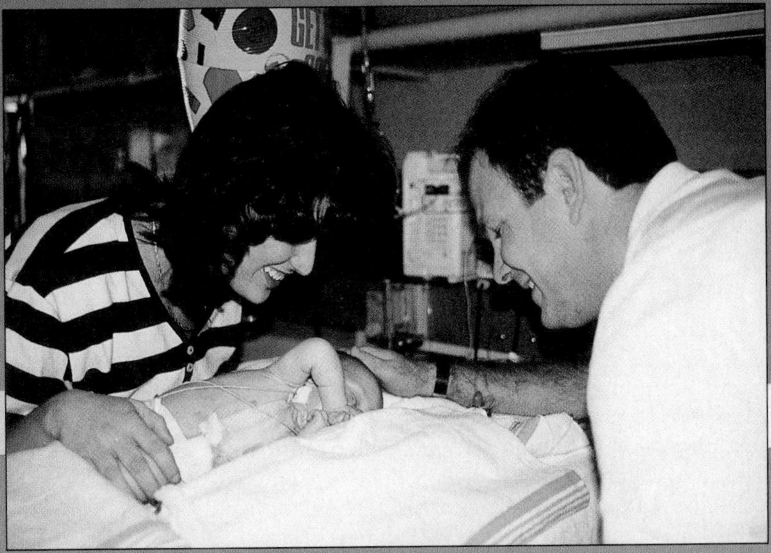

20

CHAPTER

Key Terms

- acyanotic heart disease
- afterload
- balloon angioplasty
- cardiac catheterization
- contractility
- cyanosis
- cyanotic heart disease
- diastole
- echocardiography
- electrocardiogram
- fluoroscopy
- heart failure
- hypertension
- innocent heart murmur
- left-to-right shunt
- organic heart murmur
- phonocardiography
- polycythemia
- postcardiac surgery syndrome
- postperfusion syndrome
- preload
- right-to-left shunt
- systole
- vasculitis

Objectives

After mastering the contents of this chapter, you should be able to:

1. Describe the common cardiovascular disorders of childhood.
2. Assess a child with cardiovascular dysfunction.
3. Formulate nursing diagnoses for the child with a cardiovascular disorder.
4. Establish appropriate outcomes based on the priority needs of the child with a cardiovascular disorder.
5. Plan nursing care for the child with a cardiovascular disorder.
6. Implement nursing care for the child with a cardiovascular disorder.
7. Evaluate outcomes for achievement and effectiveness of care.
8. Identify National Health Goals related to cardiovascular disorders and children that nurses could be instrumental in helping the nation achieve.
9. Identify areas related to the care of children with cardiovascular problems that could benefit from additional nursing research.
10. Use critical thinking to analyze ways that nursing care of children with cardiovascular disorders could be more family centered.
11. Integrate knowledge of cardiovascular disorders with nursing process to achieve quality child health nursing care.

Megan is a newborn who was born with tetralogy of Fallot. By 1 hour of age, she developed rapid respirations, tachycardia, and became cyanotic. An echocardiogram revealed the typical four structural defects of the syndrome. Megan's parents will be taking her home for a month to await for cardiac surgery. They tell you their doctor told them to "watch her carefully" during that time. "What does that mean?" they ask you. Will they be able to take her outside in a stroller? Exactly what should they watch for? What advice would you give them?

In previous chapters, you learned about the well child. In this chapter, you'll add information about the child who is ill with heart disease and the stress such a serious diagnosis places on a family. This is important information because it builds a base for care and health teaching for children with these disorders.

After you've studied the chapter, turn to the Critical Thinking Exercises at the end of the chapter to sharpen your skills and test your knowledge.

The cardiovascular system, the body system on which all other systems depend, consists of the heart, which acts as a reliable pump; the blood, which provides the fluid for transport; and the blood vessels. Through the regular pumping of the heart, oxygen and needed nutrients are delivered to cells and tissue waste products are removed from cells throughout the body. The cardiovascular system also transports regulatory materials such as hormones, enzymes, and antibodies to the body systems. It can adapt to changes in the body by adjusting the rate and force of heart pumping, changing the size of the blood vessels, and altering the volume and composition of the blood.

Most cardiovascular disorders in children occur as a result of a congenital anomaly; either the heart has developed inadequately in utero or the system is unable to adapt to extrauterine life. Open heart surgery is often the only treatment that will correct the primary congenital problem. Children also may experience acquired cardiovascular disorders, such as rheumatic fever or Kawasaki disease. All these disorders can lead to heart failure or infection or inadequate heart function.

Cardiovascular disorders are frightening for children and adults alike. Even small children realize the importance of the heart in sustaining life, and they recognize the seriousness of any illness that undermines the heart's activity. For the families of children who are experiencing a cardiovascular disease, understanding the functioning of the heart and circulation is an important first step toward coping with the illness. Cardiac disorders are a major focus of health promotion and disease prevention measures in both adults and children. National Health Goals related to cardiovascular illness and children are shown in Focus on National Health Goals.

FOCUS ON NATIONAL HEALTH GOALS

Cardiovascular illness is a major health problem in adults, which makes it important to begin to take preventive measures early in childhood. A number of National Health Goals address ways children should modify nutrition or exercise to achieve cardiovascular health:

- Increase to at least 75% from a baseline of 65% the proportion of children and adolescents ages 5 through 17 who engage in vigorous physical activity that promotes the development and maintenance of cardiorespiratory fitness 3 or more days per week, for 20 or more minutes per occasion.
- Reduce dietary fat intake to an average of 30% of calories or less, and average saturated fat intake to less than 10% of calories, among people age 2 years and older (DHHS, 1995).

Nurses can be instrumental in helping the nation achieve these goals by educating parents and children about the importance of planned exercise and sound nutrition programs. It is equally important for nurses to caution parents not to begin reduced fat diets until their children are 2 years old to allow for myelination of nerve cells.

Nursing research is needed to determine what type of reduced fat foods makes the best finger foods for preschoolers, what type of snacks schools could provide in snack machines that would have a reduced fat content and would also be eaten by children, and how to increase physical activity in adolescents who do not participate in any type of organized sport or exercise programs.

NURSING PROCESS OVERVIEW

for Care of the Child With a Cardiovascular Disorder

Assessment

Assessment of the child with a cardiac disorder includes both careful history taking and physical examination, because many of the signs and symptoms of heart disease in children are subtle. A variety of diagnostic studies may be used to confirm the diagnosis and prepare for surgery. Teaching and providing psychological support to children and their families are two major responsibilities of nurses throughout the assessment process.

Nursing Diagnosis

Examples of nursing diagnoses established for children with heart disease may include the following:

- Decreased cardiac output related to congenital structural defect
- Altered tissue perfusion related to inadequate cardiac output
- Knowledge deficit related to care of the child pre- and postoperatively
- Fear related to lack of knowledge about child's disease
- Altered family processes related to stresses of the diagnosis and care responsibilities

- Ineffective individual or family coping related to lack of adequate support
- Altered parenting related to inability to bond with critically ill newborn

If the concerns in the latter three diagnoses are not identified when the child is ill, they may continue long after the child is treated and returns home.

If the child will be undergoing surgery or cardiac catheterization, nursing diagnoses will focus on psychological needs of the child and family for preparation and postprocedure care in addition to physical concerns after the procedure (e.g., Hypothermia related to cooling during surgery).

Outcome Identification and Planning

A great deal of nursing planning is necessary to help parents understand the necessity for diagnostic studies and to teach them to conscientiously administer cardiac drugs. An important nursing responsibility is to establish outcomes to help the child and parents, now and in the future (e.g., coping with their present fears and caring for the child at home).

Implementation

Nursing interventions in the care of the child with a cardiovascular disorder include teaching, providing an opportunity for children and their families to express fears about the child's illness and treatment plan, psychological support, and comfort measures for the child, such as helping the child find a position that is comfortable, administering oxygen, caring for the child in cardiac failure, and providing care after cardiac surgery. An equally important role is teaching prevention of heart disease. Measures such as promoting nonsmoking and exercise, maintaining an appropriate weight, and eating a low-fat diet are discussed in Chapter 11 with care of the school-age child. For additional help, parents may wish to contact the American Heart Association, 7272 Greenville Avenue, Dallas, TX 75231-4596, for educational materials and to look for family support groups in their area.

Outcome Evaluation

Outcome evaluation should be both long term and short term for the child and family. Once treatment is completed, and even if long-term care is necessary, it is essential to evaluate whether the family is able to think of their child, not in terms of illness, but in terms of wellness. Providing the opportunity for parents to express their concerns about their child at follow-up visits may allow you to address any misconceptions about the child's future that may exist.

Expected outcomes may include the following:

- Child's heart rate remains within accepted parameters for age.
- Child demonstrates age-appropriate coping skills related to diagnosis and possible surgery.
- Parents demonstrate competence with procedures required for care of the child.
- Parents exhibit positive coping skills related to child's diagnosis and required care to foster optimal growth and development in the child.
- Parents verbalize positive aspects about the child.

THE CARDIOVASCULAR SYSTEM

Cardiac adaptations at birth are described in Chapter 5. After these adaptations, the heart can be thought of as consisting of two pumps: the right side pumps blood to the lungs, where it is oxygenated before returning to the left side of the heart; the left side pumps the oxygenated blood to the peripheral tissues through systemic arteries. After supplying nutrients and collecting wastes, the blood returns through the veins to the right side of the heart where the cycle begins again. Contraction of the chambers is termed **systole;** relaxation is termed **diastole.** Normal heart anatomy is reviewed in Figure 20-1.

Cardiac output (CO) is the volume of blood pumped by the ventricles per minute. It is calculated by multiplying stroke volume (the volume of blood a ventricle ejects during systole) by the heart rate (beats per minute). Cardiac output is affected by three main factors: preload, contractility, and afterload. **Preload** is the volume of blood in the ventricles at the end of diastole (the point just before contraction). **Afterload** refers to the resistance against which the ventricles must pump. **Contractility** is the ability of the ventricles to stretch and refers to the force of contraction generated by the myocardial muscle. The Frank-Starling law predicts that the stroke volume can be increased by increasing the stretch of the fibers. Excessive stretch, however, results in a decrease in cardiac output. Much of the therapy of heart disease is aimed at reducing preload and afterload and increasing contractility.

Most heart disease in children occurs because embryonic structures did not close at birth or the heart originally formed inappropriately. For example, a septal defect between the right and left sides of the heart may remain open. Because pressure and volume on the left side of the heart are greater than on the right side, blood will flow through the connective structure left to right, or from the area of stronger heart action to the area of weaker heart action, compromising function.

ASSESSMENT OF HEART DISORDERS IN CHILDREN

The assessment of heart disease in children begins with a thorough history and a physical assessment. More specific diagnostic studies, such as electrocardiography or echocardiography, are ordered as indicated. Because all children with heart disorders have an increased risk of poor tissue perfusion, which may affect growth and development, developmental testing should be incorporated into the assessment (Bellinger et al, 1997).

History

Heart disease is becoming increasingly recognized because of prenatal ultrasound, which shows poor heart action or a distended heart. In the newborn period, because the newborn heart rate is so rapid that extra sounds of abnormal circulation cannot be heard, heart disease may not be detected. Because of relatively high pulmonary resistance, defects of the septum may not be readily apparent at birth. The infant may be brought to a primary care set-

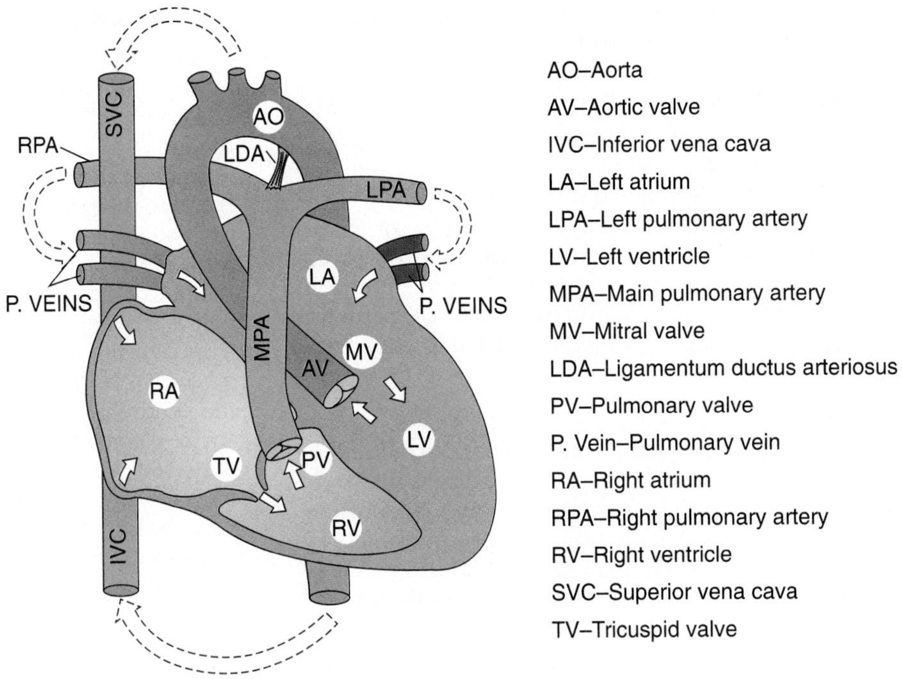

FIGURE 20.1 Circulation in the normal heart.

ting at 1 week of age by parents because the child is having difficulty feeding. Infants with heart disease generally have tachycardia and tachypnea. The infant who is breathing rapidly has to stop sucking on the bottle or breast frequently to breathe. The infant becomes easily fatigued because of ineffective heart action and has to stop sucking to rest before finishing a feeding.

The history should include a thorough pregnancy history to try to determine whether an intrauterine insult occurred. Some cardiac anomalies may occur as a result of an infection such as toxoplasmosis, cytomegalovirus, or rubella in intrauterine life. Ask if any medication was taken during pregnancy, if nutrition was adequate, or whether the client was exposed to any radiation because these may also contribute to congenital heart disorders.

Older children with heart disease also are easily fatigued. Ask in history taking: How much activity does it take before the child becomes tired? An hour of strenuous play? A short walk? Be sure parents are not confusing sedentary activities (the child who prefers to sit and read) with activities that are the result of fatigue (e.g., coming home from school and falling asleep day after day).

Ask about the child's usual position when resting. Some infants with congenital heart disease often prefer a knee-chest position, whereas older children often voluntarily squat. These positions trap blood supply in the lower extremities because of the sharp bend at the knee and hip and, therefore, allow the child to oxygenate the blood supply remaining in the upper body more fully and easily. Ask about frequency of infections, because children with heart disease have a higher incidence of lower respiratory tract infections than do other children. Children with left-to-right shunts tend to perspire excessively because of sympathetic nerve stimulation. Is there an indication of this? Edema is a late sign of heart disease in children. If it does occur, periorbital edema generally occurs first. Urine is only produced when kidney perfusion is adequate. Ask if the infant is wetting diapers or if the older child is voiding normally. **Cyanosis** (a blue tinge to the skin) may occur if a shunt allows deoxygenated blood to enter the arterial system. Such infants generally fail to thrive and are below normal height and weight on a standard growth chart. Children with coarctation of the aorta who have high blood pressure in the head and upper extremities have a history of nosebleeds and headaches. Because of corresponding low blood pressure in the lower extremities, such children may have pain in the legs on running (reported as "growing pains").

Some congenital heart disorders such as atrial septal defects may have a polygenic inheritance pattern. Ask if other family members have an incidence of heart disease. Cardiac anomalies often occur in conjunction with other disorders such as cognitive impairment and renal disease.

Physical Assessment

Physical assessment of the child with a suspected heart disorder begins with measurement of height and weight and comparing these findings against standard growth charts. A thorough physical examination should then be done, with particular emphasis on certain body parts or systems (see Assessing the Child With a Cardiovascular Disorder).

General Appearance

Inspect the toes and fingers (particularly the thumbs) for clubbing and for color. If you press on a fingernail, it will blanch white and then quickly pinken in a child with good circulation and oxygenation. In a child with poor tissue perfusion, the pink color returns slowly—taking over 5 seconds. Inspect mucous membranes of the mouth for color and evidence of cyanosis.

Cyanosis can best be recognized in the tongue and mucous membrane of the newborn. Cyanosis persisting for over 20 minutes after birth (except for acrocyanosis) suggests serious cardiopulmonary dysfunction. If the cyanosis increases with crying, cardiac dysfunction is suggested because the child is unable to meet the increased circulatory demands. If the cyanosis decreases with crying, pulmonary dysfunction is suggested because crying deepens respirations and aerates more lung tissue. Because cyanosis is difficult to detect in African-American children, inspect the buccal membrane. If the hemoglobin is reduced below 4 to 6 g/100 mL, cyanosis may not be present because severe anemia masks cyanosis.

A ruddy complexion may be present in some children with heart disease because the body overproduces red blood cells in an attempt to better oxygenate body cells. Observe children for lethargy, rapid respirations, or abnormal body posture, symptoms that the heart is an ineffective pump.

ASSESSING the Child With a Cardiovascular Disorder

History

Chief concern: fatigue, cyanosis, frequent upper respiratory infections, feeding difficulty, poor weight gain, growth failure
Past medical history: infection during pregnancy; difficulty with resuscitation at birth
Family medical history: Other members with heart disorders

Physical examination
Decreased height and weight
Easily fatigued

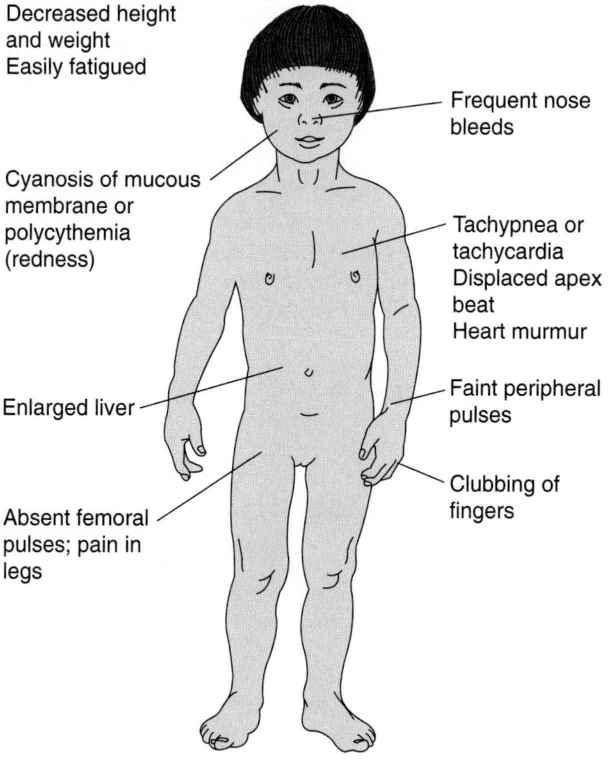

TABLE 20.1 Abnormal Pulse Patterns

PULSE PATTERN	DESCRIPTION
Water hammer	Very forceful and bounding pulse (Corrigan's pulse) and capillary pulsations may be apparent even in the fingernails; suggests cardiac insufficiency, as in patent ductus arteriosus
Pulsus alternans	A pulse of one strong beat and one weak beat; suggests myocardial weakness
Dicrotic	A double radial pulse for every apical beat; symptomatic of aortic stenosis
Thready	Weak and usually rapid pulse; suggests ineffective heart action

Because a major part of the physical assessment will include inspection, palpation, and auscultation of the chest for heart function, children must be relaxed and not crying. Provide age-appropriate toys that will distract readily. Provide a bottle of glucose water in case an infant grows hungry. Play with children before the examination so they know you.

Inspection of the chest may reveal a prominence of the left side and an obvious heart movement (apex beat, or point of maximum impulse). If a chest is extremely flat, loud innocent murmurs, accentuated heart sounds, and palpable cardiac activity may be very noticeable because of the proximity of the heart to the chest wall.

Pulse, Blood Pressure, and Respirations

The techniques for assessing pulse and blood pressure are described in Chapter 33. Normal findings for children of different ages are shown in Appendix G. *Tachycardia* is a pulse rate more than 160 bpm in an infant and more than 100 bpm at 3 years of age. An increase in pulse rate over these standards needs further investigation. Tachycardia is particularly significant if it persists during sleep, when the possibility of excitement is removed. Abnormal pulse patterns that tend to occur in children with heart disorders are shown in Table 20-1.

Murmurs. Murmurs of no significance are termed *functional, insignificant,* or *innocent murmurs.* In discussing such murmurs with parents, the term **innocent heart murmur** is preferred, because it describes that the sound heard is insignificant. It also helps to reassure parents that this is nothing to worry about. Innocent murmurs may become more pronounced during febrile illness, anxiety, or pregnancy. Hence, they may become audible for the first time at a hospital admission or with a sick-child visit. Such murmurs probably reflect a normal variation of vibration in the heart or pulmonary artery.

Parents should be told when children have innocent murmurs, because these sounds will undoubtedly be discovered again at a future health assessment. Teach parents that, although an innocent murmur is present, it is normal and is not a sign of any heart disease. Activities

TABLE 20.2 Comparison of Innocent and Organic Murmurs

CHARACTERISTIC	INNOCENT	ORGANIC
Timing	Systolic	Systolic or diastolic
Duration	Short	Longer
Quality	Soft, musical	Harsh, blowing
Intensity	Soft	Loud
Position in which heard	Usually supine positions	Heard in all positions
Affected by exercise	Yes	Constant

need not be restricted, and the child will require no more frequent health appraisals than other children. It is also important to teach parents that innocent murmurs do not turn into serious murmurs; otherwise, some parents see them as a prelude to future heart disease. At future health assessments, parents may need to be reassured again that the murmur is innocent.

If a murmur is the result of heart disease or a congenital defect, it is termed an **organic heart murmur.** The usual characteristics of innocent and organic murmurs are compared in Table 20-2.

For assessment, any murmur heard should be described according to its position in the cardiac cycle (early systolic, midsystolic, late diastolic, etc.), duration, quality (blowing, rasping, rumbling), pitch, intensity, location where it is heard best (the point of maximum intensity), whether a thrill (a palpable purring sensation) is present, and the response of the murmur to exercise or change of position.

CHECKPOINT QUESTIONS

1. What two signs are typically present in infants with heart disease?
2. What term is used to denote a murmur resulting from heart disease?

Diagnostic Tests

The diagnostic studies performed on a child with suspected heart disease will vary with the specific lesion suspected.

Electrocardiogram

An **electrocardiogram** (ECG) provides information about heart rate, rhythm, state of the myocardium, presence or absence of hypertrophy (thickening of the heart walls), ischemia or necrosis, and abnormalities of conduction. It also can provide information about the presence or effect of various drugs and electrolyte imbalances.

An ECG is a written record of the rising and falling voltages generated by the contracting heart. An upward tracing indicates a positive voltage, whereas a downward tracing indicates a negative voltage. The heart beat is initiated by the sinoatrial (SA) node in the right atrial wall near the entrance of the superior vena cava. From the SA node, the electrical impulse spreads over the atria reaching the atrioventricular (AV) node, located in the lower right atrium. From there, it spreads through the AV bundle (bundle of His) and the Purkinje fibers to the wall and septum of the ventricles. At the point that the ventricles have filled, the electrical flow has reached a peak, causing the ventricles to contract.

A normal ECG consists of an atrial wave (the P wave), a brief inactive period, then the prominent ventricular peak (the QRS spike), a large slow wave caused by ventricular recovery (the T wave), and often an incompletely understood slow wave (the U wave; Figure 20-2). A long P wave suggests that the atria are hypertrophied and it is taking longer than usual for the electrical conduction to spread over the atria. A lengthened PR interval suggests that there is difficulty in coordination between the SA and AV nodes (first-degree heart block). A heightened R wave indicates that ventricular hypertrophy is present. An R wave that is decreased in height means that the ventricles cannot contract fully, as happens if they are surrounded by fluid (pericarditis). Elongation of the T wave occurs in hyperkalemia; depression of the T wave is associated with anoxia, and depression of the ST segment is associated with abnormal calcium levels.

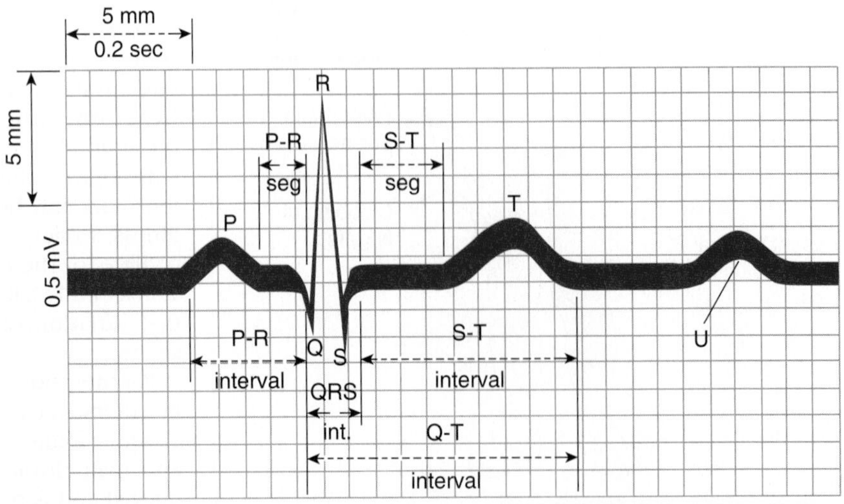

FIGURE 20.2 A normal ECG configuration.

Radiography

Radiography (x-ray) examination furnishes an accurate picture of the heart size and contour and size of heart chambers. It can reveal fluid collecting in the lungs from cardiac failure. It also can be used to confirm the placement of pacemaker leads. In a posteroanterior view, if the cardiac width is more than half the chest width, the heart is usually enlarged. This measurement does not apply to infants, because the more horizontal position of the infant heart increases this ratio to more than half. Prominence of pulmonary blood flow also may be evident.

Fluoroscopy, a form of radiography, provides important information about the size and configuration of the heart and great vessels, lungs, thoracic cage, and diaphragm. Because prolonged observation is necessary, however, special precautions must be taken to protect the child and health care personnel from radiation. Fluoroscopy provides a permanent motion picture record. The esophagus is so closely related to cardiac chambers that its visualization with barium also enhances cardiovascular structures. Interpretation of atrial or ventricular hypertrophy in infants and children by radiographic means is difficult. X-ray findings are, therefore, usually complemented by an ECG, a more sensitive and accurate measure of ventricular enlargement.

In *radioangiocardiography,* a radioactive substance such as technetium is injected intravenously into the bloodstream. As the substance circulates through the heart, it may be traced and recorded on videotape. The procedure involves a low dose of radiation and may be used to demonstrate, in particular, septal shunts.

Generalized *angiography,* or instillation of dye followed by radiographs, has little value in demonstrating pediatric heart defects. Selected *angiocardiography,* however, done as part of a cardiac catheterization, allows identification of specific abnormalities if followed by serial x-ray films. After a contrast medium has been introduced into a specific heart chamber, closed-circuit video equipment records the fluoroscopy pictures. Angiocardiography is not without hazard. Deaths have been reported from iodine sensitivity to the dye used, cardiac arrhythmias, and pulmonary edema.

Echocardiography

Echocardiography is ultrasound cardiography, which has become the primary diagnostic test for heart disease. High-frequency sound waves, directed toward the heart, are used to locate and study the movement and dimensions of cardiac structures, such as the size of chambers, thickness of walls, relationship of major vessels to chambers, and the thickness, motion, and pressure gradients of the valves. It is referred to as M-mode, a single beam that reveals chamber contractility; two-dimensional, which is used to reveal chamber and vessel size; and Doppler technique, which reveals velocity of blood flow. Remind parents that echocardiography does not use x-rays. Thus it can be repeated at frequent intervals without exposing children to the possible risk of radiation. It may be done using a transesophageal probe to better reveal heart chambers. Fetal echocardiography can reveal heart anomalies as early as 18 weeks into a pregnancy. This can alert staff to be prepared with immediate resuscitation or other needed equipment at the baby's birth.

Phonocardiography and Magnetic Resonance Imaging

A **phonocardiogram** is a diagram of heart sounds translated into electrical energy by a microphone placed on the child's chest and then recorded as a diagrammatic representation of heart sounds. The technique can measure the timing of heart sounds that occur too quickly or at too high or too low a sound frequency for the human ear to detect by direct auscultation. Magnetic resonance imaging (MRI) may also be used to evaluate heart structure, size or blood flow.

Exercise Testing

Exercise tests using treadmill walking to demonstrate that the pulmonary circulation can increase to meet the increased respiratory demands of exercise may be performed with children. With heart defects that obstruct the flow of blood to the lungs (such as pulmonary stenosis), such accommodation is not possible, and the child will evidence exertional dyspnea. Such tests are difficult to perform with children because they require the child's cooperation.

Laboratory Tests

Children with heart disease usually have a number of blood tests done to support the diagnosis of heart disease or to rule out anemia or clotting defects. Hematocrit or hemoglobin studies are performed to assess the rate of erythrocyte production, which may be increased in the body's attempt to produce more oxygen-carrying red blood cells. If the increase in the number of red blood cells is extreme (termed **polycythemia**), there will be a corresponding increase in blood volume and possibly a decrease in blood viscosity. Newborns are normally slightly polycythemic. In a newborn, polycythemia may be defined as a hemoglobin over 25 g/100 mL or a hematocrit over 70%. In an older child, polycythemia may be defined as a hemoglobin over 16 g/100 mL or a hematocrit over 55%. An elevated erythrocyte sedimentation rate (ESR) denotes inflammation and is useful in documenting that an inflammatory process such as occurs with rheumatic fever, Kawasaki disease, or myocarditis is present.

Blood gas levels are also determined. To test for this, a child can be administered 100% oxygen for 15 minutes. If the infant still has a PaO_2 less than 150 mm Hg after this time, a shunt directing deoxygenated blood into oxygenated blood is suspected. Oxygen saturation levels also are assessed; children with a deoxygenated to oxygenated shunt have a lower-than-normal oxygen saturation level in arterial blood. Normally, arterial blood oxygen saturation is 96% to 98%; oxygen saturation is under 92% when venous arterial shunts are present.

Before cardiac catheterization or surgery, blood clotting must be assessed. Expect prothrombin, partial thromboplastin, and platelet count studies to be completed before the procedure. Some children with polycythemia from heart disease have an associated reduced platelet count (thrombocytopenia). Because platelet formation is necessary for blood coagulation, the state of the platelet count must be corrected before cardiac surgery.

In children with heart failure, to ensure that an increased sodium level is not compounding edema, serum sodium level is obtained. All children receiving diuretics also should have serum potassium levels determined, because diuretics tend to deplete the body of potassium. Low serum potassium levels potentiate the effect of digitalis glycosides. Thus, serum potassium levels must also be obtained in children receiving these medications.

HEALTH PROMOTION AND RISK MANAGEMENT

Cardiac disease prevention in adults has received extensive attention in health literature. Because the risk factors that lead to adult heart disease such as obesity, high cholesterol serum levels, and lack of consistent exercise are health habits that begin in childhood, prevention of cardiac disease has shifted from an adult to a child focus. Early interventions to reduce risk factors in early life should have a major impact on reducing the incidence of heart disease in the next generation.

Risk Management for Congenital Heart Disease

The cause of congenital heart disease often cannot be documented although it is associated with familial inheritance and infection during pregnancy. All women of childbearing age should be immunized against rubella (German measles) and varicella (chickenpox) because these viruses are known specifically to cause heart damage to a fetus if the mother contracts them during pregnancy. Because some types of congenital heart defects have a familial incidence, parents who have a family member who was born with a heart defect need to alert their primary care provider so their children can be carefully screened at birth for the possibility of a like defect.

Risk Management for Acquired Heart Disease

Acquired heart diseases in children that have identified risk factors include rheumatic fever, hypertension, and hyperlipidemia. Rheumatic fever is an autoimmune response that follows a group A beta-hemolytic streptococcus infection. Ensuring that all parents know that children with streptococcal infections from otitis media, streptococcal pharyngitis and impetigo should receive adequate antibiotic therapy is essential for disease prevention (Scaglione et al, 1997).

Although **hypertension** (elevated blood pressure) occurs mainly because of a genetic predisposition, a high intake of sodium such as that in table salt, lack of exercise, and obesity increase the chances of developing the disorder in susceptible children by the time they reach late childhood. If infants are never introduced to high-sodium foods, perhaps by the time they are selecting their own meals they may continue to eat a diet prudent in sodium amount and prevent the development of hypertension in later life. For this reason, baby food manufacturers have stopped adding salt and mono-sodium glutamate to infant food. Urging school-age children and adolescents to reduce their intake of canned soups, cheese, luncheon meat, and hot dogs, all foods with high sodium contents, can effectively reduce salt intake in these age groups. School nurses can play an important role in this effort by monitoring the foods served daily in school cafeterias and advocating for more nutritious menus. Beginning when a child is 3 years of age, blood pressure should be included as part of routine child assessment to detect hypertension as early as possible (Novak, 1998).

A diet high in saturated fat has been implicated in the development of hypercholesterolemia and hyperlipedemia. It is important that fat intake not be restricted in infants because they need calories and fat for brain growth. School-age children and adolescents, however, should reduce their fat intake to 30% of total calories. The use of vegetable oils in place of saturated fat should begin when children begin solid food. Children from high-risk families (a family member has had an early myocardial infarction) should be regularly screened for cholesterol beginning at 3 years. Children with values above 170 mg/dL should receive dietary counseling and should be instructed in a regular exercise program.

✔ **CHECKPOINT QUESTIONS**

3. How do blood tests help in the diagnosis of heart disease?
4. At what age should routine blood pressure screening begin?

NURSING CARE OF THE CHILD WITH A HEART DISORDER

Taking home an infant born with a heart defect is difficult for most parents. Often, they have many questions that need to be answered fully before they feel confident enough to do this. Encourage parents to handle and feed their infant in the hospital so they can feel secure in caring for him or her at home. It is important for parents to understand as much as possible about their child's disorder. The more they know, the less they will assume that all children with congenital heart disease have the same disease. If this is not made clear to parents, they may unnecessarily limit a child's activity, assuming that because a neighbor's child was told not to do some activity, their child should not do it either.

NURSING DIAGNOSES AND RELATED INTERVENTIONS

Nursing Diagnosis: Parental health-seeking behaviors related to lack of knowledge about child's disorder

Outcome Identification: Parents will demonstrate a full understanding of child's illness and treatment plan before discharge.

Outcome Evaluation: Parents state accurately the nature of the illness and unique needs of their baby; are able to name primary care providers who will be following child's progress and can be telephoned for emergencies.

Provide Information About Care. Parents generally ask, *"Can we let the baby cry?"* If infants have tetralogy of Fallot or another heart disorder in which cyanotic spells tend to develop, or if they have a severe aortic stenosis, they should not be allowed to cry for long periods of time (no baby should). Crying for a few minutes while a parent warms formula or fully awakens at night will, as a rule, not harm them.

"What do we feed him?" Babies with cardiac disorders are generally able to tolerate a normal diet. Only rarely is salt restricted during this period because infants need sodium to regulate water balance. Because anemia stresses the heart, infants are generally given an iron supplement, either with formula or separately, to prevent iron deficiency anemia during the first year. Like any infant, they should receive supplemental vitamins with formula when breastfeeding is stopped. Because some infants with congenital heart disease tire readily, frequent, small feedings during the day rather than the usual every 3- to 4-hour pattern of other newborns may be necessary. If children are extremely poor eaters, a high-calorie formula or enteral or gastrostomy feedings may be necessary.

"How much activity can we allow the baby?" The answer to this question depends on the type and extent of the heart disorder. As a rule, infants or young children naturally limit their own activity. Parents need guidance, however, in setting limits of activity. Roughhousing with infants, such as tossing them up in the air and watching them squeal and laugh or playing games such as chasing a ball may not be advised. Encourage parents to observe the infant carefully to learn to recognize the first signs of respiratory distress and the point at which their child's activity is beginning to exceed his or her tolerance. Caution parents to observe the child carefully and thoughtfully as new activities are introduced and new interests are gained, so the child's activity is limited to what the heart can accommodate.

"What do we do if he becomes ill?" Although children with congenital heart disorders are usually seen by a cardiologist for health supervision, it is important that they are also seen by health care personnel who can ensure that they are receiving normal childhood immunizations and health guidance. As a rule, infants with heart disorders need prompt treatment for minor illnesses. The fever that accompanies a cold, for instance, can increase the metabolic rate of a child who has a severe congenital heart defect to beyond the point at which the child's heart can compensate. Dehydration must be avoided in children with polycythemia or the polycythemia may become so severe that clotting or thrombophlebitis may result. It is important that infections be treated vigorously so infectious endocarditis does not develop.

Children with congenital heart defects or rheumatic fever need prophylactic antibiotic therapy before they have oral surgery (tooth extractions or tonsils removed), because streptococcal organisms generally present in the mouth are often involved in infectious endocarditis. It is a good rule for children to be placed on prophylactic antibiotic therapy before they visit a dentist at all, because parents cannot always anticipate what dentists will do at any one visit. Penicillin is the preferred prophylactic antibiotic; erythromycin is used when a child is sensitive to penicillin. Many parents need frequent reassurance that a child will not become immune to penicillin if it is taken over long periods of time. Children with congenital heart disease should receive routine immunizations and be considered for pneumonia and influenza vaccines.

Review Steps for Follow-Up Care and Emergencies. Before parents leave the hospital with their newborn, be certain they have the name and number of the person to call if they have a question regarding the infant's health (their primary care provider and an emergency telephone number as a back-up.) Review with them the steps to take if their child becomes cyanotic, such as placing him or her in a knee–chest position. Be certain they have an appointment for a first health assessment, so they can be reassured that the responsibility of caring for this child is not being placed solely on their shoulders but will be shared by concerned health care personnel through all the child's growing years. They need to be told that, if they are unsure whether their child is in distress or ill, it is better to err on the side of caution by bringing the child to their primary care setting. Everyone who cares for infants with heart disease appreciates the responsibility the parents feel and the difficulty they have in making health judgments about their child. In many instances, they not only are the parents of this particular child but they also are new parents.

In most children, a referral for home care follow-up is essential. In addition to providing opportunities for child and family assessment, this also allows parents to discuss the sometimes frightening responsibility they feel and to obtain a second opinion of their child's health. They need to learn cardiopulmonary resuscitation (CPR) and how to activate their community's emergency medical system (EMS). A visit to the closest EMS station may be helpful for the parents so the staff will be acquainted with the child should an emergency call be necessary.

✔ CHECKPOINT QUESTIONS

5. Why is an iron supplement prescribed for an infant with congenital heart disease?
6. What is the rationale for prophylactic antibiotic administration before oral surgery for the child with heart disease?

The Child Undergoing Cardiac Catheterization

Cardiac catheterization helps to evaluate cardiac function. Diagnostic cardiac catheterization is a procedure used to help diagnose specific heart defects in anticipation of surgery. Interventional cardiac catheterization is a procedure to correct an abnormality such as dilating a narrowed valve by the use of a balloon catheter or other device. A small radiopaque catheter is passed through a major vein in the arm, leg, or neck into the heart to secure blood samples or inject dye. This allows the pressure of blood flow in any heart chamber and total cardiac output to be evaluated. Blood specimens can be obtained from the catheter to determine oxygen saturation levels, or a contrast dye can be injected for angiography. Electrodes can be introduced to record electrical activity and diagnose arrhythmias.

Cardiac catheterization may be done on an outpatient basis. Generally, children are kept NPO for 2 to 4 hours before the procedure to reduce the danger of vomiting and aspiration during the procedure. They must have had a recent chest x-ray and ECG recorded and have blood typed and cross-matched ready for use. Height and weight need to be recorded to help select catheter size. Because it is vitally important that the vessel site chosen for catheterization not be infected at the time of catheterization (or obscured by a hematoma), blood should not be drawn from the projected catheterization entry site before the procedure. Pedal pulses should be recorded for a baseline assessment. Most children are prescribed a sedation before the procedure to reduce their anxiety and help them lie still for a potentially long procedure.

In the cardiac catheterization room, ECG and pulse oximetry leads are attached. The site for catheterization is locally anesthetized with EMLA cream or intradermal lidocaine, and a catheter is threaded through a large-bore needle inserted into the site. The vessel used will differ according to the individual technique being planned. In neonates, an umbilical artery can be catheterized. Right-side heart catheterization is done by a venous approach. A right femoral vein or a vein in the antecubital fossa is used. Left-side heart catheterization can be performed by either a venous or an arterial approach. If done by the arterial route, a catheter is inserted into either the femoral or brachial artery. If a venous route is used, the catheter is inserted into the right femoral vein. Under fluoroscopy, the catheter is advanced to the right atrium and through the heart septum. Once the catheter is in a heart chamber, radiopaque dye is injected and films are taken (Figure 20-3).

Cardiac catheterization has a mortality rate of about 0.5%, so it is not without risk. Most fatalities with the procedure occur in infants under 7 months of age, usually because of cardiac perforation and arrhythmia. Transient arrhythmias may occur during passage of the catheter through the heart chambers or during injection of a contrast medium. Such arrhythmias generally stop abruptly with withdrawal of the catheter. Perforation of the heart may occur during passage of the catheter. Other complications include bleeding from the insertion site, because of heparin introduced into the catheter to reduce the possibility of clot formation, and thrombophlebitis from irritation by the catheter (a foreign body). Because cardiac catheterization is necessary for the heart surgeon to visualize and plan a cardiac repair, however, the benefit of the procedure outweighs the risks.

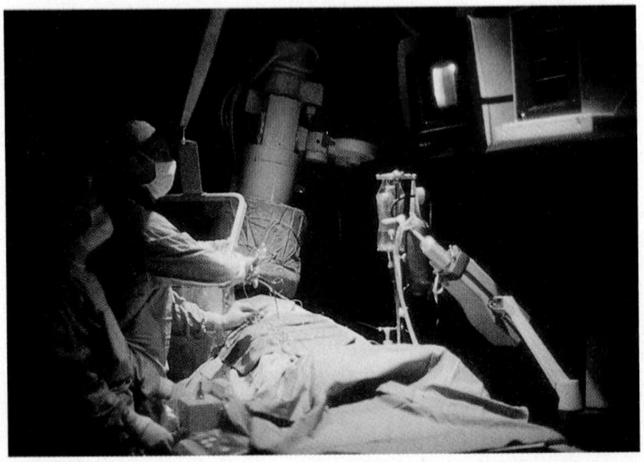

FIGURE 20.3 A child undergoing a cardiac catheterization.

NURSING DIAGNOSIS AND RELATED INTERVENTIONS: PREPROCEDURE PHASE

Nursing Diagnosis: Anxiety related to lack of knowledge about cardiac catheterization procedure

Outcome Identification: Parents and child will demonstrate reduced anxiety with increased knowledge before procedure; will express confidence about need for and outcome of procedure.

Outcome Evaluation: Parents and child (when possible) state goal of procedure and reasons for preparation and aftercare measures; state that anxiety is less after teaching.

Because most cardiac catheterizations are done with children awake but sedated with a combination of drugs such as chlorpromazine, promethazine, and meperidine, they may need more information about what is going to happen during the procedure than they would normally need for cardiac surgery. It is best to provide explanations for the children with parents present. Parents will then be able to help reinforce the information. After this explanation, parents often prefer a more detailed explanation of the procedure for themselves and time to ask their own questions.

Be aware that consenting to a cardiac catheterization experience arouses the realization that cardiac surgery may be necessary. Parents may be so concerned with what the procedure may reveal that they are unable to listen well to explanations. Allow them to accompany their children to the catheterization room and, if possible and appropriate, remain there for support during the procedure if they so choose.

Prepare children for what they will see in the catheterization room. Because they may be overwhelmed by the sight of the actual equipment, it may help if you build a facsimile room out of small cardboard boxes (representing the x-ray machine, the fluoroscopy screen, the ECG machine, and so forth). A puppet or small doll might serve as the patient in the miniature room. Dress the puppets in "sterile surgery suits" and "masks" like those worn by cardiac catheterization personnel. Older children may prefer to tour the room.

If children have never seen ECG leads or restraints before, let them touch and feel the equipment. Tell them that the procedure may be as long as 3 hours and that they will need to lie very still during this time. Help them master imagery or another stress-reduction technique (Pederson, 1995).

Do not underestimate what children know about their heart's purpose and function; even preschoolers recognize that the heart is vital to the body. Reassure them that the doctors are only taking a look at their heart, not cutting it or removing any part of it.

Teach children that when the catheter is inserted, it will not hurt, but their heart may momentarily speed up, a feeling that is uncomfortable. When dye is inserted, they may feel a stinging sensation. Do not use the word "dye," which may frighten young children who may think that dying is exactly what this procedure is all about. Instead, say "medicine." Caution them that lights will be turned off after the medicine is injected so the doctor can watch the medicine on a television screen (fluoroscopy) as it passes through the heart. Let the child know that after the procedure, a pressure dressing will be placed over the catheter insertion site to reduce the risk of bleeding. They will need to keep the extremity flat and unbent to prevent loosening the dressing.

Parents often need to have a review of heart anatomy. Although the cardiologist may have already done this, many parents appreciate being shown again the pathway the catheter takes during the procedure.

NURSING DIAGNOSES AND RELATED INTERVENTIONS: POSTPROCEDURE PHASE

Nursing Diagnosis: Risk for altered tissue perfusion related to cardiac catheterization

Outcome Identification: Child will maintain adequate tissue perfusion during the recovery period.

Outcome Evaluation: Child's vital signs are within normal limits; absence of arrhythmia; absence of bleeding or hematoma formation at catheterization site; pedal pulse is present distal to catheterization site.

When children return from the procedure, move them gently to their bed. Assess the pressure dressing over the catheterization site to see that it is snug and intact and that there is no bleeding present. Explain not to bend hip (if femoral site) or elbow (if brachial site) was used to keep the pressure dressing secure and prevent hematoma formation. This is particularly important when an artery was used for catheterization; a loose dressing on an artery will cause a large blood loss in a very short time. Also check the insertion site for signs and symptoms of infection because any opening in the skin is a portal of entry for bacteria. Palpate pulses distal to the insertion site to ensure unobstructed blood flow in the extremity is present. Also assess the extremity distal to the insertion site for color, temperature, and circulation (blanch the toe or fingernail and watch to see that it pinkens again readily). If there is bleeding at the insertion site, apply firm, continuous pressure and notify the physician immediately.

To reduce anxiety, children need an opportunity to describe their experience. Saying out loud how frightened they were—by the x-ray machine being pushed in over them, by the thought of a tube going all the way into their heart, by a comment made by one of the personnel in the room—helps alleviate their fear and allows better acceptance of the procedure. They need to be praised for their cooperation.

Keep the child flat in bed for 3 to 4 hours. This helps to prevent oozing at the insertion site and to prevent postural hypotension, which may occur when rising suddenly after lying flat for a long period of time. Assess pulse, blood pressure, and respirations at frequent intervals (about every 15 minutes) for the first several hours. In the immediate postcatheterization period, the blood pressure may be 10% to 15% lower than the child's precatheterization level because of the hypotensive effect of the radiopaque dye injected.

Cardiac arrhythmias and bradycardia may result from the mechanical action of the catheter having touched the conduction nodes of the heart. Assess pulse and blood pressure every 15 minutes. Monitor the pulse for a full minute to aid in recognizing abnormalities. Small children are unable to describe the feelings that accompany an arrhythmia. An older child might describe it as "heart fluttering" or "skipping beats." Therefore, increasing anxiety in the child after a catheterization is an important observation to report. It may be the child's way of reporting these feelings. Arrhythmias are serious complications and need to be reported immediately.

Infants may need fluid replacement to counteract the transient dehydration that results from being NPO for a period of time. If the infant is polycythemic, the increased fluid intake helps to avoid vessel thrombi. Some infants may require intravenous (IV) fluid during the procedure and for a number of hours afterward to prevent dehydration. Regulate this carefully to prevent heart failure from a fluid overload.

Adverse effects of cardiac catheterization may also be manifested by spells of apnea, sternal retractions, or dyspnea. If oxygen was administered during the catheterization procedure, it may be continued for a period of time after the procedure to reduce the stress of respirations. Like arrhythmias, dyspnea, bradycardia and blood pressure anomalies may be transient, but they should be reported so they can be evaluated further.

Nursing Diagnosis: Risk for infection related to presence of cardiac catheterization incision site

Outcome Identification: The child will remain free of signs and symptoms of infection after the procedure.

Outcome Procedure: The child's temperature is not above 38.0°C axillary; the catheter insertion site is free of erythema and foul drainage.

If the dressing is over the femoral artery or vein, keep it clean of stool and urine. Waterproofing the dressing with plastic may be necessary. Assess temperature immediately and then hourly for several hours after the procedure. Some children will have a transient elevation in temperature due to physiologic dehydration as a result of having been NPO. Some children react to the injection of the dye with a rise in temperature. Continuing to assess temperature helps to differentiate an elevated temperature caused by infection by the introduction of pathogens at the time of the procedure from a temporary cause. Alert parents to observe the insertion site daily for redness. Most are advised to omit tub baths and strenuous exercise for their child for 2 to 3 days to aid healing.

Nursing Diagnosis: Hypothermia related to cooling during procedure

Outcome Identification: Child's temperature will return to normal soon after the procedure.

Outcome Evaluation: Child's temperature is above 36.0°C axillary 1 hour after the procedure.

Some children, especially infants, may have hypothermia after cardiac catheterization from being uncovered during the procedure. This quickly compromises respiratory and heart action because, to raise body temperature, the infant has to increase his or her metabolic rate. This requires rapid breathing and increased heart action, which can lead to exhaustion. Infants may need to be placed under radiant heat warmers to help regain and maintain normal body temperature.

CHECKPOINT QUESTIONS

7. What might the child feel when a cardiac catheter is inserted?
8. Why might a child develop cardiac arrhythmias after cardiac catheterization?

The Child Undergoing Cardiac Surgery

Open heart surgery is made possible by the use of cardiopulmonary bypass (CPS) technique. The venous return to the heart is diverted from the right atrium or inferior and superior vena cava to a heart–lung machine, where it is artificially oxygenated. It is returned to the body's arterial system by way of the aorta bypassing the heart. The heart, practically bloodless, now can be opened and operated on. Blood returns to the coronary and pulmonary capillary beds from the aorta so that, even though the heart is not pumping, it still receives an adequate blood supply for self-maintenance during the bypass procedure. During surgery, hypothermia (reducing the child's body temperature to 20° to 26°C) is used to reduce the child's metabolic needs. If extreme hypothermia is used (15° to 20°C [usually on an infant]), the body temperature drops so low that the heart stops beating and the surgeon can work in a quiet and bloodless field. Very ill infants may be maintained by extracorporeal membrane oxygenation (ECMO) at the bedside after surgery.

Preoperative Care

Before surgery, vital signs (blood pressure, temperature, pulse, and respirations) need to be taken to establish a baseline. Some children may have pulse determinations done at several pulse points or blood pressures of both upper and lower extremities taken. Before obtaining a blood pressure, have the child rest for about 15 minutes prior and do the actual recording with the child lying down. Be sure to count pulse and respiratory rates for a full minute for accuracy. In addition, height and weight need to be recorded, because these parameters are necessary for the estimation of blood volume for the heart–lung machine and for medication dosages. Weighing will also be helpful in estimating blood loss or edema after surgery. Children who are receiving digitalis usually have their dose withheld 24 hours before surgery, because cardiac surgery may cause arrhythmias in the presence of digitalis.

The immediate surgical preparation of children varies from one institution to another but usually includes an enema to keep children from straining to pass stool in the immediate postoperative period and thus adding strain on the heart.

NURSING DIAGNOSES AND RELATED INTERVENTIONS: PREOPERATIVE PHASE

Nursing Diagnosis: Knowledge deficit related to cardiac surgery and its outcome

Outcome Identification: Parents and child will demonstrate increased knowledge before procedure and confidence in their health care team.

Outcome Evaluation: Parents and child accurately state the reason for surgery and expected outcome.

Bringing a child to the hospital for cardiac surgery is a large responsibility for parents. They want their child to be made well, yet they are aware that there is a definite risk from this surgery. They may have been protecting and guarding their child for months or years. They feel no less protective this morning than usual. Many procedures are done on an outpatient basis. Parents of children being readied for cardiac surgery may watch these procedures carefully. They may be anxious to help with preoperative measures to be sure that nothing is being done incorrectly. Review with them what they already know about the surgery to correct any misconceptions and what laboratory tests will be scheduled. Be certain to prepare them for the amount of equipment that will surround their child after surgery such as cardiac monitors, oxygen equipment, IV equipment, chest tubes, and a ventilator. Parents usually appreciate visiting the intensive care unit (ICU) where their child will go after surgery. Be certain that they have an opportunity to meet the ICU staff, especially if these nurses are not the same ones who are caring for the child preoperatively.

Explain Procedures to Parents and Child. Do not underestimate how much children know about the importance of their heart or the seriousness of this surgery (Figure 20-4). Some parents believe that children will be frightened by explanations about the surgery and do not want them to be told anything about it. This may stem from the protectiveness the parents have developed during the time while waiting for surgery. If you give these parents a clear, calm explanation of what is going to happen to their child, they usually find this step-by-step explanation a relief, and realize that so, probably, will their child. Remember when caring for these children preoperatively (or any time) not to make careless remarks, such

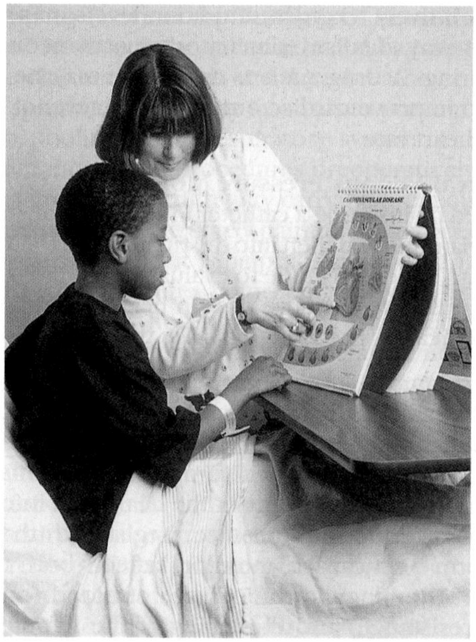

FIGURE 20.4 Orientation for cardiac surgery includes time for talking and learning more about the heart.

as "These syringes never work right" (when all you mean is that you prefer another brand) or "Amy (an ICU nurse) is a real clown" (when you mean she is not only a competent nurse but has a good sense of humor besides). Anxious parents may interpret such statements to mean their child is in less than competent hands. Because many children having cardiac surgery have had previous cardiac catheterizations, they need time to talk about their previous hospitalization experiences. Talking will reveal those things that they are most afraid of this time. Any misconceptions that they have about past experiences can be discussed and cleared away.

Prepare Child for Surgery and Postoperative Care. It is best if children are prepared for surgery with their parents present. This allows parents the opportunity to reinforce your teaching and shows children that their parents approve and feel secure with these surgery plans. Parents will then need additional time to discuss the surgical procedure with you and ask questions they might not have wished to ask in the presence of their child.

Both parents and the child may have questions about the difference between cardiac catheterization and cardiac surgery. One important difference is that children are sedated but awake for the former, but anesthetized for the latter. For some children, being awake is more reassuring; for others, it is more frightening. With the catheterization, they were aware the entire time that they were all right; asleep, how can they know? They need to express these feelings and receive reassurance that anesthetized sleep is a special sleep from which they will have no difficulty waking. Meeting the anesthesiologist and receiving reassurance directly from him or her that they will be watched over while they are asleep is often helpful.

As with cardiac catheterization, it may help to make models of the equipment that will surround the child postoperatively. Older children can be taken to the ICU where they will return after surgery and be shown the actual equipment (Stinson & McKeever, 1995).

After surgery, the child will need to cough and deep-breathe to help the lungs expand. It is good to introduce these exercises preoperatively to let the child know what is expected. Having children blow up a balloon is a helpful means of encouraging those who do not deep-breathe to do this well. In addition, introduce children to the form of oxygen therapy they will receive after surgery (mask, cannula, or ventilator). Orienting children to oxygen equipment is discussed in Chapter 19.

Familiarize children with chest tubes. Caution both children and parents that chest tubes must stay in place until it is time for them to be removed. If they want to turn over with tubes in place, they should ask for help to prevent the tubes from being pulled out. Caution parents that a chest-tube drainage reservoir must remain below the level of the child's chest and must not be raised for any reason. If children are not familiar with ECG leads, introduce these to them as part of the preoperative preparation. Comparing these tubes or leads to being "hooked up" like an astronaut is often appealing to children.

Postoperative Care

After surgery and before leaving the operating room, an x-ray film is taken and the child is weighed. Future estimates of lung expansion and weight will be checked against these two measurements.

NURSING DIAGNOSES AND RELATED INTERVENTIONS: POSTOPERATIVE PHASE

Nursing Diagnosis: Risk for altered cardiopulmonary tissue perfusion related to cardiac surgery

Outcome Identification: Child will maintain adequate tissue perfusion during the recovery period.

Outcome Evaluation: Vital signs are within normal limits; central venous pressure (CVP) or pulmonary artery wedge pressure are within acceptable parameters.

Taking accurate vital signs, as often as every 15 minutes, is essential in the immediate postoperative period. Continuous cardiac monitoring and assisted ventilation with endotracheal intubation are usually necessary. Blood pressure will probably be monitored directly by means of an intra-arterial catheter and indirectly with an automated blood pressure recording device. Hemodynamic monitoring by way of pulmonary artery or central venous catheter reveals information on chamber pressures and oxygen saturation (Figure 20-5).

Adequate voiding after surgery indicates that the kidneys are receiving adequate circulation. An indwelling urinary (Foley) catheter is usually inserted at the time of surgery so urine output can be carefully recorded postoperatively (it should be 1 mL/kg/h). Individual samples may be tested for specific gravity and pH. A specific gravity below 1.010 implies that the kidneys are not concentrating urine well, perhaps because of the stress of surgery. The pH should

forming the compressions. If the attempt is successful, the child's color will improve (especially the oral mucous membrane, which is readily visible) and the carotid pulse will become palpable. If two rescuers are working, continue to use a 1:5 ratio of ventilations to compressions in the infant and children less than 8 years of age or a 2:15 ratio in the older child (Chandra & Hazinski, 1994).

These three techniques (clearing the airway, ventilating the lungs, and circulating blood by cardiac compression) will provide adequate oxygenation to major body organs for several minutes until additional personnel arrive who can initiate further measures of resuscitation. The outcome of these secondary measures depends on how well and promptly the initial measures were performed.

Secondary Measures

IV access must be accomplished for drug administration. If this is not possible in about a minute's time span, an intraosseous catheter should be inserted. Drugs administered through an intraosseous route reach the circulation as rapidly as IV administration because of the rich blood supply in bone. Drugs such as epinephrine, lidocaine and atropine also may be given by way of an endotracheal tube. An endotracheal dose is calculated by multiplying the IV dose by 2 or 3. The drug is then diluted with normal saline, administered by a catheter inserted deeply into the tube, and followed by an additional 1 or 2 mL of normal saline and several positive-pressure breaths.

A number of drugs are helpful in resuscitation procedures and should be available on an emergency resuscitation cart. These may include:

- Atropine: Reduces bronchial secretions, keeping the airway clear during resuscitation attempts. It also reduces vagus nerve effects, relieving bradycardia.
- Calcium chloride: Increases heart contractility. A contraindication to its use is the presence of digitalis toxicity.
- Epinephrine: Strengthens or initiates cardiac contractions; increases heart rate and blood pressure.
- Adenosine: Relieves arrhythmias.
- Bretylium tosylate: Like lidocaine, counteracts ventricular arrhythmias.
- Dopamine: Increases cardiac output. It acts on alpha receptors to cause vasoconstriction.
- Dobutamine: Acts as a direct-acting beta-agonist that increases contractility and heart rate.
- Lidocaine: Counteracts ventricular arrhythmias.

Psychological Support

A cardiopulmonary arrest is an acute emergency, and everyone who arrives at the scene should know what course of action to take. Even after heart action has been initiated, ventricular fibrillation may occur requiring defibrillation. As soon as children begin to respond to resuscitation, be aware that they begin to hear. They are obviously frightened by the number of people and all the equipment surrounding them such as cardiac monitor leads, IV tubing, and possible endotracheal tube. They may have vivid memories of frightening body sensations just before going into cardiac arrest. They may regain consciousness struggling and fighting. They need to be assured that everyone is there to help them. They need to help by lying still. Someone on the cardiac arrest team should take the role of comforting the child and providing reassurance. Yet another person should assist, inform, and comfort the child's parents. It is extremely frightening for parents to see their child suddenly cease breathing. Although it is comforting to see emergency personnel arrive promptly and efficiently, parents are frightened to realize their child is ill enough to need such skilled personnel.

Be sure to provide specific information on their child's condition as soon as it is available and update them often. Allow them to see the child as soon as possible after the resuscitation attempt is complete to assure themselves that their child is breathing and has heart function. They should be reassured that follow-up procedures such as ECG monitoring or blood-gas measurements are being undertaken to prevent another emergency. Offer support to help them begin grieving if the child doesn't survive.

CHECKPOINT QUESTIONS

26. What is the most frequent cause of cardiac arrest in children?
27. What is the ratio of ventilations to compressions used for resuscitation of an infant?

KEY POINTS

Cardiovascular disorders in children may be either structural, such as congenital heart disease (the most frequent type of congenital anomaly), or acquired, such as Kawasaki disease and rheumatic fever. Assessment of children with heart disease includes history and physical examination. Echocardiogram and cardiac catheterization are procedures used frequently for diagnosis

Children with cardiac disease may fall behind in developmental progress, because they do not have the energy to play the usual childhood games. Help parents to think of games that are intellectually or developmentally stimulating without being physically exhausting.

Limiting salt and saturated fat intake are important strategies for preventing heart disease in later life.

There are a number of treatment possibilities for children with cardiac disease. For example, children born with a septal defect have open heart surgical repairs; those with hypoplastic left heart syndrome may undergo cardiac transplant. Children born with ineffective SA node function may have pacemakers implanted to improve heart function.

The families of children undergoing cardiac surgery need a great deal of support so they can cope well enough with this major event to be a support for the child.

Postcardiac surgery syndrome and postperfusion syndrome are two complications that may occur after cardiac surgery. They are related to the extracorporeal circulation used during the procedure.

Congenital heart defects are classified as those associated with increased pulmonary blood flow, decreased pulmonary blood flow, obstruction to blood flow and mixed blood flow.

Common signs of heart failure seen in children are tachycardia, tachypnea, enlarged liver, dyspnea, and cyanosis. Signs tend to be subtle in infants and may be manifested chiefly by difficulty in feeding from exhaustion and dyspnea.

Rheumatic fever is an autoimmune disease that occurs after a group-A beta-hemolytic streptococcus infection. Common signs and symptoms are fever, chorea, arthralgia, polyarthritis, erythema marginatum, subcutaneous nodules, and an elevated sedimentation rate. Helping parents (and the child) remember to administer prophylactic penicillin after the illness until age 18 helps prevent further recurrence and cardiac involvement. Children with congenital heart disease may also need to maintain this same protective routine.

Kawasaki disease results from altered immune function. An inflammation of blood vessels leads to platelet accumulation and the formation of thrombi.

Infectious endocarditis is infection of the endocardium of the heart. It may be a complication of congenital heart disease.

Hypertension in children usually occurs as a result of a secondary disorder. A moderate cholesterol diet, regular exercise, and maintenance of a weight proportional to height are important. Counseling children to follow these "heart healthy" guidelines calls for tact and persistence.

Children with heart disease are at high risk for cardiopulmonary arrest. Nurses and parents need to know how to perform cardiopulmonary resuscitation.

CRITICAL THINKING EXERCISES

1. Megan is the newborn with tetralogy of Fallot you met at the beginning of the chapter. Her parents are taking her home for a month while they wait for cardiac surgery to be scheduled. They asked you what "watch her carefully" meant and how much exercise they should allow her. What advice would you give them for how to care for Megan at home?
2. You are caring for a 6-month-old child who has heart failure. Her most important need is to have sustained periods of rest. How would you schedule your nursing care to avoid tiring her? What advice would you give to her parents at hospital discharge about home care?
3. A 10-year-old girl is recovering from rheumatic fever. She lives during the week with her mother and visits her father on the weekends. She will need to continue to take penicillin daily for the next 8 years. What steps would you take to ensure compliance over this long period of time?
4. You have been asked to prepare a class for a group of parents on cardiopulmonary resuscitation for infants. Develop a teaching plan for these parents.

REFERENCES

Adebajo, A. O. (1997). Rheumatic manifestations of infectious diseases in children. *Current Opinion in Rheumatology, 9*(1), 68.

Allan, L. D. et al (1998). Outcome after prenatal diagnosis of hypoplastic left heart syndrome. *Heart, 79*(4), 371.

American Heart Association. (1992). Pediatric basic life support. *Journal of the American Medical Association, 268*(12), 2251.

Beiser, A. S. et al. (1998). A predictive instrument for coronary artery aneurysms in Kawasaki disease. *American Journal of Cardiology, 81*(9), 111.

Bellinger, D. C., et al. (1997). Patterns of developmental dysfunction after surgery during infancy to correct transposition of the great arteries. *Journal of Developmental and Behavioral Pediatrics, 18*(2), 75.

Chandra, N. C., & Hazinski, M. F. (Eds.).(1994). *Textbook of basic life support for healthcare providers.* Dallas: American Heart Association.

Coody, D. K., et al. (1995). Hypertension in children. *Journal of Pediatric Health Care, 9*(1), 3.

Department of Health and Human Services. (1995). *Healthy People 2000: midcourse review.* Washington, D.C.: DHHS.

Feigin, R. D., Checchin, F., & Randolph, G. (1997). Kawasaki disease. In Johnson, K. B., & Oski, F. A. *Oski's essential pediatrics.* Philadelphia: Lippincott.

Fixler, D. E., & Talner, N. S. (1997). Epidemiology of congenital heart disease. In Johnson, K. B., & Oski, F. A. *Oski's essential pediatrics.* Philadelphia: Lippincott.

Friedman, R. A., & Starke, J. R. (1997). Infective endocarditis. In Johnson, K. B., & Oski, F. A. *Oski's essential pediatrics.* Philadelphia: Lippincott.

Higgins, S. S., & Kayser-Jones, J. (1996). Factors influencing parent decision making about pediatric cardiac transplantation. *Journal of Pediatric Nursing, 11*(3), 152.

Kohr, L. M., & O'Brien, P. (1995). Current management of heart failure in infants and children. *Nursing Clinics of North America, 30*(2), 261.

Kumar, V. R., Bachman, D. T., & Kiskaddon, R. T. (1997). Children and adults in cardiopulmonary arrest: are advanced life support guidelines followed in the prehospital setting? *Annals of Emergency Medicine, 29*(6), 743.

Martin, J. M., Neches, W. H., & Wald, E. R. (1997). Infectious endocarditis: 35 years of experience at a children's hospital. *Clinical Infectious Diseases, 4*(4), 669.

McNamara, D. M., et al. (1997). Intravenous immune globulin in the therapy of myocarditis and acute cardiomyopathy. *Circulation, 95*(111), 2476.

Mullins, C. E. (1997). Patent ductus arteriosus. In Johnson, K. B., & Oski, F. A. *Oski's essential pediatrics.* Philadelphia: Lippincott.

Neches, W. H., & Ettedgui, J. A. (1997). Tetralogy of Fallot. In Johnson, K. B., & Oski, F. A. *Oski's essential pediatrics.* Philadelphia: Lippincott.

Neches, W. H., Park, S. C., & Ettedgui, J. A. (1997). Cyanotic congenital heart disease. In Johnson, K. B., & Oski, F. A. *Oski's essential pediatrics.* Philadelphia: Lippincott.

Novak, J. C. (1998). Cardiovascular problems. In Burns, C. E., et al. *Pediatric primary care.* Philadelphia: W. B. Saunders.

Paquet, M., & Hanna, B. D. (1997). Cardiomyopathy. In Johnson, K. B., & Oski, F. A. *Oski's essential pediatrics.* Philadelphia: Lippincott.

Pederson, C. (1995). Effect of imagery on children's pain and anxiety during cardiac catheterization. *Journal of Pediatric Nursing, 10*(6), 365.

Peterson-Sweeney, K. L. (1995). Systemically induced vasculitis in children. *AACN Clinical Issues, 6*(4), 657.

Porkka, K. V., & Raitakari, O. T. (1996). Serum lipoproteins in children and young adults: determinants and treatment strategies. *Current Opinion in Lipidology, 7*(4), 183.

Sadeghi, A. M., Laks, H., & Pearl, J. M. (1997). Primum atrial septal defect. *Seminars in Thoracic and Cardiovascular Surgery, 9*(1), 2.

Scaglione, F., et al. (1997). Optimum treatment of streptococcal pharyngitis. *Drugs, 53*(1), 86.

Stinson, J., & McKeever, P. (1995). Mothers' information needs related to caring for infants at home following cardiac surgery. *Journal of Pediatric Nursing, 10*(1), 48.

Valdes, P., & Boudreau, S. A. (1996). Video-assisted thoracoscopic ligation of patent ductus arteriosus in children. *AORN Journal, 64*(4), 526.

Vick, G. W., & Titus, J. L. (1997). Defects of the atrial septum including the atrioventricular canal. In Johnson, K. B., & Oski, F. A. *Oski's essential pediatrics.* Philadelphia: Lippincott.

Ward, E. E. (1997). Anomalous pulmonary venous connections. In Johnson, K. B., & Oski, F. A. *Oski's essential pediatrics.* Philadelphia: Lippincott.

Williams, C. L., & Bollella, M. (1995). Guidelines for screening, evaluating, and treating children with hypercholesterolemia. *Journal of Pediatric Health Care, 9*(4), 153.

Wilson, M. D. (1997). Hypertension. In Johnson, K. B. & Oski, F. A. *Oski's essential pediatrics.* Philadelphia: Lippincott.

Wood, M. K. (1997). Acyanotic lesions with increased pulmonary blood flow. *Neonatal Network, 16*(3), 17.

SUGGESTED READINGS

Baker, A. (1994). Acquired heart disease in infants and children. *Critical Care Nursing Clinics of North America, 6*(1), 175.

Bircher, N., et al. (1996). Future directions for resuscitation research. *Resuscitation, 32*(1), 63.

Brown, V. E. et al. (1998). Echocardiographic spectrum of supracardiac total anomalous pulmonary venous connection. *Journal of the American Society of Echocardiography, 11*(3), 289.

Bush, C. M., et al. (1996). Pediatric injuries from cardiopulmonary resuscitation. *Annals of Emergency Medicine, 28*(1), 40.

Diem, S. J., Lantos, J. D., & Tulsky, J. A. (1996). Cardiopulmonary resuscitation on television. Miracles and misinformation. *New England Journal of Medicine, 334*(24), 1578.

Harris, M. A., & Valorida, J. N. (1997). Neonates with congenital heart disease. *Neonatal Network, 16*(2), 59.

Lester, C., et al. (1996). Teaching school children cardiopulmonary resuscitation. *Resuscitation, 31*(1), 33.

Napoli, K. L., Ingall, C. G., & Martin, G. R. (1996). Safety and efficacy of chloral hydrate sedation in children undergoing echocardiography. *Journal of Pediatrics, 129*(2), 287.

Sparacino, P. S., et al. (1997). The dilemmas of parents of adolescents and young adults with congenital heart disease. *Heart and Lung, 26*(3), 187.

Suddaby, E. C., Flattery, M. P., & Luna, M. (1997). Stress and coping among parents of children awaiting cardiac transplantation. *Journal of Transplant Coordination, 7*(1), 36.

Nursing Care of the Child With an Immune Disorder

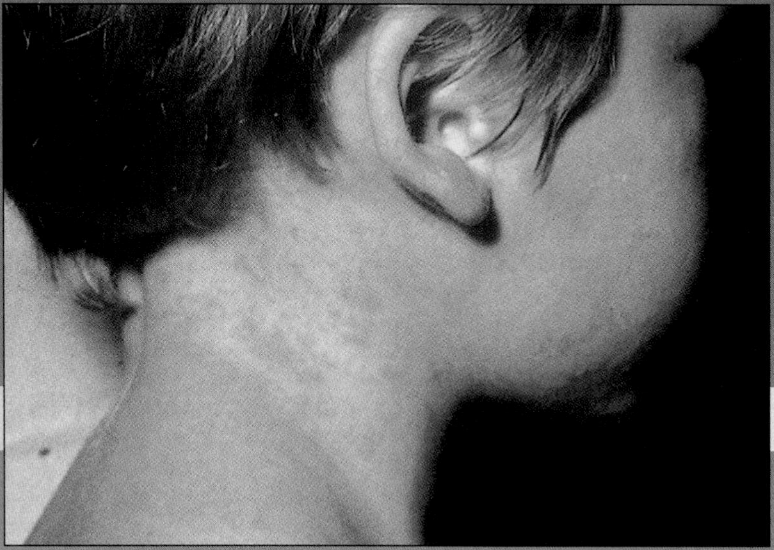

21

CHAPTER

Key Terms

- allergen
- anaphylaxis
- angioedema
- antigen
- atopy
- autoimmunity
- B lymphocyte
- cell-mediated immunity
- chemotaxis
- complement
- contact dermatitis
- cytotoxic response
- cytotoxic T cells
- delayed hypersensitivity
- environmental control
- hapten formation
- helper T cells
- humoral immunity
- hypersensitivity response
- hyposensitization
- immune response
- immunity
- immuno-competent
- immunogen
- immunoglobulins
- lymphokines
- lysis
- macrophage
- memory cell
- phagocytosis
- plasma cell
- suppressor T cells
- T lymphocyte
- tolerance
- urticaria

Objectives

After mastering the contents of this chapter, you should be able to:

1. Describe the immune process as it relates to childhood illness.
2. Assess the child with a disorder of the immune system.
3. Formulate nursing diagnoses for the child with a disorder of the immune system.
4. Establish appropriate outcomes for the child with a disorder of the immune system.
5. Plan nursing care pertinent to the child with an immune system disorder.
6. Implement nursing care for the child with an immune disorder.
7. Evaluate outcomes for achievement and effectiveness of care of the child with an immune disorder.
8. Identify National Health Goals related to immune disorders and children that nurses could be instrumental in helping the nation achieve.
9. Identify areas related to care of the child with an immune disorder that could benefit from additional nursing research.
10. Use critical thinking to analyze ways that nursing care for the child with an immune disorder can be more family centered.
11. Integrate knowledge of immune disorders and nursing process to achieve quality child health nursing care.

Dexter Goodenough is a 6-year-old boy you see in an ambulatory setting. His eyes are reddened and watering, and his nose is draining a clear discharge. His mother tells you he is constantly listless. Other children make fun of him because of his appearance. His grades are "terrible" because the minute he gets to school, his symptoms begin. Dexter is diagnosed as having atopic rhinitis (hay fever). "Thank heavens," his mother exclaims. "I thought he had something serious. What a relief to know it's only allergy."

In light of the effect this condition is having on Dexter's life, is this "only" an allergy? What additional information would you want his mother to know about the condition? Knowing this problem is worse at school, what environmental control measures would you want to suggest for Dexter?

In previous chapters, you learned about normal growth and development of children. In this chapter, you'll add information about the dramatic changes, both physically and psychosocially, that occur when a child is born with or develops a disorder of the immune system. This is important information because it builds a base for care and health teaching for children with these diseases.

After you've studied the chapter, turn to the Critical Thinking Exercises at the end of the chapter to sharpen your skills and test your knowledge.

The immune system consists of a complex network of cells interacting to protect the body against invasion by foreign substances. The study of the immune system has grown immensely during the past decade, and almost every day brings a new finding. More diseases are being attributed at least in part to a malfunctioning of the immune system, all of which makes an understanding of how the immune system works in health and disease essential for safe nursing care.

Disorders of the immune system include deficiencies of immune substances and function that affect the body's ability to ward off infection (immunodeficiency disorders); abnormal and excessive immune response to foreign substances (hypersensitivity disorders, or allergies); and abnormal and excessive immune response to self (autoimmune disorders). Immunodeficiencies and examples of allergic disorders are described in this chapter. Autoimmune disorders, which include a wide range of illnesses affecting many body systems, are addressed in those chapters that discuss the affected system (e.g., rheumatoid arthritis, which affects the joints, is discussed in Chapter 30).

Immune disorders in children are a focus of much research and study because they may hold the key to understanding major illnesses such as cancer and HIV/AIDS. National Health Goals related to immune disorders and children are shown in Focus on National Health Goals.

FOCUS ON NATIONAL HEALTH GOALS

Of the immunologic disorders, human immunodeficiency virus (HIV) is the most serious, not only because it is still ultimately fatal but also because its spread has been so difficult to stop. A number of National Health Goals address this problem:

- Increase to at least 60% from a baseline of 26% the proportion of sexually active, unmarried young women aged 15 to 19 whose partner used a condom at last sexual intercourse.
- Increase to at least 75% from a baseline of 57% the proportion of sexually active young men aged 15–19 who used a condom at last sexual intercourse.
- Increase to at least 50% from a baseline of 11% the estimated proportion of intravenous drug abusers who are in drug abuse treatment programs.
- Increase to at least 95% from a baseline of 5% the proportion of schools that have age-appropriate HIV education curricula for students in 4th through 12th grade (DHHS, 1995).

Nurses can be instrumental in helping the nation achieve these goals by educating children about the way the disease is spread (sexual relations and unclean intravenous needles) and protective measures they can take to avoid contracting the disease (using safer sex practices and not using intravenous drugs).

Nursing research that could add helpful information to the area includes research that attempts to answer the following questions: how can parents of school-age children best be convinced that safer sex practices should be part of usual school-age health awareness curricula? What methods used to educate adolescents about the danger of unprotected sex work best?

NURSING PROCESS OVERVIEW

for the Child With an Immune Disorder

Assessment

The immune system provides protection for the body from invading organisms (antigens). A deficiency of **immunocompetent** cells (cells capable of resisting foreign invaders) or alteration in their function may limit this protection. Assessment focuses on analysis of blood components, particularly the white blood cells, to determine exactly what components are altered, missing or are not functioning properly. When the immune system operates excessively or inappropriately to the invasion of certain antigens, a thorough history and analysis of presenting symptoms are usually the best way to identify the problem and develop appropriate interventions (see Assessing the Child With an Immune Disorder).

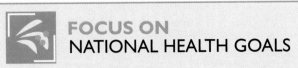

Nursing Diagnosis

Risk for infection related to altered immune response is the most relevant diagnosis with immune dysfunction. Nursing diagnoses for children experiencing allergic responses focus on their particular allergic symptoms. These may include:

ASSESSING the Child With an Immune Disorder

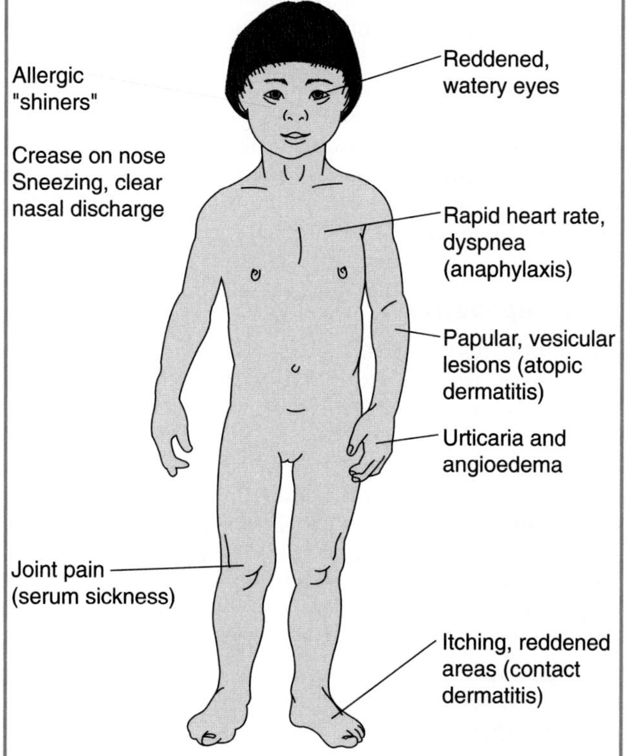

- Self-esteem disturbance related to effects of contact dermatitis
- Ineffective breathing pattern related to bronchospasm of anaphylaxis
- Anxiety related to continued allergic response
- Powerlessness related to difficulty determining cause of allergy
- Risk for altered growth and development related to chronicity of HIV/AIDS

Outcome Identification and Planning

Outcome identification and planning for the child with an immune disorder must focus both on present and future concerns. Relief of immediate symptoms is the first priority. This is followed by planning for long-term care and prevention of future problems. Looking into possible organizations for information or support could be key.

Implementation

A major nursing intervention in the care of children with immune disorders is client and family teaching. The family of the child with an immunodeficiency may need help in identifying ways to keep a child from contracting life-threatening infections while at the same time providing enough stimulation and social contact to promote normal growth and development. A similar teaching goal must be established for the child with a chronic allergic disorder. Parents need to learn ways to help their child avoid triggers or situations that provoke allergy. Yet they must not keep the child so isolated or fearful that the child misses out on important experiences. A referral to informational and support organizations may be helpful, including the following:

Asthma and Allergy Foundation of America
1125 15th Street NW. Suite 502
Washington, DC 20005

National Allergy and Asthma Network
3554 Chain Bridge Road, Suite 200
Fairfax, VA 22030-2709

Pediatric AIDS Foundation
2210 Wilshire Boulevard
Santa Monica, CA 90403-5784

Ryan White National Teen Education Program for AIDS
c/o Athletes and Entertainment for Kids
P.O. Box 191, Building B
Gardena, CA 90248-0191

National AIDS Hotline
1-800-342-2437

Outcome Evaluation

Examples of outcomes that might be established may be:

- Child voices high self-esteem even if contact dermatitis rash has not completely faded.
- Child's respiratory rate is reduced to 20/min with minimal wheezing.
- Child and parents state they are able to cope with their present level of anxiety.
- Child lists three actions he or she takes daily to help feel in control.
- Child demonstrates achievement of developmental milestones within age-acceptable parameters.

Because the field of immunology is always evolving, theories about immune diseases and associated treatment may change from visit to visit. Be certain that parents are kept abreast of new developments in the field, especially those that will affect their ability to provide an environment that is safest for their child.

THE IMMUNE SYSTEM

The purpose of the immune system is to protect the body from invasion by foreign substances. First, body surfaces such as the skin, cilia, and mucous membrane act as physical protective barriers. When an invading pathogen does get through this barrier, the process of **phagocytosis** (destruction of invaders) begins. **Macrophages** (a type of white blood cell) engulf, ingest, and neutralize the pathogen. At the same time, an inflammatory response creates vascular and cellular changes that help to rid the body of dead tissue and the inactivated antigens. The immune system maintains cells ready to attack this way whenever necessary, directing the efforts of macrophages and supplementing the inflammatory response as necessary. It also singles out specific antigens for interactions (antibody-antigen reactions). This immune response not only furnishes immediate protection but creates a template for how to destroy that particular antigen again in the future.

Immune Response

The **immune response** is the body's ability to combat outside invading organisms or substances by leukocyte and antibody activity. An **antigen** is any foreign substance (molecule) capable of stimulating an immune response. Most antigens are proteins, but other large molecules such as polysaccharides may also function as antigens. Penicillin, although not antigenic by itself, may become antigenic when it combines with a higher weight molecule, usually a protein (a process called **hapten formation,** which explains why penicillin reactions occur). If an antigen is one that can be readily destroyed by an immune response, and **immunity** (the ability to destroy like antigens) results, the antigen may be referred to as a simple **immunogen.** If, in the course of the immune response, mediating substances are released that cause tissue injury and allergic symptoms, the antigen is termed an **allergen.** Allergens may enter the body through a variety of routes. They may be ingested (e.g., foods such as eggs or wheat), inhaled (e.g., pollen, dust, or mold spores), injected (e.g., drugs), or absorbed across the skin or mucous membranes (e.g., poison ivy).

Immune System Organs and Cells

The organs of the immune system consist of the lymph nodes, bone marrow, thymus, spleen, and tonsils. Bone marrow produces lymphocytes, which are divided into **B lymphocytes** and **T lymphocytes.** Lymphocytes leave the bone marrow and locate in the lymph nodes and spleen, but travel throughout the lymphoid system. T and B lymphocytes recognize invading organisms and provide for attack of specific antigens (Figure 21-1).

B Lymphocytes

Originating in the bone marrow (the reason for their name), the B lymphocytes divide into **plasma cells** and **memory cells** when exposed to antigens. Plasma cells secrete large quantities of **immunoglobulins** or antibodies, which bind to and destroy specific antigens. When an antibody is formed in response to a particular antigen this way, it is specific to that antigen. An antibody against the pertussis antigen, for instance, will not have any effect on the tetanus antigen. Memory cells are responsible for retaining the formula or ability to produce specific immunoglobulins. Immunoglobulins are classified as IgG, IgA, IgM and IgE. Those involved in immunity are IgG, IgA, and IgM. IgM reaches adult levels at approximately age 1 year, IgG at age 4 years, and IgA at adolescence. IgE is primarily responsible for allergic or hypersensitivity responses. It is present at proportions capable of extreme response early in infancy. The functions of the immunoglobulins are summarized in Table 21-1.

T Lymphocytes

T lymphocytes account for 70% to 80% of blood lymphocytes. They are also produced by the bone marrow but mature under the influence of the thymus gland (hence the term *T cells*). When mature, T lymphocytes leave the thymus to enter specific body regions (thymus-dependent zones) mostly in the lymph nodes and spleen. They enter the blood circulation or extravascular spaces to contact antigens. They react specifically to viruses, fungi, parasites, but have an effect on all antigens. When a T cell meets an antigen, it divides until there are enough cells to destroy the antigen. T cells can be differentiated into three subtypes.

The first type, **cytotoxic** (killer) **T cells,** are T lymphocytes that have the specific feature of binding to the surface of antigens and directly destroying the cell membrane and therefore the cell. As a part of this process, cytotoxic cells secrete **lymphokines,** a substance that contains or prevents migration of antigens. Interferon is an example of a lymphokine important in preventing viral spread and helping to call leukocytes into the area (the property of chemotaxis).

The second type, **helper T cells** (CD4 cells), stimulate B lymphocytes to divide and mature into plasma cells and begin secretion of immunoglobulins. IgA antibody response depends on stimulation by helper T cells. Helper T cells can be identified in blood because of specific mark-

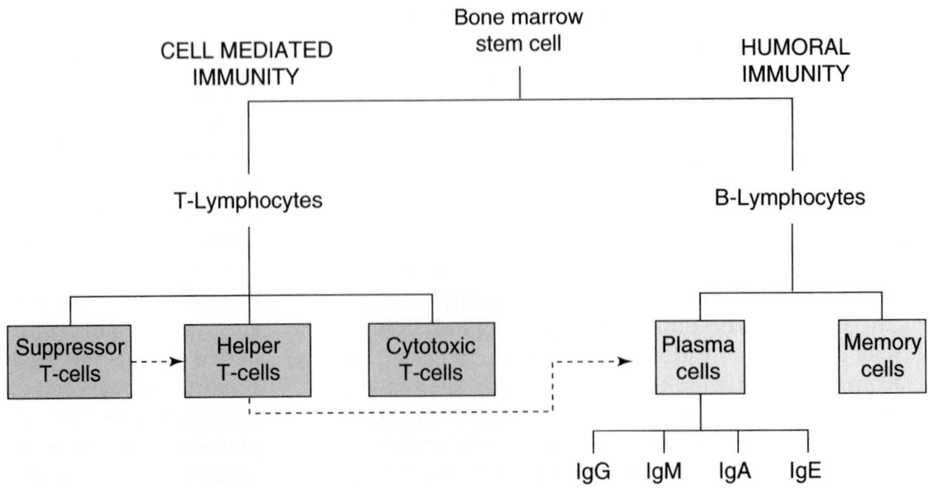

FIGURE 21.1 Lymphocyte production. From the bone marrow stem cell, T- and B-lymphocytes are formed. T-lymphocyte action leads to cell-mediated immunity. B-lymphocyte action results in humoral immunity.

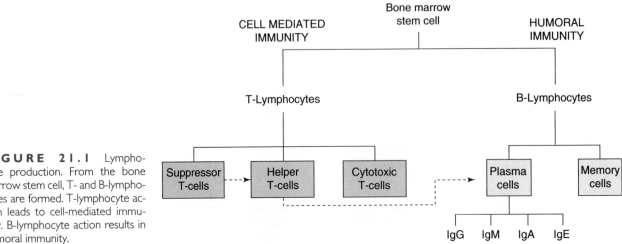

TABLE 21.1 Location and Function of Immunoglobulins

IMMUNOGLOBULIN	DESCRIPTION
IgM	Effective in agglutinating antigen as well as lysing cell walls; discovered early in the course of an infection in the bloodstream
IgG	Most frequently occurring antibody in plasma; during secondary response, it is the major immunoglobulin to be synthesized; it freely diffuses into extravascular spaces to contact antigens; in prenatal life, it diffuses across the placenta to supply passive immune protection to the fetus and until the infant can effectively produce immunoglobulins; it has the major responsibility for neutralizing bacterial toxins and in activating phagocytosis (destruction of bacteria)
IgA	Found in external body secretions such as saliva, sweat, tears, mucus, bile, and colostrum; provides defense against pathogens on exposed surfaces, especially those of the gastrointestinal tract and respiratory tract apparently by preventing adherence of pathogens to mucosal cells
IgD	Found in plasma; may be the receptor that binds antigens to lymphocyte surfaces
IgE	Involved in immediate hypersensitivity reactions; exists bound to mast cells on tissue surfaces; when contacted by an antigen, cellular granules are released; associated with allergy and parasitic infections

ers on their surface. Analysis of these (CD4 counts) is an important assessment of the competency of the immune system.

The third type, **suppressor T cells,** are T cells that reduce the production of immunoglobulins against a specific antigen and prevent their overproduction.

Types of Immunity

The action of B lymphocytes and T lymphocytes leads to two different types of immunity.

Humoral Immunity

Humoral immunity refers to immunity created by antibody production or B-lymphocyte involvement. Helper T cells recognize the antigen and cause activation of B lymphocytes (possibly by an intermediary macrophage). The specific B cells differentiate into plasma cells and begin secretion of specific immunoglobulins to mark the antigen for destruction (Figure 21-2*A*). A few antigens (e.g., *Escherichia coli*) are capable of activating B-cell response without recognition by T cells (Lederman, 1997).

Primary Response. The first time a specific antigen enters the body, B-cell differentiation and growth begin. Within 6 days, IgM antibodies specific to the antigen can be measured in the bloodstream. The production of IgM antibodies peaks at 14 days and then declines until, within a few weeks, there are few present. At approximately day 10, IgG production begins and remains high for several weeks (Figure 21-3).

Secondary Response. When a specific antigen enters the body a second or additional time, antibody production begins immediately because of memory cells. The type of immunoglobulin mainly produced in a secondary response is IgG (see Figure 21-3).

Complement Activation. Complement is comprised of 20 different proteins that are normally nonfunctional molecules; however, when activated by an antigen-antibody contact, these molecules begin a cascade response that leads to increased vascular permeability, smooth muscle contraction, **chemotaxis** ("calling" leukocytes into the area), phagocytosis, and **lysis** (killing) of the foreign antigen. The area feels warm and looks reddened and swollen (an inflammatory reaction). Although an inflammatory reaction causes some local injury to tissue around the antigen, it is helpful overall because it produces an environment harmful to the antigen. Complement reactions that persist beyond the usual inhibition may be responsible for many of the autoimmune disorders.

Cell-Mediated Immunity

Cell-mediated immunity is the type of immune response due to T-lymphocyte activity. Cytotoxic T cells attack and destroy invading antigens through either the release of chemical compounds on the antigen membrane, injection of a toxin directly into the antigen, or secretion of lymphokines. A wheal and flare response occurs due to accumulation of lymphocytes around small blood vessels, resulting in minor destruction to blood vessels (see Figure 21-2*B*). This response is termed **delayed hypersensitivity** if the T-cell activity occurs solely without an accompanying humoral response. It is this response that causes transplant rejection.

Autoimmunity

Autoimmunity results from an inability to distinguish self from nonself, causing the immune system to carry out immune responses against normal cells and tissue. Autoimmune responses may be organ specific (i.e., limited to one organ), as in Hashimoto's disease (see Chapter 27) or generalized and systemic (non-organ-specific), as in rheumatoid arthritis and systemic lupus erythematosus (see Chapter 25). There is currently much research oriented toward the study of autoimmune responses and their possible implication in a wide variety of disorders, including multiple sclerosis and hepatitis. Females are more likely than males to suffer from autoimmune disor-

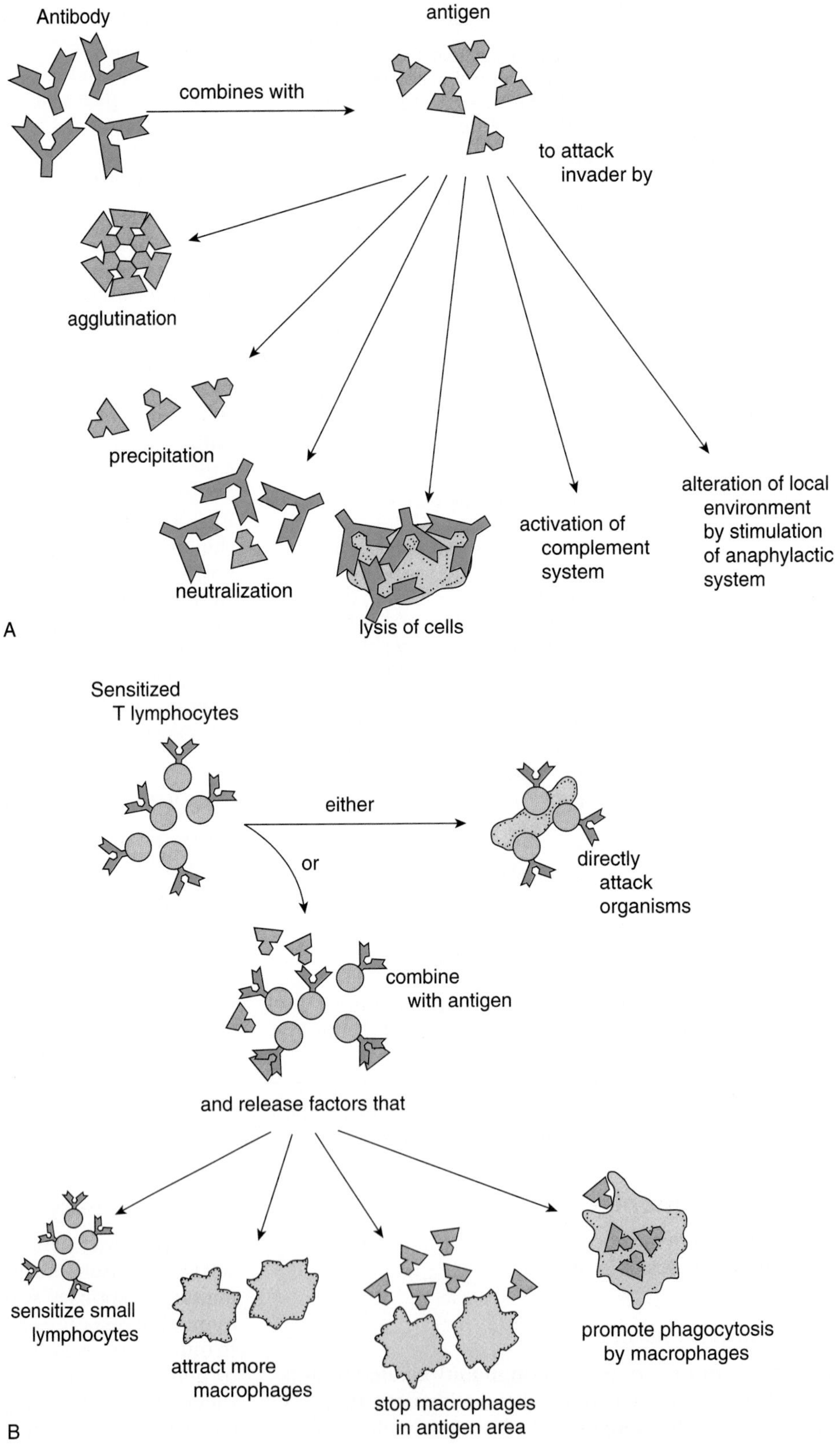

FIGURE 21.2 Mechanism of immunity response. (**A**) Humoral immunity. (**B**) Cell-mediated immunity.

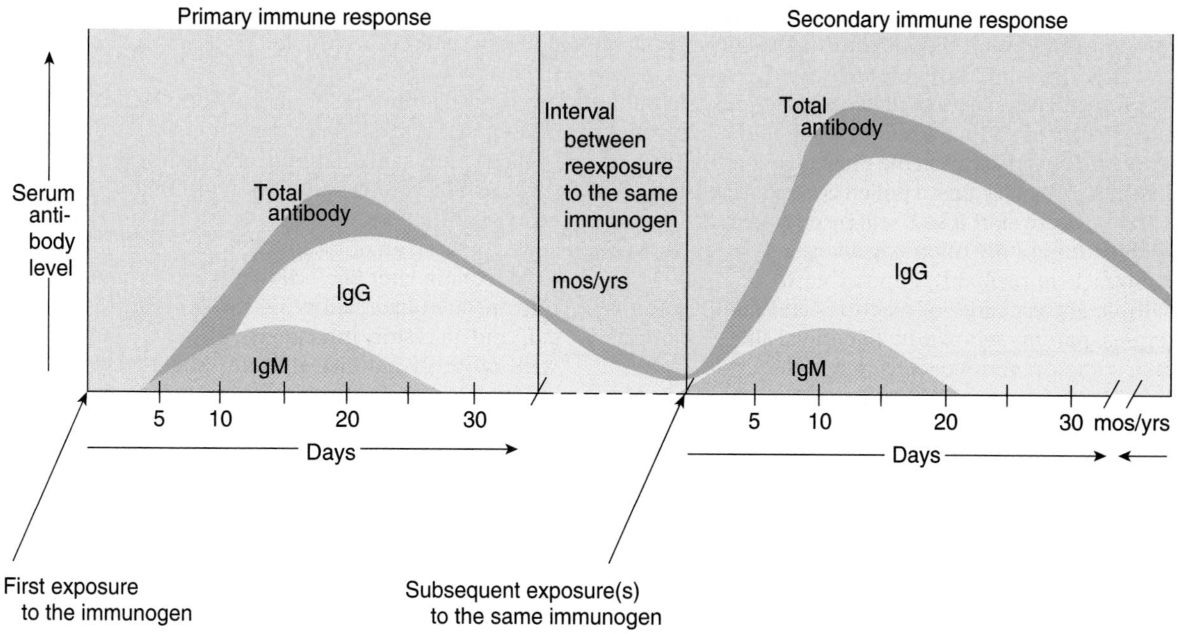

FIGURE 21.3 Primary and secondary humoral responses. IgM is the first immunoglobulin to appear in the serum.

ders, which may indicate a relationship between sex hormones and the immune response.

> **CHECKPOINT QUESTIONS**
>
> 1. What type of white blood cell is responsible for engulfing, ingesting and neutralizing a pathogen?
> 2. What are the two types of lymphocytes produced by the bone marrow?

HEALTH PROMOTION AND RISK MANAGEMENT

As many as 20% of children have some form of allergy. Preventing allergies, therefore, could have a major impact on the health of children. Early prevention can begin with encouraging women to breastfeed. Urging parents to delay the introduction of solid food until at least after 6 months of age can also delay exposure to foreign proteins. In families where there is a tendency for allergies (atopic families), parents can be encouraged to begin environmental control measures before their children are born (buying only stuffed toys with synthetic filling, removing dust collectors such as venetian blinds and shag rugs; see Focus on Cultural Competence).

Health promotion is also important to prevent HIV/AIDS. Teaching children safer sex practices is an important part of this. All health care providers can help prevent the spread of HIV/AIDS by using standard precautions. The parents of children with immune deficiencies may need to be reminded periodically to take measures to keep their children free of disease (keep immunizations updated; seek help immediately for infections).

Health Teaching

Allergies are not the type of disorders people typically think of as causing acute symptoms. Children with allergies and their parents must understand how allergic reactions lead to symptoms and how important it is for children to play a role in their own therapy. For this reason, children who develop allergies often need to be encouraged to conscientiously take their medicine. For the same reason, once parents begin a child on an immunotherapy program, they may need to be encouraged to continue it.

If parents are going to prepare an allergy-free diet, they need to consider the child's likes and dislikes and to think through the child's weekly intake to ensure that the child receives all essential nutrients. If a child eats at school or has a meal prepared every day by a child care center, parents must be certain that the center, babysitter, or school dietitian are aware of the child's allergies. If a child is al-

> **FOCUS ON CULTURAL COMPETENCE**
>
> Because families with atopy have more allergies than others, some communities have a higher incidence of children with allergies than others. As a result, these communities may have more services and specialists to treat these children, thus developing a "community culture" of allergy treatment. Children typically may leave school early for immunotherapy. School cafeterias commonly offer allergy-free foods. In other communities with fewer children with allergies, a child with an allergy is viewed as unique and needs additional support.

lergic to wheat products and cannot eat bread, preparing a bag lunch for school may be a difficult daily problem that only good planning can eliminate.

If a child's allergies involve pollen sensitivities, planning activities such as vacations at a time when the pollen count is low may make the vacation the most pleasant for the family. If desensitization against a pollen is necessary, assist parents in planning to start it so it will be effective by the time the pollen count of the offending allergen rises.

Although it is probably impossible to keep children with atopic allergies free of reactions and manifestations of allergies, parents who know of familial allergy patterns can take some preventive steps in this direction.

In families where there are allergies, infants should be breastfed if at all possible. Parents should delay beginning solid food until 6 months of age and introduce foods singly so food allergies can be detected and offending foods eliminated from the child's diet. They should omit eggs and chocolate from the child's diet for the first year. They should begin environmental control when they first choose furniture for the child's room by eliminating wool blankets, choosing toys carefully, and keeping them free of dust. Teach parents to use a minimum of washing compounds to expose children to as few chemical products as possible and not to introduce pets into the house. Avoiding spray products such as perfumes and air fresheners and discontinuing cigarette smoking also help.

These are sensible rules for parents to follow rather than waiting for a child to develop allergic rhinitis or atopic dermatitis and then having to put more extreme measures into effect.

IMMUNODEFICIENCY DISORDERS

The immune system is a complex, interlocking network of cells with specific functions. When any one portion is not functioning adequately, an immunodeficiency results. The entire system may fail in its goal to protect the body from invading organisms. The immunodeficiency disorders may be primary (congenital) or acquired (secondary to viral invasion or exposure to a toxic substance).

Primary Immunodeficiency

Children with primary congenital immunodeficiencies are born without an essential immune substance or function or with inadequate amounts of immune substances. Usually these deficiencies become apparent relatively early in life, although it may take a few months for B-cell deficiencies to produce symptoms because a newborn is born with enough maternal IgG (which crosses the placenta during pregnancy) to supply protection for approximately the first 6 months of life. It is important for parents and children to understand that primary disorders are not the same as acquired immunodeficiency (AIDS).

B-Cell (B-Lymphocyte) Deficiencies

B-cell deficiencies create abnormally low levels of immunoglobulins either selectively (as in an IgA deficiency) or totally, which is referred to as *hypogammaglobulinemia* (Lederman & Winkelstein, 1997).

Hypogammaglobulinemia. Hypogammaglobulinemia is an inherited X-linked recessive defect in the maturation of B lymphocytes. It results in abnormally low levels of all immunoglobulins. At approximately 6 months of age, at the point passively transferred maternal antibodies fade, male infants begin to show susceptibility to bacterial infections and develop frequent respiratory, digestive, and throat infections. Autoimmune diseases such as rheumatoid arthritis and systemic lupus erythematosus may occur in later life. Cellular or T-lymphocyte response remains adequate, allowing the child to resist viral, fungal, and parasitic infections. This deficiency is treated with monthly gamma globulin injections to supply immunoglobulins. Bone marrow transplantation may be successful in restoring immune competency. Parents, and the child as he or she grows older, need to be taught the importance of recognizing infection early. Also, assist them with setting up a schedule for gamma globulin injections so these are not forgotten.

Common Variable Immunoglobulin Deficiencies. The most common disorder in this group is deficiency of IgA in surface secretions. The overall level of B lymphocytes is normal, but IgA production is reduced or absent, perhaps due to an increase of IgA suppressor cells or a defect in T helper cells important for IgA synthesis. Without IgA, infection of surfaces exposed to the external environment and normally protected by mucus become common. Sinusitis, upper respiratory tract illness, and inflammatory bowel disease are apt to occur. There are associated atopic diseases (allergies) because without IgA on the surface mucosa, many more antigens than usual enter the body, permitting more antigens to interact with IgE and produce allergic symptoms. Chronic irritation due to these large numbers of antigens predispose exposed tissue to malignant transformation so malignancy of the respiratory, gastrointestinal, and lymphoid systems occurs. There is an increased risk that an antibody will cross-react with a self-antigen to cause autoimmune illness so systemic lupus erythematosus and rheumatoid arthritis also occur at increased rates. IgA deficiency can occur as a secondary type due to treatment with phenytoin and penicillamine. Gamma globulin contains little IgA so therapy with this does not greatly reduce symptoms. Parents need to be conscientious about preventing infections (Winkelstein, 1997).

T-Cell (T-Lymphocyte) Deficiencies

T-cell immunodeficiencies involve inadequate numbers or inadequate functioning of the T cells, which affects cell-mediated immunity and which can also affect humoral immunity. DiGeorge anomaly (which includes failure of the thymus to develop) and chronic mucocutaneous candidiasis are two disorders caused by T-cell deficiency or malfunction.

Combined T- and B-Cell Deficiency

Severe combined immunodeficiency syndrome (SCIDS) is the most frequently seen disorder characterized by an absence or reduction of both humoral and cell-mediated immunity. SCIDS occurs as either an X-linked or autosomal recessive disorder. It is caused by a developmental abnormality (sometimes but not always related to an absence of a particular enzyme), which prevents the formation of T lymphocytes (a stem cell abnormality). This, in turn, prevents the maturation of both T and B lymphocytes. Children are unable to respond to antigen invasion, and no antibodies are produced. Bone marrow transplantation has proven to be an effective treatment for this disorder. Gene therapy, or replacing the child's own cells with those able to produce T cells, is also now possible (Hong, 1997).

Secondary Immunodeficiency

Secondary immunodeficiency or loss of immune system response can occur from factors such as severe systemic infection, cancer, renal disease, radiation therapy, stress, malnutrition, immunosuppressive therapy, and aging. There can be complete or partial loss of both B- and T-lymphocyte response.

Stress appears to alter the immune response by interrupting a hypothalamus response. This decreases the function of the thymus gland. Stress also increases production of corticosteroids. These suppress the inflammatory response by inhibiting macrophage action. Immunosuppressive drugs and radiation act to limit or destroy rapidly growing cells. However, because both T- and B-cell lymphocytes are rapidly growing and dividing cells, they are killed by these drugs or radiation. Extreme infection can result in a decreased immune response because it exhausts the body's continued ability to combat infection.

Malnutrition causes changes because rapidly growing cells need protein for synthesis; renal disease with protein loss will deplete the amount of protein available for new lymphocyte production.

Acquired Immunodeficiency Syndrome

Acquired immunodeficiency syndrome (AIDS) is an acquired immunodeficiency caused by the RNA cytopathic human immunodeficiency retrovirus HIV (Gibbons, 1997). The virus has at least two subtypes: HIV-1 and HIV-2. It is contracted through blood and body secretions. The virus acts by attacking the lymphoreticular system, in particular CD4 bearing helper T lymphocytes. The virus enters and replicates in these lymphocytes and, in the process, destroys them. There is no defense against the virus remaining in the body for life. This results in loss of CD4 lymphocytes and the ability to initiate a B-lymphocyte response. The final result is that the immune response and the ability to screen and remove malignant cells from the body are lost. Because B cells or humoral immune function, which initiates the production of antibodies, is affected, antibody formation will be decreased (hypogammaglobulinemia). When monocytes and macrophages become affected as well, the person with HIV infection is unable to resist normal infection and is susceptible to opportunistic infections (Scott & Parks, 1997; Kuhn et al, 1998).

Transmission. HIV/AIDS infection is spread by exposure to blood and other body secretions through sexual contact, sharing of contaminated needles for injection, transfusion of contaminated blood or blood products, perinatal spread from mother to fetus/newborn, and through breastfeeding. Transmission of HIV/AIDS from mother to child by placental spread is the most common reason for childhood HIV/AIDS. This transmission can occur during pregnancy, at delivery, and possibly during breastfeeding. The incidence of transmission can be reduced to as low as 8% if an HIV-positive woman receives Zidovudine (AZT) during pregnancy (Scott & Layton, 1997). In the past, children with hemophilia, because they receive so many blood product transfusions, received contaminated blood and were infected. This source of transmission now almost never occurs. A small number of children have acquired the infection through sexual abuse. HIV is not transmitted by animals or through usual casual contact, such as shaking hands or kissing or in households, day care centers or schools.

The increasing rate of sexual activity and rapidly rising rate of sexually transmitted disease among adolescents are making this group vulnerable to growing rates of HIV/AIDS. Pediatric HIV/AIDS accounts for 1% to 2% of total AIDS disease. It is the leading cause of death in children 1 to 4 years of age, and in some areas the number one cause of death in adolescents.

Assessment. HIV has a long incubation period of about 10 years in adults. Children who receive the virus through placental transmission are usually HIV positive by 6 months, developing clinical signs by 3 years of age. Children who receive the virus from another source usually convert to being HIV positive by 2 to 6 weeks, or at least by 6 months. During this preconversion time, the child may have poor resistance to infection such as fever, swollen lymph nodes, respiratory tract infections and thrush.

All infants born to infected mothers test positive for antibodies to the virus at birth because of passive antibody transmission. This persists for about 18 months. The disease is diagnosed, therefore, by recovery of the HIV antigen in children under this age and antibodies to the virus in children over this age. Tests for detection of the antigen are termed p24 for PCR (polymerase chain reaction) tests; those for the antibody are termed ELISA and Western Blot confirmation. CD4 counts are used to document the disease status and predict disease progression. Normal counts vary according to children's ages as the lymphocyte count normally varies according to age. Table 41-2 shows the use of CD4 counts to determine disease progress. Severe suppression indicates a condition serious enough to cause life-threatening infections.

The CDC classification of HIV/AIDS in children is based on three categories: Mildly, Moderately and Severely Symptomatic.

- Category A: Mildly Symptomatic when they have two or more symptoms such as enlarged lymph nodes, liver, or spleen, or recurrent or persistent upper respiratory infections, sinusitis or otitis media.
- Category B: Moderately Symptomatic if they have developed more serious illnesses such as oropharyngeal candidiasis, bacterial meningitis, pneumonia, or sepsis, cardiomyopathy, cytomegalovirus

TABLE 21.2 CD4 Cell Counts Related to Progress of Disease in Children

	AGE OF CHILD		
	Under 12 Months	**1–5 Years**	**6–12 Years**
No evidence of suppression	>1,500 cells/uL	>1,000 cells/uL	>500 cells/uL
Evidence of moderate suppression	750–1,499 cells/uL	500–999 cells/uL	200–499 cells/uL
Severe suppression	<750 cells/uL	<500 cells/uL	<200 cells/uL

Centers for Disease Control. (1997). 1997 USPHS/IDSA guidelines for prevention of opportunistic infections in persons infected with HIV. *Morbidity and Mortality Weekly Report, 46*(12), 1.

infection, hepatitis, herpes simplex virus (HSV) bronchitis, pneumonitis, or esophagitis, herpes zoster (shingles), lymphoid interstitial pneumonia (LIP), pulmonary lymphoid hyperplasia complex, or toxoplasmosis.

- Category C: Severely Symptomatic if they have developed infections such as serious bacterial infections such as septicemia, pneumonia, meningitis, bone or joint infection or abscess of an internal organ or body cavity; candidiasis (esophageal or pulmonary), encephalopathy, herpes simplex lasting over 1 month, histoplasmosis, lymphoma, mycobacterium (tuberculosis) or *Pneumocystis carinii* pneumonia. Unlike adults, children rarely develop Kaposi's sarcoma.

Therapeutic Management. Many perinatally infected infants, whose life expectancy was thought at one time to be much shorter, now have an opportunity for long-term survival. Therapy is a complex regimen of nutrition supplements to prevent loss of weight, vaccines to prevent infections, and antiviral and antibacterial agents to combat HIV virus and opportunistic infections.

NURSING DIAGNOSES AND RELATED INTERVENTIONS

Nursing Diagnosis: Risk for Infection related to decreased immune function.

Outcome Identification: Child will remain free of infection.

Outcome Evaluation: Child's temperature is within normal parameters; no cough or skin lesions are present.

Children with HIV/AIDS and their families must maintain strict personal hygiene (e.g., frequent handwashing) and avoid close contact with anyone who has a respiratory infection to try and prevent the child from contracting dangerous opportunistic infections. When infections do occur, antibiotic and antifungal treatment should be prompt and aggressive. Prophylactic use of the antiviral drug zidovudine (AZT) increases growth and prolongs life (see Drug Highlight: Zidovudine). Many children are placed on prophylactic therapy for *Pneumocystis carinii* pneumonia (trimethoprim-sulfamethoxazole (TMP-SMZ), or aerosolized pentamidine beginning at 6 months of age. Therapy for tuberculosis is by standard antituberculosis drugs: isoniazid or rifampin. Preventing tuberculosis is becoming more difficult than formerly because more strains of tuberculosis have become resistant to these usual drugs.

Children should receive routine immunizations with the killed virus vaccines (all except oral polio and varicella vaccines). If they are exposed to varicella, intravenous varicella zoster immune globulin (VZIG) is prescribed in an attempt to prevent this disease. Yearly influenza vaccinations should begin at 6 months of age. They should receive pneumococcal vaccine at 2 years of age.

Nursing Diagnosis: Risk for ineffective family coping: compromised, related to diagnosis of HIV/AIDS in child.

DRUG HIGHLIGHT

Zidovudine (AZT)

Action: Zidovudine is a thymidine analogue that inhibits the replication of some retroviruses, including HIV.

Pregnancy risk category: C

Dosage: 2 mg/kg every 6 h to infants born to HIV-positive mothers, starting within 12 h of birth to 6 wk of age. 180 mg/m² (720 mg/m²/dose) orally or intravenously every 6 h to children ages 3 mo to 12 y (dosage not to exceed 200 mg every 6 h)

Possible adverse effects: Nausea, loss of appetite, change in taste, paresthesia, headache, fever, agranulocytopenia, and rash

Nursing Implications:

- When administering the drug intravenously, infuse the drug over 60 min to avoid too rapid an infusion.
- Administer the drug around the clock for maximum effectiveness.
- Monitor blood studies frequently for changes.
- Advise child to eat frequent small meals to counteract change in taste and loss of appetite.
- If the child experiences paresthesias, institute safety precautions and instruct the child and parents in measures to prevent injury related to loss of feeling.
- Caution child and parents that AZT does not reduce the risk of HIV transmission. Reinforce hygiene and infection control measures.

Outcome Identification: Family will demonstrate ability to care for child and maintain family functioning within 1 month.

Outcome Evaluation: Parents state ability to continue providing child's physical care; identify outside resources for help with care and decision making.

The diagnosis of HIV/AIDS in an infant or child can prove devastating for a family. When the disease is transmitted maternally, this diagnosis may be the first indication of the existence of HIV/AIDS in the mother and, as such, signals tragedy for the whole family. If the child contracted HIV/AIDS from a contaminated blood transfusion or organ donation (an occurrence less likely now with current protocols for donor screening), the family will feel betrayed and angry. Parents may be unwilling to cooperate with health care providers who, in their minds, are responsible for their child's illness. In any case, the family's coping skills, even if previously healthy, are sure to be seriously compromised. Siblings may be lost in the shuffle of health care appointments and left alone with their fears of contracting the disease themselves. The family's decision about whether to disclose that the child has HIV becomes a major problem. One of the first nursing priorities in the care of such a family should be to help the family reestablish their previous level of functioning so they can turn their attention to their child's emotional and physical care needs and to their own needs as well (Havens et al, 1997).

Physical care requirements for the child with HIV/AIDS may be extensive, depending on the child's symptoms and disease progression. No matter what the child's physical needs, however, love and emotional support are essential to his or her well-being and psychological health. Encourage parents to seek medical care for their child at the first sign of illness or infection to prevent unnecessary hospitalization and pain. Parents or caregivers will need extensive support, education, and anticipatory guidance from nurses and other members of the health care team.

✓ CHECKPOINT QUESTIONS

3. What is the transmission method by which most children acquire HIV/AIDS?
4. Why are many HIV-positive children begun on prophylactic TMP-SMZ?

ALLERGY

Allergic diseases occur as a result of an abnormal antigen-antibody response. Approximately 1 in every 5 children suffer from some form of allergy. Allergic symptoms can be chronic and minor, such as those that occur with seasonal rhinitis, or acute and severe as in an anaphylactic reaction. They can disrupt a child's life and development and the life of the family. When the cause of an allergic response is difficult to pinpoint, the child and parents often become frustrated. Even when the child has a known allergy, symptoms can vary from minor to acute without warning, ultimately disrupting family functioning.

Hypersensitivity

The underlying cause of all allergic disorders appears to be an excessive antigen-antibody response when the invading organism is an allergen rather than a simple immunogen. This is termed a type I response or a **hypersensitivity response** when it happens immediately. It can also occur as a type II, III, or IV response (Table 21-3). Types I, II, and III are mediated by antibodies (humoral response), whereas type IV is mediated by the T cells (cell-mediated response).

Type I: Atopy or Anaphylaxis

Atopy is a hypersensitivity state that is inherited and results in a range of typical illnesses. In atopic disorders, the immune response is activated when IgE antibodies attached to the surface of mast cells bind to an antigen. Mast cells are

TABLE 21.3 Classification of Hypersensitivity Reactions

TYPE	INVOLVED CELL	MECHANISM	EFFECT
I Anaphylaxis	IgE	IgE attached to surface of mast cell triggers release of intracellular granules from mast cells on contact with antigens	Allergies, asthma, atopic dermatitis, anaphylaxis
II Cytotoxic	IgG or IgM	Antigen-antibody reaction leading to antigen destruction; complement is activated	Hemolytic anemia, transfusion reaction, erythroblastosis fetalis
III Immune complex disease	IgG or IgE	Antigen-antibody complexes precipitate; complement is activated leading to inflammatory response	Rheumatoid arthritis, systemic lupus erythematosus
IV Delayed	T lymphocyte	T cells combine with antigen to induce inflammatory reactions by direct cell involvement or release of lymphokines	Contact dermatitis, transplant graft reaction

specialized cells found in connective tissue, the mucous membranes, and skin. The IgE molecule triggers these to release intracellular granules. These contain histamine, a slow-reacting substance of anaphylaxis (SRS-A), and chemotaxic substances (substances to draw leukocytes into the area). Histamine causes peripheral vasodilation and permeability of blood vessels. This leads to vascular congestion and edema. SRS-A causes extreme bronchial constriction and reduced vasodilation and permeability. **Anaphylaxis** is an acute reaction characterized by extreme vasodilation that leads to circulatory shock.

Type II: Cytotoxic Response

In a **cytotoxic** (cell-destroying) **response,** cells are detected as foreign and immunoglobulins directly attack and destroy the cells without harming surrounding tissue. Tumor cells may be destroyed by this process. Why this immune response fails when malignant cells begin to proliferate is not understood. Current research is attempting to devise ways to activate the natural immune response as a method of destroying malignant cells. Care of the child with a malignancy (neoplasm) is discussed in Chapter 32.

Type III: Immune Complex

A type III response is an IgG- or IgE-mediated antigen-antibody complex reaction that involves complement and initiates the inflammatory response. Complement reactions that persist beyond the usual inhibition may serve as the basis for many of the autoimmune illnesses such as glomerulonephritis and systemic lupus erythematosus (see Chapter 25). Serum sickness also occurs as a result of a type III response.

Type IV: Cell-Mediated Hypersensitivity

In a delayed hypersensitivity response, T cells react with antigens and release lymphokines to call macrophages into the area. An inflammatory response occurs that helps to destroy the foreign tissue. A tuberculin test is an example of this. Redness and induration of the site do not begin initially but only after approximately 12 hours from the injection. The reaction peaks in 24 hours to 72 hours (a delayed response).

Contact dermatitis is another example of a delayed hypersensitivity response. Certain substances such as cosmetics, household products, or cured leather alter the protein of skin cells so that they become an antigen, or the foreign substance combines with the protein (hapten formation) to become an antigenic protein. Lymphocytes and macrophages infiltrate the area and attempt to destroy the offending protein. Redness and vesicles may occur. Pruritus may be intense.

Assessment of Allergy in Children

History

Taking a health history of an allergic child is time consuming because many factors must be considered. A family history is important because there are familial tendencies with allergic diseases. Also, the exact symptoms of the allergy are important in helping to identify the allergen—rhinitis is probably due to an airborne antigen; **urticaria** (swelling and itching) is often caused by ingested antigens; and atopic dermatitis (often a rash) must be from something that contacts the skin in that area. The time of the year that the allergy occurs also may give a clue to its cause. If the child's allergy exists all year, the antigen must be one that is present all year (house dust, pet dander, or a common food). If it occurs in the spring, it may be due to a tree pollen; in summer, a grass pollen; if it occurs just in August, ragweed is a prime suspect as the offending antigen.

Many symptoms of allergy are vague, described as "colds all winter," "itching," or "runny nose." Listen carefully to recognize that, although no one symptom is acute, together such symptoms can interfere with a child's comfort, school experience, and long-term health (see Managing and Delegating Unlicensed Assistive Personnel). Helping parents and the child to keep a chart of when symptoms are worse and better is often an aid to identifying a specific allergen. Children with allergic rhinitis (hay fever), for example, have more symptoms on a day when the wind is blowing than when it is not, and fewer symptoms after a rainstorm than before (the rain washes pollen out of the air). Children are often poor reporters because they cannot remember clearly whether they had the same rhinitis and watery eye symptoms last summer as they do this summer. A record that details when symptoms start—for example, on arising, or only after the child reaches school—may help to identify an allergen.

Laboratory Testing

Few laboratory tests are helpful in establishing a diagnosis of allergy. A determination of IgE serum antibodies can be made. Most children with an allergy will have an increased eosinophil count. Five percent or more of eosinophils on a differential count, or an eosinophil count of 250 or more cells per cubic millimeter, is significant. Another main cause of an increased eosinophil count is invasion by ova or para-

MANAGING AND DELEGATING UNLICENSED ASSISTIVE PERSONNEL

Unlicensed assistive personnel often take children's vital signs in acute care and ambulatory settings. While doing so, they often talk to the parents about the reason the child is being seen. In many instances, a child's allergic symptoms are not the reason the child is being seen or treated. These symptoms are a major concern for the parents and child, however. Teach unlicensed assistive personnel to report these secondary concerns to primary health care providers so therapy for them can be instituted. Helping parents understand environmental control measures can be an important role for unlicensed assistive personnel as long as they are instructed in this area. In addition, be sure unlicensed assistive personnel understand the importance of using standard precautions, especially when caring for the child with HIV/AIDS.

site. Thus, a stool specimen for ova and parasites is generally collected to rule out these problems as the cause of the increased eosinophil count. A radioallergosorbent test (RAST) may be ordered. This is an indirect radioimmunoassay in which the child's serum IgE is allowed to react with specific allergens impregnated in laboratory disks.

Skin Testing

Skin testing is done to detect the presence of IgE in the skin, or to isolate an antigen (allergen) to which a child is sensitive. When an allergen is introduced into the child's skin, and the child is sensitive to that allergen, a wheal or flare response appears at the site of the test. This is due to the release of histamine, which leads to local vasodilation. Because this reaction appears quickly, the test should be read in 20 minutes. Systemic or aerosol administration of an antihistamine or a theophylline derivative will inhibit the flare response, so the child should not receive these drugs for 8 hours before skin testing. Corticosteroid therapy does not affect immediate skin reactivity and so may be continued during skin testing.

Skin testing may be done by either a scratch or an intracutaneous injection technique. Scratch testing is done by placing a drop of allergen solution on the skin after the area has been washed with alcohol. The skin under the drop of liquid is then scratched with a sterile needle. A relatively concentrated extract of allergen must be used for scratch testing because little allergen enters the child's skin. This makes it the safest form of skin testing and is used with children who are thought to be highly sensitive to the solution being tested.

Intracutaneous injections are done by injecting a small amount of an aqueous solution of allergen below the epidermis of the child's skin. This is usually done on the child's forearm, so that if a sensitivity reaction does occur, a tourniquet can be applied proximal to the test site to prevent further absorption of the antigen. If the categories to be tested are extensive, the back can be used. Solutions used for intracutaneous injections are more dilute than those used for scratch testing (1:500 dilution compared with 1:5 for scratch testing). This means that the allergen extracts are not interchangeable from a group prepared for scratch testing to a group prepared for intracutaneous injections (or vice versa).

Because intracutaneous injections are given just below the epidermal layer of skin, they are almost painless. This is the same phenomenon as passing a needle or pin under the top layer of skin of a fingertip, a trick every school-age child does at least once to the horror of friends. The child needs a great deal of support for skin testing, however, because it looks as if it will be painful and the sight of an injection is frightening.

After both scratch and intracutaneous testing, if the child is allergic to the test solution, a wheal and erythema (redness) will occur at the test site (Figure 21-4). The size of the reaction is measured and graded as 1+ to 4+ or as slight, moderate, or marked. The allergens chosen for skin testing will depend on the child's individual symptoms. Few children need more than 30 test media tried. This is because most allergies are worse at certain times of the year, and only those allergens prevalent at that time of year need to be evaluated.

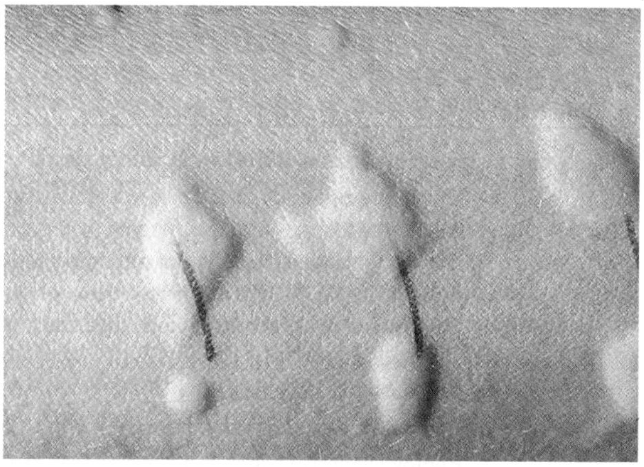

FIGURE 21.4 Allergy skin testing. Note the positive reaction.

Have a syringe filled with 1 mL of epinephrine (Adrenalin) 1:1000 on hand to counteract an unexpected, but entirely possible, anaphylactic reaction from skin testing. Epinephrine is given subcutaneously in doses of 0.01 mg/kg, up to 0.5 mg. Be sure the epinephrine is drawn up and readily available should an anaphylactic reaction occur. Be certain all children stay in the health care setting for at least 30 minutes after skin testing so they are there during the time a reaction to the injected allergen is most apt to occur.

Skin testing with food extracts is ineffective. Food allergies are best identified by eliminating a suspected food from the diet and observing the child to see if there is an improvement in symptoms. After a time of improvement, the food is reintroduced. If it is one to which the child is allergic, symptoms, absent while it was omitted, will return with its reintroduction (often called "rechallenging").

Therapeutic Management

No matter what the symptoms of a child's allergy, there are three goals for therapy: (1) reduce the child's exposure to the allergen, (2) hyposensitize the child to produce a state of increased clinical **tolerance** (a state of not responding) to the allergen, and (3) modify the child's response to the allergen with a pharmacologic agent.

Reducing the child's exposure to the allergen is possible when the offending allergen is a drug, a food, or an irritant. Reducing exposure is much more difficult when children are found to be allergic to allergens such as molds, dust, feathers, or other substances found almost everywhere.

Environmental Control

Environmental control means that as many allergens as possible that are found almost everywhere are removed from children's environment. Common measures of environmental control are shown in Table 21-4 and Empowering the Family. Some parents carry out instructions to reduce potential allergens in their house without difficulty. For others, the process seems too involved to undertake. Parents need to understand that environmental control can make a great deal of difference in their child's symptoms (see Enhancing Communication). If just environmental control is effective with their child, this will be preferable to hy-

Graft, D. F. (1996). Stinging insect hypersensitivity in children. *Current Opinion in Pediatrics, 8*(6), 597.

Havens, P. L., et al. (1997). Structure of a primary care support system to coordinate comprehensive care for children and families infected/affected by human immunodeficiency virus in a managed care environment. *Pediatric Infectious Disease Journal, 16*(2), 211.

Hollingsworth, H. (1997). Preventing insect sting anaphylaxis. *Journal of the American Medical Association, 277*(15), 1196.

Hong, R. (1997). Combined immunodeficiency diseases. In Johnson, K. B., & Oski, K. A. *Oski's essential pediatrics.* Philadelphia: Lippincott.

Kerner, J. A. (1995). Formula allergy and intolerance. *Gastroenterology Clinics of North America, 24*(1), 1.

Knowles, S., Shapiro, L., & Shear, N. H. (1997). Serious dermatologic reactions in children. *Current Opinion in Pediatrics, 9*(4), 388.

Kuhn, L. et al. (1998). Long-term survival of children with human immunodeficiency virus infection in New York City. *American Journal of Epidemiology, 147*(9), 846.

Lederman, H. M. (1997). Disorders of humoral immunity. In Johnson, K. B., & Oski, K. A. *Oski's essential pediatrics.* Philadelphia: Lippincott.

Lederman, H. M., & Winkelstein, J. A. (1997). The primary immunodeficiency diseases. In Johnson, K. B., & Oski, K. A. *Oski's essential pediatrics.* Philadelphia: Lippincott.

Mudd, K. E., & Noone, S. A. (1995). Management of severe food allergy in the school setting. *Journal of School Nursing, 11*(3), 30.

Roul, S., et al. (1996). Footwear contact dermatitis in children. *Contact Dermatitis, 35*(6), 334.

Sampson, H. A. (1997a). Atopic dermatitis. In Johnson, K. B., & Oski, K. A. *Oski's essential pediatrics.* Philadelphia: Lippincott.

Sampson, H. A. (1997b). Food allergies. In Johnson, K. B., & Oski, K. A. *Oski's essential pediatrics.* Philadelphia: Lippincott.

Schuberth, K. C. (1997). Insect sting allergy. In Johnson, K. B., & Oski, K. A. *Oski's essential pediatrics.* Philadelphia: Lippincott.

Scott, G. P., & Parks, W. P. (1997). Pediatric AIDS. In Johnson, K. B., & Oski, K. A. *Oski's essential pediatrics.* Philadelphia: Lippincott.

Scott, G. S., & Layton, T. L. (1997). Epidemiologic principles in studies of infectious disease outcomes: pediatric HIV as a model. *Journal of Communication Disorders, 30*(4), 303.

Simons, F. E. (1997). Allergic rhinitis and associated disorders. In Johnson, K. B., & Oski, K. A. *Oski's essential pediatrics.* Philadelphia: Lippincott.

Weston, W. L. (1997). Contact dermatitis in children. *Current Opinion in Pediatrics, 9*(4), 372.

Winkelstein, G. A. (1997). Complement deficiencies. In Johnson, K. B., & Oski, K. A. *Oski's essential pediatrics.* Philadelphia: Lippincott.

SUGGESTED READINGS

Chandra, R. K. (1997). Food hypersensitivity and allergic disease: a selective review. *American Journal of Clinical Nutrition, 66*(2), 526.

Duggan, C. (1996). HIV infection in children. *Paediatric Nursing, 8*(10), 32.

Dykewicz, M. S. (1996). Anaphylaxis and stinging insect reactions. *Comprehensive Therapy, 22*(9), 579.

Fireman, P. (1997). Otitis media and its relation to allergic rhinitis. *Allergy Asthma Proceedings, 18*(3), 135.

Koblenzer, P. J. (1996). Parental issues in the treatment of chronic infantile eczema. *Dermatologic Clinics, 14*(3), 423.

Moss, H. et al. (1998). A preliminary study of factors associated with psychological adjustment and disease course in school-age children infected with the human immunodeficiency virus. *Journal of Developmental and Behavioral Pediatrics, 19*(1), 18.

Mudd, K. E. (1995). Indoor environmental allergy: a guide to environmental controls. *Pediatric Nursing, 21*(6), 534.

Oehling, A., et al. (1997). Skin manifestations and immunological parameters in childhood food allergy. *Journal of Investigational Allergology and Clinical Immunology, 7*(3), 155.

Storms, W. W. (1997). Treatment of allergic rhinitis: effect of allergic rhinitis and antihistamines on performance. *Allergy Asthma Proceedings, 18*(2), 59.

Zhai, H., et al. (1997). Patch testing versus history in poison ivy/oak dermatitis. *Contact Dermatitis, 36*(4), 226.

Nursing Care of the Child With an Infectious Disorder

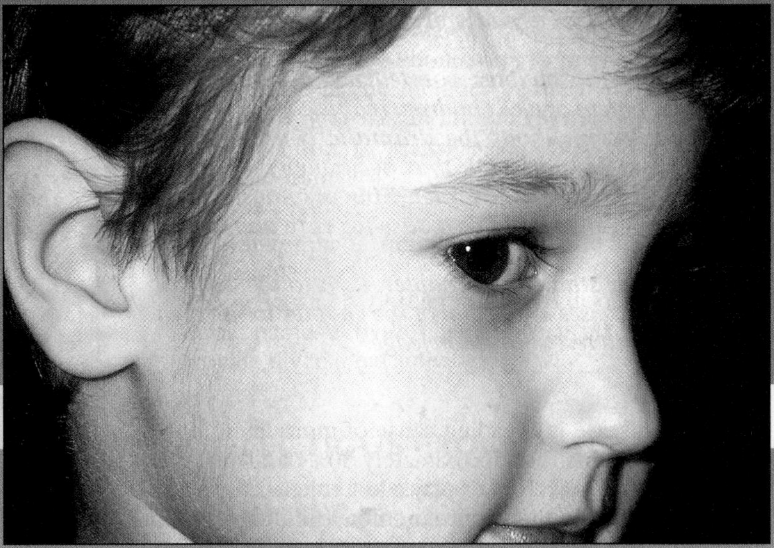

22

CHAPTER

Key Terms

- anaerobic
- antitoxin
- catarrhal stage
- chain of infection
- communicability
- complement
- convalescent period
- enanthem
- exanthem
- exotoxin
- fomites
- gamma globulin
- immune serum
- incubation period
- interferon
- Koplik's spots
- means of transmission
- pathogen
- portal of entry
- portal of exit
- prodromal period
- reservoir
- septicemia
- toxoid

Objectives

After mastering the contents of this chapter, you should be able to:

1. Describe the causes and course of common infectious disorders of childhood.
2. Assess the child with an infectious disorder.
3. Formulate nursing diagnoses for the child with an infectious disorder.
4. Establish appropriate outcomes for the care of a child with an infectious disorder.
5. Plan nursing care for the child with an infectious disorder.
6. Implement nursing care specific to the child with an infectious disorder.
7. Evaluate outcomes for achievement and effectiveness of care for the child with an infectious disorder.
8. Identify National Health Goals related to infectious disorders in children that nurses could be instrumental in helping the nation achieve.
9. Identify areas of nursing care related to children with infectious disease that could benefit from additional nursing research.
10. Use critical thinking to analyze ways that care of the child with an infectious disorder be more family centered.
11. Integrate knowledge of infectious diseases and nursing process to achieve quality child health nursing care.

Systemic infections usually have a **prodromal period,** or a time between the beginning of nonspecific symptoms and specific symptoms. Nonspecific symptoms include lethargy, low-grade fever, fatigue, and malaise. During a prodromal period, infectious diseases spread readily through communities to any susceptible children. Children are infectious (capable of spreading the microorganisms to others) during this time, and because their symptoms are so vague, they do not generally take any precautions against spreading disease. Prodromal stages are generally short, ranging from hours to a few days.

Illness is the stage during which specific symptoms are evident. Most illnesses have local symptoms related to the body organ affected, and also systemic symptoms that affect the entire body, such as fever, increased white blood cell count, or headache. Many childhood infections have an accompanying rash on the skin (exanthem) or mucous membrane (**enanthem**).

The **convalescent period** is the interval between when symptoms begin to fade and the return to full wellness. Because fatigue is often an accompanying symptom of infection, the convalescent period, or the time until full energy is restored, is often longer than anticipated.

Chain of Infection

Chain of infection refers to the method by which organisms are spread and enter a new individual to cause disease. An important method of preventing infection is to break a chain of infection. Nurses are instrumental in teaching parents how to prevent the spread of infection in homes and how to carry out safe practices so infection does not spread in health care facilities.

Reservoir

The **reservoir** is the container or place in which organisms grow and reproduce. The source of a human pathogen could be another human with the disease, a human carrying the disease, or an animal. Immunizations are helpful in limiting the use of children as reservoirs for organism growth.

Portal of Exit

The **portal of exit** is the method by which organisms leave a child's body. This could be by upper respiratory excretions, secretions, feces, vomitus, saliva, urine, vaginal secretions, blood, or lesion secretions (Table 22-1). To break a chain of infection at this point, follow good aseptic technique and prescribed transmission-based precautions such as wearing a gown, gloves, or mask as appropriate. Teach parents good handwashing technique after the use of a bathroom or after handling diapers. Supply an adequate number of disposable tissues so children can limit droplet or airborne spread.

Means of Transmission

The **means of transmission** of pathogens can be by direct or indirect contact; by **fomites,** or common vehicle transmission (i.e., inanimate objects such as soil, food, water, bedding, towels, combs, or drinking glasses); or by insects, rats, or other vermin (*vectors*). Direct contact implies body-to-body touching. Sexually transmitted diseases (STDs) and skin disorders are spread this way. The most common means of indirect contact is the spread of mouth and nose secretions (*droplet infection*) through talking, sneezing, coughing, breathing, and kissing. Some droplets containing pathogenic organisms are spread immediately to another individual in this way. Some droplets fall to the ground, where the organisms dry and then are spread by dust. If small, the organisms become suspended in the air (airborne transmission) and can infect people from a distance. The major childhood exan-

TABLE 22.1 Methods by Which Infections Spread

PORTAL OF EXIT	MEANS OF TRANSMISSION	PORTAL OF ENTRY	PREVENTION MEASURES
Blood	Arthropod vectors	Injection into bloodstream	Decreasing vector incidence
	Blood sampling		Careful handling of blood sampling equipment
	Transfusion		Screening of transfused blood for organisms such as human immunodeficiency virus (HIV) or hepatitis B
Respiratory secretions	Airborne droplets	Respiratory tract	Wearing mask
	Fomites		Droplet precautions
			Airborne precautions
			Hand washing
Feces	Water, food	Gastrointestinal tract	Hand washing before eating, after using bathroom or handling diapers
	Fomites		
	Vectors such as flies		
Exudate from lesions	Direct contact	Skin, mucous membrane	Contact precautions
	Contact with soiled dressings		Self-screening for sexual contacts
			Gloves

FOCUS ON CULTURAL COMPETENCE

Some cultures are much more aware of the role of communicable disease in childhood illnesses than others, so advocate for all children to be immunized against these disorders. Even if awareness about the danger of disease spread exists, however, it doesn't mean that all people in a community are conscientious about having their children immunized. Other factors such as cost and convenience and ethical beliefs are also important.

Some religious groups, such as the Amish, discourage immunizations. In these communities, the prevalence of illnesses such as measles can rise to high numbers. Being aware that immunization rates are not consistent from place to place aids in understanding the importance of planning health education and health surveillance based on individual community needs.

passive immunity). Like naturally acquired passive antibodies, these last only approximately 6 weeks. A child who is susceptible to tetanus, for example, would receive tetanus antibodies after a stab wound.

Types of Immunizations

Vaccines are the solutions used to immunize children to provide artificially acquired active or passive immunity. They are prepared in a number of forms.

Attenuated vaccines are made from live organisms that have been reduced in virulence to a point where they will not cause active disease but will ensure a good antibody response. Because they are strong and effective solutions, a single dose usually provides a good degree of active immunity.

Because some bacteria, such as diphtheria, cause disease by producing a toxin, the vaccine against such a disease, a **toxoid,** is actually an extract of the toxin with reduced virulence. The antibodies for toxin-producing bacteria are **antitoxins.** A solution given for passive immunity against diphtheria is an antitoxin.

Gamma globulin is serum obtained from the pooled blood of many people. Because it comes from many people, it contains the antibodies of many people and probably has antibody protection against measles, rubella, poliomyelitis, varicella, and infectious hepatitis among many other infectious diseases. It offers artificially acquired passive immunity.

Immune serum is serum removed from horses that have been given a disease. The usual preparations used are those against diphtheria, tetanus, the pit viper snake, and the black widow spider. Because these antibodies are prepared from horse serum, before administration, be certain to skin-test a child to ensure he or she is not allergic to horse serum. Equine serums are being replaced by synthetic preparations to avoid exposure to horse serum and still provide passive immunity.

Administration of Vaccines

The schedule of immunizations for children recommended by the American Academy of Pediatrics (AAP) is shown in Table 22-3.

Diphtheria, Tetanus, Pertussis (DTaP) Vaccines. Diphtheria, tetanus toxoid, and acellular pertussis (whooping cough) vaccine are supplied in a single vial as DTaP and given in one intramuscular injection. It is recommended that children receive a primary series of four immunizations with the vaccine (2, 4, 6 and 15 months). A booster is then given between ages 4 and 6 years, or before entry into school. Diphtheria and tetanus toxoid (Td vaccine) is given at 11 to 12 years, then every 10 years thereafter.

In the past, there was a great deal of controversy about the safety of the diphtheria-tetanus-pertussis vaccine, most of it directed at the pertussis component. Severe reactions, such as high fever, persistent crying, and, rarely, seizures were reported. For this reason, the former DTP vaccine has been modified to DTaP or contains a less reactive pertussis component. Side effects can still include drowsiness, fretfulness, low-grade fever, and redness and pain at the injection site.

Some parents, alerted by hearing about reactions to the former vaccine, refuse immunizations for their children. This is their right. However, children who are not immunized against pertussis (unless there is a medical or moral contraindication) may be refused admittance to preschool or beginning school programs. Parents should be informed of this when they refuse to sign consent for immunization.

Pertussis vaccination is contraindicated in children who have a progressive or unstable neurologic disorder or who have had a severe allergic reaction to pertussis in a previous DTP vaccination. If pertussis immunization is contraindicated, the DT, or diphtheria-tetanus vaccine is substituted.

Pertussis is not generally given after age 6 because the side effects of the vaccine may be more common in older children. The diphtheria toxoid is still given to children older than age 6 years, but the adult or more diluted form (d) is used after this age. After the fifth dose of DTaP, the tetanus and diluted form of diphtheria (Td) is recommended to be given every 10 years.

Polio Vaccines. Oral polio vaccine (OPV) and inactivated polio vaccine (IPV) contain all three strains of poliovirus and are both available for use in the United States. The oral form of polio vaccine (Sabin's vaccine or OPV) is preferred for routine immunization, not for its convenience as most parents believe, but because it produces longer-acting immunity than the killed injectable type (Salk vaccine). However, OPV, which consists of live attenuated poliovirus, should never be administered to any child who is immunosuppressed; this could cause a rare form of paralytic poliomyelitis. Because OPV is shed in the stools, it should not be given to any child who may come in close contact with an immunosuppressed per-

TABLE 22.3 Recommended Childhood Immunization Schedule, United States, January–December 1998[1]

Vaccines are listed under the routinely recommended ages. Bars indicate the range of acceptable ages for immunization. Catch-up immunizations should be done during any visit when possible. Shaded ovals indicate vaccines to be given (if not previously done so) during the early adolescent visit.

	AGE										
VACCINE	*Birth*	*1 mo*	*2 mos*	*4 mos*	*6 mos*	*12 mos*	*15 mos*	*18 mos*	*4–6 yrs*	*11–12 yrs*	*14–16 yrs*
Hepatitis B[2,3]	Hep B-1 (bar: birth–2 mos)										
		Hep B-2 (bar: 1–4 mos)			Hep B-3 (bar: 6–18 mos)					Hep B[3] (oval)	
Diphtheria, Tetanus, Pertussis[4]			DTaP or DTP	DTaP or DTP	DTaP or DTP		DTaP or DTP[4] (bar: 15–18 mos)		DTaP or DTP	Td (bar: 11–16 yrs)	
H influenzae type b[5]			Hib	Hib	Hib	Hib (bar: 12–15 mos)					
Polio[6]			Polio[6]	Polio	Polio[6] (bar: 6–18 mos)				Polio		
Measles, Mumps, Rubella[7]						MMR (bar: 12–15 mos)			MMR[7]	MMR[7] (oval)	
Varicella[8]						Var (bar: 12–18 mos)				Var[8] (oval)	

[1] This schedule indicates the recommended age for routine administration of currently licensed childhood vaccines. Some combination vaccines are available and may be used whenever administration of all components of the vaccine is indicated. Providers should consult the manufacturers' package inserts for detailed recommendations.

[2] *Infants born to HBsAg-negative mothers* should receive 2.5 μg of Merck vaccine (Recombivax HB) or 10 μg of SmithKline Beecham (SB) vaccine (Engerix-B). The second dose should be administered at least 1 mo after the first dose. The third dose should be given at least 2 mo after the second, but not before 6 mo of age.

Infants born to HBsAg-positive mothers should receive 0.5 mL of hepatitis B immune globulin (HBIG) within 12 h of birth, and either 5 μg of Merck vaccine (Recombivax HB) or 10 μg of SB vaccine (Engerix-B) at a separate site. The second dose is recommended at 1–2 mo of age and the third dose at 6 mo of age.

Infants born to mothers whose HBsAg status is unknown should receive either 5 μg of Merck vaccine (Recombivax HB) or 10 μg of SB vaccine (Engerix-B) within 12 h of birth. The second dose of vaccine is recommended at 1 mo of age and the third dose at 6 mo of age. Blood should be drawn at the time of delivery to determine the mother's HBsAg status; if it is positive, the infant should receive HBIG as soon as possible (no later than 1 wk of age). The dosage and timing of subsequent vaccine doses should be based on the mother's HBsAg status.

[3] Children and adolescents who have not been vaccinated against hepatitis B in infancy may begin the series during any visit. Those who have not previously received three doses of hepatitis B vaccine should initiate or complete the series during the 11- to 12-y visit, and unvaccinated older adolescents should be vaccinated whenever possible. The second dose should be administered at least 1 mo after the first dose, and the third dose should be administered at least 4 mo after the first dose and at least 2 mo after the second dose.

[4] DTaP (diphtheria and tetanus toxoids and acellular pertussis vaccine) is the preferred vaccine for all doses in the vaccination series, including completion of the series in children who have received one or more doses of whole-cell DTP vaccine. Whole-cell DTP is an acceptable alternative to DTaP. The fourth dose (DTP or DTaP) may be administered as early as 12 mo of age, provided 6 mo have elapsed since the third dose, and if the child is unlikely to return at 15–18 mo. Td (tetanus and diphtheria toxoids) is recommended at 11–12 y of age if at least 5 y have elapsed since the last dose of DTP, DTaP or DT. Subsequent routine Td boosters are recommended every 10 y.

[5] Three *H influenzae* type b (Hib) conjugate vaccines are licensed for infant use. If PRP-OMP (PedvaxHIB [Merck]) is administered at 2 and 4 mo of age, a dose at 6 mo is not required.

[6] Two poliovirus vaccines are currently licensed in the United States: inactivated poliovirus vaccine (IPV) and oral poliovirus vaccine (OPV). The following schedules are all acceptable to the ACIP, the AAP, and the AAFP. Parents and providers may choose among these options:

1. Two doses of IPV followed by two doses of OPV.
2. Four doses of IPV.
3. Four doses of OPV.

The ACIP recommends two doses of IPV at 2 and 4 mo of age followed by two doses of OPV at 12–18 mo and 4–6 years of age. IPV is the only poliovirus vaccine recommended for immunocompromised persons and their household contacts.

[7] The second dose of MMR is recommended routinely at 4–6 y of age but may be administered during any visit, provided at least 1 mo has elapsed since receipt of the first dose and that both doses are administered beginning at or after 12 mo of age. Those who have not *previously* received the second dose should complete the schedule no later than the 11- to 12-y visit.

[8] Susceptible children may receive varicella vaccine (Var) at any visit after the first birthday, and those who lack a reliable history of chickenpox should be immunized during the 11- to 12-y visit. Susceptible children 13 y of age or older should receive two doses, at least 1 mo apart.

Approved by the Advisory Committee on Immunization Practices (ACIP), the American Academy of Pediatrics (AAP), and the American Academy of Family Physicians (AAFP).

son, because of the possible risk, although small, for these contacts to develop the same OPV-paralytic disease.

OPV or IPV is administered in a primary series of three doses and given along with DTaP at 2, 4, and 6 to 18 months of age. A fourth booster dose is given between the ages of 4 and 6 years, before school entry.

Measles, Mumps, Rubella (MMR) Vaccines. Measles-mumps-rubella vaccine is furnished in one vial and routinely administered as a single injection. A first dose is given around the time of the 15-month checkup. A second dose of MMR is generally given between the ages of 4 to 6 years or, if they did not receive the 4- to 6-year dose, at 11 to 12 years. It is usually recommended that the measles vaccine not be administered to children younger than age 15 months because children receive a great deal of passive immunity to this disease from their mothers across the placenta. Until this passive immunity has faded, the injected vaccine will be neutralized by passive antibodies and no immunity will result. For the same reason, children who have recently received immune globulin or other blood products that contain antibodies should defer the MMR for 3 months because the passively acquired antibodies could interfere with the child's immune response to the vaccine.

Side effects of the vaccine include transient rashes and a fever, which may begin 5 to 12 days after vaccination and last several days. Adverse reactions include joint pain, low-grade fever, rash, and lymphadenopathy 5 to 12 days after vaccination.

Children should be skin-tested for tuberculosis before measles vaccine administration because measles virus can cause tuberculosis to become systemic. Tuberculosis skin tests may show false-negative reactions if given shortly after measles immunization (a child who has active tuberculosis will be wrongly identified as not having it).

Hepatitis Vaccine. The vaccine for hepatitis B (HBV) is recommended for all infants in the United States. Those born of HBsAg-negative mothers should receive the first dose in the newborn period, a second dose at 1 month and a third dose after 6 months of age. Those infants born of HBsAg-positive mothers receive hepatitis B immune globulin within 12 hours of birth plus HBV. A second dose of HBV is given at 1 to 2 months and a third dose at 6 months. If the mother's HBsAg status is unknown, infants should receive the vaccine within 12 hours of birth with the second dose at 1 month of age, and the third dose at 6 months of age. Children who did not receive the vaccine at birth may begin the series at any well-child visit. In addition, HBV immunization is recommended for those population groups who are at increased risk for contracting hepatitis B infection, including (but not limited to) health care workers with significant exposure to blood, clients receiving hemodialysis, those with hemophilia and others receiving clotting factor concentrates, illicit injectable drug users, and sexually active individuals with multiple sexual partners.

Two hepatitis B vaccines are licensed for use in the United States (Recombivax and Engerix-B). The dose varies depending on the formulation being used and the age and immune status of the recipient.

***Haemophilus influenzae* Type B Vaccines.** *H. influenzae* type b conjugate vaccines (Hib) protect against *H. influenzae* bacteria. Several formulations of this vaccine are available, and three of them are currently licensed for use in infancy. Depending on the individual vaccine, they are administered in a three-dose regimen at 2, 4, and 15 months or in a four-dose regimen, ordinarily at 2, 4, 6, and 12 to 15 months. Local reactions include tenderness at the injection site. Systemic reactions such as crying and fever have been reported (Kaplan, 1997).

Varicella Vaccine. Varicella (chickenpox) vaccine was a difficult vaccine to develop because of the complex structure of the herpes-zoster virus. It is an important vaccine because, once a generation of children has been successfully immunized, it will mark the end of common childhood diseases. Infants may receive varicella vaccine at any visit after their first birthday (usually scheduled at 12 to 18 months). Those who lack a reliable history of chickenpox should be immunized during the 11- to 12-year visit. Children 13 years of age or older should receive two doses, at least 1 month apart.

Assessment. Children who are seriously ill should not receive immunizations. A slight upper respiratory tract infection (a stuffy nose with no fever), however, is not a contraindication. So many infants and preschoolers have common cold symptoms (the average toddler has 10 to 12 colds a year) that if children are not immunized at health maintenance visits when they have slight cold symptoms, they will never receive basic immunizations.

Assess well children at health maintenance visits and assess the immunization status of ill children at clinic or hospital admission to identify those who need immunizations updated. Because children with chronic illness may be hospitalized when an injection is due, such children often fall behind schedule. Children who miss the scheduled time for an immunization do not have the series started over but are simply continued where they left off.

Primary care providers may choose to alter the sequence of immunization schedules if specific infections are prevalent at the time. For example, measles vaccine might be given on a first health maintenance visit (providing a child is older than age 14 months) if an epidemic were currently underway in the community.

Be sure to assess each child's health status before administering any vaccine. Children who are immunosuppressed, who are receiving corticosteroids, or who are receiving chemotherapy or radiation therapy should not receive live virus vaccines. The live attenuated viruses such as measles, rubella, oral polio, and mumps also must not be given to girls who are pregnant because these vaccines could cross the placenta causing actual disease in the fetus.

Preparation and Storage. Be careful to follow manufacturer's recommendations for storage and handling of vaccines (e.g., whether to expose to light or whether to refrigerate). Failure to follow these precautions may significantly reduce the potency and effectiveness of vaccines.

Although measles, mumps, and rubella vaccines are prepared from chick embryo cultures, egg sensitivities are not likely to occur because egg albumin and yolk components of the egg are absent from the culture. Children with egg allergy should have their allergist's permission for immunization, however, to rule out the possibility of a hypersensitivity reaction (Bruno et al, 1997).

Parent Education. A major reason that parents do not bring children for routine immunizations is that they do not know what is required. Fully inform the parents and, when old enough, the children about what immunizations they are being given and what side effects may be expected. Children may develop a low-grade fever after immunization. Counsel parents to give acetaminophen (Tylenol) or children's ibuprofen for a fever of more than 101°F (38.4°C).

Parents should report any untoward symptoms of immunization, such as high fever. Unfavorable reactions are most likely to occur within a few hours or days of administration. With live attenuated virus vaccines, viruses can multiply, so reactions may occur up to 30 days later. With rubella vaccine, a reaction (serum sickness) may occur up to 60 days later.

The date, type of vaccine, vaccine manufacturer, lot number, and name and address of the provider must be recorded so that, if a vaccine reaction should occur, the instance can be investigated. Make a copy and urge parents to keep such records at home as well. They will need this information to admit their child to school and in the event of an epidemic of a particular disease. They will need to know their child's record of tetanus immunization if their child should receive a puncture wound so the correct therapy can be given (Ferson, 1995).

✔ **CHECKPOINT QUESTIONS**

3. At what months do children typically receive DTaP vaccine?
4. What is the usual time for varicella immunization?

Preventing the Spread of Infections

Nosocomial infections, or infections that are contracted while in the hospital, represent a major threat to hospitalized children, a threat that nurses can play a major role in combating. Nurses and other health care providers must also take precautions to protect themselves from acquiring communicable diseases, including HIV and hepatitis. Standard precautions recommended by the Centers for Disease Control (CDC) are summarized in Table 22-4.

The overall rate of nosocomial, or hospital-acquired, infection in children is between 0.2% and 7%. Children younger than age 2 years, children with a nutritional deficit, those who are immunosuppressed, those who have indwelling vascular lines or catheters, those on multiple antibiotic therapy, or those who remain in the hospital for longer than 72 hours are at highest risk for contracting a nosocomial infection. Nurses provide a line of defense against infection when they always adhere to strict aseptic techniques, such as frequent and thorough handwashing, and by following protective transmission-based precautions when indicated (Box 22-1).

TABLE 22.4 Standard Precautions to Prevent Infection

OBJECT	PROCEDURE
Hands	Hands should always be washed before and after contact with clients, even when gloves have been worn; hands should be washed immediately after removing gloves. If hands come in contact with blood, body fluid, secretions, excretions and contaminated items, they should be washed immediately with soap and water. It may be necessary to wash hands between tasks and procedures on the same client to prevent cross-contamination
Gloves	Gloves should be worn when contact with blood, body fluid, secretions, excretions, or contaminated items is anticipated
Gowns	Gowns or plastic aprons are indicated if blood spattering is likely
Masks, goggles and face shields	These should be worn if aerosolization or splattering is likely to occur, such as in certain dental and surgical procedures, wound irrigations, postmortem examinations, and bronchoscopy
Sharp objects	Sharp objects should be handled in such a manner to prevent accidental cuts or punctures; used needles should not be bent, broken, reinserted into their original sheath, or unnecessarily handled; they should be discarded intact immediately after use into an impervious needle-disposal box, which should be readily accessible; all needle-stick accidents, mucosal splashes, and contamination of open wounds with blood or body fluids should be reported immediately to the department supervisor and an accident report should be filed with employee health
Blood spills	Blood spills should be cleaned up promptly with an agency-designated disinfectant solution such as 5.25% sodium hypochlorite diluted 1 : 10 with water
Blood specimens	Blood specimens should be considered biohazardous and be so labeled
Resuscitation	To minimize the need for emergency mouth-to-mouth resuscitation, mouthpieces, resuscitation bags, and other ventilatory devices should be located strategically and available for use in areas where the need for resuscitation is predictable

Garner, J. S. (1996). Guidelines for isolation precautions in hospitals. *Infection Control and Hospital Epidemiology, 17*(1), 66.

BOX 22.1

STANDARD AND TRANSMISSION-BASED PRECAUTIONS

Standard precautions reduce the risk of transmission of bloodborne or other body fluid pathogens. They should be used during the care of all patients.

Transmission-Based Precautions

Transmission-based precautions are designed for patients documented or suspected of being infected with transmissible pathogens for which additional precautions beyond standard precautions are needed. There are three categories: Airborne, Droplet and Contact Precautions. The three categories can be combined for diseases that have multiple routes of transmission.

Airborne Precautions
Airborne precautions reduce the risk of small particle organisms being transmitted through the air. Microorganisms carried by this route can be carried widely. Examples of such illnesses include measles, tuberculosis and varicella (chickenpox).

Droplet Precautions
Droplet precautions reduce the risk of pathogens being spread through large particle droplet contact. Acts such as coughing, sneezing and talking are common means by which droplets are spread. They can be spread also during procedures such as suctioning or bronchoscopy. This type of transmission requires close proximity because large droplets do not remain suspended in the air and generally travel only short distances. Examples of diseases spread this way include diphtheria, parotitis (mumps), and pertussis (whooping cough).

Contact Precautions
Contact precautions reduce the risk of transmission of pathogens by direct or indirect contact. Direct contact transmission involves skin-to-skin contact (such as shaking hands). Indirect contact transmission involves contact of a susceptible host with an intermediate object such as a comb or soiled dressing. A skin infection such as impetigo is an example of an illness spread by this means.

CARING FOR THE CHILD WITH AN INFECTIOUS DISEASE

NURSING DIAGNOSES AND RELATED INTERVENTIONS

Nursing Diagnosis: Pain related to pruritus from skin lesions

Outcome Identification: Child reports pain is within tolerable limits during course of illness.

Outcome Evaluation: Child states that he or she is more comfortable; child reports less itching; is not seen scratching rash; no signs of excessive scratching or bleeding present.

Providing comfort for the pruritus of skin lesions is important for many childhood infections. No matter what agent is causing the disease, a rash tends to be extremely itchy and uncomfortable. Fortunately, a number of remedies are available for reducing the discomfort. Because pruritus is a minimal form of pain, an analgesic, such as acetaminophen (Tylenol), may be helpful to reduce discomfort. An antihistamine, such as diphenhydramine hydrochloride (Benadryl), is extremely helpful. Calamine lotion is a nonprescription lotion that is cooling and soothing and often helps to relieve itching. Colloidal baths, such as baking soda or oatmeal, approximately 1 cup to 3 inches of bath water, are soothing for some children. Be sure to warn parents to take precautions to prevent clogging the drain with oatmeal if it is used. Caution parents to use only lukewarm water, not hot, because heat usually increases the sensation of itching. Bathing serves two purposes. It can be soothing and also distracting. The child, especially a preschooler, may splash for 15 minutes to 20 minutes in a bathtub without noticing the discomfort of a rash.

Many parents bundle up children with rashes, believing that the extra clothing brings out the rash, and that if a rash does not come out, it will go in and affect a child's heart or brain. In reality, bundling up only serves to make a rash more uncomfortable and probably increases any accompanying fever. Instead, dress the child in light cotton clothing. Remove wool blankets from the bed. Cut the child's fingernails short so scratching will not open up lesions, causing secondary infection. Placing cotton gloves on the child, especially at night may help. Comfort measures for relieving the discomfort of rashes are summarized in Empowering the Family.

None of these measures is foolproof. Some measures may provide great relief to some children and little or no relief to others. Regardless of whether they offer direct relief, they do give a parent a constructive and comforting activity, providing parents with an opportunity to soothe their children and themselves. This is, in part, how a sense of trust develops.

Most infectious diseases also involve fever. Measures to combat fever in children are discussed in Chapter 16.

Nursing Diagnosis: Social isolation related to required activity restrictions associated with precautions to prevent transmission

Outcome Identification: Child will participate in activities to keep himself occupied.

Outcome Evaluation: Child states reasons for restrictions. Expresses interest in activities proposed by nurses or parents.

A child who is restricted from others because of infection control precautions can begin to feel lonely and depressed unless stimulation and social needs are also met.

It is easy for children to associate isolation and restriction with being punished, and it is easy for them to become lonely in a room by themselves. In a hospital setting, make as few trips as possible in and out of the room

EMPOWERING THE FAMILY: Relieving the Itch of a Rash

- Dress your child in light cotton clothing so overheating and perspiration do not occur. Perspiration can make itching worse.
- Avoid wool clothing because this can irritate skin and increase itching.
- Offer adequate fluid to maintain good hydration because dry skin increases discomfort.
- Keep your child's fingernails short to avoid injury to the skin from scratching.
- Teach your child to press on an itchy area rather than scratch to relieve discomfort; cold cloths applied to an area can also be helpful.
- Administer an analgesic such as acetaminophen as needed for comfort.
- Adding a few teaspoonfuls of baking soda to bath water can be soothing. Use lukewarm rather than hot water.
- Keep in mind that some children need an antihistamine such as diphenhydramine (Benadryl) to reduce itching. Ask your primary care provider about using it.

to limit the possibility of pathogen spread; on the other hand, do not make care visits seem hurried. If there is a procedure scheduled at 9:00 AM and another at 9:30 AM, stay in the room rather than leave and return again, if possible. Use the time to read a story to the child, play a card game, or talk about how strange and lonely it feels to be separated from other people.

When the child is hospitalized, the parents may be required to follow infection control precautions. Many parents feel so self-conscious about having to gown and wash that they tend to stay away rather than visit. Remember that when children are admitted to a hospital, parents may not hear all of what is being said to them because of their anxiety over the admission. If gowning technique is explained on admission, therefore, do not expect parents to remember the next day what was said. Explain technique as many times as necessary.

Parents may be reluctant to give children who require transmission-based precautions their favorite toy, thinking that the hospital will insist on destroying it after the precautions are discontinued. There are few pathogens that are not destroyed by exposure to sunlight, and there are few articles that cannot be gas sterilized to ensure that pathogens have been removed from them. Check children's rooms for favorite toys the same as in all rooms. Never leave children in a room before checking that they have a toy to play with or an activity that will keep them busy for the length of time the child will be alone. Diversional activity deficit related to monotony of confinement is another nursing diagnosis associated with transmission-based precautions. See Chapter 15 for a discussion of interventions that can be used to promote adequate stimulation for the child requiring transmission-based precautions.

VIRAL INFECTIONS

Viruses are the smallest infectious agents known, so small they cannot be seen through an ordinary microscope. A virus is not a true cell because it contains either ribonucleic acid (RNA) or deoxyribonucleic acid (DNA), but not both. Viruses increase in number by replication inside bacteria, plant, animal, or human cell using the biochemical products of living cells to function. A cell may not be outwardly altered by a virus invasion or may die because of lysis or rupture. Symptoms usually do not become apparent until many cells have been interrupted in function. Some viruses are capable of invading only specific cells. The Epstein-Barr virus, for example, invades only B lymphocytes, HIV viruses invade T lymphocytes and tracheal cells have receptor sites specific for influenzae viruses.

Viral Exanthems

The majority of childhood exanthems (rashes) are caused by viruses. Each of these diseases has specific symptoms and a specific distribution or pattern to the rash that allows it to be identified (Figures 22-2 and 22-3). Typically the child will be cared for at home. In some instances, however, the child may develop the viral exanthem while hospitalized. If this is the case, specific transmission-based precautions may be necessary.

Exanthem Subitum (Roseola Infantum)

- Causative agent: Human herpesvirus 6 (HHV-6)
- Incubation period: Approximately 10 days
- Period of communicability: During febrile period
- Mode of transmission: Unknown
- Immunity: Contracting the disease offers lasting natural immunity; no artificial immunity is available.

Assessment. Roseola is a disease whose symptoms appear more severe than the disease actually is. It generally occurs in children ages 6 months to 3 years, mainly in the spring and fall, although it can occur any time of the year. The first symptom is a high fever (104°F to 105°F [40.0°C to 40.6°C]). Infants may be irritable and anorexic but rarely appear as ill as this high fever suggests. They usually remain playful and alert. The pharynx may be slightly inflamed. There may be enlargement of the occipital, cervical, and postauricular lymph nodes. The white blood count is usually decreased with the proportion of lymphocytes present increased (75% to 85%; McMillan & Grose, 1997).

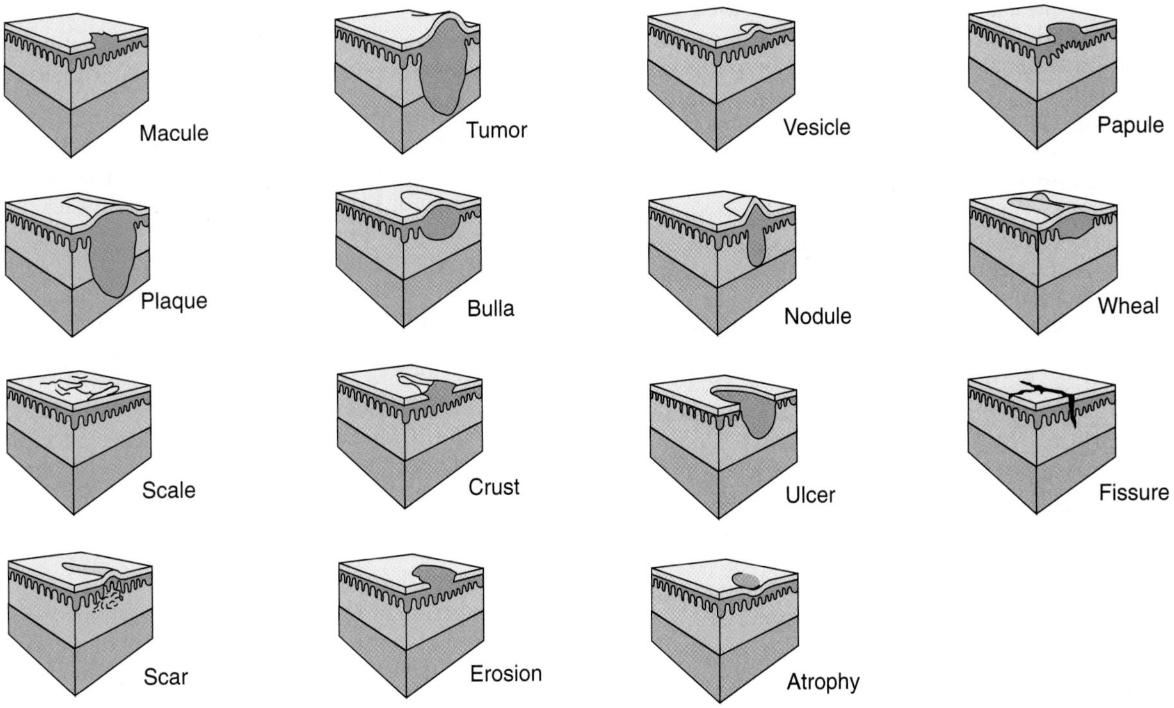

FIGURE 22.2 Primary and secondary skin lesions and their characteristics.

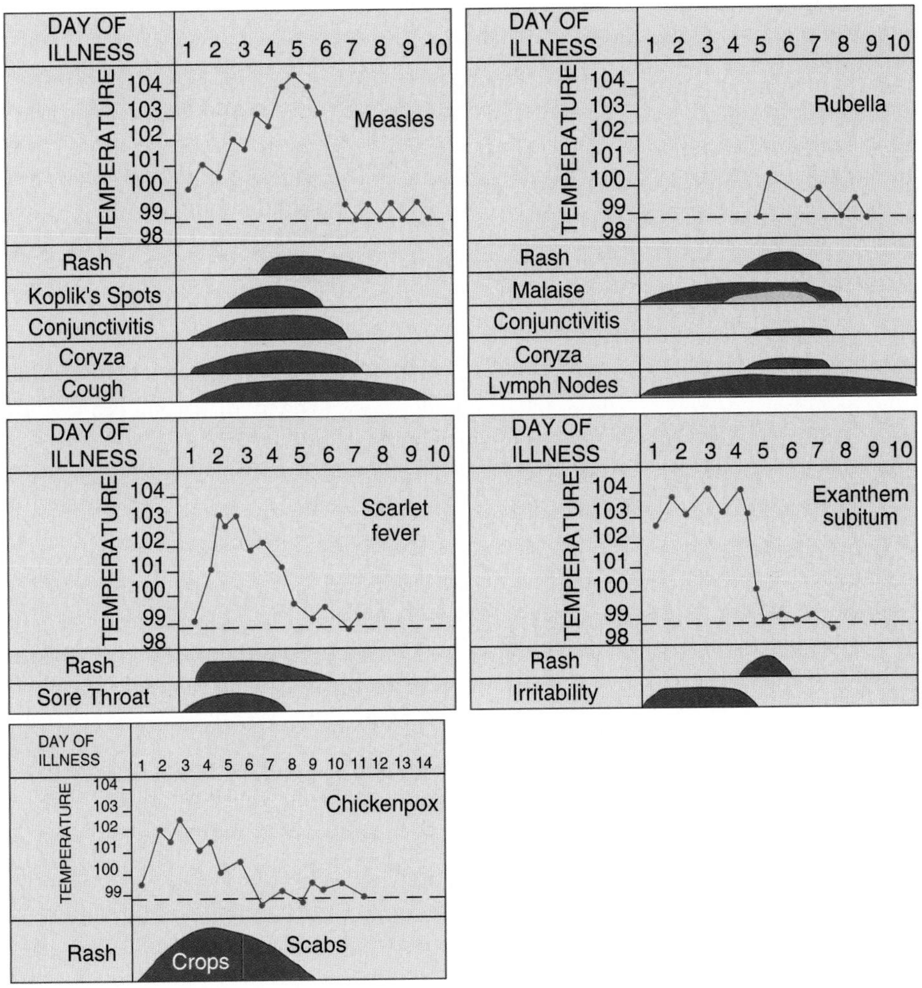

FIGURE 22.3 Differences between five acute exanthems characterized by rash.

After 3 or 4 days, the fever falls abruptly and a distinctive rash appears (see Figure 22-3). The lesions are discrete, rose-pink macules approximately 2 mm to 3 mm in size. They fade on pressure and occur most prominently on the trunk. The rash resembles that of rubella or measles, but it is darker in color, and children have no accompanying coryza (cold symptoms), conjunctivitis, or cough. Because it occurs mainly on the child's trunk, parents may report it as a heat rash. The rash lasts 1 to 2 days. The diagnosis of roseola is based on the physical signs and symptoms. The hallmark of roseola is the appearance of a rash immediately after the sharp decline in fever.

Therapeutic Management. Treatment focuses on measures to reduce the discomfort of the rash and fever. The fever will respond to acetaminophen (Tylenol), but after 4 hours is apt to rise again to the high level. If the infant develops this exanthem in the hospital, follow standard precautions. The most frequent complication of roseola is a febrile convulsion with the onset of the disease because the temperature rises so rapidly. Management of this type of convulsion is discussed in Chapter 28.

Rubella (German Measles)

- Causative agent: Rubella virus
- Incubation period: 14 to 21 days
- Period of communicability: 7 days before to approximately 5 days after the rash appears
- Mode of transmission: Direct and indirect contact with droplets
- Immunity: Contracting the disease offers lasting natural immunity
- Active artificial immunity: Attenuated live virus vaccine
- Passive artificial immunity: Immune serum globulin is considered for pregnant women

Assessment. Rubella is a disease of older school-age and adolescent children; it occurs most commonly during the spring. The incidence is greatly decreased because of the number of children who now receive MMR vaccine. The symptoms begin with a 1- to 5-day prodromal period, during which children have a low-grade fever, headache, malaise, anorexia, mild conjunctivitis, possibly a sore throat, a mild cough, and lymphadenopathy. The nodes most noticeably affected are the suboccipital, postauricular, and cervical (Taber & Demmler, 1997).

After the 1 to 5 days of prodromal signs, a discrete pink-red maculopapular rash appears (see Figure 22-3). Many children have such slight prodromal symptoms that the rash often is the first sign parents notice. It begins first on the face, then spreads downward to the trunk and extremities. On the second day, the rash begins to fade from the face. It is still prominent on the trunk, however, and may even be intensified or coalesce (fuse together) on the trunk. On the third day, the rash disappears. There is generally no desquamation (peeling); if present, it is only fine flakes.

Fever with rubella is not marked. Arthritis (joint pain) with effusion into the joints may occur in some children on the second or third day of the rash. These symptoms may last as long as 5 to 10 days. Rubella is diagnosed on clinical signs and symptoms. A high rubella antibody titer will reveal that children have recently had rubella.

Therapeutic Management. Children need comfort measures for the rash, and an antipyretic such as acetaminophen if a marked fever occurs. If arthritis occurs, acetaminophen or ibuprofen also helps to control this discomfort. If weight-bearing joints are affected, bedrest is generally advised until the discomfort subsides (2 to 3 days). If the child develops rubella while in the hospital, follow droplet precautions for 7 days after the onset of the rash in addition to standard precautions.

If rubella occurs during pregnancy, it is capable of causing extensive congenital malformation (see Chapter 6). Because of this, it can never be considered a simple disease. It is important that girls be immunized against it.

Measles (Rubeola)

- Causative agent: Measles virus
- Incubation period: 10 to 12 days
- Period of communicability: Fifth day of incubation period through the first few days of rash
- Mode of transmission: Direct or indirect contact with droplets
- Immunity: Contracting the disease offers lasting natural immunity
- Active artificial immunity: Attenuated live measles vaccine
- Passive artificial immunity: Immune serum globulin

Assessment. Measles is sometimes called brown or black, regular, or 7-day measles to differentiate it from rubella (German, or 3-day, measles). It formerly occurred most frequently in children ages 5 to 10 years. Because most children of preschool and school age have now been immunized against measles, outbreaks currently most often occur in the college-age population. Incidence of the disease is highest in the winter and spring months.

Measles has a 10- to 11-day prodromal period. During this time, lymphoid tissue, particularly postauricular, cervical, and occipital lymph nodes, becomes enlarged. Children have a high fever (103°F to 104°F [39.5°C to 40.0°C]) for 5 or 6 days. They have malaise and appear ill. By the second day of the prodromal period, there is coryza (rhinitis and a sore throat); conjunctivitis with photophobia (sensitivity to light); and a cough. **Koplik's spots,** small, irregular, bright red spots with a blue-white center point, are present on the buccal membrane. The coryza of measles is indistinguishable from that of a common cold. Children have nasal congestion and a mucopurulent discharge. Their eyes water with the conjunctivitis; they blink at bright lights. Their cough is a deep, brassy, bronchial cough caused by an inflammation reaction extending into the respiratory tract. Many children with measles are diagnosed as having a simple upper respiratory infection at this point.

Koplik's spots appear first on the buccal membrane opposite the molars, and then extend to cover the entire buccal surface (Figure 22-4). The raised base of the spots may coalesce so that the blue-white centers stand out as grains of salt on the erythematous membrane. Koplik's

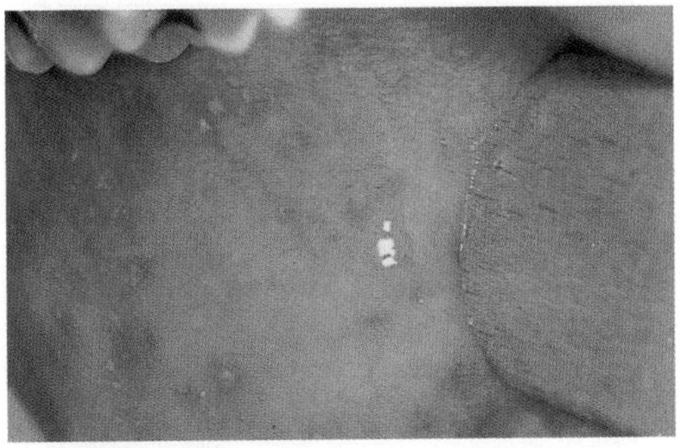

FIGURE 22.4 Koplik's spots on the oral mucous membrane.

spots are diagnostic of measles. None of the other exanthems has this finding.

On the fourth day of fever, the rash appears. On the fifth day, the fever drops and the Koplik's spots fade. The rash of measles is a deep-red maculopapular eruption. It begins first at the hairline of the forehead, behind the ears, and at the back of the neck. It then spreads to include the face, the neck, upper extremities, trunk, and, finally, the lower extremities. The rash on the upper part of the body, particularly the face, may be so intense that it coalesces (Figure 22-5). The rash on the lower extremities generally remains discrete. After several days, the rash turns from a red to a brown color. While the rash is red, it fades on pressure; when it is brown, it does not fade. This differentiates it from the rash of scarlet fever, which always fades on pressure. The rash lasts 5 to 6 days, then fades. There is a fine desquamation after this. However, the skin of the hands and feet does not desquamate, a feature differentiating it from scarlet fever.

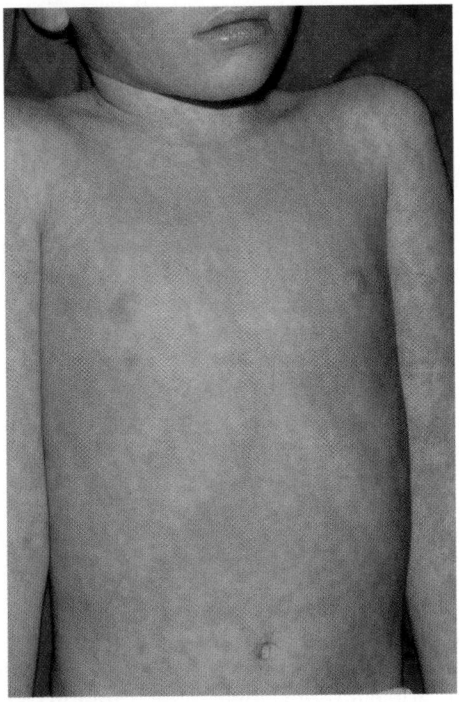

FIGURE 22.5 The typical rash of measles on a child's upper body.

Children with measles appear very ill approximately the second day of the rash. Their cough is loud and frequent, the coryza is acute, the fever is high, and the rash is pruritic. On the third or fourth day of rash, when the temperature begins to fall, the other symptoms clear quickly and children begin to feel better. Fever that lasts beyond the third or fourth day of rash generally suggests that a complication of measles, such as pneumonia, has occurred.

Therapeutic Management. Children with measles need comfort measures for the rash, and an antipyretic for the fever. The coryza, which does not respond to decongestants, fortunately lasts only for a few days. The child's skin below the nose may become excoriated from the constant nasal drainage. Applying a lubricating jelly or an emollient (A and D ointment) to the area may help prevent excoriation. The child may need a cough suppressant to control the cough; otherwise, the throat can become painful from frequent irritation. Because children with measles have photophobia, it is painful for them to look at bright lights; it may be painful for them to watch television. They are often more comfortable with the shades or curtains drawn or wearing dark glasses, so these measures should be instituted. If the child is in the hospital, follow airborne precautions for the duration of the illness in addition to standard precautions.

WHAT IF? What if a parent insists that her child has to be kept in a completely dark room until he recovers from measles? What suggestions would you make to her?

Complications. The complications of measles include otitis media (middle ear infection); pneumonia; airway obstruction; and acute encephalitis. Symptoms of otitis media are ear pain in the older child, and irritability and ear pulling in the infant. Pneumonia is revealed by a chest x-ray and by dullness to percussion, the sound of rales, and diminished breath sounds on auscultation. Some degree of hoarseness and a cough are inevitable symptoms of measles. If the inflammation process of the respiratory tract becomes acute and there is airway obstruction, children will have increased hoarseness, a bark-like cough, inspiratory stridor, dyspnea, and tachycardia. Children with airway obstruction may require endotracheal intubation to provide a patent airway. Administration of vitamin A may reduce the severity of complications such as pneumonia in such children.

Approximately 1 in 1000 children with rubeola develops measles encephalitis. Symptoms of acute encephalitis are increased fever, headache, vomiting, drowsiness, convulsions, and coma. Children may have a stiff neck or a positive Kernig's sign (pain on extending the leg after it has been flexed on the abdomen), which are signs of meningeal irritation. A lumbar puncture will reveal increased protein in the cerebrospinal fluid (CSF). The encephalitis of measles tends to be a severe fulminating type. Approximately 15% of children with this complication die. Another 25% will be left with permanent brain damage, such as cognitive disturbances, nerve deafness, hemiplegia, or paraplegia.

Chickenpox (Varicella)

- Causative agent: Varicella-zoster virus
- Incubation period: 10 to 21 days
- Period of communicability: 1 day before the rash to 5 to 6 days after its appearance, when all the vesicles have crusted
- Mode of transmission: Highly contagious; spread by direct or indirect contact of saliva or vesicles
- Immunity: Contracting the disease offers lasting natural immunity to chickenpox; because the same virus causes herpes zoster, it may be reactivated at a later time as herpes zoster.
- Active artificial immunity: An attenuated live vaccine is available.
- Passive artificial immunity: There is little passive placental immunity to chickenpox. Children who are immunosuppressed such as those with leukemia, HIV/AIDS, or who are being treated with corticosteroids are given varicella-zoster immune globulin (VZIG). This may prevent or modify chickenpox if given within 72 hours of exposure.

Assessment. Chickenpox occurs most often in the preschool or early school-age child (ages 2 to 8 years). Children first develop a low-grade fever, malaise, and, in 24 hours, the appearance of a rash (see Figure 22-3). The lesion begins as a macula, then progresses rapidly within 6 to 8 hours to a papule, then a vesicle that first becomes umbilicated and then forms a crust. Each lesion is approximately 2 mm to 3 mm in diameter and is surrounded by an erythematous area. When the first crop of lesions appears, children's temperature may rise markedly to 104°F or 105°F (40.0°C or 40.6°C).

The greatest concentration of chickenpox lesions are on the trunk, although the face, scalp, palate, and neck also may be involved. Lesions on the extremities are generally scant in number. Lesions appear in approximately three separate series. New lesions move each time through progressive stages (Figure 22-6). At one time, all four stages of lesions—(1) macule, (2) papule, (3) vesicle, and (4) crust—will be present.

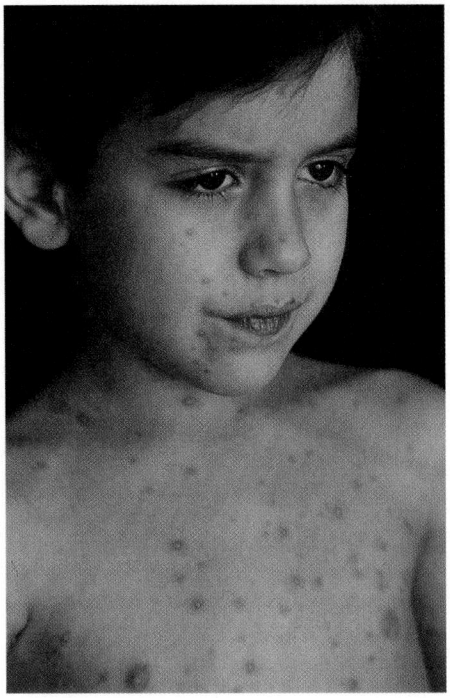

FIGURE 22.6 A school-age boy with varicella.

Therapeutic Management. If the scab from crusting is allowed to fall off naturally and lesions do not become secondarily infected, no scarring will result. Scabs removed prematurely may leave a white, round, slightly indented scar at the site. The rash of chickenpox is extremely pruritic. Because it is important that children not scratch and remove scabs, preventing scratching becomes a difficult problem for parents. A prescribed antihistamine usually helps to reduce the itchiness to a bearable level, and an antipyretic will counteract the high fever. Acyclovir may be prescribed to reduce the number of lesions and shorten the course of the illness (Grose, 1997). If the child is in the hospital, follow airborne and contact precautions until all lesions are crusted in addition to standard precautions (Erlich, 1997).

Chickenpox is extremely serious if it occurs in immunosuppressed children such as those with leukemia. Complications include secondary infections of the lesions, pneumonia, and encephalitis. The encephalitis of chickenpox generally has a lower mortality associated with it than does measles encephalitis. The development of Reye's syndrome has been associated with aspirin use during varicella and influenza virus illness (see Chapter 28). Caution parents when treating all childhood exanthems to avoid aspirin and use acetaminophen or children's ibuprofen to control fever instead.

Although chickenpox is not as serious a disease as measles, it often seems to be a more severe disease because of the extreme itchiness accompanying it (Yawn et al, 1997). Reviewing comfort measures for rashes is important. Children may return to school as soon as all lesions are crusted. The crusts are not infectious.

Herpes Zoster

Herpes zoster is caused by the varicella-zoster virus, the same virus as chickenpox. Apparently, the first time children are invaded by the virus, they have symptoms of chickenpox. Thereafter, herpes zoster symptoms may appear, due to reactivation of a latent virus or possibly due to a second or third exposure. Chickenpox tends to be a disease of preschoolers or of younger school-age children. Herpes zoster tends to occur in older children, although it can occur even in infants.

The first manifestations of herpes zoster are pruritus and cutaneous vesicular lesions on erythematous bases that follow the distributions of the lumbar and thoracic nerves (usually on the trunk, face, or upper back; Figure 22-7).

Therapeutic Management. Treatment for herpes zoster is basically symptomatic and usually includes an analgesic for pain. Acyclovir, which inhibits viral DNA synthesis, may be effective in limiting the disease. VZIG may minimize symptoms.

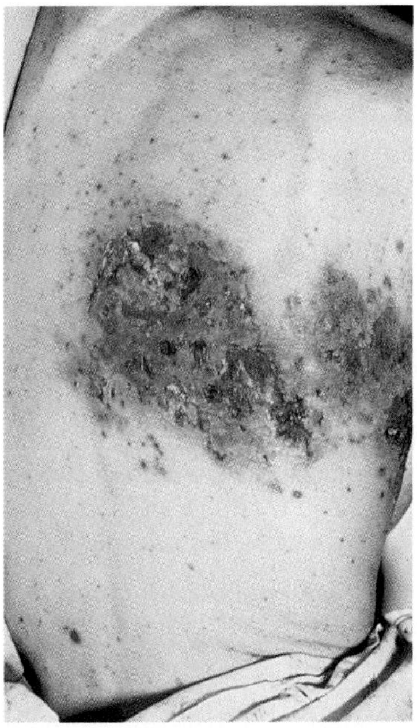

FIGURE 22.7 Herpes zoster on a child's lower back.

Erythema Infectiosum ("Fifth Disease")

- Causative agent: Parvovirus B19
- Incubation period: 6 to 14 days
- Period of communicability: Uncertain
- Mode of transmission: Droplet
- Immunity: None

Assessment. Erythema infectiosum (the fifth important childhood exanthem) occurs most often in children ages 2 to 12 years. The first phase includes fever, headache and malaise. A week later, a rash, which erupts in three stages, appears. It is intensely red and appears first on the face. The lesions are maculopapular and coalesce on the cheeks to form a "slapped face" appearance (Figure 22-8). The circumoral area appears pale next to the reddened area. The facial lesions fade in 1 to 40 days.

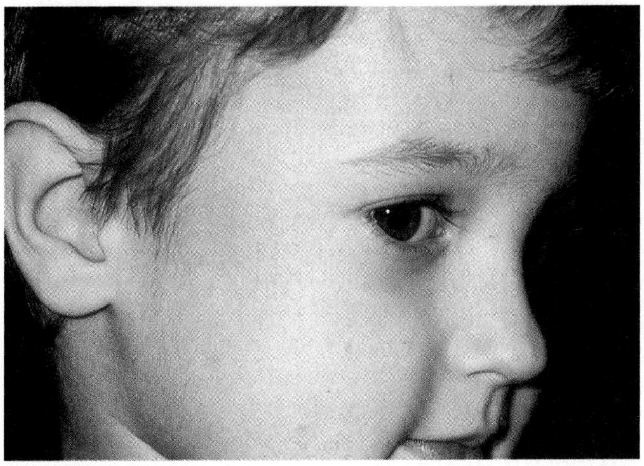

FIGURE 22.8 Fifth's disease. Note the "slapped cheek" appearance.

A day after the facial lesions appear, a rash appears on the extensor surfaces of the extremities. One day later, it invades the flexor surfaces and the trunk. These lesions last for 1 week or more. When they fade, they fade from the center outward, giving the lesions a lacelike appearance. After the rash has faded, it may reappear if precipitated by skin irritation, such as trauma, sunlight, hot, or cold. Some children develop a persistent arthritis. Children with a hemolytic anemia such as sickle-cell or thalassemia can experience a severe aplastic anemia.

Therapeutic Management. Children may need comfort measures for the rash (see Empowering the Family earlier in this chapter). There are no known complications of fifth disease for the child; it is teratogenic for a fetus, however (Cherry, 1997).

Pityriasis Rosea

- Causative agent: Probably a virus
- Incubation period: Unknown
- Period of communicability: Unknown
- Mode of transmission: Unknown
- Immunity: Apparently none

Assessment. Pityriasis rosea occurs in school-age and older children. Children may have a short, mild prodromal period of fever and sore throat. A herald patch, an erythematous round lesion with a scaly border, usually appearing on the trunk, is the first obvious lesion (Figure 22-9). Approximately 1 week after the appearance of the herald patch, a generalized rash of papules, vesicles, or urticaria appears. This is generally also confined to the trunk. It follows skin lines, giving it the unique configuration of a Christmas tree.

The rash lasts for 6 to 8 weeks. It is pruritic and, because it lasts so long, is particularly worrisome to children and parents. Because the lesions, particularly the herald patch, are scaly at the edges, they are often confused with tinea corporis (ringworm). Treatment is limited to oral antihistamines and other comfort measures for rash.

Pityriasis rosea appears to have no sequelae or complications; in fact, it is difficult to demonstrate in what manner it is infectious. It is a baffling rash of childhood and should be differentiated from serious (severe) exanthems.

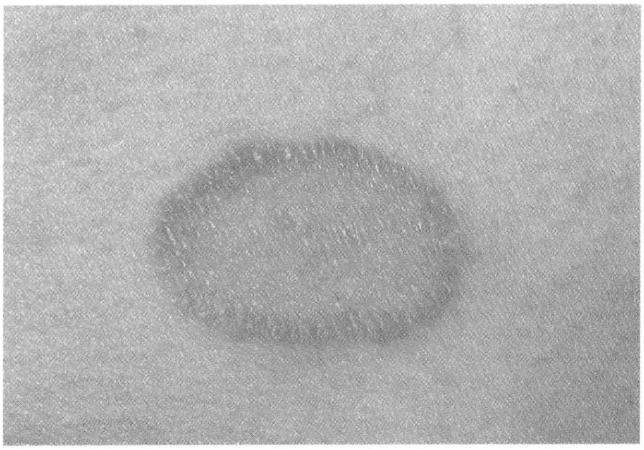

FIGURE 22.9 The "herald patch" of pityriasis rosea.

CHECKPOINT QUESTIONS

5. What is the association between the rash and fever in roseola infantum?
6. What is the first sign typically noticed by parents for the child who develops rubella?
7. What finding is found only with rubeola?
8. What are the four stages of chickenpox lesions?

Enteroviruses

There are three main types of enteroviruses: echoviruses (33 subdivisions), coxsackievirus A (24 subdivisions) and coxsackievirus B (6 types), and polioviruses (3 subdivisions).

Echovirus Infections

The echoviruses are responsible for a number of childhood diseases, including aseptic meningitis, diarrhea, acute respiratory illness, and maculopapular rashes. Such infections are usually benign and self-limiting. Treatment is aimed toward supportive measures. If the child is in the hospital, follow contact precautions for the duration of the illness in addition to standard precautions.

Coxsackievirus Infections

The coxsackievirus groups are responsible, like the echovirus groups, for a variety of diseases. One of the most frequently found diseases of children caused by coxsackievirus A is herpangina. With herpangina, children have an abrupt elevation of temperature, up to 104°F or 105°F (40.0°C or 40.6°C) for 1 to 4 days. Anorexia, difficulty swallowing, sore throat, and vomiting may be present. Children may have headaches and abdominal pain. Small lesions, generally discrete grayish vesicles, pinpoint in size, appear on the tonsillar fauces, soft palate, and uvula. They may be present elsewhere in the mouth or throat as well. The lesions gradually change to shallow ulcers surrounded by a red areola. They disappear within a few days after the temperature returns to normal. There are generally no complications.

Children need to be maintained on soft or liquid foods while their mouth and throat are sore. They may need an antipyretic for the fever. A local anesthetic (Xylocaine Viscous) may be applied to ulcers by a cotton-tipped applicator to relieve local pain. Children must not swallow the anesthetic liquid. If they do, their throat will become anesthetized and they may then aspirate with swallowing. Therefore, this agent should not be used in children under 6 years of age. If the child is in the hospital, follow contact precautions for the duration of the illness in addition to standard precautions.

Poliovirus Infections: Poliomyelitis (Infantile Paralysis)

- Causative agent: Poliovirus
- Incubation period: 7 to 14 days
- Period of communicability: Greatest shortly before and after onset of symptoms when virus is present in the throat and feces (1 week to 6 weeks)
- Mode of transmission: Direct and indirect contact
- Immunity: Contracting the disease causes active immunity against the one strain of virus causing the illness.
- Active artificial immunity: Live attenuated virus vaccine
- Passive artificial immunity: None

Poliomyelitis may be caused by any of the three strains of poliovirus, which is why children must be immunized with trivalent (three-strain) vaccine. Fortunately, because of effective immunization programs against the disease, it currently is rare. The World Health Organization has set a goal to make it extinct by the year 2000 (CDC, 1998).

Assessment. The poliovirus enters children's gastrointestinal tract, where it multiplies. Children may develop symptoms such as fever, headache, nausea, vomiting, or abdominal pain. Slight erythema of the throat may be present. Children have pain and stiffness of the neck, back, and legs. The CSF will generally show increased protein and lymphocytes.

These initial symptoms are followed by intense pain and tremors of extremities, and then paralysis, occurring either immediately or over a period of 1 to 7 days as the virus invades the central nervous system. Kernig's sign will be positive. Children show a tripod sign—when sitting on the floor or on an examining table, they are unable to sit without placing both their arms and hands behind them to brace themselves. Their deep tendon reflexes are hyperactive at first and then diminish.

Paralysis is generally asymmetric, with legs appearing to be more susceptible than the arms. Respiratory problems occur when there is damage to the cells of the cervical and thoracic segments of the spinal cord. Bulbar paralysis involves the cranial nerves. With bulbar poliomyelitis, laryngeal paralysis occurs and may be accompanied by difficulty swallowing or talking. Respiration halts as the respiratory center of the brain is involved.

Therapeutic Management. Treatment for poliomyelitis is bedrest. For the pain, moist hot packs are helpful. Passive range of motion as soon as the pain and spasm are gone will offer best results. For long-term care, children need bracing to strengthen atrophied muscles. They may need muscle transplant operations to achieve better muscle function. Poliomyelitis, in its severest form, is such a crippling disease that it is mandatory that children receive immunization against it. If respiratory muscles were involved, long-term ventilation is necessary. Survivors tend to develop progressive muscle atrophy (postpoliomyelitis muscular atrophy syndrome) in late adulthood, further compounding their ability to be self-sufficient (Cherry, 1997).

Viral Infections of the Integumentary System

Viral infections of the skin include the herpes infections and warts (verrucae).

Herpesvirus Infections

Herpesviruses are responsible for a number of infections in children.

- Causative agent: Herpes simplex or herpes type 1 or type 2 virus
- Incubation period: 2 to 12 days
- Period of communicability: Greatest early in the course of the infection
- Mode of transmission: Direct contact
- Immunity: Immunity to a primary herpes response is gained after one incident. There is no immunity to recurrent herpes infections because the virus lies dormant in the body until it is activated by stress, sun exposure, fever, other illness, or menstruation.

Assessment. When children are first invaded by a herpesvirus, they have no antibodies against the virus, so a primary form of the disease such as herpetic gingivostomatitis occurs. The virus remains latent in the neurons of local sensory ganglia or children become permanent carriers of herpes simplex (Kohl, 1997).

Acute Herpetic Gingivostomatitis. Acute herpetic gingivostomatitis is the most common form of herpes simplex invasion in children. It is an example of the primary, not the recurrent, response. It occurs in children ages 1 to 4 years. Children have a high fever (104°F to 105°F [40.0°C to 40.6°C]), are restless, and have anorexia and a sore mouth. Their gumline is swollen and reddened and bleeds easily. White plaques or shallow ulcers with red areolae appear on the buccal mucosa, tongue, palate, and perhaps on the tonsillar fauces. The anterior cervical lymph nodes are enlarged and tender. The disease runs its course in 5 to 7 days.

Therapeutic Management. Children need an antipyretic to reduce fever. Oral acyclovir helps with healing. Children need soft, acid-free foods that they can eat with minimum irritation or abrasion.

Children with gingivostomatitis are often very ill. Do not dismiss it as just a reaction to herpes simplex. It can become very serious if children's mouths are so sore that they cannot swallow readily and they become malnourished and dehydrated.

Herpes Simplex (Herpes Labialis). Herpes simplex infection is popularly known as a cold sore or fever blister. It represents the recurrent form of a type 1 herpesvirus invasion that has remained dormant in ganglia of the trigeminal or 5th cranial nerve. Herpes simplex typically appears as clusters of painful, grouped vesicles found on the lips or skin surrounding the mouth. After 2 or 3 days, vesicles crust, then gradually dry. Keeping lesions dry helps them to fade sooner, but keeping them lubricated with an ointment reduces pain. Application of topical or oral acyclovir reduces pain and increases healing. Children feel conspicuous about the appearance of herpes simplex lesions. They may need counseling to assure them that the lesions are not as obvious to others as they imagine.

Acute Herpetic Vulvovaginitis (Genital Herpes). Genital herpes is caused by the herpesvirus type 2, which remains dormant in the ganglia of the sacral nerves. Because this form is spread primarily by sexual contact, it is discussed in Chapter 26 with other STDs.

Eczema Herpeticum. Children with atopic dermatitis (infantile eczema) may have a generalized reaction if they contract a herpes infection. They develop a fever as high as 104°F to 105°F (40.0°C to 40.6°C), irritability, and crops of vesicles that erupt at the sites of eczematous skin lesions. Lesions may occur at different times during the disease course of 7 to 9 days. Generally by day 10, all lesions are crusted.

In children with severe eczema, the number of lesions that appear may be extreme. Enough body fluid can be lost through the oozing of the vesicles to cause serious fluid loss. Pain can be intense. The extent of the involvement can make children gravely ill.

Warts (Verrucae)

Warts are one of the most common dermatologic diseases in children. They are caused by the papilloma virus that has an incubation period of between 1 month and 6 months. The mode of transmission is unknown, but it is probably by direct contact.

Warts are flesh-colored, dirty-appearing papules. They generally occur on the dorsal surface of the hands, although they may occur anywhere. Plantar warts appear on the soles of the feet and are painful when children walk. They may be differentiated from calluses in that they obliterate skin lines as they grow, whereas calluses do not.

Warts on the hands or the face are generally removed if they are cosmetically unattractive to children. Plantar warts may have to be removed because of the discomfort they cause. Application of 10% salicylic acid, relatively painless, is usually effective in causing warts to atrophy. Parents can use over-the-counter wart remover preparations, such as Compound W, to apply to warts and dissolve them. Carbon dioxide snow, liquid nitrogen, electrodesiccation, and curettage are also effective for removal, but these methods are painful.

Children need some reassurance that people do not catch warts from frogs or toads. If left without any treatment, warts eventually fade by themselves (Tunnessen, 1997).

Viruses Causing Central Nervous System Diseases

Viruses are also responsible for causing central nervous system disorders. Both encephalitis and meningitis may be caused by a number of viruses of the arbovirus group or by certain bacteria. These are discussed in Chapter 28. Rabies is discussed below.

Rabies

- Causative agent: Rabies virus
- Incubation period: 2 to 6 weeks and possibly as long as 12 months
- Period of communicability: 3 to 5 days before the onset of symptoms through the course of the disease

- Mode of transmission: The bite of rabid animals; rarely through saliva from infected animals being transferred to open lesions on a child's skin
- Immunity: Contracting the disease apparently offers active immunity (few people have ever survived the illness to verify this)
- Active artificial immunity: Human diploid cell rabies vaccine
- Passive artificial immunity: Rabies immune globulin (RIG)

Any warm-blooded animal can contract rabies. Wild animals, such as skunks, squirrels, and bats, constitute the most important sources of infection from rabies in the United States. However, children receive more bites and, therefore, more treatments for rabies from bites of dogs or cats. Bites of rodents are seldom found to be rabid. Bites from other children are not rabid, although therapy is required because such bites usually contain streptococci. In the animal infected with rabies, the virus can be cultured from the central nervous system, saliva, urine, lymph, and blood. When a child is bitten by an infected animal, the virus migrates from the bite area to the child's central nervous system. Cranial nerve and spinal cord nuclei become acutely damaged. Negri bodies (cytoplasmic inclusion bodies) can be isolated from nerve cells.

Assessment. The diagnosis of rabies is established largely from the history of an animal bite and the clinical symptoms. After the long incubation period of the virus, children begin to show prodromal signs of malaise, fever, anorexia, nausea, sore throat, drowsiness, irritability, and restlessness. They may notice numbness or hyperesthesia at the area of the bite and along the course of the involved nerves. The white blood cell count (WBC) will show slight leukocytosis. CSF is usually normal, with perhaps only a slight elevation in protein and cells. As the symptoms increase, there is high fever, anxiety, and hyperexcitability. Involuntary twitching movements and generalized convulsions may occur. When children try to drink, there are violent contractions of the muscles of the mouth. They may drool saliva rather than swallow it because swallowing is extremely painful. These two phenomena give the disease its popular name, hydrophobia ("water-fear").

As symptoms progress, children become comatose with possible total body paralysis. Peripheral vascular collapse and death follow quickly in only 5 or 6 days. Postmortem examination will reveal the diagnostic Negri bodies in brain cells.

Therapeutic Management. Once the disease process begins, rabies is invariably fatal. The key is preventing the active process. All children who receive an animal bite should be seen by a primary care provider to evaluate the circumstances surrounding the bite and decide whether to begin rabies prevention measures. The decision to treat must be made immediately if treatment is to be effective.

Taking a history of the incident to determine the type of animal is of primary importance. Most children are sure they know the type of animal if it was a dog; they may be unsure if it was a wild animal. Do not lead children into naming an animal just to please. If asked, "Was it a skunk? A raccoon? A squirrel?" children may choose an animal name because they think that is the answer expected. Instead, ask the child to describe the animal, and then, from that description, establish the kind of animal that bit them. It helps in rural health facilities if there is a picture book of animals handy so preschoolers, especially, can identify the animal in the book that looks like the one that bit them. A rabid animal usually does not act normally. It runs blindly, often staggering; it may dribble saliva rather than swallow it. It is easy to assess whether a household pet is acting this way. It is sometimes difficult to assess the actions of a wild animal because the fear it experiences at being trapped or cornered may make it run about frantically (Dinman & Jarosz, 1996).

An unprovoked attack is highly suggestive that the animal is rabid rather than if the bite happens during a provoked attack. Let children know that they are not going to be punished if they were provoking an animal so they feel free to say so. Statements such as "I was only hugging him or feeding him" may sound innocent but may have constituted a provoked attack to the animal.

The kind of wound that children receive also is instrumental in deciding whether to begin treatment. A bite mark is much more serious than a scratch from an animal's claws. The immunization status of the animal should be checked if available. An animal that has been properly immunized against rabies will rarely transmit the virus. Whether rabies exists in the community at the time of the attack will also influence the decision. If there have been no other reported instances in domestic animals, the chance that this dog bite is serious in terms of rabies is smaller than if other dogs with rabies have been reported in the area.

When children are seen at health care facilities for bites, inspect the wound carefully to see whether it was caused by teeth marks or scratch marks. Wash the wound well with soap and water and a suitable antiseptic. If puncture wounds are present, the wound must not be sutured and closed, because tetanus may result. (Tetanus organisms are anaerobic and grow in deep, closed wounds where oxygen does not reach.) The animal that caused the bite must be located if at all possible and then confined for 5 to 10 days. If it develops any signs of rabies during this period, it will be destroyed and the brain examined for evidence of rabies. It is important that people understand that domestic animals are not destroyed unless the animal shows signs of rabies. Not knowing this, they may resist surrendering an animal for observation.

If the animal is found to be rabid, children receive both rabies vaccine and antirabies serum (R1G). This applies also if the animal escapes and its condition is unknown (it is assumed to be rabid; Dutta, 1998). Routine active immunization procedure involves 5 days of injections given into the deltoid muscle on days 1, 3, 7, 14, and 28. RIG is used in addition to the active immunization procedure. A portion of the dose is injected into the wound site. The remainder is given intramuscularly.

It may seem contradictory to give an active immunization serum (administering antigen to children) when they have received an animal bite (which administers antigen to them). This is done because rabies virus has a long incubation period before antibody production is stimulated; serum that is administered causes children to begin to form antibodies against the rabies virus immediately. By the time the rabies virus from the bite begins to have an effect (2 to 6 weeks after the bite), children have developed sufficient antibodies to combat it and prevent the illness.

Other Viral Infections

Mumps (Epidemic Parotitis)

- Causative agent: Mumps virus
- Incubation period: 14 to 21 days
- Period of communicability: Shortly before and after onset of parotitis
- Mode of transmission: Direct or indirect contact
- Immunity: Contracting the disease gives lasting natural immunity
- Active artificial immunity: Attenuated live mumps vaccine
- Passive artificial immunity: Mumps immune globulin

Assessment. Mumps is now a rare disease due to successful immunization programs. Mumps generally begins with fever, headache, anorexia, and malaise. Within a 24-hour period, children begin to complain of an "earache." When they point to the site of the pain, however, they point not to their ear, but to the jaw line just in front of the ear lobe. Chewing movements aggravate the pain. By the next day, the parotid gland (located just in front of the ear lobe) is swollen and tender. As the parotid gland swells, typically lasting for 1 to 6 days, it displaces the ear upward and backward.

It is often difficult to differentiate mumps from submaxillary adenitis (swelling of lymph nodes). The best method of differentiation is to place a hand along the child's jaw line. If the major amount of swelling is above the hand, it is probably mumps. If the largest amount of swelling is below the hand line, it is probably adenitis (Figure 22-10).

Therapeutic Management. Children may need to be kept on soft or liquid foods until the major portion of the swelling recedes, because chewing movements are so painful. It is also more difficult for them to swallow sour foods than sweet ones. They may need an analgesic for pain and an antipyretic for fever. If the child is in the hospital, follow droplet precautions for 9 days after the onset of swelling in addition to standard precautions.

It is important to remember that one attack of mumps gives lasting immunity. Some parents report that children had mumps only on one side 1 year ago so they are afraid the child will develop mumps on the opposite side. Children who appear to have had mumps twice are children whose diagnosis was probably confused with cervical adenitis one of the two times.

Complications. A number of serious complications can arise from mumps. Between 20% and 30% of males older than the age of puberty who develop mumps will develop the complication of orchitis (inflammation of the testes). Fortunately, mumps orchitis is generally unilateral. A single testis swells rapidly and is painful and tender. When the fever declines, testicular swelling also decreases, but the tenderness may exist for weeks. Atrophy of the testis may result. The chance that mumps orchitis will lead to complete sterility is exaggerated, however, because the condition is usually unilateral. All children should receive active immunization against epidemic parotitis at 12 to 15 months of age (Casella et al, 1997).

Meningoencephalitis may occur in a small number of children. The symptoms are increased fever, headache, vomiting, neck rigidity, and a positive Kernig's sign. Unlike the encephalitis of measles or chickenpox, this sequela rarely leaves lasting damage. Severe permanent

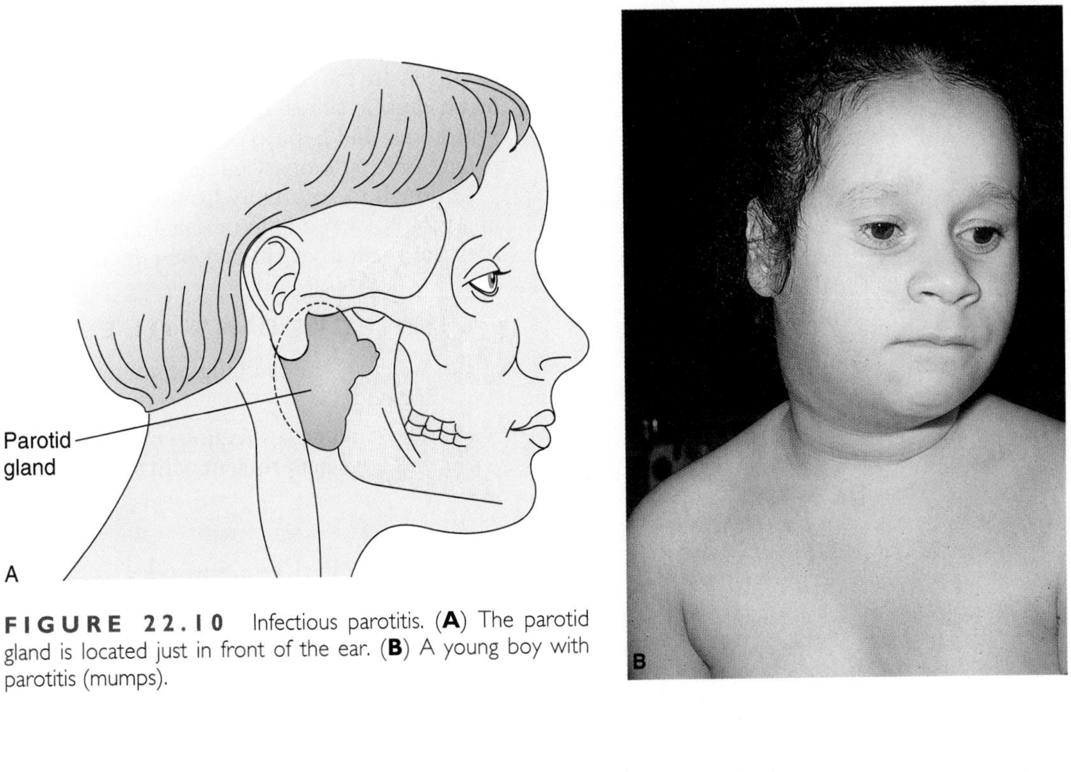

FIGURE 22.10 Infectious parotitis. (**A**) The parotid gland is located just in front of the ear. (**B**) A young boy with parotitis (mumps).

hearing impairment is a rare complication occurring because of neuritis of the auditory nerve.

Infectious Mononucleosis

- Causative agent: Epstein-Barr virus
- Incubation period: Unknown; probably 2 to 8 weeks
- Period of communicability: Unknown; probably only during acute illness
- Mode of transmission: Direct and indirect contact
- Immunity: One episode apparently gives lasting immunity. No vaccination is available.

Infectious mononucleosis is also known as glandular fever or, because it was first discovered as a disease that is transferred readily from one person to another by kissing, the kissing disease. It occurs most commonly in adolescents, although it may occur in any age child (Sumaya, 1997).

Assessment. The beginning symptoms include chills, fever, headache, anorexia, and malaise. Children develop lymphadenopathy and a severe sore throat. The fever is generally high (103°F [39.5°C]), although young children may have a low-grade fever or no fever. The fever lasts approximately 6 days.

The cervical lymph nodes, most markedly affected, are firm and tender to the touch. The tonsils are painful, enlarged and erythematous. There may be a thick, white membrane covering the tonsils (Figure 22-11). Often petechiae appear on the palate. When mesenteric lymph nodes are enlarged, children may have abdominal pain so sharp it simulates appendicitis. The spleen is enlarged, placing the child at risk for spontaneous rupture. Hepatitis, skin manifestations (such as a maculopapular eruption similar to the rash of rubella), pneumonitis, and central nervous system involvement (e.g., encephalitis, meningitis, or polyneuritis) may occur.

With infectious mononucleosis, lymphocytosis with lymphocytes comprising more than 50% of the total WBC occurs. Of these lymphocytes, a significant number (more than 20%) are atypical; they are larger-than-normal, mature lymphocytes, and their nuclei are somewhat less dense. A serologic test, known as the heterophil antibody test, is based on the fact that the antibody produced in infectious mononucleosis will agglutinate sheep red blood cells. A technique known as the monospot test has also been developed, using horse red blood cells. This test can be performed in a matter of minutes. A positive test, along with the increased number of atypical lymphocytes apparent on a blood slide, confirms a diagnosis of infectious mononucleosis. Epstein-Barr virus antibodies can be recovered from blood serum for a final diagnosis.

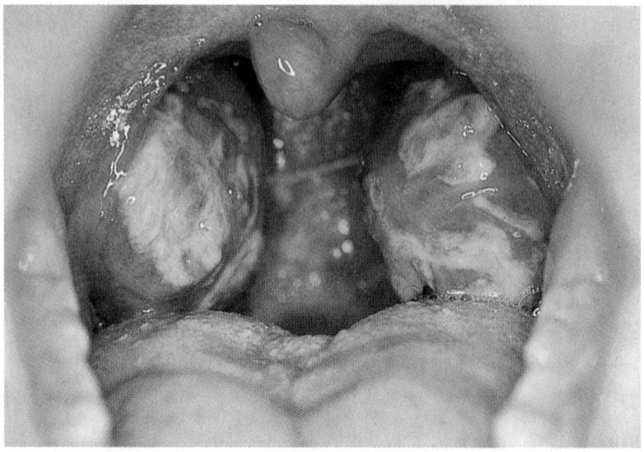

FIGURE 22.11 Appearance of the tonsils in a child with infectious mononucleosis. Note the degree of erythema, enlargement, and purulent covering.

Therapeutic Management. Children with infectious mononucleosis are kept on bedrest during the acute stage of the illness (7 to 10 days), because with the splenomegaly, there is a danger of spleen rupture with any trauma to that area. If a child is hospitalized, be sure to follow standard precautions. Be careful in helping children with this disease turn in bed so that no pressure is placed over the splenic area. When palpating the spleen, do so gently to avoid possible inadvertent rupture.

Teach children and parents the importance of maintaining a good fluid intake despite the sore throat. Cool, nonacidic fluids are often tolerated best.

Children may notice weakness and general fatigue for up to 6 weeks after the illness. Caution them to avoid contact sports as long as the spleen is enlarged. Because infectious mononucleosis occurs primarily in young adults, it may interrupt school or career plans. Help these young adults to voice their frustration with this illness. Offer support to help them through this unexpected interruption in their life.

Hantavirus Pulmonary Syndrome Infection

The hantavirus is a member of the arbovirus group. The virus infects small rodents and perhaps cats who have eaten mice. In the Far East, the virus produces an illness marked by extreme purpura from thrombocytopenia and severe gastrointestinal symptoms. In 1993, an outbreak of severe illness from a previously undiscovered hantavirus occurred in the United States; major symptoms were fever, muscle aches, thrombocytopenia, gastrointestinal symptoms, and hypotension. Death occurred from rapid progressive pulmonary edema (CDC, 1997).

Although the mortality from this particular hantavirus infection has been high (about 75%), treatment with the antiviral agent ribavirin may be effective.

✔ CHECKPOINT QUESTIONS

9. Where is the swelling of mumps typically located?
10. The child with infectious mononucleosis is at risk for what problem with abdominal palpation?

BACTERIAL INFECTIONS

Bacteria are usually single-celled organisms. They reproduce by fission, in which one cell enlarges and duplicates itself, then divides into two equal parts. Bacteria have three main shapes: (1) spheres (cocci), (2) rods (bacilli), and (3) corkscrews (spirochetes). Bacteria are independent, living organisms. They have a nucleus, cytoplasm, and a cell wall, and they contain both DNA and RNA.

Bacteria are most commonly observed under a microscope after being fixed to a slide by heating followed by staining. Those bacteria that stain violet are gram-positive organisms; those that stain red are gram-negative organisms. Those that cannot be decolorized with acid after being stained are acid-fast. As some bacteria grow, they produce **exotoxin,** or poison. Disease symptoms arise not from the bacteria themselves but from the effect of these toxins on the body. Tetanus, botulism, and diphtheria are diseases caused by the systemic spread of toxins produced by bacteria.

Some bacteria are capable of producing enzymes as they grow. Hemolytic streptococci, for example, produce streptokinase, which allows the bacteria to pass through blood clots. Penicillinase, an enzyme produced by certain bacteria, can destroy penicillin. Penicillin will be ineffective, therefore, against such organisms.

Streptococcal Diseases

Streptococci are gram-positive organisms. They are found normally in the respiratory, alimentary, and female genital tracts. The majority of severe diseases in children result from infection with *Streptococcus pyogenes* (beta-hemolytic streptococci, group A). Streptococcal pharyngeal infection is discussed in Chapter 19. Rheumatic fever, which may result as an autoimmune response, is discussed in Chapter 20.

Scarlet Fever

- Causative agent: Beta-hemolytic streptococci, group A
- Incubation period: 2 to 5 days
- Period of communicability: Greatest during acute phase of respiratory illness; 1 to 7 days
- Mode of transmission: Direct contact and large droplets
- Immunity: One episode of disease gives lasting immunity to scarlet fever toxin

Assessment. Scarlet fever occurs most commonly in the 6- to 12-year-old age group, although it may be seen in the preschooler. The incidence is highest in temperate climates, and it occurs usually in late winter or early spring months.

The symptoms of scarlet fever begin abruptly and are those of a streptococcal pharyngitis: fever, sore throat, perhaps headache, chills, and malaise. As the beta-hemolytic, group A streptococcus grows in children's bodies, it produces a number of toxins: erythrogenic toxin is the one that is responsible for the rash of scarlet fever. The rash appears 12 to 48 hours after the onset of the pharyngeal symptoms (see Figure 22-3). The fever is high (103°F to 104°F [39.5°C to 40.0°C]) on the first day of throat symptoms, again on the day the rash appears, and then gradually returns to normal. The child's pulse rate may be increased out of proportion to the fever.

The rash of scarlet fever is both enanthematous and exanthematous (on both mucous membrane and skin). The tonsils are inflamed and enlarged and usually covered with white exudate. The uvula and pharynx are beefy red. The palate is usually covered with erythematous punctiform (pinpoint) lesions and perhaps scattered petechiae. The tongue, during the first 2 days of the illness, is white and furry-appearing. By day 3, papillae enlarge and protrude through the white coat, giving the tongue a white strawberry appearance. By day 4 or 5, the white coat disappears and the prominent papillae of the tongue give it a red strawberry appearance. A "strawberry tongue" is distinctive for scarlet fever and helps to differentiate the disease from other rashes.

The skin rash comprises red, pinpoint lesions that blanch on pressure. Lesions are most dense on the trunk and in skin folds. Few lesions appear on the face. The area around the mouth tends to be abnormally pale (circumoral pallor). There are areas of hyperpigmentation in the folds of the joints (Pastia's sign). The rash persists for approximately 1 week. It desquamates with large areas of skin peeling off in fine flakes. A throat culture reveals streptococcus.

A particularly virulent form of group A streptococcus has been identified. Caution parents not to "self-treat" children with scarlet fever in case the streptococcus involved is this virulent strain. The child should be seen by a primary care provider.

Therapeutic Management. Children with scarlet fever usually appear ill. They need a soft or liquid diet for a few days until their throat soreness has diminished. They may need an analgesic and antipyretic, such as acetaminophen (Tylenol) or children's ibuprofen for pain and fever. The rash of scarlet fever tends to be pruritic, so comfort measures are necessary. Because the underlying cause of the illness is a streptococcus infection, a 10-day course of penicillin is usually prescribed. Caution parents to give the full amount prescribed for the full course to prevent the complications of beta-hemolytic, group A streptococcal infections (acute glomerulonephritis or rheumatic fever). If the child is in the hospital, follow droplet precautions until 24 hours after therapy is started in addition to standard precautions (see the Nursing Care Plan).

Children who receive penicillin do not have the typical extreme rash, and obviously do not have as severe a systemic illness as those who do not receive penicillin. As a result, scarlet fever is currently popularly termed *scarlatina* (a small, scarlet rash). Caution parents that, regardless of the name applied to the disorder, the consequences of it can be grave and penicillin therapy is necessary.

Rheumatic fever and acute glomerulonephritis occur as sequelae to scarlet fever in only approximately 2% to 3% of children. This occurs 1 week to 3 weeks after the rash. The occurrence seems to be related not to the severity of the scarlet fever but to the body reaction to the toxins produced at the time of the illness.

Impetigo

- Causative agent: Formerly beta-hemolytic streptococcus, group A; now usually *Staphylococcus aureus*
- Incubation period: 2 to 5 days

Nursing Care Plan

THE HOSPITALIZED CHILD WITH SCARLET FEVER

A 7-year-old female who is hospitalized following abdominal surgery develops a fever of 103°F (39.5°C) and a red, macular rash on her chest and abdomen on her second postoperative day. She states, "My throat hurts."

Assessment: Macular, pinpoint erythematous rash on abdomen, groin folds, and chest. Lesions blanch with pressure. Groin fold areas hyperpigmented. "This rash itches so much it hurts." Child states that lesions are very "itchy" and seen scratching lesions constantly. Uvula and pharynx beefy red. Tonsils inflamed and enlarged with white exudate. Pinpoint lesions with two to three scattered petechiae noted on palate. Tongue white and furry. Throat culture positive for streptococcus. Other physical examination findings within normal limits for postoperative course. A diagnosis of scarlet fever is made.

Child upset and crying. "I wish my mommy were here to stay with me. I'm all by myself. I can't even go to the play room." Mother is single parent with two smaller children, ages 4 years and 1 year, at home. Usually visits once a day in the late afternoon.

Nursing Diagnosis: Social isolation related to required restrictions associated with infection control precautions

Outcome Identification: Child participates in stimulating activities while hospitalized.

Outcome Evaluation: Child states reason for restrictions; identifies time when restrictions will be lifted; expresses interest in activities proposed.

Interventions	Rationale
1. Explain the reasons for restrictions and infection control precautions. Inform child about the length of time restrictions will be enforced.	1. Child may associate precautions and restrictions with feelings of being punished. Explanations help to increase understanding and decrease anxiety about unfamiliar events. Information about duration of restrictions provides the child with an end point to work towards.
2. Allow the child to see caregivers' faces before putting on necessary barriers such as masks prior to entering the room.	2. Being able to identify the person coming into the room helps to minimize the child's anxieties about strangers and the unknown.
3. Visit the child frequently, at least every hour, and provide her with opportunities for therapeutic play.	3. Frequent visits help to decrease feelings of being alone. Therapeutic play helps the child deal with feelings associated with her condition.
4. Plan age-appropriate activities that the child can engage in with health care personnel and when alone.	4. Participation in age-appropriate activities fosters growth and development. Joint activities help to decrease feelings of loneliness. Solo activities help to occupy time when child is alone.
5. Encourage the child to talk about how she feels about being separated from others.	5. Talking with the child allows her to share feelings and concerns openly and safely, possibly increasing the child's awareness of them and helping to diminish feelings of loneliness.
6. Encourage the child and mother to telephone each other if possible throughout the day.	6. Telephone contact helps to increase feelings of safety and security.
7. Encourage the child's mother to bring in the child's favorite toy.	7. Having a favorite toy nearby provides the child with a sense of security.
8. Begin antibiotic therapy as ordered.	8. Droplet precautions are followed until 24 hours after the initiation of therapy, minimizing the time required for the child to be restricted and separated from others.

(continued)

Nursing Diagnosis: Pain related to pruritus from the skin lesions and sore throat

Outcome Identification: Child reports pain is within tolerable levels.

Outcome Evaluation: Child states she is comfortable; reports itching is less severe; is observed not scratching lesions. Absence of further irritation or excoriation.

Interventions	Rationale
1. Administer analgesics and antihistamines as ordered.	1. Analgesics act to decrease pain. Antihistamines act to block histamine release associated with the inflammatory process.
2. Apply calamine lotion or use colloidal baths in lukewarm water as indicated.	2. Calamine lotion and colloidal baths help soothe the skin and decrease itching. Heat causes vasodilation and increases the sensation of itching.
3. Instruct the child to press on the itchy area rather than scratch.	3. Pressing on the area may help to diminish the itching sensation without further irritation and possible subsequent skin breakdown from excessive scratching.
4. Apply cool compresses to the area. Encourage the child to participate with applying the dressings.	4. Cool compresses cause vasoconstriction, decrease inflammation, and help soothe the itching sensation. Participation by the child provides a purposeful activity and helps to promote a feeling of control.
5. Provide diversional activities.	5. Diversional activities help to focus the child's attention on other things rather than the itch.
6. Dress the child in cool, lightweight, cotton clothing.	6. Appropriate clothing allows for evaporation of perspiration and heat. Perspiration and overheating worsen itching, further irritating the skin.
7. Provide frequent fluids with a soft or liquid diet.	7. Adequate fluid intake is important to prevent skin dryness, which increases discomfort. A soft or liquid diet is less irritating to the child's sore throat.
8. Cut the child's fingernails short and use cotton gloves as necessary.	8. Keeping fingernails short and using cotton gloves help to minimize the risk for injury from excessive scratching.

- Period of communicability: From outbreak of lesions until lesions are healed
- Mode of transmission: Direct contact with lesions
- Immunity: None

Impetigo is a superficial infection of the skin. It begins as a single papulovesicular lesion surrounded by localized erythema. As more vesicles appear, they become purulent, ooze, and form honey-colored crusts (Figure 22-12). They are found most commonly on the face and extremities. They are often seen as secondary infections of insect bites or in children who have pierced ears. If there are a number of lesions, children may have local adenopathy.

Impetigo is only mildly infectious because it seems to be transmitted only by direct contact. It is not uncommon to see several children in a family with identical lesions, however. Parents may be upset at being told their child has impetigo, because at one time the lesions (dirty and crusty appearing) were associated with poor hygiene. Parents' first statement at being told the diagnosis may be, "But our children take baths every day." They can be assured that microorganisms are so numerous that the cleanest child can contract disease. The presence of the infection reflects on the number of organisms available, not on their child care.

Caution parents to seek health supervision for any lesion that appears reddened or filled with pus (infected), because the causative agent may be a particularly virulent form.

Therapeutic Management. Treatment is oral administration of penicillin or erythromycin or the application of mupirocin (Bactroban) ointment for a full 10 days (see Drug Highlight: Mupirocin [Bactroban]). The application of local antibiotic ointment is not as effective because it does not reduce the number of organisms and, therefore, does not reduce the toxin level as effectively. The lesions heal most quickly if a parent or the child washes the crusts daily with soap and water.

Although rare, complications of rheumatic fever or acute glomerulonephritis may occur after impetigo as they may after other streptococcal infections. If the child develops impetigo while in the hospital, follow contact precautions until 24 hours after initiation of therapy.

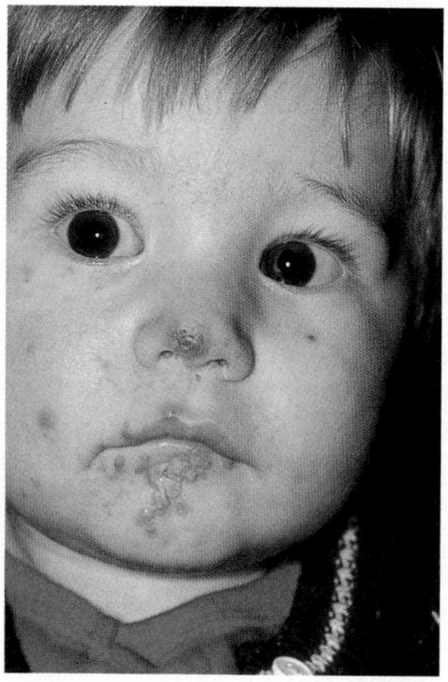

FIGURE 22.12 Impetigo in a toddler. Note the honey-colored crust appearance of some of the lesions.

Cat-Scratch Disease

- Causative agent: *Bartonella henselae* bacteria
- Incubation period: 3 to 10 days
- Period of communicability: Unknown
- Mode of transmission: Bite or scratch from a cat or kitten
- Immunity: One episode of disease gives lasting immunity; no passive artificial immunity

Cat-scratch disease occurs most commonly in preschool children because children at that age play roughly with cats or pick them up against their will and thus receive scratches. At the time the child contracts the disease, the cat does not appear to be ill.

The first symptom for the child is a single skin papule or pustule that lasts 1 to 3 weeks. Approximately 2 weeks after the scratch, severe local lymphadenopathy develops. The nodes most markedly involved are those of the head, neck, and axilla. The node enlargement generally lasts 2 to 3 months. In some children, there is node suppuration (a node breaks open to the skin and drains sterile pus).

Some children have a low-grade fever and malaise. Occasionally, central nervous system involvement, such as encephalitis or meningitis, occurs. A positive reaction to a skin test of cat-scratch disease antigen will be present. This, along with the history of a cat scratch and the aspiration of sterile pus from enlarged lymph nodes, is diagnostic. Treatment is symptomatic, although an antibiotic may be prescribed to help shorten the course of the disease. Children may need an analgesic for painful adenopathy. Aspiration of involved nodes may be necessary to relieve pain.

Parents may ask if the cat should be destroyed. Because an attack of cat-scratch disease gives lifetime immunity and fewer than 10% of children scratched by the same cat contract cat-scratch disease, there is no need to destroy the cat (Boyer, 1997).

DRUG HIGHLIGHT

Mupirocin (Bactroban)

Action: Mupirocin is a topical antibiotic treatment for impetigo caused by *Staphylococcus aureus* and *Streptococcus pyogenes.*

Pregnancy risk category: B

Dosage: Small amount applied two to five times a day to the affected areas for 10 days.

Possible adverse effects: Erythema, dry skin, pruritus, burning, stinging

Nursing Implications:

- Advise parents to wash the lesions with soap and water, and pat dry before applying ointment to soften crusts for better absorption.
- Caution parents that causative organisms are infectious by direct contact. Instruct them to wash their own hands before and after applying the ointment.
- Urge parents to continue to use the ointment to ensure complete eradication of the causative germs. The lesions may begin to improve before 10 days have elapsed.
- Instruct the parents to use caution when applying the ointment around the eyes. Ointment is irritating to the eyes.
- Teach the parents about the signs and symptoms of possible fungal infection that may occur and to notify a health care provider should any occur.

Staphylococcal Infections

The staphylococcal organisms are gram-positive. Colonies of staphylococci are normally found on the skin, so they are generally the organisms involved in skin infections (pyodermas). Because the organisms grow rapidly in cream foods that are not well refrigerated, such as potato salad or cream pies, they are often the organisms involved in food poisoning episodes during the summer months. Food poisoning leads to gastrointestinal symptoms (see Chapter 24).

Furunculosis (Boils)

A furuncle is a staphylococcal infection of the hair follicle. A yellow pustule forms at the site. There is localized redness, pain, and edema of the surrounding skin. Children must be urged not to rupture these lesions but to allow them to run their self-limiting course so the infection is not spread to surrounding tissue and does not become a cellulitis.

Cellulitis

Cellulitis is a staphylococcal inflammation of the deeper layers of skin. It occurs generally on the extremities or face, or surrounding wounds. The skin feels warm to the touch and is edematous and reddened. Cellulitis is treated with a systemic antibiotic. Warm soaks relieve pain and inflammation.

Scalded Skin Disease

Scalded skin disease (Ritter's disease) is a staphylococcal infection seen primarily in newborns. Children develop rough textured skin and general erythema. Large bullae (vesicles), filled with clear fluid, form. The epidermis separates from children in large sheets, leaving a red, glistening, scalded-looking surface. Children need intensive therapy with an intravenous antibiotic to survive this extreme infection.

✔ **CHECKPOINT QUESTIONS**

11. What organism is responsible for scarlet fever?
12. What organism is often the cause of food poisoning episodes during the summer months?

Other Bacterial Infections

Diphtheria

- Causative agent: *Corynebacterium diphtheriae* (Klebs-Löffler bacillus)
- Incubation period: 2 to 6 days
- Period of communicability: Rarely more than 2 weeks to 4 weeks in untreated persons; 1 to 2 days in patients treated with antibiotics
- Mode of transmission: Direct or indirect contact
- Immunity: Contracting the disease gives lasting natural immunity
- Active artificial immunity: Diphtheria toxin given as part of DTaP vaccine
- Passive artificial immunity: Diphtheria antitoxin

Assessment. When diphtheria bacilli invade and grow in the nasopharynx of children, they produce an exotoxin (a potent protein poison) that causes massive cell necrosis and inflammation. The necrosing material lends itself well to the growth of the bacilli, so the bacilli reproduce rapidly. The inflammation and necrosing cells form a characteristic gray membrane on the nasopharynx. It may extend up into the nose and down into the major bronchi, causing a purulent nasal discharge and a brassy cough. The toxin is absorbed from the membrane surface and spread systemically by the bloodstream to affect the heart causing myocarditis with heart failure and conduction disturbances on approximately day 10 to 14 of the illness and the nervous system (severe neuritis with paralysis of the diaphragm and pharyngeal and laryngeal muscles) on day 3 to week 7 of the illness. Airway obstruction from inflammation and membrane formation is a possibility from the time it first forms. The diagnosis of diphtheria is made on clinical appearance and on a throat culture, which reveals the presence of the bacilli.

Therapeutic Management. Treatment involves intravenous administration of antitoxin in large doses. The antitoxin of diphtheria is grown from a horse-serum base. Before it is administered, therefore, children must be given a skin or conjunctiva test to rule out a reaction to horse serum. For a conjunctiva test, a drop of the diphtheria antitoxin well diluted with saline is instilled inside the lower lid of one eye. A drop of saline is placed in the other eye as a control. In 20 minutes, both eyes are examined. If lacrimation or conjunctivitis is present in the eye that received the serum, it suggests the child is hypersensitive to horse serum. The antitoxin cannot be administered until the child is desensitized. For a skin test, a small amount of diluted diphtheria antitoxin is administered intracutaneously. After 20 minutes, a wheal 1 cm or more in diameter reveals sensitivity to horse serum. Again, the antitoxin cannot be given until the child is desensitized. Have a syringe of epinephrine readily available before horse-serum antitoxin testing or administration is begun in case a sudden anaphylactic reaction occurs with the serum administration.

In addition to the antitoxin, children are given penicillin or erythromycin intravenously. They need to be maintained on bedrest for the acute stage of the illness, and droplet precautions must be followed until antibiotic therapy is completed and cultures are negative. They need careful observation to prevent airway obstruction. If this does occur, endotracheal intubation may be necessary.

Because diphtheria vaccine is included in routine immunizations for infants, it is almost an extinct disease in the United States. However, isolated instances do occur, and when they do, prompt recognition and treatment are necessary (Feigin, 1997).

Whooping Cough (Pertussis)

- Causative agent: *Bordetella pertussis*
- Incubation period: 5 to 21 days
- Mode of transmission: Direct or indirect contact
- Period of communicability: Greatest in **catarrhal** (respiratory illness) **stage**
- Immunity: Contracting the disease offers lasting natural immunity
- Active artificial immunity: Pertussis vaccine given as part of DTaP vaccine
- Passive artificial immunity: Pertussis immune serum globulin

Pertussis is a serious disease of childhood, particularly in the infant period. It occurs most often in children up to age 9 years. African-American and Native American children seem to be most susceptible. In older children, more girls than boys contract the infection. It occurs with no seasonal variation.

Assessment. Pertussis manifests itself in three stages: (1) catarrhal, (2) paroxysmal, and (3) convalescent. The catarrhal stage begins with upper respiratory symptoms such as coryza, sneezing, lacrimation, cough, and a low-grade fever. Children are irritable and listless. In some children, a mild cough is the only symptom during this stage. It lasts from 1 to 2 weeks.

The paroxysmal stage lasts 4 to 6 weeks. During this time, the cough changes from a mild one to a paroxysmal one, involving five to ten short, rapid coughs, followed by a rapid inspiration, which causes the "whoop," or high-pitched crowing sound, of whooping cough. Children are in obvious distress while coughing. They may become cyanotic or red faced, and their nose may drain thick, tenacious mucus. They often vomit after a paroxysm of coughing, and they are exhausted afterward from the effort. Attacks of coughing tend to be more severe at night than during the daytime.

WHAT IF? What if a child with pertussis vomits after an episode of coughing? Would you want to refeed the child, or do you think that he or she would be too nauseated to eat again?

During the convalescent stage, there is a gradual cessation of the coughing and vomiting. The cough may be present for some time, but as single, not paroxysmal coughs. During the next year, if children develop an upper respiratory infection, they may again have a return of the paroxysmal coughing with vomiting.

Pertussis is diagnosed by its striking symptoms, although in children younger than age 6 months the "whoop" of the cough may be absent, making it more difficult to diagnose. The *B pertussis* bacillus may be cultured from nasopharyngeal secretions during the catarrhal and paroxysmal stages. WBC, particularly the lymphocyte count, rises with whooping cough. WBC may be as high as 20,000 to 30,000 mm^3 at the end of the catarrhal stage (normal is 5,000 to 10,000 mm^3).

Therapeutic Management. Children with pertussis must be maintained on bedrest until the paroxysms of coughing subside. They need to be secluded from external factors such as cigarette smoke, dust, and strenuous activity that initiate coughing episodes. Nutrition may be a problem if the child is constantly coughing and vomiting. There is no nausea with this form of vomiting, so children can be fed again immediately after vomiting. As a rule, frequent small meals are vomited less than larger meals. Infants with pertussis may be admitted to a health care facility for observation because they may have such tenacious secretions with coughing episodes that they need airway suction. Placing an intercom in the infant's room allows personnel to listen for paroxysms of coughing even when not immediately near the child.

A full 10-day course of erythromycin or penicillin may be prescribed. These drugs have the potential to shorten the period of communicability and may shorten the duration of symptoms. Droplet precautions are used until 5 days after child is placed on effective therapy.

Complications of pertussis include pneumonia, atelectasis, or emphysema from plugged bronchioles. Convulsions from asphyxia as a result of severe paroxysms of coughing may occur. Epitaxis, subconjunctival and subarachnoid bleeding from the forcefulness of coughing, may occur. If sufficient fluid intake cannot be maintained, alkalosis and dehydration from persistent vomiting can occur.

Prevention. Little passive immunity is transferred to the newborn, so children in their early months are particularly susceptible to this disease. Infants who are exposed may be administered pertussis immune serum globulin to protect them from contracting the disease.

Tetanus (Lockjaw)

- Causative agent: *Clostridium tetani*
- Incubation period: 3 days to 3 weeks
- Period of communicability: None
- Mode of transmission: Direct or indirect contamination of a closed wound
- Immunity: Development of the disease gives lasting natural immunity.
- Active artificial immunity: Tetanus toxoid contained in DTaP vaccine
- Passive artificial immunity: Tetanus immune globulin

Tetanus, a highly fatal disease with a mortality rate as high as 35%, is caused by an anaerobic, spore-forming bacillus. The bacillus, found in soil and the excretions of animals, enters the body through a wound. If the wound is deep, such as a puncture wound, where the distal end of the wound is shut off from an oxygen source, the tetanus bacilli begins to reproduce. The organism may also enter through a burn site, which crusts, creating an anaerobic environment. As the bacilli grow, they produce exotoxins that cause the disease symptoms by affecting the motor nuclei of the central nervous system.

The entrance site of the bacillus does not appear infected (no pus or reddened area is present unless a secondary infection also exists). After the incubation period, the exotoxins have developed to such an extent, however, that they are capable of disrupting the nervous system.

Assessment. The first symptoms that are noticeable are stiffness of the neck and jaw (lockjaw). Within 24 to 48 hours, muscular rigidity of the trunk and extremities develops. Children's backs become arched (opisthotonos); their abdominal muscles are stiff and boardlike; and their faces assume an unusual appearance with wrinkling of the forehead and distortion of the corners of the mouth (a "sardonic grin" sign). Any stimulation such as a sudden noise, a bright light, or someone touching them causes children to have painful, paroxysmal spasms. Children's sensoriums are clear throughout the course of the disease, so they are aware of the pain associated with muscle spasms. As these spasms begin to include laryngospasm, respiratory obstruction, and a collection of secretions in the respiratory tract, they may lead ultimately to death by asphyxiation (Dunkle, 1997).

Fever is an ominous sign accompanying tetanus. Those children who survive the disease rarely have more than a low-grade fever.

Therapeutic Management. Children need to be cared for in a quiet, stimulation-free room. If the wound has necrotic tissue, it may be debrided to ensure that no secondary infections arise. Enteral or total parenteral nutrition may be necessary to prevent aspiration from laryngeal spasm. Tetanus immune globulin (human) is administered to supply passive antitoxins to combat the extent of the disease involvement.

Parenteral penicillin G or a form of tetracycline is administered to reduce the number of growing forms of the bacillus. Sedation and a muscle relaxant may be necessary to reduce the severity and pain of the muscle spasms. Children need to be intubated, and mechanical ventilation is begun to maintain respiratory function after administration.

Prevention. Tetanus is a serious disease, but is also a preventable one through active immunization and suitable booster immunization. Children routinely receive tetanus immunization as part of routine DPT immunization and a booster dose at school age; thereafter they should receive a booster dose every 10 years. At the time of a wound, the wound site should be cleaned well with soap and water and a suitable antiseptic. If the wound is deep, such as a knife stab, a nail puncture, or a dog bite, it should not be sutured but, rather, left open to heal by secondary intention. This reduces the possibility of an anaerobic pocket forming in the wound. If children received their basic immunization against tetanus (five doses) and it has been fewer than 10 years since the last injection, they need no booster or antitoxin management at the time of the wound.

If a child's immunization record cannot be obtained, or if it has been more than 10 years since the child received a booster injection or an initial injection for tetanus, the child will probably be treated with a booster injection and tetanus immune globulin. A booster injection provides tetanus antigen to the child. If children received their initial immunization for this disease, the booster will cause their bodies to "remember" how to make tetanus antibodies, and their body will begin to produce them rapidly. By the time the invading tetanus organisms from the wound have passed their long incubation period (3 days to 3 weeks), children have antibodies in their system prepared to eradicate the organisms. If their initial immunizations were incomplete or are unknown, in addition to tetanus antigen they will also receive the passive antibodies included in tetanus immune globulin.

Lyme Disease

Lyme disease is caused by a spirochete, *Borrelia burgdorferi*, that is transmitted by a tick often carried on deer. The disease is the most frequently reported vector-borne infection in the United States, occurring most often in the summer and early fall. Almost immediately after the tick bite, an erythematous papule is noticeable at the site, which spreads over the next 3 to 30 days (the incubation period) to become a large, round ring with a raised swollen border (erythema chronicum migrans; Figure 22-13). This is followed by systemic involvement that leads to cardiac, musculoskeletal, and neurologic symptoms. Cardiac involvement may be so severe that it includes heart block from atrioventricular conduction abnormalities. Neurologic symptoms commonly include stiff neck, headache, and cranial nerve palsy. Musculoskeletal symptoms occur in 50% of children and include painful swollen arthritic joints, particularly the knee.

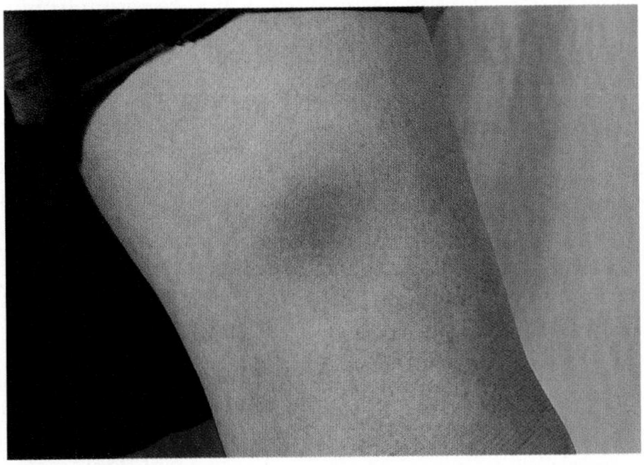

FIGURE 22.13 The rash of Lyme disease.

BOX 22.2

TIPS FOR AVOIDING EXPOSURE TO LYME DISEASE

- Wear protective clothing when hiking in wooded areas: long sleeves, high necklines, long slacks. Tuck bottom of slacks into socks or boots.
- Wear light-colored clothing so any tick present on clothing can be readily observed.
- Inspect skin for ticks after hiking in woody areas. Remove any present with tweezers.
- Report any area of inflammation that might be a tick bite to a health care provider for early diagnosis.

Oral penicillin is administered at the time of the bite to young children. Tetracycline is given to those older than age 8 years. Anti-inflammatory agents and daily corticosteroids, such as prednisone, may be necessary to reduce the cardiac and arthritic effects.

Parents should be cautioned to inspect the skin of children who have been playing in wooded areas for possible tick bites when they return from play to aid in identifying the disorder before debilitating symptoms occur. Other suggestions for avoiding Lyme disease are shown in Box 22-2.

✓ CHECKPOINT QUESTIONS

13. What is the result of exotoxin production by diphtheria bacilli?
14. What is the major complication of pertussis?

OTHER INFECTIOUS PATHOGENS

Rickettsial Diseases

Rickettsiae are organisms that resemble viruses both in size and in their inability to reproduce except inside the cells of a host organism. They reproduce by fission, however, as bacteria do; like bacteria, they are complete organisms containing both RNA and DNA. They multiply inside ticks, lice, mites, or fleas (arthropods) without causing disease. They are transmitted to humans through the bite or feces of the infected arthropod. An exception is Q fever, which is spread by droplet infection. All rickettsial diseases include fever and almost all include a rash caused by rickettsial multiplication in the endothelial cells of small blood vessels. Rickettsiae invasion triggers an immune response.

Rocky Mountain Spotted Fever

- Causative agent: *Rickettsia rickettsii*
- Incubation period: 3 to 12 days

- Period of communicability: Not communicable from one person to another
- Mode of transmission: Wood, dog, or rabbit tick
- Active artificial immunity: Rocky Mountain spotted fever vaccine

This is the most common rickettsial disease seen in the United States, most prevalent in the eastern United States, transmitted by a tick. It is seen most often during the spring and early summer when ticks are most commonly seen. A reddened area develops at the site of the tick bit. In 2 to 8 days, a typical rash, persistent headache, fever (as high as 40°C), and mental confusion begin. The rash is distinctive, beginning with reddened macules, then changing to petechiae. It begins on the wrists and ankles, then spreads up the arms and legs onto the trunk. Unlike most rashes, it can cover the palms of the hands and soles of the feet (Figure 22-14).

In untreated children, symptoms worsen to include symptoms of central nervous system involvement (stiff neck, seizures), cardiac and pulmonary symptoms such as heart failure and pneumonia. Nitrogen loss in the urine becomes extreme. An accompanying hyponatremia may also be present.

Therapy is with chloramphenical or tetracycline for 7 to 10 days. Caution parents to administer the drug for the full course of therapy to ensure disease eradication and prevent the risk of complications. Rocky Moutain spotted fever was a serious childhood illness before antibiotic therapy was available. It still has the potential to be serious if the symptoms are not reported when they first occur.

Rickettsialpox

Rickettsialpox is a disease of crowded urban areas because it is carried by a mouse mite. There is a local lesion at the site of the bite and a generalized rash over the entire body with the exception of the palms and soles. The illness responds to tetracycline.

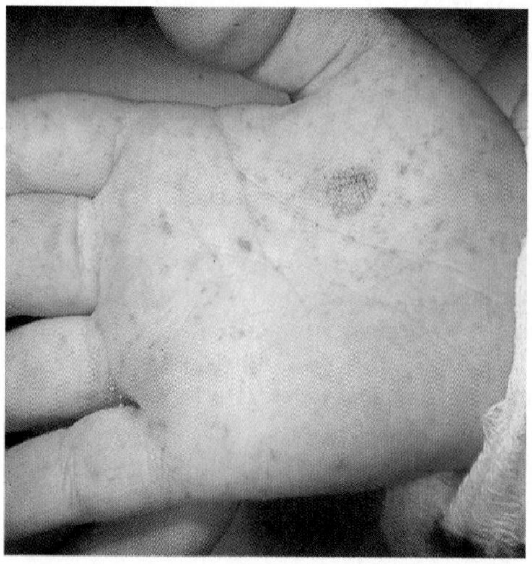

FIGURE 22.14 Typical rash of Rocky Mountain spotted fever.

Murine Typhus

Murine typhus is seen almost exclusively in the southern United States. It is transmitted by mites and fleas that live on rats. It is almost identical in symptoms to Rocky Mountain spotted fever. It responds to tetracycline or a third-generation antibiotic such as ciprofloxacin.

Chlamydial Infections

Chlamydiae are gram-negative nonmotile organisms similar to rickettsiae. Chlamydial pneumonia or vaginitis may occur (see Chapters 19 and 26). Psittacosis is a chlamydial infection commonly found in children.

Psittacosis

Psittacosis is caused by *Chlamydia psittace*. It is a disease transmitted to children by birds, such as parakeets, lovebirds, parrots, chickens, turkeys, and pigeons. The bird has no apparent symptoms of illness. Children develop symptoms of an upper respiratory infection, possibly accompanied by a low-grade fever, a dry cough, weakness, and anorexia out of proportion to the fever. An enlarged spleen may also be present. Children may develop patchy bronchopneumonia. The course of the disease is as long as 3 to 4 weeks. Treatment is with tetracycline.

Parasitic Infections

Parasites are organisms that live and obtain their food supply from other organisms. Frequently seen parasites in children include head lice and scabies (Table 22-5). Parents are often embarassed when they learn that their child has lice. Reassure them that this infestation can happen to any child (see Enhancing Communication).

Helminthic Infections

Helminth means worm and refers to pathogenic or parasitic ones. They may be roundworms (nematodes), flukes (trematodes), or tapeworms (cestodes). Most helminths begin life when the eggs or larvae are eliminated in feces or urine of humans. They are then transmitted to the oral cavity by unclean foods or hands. Because children tend to be careless about washing hands before eating or tend to suck their thumbs, they are prone to these infections.

Roundworms (Ascariasis)

The roundworm parasite lives in the intestinal tract. Eggs are excreted in the feces. If children eat food or have hands that are improperly washed, eggs may be ingested by them along with soil. Larvae, which hatch from the ingested eggs, penetrate the intestinal wall and enter the circulation. From there, they may migrate to any body tissue. Children have a loss of appetite and perhaps nausea and vomiting. Intestinal obstruction may occur from a mass of roundworms in the intestinal tract. Ascariasis can be prevented by the sanitary disposal of feces so this does not contaminate soil. A single dose of an anthelmintic such as pyrantel pamoate (Antiminth) controls the infection.

TABLE 22.5 Common Parasitic Infections

INFECTION	ORGANISM	SYMPTOMS	TREATMENT
Pediculosis capitis	Head lice	Small, white flecks on hair shaft (nits or eggs of lice) Extremely pruritic	Wash hair with shampoo such as lindane (Kwell) Comb nits from hair with fine-toothed comb Wash bed sheets, recently worn clothes Vacuum pillows, mattresses or other items unable to be washed Teach children not to exchange combs, hair barrettes, or other personal items
Pediculosis pubis	Pubic lice	Same as for head lice except on pubic hair	Same as head lice Warn client that it might be spread by physical intimacy
Scabies	Female mite (acarus scabiei)	Black burrow filled with mite feces ½ inch long, usually between fingers and toes, on palms, or in axilla or groin	Wash area with lindane (Kwell) lotion or permethrin

Hookworms

Hookworm eggs, like roundworm eggs, are found in human feces. They enter children's bodies through the skin and then migrate to the intestinal tract, where they attach themselves onto the intestinal villi. They suck blood from children's intestinal wall to sustain themselves. If a great number of hookworms are present, severe anemia may result. Treatment is with anthelmintics to destroy the worms. Children may also need therapy for the anemia.

Pinworms

Pinworms are small, white, threadlike worms that live in the cecum. At night, the female pinworm migrates down the intestinal tract and out the anus to deposit eggs in the anal and perianal region. The anal area itches, and the child wakes at night crying and scratching. Some of the eggs are then carried from their fingernails to their mouths. They hatch in children's intestinal tract, and the cycle is repeated.

The worms are large enough that they can be seen if children's buttocks are separated when they are sleeping. Pressing a piece of cellophane tape against the anus and then looking at it under a microscope will generally reveal pinworm eggs.

Treatment is with a single dose of mebendazole (Vermox) or pyrantel pamoate (Antiminth). Both drugs destroy pinworms effectively. All family members are treated for pinworm infestation because such worms are easily transmitted from person to person. Underclothing, bedding, towels, and nightclothing should be washed before reuse. Teach children to avoid nailbiting and to wash hands before food preparation or eating to avoid transfer of pinworm eggs to the gastrointestinal tract.

Protozoan Infections

Protozoa are unicellular organisms. They absorb fluid through the cell membrane and are able to move from place to place by pseudopod, flagella, or cilia action. They are most pathogenic in the gastrointestinal, genitourinary, and circulatory systems. Some protozoa reproduce by simple binary fission; other forms have complex life cycles. Protozoa have the ability to form cysts or surround themselves with a resistant membrane. This makes them resistant to destruction.

Giardia lamblia

Giardia lamblia is a protozoan infection that is responsible for epidemic outbreaks of diarrhea, particularly in travelers to Europe and in United States day care centers.

Transmission occurs when the child ingests the cysts of the organism on unclean hands. In the intestine, the cysts develop into the mature form of the organism causing symptoms such as diarrhea, weight loss, abdominal cramps, and nausea.

Diagnosis is made by history and recognition of the mature form of the organism in the stool or on duodenal aspiration. Therapy is with quinacrine hydrochloride (Atabrine) for 5 to 7 days or metronidazole (Flagyl) for 5 days. Be certain that parents of children know that Flagyl is contraindicated during pregnancy so a pregnant mother does not self-medicate.

Fungal Infections

Fungi are larger than bacteria; some are unicellular (yeasts), but generally they are multicellular (molds). Fungal infections are most often divided into groups according to the body tissue they infect. Deep mycoses invade internal organs. Transmission is by the inhalation of spores. Subcutaneous mycoses invade skin, subcutaneous tissue, and bone. Infections usually occur from introduction of the fungi into a wound. Superficial mycoses invade only the hair, skin, or nails.

Superficial Fungal Infections

Four superficial fungal infections are seen frequently in children.

ENHANCING COMMUNICATION

Joshua is a 1-year-old boy you see in an ambulatory clinic. He has scratch marks on his neck and forehead. His hair shafts are covered by sandlike particles. He is diagnosed as having pediculosis capitis.

Less Effective Communication

Nurse: Hello, Mrs. Ireland. Did the doctor tell you what is wrong with Joshua?
Mrs. Ireland: No.
Nurse: I heard him tell you that Joshua has head lice. I have the prescription for you that you need for shampoo.
Mrs. Ireland: The doctor hasn't done any tests yet.
Nurse: There aren't any tests for head lice. Take the prescription to your drugstore and buy the shampoo.
Mrs. Ireland: What about the itchiness? Or these white marks?
Nurse: The shampoo will take care of it.
Mrs. Ireland: I'm not putting anything on his head for lice.
Nurse: Okay. I'll leave the prescription and you can think about it.

More Effective Communication

Nurse: Hello, Mrs. Ireland. Did the doctor tell you what is wrong with Joshua?
Mrs. Ireland: No.
Nurse: I heard him tell you Joshua has head lice.
Mrs. Ireland: The doctor hasn't done any tests yet.
Nurse: Do you have any questions about what he said?
Mrs. Ireland: He said Joshua has head lice. But we're not that poor.
Nurse: Let's talk about head lice, and how easy it is for anyone to get them.

The above scenario is an example of what can happen if people believe one of the community stories that circulate related to communicable diseases. By allowing the mother to explain why she thinks the diagnosis could not be right rather than just proceeding with instructions, the nurse makes it possible for her to learn correct information and should increase compliance.

Tinea Cruris. *Tinea cruris* (jock itch) occurs on the inner aspects of the thighs and scrotum. It is pruritic. Local application of tolnaftate liquid or powder is effective in destroying the infection.

Tinea Pedis. *Tinea pedis* (athlete's foot) produces skin lesions between toes and on the plantar surface of the foot. Pruritic, pinpoint vesicles and fissuring, especially between the toes, may occur. It is treated with liquid preparations of tolnaftate.

Tinea Capitis. *Tinea capitis* (ringworm) is a fungal infection that begins as an infection of a single hair follicle but spreads rapidly in a circular pattern to produce a lesion usually approximately 1 inch in diameter (Figure 22-15). The hairs involved in the lesion generally break off. The circle becomes filled with dirty-appearing scales. Some strains of tinea capitis may be detected because they glow green under a Wood's light. Newer strains of the organism do not do this, so the test is losing its accuracy. Treatment is with griseofulvin given orally. Teach adolescents not to use alcohol while taking this drug; this may cause tachycardia. Safety during pregnancy is not established. Children need to avoid strong sunlight during therapy, because photosensitivity may occur. Tinea capitis is not as contagious as was once assumed. Children need not be kept home from school, although they should be cautioned not to exchange towels or combs or other potential fomites. The course of the disease may be long; it may be 3 months before all lesions have faded.

Tinea Corporis. *Tinea corporis* is fungal infection of the epidermal layer of the skin. It presents as a scaly ring of inflammation with a clear area in the center. Treatment is with a topical antifungal agent such as clotrimazole (Tunnessen, 1997).

Candidiasis

Candida albicans is the fungus that is responsible for candidal (monilial infections). *Candida* organisms grow in the vagina of many adult women (candidal vaginitis). Newborns delivered vaginally may develop an infection of the mucous membrane of the mouth (thrush or oral *Candida* infection). Thrush is characterized by white plaques on an erythematous base on the buccal membrane and the surface of the tongue. It resembles milk curd left from a recent milk feeding. Thrush plaques do not scrape away, however, whereas milk curds do. The child's mouth is painful, and he or she does not eat well due to the inflammation and local pain. Adolescent girls may develop candidal vaginitis.

C. albicans also causes a severe, bright red, sharply circumscribed diaper-area rash (Figure 22-16). Satellite lesions also may appear. The rash is marked by its intense color, and it does not improve with the usual diaper-rash measures, such as Desitin, frequent changing of diapers, or exposure to air.

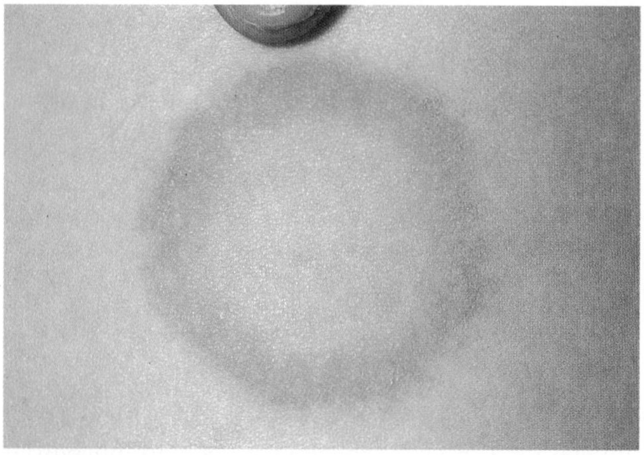

FIGURE 22.15 Ringworm. The fungus spreads rapidly, producing a circular, ringlike lesion.

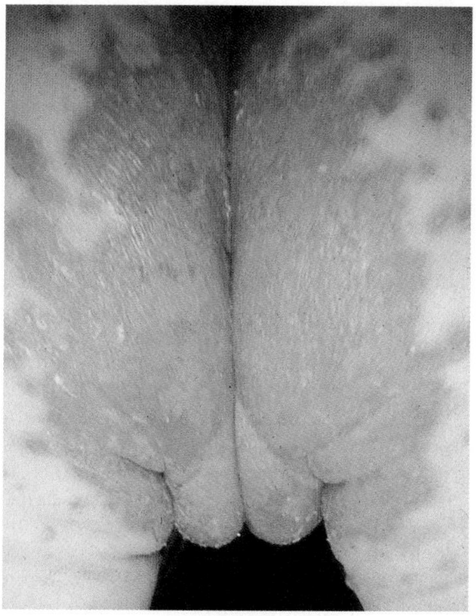

FIGURE 22.16 Monilial diaper rash. Note the intense red color of the rash.

Nystatin is an effective antifungal drug. For thrush, it is generally administered orally approximately four times a day. It should be dropped into infants' mouths after feedings so it will remain in contact with lesions for a time rather than being washed away immediately by a feeding. For diaper rash, a nystatin ointment is prescribed. For candidal vaginitis in the adolescent, vaginal suppositories of nystatin may be ordered. Teach adolescents to continue use through the menstrual period. A sexual partner should use a condom to avoid reinfection. Itraconazole may be prescribed if the infection is persistent.

Candidiasis can become a generalized infection, especially in a newborn. There is a tendency to think of thrush as a common—almost something to be expected—disease of infants. It needs treatment, however, to prevent it from becoming more serious or systemic.

✔ CHECKPOINT QUESTIONS

15. How are helminthic infections transmitted?
16. What organism is responsible for thrush?

KEY POINTS

The incubation period of infectious disease is the time between the invasion of an organism and the onset of symptoms. A prodromal period is the time between the beginning of nonspecific symptoms and specific symptoms. Children are infectious during the prodromal period. Illness is the stage during which specific symptoms are evident. The convalescent period is the interval between the time symptoms begin to fade and the child returns to full wellness.

The chain of infection depends on the presence of a reservoir, a portal of exit, a means of transmission, a portal of entry, and a susceptible host. To reduce the spread of infection, use standard precautions. Transmission-based precautions—airborne, droplet and contact—also may be necessary.

Immunization depends on the activation of the immune system. Both B-cell (humoral immunity) and T-cell (cell-mediated immunity) lymphocytes are involved. Immunity may be active (the child has developed the disease or had antigens of the disease administered), or passive (antibodies against the disease are administered to the child by vaccines or placental transfer).

Common viral infections of childhood are exanthem subitum (roseola), rubella (German measles), measles (rubeola), chickenpox (varicella), herpes zoster, erythema infectiosum (fifth disease), pityriasis rosea, mumps (epidemic parotitis), infectious mononucleosis, and cat-scratch disease. Other important viral infections include poliomyelitis (now almost extinct), herpesvirus infections, verrucae (warts) and rabies.

Streptococcal diseases seen include scarlet fever and impetigo. Staphylococcal infections seen include furunculosis (boils), cellulitis, and scalded skin disease. Outbreaks of diphtheria, whooping cough (pertussis), and tetanus (lockjaw) still occur.

Important rickettsial diseases are Rocky Mountain spotted fever and Lyme disease. Parasitic infections are pediculosis capitis (head lice), pediculosis pubis, and scabies. Helminthic infections are roundworms, hookworms, and pinworms. Fungal infections are tinea capitis and tinea corporis (ringworm).

Teaching parents and children about infection control measures and immunizations is essential to reduce the risk and prevent infectious disorders.

CRITICAL THINKING EXERCISES

1. Marty is the 6-year-old boy you met at the beginning of the chapter. He was diagnosed as having chickenpox (varicella) the morning after surgery for appendicitis. Is it most likely that Marty contracted this infection while he was hospitalized or is it most likely that the contact occurred before hospitalization? What is the typical pattern of chickenpox lesions? What would you recommend to his parents to help reduce the itchiness of the rash?
2. A 2-year-old boy is found to have pediculosis on a routine health examination. His mother tells you she can't believe the diagnosis because she thought only poor children developed head lice. She is also very concerned that her son will have his head shaved to cure him. How would you advise her?

3. A mother tells you that she doesn't intend to have her newborn immunized because she feels the risk of developing a complication from vaccine administration is higher than letting her child contract simple childhood illnesses. How would you counsel her?

REFERENCES

Boyer, K. M. (1997). Cat-scratch disease. In Johnson, K. B., & Oski, F. A. *Oski's essential pediatrics.* Philadelphia: Lippincott.

Bruno, G., et al. (1997). Measles vaccine in egg allergic children. *Pediatric Allergy and Immunology, 8*(1), 17.

Casella, R. et al. (1997). Mumps orchitis: report of a mini-epidemic. *Journal of Urology, 158*(6), 2158.

Centers for Disease Control. (1997). Hantavirus pulmonary syndrome. *MMWR: Morbidity and Mortality Weekly Report, 46*(40), 94.

Centers for Disease Control. (1998). One thousand days until the target date for global poliomyelitis eradication. *MMWR: Morbidity and Mortality Weekly Report, 47*(12), 234.

Cherry, J. D. (1997). Parvoviruses. In Johnson, K. B., & Oski, F. A. *Oski's essential pediatrics.* Philadelphia: Lippincott.

Christy, C., McConnochie, K. M., Zernik, N., & Brzoza, S. (1997). Impact of an algorithm-guided nurse intervention on the use of immunization opportunities. *Archives of Pediatrics and Adolescent Medicine, 151*(4), 384.

Department of Health and Human Services. (1995). *Healthy people 2000: midcourse review.* Washington, D.C.: DHHS.

Dinman, S., & Jarosz, D. A. (1996). Managing serious dog bite injuries in children. *Pediatric Nursing, 22*(5), 413.

Dunkle, L. A. (1997). Anaerobic infections. In Johnson, K. B., & Oski, F. A. *Oski's essential pediatrics.* Philadelphia: Lippincott.

Dutta, J. K. (1998). Index of suspicion: Rabies. *Pediatrics in Review, 19*(5), 173.

Erlich, S. (1997). Management of herpes simplex and varicella-zoster virus infections. *Western Journal of Medicine, 166*(3), 211.

Feigin, R. D. (1997). Diphtheria. In Johnson, K. B., & Oski, F. A. *Oski's essential pediatrics.* Philadelphia: Lippincott.

Feigin, R. D., & Boom, M. C. (1997). Rickettsial diseases. In Johnson, K. B., & Oski, F. A. *Oski's essential pediatrics.* Philadelphia: Lippincott.

Ferson, M. J., et al. (1995). School health nurse interventions to increase immunization uptake in school entrants. *Public Health, 109*(1), 25.

Garner, J. S. (1996). Guidelines for isolation precautions in hospitals. *Infection Control and Hospital Epidemiology, 17*(1), 66.

Grose, C. (1997). Varicella-zoster virus infections. In Johnson, K. B., & Oski, F. A. *Oski's essential pediatrics.* Philadelphia: Lippincott.

Kaplan, S. L. (1997). *Haemophilus influenzae.* In Johnson, K. B., & Oski, F. A. *Oski's essential pediatrics.* Philadelphia: Lippincott.

Kohl, S. (1997). Postnatal herpes simplex virus. In Johnson, K. B., & Oski, F. A. *Oski's essential pediatrics.* Philadelphia: Lippincott.

McMillan, J., & Grose, C. (1997). Roseola and human herpesvirus type 6. In Johnson, K. B., & Oski, F. A. *Oski's essential pediatrics.* Philadelphia: Lippincott.

Sanchez, P. J., & Siegel, J. D. (1997). Congenital and perinatal infections. In Johnson, K. B., & Oski, F. A. *Oski's essential pediatrics.* Philadelphia: Lippincott.

Sumaya, C. V. (1997). Infectious mononucleosis. In Johnson, K. B., & Oski, F. A. *Oski's essential pediatrics.* Philadelphia: Lippincott.

Taber, L. H., & Demmler, G. J. (1997). Rubella (German measles). In Johnson, K. B., & Oski, F. A. *Oski's essential pediatrics.* Philadelphia: Lippincott.

Tunnessen, W. (1997). Pediatric dermatology. In Johnson, K. B. & Oski, F. A. (Eds.). *Oski's essential pediatrics.* Philadelphia: Lippincott.

Yawn, B. P., Yawn, R. A., & Lydick, E. (1997). Community impact of childhood varicella infections. *Journal of Pediatrics, 130*(5), 759.

SUGGESTED READINGS

Clayton, D., et al. (1995). Measles pneumonia in the critically ill child: application of alternative ventilation strategies. *Critical Care Nurse, 15*(2), 39.

Mandelbrot, L. (1998). Vertical transmission of viral infections. *Current Opinion in Obstetrics and Gynecology, 10*(2), 123.

Salsberry, P. J., Nickel, J. T., & Mitch, R. (1994). Inadequate immunization among 2-year-old children: a profile of children at risk. *Journal of Pediatric Nursing, 9*(3), 158.

Saphire, L. S., & Doran, B. (1996). International travel preparedness: a guideline for occupational health professionals. *AAOHN Journal, 44*(3), 123.

Simpson, D. M., Suarez, L., & Smith, D. R. (1997). Immunization rates among young children in the public and private health care sectors. *American Journal of Preventive Medicine, 13*(2), 84.

Strassels, S. A., & Sullivan, S. D. (1997). Clinical and economic considerations of vaccination against varicella. *Pharmacotherapy, 17*(1), 133.

Suarez, L., Simpson, D. M., & Smith, D. R. (1997). The impact of public assistance factors on the immunization levels of children younger than 2 years. *American Journal of Public Health, 87*(5), 845.

Weber, D. J., Rutala, W. A., & Hamilton, H. (1996). Prevention and control of varicella-zoster infections in healthcare facilities. *Infection Control and Hospital Epidemiology, 17*(10), 694.

Nursing Care of the Child With a Hematologic Disorder

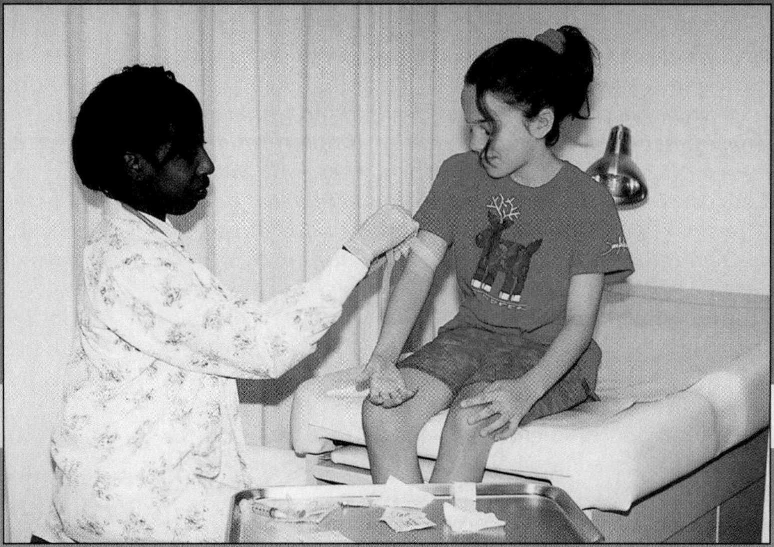

23

CHAPTER

Key Terms

- agranulocytes
- allogeneic transplantation
- aplastic anemias
- autologous transplantation
- blood dyscrasias
- blood plasma
- direct bilirubin
- erythroblasts
- erythrocytes
- erythropoietin
- granulocytes
- Heinz bodies
- hemochromatosis
- hemoglobin
- hemolysis
- hemosiderosis
- hypodermoclysis
- leukocytes
- leukopenia
- megakaryocytes
- normoblasts
- pancytopenia
- petechiae
- plethora
- poikilocytic
- polycythemia
- priaprism
- purpura
- reticulocytes
- sickle-cell crisis
- sickle-cell trait
- synergeneic transplantation
- thrombocytes
- thrombocytopenia

Objectives

After mastering the contents of this chapter, you should be able to:

1. Describe the major hematologic disorders of childhood.
2. Assess the child with a hematologic disorder.
3. Formulate nursing diagnoses for the child with a hematologic disorder such as sickle-cell anemia.
4. Identify appropriate outcomes for the child with a hematologic disorder.
5. Plan nursing care for the child with a hematologic disorder.
6. Implement nursing care related to the child with a hematologic disorder.
7. Evaluate outcomes for achievement and effectiveness of care.
8. Identify National Health Goals related to children with hematologic disorders that nurses could be instrumental in helping the nation achieve.
9. Identify areas related to care of children with hematologic disorders that could benefit from additional nursing research.
10. Use critical thinking to analyze ways that nursing care for a child with a hematologic disorder could be more family centered.
11. Integrate knowledge of hematologic disorders in children with nursing process to achieve quality child health nursing care.

Heather is a 2-year-old girl diagnosed with thalassemia major. She has a prominent mandible and wide-spaced upper teeth from the overgrowth of bone marrow centers. Her skin is bronze colored from the number of transfusions (64) she has received in her short lifetime. Joey is a 4-year-old boy seen at the same clinic. He is diagnosed as having thalassemia minor. He has no facial deformities or skin discoloration. "Why did this happen?" Heather's mother asks you. "How can two children with the same disease look so different?" What additional health teaching about thalassemia does Heather's parent need to help her better understand her daughter's disease?

In previous chapters, you learned about growth and development of well children. In this chapter, you'll add information about the dramatic changes, both physical and psychosocial, that occur when children have a hematologic disorder. This is important information because it builds a base for care and health teaching.

After you've studied the chapter, turn to the Critical Thinking Exercises at the end of the chapter to sharpen your skills and test your knowledge.

FOCUS ON NATIONAL HEALTH GOALS

A National Health Goal that addresses iron deficiency anemia, the most common blood disorder in children, is:

- Reduce iron deficiency in low-income children aged 1 to 2 years to less than 10% and among women of childbearing age to less than 3% from baselines of 21% and 5% (DHHS, 1995).

Nurses can be instrumental in helping the nation achieve this goal by educating parents about the importance of adding iron-rich cereal to infants' diets and women taking an iron supplement during pregnancy. Nursing research questions that could add important information for prevention include: what are ways of increasing compliance in pregnant women that would help ensure that all women take an iron supplement during pregnancy; and do infants maintain higher iron levels when cereal is eaten with milk or orange juice?

The blood and blood-forming tissues that make up the hematologic system play a vital role in body metabolism—transporting oxygen and nutrients to body cells, removing carbon dioxide from cells, and initiating blood coagulation when vessels are injured. As a result, any alteration in the substance or function of blood or its components can have immediate and life-threatening effects on the functioning of all body systems. For instance, an alteration in the process of coagulation can result in death from acute and uncontrollable blood loss. Inadequate red cell formation results in decreased oxygenation in tissues.

Hematologic disorders, often called **blood dyscrasias,** occur when components of the blood either increase or decrease in amount beyond normal ranges or are formed incorrectly. Most blood dyscrasias originate in the bone marrow where blood cells are formed.

A common hematologic disorder in children is iron-deficiency anemia. National Health Goals related to this disorder and children are shown in Focus on National Health Goals.

NURSING PROCESS OVERVIEW

for the Child With a Blood Disorder

Assessment

Many of the symptoms of hematologic disorders begin insidiously, with pallor, lethargy, and bruising (see Assessing the Child With Symptoms of Hematologic Disorders). These seem to be such minor symptoms that parents may not bring their child to a health care facility for some time. They are surprised to learn that subtle symptoms such as these can signify the presence of a serious disease.

Many hematologic disorders are inherited. When one is diagnosed, parents may feel guilty or blame themselves or their partner for the child's disease. It is difficult for parents to support a child during an illness when they themselves need intensive support. Be certain the parents and children receive the support and comfort they need.

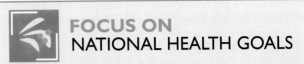

Asking at routine checkups about a child's dietary intake often reveals iron-deficiency anemia. Many babies with this problem have been drinking too much milk and not enough iron-containing foods. This makes them iron deficient, but aside from paleness and irritability, they appear plump and "healthy." Their parents have not suspected that their baby's appearance masks a nutritional deficiency.

Nursing Diagnosis

Nursing diagnoses that might be used with children who have hematologic disorders may include:

- Knowledge deficit related to cause of illness
- Altered nutrition: less than body requirements related to parental lack of knowledge of need for iron-rich diet
- Anxiety related to frequent blood-sampling procedures
- Pain related to tissue ischemia
- Family coping, compromised, ineffective related to long-term care needs of child with chronic hematologic disorder

Outcome Identification and Planning

Be certain in helping parents plan outcomes that they are realistic. The number of blood-sampling procedures, for example, cannot be reduced, but the child can be helped to deal with the pain and anxiety the procedures cause through individual distraction techniques.

Children with hematologic disorders often are placed on long-term medication such as a corticosteroid. When a child is very ill, parents are usually very conscientious about giving such medicine.

ASSESSING the Child With Symptoms of Hematologic Disorders

History

Chief concern: Fatigue, easy bruising, epistaxis.
Pregnancy history: Low birth weight; blood loss at birth; lack of vitamin K administration at birth.
Nutrition: "Picky eater" or presence of pica. Increased milk intake.
Past illnesses: History of recent illness; history of recent medicine ingestion.
Family history: Inherited blood disorder; parents known to have sickle cell trait or thalassemia minor; hemophilia in family.

Physical assessment

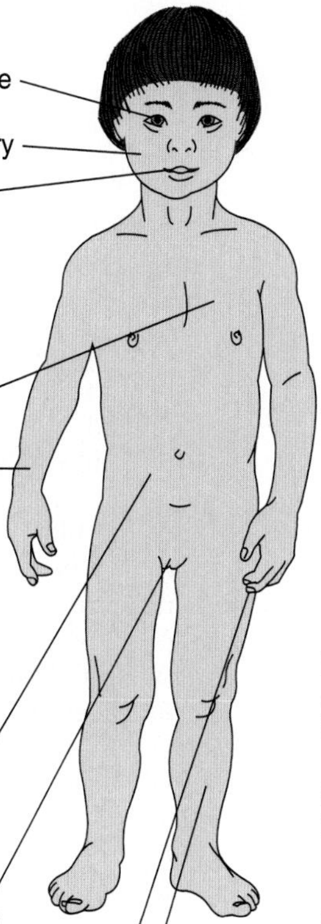

	Possible significance
General appearance	
Obese infant	Iron-deficiency anemia
Fatigue	Anemia
Eyes	
Retinal hemorrhage	Sickle cell anemia
Face	
Bossing of maxillary bone	Thalassemia
Mouth	
Pale mucous membrane	Iron-deficiency anemia
Ecchymotic or bleeding gumline	Decreased coagulation ability
Heart	
Increased rate, possible murmur	Anemia
Skin	
Petechiae, ecchymosis	Decreased coagulation ability
Blood oozing from wound or injection point	
Jaundice	Hemolytic anemia
Pallor	Anemia
Bronze color	Frequent blood transfusion
Abdomen	
Pain on palpation	Sickle cell anemia
Increased liver or spleen	Hemolytic anemia
Genitourinary	
Delayed secondary sex characteristics	Sickle cell anemia
Extremities	
Spoon nails	Iron-deficiency anemia
Joint swelling, pain	Hemophilia, sickle cell crisis
Neurologic	
Weak muscle tone	Iron-deficiency anemia

When a child has a disorder with few symptoms, however, it is easy for parents to forget to give medication. In addition, the child may refuse to take the medication because it tastes bad or upsets the stomach. Planning includes helping the parents devise ways to disguise the taste or remember to give the medication over a long period.

Nutritional planning is another area that needs consideration. Parents of children with iron-deficiency anemia, for example, may need to modify meal plans not only for the child but also for the entire family. Remember that iron-rich foods often are the most expensive foods. A parent planning on a limited budget may have difficulty, therefore, providing meals rich in iron content. If children are "fussy eaters," parents may need a great deal of support to insist on foods containing iron rather than giving children what they want. If children will be restricted for long periods because their immune system is compromised as a part of their illness, planning must include ways to keep the child interested in activities to promote development. Investigate possible resources for parental and child support and education.

Implementation

Nursing interventions for children with hematologic disorders include helping with blood sampling and assisting with blood or bone marrow transfusions. Remember that a finger stick for blood is often as painful as a venipuncture (and more painful afterward because the fingertip is irritated every time the child attempts to use it). Suggesting that blood be drawn by means of an intermittent device such as a heparin lock may help to reduce the number of times a child is subjected to venipuncture. Applying EMLA cream before finger sticks or venipunctures also helps to reduce pain and improve compliance with procedures. Even so, children may need some therapeutic play time with a syringe and a doll to express angry feelings about constant invasion by needles.

Because of the chronicity of some of the hematologic disorders, parents and children often need the support of outside agencies. Three organizations helpful for referral are:

Aplastic Anemia Foundation of America
P.O. Box 22689
Baltimore, MD 21203

National Association for Sickle Cell Disease, Inc.
3345 Wilshire Boulevard, Suite 1106
Los Angeles, CA 90010-1880

National Hemophilia Foundation
110 Greene Street, Suite 303
New York, NY 10012

Outcome Evaluation

Evaluation will focus on the achievement of short-term outcomes (such as the moderation of pain or elimination of anxiety in the child undergoing testing or treatment) and progress toward the achievement of long-term outcomes (such as improving the ability of the family to manage the stress of raising a child with a chronic illness or deal with frequently occurring health crises [e.g., the family with a child who has sickle-cell anemia]).

Examples of possible outcomes may include:

- Parents state increased knowledge of cause of iron-deficiency anemia.
- Child states he or she feels better able to cope with blood-sampling procedures through the use of imagery.
- Parents describe realistic plans to ensure compliance with long-term medication administration.

STRUCTURE AND FUNCTION OF BLOOD

Blood Formation and Components

The formation of blood cells begins as early as week 2 of intrauterine life. The yolk sac is responsible for this early blood formation. By month 2 of intrauterine life, the liver and spleen begin forming blood components. At approximately month 4, the bone marrow becomes and remains the active center for the origination of blood cells. As in extrauterine life, the spleen serves as the organ for the destruction of blood cells once their normal lifetime has passed.

The total volume of blood in the body is roughly proportional to body weight: 85 mL/kg at birth, 75 mL/ kg at age 6 months, and 70 mL/kg after the first year. The **blood plasma** (liquid portion containing proteins, hormones, enzymes, and electrolytes) is in equilibrium with the fluid of the interstitial tissue spaces. Although important in diseases causing vomiting and diarrhea (when it may become depleted, leading to dehydration), plasma is not a major site of hematologic disease. The formed elements, the **eryth-rocytes** (red blood cells); **leukocytes** (white blood cells); and **thrombocytes** (platelets), are the portions most affected by hematologic disorders in children.

Erythrocytes (Red Blood Cells)

Erythrocytes function chiefly to transport oxygen to and carry carbon dioxide from body cells. Red blood cells are formed under the stimulation of **erythropoietin,** a hormone produced by the kidneys. An increase in erythropoietin is stimulated whenever a child has tissue hypoxia. **Polycythemia,** or an overproduction of red blood cells, is chronically present in children who experience prolonged systemic hypoxia. Children with kidney disease often have a low number of red blood cells because erythropoietin secretion is inadequate in diseased kidneys.

Red blood cells form first as **erythroblasts** (large, nucleated cells), then mature through **normoblast** and **reticulocyte** stages to mature, nonnucleated erythrocytes. Approximately 1% of red blood cells are in the reticulocyte stage at all times. An elevated reticulocyte count in children indicates rapid production of red blood cells. This is seen in children with iron-deficiency anemia once iron therapy is begun and the body is again able to produce red blood cells. The absence of a nucleus in the mature cell allows for increased space for oxygen transport; it also, unfortunately, limits the life of cells because metabolic processes are limited. At the end of their life span, erythrocytes are destroyed through phagocytosis by reticuloendothelial cells, found in the highest proportion in the spleen.

In infants, the long bones of the body are filled with red marrow actively producing disc-shaped red blood cells. In early childhood, yellow marrow begins to replace this in long bones so blood element production is then carried out mainly in ribs, scapulas, vertebrae, and skull bones. The yellow marrow remaining in the extremities can be activated if necessary to produce additional blood products.

At birth, an infant has approximately 5 million red blood cells per cubic millimeter of blood. This concentration diminishes rapidly in the first months, reaching a low of approximately 4.1 million per cubic millimeter at age 3 to 4 months. The number then slowly increases until adolescence, when adult values of approximately 4.9 million per cubic millimeter are reached.

Hemoglobin. The component of red blood cells that allows them to carry out the transport of oxygen is **hemoglobin,** a complex protein. Hemoglobin comprises globin, a protein dependent (like all protein) on nitrogen metabolism for its formation, and heme, an iron-containing pigment. Deficiency of either iron stores or nitrogen will interfere with the synthesis of hemoglobin. It is the heme portion that combines with oxygen and carbon dioxide for transport.

The hemoglobin in erythrocytes during fetal life is different from that formed after birth. Fetal hemoglobin serves the fetus well because it can absorb oxygen at the low oxygen tension that exists in utero. It comprises two alpha and two gamma polypeptide chains. At birth, between 40% and 70% of the child's hemoglobin is fetal hemoglobin (hemoglobin F). Fetal hemoglobin is gradually replaced by adult hemoglobin (hemoglobin A) during the first 6 months of life. Hemoglobin A comprises two alpha and two beta chains. This is the reason that diseases such as sickle-cell anemia or the thalassemias, which are defects of the beta chains, do not become apparent clinically until this hemoglobin change has occurred (at approximately age 6 months). However, because from early intrauterine life, some hemoglobin A is present, they can be diagnosed prenatally.

The hemoglobin level of blood varies according to the number of red blood cells present and the average amount of hemoglobin each cell contains. Hemoglobin levels are highest at birth (between 13.7 and 20.1 g/100 mL); reach a low at approximately age 3 months (between 9.5 and 14.5 g/100 mL); and gradually rise again until adult values are reached at puberty (between 11 and 16 g/100 mL).

Bilirubin. Red blood cells have a life span of approximately 120 days. After this time, they disintegrate and their components are preserved by specialized cells in the liver and spleen (reticuloendothelial cells) for further use. Iron is released for reuse by the bone marrow to construct new red blood cells. As the heme portion is degraded, it is converted into protoporphyrin. Protoporphyrin is then further broken down into indirect bilirubin. Indirect bilirubin is fat soluble and cannot be excreted by the kidneys in this state. It is therefore converted by the liver enzyme glucuronyl transferase into **direct bilirubin,** which is water soluble and is combined and excreted in bile.

In the newborn infant, liver function is generally so immature that the conversion to direct bilirubin cannot be made. Therefore, bilirubin remains in the indirect form. When the level of indirect bilirubin in the blood rises to more than 7 mg/100 mL, it permeates outside the circulatory system, and the infant shows signs of yellowing from physiologic jaundice. If excessive **hemolysis** (destruction) of red blood cells occurs, the child will also show signs of jaundice.

Leukocytes (White Blood Cells)

Leukocytes are nucleated cells, few in number when compared with red blood cells (there is only approximately 1 white blood cell to every 500 red blood cells). Their primary function is defense against antigen invasion. There are two main forms of white blood cells: (1) **granulocytes** (those with granules in the cell cytoplasm) and (2) **agranulocytes** (those without granules in the cell cytoplasm). Granulocytes (often referred to as polymorphonuclear forms) are further differentiated as neutrophils, basophils, and eosinophils. The agranulocytic leukocytes are further differentiated as lymphocytes and monocytes.

The total white blood cell count in newborns is approximately 20,000 per cubic millimeter, a high level caused by the trauma of birth. In the newborn, granulocytes are the most common white blood cells. By 14 days to 30 days of life, the total white blood cell count falls to approximately 12,000 per cubic millimeter, and lymphocytes become the dominant type. By age 4 years, the white blood cell count reaches the adult level, and granulocytes are again the dominant type. Leukocytes are produced in response to need. The life span of leukocytes varies from approximately 6 hours to unknown intervals.

Thrombocytes (Platelets)

When blood is centrifuged in a test tube, plasma rises to the top as a clear yellow fluid; red cells sink to the bottom as a dark red paste. Between these two layers forms a thin white strip (often termed a buffy coat) that comprises the white blood cells and platelets. Thrombocytes are round, nonnucleated bodies formed by bone marrow. Their function is capillary hemostasis and primary coagulation. The normal range is 150,000 to 300,000 per cubic millimeter after the first year. Immature thrombocytes are termed **megakaryocytes.** If large numbers of these are present in serum, it indicates rapid production of platelets is occurring.

Blood Coagulation

Effective blood coagulation depends on a complex series of events including a combination of blood and tissue factors released from the plasma (the intrinsic system) and from injured tissue (the extrinsic system). The factors released from the plasma are factors VIII, IX and XII. Factors released from injured tissues are a tissue factor (an incomplete thromboplastin or factor III), plus factors VII and X. Together, the pathways form factor V. The names for coagulation factors are given in Box 23-1.

When a vessel is injured, vasoconstriction occurs in the area proximal to the injury, narrowing the vessel lumen and reducing the amount of blood to the injured area. Platelets begin to adhere to the damaged vessel site and to one another, forming a platelet plug. This is the first stage, or phase, of clotting (Figure 23-1).

In a second stage, factors from either the intrinsic or the extrinsic system combine with platelet phospholipid to form complete thromboplastin.

In a third stage, thromboplastin converts prothrombin (factor II) to thrombin if ionized calcium is present. The production of prothrombin and factors VII, IX, and X depends on the presence of vitamin K. This stage will be in-

TABLE 23.2 Common Blood Transfusion Reaction Symptoms

SYMPTOMS	CAUSE	TIME OF OCCURRENCE	NURSING INTERVENTION
Headache, chills, back pain, dyspnea, hypotension, hemoglobinuria (blood in urine)	Anaphylactic reaction to incompatible blood; agglutination of red blood cells occurs; kidney tubules may become blocked, resulting in kidney failure	Immediately after start of transfusion	Discontinue transfusion; maintain normal saline infusion for accessible intravenous line; administer oxygen as necessary; physician may order diuretic to increase renal tubule flow and reduce tubule plugging; heparin to reduce intravascular coagulation
Pruritus, urticaria (hives), wheezing	Allergy to protein components of transfusion	Within first hour after start of transfusion	Discontinue transfusion temporarily; give oxygen as needed; physician may order antihistamine to reduce symptoms
Increased temperature	Possible contaminant in transfused blood	Approximately 1 hour after start of transfusion	Discontinue transfusion; blood culture may be obtained to rule out bacterial invasion
Increased pulse, dyspnea	Circulatory overload	During course of transfusion	Discontinue transfusion; give oxygen as needed; supportive care for pulmonary edema and congestive heart failure; physician may order diuretic to increase excretion of fluid
Muscle cramping, twitching of extremities, convulsion	Acid-citrate-dextrose anticoagulant in transfusion is combining with serum calcium and causing hypocalcemia	During course of transfusion	Discontinue transfusion; physician may order calcium gluconate administered intravenously to restore calcium level
Fever, jaundice, lethargy, tenderness over liver	Hepatitis from contaminated transfusion	Weeks or months after transfusion	Obtain transfusion history of any child with hepatitis symptoms; refer for care of hepatitis
Bronze-colored skin	Hemosiderosis or deposition of iron from transfusion in skin	After repeated transfusions	Support self-esteem with altered body image; iron-chelating agent (deferoxamine) may be ordered to help reduce level of accumulating iron

usually a sibling, (obtained through aspiration) and its intravenous infusion to the recipient. The term **synergeneic transplantation** is used when the donor and recipient are genetically identical (i.e., identical twins). In **autologous transplantation,** the child's own marrow is used. The marrow is aspirated, treated to remove abnormal cells, and then reinfused.

Bone marrow transplantation has become a relatively common procedure for children with blood disorders such as acquired aplastic anemia, sickle cell, thalassemia, and leukemia and some forms of immune dysfunction. Bone marrow transplants are most successful when the recipients have not already received multiple blood transfusions that have sensitized them to blood products. Success also depends on the compatibility of donated marrow to a child's blood. An identical twin is the ideal donor; a parent or sibling may be next best, although compatibility is not guaranteed. Siblings have a 25% chance of being compatible. Donors registered with regional or national bone marrow "banks" have provided closer matches in some instances.

All potential donors are typed for human leukocyte antigen (HLA) compatibility. Parents who are found to be incompatible often feel guilty and frustrated that they could not do more for their child. If the most compatible person is a young sibling, health care personnel and parents alike may have some reservations about submitting a child to bone marrow aspiration. There is no guarantee that the graft will be accepted by the recipient child, or that improvement will occur. Although with good tissue compatibility in the absence of infection, this can be effective in 80% to 90% of children.

To prevent a child rejecting newly transplanted marrow by the T lymphocytes, a drug such as cyclophosphamide (Cytoxan) is administered intravenously to the child to suppress marrow and T lymphocyte production. This may cause nausea and vomiting. Total body irradiation to destroy the child's marrow also may be done. This is a difficult time for the child because total body irradiation causes extreme nausea, vomiting, and diarrhea.

WHAT IF? What if a child donates bone marrow to a sibling but the transplant doesn't take? How would you explain to the donor child that he or she did not fail?

On the day of the procedure, the donor receives a general anesthetic or conscious sedation and samples of bone marrow are obtained by multiple aspirations. The marrow is strained to remove fat and bone particles and any other unwanted cells. An anticoagulant is added to prevent clotting. It is infused intravenously into the recipient child's bloodstream. Because the infused solution is fairly thick, this infusion takes 60 to 90 minutes. Do not use a filter that is normally used for infusion of blood products because this would filter out marrow tissue. Monitor the child's cardiac rate and rhythm during the infusion to detect circulatory overload or pulmonary emboli from unfiltered particles.

Fever and chills are common reactions to bone marrow transplant infusion. Acetaminophen (Tylenol), diazepam (Valium), and diphenhydramine hydrochloride (Benadryl) may be prescribed to reduce this reaction.

After the infusion, take the child's temperature at 1 hour and then every 4 hours to detect infection that could occur because of nonfunctioning white blood cells from radiation. Reinforce strict handwashing and limit diet to cooked foods to reduce the presence of bacteria. White blood cell count must be measured daily; bone marrow aspirations or venous blood samples are scheduled at regular intervals to assess the growth of the new marrow.

Almost immediately after the infusion, marrow cells begin to migrate from the child's bloodstream into the marrow. If engraftment occurs (the transplant is accepted), red blood cells can be detected in peripheral blood in approximately 3 weeks. White blood cells and platelet cells may not return to normal for up to 1 year posttransplant.

NURSING DIAGNOSES AND RELATED INTERVENTIONS

Nursing Diagnosis: Anxiety related to lack of knowledge about procedure for and expected outcome of transplant

Outcome Identification: Parents and child will demonstrate an understanding of transplant procedure and uncertainty of outcome during therapy by 24 hours.

Outcome Evaluation: Parents state the reasons for the transplant; verbalize that they know transplant may not work, depending on immunologic factors that are not totally known to science, but are agreeable to procedure.

Bone marrow transplantation is an emotional experience not only for the child but for the parents and for the marrow donor as well. Be certain that the child who receives the transplant and the donor understand that they are not responsible for the outcome of the transplant. Its success does not depend on their behavior or what kind of person they are but on immunologic factors over which they have no control. If a sibling was the donor, he or she may become jealous of the recipient child who is the center of attention. Be certain that donors know that donor sites will feel tender afterward. General anesthesia or conscious sedation will leave them feeling exhausted for several days. Donors generally return to the hospital in 24 hours to 48 hours for evaluation that the aspiration sites are not infected (no local swelling, redness or intense pain, or elevated temperature is present).

Nursing Diagnosis: Risk for altered growth and development related to extended restrictions and infection control precautions in hospital or at home

Outcome Identification: Child will demonstrate age-appropriate growth in motor skills and social, cognitive, and emotional behaviors during course of therapy.

Outcome Evaluation: Parents express satisfaction with child's ongoing development. Objective tests of developmental stage show child within age-appropriate ranges.

Children may be restricted from others to prevent them from contracting an infection. Be certain that children are not socially isolated as well. Visit the room frequently; provide gas-sterilized play materials. Most children grow tired of a restricted diet and may crave fresh fruits and vegetables that are usually not their favorite food. Thick-skinned fruits such as bananas and oranges can be given soon after the procedure. Unwashed foods should be avoided (see Managing and Delegating Unlicensed Assistive Personnel).

Be certain that children are well prepared for all procedures. Allow them to make as many choices as they can about their care to help them preserve a sense of control over their life. Children who receive a transplant need periods of therapeutic play incorporated into care so they can begin to express their anger and frustration at the number of intravenous therapies or follow-up bone marrow aspirations they require. Measures to help children

MANAGING AND DELEGATING UNLICENSED ASSISTIVE PERSONNEL

Unlicensed assistive personnel may be assigned to care for children after bone marrow transplants. Measures to minimize the child's risk for infection are paramount. Be certain unlicensed assistive personnel understand that until these children's immune response returns to normal, they should not be offered foods such as unwashed fruit that could carry microorganisms. Review specific infection control precautions and reinstruct unlicensed assistive personnel in measures to prevent infection. Be certain too that they understand that, if they have an infection such as herpes simplex or an upper respiratory infection, they should not care for a child after a bone marrow transplant.

cope with pain, such as imagery, can help a child to accept one more painful procedure. Encourage parents to spend time with their child during long periods of hospitalization and also with other children at home.

Provisions for completing schoolwork need to be made as soon as the child has a return of red blood cells in peripheral blood (approximately 3 weeks). If children are prepared adequately for these painful procedures and supported throughout, they should have no long-term consequences. Not all transplants are successful, however, and some children will die of the original disease that required the transplant. Some children develop an infection despite all precautions and die in the weeks immediately after the transplant.

On the day of hospital discharge, parents may be surprised that the child's blood replacement is not totally complete and that they will need to continue infection control measures and restrictions at home. Help them locate a support group in the community if possible. Be certain that they feel free to call the transplant center after discharge if they have any problems. Once the danger of infection has passed and the restriction can be discontinued, parents may still be reluctant to allow their child outside, fearing that the child may still be susceptible to infection. Frequent follow-up for the next year is necessary to ensure that the child is free of infection until white blood cells have risen to normal levels. Follow-up should also address the parents' commitment to allowing their child to pursue age-appropriate activities and avoiding overprotecting him or her.

Graft-Versus-Host Disease

Graft-versus-host disease (GVHD) is a potentially lethal immunologic response of donor T cells against the tissue of the recipient. The symptoms ranging from mild to severe include a rash and general malaise beginning 7 to 14 days posttransplant. Latent virus infections may become active. Severe symptoms include high fever and diarrhea, and liver and spleen enlargement as cells are destroyed.

Because there is no known cure for GVHD, prevention is essential. Careful tissue typing, intravenous administration of methotrexate or cyclosporine, and irradiation of blood products (which helps to inactivate mature T cells) before bone marrow infusion all can contribute to the reduction of this complication. Drugs such as methotrexate and cyclosporine kill all rapidly growing cells, including white blood cells and T lymphocytes, so administration of these drugs after transplantation cannot be continued because they would also slow the growth of the host's bone marrow. Depletion of mature T cells from donor bone marrow before infusion into the child seems to have the best results.

Splenectomy

One of the purposes of the spleen is to remove damaged or aged blood cells. This poses a difficulty with diseases such as sickle-cell anemia and the thalassemias because the spleen recognizes the typical cells of these diseases as damaged and destroys them. This causes these children to have a continuous anemia, with hemoglobin as low as 5 to 9 g/mL. In some children, therefore, removal of the spleen or splenectomy, will not cure the basic defect of the blood cells, but will limit the degree of anemia.

Splenectomy is major surgery because in most instances it involves an abdominal incision. Newer techniques allow it to be done by laparoscopy (Esposito, 1997).

A second function of the spleen is to strain the plasma for invading organisms so phagocytes and lymphocytes can destroy them. Children with their spleen removed appear to be very susceptible to the pneumococcal infections. After surgery, children are kept on prophylactic antibiotics for a year or two. They should receive pneumococcal and meningococcal vaccines as well as routine immunizations (Martin & Pearson, 1997a). Parents need to be instructed about signs of infection (cough, fever, general malaise), and encouraged to report them immediately.

✔ CHECKPOINT QUESTIONS

3. Where is the preferred site for bone marrow aspiration in a child?
4. All bone marrow donors are screened for what type of compatibility?

HEALTH PROMOTION AND RISK MANAGEMENT

Many hematologic disorders such as sickle-cell anemia and hemophilia are inherited disorders. Thus health promotion and disease prevention begin with ensuring families access to genetic counseling so they can be aware of the incidence of the disorder in their family and, therefore, the potential for the disease to develop in their child.

The most frequently occurring anemia in children, iron-deficiency anemia, is preventable. This condition could be eradicated in infants if all bottle-fed infants were fed iron-fortified formula for the first year and when cereal is introduced, iron-fortified types are used. The disorder occurs again at a high incidence in adolescents because their diets tend to be low in meat and green vegetables, the chief dietary sources of iron. Adolescents who begin vegetarian diets become especially prone to developing the disorder. Counseling adolescents to ingest iron-rich food sources could have a major impact on decreasing the disorder at this age as well.

Aplastic anemia, or the inability to form blood elements, can be acquired if a child is exposed to a toxic drug or chemical. Educating parents about the importance of keeping poisons locked and out of the reach of children could have a major impact on decreasing the incidence of this disorder.

Because many of the disorders are inherited, nurses cannot play a role in prevention. However, nurses can be instrumental in making the therapy for these disorders much less painful and distressful than it was in the past. All hematologic disorders require blood specimen withdrawal for diagnosis and continued testing for follow-up. Many therapies include blood product transfusion. The use of EMLA cream, a topical anesthetic, can greatly reduce the pain of venipuncture. Helping a child to use a distraction technique such as imagery can greatly reduce any apprehension or fear associated with the procedures or treatments.

DISORDERS OF THE RED BLOOD CELLS

Most red blood cell disorders fall into the category of the anemias, or a reduction in the number or function of erythrocytes. Polycythemia, or an increase in the number of red blood cells, can also occur, and may be as dangerous to the child as a reduction in red blood cell production (see Focus on Cultural Competence).

Anemia occurs when the rate of red blood cell production falls below that of cell destruction, or when there is a loss of red blood cells, causing their number, or the hemoglobin level, to fall below the normal value for a child's age. Anemias are classified either according to the changes seen in red blood cell numbers or configuration, or according to the source of the problem. Although any reduction in the amount of circulating hemoglobin lessens the oxygen-carrying capacity, clinical symptoms of this are not apparent until hemoglobin reaches 7 to 8 g/100 mL. Average values for hemoglobin and red cell number are shown in Appendix F.

Normochromic, Normocytic Anemias

Normochromic, normocytic anemias are marked by impaired production of erythrocytes by the bone marrow, or by abnormal or uncompensated loss of circulating red blood cells such as in acute hemorrhage. The remaining red blood cells are normal in both color and size, simply too few in number.

Acute Blood-Loss Anemia

Blood loss sufficient to cause anemia might occur from trauma such as an automobile accident with internal bleeding; acute nephritis in which blood is being lost in the urine; or, in the newborn, from disorders such as placenta previa, premature separation of the placenta, maternal–fetal or twin-to-twin transfusion, or trauma to the cord or placenta as might occur with cesarean birth.

> **FOCUS ON CULTURAL COMPETENCE**
>
> Blood dyscrasias do not occur at equal rates in all countries because many of them are inherited. Sickle-cell anemia occurs mainly in African Americans; thalassemia occurs in children from Mediterranean countries. Iron deficiency anemia, an example of a noninherited disorder, tends to occur in children from lower socioeconomic areas of many countries because iron-rich foods are the most expensive foods for families to buy. Being aware of the differences in the incidence of blood dyscrasias can be helpful in planning care and health care services for an individual community.
>
> Blood transfusions are often the therapy for blood disorders. Clients who are Jehovah's Witnesses may refuse such transfusions as a religious stipulation.

Children are in shock from acute blood loss, and appear pale. As the heart attempts to push the reduced amount of blood through the body more rapidly, tachycardia will occur. Loss of red blood cells needed for oxygen transport causes body cells to register an oxygen deficit, and children experience tachypnea. Newborns may have gasping respirations, sternal retractions, and cyanosis. They will not respond to oxygen therapy because they lack red blood cells to transport and use the oxygen. Such infants will be listless and inactive.

This type of acute blood-loss anemia generally is transitory because sudden reduction in available oxygen stimulates a regeneration response in the bone marrow. The reticulocyte count becomes elevated, evidence that the bone marrow is trying to increase production of erythrocytes to meet the sudden shortage.

Treatment involves control of bleeding by addressing its underlying cause. The child or infant should be placed in a supine position to provide as much circulation as possible to brain cells. Keep the child warm with blankets; place an infant in an incubator. Blood transfusion may be necessary for an immediate increase in the number of erythrocytes. Until blood is available for transfusion, a blood expander such as plasma, or intravenous fluid such as normal saline or Ringer's lactate, may be given to expand blood volume and improve blood pressure.

Anemia of Acute Infection

Acute infection or inflammation, especially in infants, may lead to increased destruction of erythrocytes and therefore to decreased erythrocyte levels. Common conditions include osteomyelitis, ulcerative colitis, and advanced renal disease. Impaired production of erythrocytes due to the infection may also contribute to the anemia. Management involves treatment of the underlying condition. When this is reversed, the blood picture will return to normal.

Anemia of Neoplastic Disease

Malignant growths such as leukemia or lymphosarcoma (common neoplasms of childhood) result in normochromic, normocytic anemias because invasion of bone marrow by proliferating neoplastic cells impairs red blood cell production. There may be accompanying blood loss if platelet formation also has decreased. The treatment of such an anemia involves measures designed to achieve remission of the neoplastic process and transfusion to increase the erythrocyte count.

Aplastic Anemias

Aplastic anemias result from depression of hematopoietic activity in bone marrow. The formation and development of white blood cells, platelets, and red blood cells are all affected.

Congenital aplastic anemia (Fanconi's syndrome) is inherited as an autosomal recessive trait. The child is born with a number of congenital anomalies, such as skeletal and renal abnormalities, hypogenitalism, and dwarfism. Between 4 and 12 years of age, children begin to manifest symptoms of **pancytopenia** (reduction of all blood cell components).

Acquired Aplastic Anemia. Acquired aplastic anemia is a decrease in bone marrow production that can occur if children have excessive exposure to radiation, drugs, or chemicals known to cause bone marrow damage. Chloramphenicol is the major drug involved in such an anemia. Other contributory drugs include sulfonamides, arsenic (contained in rat poison, sometimes eaten by children), hydantoin, benzene, and quinine. Exposure to insecticides also may cause such bone marrow dysfunction. Chemotherapeutic drugs temporarily reduce bone marrow production. A serious infection such as mennococcal pneumonia might cause autoimmunologic suppression of bone marrow.

Assessment. As symptoms begin, children appear pale; they fatigue easily and have anorexia. These symptoms reflect the lower red blood cell count (anemia) and tissue hypoxia. Because of reduced platelet formation (thrombocytopenia), children bruise easily or have **petechiae** (pinpoint, macular, purplish-red spots caused by intradermal or submucous hemorrhage). They may have excessive nose bleeds or gastrointestinal bleeding. As a result of a decrease in white blood cells, termed **leukopenia,** children may contract an increased number of infections and respond poorly to antibiotic therapy. Observe closely for signs of cardiac decompensation (e.g., tachycardia, tachypnea, shortness of breath, or cyanosis) from the long-term increased workload on the heart (see Assessing the Child With Symptoms of Hematologic Disorders earlier in this chapter). Ask about exposure to drugs, chemicals or recent infection.

Bone marrow samples will show a reduced number of hematopoietic forms; blood-forming spaces are infiltrated by fatty tissue.

Therapeutic Management. The goal of treatment for aplastic anemia is bone marrow transplantation. If a donor cannot be located, the child is managed by procedures to suppress T-cell-dependent autoimmune responses with antithymocyte globulin (ATG) or antilymphocyte globulin (ALG) and to supplement blood elements being formed in abnormally low numbers. Any drug or chemical suspected of causing the bone marrow dysfunction must be discontinued at once. Both ATG and ALG are given intravenously and must be administered cautiously because of the high risk for anaphylaxis. Packed red blood cell and platelet transfusions are generally necessary to maintain adequate blood elements. A red cell-stimulating factor (erythropoietin) may be helpful. Colony-stimulating factors (CSFs) may also improve bone marrow function.

Some children with congenital aplastic anemia show improvement with a course of an oral corticosteroid (prednisone) and testosterone (oxymetholone). The testosterone acts to increase erythrocyte production in the bone marrow. Prednisone acts to decrease erythrocyte destruction and prolong closure of the epiphyseal lines of the long bones. This reverses the early closure that would normally occur with administration of testosterone. Such therapy must be given for an extended period, usually approximately 1 year.

If children survive the first 6 months of aplastic anemia that is drug or chemical induced, their chances for complete recovery are good. A decreased platelet count may persist for years after other blood elements have returned to normal. Hence, bleeding, especially petechiae or purpura, may be a long-term problem. If the disease was caused by exposure to a drug or chemical, children must never be exposed to that substance again.

Be certain, when discussing with parents the outcome of this disease, to be conservatively optimistic. For some children, the outcome will be fatal. It may be easier for parents to deal with this problem if they face only 1 day or one blood test at a time, rather than trying to predict the outcomes of all the blood tests to come. They need to feel that they can discuss with health care personnel their frustration and bitterness about continual abnormal results. Establishing good communication with these parents does much to reestablish their trust in everyone caring for their child.

NURSING DIAGNOSES AND RELATED INTERVENTIONS

Children with aplastic anemia are apt to be irritable because of their fatigue and recurring symptoms. Their parents may feel responsible for causing the illness if it originated from exposure to a chemical such as an insecticide. Many parents will have less confidence in health care personnel if the illness followed treatment with a drug such as chloramphenicol. They feel that if one drug caused this illness, how can they trust another to cure it? How can they trust that their child will not be harmed further?

Nursing Diagnosis: Risk for infection related to dramatic decrease in number of white blood cells

Outcome Identification: Child will remain free of any signs and symptoms of infection during treatment period.

Outcome Evaluation: Child's temperature is below 38.0°C (100°F) axillary; symptoms such as cough, vomiting, or diarrhea are absent.

Exposure to other children must be limited as long as white cell production is inadequate to prevent infection. Remind parents of the signs and symptoms of infection and advise them to come for treatment promptly if the child shows any of these symptoms. In the absence of granulocytes, however, antibiotic therapy may be ineffective, and severe septicemia can result. White blood cells (granulocytes) may be transfused for a severe infection.

Nursing Diagnosis: Risk for body image disturbance related to changed appearance occurring as medication side effect

Outcome Identification: Child will demonstrate adequate self-esteem during therapy interval.

Outcome Evaluation: Child voices that he or she thinks of himself or herself as a worthwhile person and is not excessively shy or reluctant to interact with peers.

Children who receive corticosteroid therapy such as prednisone for a long period almost certainly will experience some of the side effects, such as a cushingoid appearance, hirsutism, hypertension, and marked weight gain. Masculinizing effects, such as growth of facial and body hair, the development of acne, and deepening of the voice, may occur as the result of long-term therapy with testosterone. Both child and parents need to be prepared that these effects may occur, that they are related to the medication being taken, and that they will remain for an extended period, but they will fade when the medication is withdrawn.

Adolescents may have an especially difficult time accepting weight gain and increased acne. They need a chance to express their feelings about their changed appearance. Reinforce and emphasize positive attributes.

Nursing Diagnosis: Risk for fluid volume deficit related to ineffective blood clotting mechanisms secondary to inadequate platelet formation

Outcome Identification: Child will remain free of excessive bleeding episodes while condition is resolving.

Outcome Evaluation: Child exhibits absence of ecchymotic skin areas, gingival bleeding, or epistaxis; stools negative for occult blood.

Inadequate platelet formation interferes with blood coagulation, placing the child at risk for bleeding. Techniques for reducing bleeding due to inadequate platelet formation include the following:

- Limit the number of blood-drawing procedures; combine samples whenever possible; use a blood pressure cuff instead of a tourniquet to reduce the number of petechiae.
- Apply pressure to any puncture site for a full 5 minutes before applying a bandage.
- Minimize use of adhesive tape to the skin (pulling for removal may tear the skin and cause petechiae).
- Pad side and crib rails to prevent bruising.
- Protect intravenous sites to avoid numerous reinsertions.
- Administer medication orally or by intravenous infusion to minimize the injection sites.
- Assess diet for foods that child can chew without irritation (e.g., avoid toast crusts).
- Urge the child to use a soft toothbrush.
- Check toys for sharp corners, which may cause scratches. Urge the child to be careful with paper. Paper cuts can bleed out of proportion to their size.
- Assess necessity of routine blood pressure determinations. Tight cuffs could lead to petechiae.
- Distract from "rough" play; suggest stimulating but quiet activities to minimize risk of injury.
- Keep a record of blood drawn; do not draw extra amounts "just in case."

These measures require conscientious nursing care.

Hypoplastic Anemias

Hypoplastic anemias also result from depression of hematopoietic activity in bone marrow; they can be either congenital or acquired. Unlike aplastic anemias, in which white and red blood cells and platelets are affected, in hypoplastic anemias, only the red blood cells are affected.

Congenital hypoplastic anemia (Blackfan-Diamond syndrome) is a rare disorder revealed in the first 6 to 8 months of life. It affects both sexes and is apparently caused by an inherent defect in red blood cell formation. There are no changes in the leukocytes or platelets. An acquired form is caused by infection with parvovirus, the infectious agent of fifth disease.

The onset of hypoplastic anemia is insidious and must be differentiated from iron-deficiency anemia. The blood cells will appear hypochromic and microcytic in iron-deficiency anemia; in hypoplastic anemia, they are normochromic and normocytic.

With acquired hypoplastic anemia, the reduction of red blood cells is transient, so no therapy is necessary. Children with the congenital form will show increased erythropoiesis with corticosteroid therapy. Long-term transfusions of packed red cells are needed to raise erythrocyte levels. So many transfusions will result in **hemosiderosis** (deposition of iron in body tissue) so an iron chelation program such as subcutaneous infusion (**hypodermoclysis**) of deferoxamine is begun concurrently with transfusions. Deferoxamine binds with iron and aids its excretion from the body in urine; it is given 5 or 6 days a week over an 8-hour period. This is one of the few times that an infusion is given subcutaneously. Parents can do this at home after careful instruction, often when the child is asleep at night. The parent must assess that voiding is present and specific gravity is normal (1.003 to 1.030) before administration. For a subcutaneous infusion, an area beside the scapula or on the thigh is cleaned with alcohol; a short 25-gauge needle is inserted at a low angle into only the subcutaneous tissue. The medication is then allowed to infuse slowly. Periodic slit-lamp eye examinations should be scheduled to check for cataract formation, a possible adverse effect of the drug.

Congenital hypoplastic anemia is a chronic condition. However, approximately one fourth of affected children will undergo spontaneous permanent remission before age 13 years. Regardless, both the child and the parents need support from health care personnel to help them accept the many procedures and tests required.

Hypersplenism

Under normal conditions, blood is filtered rapidly through the spleen. If the spleen is enlarged and functioning abnormally, blood cells pass through more slowly, with more cells being destroyed in the process. The increased destruction of red blood cells causes anemia and may lead to pancytopenia (deficiency of all cell elements of blood). Virtually any underlying splenic condition can cause this syndrome.

Therapeutic management consists of treating the underlying splenic disorder, including possible splenectomy. Although the spleen's role in the body's defense mechanisms against infection is not well documented, the organ appears to be relatively important in early infancy. Its function decreases as the child grows older and may serve no function at all in adulthood. If the spleen is removed, there is no decrease in general immunity or in gamma globulin or antibody formation. With the removal of the spleen's filtering function, however, there seems to be an increased susceptibility to meningitis due to pneumococci (Martin & Pearson, 1997a). For this reason, a splenectomy may be delayed until after age 2 years, when the risk of meningitis decreases. Such children should receive immunization against pneumococci, in addition to prophylactic penicillin for 2 years after the splenectomy.

✔ CHECKPOINT QUESTIONS

5. What blood cells are affected with aplastic anemia?
6. What problem indicates the need for iron chelation therapy?

Hypochromic Anemias

When hemoglobin synthesis is inadequate, the erythrocytes appear pale (hypochromia). Hypochromia is generally accompanied by a reduction in the diameter of cells (red blood cells are also microcytic).

Iron-Deficiency Anemia

Iron-deficiency anemia is the most common anemia of infancy and childhood, occurring when the intake of dietary iron is inadequate (Richer, 1997). This lack prevents proper hemoglobin formation. Most iron in the body is incorporated in hemoglobin, but an additional amount is stored in the bone marrow to be available for hemoglobin production. With iron-deficiency anemia, red blood cells are both small in size (hypocytic) and pale (hypochromic) due to the stunted hemoglobin.

Children are at high risk for iron-deficiency anemia because they need more daily iron in proportion to their body weight to maintain an adequate iron level than do adults. A daily intake of 6 to 15 mg of iron is necessary. Iron-deficiency anemia occurs most often between ages 6 months and 2 years; its frequency rises again in adolescence when iron requirements increase for girls who are menstruating. As many as 25% of adolescent girls and 40% of infants are anemic (Rapetti et al, 1997).

Prevention. Iron-deficiency anemia can be prevented in formula-fed infants by giving them iron-fortified formula. If an infant is breastfed, iron-fortified cereal should be introduced when solid foods are introduced in the first year. Fortunately, these cost no more than non-fortified foods. Occasionally, an infant will become constipated on iron-rich formula, but this is the exception rather than the rule.

Causes in Infants. When an infant's diet lacks sufficient iron, he or she usually has enough in reserve to last for the first 6 months. After that, if the infant continues to be iron deficient, he or she will have difficulty forming the red cells needed. Infants of low birth weight have fewer iron stores than those born at term because the iron stores develop near the end of gestation. Because low-birth-weight infants grow rapidly and their need for red blood cells expands accordingly, they will develop an iron-deficiency anemia before 5 to 6 months. They are given an iron supplement at the time of hospital discharge or at the age they would have reached term to prevent this from happening.

Women with iron deficiency during pregnancy tend to give birth to iron-deficient babies, because of their lack of iron stores. Low hemoglobin levels from iron-deficiency anemia lead to diffusion of plasma proteins such as albumin and gamma globulin out of the bloodstream by osmosis. The loss of transferrin, a plasma protein responsible for binding iron to protein to facilitate its transportation to bone marrow after absorption from the gastrointestinal tract, further depletes this system of iron transport.

Infants born with structural defects of the gastrointestinal system, such as gastroesophageal reflux (chalasia—immature valve between esophagus and stomach resulting in regurgitation) or pyloric stenosis (narrowing between stomach and duodenum resulting in vomiting), are particularly prone to iron-deficiency anemia. Although their diet is adequate, they are unable to make use of the iron because it is never adequately digested. Infants with chronic diarrhea are also prone to this form of anemia, due to inadequate absorption.

Causes in Toddlers and Older Children. In children older than age 2 years, chronic blood loss is the most frequent cause of iron-deficiency anemia. This results from gastrointestinal tract lesions such as polyps, ulcerative colitis, Crohn's disease, protein-induced enteropathies, parasitic infestation, or frequent epistaxis.

Many adolescent girls are iron deficient because their frequent attempts to diet combined with overconsumption of snack foods results in low iron intake. Without sufficient iron, their body cannot compensate for the iron lost with menstrual flow.

Assessment. Common symptoms of iron-deficiency anemia are shown in Assessing the Child With Iron-Deficiency Anemia. Children with iron-deficiency anemia appear pale. Because the pallor develops slowly, however, parents may not realize how extensive it is. They may describe their child as "fair skinned" even though the child's pallor is so extreme that his or her skin is transparent. In dark-skinned infants, pale mucous membranes may be the most significant finding.

Infants may show poor muscle tone and reduced activity. They are generally irritable from fatigue. The heart may be enlarged, and there may be a soft systolic precordial murmur as the heart increases its action, attempting to supply blood cells better. The spleen may be slightly enlarged. Fingernails become typically "spoon-shaped" or depressed in contour.

A dietary history generally reveals an abnormally high milk intake. As a rule, infants should not ingest more than 32 oz of milk a day. Infants with iron-deficiency anemia may be drinking up to 50 oz a day. One quart of milk provides only approximately 0.5 mg of iron. In contrast, 1 tablespoon of iron-fortified baby cereal supplies 2.5 to 5.0 mg of iron.

With iron-deficiency anemia, laboratory studies reveal decreased hemoglobin (defined as a hemoglobin level less than 11 g per 100 mL of blood) and hematocrit levels

ASSESSING the Child With Iron-Deficiency Anemia

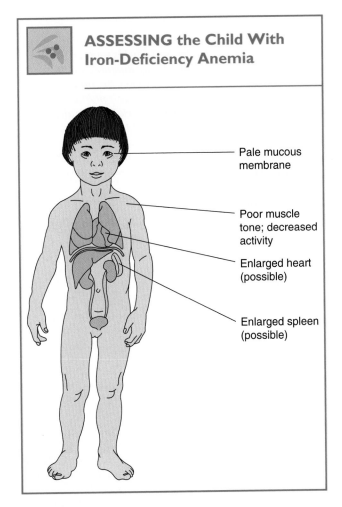

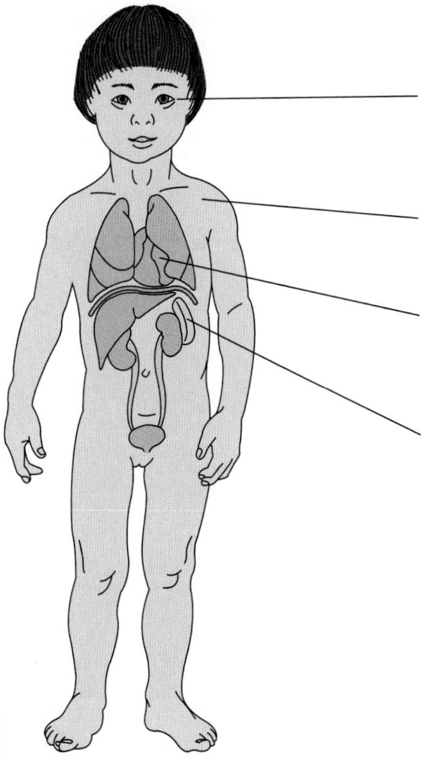

(a level below 33%). The red blood cells are microcytic and hypochromic and possibly **poikilocytic** (irregular in shape). The mean corpuscular volume (MCV) will be low. The mean corpuscular hemoglobin (MCH) may be reduced. Serum iron levels are normally 70 μg/100 mL; with iron-deficiency anemia the level is often as low as 30 μg/100 mL with an increased iron-binding capacity (more than 350 μg/100 mL). The level of serum ferritin reflects the extent of iron stores and will be less than 10 μg/100 mL (normal is 35 μg/mL). Without iron, heme precursors cannot be used, so free erythrocyte protoporphyrins increase to more than 10 μg/g from a normal of 1.9 μg/g.

Monoamine oxidase (MAO) is an enzyme important for central nervous system maturation. Iron is incorporated into MAO, so without iron, this necessary enzyme is absent and CNS maturation may be affected.

Iron-deficiency anemia is associated with infants who are more fearful, less active, and less persistent (deAndraca et al, 1997). School-age children with iron-deficiency anemia score less well on tests than their healthy counterparts and tend to be more inattentive and disruptive in class. Iron-deficiency anemia is also associated with pica (the eating of inedible substances such as dirt and paper). Eating ice cubes is common in adolescents. Until the anemia is corrected, parents need to supervise the child's environment to keep inedible materials out of the child's reach.

Therapeutic Management. Treatment of iron-deficiency anemia focuses on the treatment of the underlying cause. Sources of gastrointestinal bleeding must be ruled out. The diet must be rich in iron and should contain extra vitamin C that will enhance iron absorption. Infants who are bottle fed should be given iron-fortified formula for a full year. Ferrous sulfate for 4 to 6 weeks is the drug of choice to improve red cell formation and replace iron stores (see the Nursing Care Plan and the Drug Highlight).

NURSING DIAGNOSES AND RELATED INTERVENTIONS

Nursing Diagnosis: Altered nutrition, less than body requirements, related to inadequate ingestion of iron

Outcome Identification: Child will demonstrate an increase in his or her oral intake of iron by 24 hours.

Outcome Evaluation: Parents report dietary intake of child includes iron-rich foods; administer ferrous sulfate as prescribed; serum iron levels increase to normal by 6 months.

When planning care for the infant with iron-deficiency anemia, minimize the child's activities to prevent fatigue, particularly at mealtime. If a child is fatigued, he won't be able to eat, let alone eat iron-rich foods.

Parents need to be counseled on measures to improve their child's diet, such as adding iron-rich foods while decreasing milk intake to maintain the iron levels and prevent recurring anemia. If the child is not fond of meat, parents can substitute cheese, eggs, green vegetables, or fortified cereal. Because iron-rich foods are often expensive, remind parents that these items are important, and that they should not substitute less expensive, high-carbohydrate foods.

Before iron therapy is started, alert parents to any possible side effects, such as stomach irritation. If oral iron is not tolerated or if there is a doubt that the child will take it, an iron-dextran injection (Imferon) can be given intramuscularly. Imferon stains skin and is extremely irritating unless it is given by deep z-track intramuscular injection.

Of all age groups, adolescents do the least well with medicine compliance. Help them plan a daily time for taking their iron supplement with a medication reminder chart. At first, they may reject this as "childish," but assure them that everyone needs these charts, not just adolescents. Review with them the iron-rich foods they will need to eat daily. An iron supplement is effective only if taken with iron-rich foods.

After 7 days of iron therapy, a reticulocyte count is usually done. If elevated, this means that the child is receiving adequate iron and that the rapid proliferation of new erythrocytes is correcting the anemia. Iron medication must be taken for at least 4 to 6 weeks after the red cell count is normal to rebuild iron levels in the blood. In some children, maintenance therapy may continue for as long as 1 year.

Chronic-Infection Anemia

Acute infection interferes with red blood cell production, producing a normochromic, normocytic anemia. When infections are chronic, anemia of a hypochromic, microcytic

Nursing Care Plan

THE CHILD WITH IRON DEFICIENCY ANEMIA

A 4-year-old is brought to the clinic by his mother after being diagnosed with iron deficiency anemia after a routine health maintenance visit. He is scheduled to start oral iron therapy. His mother states, "How could this have happened?"

Assessment: Thin, black male whose weight is at approximately 25th percentile for age. Has a history of frequent nosebleeds. "Sometimes he has three or four in one day." Mucous membranes and conjunctiva pale. Mother reports child is a "picky eater but loves cheese and yogurt."

Hemoglobin 10 g/100 mL; hematocrit 31%; serum iron level 50 μg/100 mL; serum ferritin 10 μg/100 mL. The physician orders ferrous sulfate elixir t.i.d. for 6 weeks. Mother is asking many questions about her son's condition and medication therapy. "I don't know how I'll get him to take this medication. I always have trouble giving him any kind of medicine."

Nursing Diagnosis: Knowledge deficit related to causes and treatment of iron deficiency anemia

Outcome Identification: Parent and child will verbalize accurate information about the disorder and its treatment.

Outcome Evaluation: Parent identifies possible causes; demonstrates proper administration methods for iron elixir; identifies signs and symptoms of iron toxicity; identifies foods high in iron; states the need for medication compliance; describes measures to involve child in medication therapy. Child states reason for iron therapy; identifies appropriate high-iron food choices; states he takes the medication three times a day.

Interventions	Rationale
1. Assess parent and child's current knowledge about iron deficiency anemia.	1. Obtaining a baseline knowledge assessment provides a foundation on which to build future teaching strategies.
2. Explore with the child and mother about possible contributing factors associated with iron deficiency anemia.	2. A dietary intake of large amounts of milk products and chronic blood loss, such as from frequent epistaxis, are common contributing factors to the development of iron deficiency anemia.
3. Question child about his food likes and dislikes.	3. Ascertaining the child's likes and dislikes provides a baseline for future suggestions for food choices that would be followed.
4. Instruct the mother in foods that are high in iron and measures to include iron-rich foods in diet. Refer for financial assistance for food purchases, if appropriate.	4. Foods high in iron provide an additional means for supplementing needed iron. These foods are typically more expensive than other foods; therefore, financial assistance may be necessary to ensure appropriate food purchases.
5. Allow the child to choose foods from a list of high-iron foods. Develop a simple contract with the child for including one high-iron food with each meal.	5. Contracting and providing the child with choices promote active participation in his care and a feeling of control, enhancing the chances for success.
6. Review the rationale for ferrous sulfate therapy.	6. Ferrous sulfate improves red blood cell formation and replaces iron stores.
7. Instruct the mother to administer the elixir 1 hour before or 2 hours after a meal, mixed with water or juice. Advise the mother to have the child drink the medication through a straw.	7. Mixing the elixir with water or juice helps to mask its taste. Using a straw prevents staining of the teeth.
8. Suggest administering the medication with a citrus juice.	8. Vitamin C enhances iron absorption.

(continued)

9. Teach the parent about possible adverse effects such as gastrointestinal upset, constipation, and black tarry stools. Encourage the addition of high-fiber foods to the diet.	9. Knowledge of possible adverse effects is important for early detection and prompt intervention should any occur. Adding fiber to the diet helps to reduce the risk of constipation.
10. Instruct the mother to give the medication exactly as prescribed and not to increase the dosage or frequency unless directed to do so by the physician. Advise the parent to call the health care provider if the child experiences any nausea, vomiting, abdominal pain, or blood in emesis or stool (signs of iron toxicity).	10. Giving iron more frequently or in greater doses than ordered can lead to iron toxicity.
11. Encourage the child to brush his teeth thoroughly and regularly after each meal.	11. Thorough, regular brushing helps to prevent staining of the teeth.
12. Reinforce the need for compliance with therapy. Arrange for follow-up appointment and blood studies within 4 weeks.	12. Follow-up is essential for assessing compliance and evaluating the effectiveness of therapy and teaching.

DRUG HIGHLIGHT

Ferrous Sulfate (Feosol)

Action: Ferrous sulfate is an iron salt that acts to supply iron for red cell production. It elevates the serum iron concentration and then is converted to hemoglobin or trapped in the reticuloendothelial cells for storage and eventual conversion to a usable form of iron.

Pregnancy risk category: A

Dosage: For severe iron deficiency anemia: 4 to 6 mg/kg/day in three divided doses. For mild iron deficiency anemia: 3 mg/kg/day in two divided doses.

Possible adverse effects: Gastrointestinal upset, anorexia, nausea, vomiting, constipation, dark stools, stained teeth (liquid preparations)

Nursing Implications:

- Instruct parents to administer the drug on an empty stomach with water to enhance absorption. If this causes GI irritation, administer it after meals. Avoid giving it with milk, eggs, coffee, or tea.
- If liquid preparation is ordered, advise parents to mix it with water or juice to mask the taste and prevent staining of teeth. Encourage the parents to have the child drink the medication through a straw to avoid staining of the teeth.
- Keep in mind that iron is absorbed best in the presence of vitamin C. Suggest parents give the iron with a citrus juice such as orange juice to help absorption. Some children may be prescribed vitamin C to take concurrently to increase absorption.
- Educate child and parents that iron may turn stools black.
- Encourage parents to include high-fiber food sources in the child's diet to minimize the risk of constipation.
- Reinforce the need for thorough brushing of teeth to prevent staining.
- Remind parents about the need for follow-up blood studies to evaluate the effectiveness of the drug.

type occurs. This is probably caused by impaired iron metabolism as well as impaired red blood cell production.

The degree of anemia is rarely as severe as that occurring with iron deficiency. Administration of iron has little effect until the infection is controlled.

Macrocytic (Megaloblastic) Anemias

A macrocytic anemia is one in which red blood cells are abnormally large. These cells are actually immature erythrocytes or megaloblasts (nucleated immature red cells). For this reason, these anemias are often referred to as megaloblastic anemias. They are uncommon in the United States.

Anemia of Folic Acid Deficiency

A deficiency of folic acid combined with vitamin C deficiency produces an anemia in which erythrocytes are abnormally large. There is accompanying neutropenia and thrombocytopenia. MCV and MCH will be increased, whereas mean corpuscular hemoglobin concentration (MCHC) will be normal. Bone marrow will contain megaloblasts, indicating inhibition of the production of erythrocytes at an early stage. Megaloblastic arrest or inability of red blood cells to mature past an early stage may occur in the first year of life from the continued use of infant food containing too little folic acid or goat's milk, which tends to be deficient in folic acid. Treatment is daily oral administration of folic acid. Response to treatment is dramatic.

Pernicious Anemia (Vitamin B_{12} Deficiency)

Vitamin B_{12} is necessary for maturation of red blood cells. Pernicious anemia results from deficiency or inability to use the vitamin. Vitamin B_{12}, found primarily in food of animal origin, including both cow's milk and breast milk, usually is readily available to infants. An adolescent may be deficient in vitamin B_{12} if he or she is on a long-term, poorly formulated vegetarian diet (Requejo et al, 1997).

For absorption of vitamin B_{12} from the intestine, an intrinsic factor must be present in the gastric mucosa. Lack of the intrinsic factor is the most frequent cause of the disorder. Symptoms of intrinsic factor deficiency generally occur in the first 2 years of life (once the intrauterine stores of vitamin B_{12} have been exhausted). The child appears pale, anorexic, and irritable, with chronic diarrhea. The tongue appears smooth and beef-red in color due to papillary atrophy. In children, neuropathologic findings such ataxia, hyporeflexia, paresthesia, and a positive Babinski reflex are less noticeable than in adults.

Laboratory findings will reveal low serum levels of vitamin B_{12}. The rate and efficiency of absorption of vitamin B_{12} can be tested by the ingestion of the radioactively tagged vitamin. The dose absorbed in the presence and absence of a dose of intrinsic factor can be measured (a Schilling test).

Pernicious anemia is treated with lifelong monthly intramuscular injections of vitamin B_{12}. Parents and the child need to understand that lifelong therapy is necessary.

CHECKPOINT QUESTIONS

7. What is the drug of choice for treating iron-deficiency anemia?
8. What must be present for vitamin B_{12} absorption?

Hemolytic Anemias

Hemolytic anemias are those in which the number of erythrocytes decreases because of increased destruction of erythrocytes. This may be caused by fundamental abnormalities of erythrocyte structure or by extracellular destruction forces.

Congenital Spherocytosis

Congenital spherocytosis is a hemolytic anemia that is inherited as an autosomal dominant trait. It occurs most frequently in the white population. The cells are small and defective, apparently due to abnormalities of the protein of the cell membrane that make them unusually permeable to sodium. The life span of erythrocytes is diminished.

The disease may be noticed shortly after birth, although symptoms may appear at any age. The hemolysis of red blood cells appears to occur in the spleen, apparently from excessive absorption of sodium into the cell. The abnormal cell swells and ruptures and so is destroyed. Chronic jaundice and splenomegaly are present. The MCHC will be increased because the cells are small. Gallstones may be present in the older school-age child and adolescent because of the continuous hemolysis, bilirubin release, and incorporation of bilirubin into gallstones.

Infections may precipitate a "crisis" involving bone marrow failure. During such a period, the anemia increases rapidly as the hemolysis continues. Blood transfusion will be necessary to maintain a sufficient number of circulating erythrocytes.

The diagnosis of the disease is based on family history, the obvious hemolysis, and the presence of the abnormal spherocytes. The medical treatment is generally splenectomy at approximately 5 to 6 years. This measure will increase the number of red blood cells present but will not alter their abnormal structure.

Glucose-6-Phosphate Dehydrogenase (G6PD) Deficiency

The enzyme G6PD is necessary for maintenance of red blood cell life. Lack of the enzyme results in premature destruction of red blood cells if the cells are exposed to an oxidant, such as acetylsalicylic acid. Deficiency of the enzyme occurs most frequently in children of African-American, Asian, Sephardic Jewish, and Mediterranean descent. The disease is transmitted as a sex-linked recessive trait. Approximately 13% of African-American males and 2% of African-American females have the disorder (Martin & Pearson, 1997b).

G6PD occurs in two identifiable forms. Children with congenital nonspherocytic hemolytic anemia have hemolysis, jaundice, and splenomegaly, and may have aplastic crises. Other children have a drug-induced form in which the blood patterns are normal until the child is exposed to fava beans or drugs such as antipyretics, sulfonamides, antimalarials, and naphthaquinolones (the most common drug in these groups is acetylsalicylic acid [aspirin]). Approximately 2 days after ingestion of such an oxidant drug, the child begins to show evidence of hemolysis.

A blood smear will show **Heinz bodies** (oddly shaped particles in red blood cells). The degree of red blood cell destruction depends on the drug and the extent of exposure to it. The child may have accompanying fever and back pain. Occasionally a newborn is seen with marked hemolysis because the mother ingested an initiating drug during pregnancy.

Drug-induced hemolysis usually is self-limiting, and blood transfusions are rarely necessary. G6PD deficiency may be diagnosed by a rapid enzyme screening test or electrophoretic analysis of red blood cells. Both parents and children must be told of the defect in the child's metabolism so they can avoid common drugs such as acetylsalicylic acid.

Because the disease is sex linked, males of high-risk groups should be screened in infancy.

Sickle-Cell Anemia

Sickle-cell anemia is the presence of abnormally shaped (elongated) red blood cells. It is an autosomal recessive inherited defect of the beta chain of hemoglobin; the amino acid valine takes the place of the normally appearing glutamic acid. The erythrocytes become characteristically elongated and crescent shaped (sickled) when they are submitted to low oxygen tension (less than 60% to 70%), a low blood pH (acidosis), or increased blood viscosity such as occurs with dehydration or hypoxia. When red blood cells sickle, they do not move freely through vessels. Stasis and further sickling occurs (a sickle-cell crisis). Blood flow halts and tissue distal to the blockage becomes ischemic, resulting in acute pain and cell destruction.

Because fetal hemoglobin contains a gamma, not a beta, chain, the disease usually will not result in clinical symptoms until the child's hemoglobin changes from the fetal to the adult form at approximately 6 months. However, the disease can be diagnosed prenatally by chorionic villi sampling or from cord blood during amniocentesis (Eboh & Van den Akker, 1997). The abnormal form of hemoglobin in this disorder is designated hemoglobin S. A child with sickle-cell disease is said to have hemoglobin SS (homozygous involvement).

Sickle-cell disease occurs almost exclusively among African Americans. Both parents of the child with the disease will have both normal adult and hemoglobin S or be carriers (heterozygous) of the **sickle-cell trait** (have hemoglobin AS). In people with the trait, approximately 25% to 50% of hemoglobin produced is abnormal. They produce enough normal hemoglobin to compensate for the defect and therefore show no symptoms. Sickle-cell trait occurs in approximately 8% to 10% of African Americans. A child with the disease (homozygous) produces no normal hemoglobin and so shows characteristic symptoms of sickle-cell anemia. Approximately 1 in 400 African Americans has the disease (Martin & Pearson, 1997b). A very few children have combinations of hemoglobin S and hemoglobin C or E leading to mild anemia.

Assessment. Screening for sickle-cell anemia is a simple finger-stick (a sickledex) procedure.

Unfortunately, all hemoglobin S cells sickle in a sickling test, so the test yields a positive result both for people with sickle-cell disease and those with sickle-cell trait. Further differentiation involves hemoglobin electrophoresis. In many states, all newborns are routinely screened for the disorder.

At approximately 6 months of age, children with sickle-cell disease will begin to show initial signs of fever and anemia. Stasis of blood and infarction may occur in any body part, leading to local disease. Some infants have swelling of the hands and feet (a hand–foot syndrome). This is probably caused by aseptic infarction of the bones of the hands and feet. Children with sickle-cell anemia tend to have a slight build and characteristically long arms and legs. They may have a protruding abdomen because of an enlarged spleen and liver. In adolescence, the spleen size may be decreased from repeated infarction and atrophy. An atropic spleen leaves a child more susceptible to infection than normal because the spleen can no longer filter bacteria. Pneumococcal meningitis and *Salmonella*-induced osteomyelitis are frequent illnesses. A chest syndrome, with symptoms similar to pneumonia may occur. To prevent infection, many children are placed on prophylactic penicillin from about 6 months to 6 years of age. The liver may become enlarged from stasis of blood flow. Eventually, cirrhosis (fibrotic degeneration) will occur from infarcts and tissue scarring. The kidneys may have subsequent scarring also, and kidney function may be decreased. The sclerae are generally icteric (yellowed) from chronic destruction of the sickled cells: small retinal occlusions may lead to decreased vision. Regular eye examinations are necessary in children with sickle-cell disease to detect this. Cell clusters in the blood vessel of the penis may cause **priapism,** or persistent, painful erection.

Sickle-Cell Crisis. **Sickle-cell crisis** is the term used to denote a sudden, severe onset of sickling. Symptoms of crisis occur from pooling of the many new sickled cells in vessels and consequent tissue hypoxia (a vaso-occlusive crisis). A sickle-cell crisis can occur when a child has an illness causing dehydration or a respiratory infection that results in lowered oxygen exchange and lowered arterial oxygen level, or after extremely strenuous exercise (enough to lead to tissue hypoxia). Sometimes no obvious cause of a crisis can be found. Symptoms are sudden, severe, and painful (Conner-Warren, 1996; see Assessing the Child With Sickle-Cell Crisis). Aseptic necrosis of the head of the femur or humerus with increased joint pain may occur. Laboratory reports reveal a hemoglobin of only 6 to 8 g/100 mL. A peripheral blood smear will demonstrate sickled cells. White blood count is often elevated to 12,000 to 20,000/mm^3. Bilirubin and reticulocyte levels will be increased.

If a cerebrovascular accident occurs from a blocked artery, the central nervous system will be affected and the child may have coma, convulsions, or even death. If there is renal involvement, hematuria or flank pain may result.

Less frequent forms of crisis may occur when there is splenic sequestration of red blood cells or severe anemia due to pooling and increased destruction of sickled cells in the liver and spleen (a sequestration crisis). This leads to shock from hypovolemia. The spleen is enlarged and tender. An aplastic crisis is manifested by severe anemia due to a sudden decrease in production of red blood cells. This form usually occurs with infection. A hyperhemolytic crisis can occur when there is increased destruc-

ASSESSING the Child With Sickle-Cell Crisis

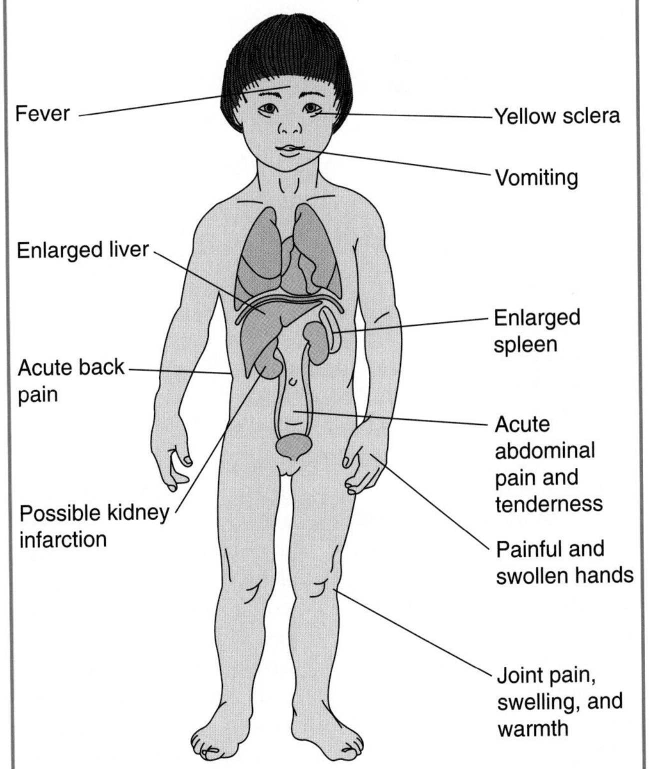

tion of red blood cells. A megaloblastic crisis may occur if the child has folic acid or vitamin B_{12} deficiency (new red blood cells cannot be fully formed due to lack of these ingredients).

Therapeutic Management. The child in sickle-cell crisis has two primary needs: (1) pain relief and (2) adequate hydration and oxygenation to prevent further sickling and halt the crisis.

Acetaminophen (Tylenol) or narcotics are usually prescribed to control pain; administer as often as allowed. Once the child is pain free, his or her agitation will decrease, reducing the metabolic demand for oxygen and ending the sickling. Hydration is generally accomplished with intensive intravenous fluid replacement therapy. Tissue hypoxia leads to acidosis. The acidosis must be corrected by electrolyte replacement. Be aware that some kidney infarction may have occurred. Do not administer potassium intravenously until kidney function has been determined. Otherwise, excessive potassium levels may occur, possibly leading to cardiac arrhythmias. Infection may precipitate a sickling crisis. If this occurs, blood and urine cultures, a chest x-ray, and a complete blood count will be taken and the infection will be treated by antibiotics.

Blood transfusion (usually packed red cells) may be necessary to maintain the hemoglobin above 12 g/dL (termed *hypertransfusion*).

If none of the above measures appears to be effective, children may be given an exchange transfusion to remove most of the sickled cells and replace them with normal cells. Exchange transfusion (see Chapter 6) must be done with small amounts of blood at each exchange. Otherwise, the pressure changes can cause such irregularities in blood volume that heart failure results. Bone marrow transplantation and gene therapy are being researched as possible treatments.

NURSING DIAGNOSES AND RELATED INTERVENTIONS

Nursing Diagnosis: Impaired tissue perfusion related to infarcts due to sickling

Outcome Identification: Child will remain free of detrimental effects of sickle-cell crisis during course of crisis.

Outcome Evaluation: Child's respiratory rate is 16/min to 20/min; cyanosis absent; arterial blood gases within acceptable parameters including $PaCo_2 = 40$ mm Hg; $PaO_2 = 80$ mm Hg to 90 mm Hg; oxygen saturation of 95%; urine output is greater than 1 mL/kg/h.

Oxygen may be administered by nasal cannula or mask if arterial blood gases reveal a low PaO_2 level. Oxygen may not reach every distal body part effectively if blood flowing to the part is obstructed by the sickled cells. When hemoglobin S is below 40%, there is adequate blood flow to body cells. High concentrations of oxygen are not used because hypoxia is a stimulant to erythrocyte production—production badly needed to replace damaged cells. Monitor the flow rate carefully and use pulse oximetry to evaluate oxygen saturation levels for changes. Encourage bedrest to relieve the pain and reduce oxygen expenditure.

It is important to maintain accurate intake and output records, test urine for specific gravity, and hematuria to detect the extent or presence of kidney damage from infarcts.

Nursing Diagnosis: Altered health maintenance related to lack of knowledge regarding long-term needs of child with sickle-cell anemia

Outcome Identification: Family will demonstrate ability to carry out necessary measures to maintain child's health in the future.

Outcome Evaluation: Mother or father accurately describes disease process and identifies special precautions necessary to prevent sickle-cell crisis.

In many children, episodes of sickling grow less severe as the child reaches adolescence. These children may live a normal life expectancy but still experience the stresses of chronic illness. Other children experience such devastating episodes in early childhood that the disease is fatal at an early age. Parents need support to supervise children carefully day by day when they are aware that, due to children's intense episodes, the children may die despite the parents' precautions.

Between crisis periods, care focuses on preventing recurring crisis. Although the hemoglobin level of children may remain as low as 6 to 9 g/100 mL, children adjust well to this chronic state. Children who are having frequent blood transfusions should not be given supplementary iron or iron-fortified formula or vitamins or they may receive too much iron; high levels of excess iron are deposited in body tissues (hemosiderosis) to a point of destroying them (**hemochromatosis**). Oral folic acid may be prescribed to help rebuild hemolyzed red blood cells.

Children with sickle-cell anemia need to be followed at regular health care visits. They must receive childhood immunizations so they are not vulnerable to common childhood infections such as measles or pertussis. They may be prescribed oral penicillin as prophylaxis for the first 5 years. They are also candidates for meningococcal and pneumococcal vaccines to prevent infection. Puberty may be delayed. Both parents and children may need counseling to accept this. Once puberty changes do occur, they are adequate, just later than normal. Parents and children with sickle-cell disease also need support and positive reinforcement to enhance the child's self-esteem (see Focus on Nursing Research).

Caution parents to bring their child to a health care facility at the first indication of infection. Some parents are reluctant to do this, afraid that they will be labeled "overprotective." Assure them that health care personnel are knowledgeable about sickle-cell anemia, and they know that a child with even a minor infection could become very ill. Respiratory illness will lead to sickling for two reasons: (1) the accompanying dehydration and (2) the lowered oxygen tension from altered oxygen–carbon dioxide exchange.

Parents must make decisions regarding children's activity levels. Children should attend regular school and be allowed to participate in all school activities except contact sports (such as football), which could result in rupture of an enlarged spleen. Long-distance running is also inadvisable because it can lead to dehydration. Caution parents to give the child fluids frequently, especially on

FOCUS ON NURSING RESEARCH

Do Children With Sickle-Cell Disease Feel Less Competent Than Their Disease-Free Siblings?

To answer this question, children were randomly selected from the case management program of the Sickle Cell Anemia Foundation. They were all African American. Children with sickle-cell anemia were compared to their disease-free siblings on issues such as hopelessness and self-perception of competence. Findings of the study revealed that children with sickle-cell disease did score lower on perceived physical competence.

The results of this study are not surprising because it is likely that children with sickle-cell disease who are having episodes of pain will feel less competent at performing physical tasks than their healthy siblings. It is an important study because it demonstrates how nurses can document feelings and experiences of children, providing scientific evidence of research-based nursing care.

Lee, E. J., Phoenix, D., Brown, W., & Jackson, B. S. (1997). A comparison study of children with sickle cell disease and their non-diseased siblings on hopelessness, depression, and perceived competence. *Journal of Advanced Nursing, 25*(1), 79.

long hikes and at the beach. Caution them against taking the child on board an unpressurized aircraft in which the oxygen concentration may fall during flight. During the summer months, parents need to be certain that they offer the child frequent drinks to prevent dehydration (Williams et al, 1997).

Some children who have had kidney infarcts and lessened ability to concentrate urine will have chronic nocturnal enuresis (bedwetting) (see Empowering the Family).

WHAT IF? What if a parent tells you she restricts her child who has sickle-cell anemia from drinking any fluid after 4 PM to prevent bedwetting? Is this a good solution to bedwetting for this child? How would you counsel this parent?

Children with sickle-cell disease are at high risk if they need surgery. The hours of being on nothing-by-mouth status, as well as being unable to eat afterward, may lead to dehydration. Anesthesia may cause a transient hypoxia leading to sickling. Parents must be cautioned that even for such a simple operation as tooth extraction, they must alert health care personnel of their child's condition.

✔ CHECKPOINT QUESTIONS

9. What is the treatment of choice for congenital spherocytosis?
10. With sickle-cell anemia, do children need less or more fluid in summer months and why?

Thalassemias

The thalassemias are anemias associated with abnormalities of the beta chain of adult hemoglobin (HgbA). Although these anemias occur most frequently in the Mediterranean population, they also occur in children of African and Asian heritage.

Thalassemia Minor (Heterozygous β-Thalassemia)

Children with thalassemia minor, a mild form of this anemia, produce both defective beta hemoglobin and normal hemoglobin. Because there is some normal production, the red blood cell count will be normal but the hemoglobin concentration will be decreased 2 to 3 g/100 mL below normal levels. The blood cells are moderately hypochromic and microcytic because of the poor hemoglobin formation.

EMPOWERING THE FAMILY: **Safety Precautions for School**

- Children with sickle-cell anemia need to maintain a high fluid intake to prevent blood from becoming thick. Be certain your child either takes fluid with him or buys adequate fluid for lunch.
- Provide additional fluid in the summer when dehydration is more apt to happen. Anticipate ways to provide fluid during long hikes or school trips; time spent on a hot beach may need to be limited.
- Learn about sources high in folic acid such as vegetables and fruit and be certain these are included in your child's diet every day.
- Encourage the child to get adequate sleep at night as a general measure to prevent illness.
- With the exception of contact sports (to avoid damage to an enlarged spleen) and long-distance running (to prevent dehydration), encourage your child to participate in normal school activities.
- Nocturnal enuresis (bedwetting) may occur as part of the illness. Encourage your child to take baths in the morning if this occurs so his clothes don't smell of urine.
- Maintain routine health care such as immunizations to prevent common childhood illnesses such as measles and mumps.
- Call your primary health care provider at the first sign of illness such as an upper respiratory infection so therapy can be begun immediately.

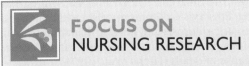

Children may have no symptoms other than pallor. They require no treatment, and life expectancy is normal. They should not receive a routine iron supplement because their inability to incorporate it well into hemoglobin may cause them to accumulate too much iron. The condition represents the heterozygous form of the disorder or can be compared with children having the sickle-cell trait.

Thalassemia Major (Homozygous β-Thalassemia)

Thalassemia major is also called Cooley's anemia or Mediterranean anemia. Because thalassemia is a beta-chain hemoglobin defect, symptoms do not become apparent until children's fetal hemoglobin has largely been replaced by adult hemoglobin during the second half of the first year of life. Effects of thalassemia major on body systems are summarized in Table 23-3. Unable to produce normal beta hemoglobin, children show symptoms of anemia: pallor, irritability, and anorexia.

Red blood cells will be hypochromic (pale) and microcytic (small). Fragmented poikilocytes and basophilic stippling (unevenness of hemoglobin concentration) will be present. The hemoglobin level will be less than 5 g/100 mL. The serum iron level will be high because iron is not being incorporated into hemoglobin; iron saturation will be 100%.

Assessment. To maintain a functional level of hemoglobin, the bone marrow hypertrophies in an attempt to produce more red blood cells. This may cause bone pain; the ineffective attempt often leads to the formation of target cells or large macrocytes that are short lived and nonfunctional. As bone marrow becomes hyperactive, this results in the characteristic change in the shape of the skull (parietal and frontal bossing) and protrusion of the upper teeth, with marked malocclusion. The base of the nose may be broad and flattened; the eyes may be slanted with an epicanthal fold as in Down syndrome. An x-ray of bone will show marked osteoporotic (lessened density) tissue, possibly resulting in fractures. The child may have hepatosplenomegaly due to excessive iron deposits and fibrotic scarring in the liver, and the spleen's increased attempts to destroy defective red blood cells. Abdominal pressure from the enlarged spleen may cause anorexia and vomiting. Epistaxis is common, as is diabetes mellitus due to pancreatic siderosis and cardiac dilatation with an accompanying murmur. Arrhythmias and heart failure are a frequent cause of death (Fuchs et al, 1997).

TABLE 23.3 Effects of Thalassemia Major

BODY ORGAN OR SYSTEM	EFFECT OF ABNORMAL CELL PRODUCTION
Bone marrow	Overstimulation of bone marrow leads to increased facial-mandibular growth
Skin	Bronze colored from hemosiderosis and jaundice
Spleen	Splenomegaly
Liver and gallbladder	Cirrhosis and cholelithiasis
Pancreas	Destruction of islet cells and diabetes mellitus
Heart	Failure from circulatory overload

Therapeutic Management. Digitalis, diuretics, and a low-sodium diet may be prescribed to prevent heart failure, which could result from the decompensation that accompanies anemia, and from myocardial fibrosis caused by invasion of iron (hemochromatosis). Transfusion of packed red cells every 2 to 4 weeks (hypertransfusion therapy) will maintain hemoglobin between 10 and 12 g/100 mL. With this level of hemoglobin, erythropoiesis is suppressed and cosmetic facial alterations, osteoporosis, and cardiac dilatation are kept to a minimum. Hypertransfusion therapy also reduces the possibility that splenectomy will be necessary. Frequent blood transfusions unfortunately increase the risk of bloodborne disease, such as hepatitis B, and deposition of iron in body tissues (hemosiderosis). Children may receive an iron chelating agent to remove this excessive store of iron, such as desferoxamine (given subcutaneously over 6 to 8 hours; Martin & Pearson, 1997b).

Splenectomy may become necessary to reduce discomfort and also reduce the rate of red cell hemolysis and the number of necessary transfusions. Bone marrow transplantation can offer a cure. Gene therapy is a future possibility (Giardini, 1997).

The overall prognosis of thalassemia is improving but still grave. Most children with the disease will die from cardiac failure during adolescence or as young adults.

NURSING DIAGNOSES AND RELATED INTERVENTIONS

Nursing Diagnosis: Risk for self-esteem disturbance related to changed physical appearance

Outcome Identification: Child will demonstrate an adequate level of self-esteem during course of illness.

Outcome Evaluation: Child states he or she can accept altered appearance and interacts with peers.

Children with thalassemia major may have delayed growth and sexual maturation. They usually develop a marked change in facial appearance because of the overgrowth of marrow-producing centers of the facial bones. This can be demoralizing because these changes will be permanent. In addition, the child who receives frequent blood transfusions may develop such hemosiderosis that his or her skin appears bronze.

Children should be allowed as much activity as possible and should attend regular school, if possible, to maintain a nearly normal childhood. Discussions about other children's reactions to their changing facial appearance can be helpful.

Autoimmune Acquired Hemolytic Anemia

Occasionally, autoimmune antibodies (abnormal antibodies of the IgG class) attach themselves to red blood cells, destroy them and cause hemolysis. This may occur at any age, and its origin is generally idiopathic, although the disorder may be associated with malignancy, viral infections, or collagen diseases such as rheumatoid arthritis or systemic lupus erythematosus. A child may recently have had an upper respiratory infection, measles, or varicella virus infection (chickenpox). Such hemolysis may occur after the administration of drugs such as quinine, phenacetin, sulfonamides, or penicillin.

The exact cause is unknown but may involve a change in the red blood cells themselves, making them antigenic, or a change in antibody production, making antibodies destructive to other substances.

Assessment. The onset of hemolytic anemia is insidious. Children have a low-grade fever, anorexia, lethargy, pallor, and icterus from release of indirect bilirubin from the hemolyzed cells. Both urine and stools appear dark because the excess bilirubin is being excreted. In some children, the illness begins abruptly with high fever, hemoglobinuria, marked jaundice, and pallor. There may be an enlarged liver and spleen.

Laboratory findings will reveal that the red cells are extremely small and round (spherocytosis), resembling hereditary spherocytosis. The reticulocyte count will be increased as the body attempts to form replacement red cells. A direct Coombs' test result will be positive, indicating the presence of antibodies attached to red cells. Hemoglobin levels may fall as low as 6 g/100 mL.

Therapeutic Management. In some children, the disease process runs a limited course and no treatment is necessary. In others, a single blood transfusion may correct the disturbance. For these children, it is difficult to cross match blood for transfusion because the red cell antibody tends to clump or agglutinate all blood tested. If cross matching is impossible, the child may be given type O Rh-blood. Observe the child carefully during any transfusion for signs of transfusion reaction.

If the anemia is persistent, corticosteroid therapy (oral prednisone) is generally effective, increasing the red blood cell count and hemoglobin concentration in a short period. If this is ineffective, splenectomy may be necessary. For some children, immunosuppressive agents (such as cyclophosphamide [Cytoxan] or azathioprine [Imuran]) are effective in reducing antibody formation.

Often it is difficult for parents to understand the process. How could a child's body turn on itself? What caused this? How long will it last? What will stop it from happening again? There are no answers to these questions. Provide the parents and child with support as they wait for this unexplainable process to run its course and for the child to be well again.

Polycythemia

Polycythemia is an increase in the number of red blood cells that results as a compensatory response to insufficient oxygenation of the blood. With this disorder, erythropoiesis is increased to attempt to supply enough red blood cells to supply oxygen to cells. Chronic pulmonary disease and congenital heart disease are the usual causes of polycythemia in childhood. Also, it may occur from twin transfusion at birth (one twin receives excess blood while a second twin is anemic).

Plethora (marked reddened appearance of the skin) occurs because of the increase in total red cell volume. The erythrocytes are usually macrocytic (large) and the hemoglobin content is high. This means that the MCH will be elevated; the MCHC, however, will be normal, indicating that, although many in number, each erythrocyte is normally saturated with hemoglobin. The red blood cell count may be as high as 7 million/mm^3. Hemoglobin levels may be as high as 23 g/100 mL.

Treatment of polycythemia involves treatment of the underlying cause. Because of the high blood viscosity from so many crowded blood cells, cerebrovascular accident or emboli may occur. The risk increases particularly if the child becomes dehydrated, such as with fever or during surgery. Exchange transfusion to reduce the red blood cell count may be necessary.

✔ CHECKPOINT QUESTIONS

11. What body appearance is associated with thalasemia major?
12. What laboratory test results would be seen with a child with autoimmune acquired hemolytic anemia?

DISORDERS OF THE WHITE BLOOD CELLS

Disorders Related to the Number or Proportion of White Blood Cells

Most disorders characterized by a decrease or increase in the number of white blood cells or specific white blood cell components occur in response to other disease (often infection or an allergic reaction) in the body. Laboratory values of white blood cells, therefore, provide one of the first objective indicators of disease, often aiding in specific diagnosis (Table 23-4).

DISORDERS OF BLOOD COAGULATION

A normal platelet level is 150,000/mm^3. **Thrombocytopenia** (decreased platelet count) may be defined as a platelet count of less than 40,000/mm^3. Because platelets are necessary for blood coagulation, platelet disorders limit the effectiveness of blood coagulation. In one disorder, children are born with thrombocytopenia and also are missing the radius bone in the forearm (TAR [thrombocytopenia-absent radius] syndrome). Thrombocytopenia leads to purpura (Casella, 1997).

Purpuras

Purpura is a hemorrhagic rash or small hemorrhages occurring in the superficial layer of skin. Two main types of purpura occur in children.

Idiopathic Thrombocytopenic Purpura

Idiopathic thrombocytopenic purpura (ITP) is the result of a decrease in the number of circulating platelets in the

TABLE 23.4 Disorders of White Blood Cells

DISORDER	DESCRIPTION	CAUSES/TREATMENT
Neutropenia	Reduced number of white blood cells	Transient phenomenon with nonpyrogenic infections such as viral disease Response to therapy with some drugs, such as 6-mercaptopurine or nitrogen mustard Possible side effect from drugs such as phenytoin sodium (Dilantin), chloramphenicol, or chlorpromazine Treatments: Possibly white blood cell transfusion; prophylactic antibiotics
Neutrophilia	Increased number of circulating white blood cells, primarily neutrophils (total number of cells increases and the proportion of mature neutrophils changes, with an increase in immature cells)	Usually in response to infection or inflammation (see Chapter 42)
Leukemia	Uncontrolled proliferation of white blood cells	Neoplastic disorder (see Chapter 52)
Eosinophilia	Increase in the number of eosinophils	Associated with many allergic disorders, such as atopic dermatitis and with parasitic invasion (see Chapters 41 and 42)
Lymphocytosis	Increase in the number of lymphocytes	Normally occurring in the preschool period when there is a marked predominance of lymphocytes in relation to neutrophils Abnormally elevated in childhood illnesses such as pertussis, infectious mononucleosis, and lymphoblastic leukemia

presence of adequate megakaryocytes (precursors to platelets). The cause is unknown, but it probably results from an increased rate of platelet destruction due to an antiplatelet antibody that destroys platelets (making this an autoimmune illness).

In most instances, ITP occurs approximately 2 weeks after a viral infection such as rubella, rubeola, varicella, or an upper respiratory tract infection. Congenital ITP may occur in the newborn of a woman who has had ITP during pregnancy. An antiplatelet factor apparently crosses the placenta and causes platelet destruction in the newborn. If it occurs in infants whose mother did not have ITP, the disease appears to develop in the same way as Rh incompatibility or hemolytic disease of the newborn. However, in ITP, the platelets, not the red blood cells, are sensitized (see Chapter 6).

Assessment. Manifestations often begin abruptly, first evidenced as miniature petechiae or as large areas of asymmetric ecchymosis most prominent over the legs, although they may occur anywhere on the body (Figure 23-3). Epistaxis or bleeding into joints may be present.

Laboratory studies reveal marked thrombocytopenia. The platelet count may be as low as 20,000/mm^3. Bone marrow examination will show a normal number of megakaryocytes. A tourniquet test may be performed. For this, the child's blood pressure is taken. Then the cuff is reinflated on the child's arm to a point halfway between systolic and diastolic pressure and left inflated for 5 minutes. In a child with normal coagulation ability, this extended pressure should result in fewer than two petechiae marks on an area of skin on the forearm 2 cm square. The child with decreased platelets will have a greater number of petechiae (George & Rashkob, 1997).

Therapeutic Management. Administration of oral prednisone is used to treat ITP. Platelet transfusion will temporarily increase the platelet count, but because the lifespan of platelets is relatively short, a platelet transfusion will have limited effect. Children with central nervous system bleeding are treated more vigorously, initially with a splenectomy and then transfusion.

If the child experiences joint pain from bleeding, do not give salicylates. Salicylates interfere with blood clotting by preventing the aggregation of platelets at wound sites.

In most children, ITP runs a limited, 1- to 3-month course. A few children develop chronic ITP. A course of immunosuppressive drugs may be attempted if the chronic state persists; intravenous gamma globulin may be used to improve the platelet count. Plasmapheresis (transfusion of plasma) may be effective in some children.

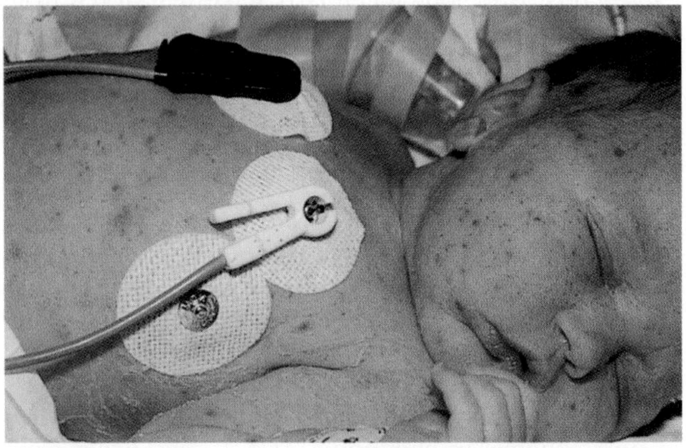

FIGURE 23.3 The infant with ITP. Notice the tiny petechiae and large ecchymotic areas.

All children need to be vaccinated against the viral diseases of childhood so that diseases such as rubella, rubeola, and varicella are eradicated and no longer lead to this defective coagulation process.

NURSING DIAGNOSES AND RELATED INTERVENTIONS

Nursing Diagnosis: Health-seeking behaviors related to injury prevention measures

Outcome Identification: Parents will demonstrate measures to prevent injury that would result in bleeding during child's illness.

Outcome Evaluation: Parents state precautions they will take to reduce possibility of bleeding injury; repeat correct dose and timing of medication therapy; child's skin is free of ecchymotic areas; platelet count rises to within normal values.

The techniques for reducing bleeding described earlier in the chapter can be used to reduce the possibility of bleeding (e.g., padding the surfaces where the child plays) for the child with ITP. Parents cannot completely eliminate the possibility of a serious bleeding injury, however, until the platelet count returns to normal. The chief danger to the child from ITP, aside from the psychological stress of a perplexing illness, is intracranial hemorrhage. Although rare, be alert for signs such as persistent headache, nuchal rigidity, and lethargy.

Nursing Diagnosis: Risk for ineffective family coping, compromised, related to diagnosis of child's illness

Outcome Identification: Parents demonstrate ability to cope with life-threatening circumstances during course of illness.

Outcome Evaluation: Parents state that they understand the nature of their child's illness and have identified ways to carry out daily activities despite the illness.

Because the symptoms (e.g., easy bruising) of ITP mimic the beginning ones of leukemia, parents may be extremely frightened. Assure them that this bruising is not leukemia. If the ITP follows a long course (2 or 3 months), reassure them that this process will not later become leukemia. A child may have so many bruises that the parents are initially suspected of child abuse. They may become very defensive and angry at health care personnel. They need time to express their anger and regain confidence in the health care team.

It is also bewildering for parents to be told that no one knows exactly what is causing their child's disease. To be convinced that health care personnel can manage their child's care without knowing the exact cause, they need careful explanations of all procedures (Yetgin et al, 1997).

Henoch-Schönlein Syndrome

Henoch-Schönlein purpura (also called anaphylactoid purpura) is caused by increased vessel permeability. Although no definite allergic correlation can be identified, Henoch-Schönlein purpura is generally considered to be a hypersensitivity reaction to an invading allergen. It occurs most frequently in children between 2 and 8 years of age, and more frequently in boys than girls. Usually, there is a history of mild infection before the outbreak of symptoms. The syndrome presents (because of the purpura) as a possible platelet disorder until a differential diagnosis is made.

Assessment. The purpural rash occurs typically on the buttocks, posterior thighs, and extensor surface of the arms and legs (Figure 23-4). The tips of the ears may be involved. The rash begins as a crop of urticarial lesions that change to pink maculopapules. These become hemorrhagic (bright red), then fade, leaving brown macular spots that remain for several weeks. The child's joints are tender and swollen. The child may have gastrointestinal symptoms such as abdominal pain, vomiting, or blood in stools. Gross or microscopic hematuria may be present from kidney involvement. A biopsy shows granulocytes in the walls of small arterioles.

Laboratory studies will show a normal platelet count. Sedimentation rate, white blood count, and eosinophil count will be elevated.

Therapeutic Management. Treatment involves steroid therapy (oral prednisone) for a short period. Nose and throat cultures rule out continuing bacterial involvement. Urine should be assessed for protein and glucose to detect kidney involvement. Typically the disease runs a course of 4 to 6 weeks. A few children will develop chronic nephritis as a complication.

Disseminated Intravascular Coagulation

Disseminated intravascular coagulation (DIC) is an acquired disorder of blood clotting that results from excessive trauma or some similar underlying stimulus.

Normal blood clotting is a balance between the hemostatic (clotting) system and the fibrinolytic (dissolving) system of the bloodstream. After a blood vessel injury, local vasoconstriction rapidly prevents additional blood

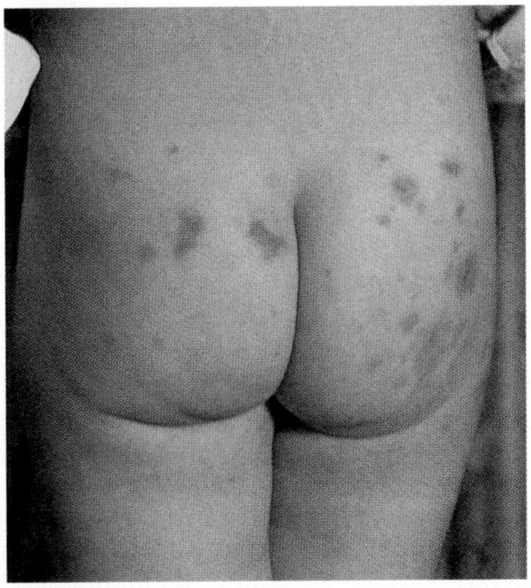

FIGURE 23.4 The distinctive purpural rash of Henoch-Schönlein syndrome appearing on the buttocks of a young child.

loss at the site. With the tear in the vessel wall, the underlying collagen is exposed. This causes platelets to swell and become adherent and irregular in shape. They release adenosine diphosphate, which attracts additional platelets and binds them together (platelet aggregation). This phenomenon results in a platelet plug to seal the vessel. The plug is strengthened by fibrin threads forming as a result of an intrinsic and extrinsic coagulation process into a firm, fixed structure. To prevent too much clotting from occurring, plasmin or fibrinolysin, a proteolytic enzyme formed from plasminogen, digests fibrin threads and causes lysis of the clot along with consumption of blood clotting factors. As plasmin, fibrinogen, and fibrin are lysed, fibrin degradation products are formed. These products prevent the laying down of further fibrin and platelet aggregation.

With DIC, an imbalance occurs between clotting activity and fibrinolysis. Extreme clotting due to endothelial damage begins at one point in the circulatory system, depleting the availability of clotting factors such as platelets and fibrin from the general circulation. A secondary initiation of fibrinolysis begins as well. A paradox exists: the person has both increased coagulation and a bleeding defect at the same time. Many of the complications of pregnancy (abruptio placenta or death of a fetus) initiate DIC, so this is a common complication seen accompanying bleeding during pregnancy. DIC can occur in children with acute infections.

Assessment. A child begins to have uncontrolled bleeding from puncture sites from injections or intravenous therapy. Ecchymosis and petechiae form on the skin. The child's toes and fingers may be pale, cyanotic or mottled and cold because small blood vessels are so filled with coagulated blood that circulation to extremities is impaired. If coagulation is acute, neurologic or renal symptoms may occur from occlusion of vessels supplying the brain and kidneys. Observe all children with a serious illness carefully for signs of increased bleeding such as skin petechiae or oozing from blood-drawing sites.

With DIC, laboratory tests usually show the following:

- Thrombocytopenia (level depends on the rate at which bone marrow is able to replace platelets)
- Large-appearing platelets on blood smear, possibly fragmented (from passing through meshes of collecting fibrin)
- Prothrombin and partial thromboplastin times prolonged
- Serum fibrinogen levels markedly low (less than 100 mg/100 mL)
- Fibrin split products elevated

Therapeutic Management. To stop DIC, the underlying insult that began the phenomenon must be halted. Intravenous heparin administration helps to interfere with the marked coagulation. Although blood transfusion may be necessary to correct blood loss, it may be delayed until after heparin has been administered so that the new blood factors are not also consumed by the coagulation process. Fresh frozen plasma, platelets, or fibrinogen may be administered.

With adequate therapy, blood coagulation studies will return to normal. If renal or brain cells were damaged from occluded capillaries, permanent injury to these areas may result.

NURSING DIAGNOSES AND RELATED INTERVENTIONS

Nursing Diagnosis: Knowledge deficit about blood clotting disorder related to its paradoxical nature

Outcome Identification: Client (or parents) will demonstrate increased knowledge of the illness by 1 hour.

Outcome Evaluation: Client (or parents) accurately state nature of illness and proposed therapy; states signs and symptoms of disease; verbalizes understanding of treatments.

Parents may be bewildered by the paradoxical problems of bleeding on one hand and clotting on the other. If they understand the action of heparin—to discourage blood coagulation—their child's need and the medication seem directly contradictory. Be certain that both children and parents are given a full explanation: The child has an increased risk of hemorrhaging because part of the coagulation system has begun coagulation; heparin is acting to stop coagulation. This effort will help parents better understand what is happening and foster trust and confidence in caregivers.

✔ CHECKPOINT QUESTIONS

13. What white blood cell disorder is commonly associated with allergies?
14. Why should salicylates be avoided for the child with ITP?

Hemophilias

Hemophilia is an inherited interference with blood coagulation. There are numerous hemophilia types, each involving deficiency of a different blood coagulation factor.

Hemophilia A (Factor VIII Deficiency)

The classic form of hemophilia is caused by deficiency of the coagulation component factor VIII, the antihemophilic factor, which is transmitted as a sex-linked recessive trait. In the United States, the incidence is approximately 1 in 10,000 white males. The female carrier may have slightly lowered but sufficient levels of the factor VIII component so that she does not manifest a bleeding disorder. Males with the disease also have varying levels of factor VIII, and their bleeding tendency varies accordingly, from mild to severe.

Factor VIII is an intrinsic factor of coagulation, so the intrinsic system for manufacturing thromboplastin is incomplete. The child's coagulation ability is not absent because the extrinsic or tissue system remains intact. Thus, the child's blood will eventually coagulate after an injury.

Assessment. Hemophilia often is recognized first in the infant who bleeds excessively after circumcision. If the disease has not shown itself for several generations in a family, the parents may be unaware of its existence. For this reason, all infants need careful and thoughtful observation after circumcision.

Because infants do not receive many injuries, the child's bleeding tendency may not become apparent until the child begins to walk. Suddenly the lower extremities (where the child bumps things) become heavily bruised. There is soft tissue bleeding and painful hemorrhage into the joints, which become swollen and warm. The child holds the injured joint stiffly. Repeated bleeding into a joint causes damage to the synovial membrane (hemarthrosis), possibly resulting in severe loss of joint mobility.

Severe bleeding may also occur into the gastrointestinal tract, peritoneal cavity, or central nervous system. Interestingly, nosebleeds are common, but are not as severe as with the platelet deficiency syndromes. The child must be identified as having hemophilia before surgery is performed for any reason; otherwise, fatal bleeding could occur (Casella, 1997).

With hemophilia, the platelet count and prothrombin time are normal. The whole blood clotting time is markedly prolonged or normal, depending on the level of factor VIII present. A thromboplastin generation test is abnormal. PTT is the test that best reveals the low levels of factor VIII.

Therapeutic Management. With even minor abrasions, bleeding must be controlled by the administration of factor VIII. This may be supplied by fresh whole blood or by fresh or frozen plasma, but it is best supplied by a concentrate of factor VIII. One bag of concentrate per 5 kg of body weight is usually sufficient. This provides protection for approximately 12 hours; another transfusion may be necessary at that time. Powdered forms of factor VIII that can be stored at home and reconstructed as needed are available. Prophylactic administration may best reduce bleeding episodes (Lusher, 1997).

In a small number of children, antibodies (termed *inhibitors*) to factor VIII develop, rendering the factor ineffective. Epsilon-aminocaproic acid, a fibrinolytic enzyme that helps to stabilize clot formation and promote wound healing, can be self-administered every 6 hours if needed. Children with inhibitors to factor VIII can also be administered a factor IX concentrate (Proplex or Konyne). This concentrate enters the coagulation cascade after factor VIII and halts bleeding. Gene therapy to replace the affected defect is a future possibility.

NURSING DIAGNOSES AND RELATED INTERVENTIONS

Nursing Diagnosis: Parental health-seeking behaviors related to strategies for protecting the child from injury

Outcome Identification: Parents will develop plan for preventing injury to the child and child will not experience major bleeding episodes during childhood.

Outcome Evaluation: Child's skin is free of ecchymotic areas; absence of frequent epistaxis; blood pressure within age-appropriate parameters; absence of swelling or warmth at joints.

Prevention of injury is the most important intervention with these children. Parents need information about how to prevent bleeding episodes and also how to respond when one occurs (see Enhancing Communication). Help parents to set appropriate limits. An active infant may

ENHANCING COMMUNICATION

Murray Harrow is an 8-year-old boy with hemophilia you see in an emergency room. His right knee is covered by a large brush burn and is swollen, discolored, and warm to touch.

Less Effective Communication

Nurse: Hello, Mrs. Harrow. I need to take a history of Murray's accident.

Mrs. Harrow: He doesn't know how he hurt it.

Nurse: It looks like he fell. Were you running, Murray? Riding a bicycle? Skateboarding?

Mrs. Harrow: He's never ridden a bicycle. I don't allow it. Or skateboarding. He better not say that he was doing that.

Nurse: Murray? How do you think you hurt your knee?

Murray: I don't know.

Nurse: You must have hit it hard to cause so much damage to the surface skin. You didn't notice hitting it so hard?

Murray: No.

Nurse: Okay. Let's get your factor replacement started and get the swelling down.

More Effective Communication

Nurse: Hello, Mrs. Harrow. I need to take a history of Murray's accident.

Mrs. Harrow: He doesn't know how he hurt it.

Nurse: It looks like he fell. Were you running, Murray?

Mrs. Harrow: He better not say that was what he was doing. He knows better than that.

Nurse: What about riding a bicycle?

Mrs. Harrow: He's never ridden a bicycle. I don't allow it.

Nurse: How about skateboarding?

Mrs. Harrow: He better not say he was doing that.

Nurse: My job, Mrs. Harrow, is to get an accurate history of what happened. Let's let Murray tell us how he thinks the accident happened. Later, we can talk about what are good rules for him to be following.

Children with bleeding disorders have to follow a great many rules to avoid bleeding episodes, such as not playing contact sports or skateboarding. Because these forbidden activities are appealing, children occasionally break the rules. In an emergency room, it is important that children and parents both recognize that the priority at the moment is obtaining an accurate history. Until they realize this, they may be so concerned with the broken rule that they are unable to move beyond that to secure adequate therapy.

need his or her crib sides padded; all toys need to be inspected for sharp edges or parts.

Parents (and the child as soon as he is approximately 10 years old) can be taught to administer a replacement factor intravenously to prevent bleeding immediately after an injury. This action, combined with immobilization of the injured extremity and an ice pack applied locally, will almost always eliminate the need for hospital admissions. Pressure should be applied to a laceration to halt bleeding directly. Suturing of lacerations is avoided whenever possible, because the sutures make additional puncture sites that may bleed.

Nursing Diagnosis: Pain related to joint infiltration by blood

Outcome Identification: Child will experience a tolerable level of pain after injury.

Outcome Evaluation: Child voices that pain is at a tolerable level.

The child with hemophiliac bleeding experiences discomfort because of the bleeding into joints and may be frightened because the parents are so frightened. Immobilization of the affected joint helps to decrease bleeding and also provide relief. Be certain that immobilized joints are in good alignment. As soon as the acute bleeding episode has halted (approximately 48 hours), perform passive range of motion as ordered to maintain function. Aspirin is not ordered as an analgesic because it may prolong bleeding. As soon as effective levels of factor VIII have been provided, the pain in the bleeding joint is generally relieved, despite the continued heat or swelling.

Nursing Diagnosis: Risk for altered family processes related to fears regarding child's prognosis and long-term nature of illness

Outcome Identification: Family members will demonstrate adequate coping behaviors by 1 month.

Outcome Evaluation: Family members voice their feelings of fear regarding illness; state that they are able to cope despite stress level; demonstrate positive coping responses.

Parents of children with hemophilia are frightened during a time of acute bleeding, not just because of what is currently happening but also because they may have seen other family members or even a previous child die of the disease. Be certain to give them a chance to talk about how the bleeding began (e.g., "I should have noticed that toy had a sharp edge," "He fell from his bike. I should have watched him more closely"). Parents need assurance that it is extremely important that they allow their child to lead a normal life, with toys and bicycle riding. Remind them that it is impossible to prevent all injuries. Assist them with measures that offer them a sense of control over the situation. As the child reaches school age, the child must learn to monitor his own activities.

Von Willebrand's Disease

Von Willebrand's disease, an inherited autosomal dominant disorder affecting both sexes, is often referred to as angiohemophilia. Along with a factor VIII defect there is also an inability of the platelets to aggregate. Additionally, the blood vessels are unable to constrict and aid in coagulation. Bleeding time is prolonged, with most hemorrhages occurring from mucous membrane sites.

Epistaxis is a major problem, because children tend to rub or pick at their noses as a nervous mechanism. In girls, menstrual flow will be unusually heavy and may cause embarrassment from stained clothing. Childbirth is obviously a risk for women with von Willebrand's disease. Bleeding is controlled with factor VIII replenishment as with hemophilia, or by administration of arginine desmopressin (DDAVP), a vasoconstricting agent (Casella, 1997).

Christmas Disease (Hemophilia B, Factor IX Deficiency)

Christmas disease, caused by factor IX deficiency, is transmitted as a sex-linked recessive trait. Only approximately 15% of people with hemophilia have this form. Treatment is with a concentrate of factor IX, available for home administration (White et al, 1998).

Hemophilia C (Factor XI deficiency)

Plasma thromboplastin antecedent deficiency, caused by factor XI deficiency, is transmitted as an autosomal recessive trait occurring in both sexes. It tends to occur in Jewish children. The symptoms are generally mild compared with those in children with factor VIII or factor IX deficiencies. Bleeding episodes are treated with the transfusion of fresh blood or plasma.

✔ CHECKPOINT QUESTIONS

15. What coagulation factor is deficient with hemophilia A?
16. What intervention is crucial for any child with hemophilia?

KEY POINTS

Bone marrow transplantation is the main therapy for a number of blood dyscrasias. Transplantation can be allogeneic (from a histocompatible donor) or autologous (using the child's own marrow). Splenectomy, another possible treatment, may increase a child's susceptibility to pneumococcal infections. Assess if children receive pneumococcal vaccine after a splenectomy.

Disorders of the red blood cells that commonly occur in children include acute blood-loss anemia and anemia of acute infection. Aplastic and hypoplastic anemias occur from depression of hematopoietic activity in bone marrow. These anemias can be congenital or acquired.

A major hypochromic anemia that develops in children is iron-deficiency anemia. Children with anemia invariably fatigue easily because they are unable to oxygenate body cells well. Their care must include measures to keep them from tiring; oxygen administration may be necessary.

Macrocytic anemias occur from folic acid deficiency and pernicious anemia (vitamin B_{12} deficiency).

Hemolytic anemias include congenital spherocytosis, glucose-6-dehydrogenase deficiency, sickle-cell anemia, thalassemia, and autoimmune acquired hemolytic anemia. Sickle-cell anemia occurs most often in African-American children.

Disorders of white blood cells that occur are neutropenia (reduced number of white blood cells) and neutrophilia (increased number). Neutropenia makes children susceptible to infection.

Disorders of blood coagulation seen are the purpuras (idiopathic thrombocytopenic purpura and Henoch-Schönlein syndrome), disseminated intravascular coagulation (DIC) and the hemophilias.

Children with blood coagulation disorders must be guarded carefully against injury. This includes monitoring types of toys and activities. It may include padding a crib or side rails.

Disorders of the blood tend to be long-term illnesses. Education of the parents and of the child is important to promote adaptation to the condition and compliance with long-term medication therapy.

CRITICAL THINKING EXERCISES

1. Heather is the 2-year-old girl with thalassemia major you met at the beginning of the chapter. Her mother asked you why Heather has developed a prominent mandible while another patient with thalassemia minor has no such facial changes. What additional health teaching does Heather's mother need to help her better understand what is happening to her daughter? How would you explain why skin color changes have happened to her daughter?
2. A 12-year-old girl has been diagnosed with sickle-cell anemia. You have noticed that every summer for the past 5 years while she has been home from school on summer vacation, she has had an acute episode of her illness. What assessments would you want to make of her family before this summer? What precautions would you want to discuss with them?
3. A 6-year-old boy has glucose-6-phosphate dehydrogenase (66PD) deficiency. He has frequent sinus headaches. What analgesic would be contraindicated for him?
4. A 5-year-old boy with hemophilia wants to join a preschool soccer program. How would you counsel his family regarding this?

REFERENCES

Casella, J. F. (1997). Disorders of coagulation. In Johnson, K. B., & Oski, F. A. *Oski's essential pediatrics*. Philadelphia: Lippincott.

Conner-Warren, R. L. (1996). Pain intensity and home pain management of children with sickle cell disease. *Issues in Comprehensive Pediatric Nursing, 19*(3), 183.

deAndraca, I., Castillo, M., & Walter, T. (1997). Psychomotor development and behavior in iron-deficient anemic infants. *Nutrition Reviews, 55*(4), 125.

Department of Health and Human Services. (1995). *Healthy people 2000: midcourse review*. Washington, D.C.: DHHS.

Eboh, W., & Van den Akker, O. (1997). Antenatal screening for couples at risk of having children with sickle cell disorders. *Midwives, 110*(1309), 26.

Esposito, C., et al. (1997). Pediatric laparoscopic splenectomy: are there real advantages in comparison with the traditional open approach? *Pediatric Surgery International, 12*(7), 509.

Fuchs, G. J., et al. (1997). Nutritional support and growth in thalassaemia major. *Archives of Disease in Childhood, 76*(6), 509.

George, J. N., & Rashkob, G. E. (1997). Clinical decisions in idiopathic thrombocytopenic purpura. *Hospital Practice, 32*(9), 159.

Giardini, C. (1997). Treatment of beta-thalassemia. *Current Opinions in Hematology. 4*(2), 79.

Lee, E. J., Phoenix, D., Brown, W., & Jackson, B. S. (1997). A comparison study of children with sickle cell disease and their non-diseased siblings on hopelessness, depression, and perceived competence. *Journal of Advanced Nursing, 25*(1), 79.

Lusher, J. M. (1997). Prophylaxis in children with hemophilia: is it the optimal treatment? *Thrombosis and Haemostasis, 78*(1), 726.

Martin, P. L., & Pearson, H. A. (1997a). The hemolytic anemias. In Johnson, K. B., & Oski, F. A. *Oski's essential pediatrics*. Philadelphia: Lippincott.

Martin, P. L., & Pearson, H. A. (1997b). Hemoglobinopathies and thalassemias. In Johnson, K. B., & Oski, F. A. *Oski's essential pediatrics*. Philadelphia: Lippincott.

Rapetti, M. C., et al. (1997). Correction of iron deficiency with an iron-fortified fluid whole cow's milk in children: results of a pilot study. *Journal of Pediatric Hematology/Oncology, 19*(3), 192.

Requejo, A. M., et al. (1997). Folate and vitamin B_{12} status in a group of preschool children. *International Journal for Vitamin and Nutrition Research, 67*(3), 171.

Richer, S. (1997). A practical guide for differentiating between iron deficiency anemia and anemia of chronic disease in children and adults. *Nurse Practitioner, 22*(4), 82.

White, G. et al. (1998). Clinical evaluation of recombinant factor IX. *Seminars in Hematology, 35*(2), 33.

Williams, R., George, E. O., & Wang, W. (1997). Nutrition assessment in children with sickle cell disease. *Journal of the Association for Academic Minority Physicians, 8*(3), 44.

Yetgin, S., et al. (1997). Retrospective analysis of 78 children with chronic idiopathic thrombocytopenic purpura: follow-up from 1976 to 1996. *Pediatric Hematology and Oncology, 14*(5), 399.

SUGGESTED READINGS

Blanco, R., et al. (1997). Henoch-Schonlein purpura in adulthood and childhood: two different expressions of the same syndrome. *Arthritis and Rheumatism, 40*(5), 859.

Cahill, M. (1996). Hematologic problems in pediatric patients. *Seminars in Oncology Nursing, 12*(1), 38.

Conlon, B., et al. (1996). ENT surgery in children with inherited bleeding disorders. *Journal of Laryngology and Otology, 110*(10), 947.

Derkay, C. S., Werner, E., & Plotnick, E. (1996). Management of children with von Willebrand disease undergoing adenotonsillectomy. *American Journal of Otolaryngology, 17*(3), 172.

Eaton, M. L., et al. (1995). Hospitalizations for painful episodes: association with school absenteeism and academic performance in children and adolescents with sickle cell anemia. *Issues in Comprehensive Pediatric Nursing, 18*(1), 1.

Gribbons, D., Zahr, L. K., & Opas, S. R. (1995). Nursing management of children with sickle cell disease: an update. *Journal of Pediatric Nursing, 10*(4), 232.

Johnson, F. L. (1996). What is the most effective treatment of children with severe aplastic anemia who lack a matched sibling donor? *Bone Marrow Transplantation, 18*(3), 839.

Lawlor, E. R., et al. (1997). Immunosuppressive therapy: a potential alternative to bone marrow transplantation as initial therapy for acquired severe aplastic anemia in childhood. *Journal of Pediatric Hematology/Oncology, 19*(2), 115.

Pastan, S. & Bailey, J. (1998). Dialysis therapy. *New England Journal of Medicine, 338*(20), 1428.

Werner, E. J. (1996). Von Willebrand disease in children and adolescents. *Pediatric Clinics of North America, 43*(3), 683.

Nursing Care of the Child With a Gastrointestinal Disorder

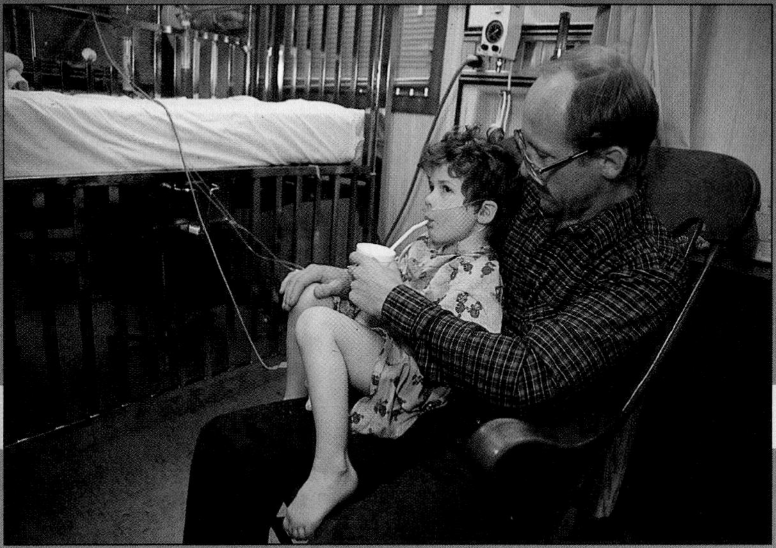

24

CHAPTER

Key Terms

- aganglionic megacolon
- anion
- appendicitis
- beriberi
- cation
- celiac disease
- chalasia
- gastroesophageal reflux (GER)
- hepatitis
- hiatal hernia
- hypertonic dehydration
- hypotonic dehydration
- inguinal hernia
- insensible loss
- intussusception
- irritable bowel syndrome
- isotonic dehydration
- keratomalacia
- kwashiorkor
- liver transplantation
- McBurney's point
- Meckel's diverticulum
- metabolic acidosis
- metabolic alkalosis
- necrotizing enterocolitis
- nutritional marasmus
- overhydration
- pellagra
- peptic ulcer
- pyloric stenosis
- rickets
- steatorrhea
- volvulus
- xerophthalmia

Objectives

After mastering the contents of this chapter, you should be able to:

1. Describe common gastrointestinal disorders seen in children.
2. Assess the child with a gastrointestinal disorder.
3. Formulate nursing diagnoses for the child with a gastrointestinal disorder.
4. Develop appropriate outcomes for the child with a gastrointestinal disorder.
5. Plan nursing care with specific goals for the child with a gastrointestinal disorder.
6. Implement nursing care for the child with a gastrointestinal disorder.
7. Evaluate outcomes for effectiveness and achievement of care.
8. Identify National Health Goals related to gastrointestinal disorders and children that nurses could be instrumental in helping the nation achieve.
9. Identify areas of care related to gastrointestinal disorders and children that could benefit from additional nursing research.
10. Analyze ways that nursing care of the child with a gastrointestinal disorder can be more family centered.
11. Integrate knowledge of gastrointestinal disorders with nursing process to achieve quality child health nursing care.

Barry is a 2-year-old diagnosed with celiac disease that you see at a birthday party. His abdomen is protuberant, yet his arms and legs seem thin and wasted. He refuses to eat a piece of birthday cake even though his mother sits beside him insisting on it. "See the problem I have with him?," she asks you. "He eats nothing. When he does, he gets diarrhea."

Does Barry's mother understand her son's disease? Is she choosing wise food selections for him?

In previous chapters, you learned about the growth and development of well children and the nursing care for children with disorders of other systems. In this chapter, you'll add information about the dramatic changes, both physically and psychosocially, that occur when children develop gastrointestinal disorders. This is important information because it builds a base for care and health teaching.

After you've studied the chapter, turn to the Critical Thinking Exercises at the end of the chapter to help sharpen your skills and test your knowledge.

The gastrointestinal (GI) system involves a long body tract with numerous organs. A multitude of possible disorders can occur in it, including both congenital defects and acquired illnesses. (Developmental physical defects that are discovered at birth are discussed in Chapter 18.) Because the GI system is responsible for taking in and processing nutrients for all parts of the body, any problem can quickly affect other systems of the body and, if not adequately treated, can affect overall health, growth, and development.

Health education is extremely important for children with gastrointestinal disorders and their families because many parents do not appreciate the seriousness of gastrointestinal illness. Often, they are surprised to find that what they thought was a simple "stomach flu" has caused serious electrolyte imbalances and possibly a life-threatening state for their child. Some gastrointestinal disorders require both parents and child to learn about a new diet. When the child is young, the parents need education concerning the diet and other care measures. As the child grows older, counseling to help the child maintain self-esteem and learn diet requirements becomes important.

Specifically, diarrhea and hepatitis B in children have received much attention as National Health Goals. These are shown in the Focus on National Health Goals.

FOCUS ON NATIONAL HEALTH GOALS

In the past, diarrhea was a major cause of death in infants. National Health Goals address this as well as hepatitis B. These goals are:

- Reduce viral hepatitis B in infants to 350/100,000 new carriers from a baseline of 500/100,000.
- Reduce infectious diarrhea by at least 25% among children in licensed child care centers and children in programs that provide an individualized education program (DHHS, 1995).

Nurses can be instrumental in helping the nation achieve these goals by serving as consultants to day care providers to reduce the spread of diarrhea in these settings and actively administering hepatitis B vaccine to infants to eradicate this illness in another generation. Nursing research on a number of areas could be helpful: Do the brand names of diapers used by children in day care influence the spread of infectious diarrhea; how many infants are not being brought for follow-up care and thus do not receive all three immunizations against hepatitis B; and do the majority of parents appreciate the devastating outcome that can result from diarrhea in infants?

NURSING PROCESS OVERVIEW

for the Child With Altered Gastrointestinal Function

Assessment

Children with gastrointestinal disorders quickly become dehydrated, especially if vomiting or diarrhea is one of the symptoms. They need to be assessed for signs of dehydration, such as poor skin turgor, dry mucous membranes, or lack of tearing (see Assessing the Child With Altered GI Function). When talking to parents about a child's symptoms, ask exactly what they mean when they say "spitting up" or "a little vomiting." Also ask how many times a child has voided or how many diapers have been wet in the past 24 hours, and whether this is less than usual. Compare current weight with past weight measurements, if available. Unless the child is an adolescent who has been actively dieting, there is never a normal reason for weight loss in children.

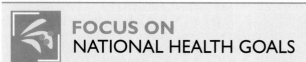

Ask parents to describe what they mean by diarrhea. Some parents mistakenly confuse normal newborn stools with diarrhea. As a rule, all children with diarrhea, especially small children, need to be seen by a health care provider because fluid and electrolyte changes occur rapidly in children because of the greater percentage of fluid held extracellularly rather than intracellularly.

For many children, a gastrointestinal tract disorder is diagnosed largely by presenting symptoms such as those just described. In other instances, x-ray studies with a contrast medium (barium) may be used to confirm the presence of an anomaly. Ultrasound or magnetic resonance imaging also may be helpful. Another important assessment area is laboratory testing for electrolyte balance through serum analysis, or fluid concentration through urinalysis.

Nursing Diagnosis

Nursing diagnoses relevant to children with gastrointestinal disorders invariably center on altered nutrition, because most gastrointestinal diseases in some way alter the kind and amount of nutrients ingested or absorbed into the body. However, gastrointestinal disorders also take an emotional toll on the ill child and family. Feeding is one of the primary ways mothers bond with their newborns, and bonding can be seri-

ASSESSING the Child With Altered GI Function

History

Chief concern: Vomiting, diarrhea, constipation, abdominal pain, abdominal distention, weight below normal standard, lethargy, paleness.
Past medical history: History of past vomiting or diarrhea or abdominal pain; hydramnios in pregnancy.
Family history: Relatives have a similar disorder; high stress level because of home or school environment.

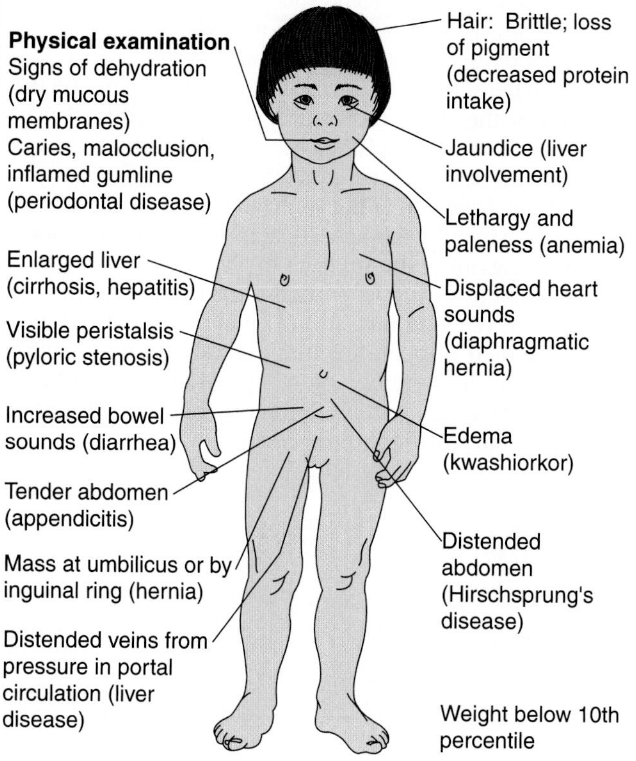

ously threatened when the infant suffers from a gastrointestinal disorder, especially when hospitalization is required. Eating and diet are also integral components of family life and culture, so any disruption caused by illness can place a strain on the entire family. Examples of nursing diagnoses may include:

- Altered parenting related to interference with establishing parent-infant bond
- Altered family processes related to chronic illness in child
- Risk for fluid volume deficit related to chronic diarrhea
- Altered nutrition, less than body requirements, related to malabsorption of necessary nutrients
- Self-esteem disturbance related to feelings of being different resulting from special dietary restrictions

Outcome Identification and Planning

Planning care for the child with a gastrointestinal disorder often includes diet planning with the child and parents. Be certain when helping to plan a diet that the person who actually prepares or supervises the child's diet is included. In many instances, part of the diet may be prepared by a baby sitter, day care center staff, the child's other parent, or a grandparent. Many children eat breakfast and lunch at school cafeterias. It may be necessary to contact school staff to ask them to make meal exceptions for the child or to supervise a choice of foods (or to see that a child eats only the packaged lunch he or she brought to school, not extra items the child trades for with friends).

Some parents are unfamiliar with the basic food groups and the importance of providing food from a food pyramid in children's diets. They may have little understanding of which foods have high or low fiber content, or which foods are "bland" or "clear." Many parents have difficulty keeping children restricted to "nothing by mouth" (NPO) for tests or to rest the gastrointestinal tract. They have been told that dehydration happens quickly in infants; they need support to follow the necessary restrictions when those restrictions are so opposed to basic parenting, which involves giving food.

If feedings will be given by nasogastric or gastrostomy tube, parents need enough practice time to be comfortable with the equipment and the technique before they are given the responsibility of doing it alone at home. If a child is going to gag or become distressed when a new tube is passed, parents need to have this happen where there are calm, supportive people nearby, not when they are by themselves at home.

Implementation

Never underestimate the difficulty family members may experience adapting to alternative nutrition methods such as total parenteral nutrition or enteric feeding tubes, or caring for a child with a colostomy. Parents need a great deal of support to adapt their busy life to these alternative methods of care.

Insertion of a nasogastric tube, enteral and parenteral nutrition, and administration of an enema are discussed in Chapter 16. Be certain to give clear, simple explanations and praise the parents and child after they demonstrate these procedures. Children can easily interpret enemas as punishment because of the extreme intrusiveness. Provide therapeutic play before and after these procedures to reduce children's anxiety.

Anticipate the need for additional support for the family and child with a chronic gastrointestinal disorder. Agencies that might be helpful for referral are:

American Celiac Society
58 Musano Court
West Orange, NJ 07052

Crohn's Disease Foundation of America
3684 Park Avenue South
New York, NY 10015

American Pseudo-Obstruction and Hirschsprung Disease Society
P. O. Box 772
Medford, MA 02155

Outcome Evaluation

Recording children's height and weight is a primary method to evaluate nutritional outcomes. Even if a diet is limited in a special way, if it is adequate, children should gain weight and maintain growth.

Because children will ultimately be responsible for their own diet, evaluation often includes making certain that children gradually learn more about their diet so they can become increasingly responsible for their own intake. Often, only when they are at this stage can their parents feel secure enough to let them stay overnight with a friend, visit a relative in a distant city, go to summer camp—activities that become important to children as they reach school age.

The saying "people are what they eat" has some relevance. Children who are on special diets need to be evaluated for self-esteem at periodic health visits. Does the child think of himself or herself as inferior to or different from others because of food restrictions? What kind of positive experiences can be offered to such a child, or what can parents do to provide the child with experiences that would improve the child's self-esteem?

Some examples of outcome criteria may include:

- Child lists examples of bland foods to select for lunch from school cafeteria menu.
- Parent states steps she will take to seek medical care if child has a second episode of severe diarrhea.
- Family members state they have adjusted to care of a child with celiac disease.

ANATOMY AND PHYSIOLOGY OF THE GASTROINTESTINAL SYSTEM

Embryonic development of the gastrointestinal tract is discussed in Chapter 8. Digestion begins in the mouth, where food is broken down into small particles and mixed with saliva from the sublingual, submandibular, and parotid glands. Both gagging and swallowing reflexes are present even in newborns to prevent aspiration with swallowing.

The esophagus serves as a passageway to the stomach. It pierces the diaphragm to do this (Figure 24-1). Occasionally, an infant is born with a portion of the bowel or stomach protruding through the diaphragm's esophageal opening (hiatal hernia). At the junction of the esophagus and the stomach is the gastroesophageal (cardiac) sphincter. In some newborns, this sphincter is so lax that fluid regurgitates into the esophagus (gastroesophageal reflux [chalasia]). At the distal end of the stomach is the pyloric sphincter. In some infants, this valve is stenosed, preventing food from flowing out of the stomach freely (pyloric stenosis).

The small intestine is divided into three sections: (1) duodenum, (2) jejunum, and (3) ileum. The large intestine is divided into the cecum, ascending colon, transverse colon, descending colon, sigmoid colon, and rectum. The appendix, which frequently becomes diseased in children, is attached to the cecum.

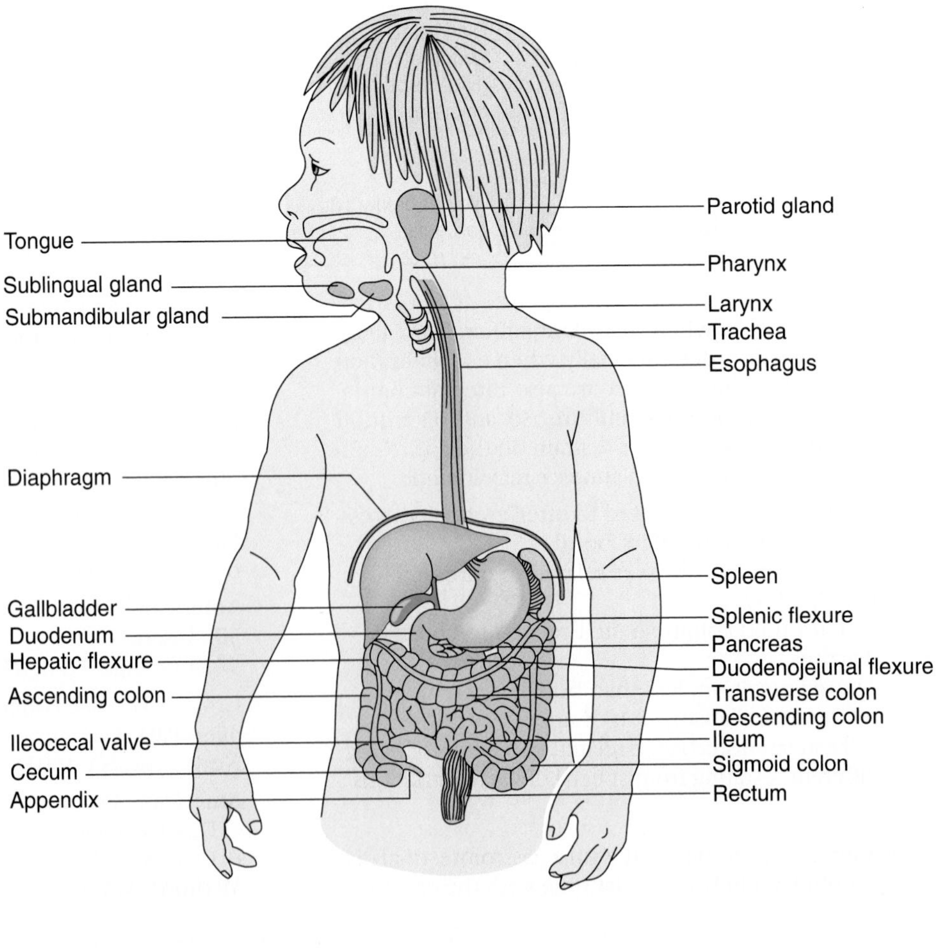

FIGURE 24.1 The gastrointestinal tract.

DIAGNOSTIC AND THERAPEUTIC TECHNIQUES

A number of typical procedures are used in the diagnosis and therapy of gastrointestinal disorders. Common diagnostic procedures used include fiberoptic endoscopy and barium enema. Children need good preparation for these procedures because they are potentially frightening. If children receive conscious sedation for endoscopy, they need preparation for this as well as the actual procedure.

Therapy may include alternative methods of feeding such as enteral(nasogastric or gastrostomy tube feedings), total parenteral nutrition, and intravenous therapy to rest the gastrointestinal tract. A colostomy or ileostomy may be created for the same reason. These tests and procedures, their meaning, impact on children, and nursing responsibilities for them are discussed in Chapter 16.

HEALTH PROMOTION AND RISK MANAGEMENT

Health promotion related to gastrointestinal disorders must cover a wide area because the causes of gastrointestinal disorders cover a wide range and are varied. Some disorders cannot be prevented because they occur for unpredictable causes—such as appendicitis. Some have genetic aspects, such as celiac disease. Some, such as Crohn's disease and ulcerative colitis, have autoimmune focuses. Vomiting and diarrhea, often caused by foods that were refrigerated improperly or spread through contaminated food from improper handwashing, can be prevented. Hepatitis can be prevented through good handwashing (hepatitis A) and routine immunization (hepatitis B). Vitamin and protein deficiency disorders can be prevented by educating parents about the food pyramid and how to select foods that fit each of the sections.

Because an interference in nutrition pervades many aspects of children's lives, families often need help with planning care. Help families plan the necessary adaptations to their lifestyle to prevent the disease from interfering with family functioning (e.g., Will day care center personnel do gastrostomy feedings? Will a nursery school accept a child with a colostomy? Can a child select a gluten-free diet at the school cafeteria?) All families should be encouraged to eat at least one meal together so they can have time to share experiences and "touch base" with each other. For the family with a child who has a special feeding problem such as a gastrostomy feeding or total parenteral nutrition, this can be difficult. Urge such families to bring the child to the table for a social time even if the child cannot eat with the family. If watching family members eat while the child cannot is too difficult, urge the family to provide a "together" time in some other way so they do not miss out on this valuable family activity.

Some gastrointestinal disorders in children such as aganglionic megacolon are diagnosed late because children's parents think the child's refusal to eat is just the sign of being a "picky eater" or a manifestation of 2-year-old autonomy. Educating parents about normal nutrition and how to distinguish such things as vomiting from illness from normal "spitting up" or severe diarrhea from a simple GI upset helps parents bring their children for care at the first possible time. Early intervention prevents the child from becoming dehydrated and seriously ill.

FLUID AND ELECTROLYTE IMBALANCE

Fluid Balance

Fluid is of greater importance in the body chemistry of infants than adults because it constitutes a greater fraction of the infant's total weight. In adults, body water accounts for approximately 60% of total weight. In infants, it accounts for as much as 75% to 80% of total weight; in children, it averages approximately 65% to 70%.

Fluid is distributed in three body compartments: (1) intracellular (within cells), 35% to 40% of body weight; (2) interstitial (surrounding cells and bloodstream), 20% of body weight; and (3) intravascular (blood plasma), 5% of body weight. The interstitial and the intravascular fluid together are often referred to as the extracellular fluid (ECF), totaling 25% of body weight. In infants, the extracellular portion is much greater, totaling up to 45% of total body weight (Figure 24-2). In young children, this is 30%; in adolescents, 25%.

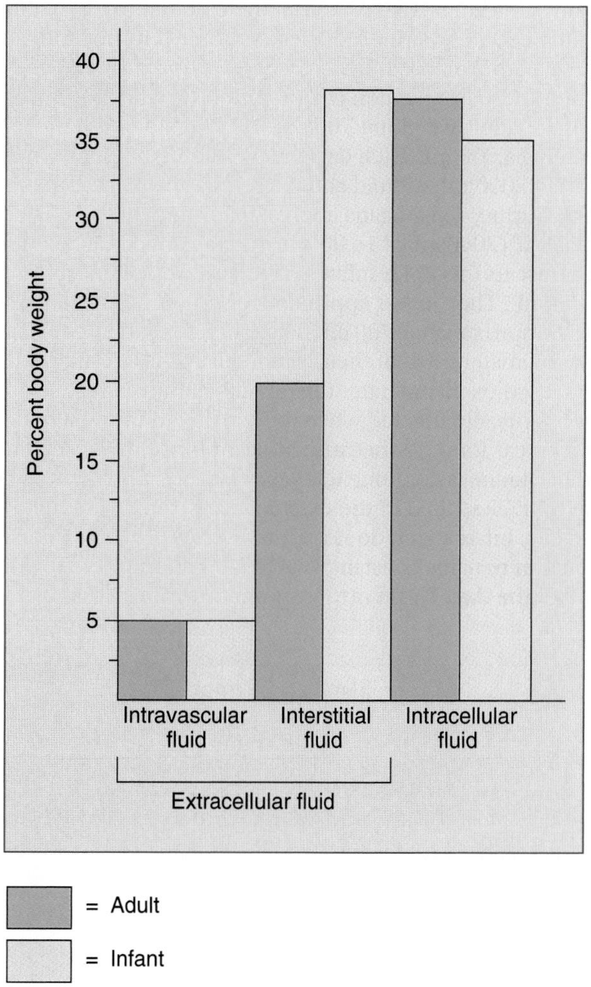

FIGURE 24.2 Distribution of fluid in body compartments.

TABLE 24.1 Maintenance Requirements of Fluid Based on Caloric Expenditure

BODY WT (kg)	CALORIC EXPENDITURE	DAILY FLUID REQUIREMENT
3–10	100 cal/kg/d	100 mL/kg
10–20	1000 cal + 50 cal/kg for each kg of body wt more than 10 kg	1000 mL + 50 mL/kg for each kg of body wt more than 10 kg
More than 20	1500 cal + 20 cal/kg for each kg of body wt more than 20 kg	1500 mL + 20 mL/kg for each kg of body wt more than 20 kg

Behrman, R. E., Kliegman, R. M., & Arvin, A. M. (1996). *Nelson's textbook of pediatrics* (15th ed.). Philadelphia: Saunders.

Fluid is normally taken into the body by oral ingestion of fluid and by the water formed in the metabolic breakdown of food. Primarily, fluid is lost from the body in urine and feces. Minor losses, **insensible losses**, occur from evaporation from skin and lungs and from saliva (of little importance except in children with tracheostomies or those requiring nasopharyngeal suction). Infants do not concentrate urine as well as adults because their kidneys are immature. As a result, they have a proportionally greater loss of water in their urine. In infants, the relatively greater surface area to body mass causes a greater insensible loss as well. Fluid intake is altered when a child is nauseated and unable to ingest fluid or vomiting and losing fluid ingested. When diarrhea occurs, or when a child becomes diaphoretic because of fever, the fluid output can be markedly increased. **Dehydration** occurs when there is an excessive loss of body water.

In an adult weighing 70 kg, the ECF volume is approximately 14,000 mL. Each day, the well adult ingests approximately 2000 mL of fluid and excretes approximately 2000 mL as urine. This means approximately 14% of his or her total ECF (2000 mL of 14,000 mL) is exchanged each day. In contrast to this, 7-kg infants have an ECF volume of only 1750 mL. They ingest approximately 700 mL daily and excrete approximately 700 mL daily. Therefore, they exchange approximately 40% of their volume daily. As a result of this increased exchange rate, the infant's fluid balance may be more critically affected when they are ill. Adults, when they do not eat for a day because of gastrointestinal upset, and whose kidneys continue to excrete at the normal rate, will have 14% less fluid in the extracellular space by the end of the day. Infants who do not eat for a day (providing kidney function remains constant) will be 40% short of ECF by the end of the day. This is obviously a more critical loss of fluid than the same loss would be in an adult; thus, dehydration is always a more serious problem in infants than in older children and adults. Maintenance requirements of fluid for infants and children are shown in Table 24-1.

Under most circumstances, water and salt are lost in proportion to each other (**isotonic dehydration**). Occasionally, water is lost out of proportion to salt (i.e., water depletion or **hypertonic dehydration**). Occasionally, electrolytes are lost out of proportion to water (**hypotonic dehydration**). Each of these abnormal states produces specific symptoms.

Isotonic Dehydration

When the body loses more water than it absorbs (because of diarrhea) or absorbs less fluid than it excretes (as in nausea and vomiting), the first result will be a decrease in the volume of blood plasma. The body compensates for this fairly rapidly by a shift of interstitial fluid into the blood vessels. The composition of fluid in these two spaces is similar, so the replacement by this fluid does not change plasma composition. However, this replacement phenomenon will only proceed until the interstitial fluid reserve is depleted—a danger point for the child because it is difficult for the body to replace interstitial fluid from the intracellular fluid (the fluids in these two compartments have different electrolyte contents). If an infant continues to lose fluid after this point, the volume of the plasma will continue to fall rapidly, resulting in cardiovascular collapse. Typical signs and symptoms are summarized in Table 24-2.

Hypertonic Dehydration

Water is apt to be lost in a greater proportion than electrolytes when there is decreased fluid intake and in-

TABLE 24.2 Signs and Symptoms of Dehydration

	ISOTONIC	HYPOTONIC	HYPERTONIC
Thirst	Mild	Moderate	Extreme
Skin turgor	Poor	Very poor	Moderate
Skin consistency	Dry	Clammy	Moderate
Skin temperature	Cold	Cold	Warm
Urine output	Decreased	Decreased	Decreased
Activity	Irritable	Lethargic	Very lethargic
Serum sodium level	Normal level	Reduced	Increased

creased fluid loss, such as might occur in a child with nausea (preventing fluid intake) and fever (increased fluid loss through perspiration); profuse diarrhea, where there is a greater loss of fluid than salt; or renal disease associated with polyuria (i.e., diabetes insipidus or nephrosis with diuresis).

When there is such an increased loss of fluid, electrolytes concentrate in the blood. Fluid shifts from the interstitial and intracellular spaces to the bloodstream (from areas of less osmotic pressure to areas of greater pressure). Dehydration in the interstitial and intracellular compartments occurs. The red blood cell count and hematocrit will be elevated because the blood is more concentrated than normally. Electrolytes (i.e., sodium, chloride, and bicarbonate) will also likely be increased. Additional signs and symptoms of this are summarized in Table 24-2.

Hypotonic Dehydration

With hypotonic dehydration, there has been a disproportionately high loss of electrolytes relative to fluid lost. The plasma concentration of sodium and chloride will be low. This could result from excessive gastrointestinal loss by vomiting or from low intake of salt associated with extreme losses through therapeutic diuresis. It also occurs when there is extreme loss of electrolytes in diseases such as adrenocortical insufficiency or diabetic acidosis. When low levels of electrolytes occur, the osmotic pressure in extracellular spaces decreases. The kidneys begin to excrete more fluid to decrease ECF volume and bring the proportion of electrolytes and fluid back into line. This may lead to a secondary extracellular dehydration. (See Table 24-2).

Overhydration

Overhydration is as serious as dehydration. It generally occurs in children who are receiving intravenous fluid. The excess fluid in these instances is usually extracellular. The condition is serious because the ECF overload may result in cardiovascular overload and cardiac failure.

When large quantities of salt-poor fluid (hypotonic solutions) such as tap water are ingested or are given by enema, the body transfers water from the extracellular space into the intracellular space to restore the normal osmotic relationships. This transfer results in intracellular edema manifested by headache, nausea, vomiting, dimness and blurring of vision, cramps, muscle twitching, and convulsions. A situation in which intracellular edema may occur is when tap water enemas are given in the presence of aganglionic disease of the intestine.

Acid–Base Balance

When acids, bases, and salts are dissolved in water, they dissociate into **cations**, positively charged particles, and **anions**, negatively charged particles. Because these particles have positive or negative electric charges, they are termed *electrolytes.* The common cations found in blood include sodium (Na^+), potassium (K^+), magnesium (Mg^{++}), and calcium (Ca^{++}). The common anions found in blood include bicarbonate (HCO_3^-), phosphate (PO_4^{---}), sulfate (SO_4^{--}), and chloride (Cl^-).

Most ions have a single positive or negative charge. Others such as calcium (Ca^{++}) and sulfate (SO_4^{--}) have a double charge. In an electrolyte solution, the number of positive charges is matched with the number of negative charges. In a healthy person, the above-mentioned cations and anions of the blood will adjust themselves so that the number of positive charges present equals the number of negative charges present.

Not only is the fluid in the body divided into different compartments, but electrolytes are compartmentalized as well. The major cation of the plasma and interstitial fluid (extracellular fluid) is Na^+; the anions in these compartments are mainly Cl^- and HCO_3^- (bicarbonate). In cell fluid, K^+ is the main cation and PO_4^{---} (phosphate) is the main anion.

pH

The abbreviation "pH" refers to two French words that mean the "power of hydrogen." Water (H_2O) can be dissociated into H^+ and OH^-. A solution is acid (pH below 7.0) if it contains more H^+ ions than OH^- ions. It is alkaline (pH above 7.0) if the number of OH^- ions exceeds that of H^+ ions. The pH of blood normally ranges from 7.35 to 7.45, or slightly alkaline, and OH^- ions and H^+ ions are at a 20:1 proportion. For example, hypothetically, if the number of anions (e.g., Cl^-) should decrease by 10 (as would occur in vomiting, when hydrochloric acid is lost), the number of H^+ ions must be decreased by 10 to keep the number of positive and negative charges in proportion. Because this makes the OH^- concentration in blood proportionately greater than the H^+ concentration, the plasma is more alkaline than normal, the typical picture in vomiting. Conversely, if the number of H^+ ions should increase by 10, the blood will become acidotic because there are then more H^+ ions present proportionately than OH^- ions. Hemoglobin is unable to carry as much oxygen in an acidic state as in a normal pH state. A low pH also leads to vascular constriction, particularly of the pulmonary vessels. The pH levels, then, affect overall circulatory and oxygenation function.

Three buffer systems in the body work to try to keep the number of OH^- and H^+ ions at 20:1 so the pH remains at the usual point of near neutrality. A pH less than 7.0 or more than 7.8 is incompatible with life. These buffer systems involve buffer salts, the respiratory system, and the kidneys.

Buffer Salts

Buffer salts are basic or acidic substances that convert strong acids or bases into weaker ones. After being buffered, an acid that normally would yield many H^+ ions is changed into one that now yields only a few H^+ ions. A strong base is converted to a substance that now yields only a few OH^- ions. By this mechanism, dramatic changes in blood pH are avoided because fewer H^+ ions or OH^- ions are added to the blood at one time.

Respiratory System

The lungs are capable of removing excess H^+ ions from the blood. Hydrogen ions (H^+) combine with bicarbonate ions (HCO_3^-) to form carbonic acid (H_2CO_3). In the lungs, carbonic acid is converted to CO_2 and H_2O. The CO_2 is excreted from the lungs. The H^- ion is tied up in the production of H_2O and no longer affects the acidity of the blood ($H^+ + HCO_3^- = H_2CO_3 = CO_2 + H_2O$). Conversely, with a rising pH level, the lungs will retain CO_2, and the reverse equation results: CO_2 and H_2O combine to form carbonic acid, which then is converted into H^+ and HCO^{3-} ($H_2O + CO_2 = H_2CO_3 = H^+ + HCO_3^-$).

Kidneys

The kidneys regulate bicarbonate to keep it available as a buffer and excrete hydrogen ions. H^+ by itself or as NH_4^+ (ammonia) can be excreted in the urine in exchange for sodium and potassium. Conversely, when the serum HCO_3^- and serum pH rise, H^+ ion secretion stops, and potassium excretion may be excessive.

Serum CO_2 as an Indicator of Blood pH

Disturbances in acid–base balance lead to acidosis or alkalosis (low or high pH, respectively). How much either of these is present is reflected in the measured serum CO_2 level.

The serum CO_2 represents all of the CO_2 present in the plasma. Most of the CO_2 content of plasma is in the form of bicarbonate, with a small amount held at the intermediary stage as carbonic acid, which is actually dissolved CO_2. The CO_2 concentration is expressed as milliequivalents per liter. The normal value is 22 to 28 mEq/L.

Metabolic Acidosis. Sodium is the major electrolyte lost through diarrhea. When excessive Na^+ ion is lost this way, the body conserves H^+ ions to keep the positive and negative charges equal in number. The child begins to become acidotic as the number of H^+ ions in the blood increases over the number of OH^- ions present. To correct the blood pH, the body can excrete H^+ ions by way of the kidney; it does this most rapidly by combining H^+ ions with HCO_3^- ions in the blood to form carbonic acid, which in turn, is broken down into CO_2 and H_2O to be eliminated by the lungs. When this continues for a time, the CO_2 level will fall lower and lower as the body uses up its store of bicarbonate. In **metabolic acidosis**, therefore, the serum CO_2 value is invariably low. The lower the serum CO_2 value, presumably the larger the number of Na^+ ions that have been lost.

The child will develop hyperpnea as the body attempts to "blow off" CO, to prevent it from combining with H_2O and releasing H^+ ions as H^+ and HCO_3^-. There is increased Cl^- (chloride ion) and ammonia formation in the urine as the kidney attempts to remove excess H^+.

Metabolic Alkalosis. With vomiting, a great deal of hydrochloric acid is lost. When Cl^- ions are lost this way with vomiting, the body decreases the number of H^+ ions present so the number of positive and negative charges remains the same. The child is now nearing alkalosis; the number of H^+ ions is smaller than the number of OH^- ions present. To compensate for this, the kidney can conserve H^+ ions; a more immediate solution is for the lungs to conserve CO_2. The child's respirations slow and become shallow (*hypopnea*). The excessive CO_2 accumulated is dissolved in the blood as carbonic acid and then is converted into H^+ and HCO_3^-. The total blood CO_2 content (HCO_3^- and carbonic acid) will rise. In **metabolic alkalosis,** therefore, the serum CO^2 level will invariably be high. The higher the number, presumably the larger the number of Cl^- ions that have been lost.

To increase the number of H^+ ions in the blood, H^+ ions are released from cells in exchange for Na^+ or K^+. The kidneys excrete K^+ into urine to reduce the intracellular load. As a result of this loss of K^+ in urine, low K^+ levels invariably accompany alkalosis.

The child will evidence hypopnea (slowed respirations) as the body attempts to retain CO_2 in the lungs to further increase H^+ ions. The serum CO_2 will be above 40 mEq/L. Tetany may also occur with alkalosis because the increased HCO_3^- may combine with calcium ions (Ca^{++}).

CHECKPOINT QUESTIONS

1. Which body fluid compartment accounts for a greater percentage of body weight in infants than adults?
2. With isotonic dehydration, how does the body compensate initially?
3. What is the major cation of the extracellular fluid?
4. What is the major cation of the intracellular fluid?

COMMON GASTROINTESTINAL SYMPTOMS OF ILLNESS IN CHILDREN

Vomiting and diarrhea in children commonly occur as symptoms of disease of the gastrointestinal tract as well as symptoms of disease in other body systems. Pneumonia or otitis media, for example, may present first with vomiting or diarrhea. The danger is that either can lead to a disturbance in hydration or electrolyte balance. In many infants, these secondary disturbances can be more threatening to the child than the primary disease (Behrman, Kliegman & Arvin, 1996).

Vomiting

Many children with vomiting are suffering from a mild gastroenteritis (infection) caused by a viral or bacterial organism. The adolescent who is pregnant may also experience vomiting. The condition is always potentially serious because a metabolic alkalosis may result.

Assessment

In describing symptoms of vomiting, be certain to differentiate between the various terms that are used (Table 24-3). It is important that vomiting be described correctly this way because different conditions are marked by different forms of vomiting, and a correct description of the child's actions can aid greatly in diagnosis (see Managing and Delegating Unlicensed Assistive Personnel).

TABLE 24.3 Differentiation Between Regurgitation and Vomiting

CHARACTERISTIC	REGURGITATION	VOMITING
Timing	Occurs with feeding	Timing unrelated to feeding
Forcefulness	Runs out of mouth with *little force*	Forceful; often projected 1 ft away from the infant; *projectile vomiting* is projected as much as 4 feet; this is most often related to increased intracranial pressure in newborns; in infants age 4–6 wk, may be caused by pyloric stenosis
Description	Smells barely sour; only slightly curdled	Smells very sour, appears curdled, yellow, green, or clear water, or black; perhaps fresh blood or old blood staining from swallowed maternal blood in newborns
Distress	Nonpainful; child does not appear to be in distress and may even smile as if sensation is enjoyable	Child may cry just before vomiting as if abdominal pain is present, and after vomiting as if the force of action is frightening
Duration	Occurs once per feeding	Continues until stomach is empty and then dry retching occurs
Amount	1–2 tsp	Full stomach contents

Therapeutic Management

The treatment for vomiting is to withhold food from the stomach for a time. If there is nothing in the stomach, vomiting cannot occur. Most parents treat vomiting in the opposite way. Every time the child vomits, they attempt to feed the child again. The child vomits again and they feed again, and so on. This prolongs the vomiting and intensifies the potential for electrolyte imbalance.

NURSING DIAGNOSES AND RELATED INTERVENTIONS

Nursing Diagnosis: Risk for fluid volume deficit, related to vomiting

Outcome Identification: Child will maintain an adequate fluid volume until vomiting ceases.

Outcome Evaluation: Skin turgor is good; specific gravity of urine is 1.003 to 1.030; urine output is more than 1 mL/kg/h; episodes of vomiting decrease in frequency and amount.

To decrease vomiting, withhold food and fluid for a time (nothing by mouth [NPO]), depending on the age of the child. On the average, 3 to 6 hours are usually sufficient. In the older child, after this period of fasting, offer a few ice chips, then water in small amounts—approximately 1 tbs every 15 minutes, four times; then 2 tbs every ½ hour, four times. Popsicles can be substituted for water. If retained, children can be given small sips of clear liquids, such as tea, ginger ale, or Gatorade. Children may become hungry and want whole glasses, but keeping the quantity to small sips prevents vomiting. If the child retains sips of clear liquids, they can be offered portions of broth, clear soup, and skimmed milk in addition to clear liquids. Dry crackers or toast will help hunger. By the second day, children can take a soft diet; by the third day, they should be back to their regular diet.

For the infant, introduce fluid after a fasting period of approximately 3 hours in the same slow manner: 1 tbs every 15 minutes for 2 hours, then 1 oz every 2 hours for the next 12 to 18 hours. Glucose water or a commercial electrolyte solution such as Pedialyte may be given as fluid during this time to help the infant maintain electrolyte balance (see Focus on Nursing Research). Infants progress, as do older children, gradually to clear liquids or breast milk, then a soft diet, then a regular diet. If vomiting is prolonged, infants need intravenous therapy to restore hydration.

Teach parents the importance of following these routines of gradually increasing fluid at intervals. Assure them that if children receive a small amount of fluid and do not vomit it they will ultimately receive more fluid than if they take a large amount but, because of a gastroenteritis, vomit that amount. Parents are capable of understanding that stomach secretions are lost along with vomitus each time, and the preservation of these stomach secretions is important to keep their child well. Antiemetics are rarely necessary for children (see Focus on Cultural Competence). Parents should not give over-the-counter preparations for vomiting to children. Instead, they should control vomiting by dietary management. Prochlorperazine (Compazine), used with adults to control vomiting, may result in bizarre behavior symptoms (toxicity) in children. Thus, it is rarely prescribed for children who have not reached adolescence.

MANAGING AND DELEGATING UNLICENSED ASSISTIVE PERSONNEL

Unlicensed assistive personnel are often asked to feed infants in hospital settings. They often change infants' diapers. Teach them to differentiate between simple "spitting up," which is normal in infants, and vomiting so they do not miss this important symptom of disease. Likewise, be certain they can distinguish between normally loose infant bowel movements and a diarrheal stool. Be certain when they are talking with parents that they do not dismiss the importance of seeking help for either vomiting or diarrhea. Teach them as well as parents that there is no such thing as "simple" diarrhea in infants.

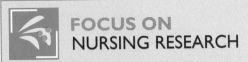

FOCUS ON NURSING RESEARCH

Can Parents Add Flavoring to Oral Rehydration Solutions to Make Them Taste Better?

It is important that parents do not change the osmolality of oral rehydration solutions or they will lose their effectiveness. To determine the effect of parents adding sweeteners to these solutions so their children will drink them more readily, the concentration of sodium, potassium, glucose, and osmolality of solutions were analyzed after they were flavored with varying amounts of unsweetened Kool-Aid powder, Jell-O powder, apple juice, or orange juice. The results of the study showed that the addition of these flavorings did not alter the electrolyte content or osmolality of solutions. The researchers conclude that small amounts of flavorings can be safely added to oral rehydration solutions without significantly altering electrolyte or osmolality.

This is an important study for nurses because nurses are often the health care providers who give instructions to parents about oral rehydration solutions. Alerting them that they can add small amounts of flavoring to these solutions can help them make them more tolerable for children.

Nijssen-Jordan, C. (1997). Can oral rehydration solutions be safely flavored at home? *Pediatric Emergency Care, 13*(6), 374.

Diarrhea

Diarrhea is the major cause of infant mortality in developing countries. Although diarrhea in infants may result from other causes, its primary cause is viral or bacterial invasion of the gastrointestinal tract. The most common viral pathogens are rotaviruses and adenoviruses. The most common bacterial pathogens are *Campylobacter jejuni, Salmonella, Giardia lamblia, and Clostridium difficile.* Diarrhea in infants is always serious because infants have such a small ECF reserve that sudden losses of water exhaust the supply quickly. The loss of extracellular sodium leads to a decrease in plasma volume (additional water is excreted) and possible circulatory collapse. Renal failure results, with irreversible acidosis and death. Breastfeeding may actively prevent diarrhea, especially that caused by *Campylobacter,* and it should be advocated. Diarrhea that is acute is usually associated with infection; that which is chronic is more likely related to a malabsorption or inflammatory cause.

FOCUS ON CULTURAL COMPETENCE

Gastrointestinal illnesses do not occur at the same incidence in all communities. Vomiting and diarrhea, for example, tend to occur in communities where refrigeration is less than optimal. Celiac disease occurs most frequently in children with north European ancestry. Because vomiting and diarrhea are so common, there are home remedies for these in every culture. To be certain that a child seen in a health care facility does not receive two forms of the same drug (one prescribed and one given in an herb form by a parent), always ask what home remedies have been given and document these on the child's nursing plan.

Assessment of Mild Diarrhea

Normal and diarrheal stool characteristics are compared in Table 24-4. In mild diarrhea, fever of 101°F to 102°F (38.4°C to 39.0°C) may be present. Children usually are anorectic, irritable, and appear unwell. The episodes of diarrhea consist of 2 to 10 loose, watery bowel movements per day.

The mucous membrane of the infant's mouth with mild diarrhea will be dry. Pulse will be rapid and out of proportion to the low-grade fever. Skin feels warm. Skin turgor is not yet decreased. Urine output is usually normal.

Therapeutic Management of Mild Diarrhea

At this stage, diarrhea is not yet serious, and children can be cared for at home (AAP, 1996). As with vomiting, treatment for diarrhea must involve resting the gastrointestinal tract, but this is only necessary for a short time. At the end of approximately 1 hour, parents can begin to offer water or an oral rehydration solution such as Pedialyte in small amounts on a regimen similar to that for vomiting. If infants are breastfed, breastfeeding should continue. Again, it may be difficult for parents to restrict fluid for a short time if they think they should overfeed children to make up for the fluid loss. Children also need measures taken to reduce the elevated temperature. Caution parents not to use over-the-counter drugs such as loperamide (Imodium) or kaolin and pectin (Kaopectate) to halt diarrhea. As a rule, these are too strong for young children. Caution them also to wash their hands after changing diapers to prevent the spread of possible infection.

Infants may develop a lactase deficiency after diarrhea. This leads to lactose intolerance. With lactose intoler-

TABLE 24.4 Differentiating Normal Infant and Diarrheal Stool

CHARACTERISTIC	NORMAL INFANT STOOL	DIARRHEAL STOOL
Frequency	1–3 daily	Unlimited number
Color	Yellow	Green
Effort of expulsion	Some pushing effort	Effortless; may be explosive
*p*H	More than 7.0 (alkaline)	Less than 7.0 (acidic)
Odor	Odorless	Sweet or foul-smelling
Occult blood	Negative	Positive, blood may be overt
Reducing substances	Negative	Positive

ance, the child is unable to take formula or breast milk or new diarrhea will begin. Such an infant will need to be introduced to a lactose-free formula initially before being returned to the usual formula or to breast milk.

Assessment of Severe Diarrhea

Severe diarrhea may result from progressive mild diarrhea, or it may begin in a severe form. Infants with severe diarrhea are obviously ill. Rectal temperature is often as high as 103°F to 104°F (39.5°C to 40.0°C). Both pulse and respirations are weak and rapid. The skin is pale and cool. Infants may appear apprehensive, listless, and lethargic. They have obvious signs of dehydration such as a depressed fontanelle, sunken eyes, and poor skin turgor. The episodes of diarrhea usually consist of a bowel movement every few minutes. The stool is liquid green, perhaps mixed with mucus and blood, and it may be passed with explosive force. Urine output will be scanty and concentrated. Laboratory findings will show an elevated hematocrit, hemoglobin, and serum protein levels due to the dehydration. Electrolyte determinations will indicate a metabolic acidosis.

It is difficult to measure the amount of fluid the child has lost, but an estimation can be derived from the loss in body weight if known. For example, if a child weighed 10.4 kg yesterday at a health maintenance visit and today weighs 8.9 kg, he or she has lost more than 10% of body weight. Mild dehydration occurs with a loss of 2.5% to 5% of body weight. In contrast, severe diarrhea quickly causes a 5% to 15% loss. Any infant who has lost 10% or more of body weight requires immediate treatment.

Therapeutic Management of Severe Diarrhea

Treatment focuses on regulating electrolyte and fluid balance, initiating rest for the gastrointestinal tract, and discovering the organism responsible for the diarrhea.

All children with diarrhea should have a stool culture taken so that definite antibiotic therapy can be prescribed. Stool cultures may be taken from the rectum or from stool in the diaper or a bedpan. Blood specimens need to be drawn for a hemoglobin level (an estimation of hydration as well as anemia); white blood cell and differential counts (to attempt to establish whether infection is present); and determinations of CO_2, Cl^-, Na^+, K^+, and pH (to establish electrolyte needs). Before these results are obtained, an intravenous solution such as normal saline or 5% glucose in normal saline is started (Figure 24-3). The solution will provide replacement of fluid, sodium, and calories. Although infants usually have a potassium depletion, potassium cannot be given until it is established that they are not in renal failure. Giving potassium intravenously when the body has no outlet for excessive potassium can lead to excessively high potassium levels and heart block. *Before this initial fluid is changed to a potassium solution, therefore, be certain that the infant or child has voided—proof that the kidneys are functioning.*

Fluid must be given to replace the deficit that has occurred, for maintenance therapy, and to replace the continuing loss until the diarrhea improves. If infants have lost less than 5% of total body weight, their fluid deficit is approximately 50 mL/kg of body weight. If infants have lost 10% of body weight, they need approximately 100 mL/kg of body weight to replace their fluid deficit. If the weight loss suggests a 12% to 15% loss of body fluid, they require 125 mL/kg of body weight to replace the fluid lost. This fluid will be given rapidly in the first 3 to 6 hours, then it will be slowed to a maintenance rate. Once infants void, a sodium lactate solution or a potassium additive may be started to replace potassium.

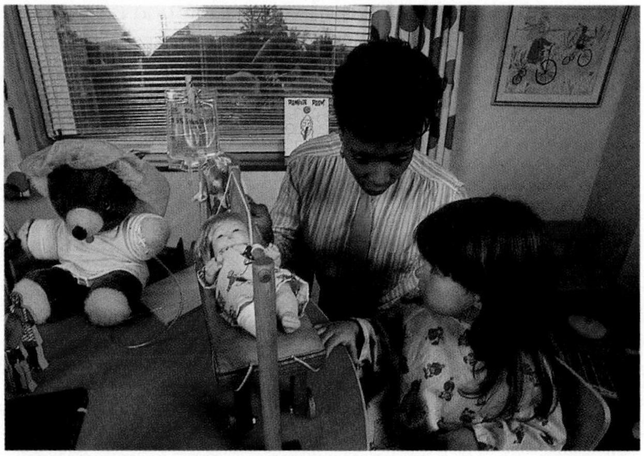

FIGURE 24.3 Play therapy is commonly used to help prepare the child for intravenous catheter insertion and fluid administration. Here a doll and bear are receiving intravenous therapy.

NURSING DIAGNOSES AND RELATED INTERVENTIONS

Nursing Diagnosis: Fluid volume deficit, related to loss of fluid through diarrhea

Outcome Identification: Child will maintain an adequate fluid balance until normal elimination pattern is restored.

Outcome Evaluation: Skin turgor is good; specific gravity of urine is 1.003 to 1.030; urine output is more than 1 mL/kg/h, bowel movements are formed and fewer than four per day. Stool tests negative for reducing substances and blood. pH = more than 7.

Promote Hydration and Comfort. For a short time, infants are NPO because vomiting at this point would compound the problem by adding to the dehydration. Wet infants' lips with a moisturizing jelly (Vaseline) if they appear to be dry. Give them a pacifier to suck if this seems to comfort them. (They want to suck because they are very thirsty, and if they have intestinal cramping with the diarrhea, they interpret this as hunger.)

After a short time, infants may be allowed small sips of clear fluid, an oral rehydration solution, or breast milk. Gradually, the infant's oral intake is increased, changing to a soft diet (sometimes called a BRAT diet because it comprises bananas, rice cereal, applesauce, and toast). If the child with severe diarrhea also has a fever, measures to reduce the fever will be necessary (see Chapter 16). Do not obtain rectal temperatures to assess fever, because stimulating the anal sphincter could initiate more diarrhea. Assess perianal skin for irritation from liquid stools and keep the skin clean and dry.

Record Fluid Intake and Output. Much of the nursing care of children with diarrhea focuses on careful recording of fluid intake and output. Because children have dehydration when first seen, their intravenous therapy tubing serves as their lifeline. Be sure to maintain proper functioning of the infusion and site. An arm board may be necessary to prevent catheter dislodgement or interference with the infusion. Instruct the child and parents about the need to refrain from touching or playing with any part of the IV setup. If the child is too young to understand, soft restraints applied to the affected and unaffected extremities may be necessary to prevent pulling, playing with, or poking at the tubing or site. If soft restraints are used, be sure to release them every hour and passively exercise the child's extremities. Give parents an explanation of why the intravenous infusion is important so that they will understand the necessity of the soft restraints.

In children who are not toilet trained, apply a disposable urine collection bag to help separate urine from feces. This makes it obvious that the child is voiding, confirming adequate kidney function. Confirmation of adequate kidney function is necessary for intravenous (IV) $K+$ replacement therapy, if ordered.

Separating urine from stools also helps to judge the appearance of stools or their water content better. For each stool passed, record its color, consistency, odor, size, and the presence of any blood or mucus. Weigh soiled diapers to reveal the number of grams of stool in the diaper (1 g = 1 mL fluid). Testing the stool for acidity and for reducing substances (sugars) indicates how quickly the stool is passing through the irritated tract. A stool positive for sugar indicates that little absorption has occurred because sugar is absorbed rapidly from ingested food. Acid stool (pH less than 7.0) shows the presence of unabsorbed sugar also (a process occurs similar to the process that causes acid to invade tooth enamel in the presence of glucose on teeth). Diarrheal stools are green from lack of time for bile to be modified in the intestine. As diarrhea improves and stool remains in the intestine for a longer period, the stool deepens in color, and the acid and sugar content fade. Testing stools for occult blood shows the extent of bowel irritation that is occurring from the acid stool. As the diarrhea improves and the irritation to the bowel lessens, occult blood disappears.

Nursing Diagnosis: Risk for altered skin integrity related to presence of diarrheal stool on skin

Outcome Identification: Child's skin will remain intact during period of diarrhea.

Outcome Evaluation: Skin in diaper area is not erythematous or with ulcerations.

Because diarrheal stool is extremely irritating to the skin, change diapers immediately after infants stool (caution older children to wipe away stool thoroughly). Wash the skin of the diaper area well after each stool and cover it with an ointment such as Vaseline or A and D to protect it from further irritation.

If infants already have skin excoriation from the number of stools they have had at home, an ointment such as Desitin or Balmex may be helpful in soothing the irritated skin. Placing infants on their abdomen and exposing their buttocks to air is generally helpful in healing irritation.

Nursing Diagnosis: Anxiety related to traumatic experience

Outcome Identification: Child will not suffer long-term effects of experience.

Outcome Evaluation: Child interacts with parents in age-appropriate way; is able to be comforted after painful procedures.

All children with diarrhea are assumed to have an infectious form of gastroenteritis and, therefore, need infection control and standard precautions. If the child is diapered, also follow contact precautions. Children usually are uncomfortable from the diarrhea, exhausted, and confused with these new body sensations. They need the security of someone to stay with them. When a child with severe diarrhea is admitted to the hospital, many emergency procedures must be performed, such as establishing the intravenous route, collecting specimens, and reducing temperature. During all of these procedures, try to remember how all of this must seem to the child in the bed. Be sure to take time during initial procedures to touch and soothe children and talk to them; once the initial admission procedures are done, sit by the bed and hold the child or gently stroke the child's head. Teach parents how to adhere to standard precautions and follow contact precautions if necessary. Encourage them to give any care possible. Children need this support to counteract the strange world into which they have suddenly been plunged.

Bacterial Infectious Diseases That Cause Diarrhea and Vomiting

Salmonella

- Causative agent: One of the *Salmonella* bacteria
- Incubation period: 6 to 72 hours for intraluminal type; 7 to 14 days for extraluminal type
- Period of communicability: As long as organisms are being excreted (may be as long as 3 months)
- Mode of transmission: Ingestion of contaminated food

Salmonella is the most common type of food poisoning in the United States and a major cause of diarrhea in children. The diagnosis of the infection can be made from stool culture. Children with a *Salmonella* infection have symptoms of diarrhea, abdominal pain, vomiting, high temperature, and headache. They are listless and drowsy. The diarrhea is severe and may contain blood and mucus. *Salmonella* infection may remain in the bowel as an intraluminal disease. When it does, it is treated, like severe diarrhea, with fluid and electrolyte replacement. It also may become systemic (extraluminal disease) and, in that instance, it is treated with an antibiotic such as amoxicillin.

Complications such as meningitis, bronchitis, and osteomyelitis may occur. Although the source of *Salmonella* generally is infected food (contaminated chicken and eggs are common sources), it may be transmitted to children by infected turtles (see Empowering the Family).

Shigellosis (Dysentery)

- Causative agent: Organisms of the genus *Shigella*
- Incubation period: 1 to 7 days

EMPOWERING THE FAMILY: Preventing Salmonella-Caused Gastroenteritis

Methods to prevent the spread include the following:

- Wash your hands well before preparing any foods, but especially chicken and eggs.
- Remember that chicken may become contaminated with salmonella at the factory where it was prepared. Wash your hands well after handling raw chicken to prevent the spread of infection to other foods being prepared.
- Clean cutting boards or food preparation surfaces with hot soapy water and dry thoroughly after use to prevent them from becoming reservoirs of infection.
- Make a habit of preparing chicken last, after other foods are prepared.
- Cook eggs well (do not use raw eggs in milkshakes; cook soft-boiled or poached eggs at least 3 minutes).
- Refrigerate chicken and eggs after preparation.
- Wash hands well after playing with, feeding a pet turtle or changing the turtle's water.

- Period of communicability: Approximately 1 to 4 weeks
- Mode of transmission: Contaminated food or milk products

Shigella organisms, like the *Salmonella* group, cause extremely severe diarrhea that contains blood and mucus. Ampicillin or trimethoprim sulfamethoxazole are typical drugs for therapy. The child needs intense fluid and electrolyte replacement. Shigella infection can be prevented by safe food handling.

Staphylococcal Food Poisoning

- Causative agent: Staphylococcal enterotoxin produced by some strains of *Staphylococcus aureus*
- Incubation period: 1 to 7 hours
- Period of communicability: Carriers may contaminate food as long as they harbor the organism
- Mode of transmission: Ingestion of contaminated food

With staphylococcal food poisoning, the child has severe vomiting and diarrhea, abdominal cramping, excessive salivation, and nausea. Organisms are most often spread through creamed foods. It is often difficult to culture the causative organism from the contaminated food because, although the staphylococci may have been destroyed by inadequate cooking, the enterotoxin that actually causes the disorder will not have been destroyed. The child needs intensive supportive therapy with fluid and electrolyte replacement. Food poisoning from this source is prevented by proper food refrigeration.

CHECKPOINT QUESTIONS

5. For approximately how long should a child be NPO if he is experiencing vomiting?
6. What are the two primary causes of diarrhea in a child?
7. What acid–base imbalance is typical with severe diarrhea?
8. What causative organism would you suspect if a child develops diarrhea from eating *raw* eggs?

DISORDERS OF THE STOMACH AND DUODENUM

Gastroesophageal Reflux (Chalasia)

Gastroesophageal reflux (GER [chalasia]) is a neuromuscular disturbance in which the gastroesophageal (cardiac) sphincter and the lower portion of the esophagus are lax and, therefore, allow easy regurgitation of gastric contents into the esophagus. It usually starts within 1 week after birth and may be associated with a hiatal hernia. The regurgitation occurs almost immediately after feeding or when the infant is laid down after a feeding. Children with cerebral palsy or other neurological involvement are at particular risk. Aspiration pneumonia or esophageal stricture from the constant reflux of hydrochloric acid into the esophagus may occur. If the reflux is large, the infant does not retain sufficient calories and will fail to thrive.

Assessment

The diagnosis is suggested by the history. Vomiting is effortless and nonprojectile, beginning much earlier than vomiting associated with pyloric stenosis. The child may be irritable and experience periods of apnea. Inserting a probe or catheter into the esophagus through the nose to the distal esophagus, and determining the pH from secretions can show whether gastric secretions are entering the esophagus (if pH is less than 7.0, then acid is present). Fiber-optic endoscopy or an esophagography (barium swallow) will show the lax sphincter and the reflux of stomach contents into the esophagus, especially if the infant's head is tilted down (Belknap & McEvoy, 1997).

Therapeutic Management

The traditional treatment of gastrointestinal reflux is to feed infants a formula thickened with rice cereal (1 tbs cereal per 1 oz of formula) while holding them in an upright position and to keep them in an elevated prone position for 1 hour after feeding so gravity helps prevent reflux. In light of the caution not to lie infants on their abdomen, however, infants may be placed on their left side (Tobin et al, 1997). An antacid or histamine 2 receptor antagonist such

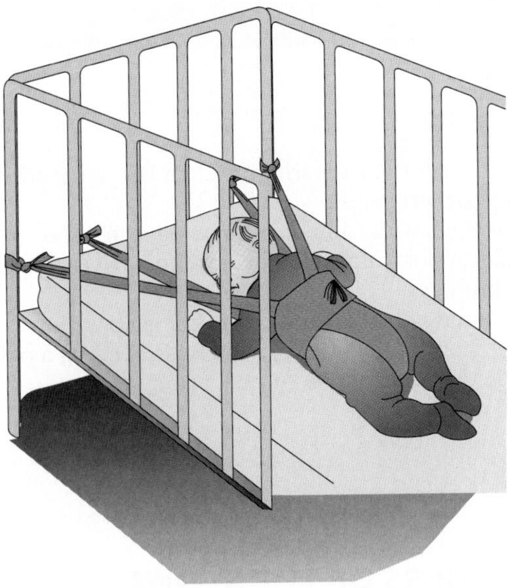

FIGURE 24.4 Positional treatment for gastroesophageal reflux.

as cimetidine may be prescribed three or four times daily to reduce the possibility of the stomach acid contents irritating the esophagus. Bethanechol or cisapride (propulsid) may be prescribed to hurry gastric emptying.

Gastroesophageal reflux is usually a self-limiting condition. As the esophageal sphincter matures and the child begins to eat solid food and is maintained in a more upright position, the problem disappears. However, it is a problem that needs treatment. Otherwise, serious consequences can result from dehydration, alkalosis, or damage to the esophagus. If medical therapy is ineffective, a surgical procedure (a Nissen fundoplication) may be scheduled to repair the sphincter. After this, the child will return from surgery with a nasogastric tube inserted and attached to low suction. It is usually irrigated with normal saline every 2 hours to ensure its patency. Assess nasogastric tube drainage for coffee-colored drainage (although this is normal for the first 24 hours) that would indicate bleeding from the incision. After surgery, infants may display symptoms of abdominal discomfort and stomach distention because food can no longer enter the esophagus. As their stomach adjusts to this, symptoms fade. Before this happens, however, the distention may be so extreme that it leads to bradycardia and dyspnea.

NURSING DIAGNOSES AND RELATED INTERVENTIONS

Nursing Diagnosis: Risk for altered nutrition, less than body requirements related to regurgitation of food with esophageal reflux

Outcome Identification: Infant will receive adequate nutrition during course of therapy.

Outcome Evaluation: Skin turgor is good; specific gravity of urine is 1.003 to 1.030; intake is 50 cal/lb/24h.

Monitor intake, output (urination), and weight. After a feeding, the infant should lie on the side or prone on a slanted surface (Figure 24-4). Use a sheepskin-like covering to prevent knee and face irritation. Be certain parents understand how much cereal to mix with formula. Mothers who are breastfeeding may manually express breast milk and mix it with rice cereal for feedings.

Help parents to understand that this feeding difficulty was in no way their fault (they are not poor nurturers; the infant had an internal problem). Encourage them to feed the infant in the hospital after surgery and give care to regain confidence in themselves as parents.

WHAT IF? What if a mother tells you she thinks its important to keep infants on their back to prevent sudden infant death syndrome? How would you explain the importance of keeping her infant with gastrointestinal reflux on his abdomen or side?

Pyloric Stenosis

The pyloric sphincter is the opening between the lower portion of the stomach and the beginning portion of the intestine, the duodenum. If hypertrophy or hyperplasia of the muscle surrounding the sphincter occurs, it is difficult for the stomach to empty, a condition called **pyloric stenosis** (Figure 24-5). With this condition, at 4 to 6 weeks of age, children begin to vomit almost immediately after each feeding. The vomiting grows increasingly forceful until it is projectile, possibly projecting as much as 3 to 4 feet. Pyloric stenosis tends to occur most frequently in first-born white male infants. The incidence is high, approxi-

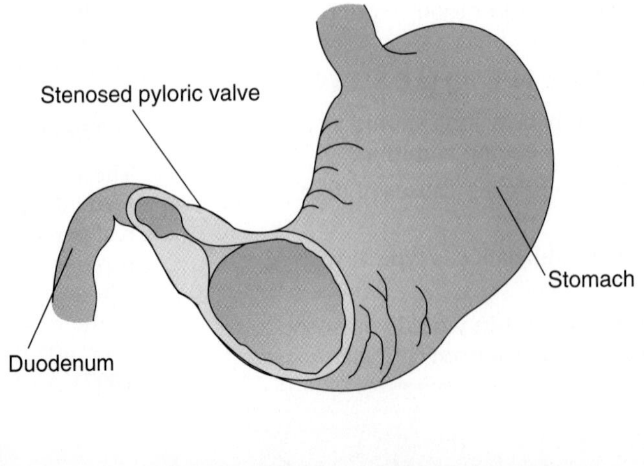

FIGURE 24.5 Pyloric stenosis. Fluid is unable to pass easily through the stenosed and hypertrophied pyloric valve.

mately 1:150 in males, 1:750 in females. The exact cause is unknown, but multifactorial inheritance is the likely cause. It occurs less frequently in breastfed infants than in formula-fed infants. Infants fed on formula who will develop the condition typically begin having symptoms at approximately 4 weeks of age. Breastfed infants begin developing symptoms at approximately 6 weeks because the curd of breast milk is smaller than that of cow's milk, and it passes through a hypertrophied muscle more easily.

Vomitus usually smells sour because it has reached the stomach and has been in contact with stomach enzymes. There is never bile in the vomiting of pyloric stenosis because the feeding does not reach the duodenum to become mixed with bile. The infant is usually hungry immediately after vomiting because he or she is not nauseated. It is difficult to assess whether nausea is present in infants, but some of its symptoms may be a disinterest in eating, excessive drooling, or chewing on the tongue.

Assessment

The diagnosis of pyloric stenosis is made primarily from the history. Whenever parents say that their baby is vomiting or spitting up, be certain to get a full description.

- What is the duration?
- What is the intensity?
- What is the frequency?
- What is the description of the vomitus?
- Is the infant ill in any other way?

Many infants have signs of dehydration from the vomiting at the time they are first seen. Lack of tears (many infants younger than age 6 weeks do not tear); dry mucous membrane of the mouth; sunken fontanelles; fever; decreased urine output; poor skin turgor; and loss of weight are common signs of dehydration seen. Alkalosis also may be present because of the excessive loss of Cl^- ions from stomach fluid along with accompanying hypochloremia, hypokalemia, and starvation. Hypopnea (slowed respirations) occurs as the body attempts to compensate for the alkalosis. This will cause the CO_2 content of plasma generally to be above 30 mEq/L (normal is 22 mEq/L to 28 mEq/L). Tetany may occur with alkalosis because the increased HCO_3^- ions may combine with Ca^{++} ions, trying to effect homeostasis and thereby lowering the level of ionized calcium. Low serum calcium leads to tetany.

A definitive diagnosis is made by watching the infant drink. Before the child drinks, attempt to palpate the right upper quadrant of the abdomen for a possible pyloric mass. If one is present, it feels round and firm, approximately the size of an olive. As the infant drinks, observe for gastric peristaltic waves passing from left to right across the abdomen. The olive-size lump becomes more prominent. The infant vomits with projectile emesis. If the diagnosis is still in doubt, the child may have an ultrasound, which will show the hypertrophied sphincter (Yamamoto et al, 1998). Endoscopy also may be used for diagnosis by directly visualizing the hypertrophied sphincter.

Therapeutic Management

Treatment is surgical correction before electrolyte imbalance from the vomiting or hypoglycemia from the lack of food intake occurs. Before surgery, the electrolyte imbalance, dehydration, and starvation must be corrected by administration of intravenous fluid, usually isotonic saline or 5% glucose in saline because this contains an excess of Cl^- ions. Oral feedings are withheld to prevent further electrolyte depletion. An infant who is receiving only intravenous fluid generally needs a pacifier to meet nonnutritive sucking needs and be comfortable. If tetany is present, intravenous calcium also must be administered. The infant usually needs additional potassium, but, as a rule, this must not be administered until it is ascertained that the child's kidneys are functioning (i.e., the child is voiding). Otherwise, the potassium buildup could cause cardiac arrhythmias.

The surgical procedure for pyloric stenosis is a pyloromyotomy (a *Fredet-Ramstedt operation*). This may be done by laparoscopy. The muscle of the pylorus is split, allowing for a larger lumen. Although the procedure sounds simple, it is technically difficult to perform, and there is high risk for infection afterward because the incision is near the diaper area. Laparoscopy is a safe and successful procedure that markedly reduces time in surgery and postoperative recovery.

The prognosis for infants with pyloric stenosis is excellent if the condition was discovered before the electrolyte imbalance occurred.

NURSING DIAGNOSES AND RELATED INTERVENTIONS

Nursing Diagnosis: Risk for fluid volume deficit related to inability to retain food

Outcome Identification: Infant will remain well hydrated until condition is corrected.

Outcome Evaluation: Skin turgor is good; specific gravity of urine is 1.003 to 1.030; vomiting episodes have ceased; weight within acceptable age-appropriate parameters.

Preoperative Care. A baseline weight is essential for establishing the extent of dehydration. Note carefully the frequency of urination, the specific gravity of the urine, and the number of stools passed to help assess dehydration and starvation. Parents may be impatient with preoperative management. They need an explanation that infants cannot go to surgery with an electrolyte imbalance; these hours before surgery are as important to the welfare of their child as the operation itself.

Postoperative Care. Infants may return from surgery or laparoscopy with an intravenous line in place. The feeding regimen postoperatively differs from one surgeon to another, but usually is based on a regimen requiring frequent feedings of small amounts of fluid, referred to as *Down's regimen.* Approximately 4 to 6 hours after surgery, children are given approximately 1 tsp of 5% glucose in saline hourly by bottle for four feedings; if no vomiting occurs, the amount is increased to 2 tsp hourly for four more feedings. Next, half-strength formula is begun every 4 hours. Finally, by 24 hours to 48 hours, infants are taking their full formula diet or being breastfed. They are usually discharged at the end of 48 hours.

It is important that infants be given no more than the amount of fluid ordered at a time so the surgical repair site is not overwhelmed. It is important that infants take these small amounts because a small quantity of fluid passing through the sphincter in the immediate postoperative days helps to keep adhesions of the incision from forming. As the amount taken orally increases, the intravenous fluid will be decreased and then discontinued. Infants should be bubbled well after a feeding so there is no pressure from air in the stomach. Lay them on their side after feeding so if vomiting does occur, there is little chance of aspiration. Laying them on their right side possibly aids the flow of fluid through the pyloric valve by gravity. Continue to monitor daily weights to confirm that children are receiving adequate intake. Usually no vomiting occurs postoperatively. However, if it does occur, report it immediately. The feeding regimen may need to be adjusted accordingly, and the infant may be kept in the hospital longer. Some infants have a short-term diarrhea after surgery because of rapid functioning of the pyloric sphincter. A number of them may be colicky and fretful.

Nursing Diagnosis: Risk for infection at site of surgical incision related to proximity of incision to diaper area

Outcome Identification: Infant's surgical incision will exhibit signs and symptoms of healing without infection.

Outcome Evaluation: Infant's temperature is below 37.0°C axillary; incision clean, dry, and intact without erythema or drainage.

The surgical incision for pyloric stenosis may be covered with collodion, a solution similar to clear nail polish, to help keep urine and feces from touching it. Keep diapers folded low to prevent the incision from being contaminated, and change diapers frequently. If the incision should be exposed to feces, wash the collodion well with soap and water.

Nursing Diagnosis: Risk for altered parenting related to infant's feeding difficulty and illness

Outcome Identification: Parents will demonstrate positive bonding behaviors with the infant both preoperatively and postoperatively.

Outcome Evaluation: Parents hold and feed infant; express positive characteristics about infant.

Encourage the parents of a baby this young who may remain overnight in the hospital to room in so that they can grow comfortable and confident in caring for their child again. When the child first began vomiting so forcefully, parents may have felt they were doing something wrong, possibly losing confidence in themselves as parents. Explain to them that the vomiting was caused by a physical problem and not by anything they did.

Hospitalization often occurs near the infant's second month, when the child would normally receive diphtheria-tetanus-pertussis, oral poliomyelitis, and *Haemophilus influenzae* immunization. Ask if this could be administered before discharge so the child's immunization status remains current. This also might serve to remind parents that getting back to normal means regular health care visits for vaccines and checkups.

CHECKPOINT QUESTIONS

9. What is the best position after feeding for a child with gastrointestinal reflux?
10. What type of vomiting is associated with pyloric stenosis?

Peptic Ulcer Disease

A **peptic ulcer** is a shallow excavation formed in the mucosal wall of the stomach, the pylorus, or the duodenum. In infants, ulcers tend to be gastric; in adolescents, usually duodenal. Such ulcers occur in a primary form caused by infection of the *H. pylori* bacteria and a secondary form that follows severe stress such as burns or chronic ingestion of medications such as acetosalicylic acid or prednisone. A small ulceration of the gastric or duodenal lining will lead to symptoms of pain, blood in the stools, and vomiting (with blood). If left uncorrected, peptic ulcer disease can lead to bowel or stomach perforation with acute hemorrhage or pyloric obstruction. A chronic ulcer condition may lead to anemia from the constant slight blood loss.

Peptic ulcer disease occurs in only 1% to 2% of children. It occurs more frequently in males than in females. In addition to infection from *H. pylori,* other associated factors may include genetic tendency and use of alcohol, caffeine, and cigarettes.

Assessment

An ulcer occurring in a neonate usually presents with hematemesis (blood in vomitus) or melena (blood in the stool). Such ulcers are usually superficial and heal rapidly, although they can lead to rupture, with symptoms of respiratory distress, abdominal distention, vomiting, and, if extensive, cardiovascular collapse. If the ulcer occurs in the toddler, the first symptoms are usually anorexia or vomiting. Bleeding follows in several weeks. If the ulcer begins when children are of preschool or early school age, pain may be the presenting symptom. Children experience pain on arising in the morning. Unlike with adults with peptic ulcer disease, the pain is not necessarily relieved by the ingestion of food as it is in adults with peptic ulcers. Children may report pain as mild, severe, colicky, or continuous. It is often poorly localized, although it may be in the epigastric area as in adult clients. It may occur in the right lower quadrant and be confused with appendicitis.

In older school-age children and adolescents, the symptoms are generally those of the adult: a gnawing or aching pain in the epigastric area before meals that is relieved by eating. Vomiting (due to spasm and edema of the pylorus) also may occur in a small number of children. On abdominal palpation, there is tenderness in the epigastric region.

Fiber-optic endoscopy, the most reliable diagnostic test to confirm the diagnosis of peptic ulcer disease, allows for visual inspection and cultures for *H. pylori.* Because childhood ulcers are shallow, they may not show well on radiographs. In many children, little increase in gastric activity is demonstrable by gastric analysis. Children with this condition must have blood tests done periodically to be monitored for hypochromic, microcytic anemia (blood loss anemia).

Therapeutic Management

Children with peptic ulcer disease are treated with a combination of medications to reduce bacterium count and suppress gastric acidity. Children are prescribed a course of antibiotics to eradicate *H. pylori* and an antacid such as Maalox, Mylanta, or an H_2-antagonist such as cimetidine. Some children may be placed on a mucosal protectant medication such as sucralfate. If a secondary ulcer with bleeding is present, a continuous nasogastric infusion of an antacid may be necessary. With current therapy, only a few children experience the potential complications of perforation, blood loss anemia, and intestinal obstruction, although up to 50% of school-age children and adolescents will have symptoms of recurrence within a year (Motil, 1997).

NURSING DIAGNOSES AND RELATED INTERVENTIONS

Having peptic ulcer disease can be difficult for children because it is painful, and remembering to take medicine daily may be difficult for children.

Be certain that outcomes planned are realistic. It may not be possible to relieve symptoms of peptic ulcer immediately. Children can be helped immediately to understand why the pain occurs, however, and what they can do to help relieve it.

Nursing Diagnosis: Pain related to ulceration in intestinal tract

Outcome Identification: Child will report pain is at an acceptable level during course of illness.

Outcome Evaluation: Child exhibits verbal and nonverbal signs of decreased pain; the infant appears comfortable without excessive crying.

Children with peptic ulcer disease should be able to eat a normal diet, avoiding heavily spiced food such as pizza or sausage if such food causes discomfort. Work with them to devise a schedule they can remember for taking their prescribed medications. Antacid compounds that contain magnesium sulfate (e.g., Maalox) are less constipating than aluminum hydroxide products (Amphojel, Gelusil, or Mylanta). For children in school, antacid tablets are less attention-getting than liquids and, although not as effective, may be taken more easily.

In addition to administering medications, explore with such children the terms on which they are asked to live at home and at school. Some children will need help in learning coping mechanisms that serve them better and reduce gastric secretions.

✓ CHECKPOINT QUESTIONS

11. What diagnostic test is the most reliable for diagnosing peptic ulcer disease?
12. For what three complications is the child with peptic ulcer disease at risk?

HEPATIC DISORDERS

Hepatic disorders include both acquired disorders, such as hepatitis or cirrhosis, and congenital disorders, such as obstruction or atresia of the biliary duct.

Liver Function

The liver lies immediately under the diaphragm on the child's right side (In infants, 1 or 2 cm of liver is readily and normally palpable.). The organ is essential for the normal metabolism of all three types of foods. It plays a role in the maintenance of normal blood sugar level by changing glucose to glycogen and storing it until needed by body cells. It then reverses the process and changes glycogen back to glucose and releases it into the blood when cells need it.

The liver assists in the catabolism of fatty acids and protein and serves as a temporary storage space for both fat and protein. The liver, by the means of the enzyme glucuronyl transferase, converts indirect (or unconjugated) bilirubin into direct (or conjugated) bilirubin so that it can be excreted in bile and eliminated from the body. This is an important function in the newborn, and jaundice can result if the enzyme glucuronyl transferase is low because of immaturity.

The liver manufactures bile, a secretion necessary for the digestion of fat; fibrinogen and prothrombin, substances essential for blood clotting; heparin, a substance necessary to keep blood from clotting in intact vessels; and blood proteins. It produces large amounts of body heat. It destroys red blood cells and detoxifies many harmful absorbed substances, such as drugs. Because the liver, a life-sustaining organ, performs all of these functions, liver disease is always serious. A number of common liver function tests are used to diagnose the nature of liver pathology. These are summarized in Table 24-5.

Hepatitis

Hepatitis (inflammation and infection of the liver) is caused by the invasion of hepatitis A, hepatitis B, hepatitis C, hepatitis D, or hepatitis E viruses.

Hepatitis A

- Causative agent: a picornavirus; hepatitis A virus (HAV)
- Incubation period: 25 days on average
- Period of communicability: Highest during 2 weeks preceding onset of symptoms
- Mode of transmission: In children, ingestion of fecally contaminated water or shellfish; day care center spread from contaminated changing tables
- Immunity: Natural; one episode induces immunity for the specific type of virus
- Active artificial immunity: HAV vaccine (recommended for workers in day care centers)
- Passive artificial immunity: Immune globulin

Hepatitis B

- Causative agent: A hepadnavirus; hepatitis B virus (HBV)
- Incubation period: 120 days on average

TABLE 24.5 Liver Function Tests

TEST	DESCRIPTION
Serum bilirubin	Indirect bilirubin found in large quantities in bloodstream indicates that the child is not converting it to direct bilirubin; hence, liver cell function may be impaired; the normal value of total bilirubin in serum is 1.5 mg per 100 mL; if large amounts of direct bilirubin are found in serum, it implies obstruction of the bile duct, preventing the excretion of the converted substance.
Stool and urine bilirubin	If bile pigments can be obtained from stool (excreted as urobilinogen in stool and urine), it is evidence that bile is being manufactured and excreted from the liver; without the presence of bile pigment stool appears light in color (clay colored). Even trace amounts of bilirubin in urine is abnormal, possibly indicating liver dysfunction.
Alkaline phosphatase	Alkaline phosphatase is an enzyme produced by the liver and bone that is excreted in the bile; with bile duct obstruction, there will be increased levels of alkaline phosphatase in the blood.
Prothrombin time	In chronic liver disease, the level of prothrombin produced by the liver may fall so severely that the prothrombin time is increased; there is little change in prothrombin time in mild or short-term liver disease.
Aspartate transaminase (AST; serum glutamic oxaloacetic transaminase [SGOT])	AST(SGOT) is an enzyme found in the heart and liver; when there is acute cellular destruction to either organ, the enzyme is released into the bloodstream from the damaged cells; the blood levels are increased by 8 hours after injury; the level reaches a peak in 24 or 36 h and then falls to normal in 4 to 6 d.
Alanine transaminase (ALT; serum glutamic pyruvic transaminase [SGPT])	ALT (SGPT) is an enzyme found mostly in the liver; it rises for the same reasons as SGOT but is not as sensitive an indicator of liver damage.
Lactic dehydrogenase (LDH)	LDH is another enzyme found in the heart and liver; it is a relatively insensitive indicator of liver destruction, however; infectious mononucleosis is the one disease in which increased levels of LDH seem to be seen frequently.
Serum proteins	Because albumin is chiefly synthesized in the liver, most acute or chronic liver disease will show decreased serum albumin.

- Period of communicability: Later part of incubation period and during the acute stage
- Mode of transmission: Transfusion of contaminated blood and plasma or semen; inoculation by a contaminated syringe or needle through intravenous drug use; may be spread to fetus if mother has infection in third trimester of pregnancy
- Immunity: Natural; one episode induces immunity for the specific type of virus
- Active artificial immunity: Vaccine for the HBV virus (recommended for routine immunization series and health care providers)
- Passive artificial immunity: Specific hepatitis B immune serum globulin

Hepatitis C, D, and E

Although hepatitis A and B are the most frequent viruses to cause hepatitis, hepatitis C, D, and E viruses may also be involved. Hepatitis C (HCV) is a single-strand RNA virus. Transmission, as with HBV, is primarily by blood or blood products, intravenous drug use, or sexual contact. The virus produces mild symptoms of disease. There is, however, a high incidence of chronic infection with the virus. Treatment with interferon for 6 months limits the symptoms and possibly prevents the disease from becoming chronic.

Hepatitis D (HDV) or the delta form is similar to HBV in transmission. It requires a coexisting HBV infection to be activated. Disease symptoms are mild, but there is a high incidence of fulminant hepatitis after the initial infection. The E form of hepatitis is enterically transmitted similarly to hepatitis A (fecally contaminated water). Disease symptoms from the E virus are usually mild, except in pregnant women, in whom they tend to be severe.

Chronic Hepatitis

Hepatitis becomes chronic when it persists over 4 months. This is most usually a result of B, D, and C infection. A liver biopsy establishes the diagnosis and can also predict the severity. With chronic hepatitis, fatty infiltration and bile duct damage are present. The disease may progress to cirrhosis and eventually liver failure. Therapy is supportive to compensate for decreased liver function.

Fulminant Hepatic Failure

Fulminant hepatic failure is present when acute, massive necrosis or sudden, severe impairment of liver function occurs leading to hepatic encephalopathy. Hepatic encephalopathy is the result of ammonia intoxication caused by the inability of the liver to detoxify the ammonia being constantly produced by the intestine in the process of digestion. Children show signs of mental aberrations such as confusion, drowsiness, or disorientation. Treatment is to reduce protein intake and administer lactulose to prevent absorption of ammonia in the colon or to administer nonabsorbable antibiotics such as neomycin, to decrease the production of ammonia by the intestinal bacteria.

Although fulminant hepatitis is usually the result of hepatitis D infection, a number of drugs, noticeably acetaminophen toxicity, may be a cause (Novak, Suchy, & Balistreri, 1997). Children need supportive therapy to compensate for decreased liver function. Liver transplantation may be necessary. Unfortunately, many children may not be able to survive the long wait for a donor organ.

Assessment

Hepatitis is a generalized body infection with specific intense liver effects. Type A occurs in children of all ages. Hepatitis B tends to occur in adolescents after intimate contact or the use of contaminated syringes for drug injection.

Clinically, it is impossible to differentiate the type of hepatitis from the signs that are present. All hepatitis viruses cause liver cell destruction, leading to increased serum aspartate transaminase (AST [glutamic-oxaloacetic transaminase—SGOT]) and alkaline phosphatase levels. There is decreased albumin synthesis and impaired bile formation and excretion. The type of virus causing the disease can be determined by the recognition of a specific antibody against the virus (anti-HAV IgM; anti-HBV IgM, etc.).

Children notice headache, fever, and anorexia. Symptoms with hepatitis A are generally mild. Jaundice occurs as liver function slows. This lasts for approximately a week, then symptoms fade with full recovery. Symptoms of hepatitis B are more marked. Children report generalized aching, right upper quadrant pain, and headache. They may have a low-grade fever. They feel ill; they are irritable and fretful from pruritus. After 3 to 7 days of such symptoms, the color of the urine becomes darker (brown) because of the excretion of bilirubin. In another 2 days, children's eye scleras become jaundiced; soon they have generalized jaundice. With the generalized jaundice, there is little excretion of bilirubin into the stool, so the stool color becomes white or gray. This icteric (jaundiced) phase lasts for a few days to 2 weeks. Some children have an anicteric form of infection, in which they develop the beginning symptoms but then never develop the jaundice. They are as infectious, however, as children with overt jaundice.

Laboratory studies will show elevations of AST (SGOT) and serum alanine transaminase (ALT [glutamate pyruvate transaminase—SGPT]). Measurement of bilirubin in the urine shows increased levels. Bile pigments in the stool are decreased. Serum bilirubin levels will be increased.

Therapeutic Management

Strict handwashing and infection control precautions are mandatory when caring for children with hepatitis. Feces must be disposed of carefully because the type A virus may be cultured from feces. Syringes and needles must be disposed of with caution because the type B virus can be transmitted by blood. Contacts should receive immune globulin (hepatitis A) or hepatitis B immune globulin (HBIG) as appropriate. All health care providers should receive prophylaxis against hepatitis by the hepatitis vaccine. Children should receive routine immunization against HBV. All women should be screened during pregnancy for hepatitis B surface antigen (HBsAg). Infants born of hepatitis-positive mothers receive both HBIG and active immunization at birth to prevent their contracting the disease.

The treatment for hepatitis A is increased rest and maintenance of a good caloric intake. Interferon may be prescribed. A low-fat diet, once recommended, is not required and in any event is difficult to enforce. Children are generally hungrier at breakfast than later in the day, so a good intake should be encouraged for breakfast. Children can be cared for at home. They should not return to school or a day care center until 2 weeks after the onset of symptoms (Novak, Suchy & Balistreri, 1997).

Of those with type B, 90% will also recover completely, but 10% will develop chronic hepatitis and become hepatitis carriers. Infants who contracted the disease at birth have an increased risk for liver carcinoma later in life (Novak, Suchy & Balistreri, 1997).

NURSING DIAGNOSES AND RELATED INTERVENTIONS

Nursing Diagnosis: Pain related to pruritus of jaundice and liver inflammation

Outcome Identification: Child will not experience extreme discomfort during course of illness.

Outcome Evaluation: Child states level of itching is tolerable; no scratch marks on skin are present; reports right upper quadrant pain is minimal.

Jaundice commonly causes pruritus, and for some children this can result in extreme discomfort. Being certain that the child is not overheated and not perspiring reduces the itching. A cool bath is often comforting. Skin moisturizers such as Eucerin or an antihistamine may be prescribed. Teach the child distractive techniques such as putting pressure on a pruritic area or trying imagery to lessen the urge to scratch.

✔ **CHECKPOINT QUESTIONS**

13. Which hepatitis viruses are spread through fecally contaminated water?
14. Which hepatitis virus is most often responsible for fulminant hepatitis?

Obstruction of the Bile Ducts

Obstruction of the bile ducts in children generally occurs from congenital atresia, stenosis, or absence of the duct. Although rare, it also can occur from a plugging of biliary secretions. When the bile duct is obstructed, bile, unable to enter the intestinal tract, accumulates in the liver. Bile pigments (direct bilirubin) enter the bloodstream and jaundice occurs, increasing in intensity daily.

Assessment

Although bile duct obstruction is a congenital disorder, the chief sign (jaundice) does not develop until approximately 2 weeks. This delay in development differentiates it clinically from physiologic jaundice, which occurs in almost all newborns on the third day of life, or the jaundice of Rh isoimmunization, which typically occurs during the first 24 hours of life. Laboratory findings will also distinguish this type of jaundice. Physiologic jaundice and Rh isoimmunization jaundice occur from a rise in indirect bilirubin, whereas the jaundice of bile duct obstruction is a result of a rise in direct bilirubin. Alkaline phosphatase levels will be elevated. AST(SGOT) is normal in the early phase and later becomes abnormal, when prolonged obstruction and backpressure cause liver cell damage. In addition, because bile salts (necessary for fat absorption) are not reaching the intestine, absorption of fat and fat-soluble vitamins (i.e., vitamins A, D, E, and K) is poor. Calcium absorption, which depends on vitamin D absorption, also is poor. Infant's stools appear light in color from lack of bile pigments. The pressure on the liver from the obstruction becomes so acute with time that cell destruction or cirrhosis occurs. Ultimately, without liver transplantation, death of liver failure will result.

Therapeutic Management

Before treatment is begun, appropriate blood work and a punch biopsy under a local anesthesia may be done to rule out hepatitis. Duodenal secretions may be collected by endoscopy to assess for bile. Radionuclide imaging, in which the infant is given an IV radioactive isotope that, when taken up by the liver, can be shown flowing through the bile ducts, also may be performed. Phenobarbital is administered at the same time to increase bile flow. If a mucus plug in the duct is suspected, children may be given a course of magnesium sulfate (installed into the duodenum to relax the bile duct) or given dehydrocholic acid (Decholin) intravenously to stimulate the flow of bile. If atresia of the bile duct appears to be the problem, surgical correction is the treatment (a Kasai procedure). With this surgery, a loop of bowel is sutured next to the liver to create a fistula for bile flow between the liver and intestine. A double-barreled colostomy is then created (enterostomy). Bile flows out of the proximal loop into a collecting bag. It is periodically returned to the distal loop of intestine by injection. After 6 to 12 weeks, the colostomy is closed when a normal bile flow has been established. Unfortunately, surgical correction is impossible in all infants with atresia because the atresia tends to occur too far back in the liver to be in an operable area. Liver transplantation is needed for those children with extensive involvement.

NURSING DIAGNOSES AND RELATED INTERVENTIONS

Nursing Diagnosis: Risk for altered nutrition, less than body requirements, related to inability to digest fat

Outcome Identification: Child will ingest adequate nutritional requirements until surgical correction is complete.

Outcome Evaluation: Infant's weight remains in same percentile on standardized growth curve; absence of vitamin deficiency (e.g., cracked lips or altered bone growth); dietary record reflects intakes of adequate nutrients.

Preoperative Care. Infants who are admitted for surgery for bile duct obstruction are placed on a low-fat, high-protein diet preoperatively. They are given water-soluble forms of vitamins A, D, and K to improve vitamin levels. If vitamin K level is too low, coagulation may be affected, increasing their surgical risk. Vitamin K may be administered parenterally until the prothrombin levels rise to normal limits. Infants will also be well hydrated with parenteral fluids.

Postoperative Care. After surgery, infants return with a nasogastric tube in place attached to low suction. Observe carefully for abdominal distention because paralytic ileus is a frequent complication of this type of surgery. The nasogastric tube will be left in place until bowel peristalsis has returned. Gradually, children will then be introduced to oral fluids and then eventually to a normal diet. If the repair is successful, the child's stools change to a yellow and then brown (normal stool) color after surgery. Description of stools is therefore an important postoperative observation.

If bile flow is inadequate after surgery, infants will remain on a low-fat, high-protein diet or receive total parenteral nutrition while they await transplant surgery.

Cirrhosis

Cirrhosis is fibrotic scarring of the liver. Cirrhosis means "yellow" or the typical color of hepatic scar tissue. It occurs rarely in children, although it may be seen as a result of congenital biliary atresia or as a complication of chronic illnesses such as protracted hepatitis, sickle cell anemia, or cystic fibrosis.

When fibrotic infiltrates replace normal liver cells, liver function is impaired, resulting in a decreased ability to detoxify toxic substances, decreased protein synthesis, inability to produce prothrombin, decreased ability to produce bile, and, possibly, hypoglycemia. Children will have large, fatty stools resulting from the decrease in bile production; avitaminosis of fat-soluble vitamins; symptoms of hemorrhage from decreased clotting ability; and anemia.

Fibrotic infiltration interferes not only with the function of liver cells but also with the hepatic blood flow. This leads to portal hypertension from the back pressure of blood that cannot flow readily through the scarred organ (Figure 24-6). Children will have compromised heart action, *ascites* (an exudate of fluid into the abdomen), possibly esophageal varices (backpressure causing them to dilate), and hypersplenism.

Once fibrotic infiltration begins, there is no way to reverse the changes. Nursing care focuses on promoting comfort, providing adequate nutrition by a high-protein, high-carbohydrate, and medium-chain-triglyceride diet, and preventing further involvement until liver transplantation can be scheduled. Cholestyramine (Questran) may be prescribed to stimulate bile flow and reduce reabsorption of bile into the circulation (this will minimize jaundice).

Esophageal Varices

Esophageal varices (distended veins) can be a frequent complication of liver disorders such as cirrhosis. They generally form at the distal end of the esophagus close to

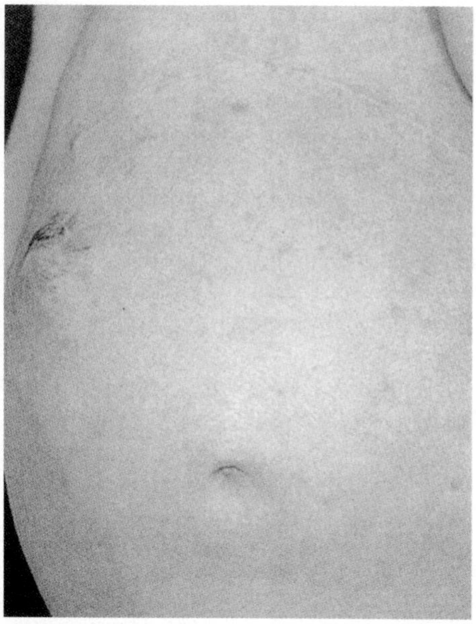

FIGURE 24.6 A child with cirrhosis of the liver. Note the abdominal distention and development of prominent, tortuous veins secondary to portal hypertension.

the stomach when there is backpressure on the veins from increased blood pressure in the portal circulation. Bleeding of varices may occur if children cough vigorously or strain to pass stool. Gastric reflux into the distal esophagus may irritate and erode the fine covering of the distended vessels, causing rupture.

Rupture of esophageal varices is an emergency situation because children can lose a large quantity of blood quickly from the ruptured, engorged vessels. Vasopressin or nitroglycerin may be given intravenously to lessen hypertension and reduce the hemorrhage. Injection of a sclerosing agent into veins may be attempted. Cold saline nasogastric lavage may be instituted to promote vasoconstriction. A Sengstaken-Blakemore tube or Linton-Nachlas catheter may be passed into the stomach. After insertion, balloons on the sides of the catheter are inflated to apply pressure against the bleeding vessels. As with an external tourniquet, the compression in such a catheter must be reduced for a 5- to 10-minute period every 6 hours to 8 hours or tissue necrosis can result.

Children must be monitored for future bleeding episodes. Frequent vital sign measurements and testing of stool and any vomitus for the presence of blood will indicate new gastrointestinal system bleeding.

ENHANCING COMMUNICATION

Baxter is a 2-year-old who was born with congenital obstruction of the bile duct. Unable to be surgically repaired, it has progressed to severe cirrhosis. Baxter's doctors spoke with her mother yesterday about the need for a liver transplant. Today, you see Mrs. Commons filling out forms by Baxter's bedside.

Less Effective Communication

Nurse: Mrs. Commons? Can I help you with anything?
Mrs. Commons: No. Baxter's going to have a transplant. With her well again, I'll be free to start back to college. I'm filling out the forms.
Nurse: Will the transplant really be that soon?
Mrs. Commons: As soon as tomorrow. Because Baxter won't be able to wait a long time.
Nurse: Do you think the doctors meant it could be that soon? But sometimes there's a long waiting period?
Mrs. Commons: No. Because Baxter can't wait long. If she has to, she'll die.
Nurse: It's lucky then a liver is available.

More Effective Communication

Nurse: Mrs. Commons? Can I help you with anything?
Mrs. Commons: No. Baxter's going to have a transplant. With her well again, I'll be free to start back to college. I'm filling out the forms.
Nurse: Will the transplant really be that soon?
Mrs. Commons: As soon as tomorrow. Because Baxter won't be able to wait a long time.
Nurse: Do you think the doctors meant it could be that soon? But sometimes there's a long waiting period?
Mrs. Commons: No. Because Baxter can't wait long. If she has to, she'll die.
Nurse: Do you think that's what they were trying to tell you?

People under stress often do not hear instructions well. When this happens, they may need them repeated several times before they truly comprehend what was said. An easy solution when you are aware that a parent has not heard potentially bad news is to ignore the loss of information, as in the first scenario above. A better solution is to explore with the parents what they did hear and help them receive more accurate information.

Liver Transplantation

Liver transplantation is the surgical replacement of a malfunctioning liver by a donor liver. Donor livers are not readily available, so the waiting time for surgery may be months (see Enhancing Communication). It may be difficult finding an acceptable child-sized liver. Adult livers can be reduced in size for transplantation. Often a child is extremely ill with ascites, gastrointestinal bleeding, extreme pruritus, hepatic encephalopathy, or renal dysfunction before the surgery can be accomplished. Nursing care after liver transplantation in a child is compounded because it involves taking care of a child who has had major surgery, and also one who normally would be categorized as too ill to undergo surgery. Despite the severity of illness and the length of surgery, children tend to recover quickly after liver transplantation. Both children and parents must have thorough preoperative preparation so that they understand the seriousness of the surgery and the possibility that the graft will be rejected. It helps to introduce the parents to others whose children have successfully undergone the procedure so they have support people available.

Surgical Procedure

Liver transplantation requires a wide subcostal incision. The vena cava is temporarily clamped during the removal of the natural liver to prevent bleeding, which means that all intravenous lines must be placed in the upper extremities (if placed in lower extremities, fluid could not return through the clamped venous circulation to the upper body). Clamping the vena cava this way can result in renal failure because of the temporary halt of blood flow to the kidneys and dramatic shifts of fluid during surgery. The total operation takes 10 to 14 hours to complete.

Postoperative Management

If a liver transplant is rejected, it is most often rejected because of the function of T-lymphocytes. Careful tissue matching (HLA matching) is necessary to reduce the possibility of stimulating T-cell rejection. To further reduce the action of T-lymphocytes, children are administered a course of an immunosuppressive drug such as cyclosporine before the transplantation.

Nursing care after liver transplantation surgery focuses on preventing complications that may arise from the surgery and postoperative medical management. Children need assisted ventilation for approximately 24 hours. Pulmonary complications such as atelectasis and pneumonia are likely to occur because the large abdominal incision makes coughing and deep breathing difficult. In addition, ascites places pressure against the diaphragm, interfering with lung expansion, and preoperative pulmonary edema may be present, further impairing gas exchange. After discontinuation of mechanical ventilation and extubation, chest physiotherapy may be started to mobilize secretions.

Assess blood pressure, capillary refilling, peripheral pulses, and skin color frequently in the postoperative period to be certain that cardiovascular function is adequate, important for good tissue perfusion of the transplanted liver. The child may have a central venous pressure line or an arterial line such as a Swan-Gantz catheter inserted to assess hemodynamic status. Assess neurologic status hourly using a modified Glasgow coma scale (see Chapter 31).

The child is positioned flat for the first 24 hours to prevent cerebral air emboli, which may result from any air remaining in the transplanted liver. Typically, children have a nasogastric tube inserted during surgery attached to low intermittent suction postoperatively. Irrigate the tube according to agency policy to maintain patency. Assess the gastric pH by aspirating stomach contents every 4 hours and, based on this assessment, administer antacids and H_2 receptor antagonists such as cimetidine or mucosal protectants as prescribed to help prevent stress ulcer. If preoperative esophageal varices are present, assess nasogastric drainage carefully for occult blood.

A T-tube inserted for drainage allows the amount of bile being produced by the new liver to be evaluated. Once bowel sounds become active, nasogastric suction is usually discontinued as liquids and then solid foods are introduced gradually. If vomiting occurs and is persistent, total parenteral nutrition may be used for 3 or 4 days to rest the intestinal tract before fluid is reintroduced.

Hypoglycemia is a danger postoperatively because glucose levels are regulated by the liver, and the transplanted organ may not function efficiently at first. Assess serum glucose levels hourly by fingerstick puncture. A 10% solution of dextrose may be necessary to prevent hypoglycemia.

Sodium, potassium, chloride, and calcium levels are evaluated approximately every 6 to 8 hours to be certain that an electrolyte balance is maintained. Even if a low potassium level is detected, potassium is rarely added to intravenous solutions because of the risk of renal failure due to the stress of surgery. If the graft begins to necrose, the breakdown of cells releases potassium, elevating the level. Continuous cardiac monitoring is usually necessary to detect hyperkalemia (hyperkalemia causes elevation of T waves or ventricular fibrillation), hypokalemia (causes small T waves and the presence of a U wave), or other arrhythmias.

Most children develop hypertension within 72 hours after surgery. This is because of alterations in the renin-angiotensin system of the transplanted liver, a side effect of cyclosporine and steroid therapy. Intravenous therapy with hypotensive agents such as hydralazine (Apresoline) and nitroprusside is usually necessary. Hypotension will occur if the transplanted liver becomes dysfunctional or there is bleeding caused by poor blood coagulation. The child has an increased risk for bleeding because of the number of anastomosis sites included in the procedure. Observe and record abdominal girth, the incision line, and drainage from incision catheters to help detect bleeding.

Take axillary, not rectal, temperatures, because many children with liver damage have rectal hemorrhoids that could rupture from the trauma of a thermometer touching them. Maintain normal body temperature by preventing the child from being unnecessarily exposed during procedures. A warming blanket may be required postoperatively to maintain normal body temperature after the long exposure of surgery.

NURSING DIAGNOSES AND RELATED INTERVENTIONS

Nursing Diagnosis: Risk for infection related to administration of immunosuppressive medication

Outcome Identification: Child will remain free of signs and symptoms of infection postoperatively.

Outcome Evaluation: Temperature remains within normal range; no presence of exudate or inflammation around abdominal incision.

Successful liver transplantation is possible because of the preoperative administration of cyclosporine A, which effectively suppresses T lymphocytes, the lymphocytes responsible for rejecting transplanted organs. In addition, cyclosporine (Sandimmune) and steroids (Solu-Medrol) are administered intravenously immediately postoperatively to prevent graft rejection. Because children are prone to infection while receiving immunosuppressive therapy, prevent their contracting an infection by using strict aseptic techniques, standard precautions, and careful handwashing. Clean the skin around any abdominal drains every 4 hours to prevent skin breakdown that opens a site for microorganisms to enter.

Serum transaminases (AST [SGOT] and ALT [SGPT]), alkaline phosphatase, serum bilirubin, and ammonia levels are assessed daily to detect rejection, although children usually do not show signs of liver rejection until 5 to 7 days after surgery. In addition to changes in these laboratory values, with liver rejection the child also may develop fever and increasing abdominal girth. Also, the urine turns orange from increased urobilinogen excretion. If signs of rejection appear to be occurring, doses of cyclosporine and steroids are increased to maximum levels.

Nursing Diagnosis: Altered family processes related to stress of surgery and uncertainty of transplant outcome

Outcome Identification: Child and family will demonstrate adequate coping techniques postoperatively.

Outcome Evaluation: Child and family state that, although waiting is difficult, they are able to do so; identify ways they have changed their family life at home to accommodate child's illness and surgery.

Children and parents need continued support during the postoperative period while they wait to see if the graft will be rejected. They appreciate continued contact with health care personnel through telephone calls and clinic visits.

After successful liver transplantation, a child should be able to function normally, attending school and enjoying age-appropriate activities. Be certain by hospital discharge that parents have a return appointment for evaluation and are aware of the symptoms of graft rejection, such as jaundice, lethargy, and fever.

CHECKPOINT QUESTIONS

15. For the child with bile duct obstruction, absorption of what substances will be impaired?
16. The child with esophageal varices secondary to cirrhosis is at high risk for what complication?
17. Why is hypoglycemia a complication of liver transplantation?

INTESTINAL DISORDERS

Intussusception

Intussusception is the invagination of one portion of the intestine into another (Figure 24-7). This generally occurs in the second half of the first year (Pokorny, 1997).

In infants younger than 1 year, intussusception generally occurs for idiopathic reasons. In infants older than age 1 year, a "lead point" on the intestine likely cues the invagination. Such a point might be a Meckel's diverticulum; a polyp; hypertrophy of *Peyer's patches* (lymphatic tissue of the bowel that increases in size with viral diseases); or bowel tumors. The point of the invagination is generally the juncture of the distal ileum and proximal colon.

This condition is a surgical emergency. Reduction of the intussusception must be done promptly by either instillation of solution (or air) or surgery before necrosis of the invaginated portion of the bowel results.

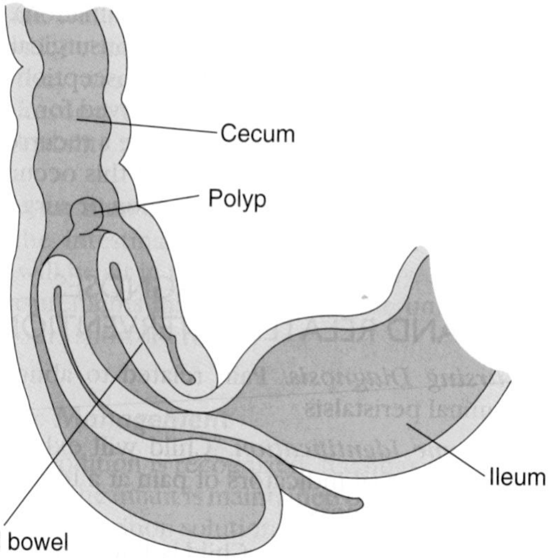

FIGURE 24.7 Intussusception. The distal ileal segment of bowel has invaginated into the cecum. A polyp serves as a lead point.

Assessment

Children with this disorder suddenly draw up their legs and cry as if they are in severe pain and possibly vomit. After the peristaltic wave that caused the discomfort, they are symptom free. They play happily. In approximately 15 minutes, the same phenomenon of intense abdominal pain strikes again. Vomitus will begin to contain bile because the obstruction is invariably below the *ampulla of Vater,* the point in the intestine where bile empties into the duodenum. After approximately 12 hours, children develop blood in stool, described as a "currant jelly" appearance. Their abdomen becomes distended as the bowel above the intussusception distends.

If necrosis has occurred, children generally have an elevated temperature, peritoneal irritation (their abdomen will feel tender; they may "guard" it by tightening their abdominal muscles), an increased white blood cell count (WBC), and often a rapid pulse.

Diagnosis is suggested by the history. Any time a parent is describing a child who is crying, be certain to ask enough questions that it is possible to recognize a history of intussusception.

- What is the duration of the pain? (It lasts a short time with intervals of no crying in between.)
- What is the intensity? (Severe.)
- What is the frequency? (Approximately every 15 to 20 minutes.)
- What is the description? (The child pulls up his or her legs with crying.)
- Is the child ill in any other way? (Yes. Vomits; refuses food; states his or her stomach feels "full.")

The presence of the intussusception is confirmed by sonogram.

Therapeutic Management

Intussusception requires surgery to straighten the invaginated portion, or reduction by a water-soluble solution,

Nursing Care of the Child With a Renal or Urinary Tract Disorder

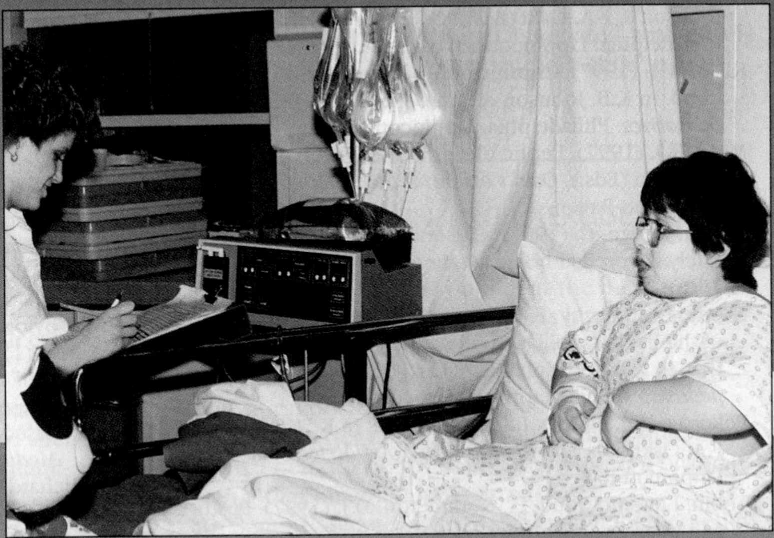

25

CHAPTER

Key Terms

- **acute transplant rejection**
- **Alport's syndrome**
- **azotemia**
- **Bowman's capsule**
- **dialysis**
- **enuresis**
- **epispadias**
- **exstrophy of the bladder**
- **glomerular filtration rate**
- **glomerulonephritis**
- **hydronephrosis**
- **hypospadias**
- **nephrosis**
- **patent urachus**
- **polycystic kidney**
- **postural proteinuria**
- **prune belly syndrome**
- **vesicoureteral reflux**

Objectives

After mastering the contents of this chapter, you should be able to:

1. Describe common renal and urinary disorders that occur in children.
2. Assess a child for a renal or urinary tract disorder.
3. Formulate nursing diagnoses related to renal or urinary disorders.
4. Establish appropriate outcomes related to the care of a child with a renal or urinary disorder.
5. Plan nursing care related to urinary or renal disorders.
6. Implement nursing care for the child with a renal or urinary disorder.
7. Evaluate outcomes for achievement and effectiveness of care.
8. Identify National Health Goals related to renal or urinary tract disorders and children that nurses can be instrumental in helping the nation achieve.
9. Identify areas related to care of the child with a renal or urinary disorder that would benefit from additional nursing research.
10. Analyze methods for making nursing care of the child with a renal or urinary disorder more family centered.
11. Integrate knowledge of renal and urinary tract disorders with the nursing process to achieve quality child health nursing care.

Carol is a 4-year-old admitted to the hospital with nephrotic syndrome. She has marked ascites and edema. "I kept asking everyone in my family how she could be gaining so much weight, yet she doesn't eat anything," her parent tells you. "My aunt said this happened because Carol drank part of a beer I left on the coffee table. I didn't give her the beer, she just picked it up and drank it. Do you think that's what caused it? What if she needs a kidney transplant? Will I be allowed to do that?"

How would you answer Carol's mother? What information does she need to better understand her child's condition?

In previous chapters, you learned about the growth and development of well children and the nursing care of children with disorders of other systems. In this chapter, you'll add information about the dramatic changes, both physical and psychosocial, that occur when children develop urinary tract or renal disorders. This is important information because it builds a base for care and health teaching.

After you've studied the chapter, turn to the Critical Thinking Exercises at the end of the chapter to help sharpen your skills and test your knowledge.

FOCUS ON NATIONAL HEALTH GOALS

Renal disease can lead to long-term illness. The following National Health Goal addresses prevention of long-term illness:

- Reduce to no more than 8% the proportion of people who experience a limitation in major activity due to chronic conditions from a baseline of 9.4% (DHHS, 1995).

Nurses can be instrumental in helping the nation achieve this goal by educating parents that children need a follow-up assessment for protein in urine after streptococcal infections. They also need to provide optimal care to children with renal disease.

Nursing research would be helpful to determine parents' or children's ability to accurately self-assess for proteinuria after streptococcal infections, the specific needs of children on ambulatory peritoneal dialysis, and ways to make low-potassium diets more appealing to children with end-stage renal disease.

Normally, the urinary system maintains the proper balance of fluid (water) and electrolytes in the blood. When disease occurs, such as with structural abnormalities or renal (kidney) malfunction, a child may be left with excessive amounts of fluid in the body or with an imbalance of electrolytes and other substances essential to the body's functioning. Disorders of the urinary system may be long term. Any urinary tract disorder can ultimately (if not originally) affect the kidneys, resulting in kidney dysfunction with potentially fatal consequences.

Unfortunately, because symptoms may be vague, or because the child or parents do not realize the seriousness of urinary disease or are embarrassed to discuss it, children may not be evaluated at the first sign of illness.

Health education to increase awareness of the symptoms of urinary tract and kidney disorders is an important area of family health teaching. National Health Goals related to renal or urinary tract disorders and children are shown in the Focus on National Health Goals.

NURSING PROCESS OVERVIEW

for Care of the Child With a Renal or Urinary Tract Disorder

Assessment

Because the symptoms of many urinary tract and renal disorders (e.g., mild abdominal pain, slowly growing edema, or low-grade fever) are subtle, parents may not bring their child for evaluation as early in the disease as they might if symptoms were more definite. School nurses play an important role in recognizing the seriousness of minor symptoms and making proper referrals for care.

Common findings from a health history and physical examination are shown in Assessing the Child for Signs and Symptoms of Urinary Tract Dysfunction. If children have a urinary tract infection or have had bladder surgery, they may experience pain on urination or pain from bladder spasms. Be sure to assess the degree of pain, including its location and intensity, before administering an analgesic or antispasmodic. Urine specimens also provide valuable assessment information. Techniques for obtaining urine samples (i.e., clean-catch, catheterization, 24-hour collections, suprapubic aspiration, and urinalysis) are described in Chapter 16.

Nursing Diagnosis

Examples of nursing diagnoses for children with urinary tract or renal disorders may include the following:

- Pain related to effects of urinary tract infection
- Fluid volume excess related to decreased kidney function and fluid accumulation
- Fear related to outcome of kidney transplantation
- Altered nutrition, less than body requirements, related to effects of dietary restrictions
- Social isolation related to immunosuppressant therapy
- Risk for injury related to body's inability to excrete waste products properly

Because the entire family becomes involved in long-term renal disease, other appropriate nursing diagnoses may include:

- Altered family processes related to the effects and stresses of the child's chronic illness
- Ineffective family coping, compromised, related to the chronicity of the child's illness

Outcome Identification and Planning

Be certain that outcomes established for care are relevant to the child's age and condition. Because renal

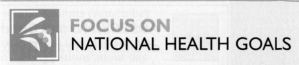

ENHANCING COMMUNICATION

Shasha is a 9-year-old recipient of a kidney transplant whom you visit at home. Her mother tells you that Shasha has "changed completely" since the transplant. She thinks this is as wonderful as the transplant itself.

Less Effective Communication

Nurse: Mrs. Maronia? In what way has Shasha changed?

Mrs. Maronia: She used to whine all the time. And constantly ask for things. Now she entertains herself. It's like heaven.

Nurse: How does she behave with her brother?

Mrs. Maronia: Perfect. She never used to share with him. Yesterday she gave him her magic markers. She even lets him watch his television programs instead of hers.

Nurse: That sounds wonderful. Let's review her medicine routine to be sure that's going well.

Mrs. Maronia: That's another thing she does perfectly. Never fusses a bit about anything she has to take.

More Effective Communication

Nurse: Mrs. Maronia? In what way has Shasha changed?

Mrs. Maronia: She used to whine all the time. And constantly ask for things. Now she entertains herself. It's like heaven.

Nurse: How does she behave with her brother?

Mrs. Maronia: Perfect. She never used to share with him. Yesterday she gave him her magic markers. She even lets him watch his television programs instead of hers.

Nurse: Do you think she's acting a little too perfect? Do you think she could be worrying that if she misbehaves, her transplant might not take?

Mrs. Maronia: I would feel better if she started to act like her old self.

What the mother above is describing is a "honeymoon" period that children may pass through after a transplant. Parents often need help seeing this for what it is so they can begin to reassure the child that behaving perfectly will not influence the transplant and because they loved them as they were, they will continue to love them regardless.

none of these factors is related to whether the child is good or bad or deserves or does not deserve to have the transplant work.

Children with end-stage renal disease usually fail to grow despite treatment. Although the rate of growth is improved after a kidney transplantation, they will probably never reach full height. Part of this growth retardation is related to the need for corticosteroid maintenance therapy.

KEY POINTS

Many urinary tract disorders such as polycystic kidneys, urethral obstruction, and bladder exstrophy are evident on fetal sonogram. Early identification allows therapy to begin immediately at birth.

Many urinary tract disorders such as polycystic kidneys or chronic renal failure are long-term conditions requiring years of therapy. Be certain that parents are well informed about the child's condition so they can continue to participate in planning the child's care.

Congenital structural abnormalities of the urinary tract include patent urachus, exstrophy of the bladder, hypospadias, and epispadias. Surgical correction is required for all of these.

Urinary tract infections tend to occur more often in girls than boys. "Honeymoon cystitis" refers to a UTI occurring with first-time sexual intercourse.

Vesicoureteral reflex is the backflow of urine into ureters with voiding. It occurs because the valve that guards the entrance to the ureters is defective. Surgical correction may be necessary to prevent repeated urinary tract infection.

Renal dysfunction can occur for structural reasons such as kidney agenesis, polycystic kidney, and renal hypoplasia. Acute poststreptococcal glomerulonephritis is inflammation of the glomeruli after a streptococcal infection. It is characterized by an acute episode of hematuria and proteinuria.

Diminished kidney function leads to both fluid and electrolyte imbalances. Creative techniques are necessary to encourage children to continue to ingest a high-protein diet to counteract protein losses in urine.

Nephrotic syndrome is an immunologic process that results in altered glomeruli permeability. Nursing diagnoses associated with this are altered nutrition, high risk for altered skin integrity, and knowledge deficit.

Renal failure can be acute or chronic. Peritoneal dialysis or hemodialysis may be used to remove body waste until kidney function can be restored.

Kidney transplantation may be a therapy option for some children with kidney disorders. This is extensive surgery and requires the child to remain on immunosuppressive therapy to counteract transplant rejection.

CRITICAL THINKING EXERCISES

1. Carol is the preschooler with nephrotic syndrome you met at the beginning of the chapter. Her par-

ent asked you whether Carol accidentally drinking beer off the coffee table could have caused the kidney disease. What would you tell her is the cause of nephrosis? What discharge instructions can you anticipate you will need to review with Carol's mother?

2. A 12-year-old comes to a pediatric clinic with her third urinary tract infection this year. Her mother asks you whether there is anything she should be doing to help prevent these. How would you answer her?
3. A child with end-stage renal disease is awaiting a kidney transplant. He tells you he hopes he has been good enough to deserve being chosen for the next kidney available. What would you want to teach him about the transplant selection process?
4. A 6-year-old is receiving continuous ambulatory peritoneal dialysis. She wants to go to her church camp this summer. Her parents ask you whether this would be a good experience for her. What factors would you want to know about the camp? About the child? About her procedure?

REFERENCES

Barber, N. (1996). Genitourinary disorders. In Burns, C.E., et al. (Eds.). *Pediatric primary care*. Philadelphia: Saunders.

Berry, P.L. & Brewer, E.D. (1997). Glomerulonephritis and nephrotic syndrome. In Johnson, K.B. & Oski, F.A. *Oski's essential pediatrics*. Philadelphia: Lippincott.

Carlson, D. & Mowery, B.D. (1997). Standards to prevent complications of urinary catheterization in children: should and should-nots. *Journal of the Society of Pediatric Nurses, 2*(1), 37.

Department of Health and Human Services (1995). *Healthy people 2000; midcourse review*. Washington, D.C.: DHHS.

Elder, J.S. (1997). Antenatal hydronephrosis: fetal and neonatal management. *Pediatric Clinics of North America, 44*(5), 1299.

Fontaine, E. et al. (1997). Long-term results of renal transplantation in children with the prune-belly syndrome. *Journal of Urology, 158*(3.1), 895.

Friedman, A.L. (1996). Etiology, pathophysiology, diagnosis and management of chronic renal failure in children. *Current Opinion in Pediatrics, 8*(2), 148.

Gabow, P., et al. (1997). Utility of ultrasonography in the diagnosis of autosomal dominant polycystic kidney disease in children. *Journal of the American Society of Nephrology, 8*(1), 105.

Hellerstein, S. (1998). Urinary tract infections in children: why they occur and how to prevent them. *American Family Physician, 57*(10), 2440.

Kantor, R., Salai, M. & Ganel, A. (1997). Orthopaedic long term aspects of bladder exstrophy. *Clinical Orthopaedics and Related Research, 335*, 240.

Lottmann, H.B. et al. (1997). Bladder exstrophy: evaluation of factors leading to continence with spontaneous voiding after staged reconstruction. *Journal of Urology, 158*(3), 1041.

Louis, P.T. (1997). Hemolytic-uremic syndrome. In Johnson, K.B. & Oski, F.A. *Oski's essential pediatrics*. Philadelphia: Lippincott.

Mariscalco, M.M. (1997). Acute renal failure. In Johnson, K.B. & Oski, F. A. *Oski's essential pediatrics*. Philadelphia: Lippincott.

Ribby, K.J. & Cox, K.R. (1997). Organization and development of a pediatric end stage renal disease teaching protocol for peritoneal dialysis. *Pediatric Nursing, 23*(4), 393.

Riley, K.E. (1997). Evaluation and management of primary nocturnal enuresis. *Journal of the American Academy of Nurse Practitioners, 9*(1), 33.

Roth, D.R. & Gonzales, E.T. (1997). Urinary tract infections. In Johnson, K.B. & Oski, F.A. *Oski's essential pediatrics*. Philadelphia: Lippincott.

Sigler, M.H. (1997). Transport characteristics of the slow therapies: implications for achieving adequacy of dialysis in acute renal failure. *Advances in Renal Replacement Therapy, 4*(1), 68.

Skoog, S.J., Stokes, A., & Turner, K.L. (1997). Oral desmopressin: a randomized double-blind placebo controlled study of effectiveness in children with primary nocturnal enuresis. *Journal of Urology, 158*(3.2), 1035.

Van der Voort, J. et al. (1997). The struggle to diagnose UTI in children under two in primary care. *Family Practice, 14*(1), 4.

Yu, T.J. & Chen, W.F. (1997). Surgical management of grades III and IV primary vesicoureteral reflux in children with and without acute pyelonephritis as breakthrough infections: a comparative analysis. *Journal of Urology, 157*(4), 1404.

Zoric, D. et al. (1997). Acute poststreptococcal glomerulonephritis in children. *Advances in Experimental Medicine & Biology, 418*, 125.

SUGGESTED READINGS

Cohen, H.A., et al. (1997). Urine samples from disposable diapers: an accurate method for urine cultures. *Journal of Family Practice, 44*(3), 290.

Feld, L.G. et al. (1997). Hematuria: an integrated medical and surgical approach. *Pediatric Clinics of North America, 44*(5), 1101.

Miller, K.L. (1996). Urinary tract infections: children are not little adults. *Pediatric Nursing, 22*(6), 473.

Naseer, S.R. & Steinhardt, G.F. (1997). New renal scars in children with urinary tract infections, vesicoureteral reflux and voiding dysfunction: a prospective evaluation. *The Journal of Urology, 158*(2), 566.

Oliveira, D.B. (1997). Poststreptococcal glomerulonephritis: getting to know an old enemy. *Clinical and Experimental Immunology, 107*(1), 8.

Pastan, S. & Bailey, J. (1998). Dialysis therapy. *New England Journal of Medicine, 338*(20), 1428.

Peritoneal dialysis: making a clean sweep. (1996). *Nursing 26*(5), 58.

Shaw, K.N. & McGowan, K.L. (1997). Evaluation of a rapid screening filter test for urinary tract infection in children. *Pediatric Infectious Disease Journal, 16*(3), 283.

Stewart, C.L. & Barnett, R. (1997). Acute renal failure in infants, children and adults. *Critical Care Clinics, 13*(3), 55.

Urine chemistry: monitoring fluids and electrolytes. *Nursing, 26*(4), 241.

Nursing Care of the Child With a Reproductive Disorder

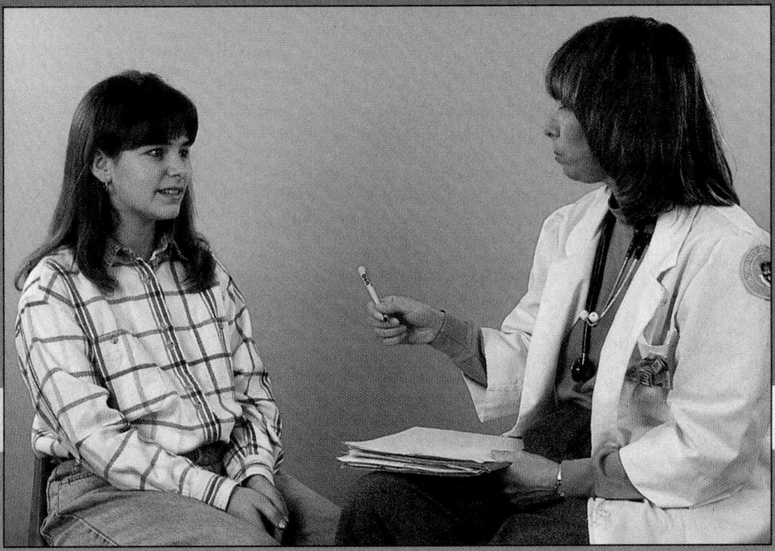

26
CHAPTER

Key Terms

- adenocarcinoma
- adenosis
- amenorrhea
- anovulatory
- cryptorchidism
- dysmenorrhea
- endometriosis
- fibrocystic breast condition
- gynecomastia
- hermaphrodite
- hydrocele
- menorrhagia
- metrorrhagia
- mittelschmerz
- orchiectomy
- orchiopexy
- pelvic inflammatory disease
- premenstrual syndrome (PMS)
- pseudohermaphrodite
- sexually transmitted disease (STD)
- toxic shock syndrome
- varicocele
- vulvovaginitis

Objectives

After mastering the contents of this chapter, you should be able to:

1. Describe common reproductive disorders in children.
2. Assess the child with a reproductive disorder.
3. Formulate nursing diagnoses related to a child's reproductive illness.
4. Develop appropriate outcomes for the child with a reproductive disorder.
5. Plan nursing care related to preventing reproductive disorders in children.
6. Implement nursing care for the child with a reproductive disorder.
7. Evaluate outcomes for achievement and effectiveness of care.
8. Identify National Health Goals related to reproductive disorders that nurses can help the nation achieve.
9. Identify areas for additional nursing research that may benefit those caring for children with reproductive disorders.
10. Analyze ways to implement more family centered nursing care for the child with a reproductive disorder.
11. Integrate knowledge of reproductive disorders in children with the nursing process to achieve quality child health nursing care.

Helen is a 15-year-old seen in a pediatric clinic. She has been diagnosed with gonorrhea. She has a purulent vaginal discharge and burning on urination. When you ask her if she is sexually active, she says no; she thinks she contracted the infection from sharing a towel in a locker room after gym class. As she leaves the clinic you hear her tell the receptionist, "I'm glad I got this early in life. Now I won't have to worry about getting it again." What kind of health education does Helen need?

In previous chapters, you learned about the growth and development of well children. In this chapter, you will add information about the dramatic changes, both physically and psychosocially, that occur when children develop reproductive disorders. This is important information because it constitutes a basis for care and health teaching.

After you have studied the chapter, turn to the Critical Thinking Exercises at the end of the chapter to help sharpen your skills and test your knowledge.

Reproductive disorders in children range from mild infections to serious anatomic malformations that can interfere with fertility. All of these disorders, however, require prompt and careful treatment so that the child will reach adulthood in reproductive health and with a positive sense of sexuality.

Parents are not always as comfortable inquiring about disorders of the reproductive tract as they are inquiring about other disorders. Unless they have clear, thorough explanations of the disease process and prescribed therapy, their reluctance to pursue the subject may leave them confused or misinformed. Even young children can sense that illness affecting genitalia or reproductive ability is viewed by some adults as different from other diseases. As they reach puberty, they need honest explanations about any effect such a condition will have on interpersonal relationships, sexual functioning, or childbearing. National Health Goals related to reproductive disorders in children are shown in the Focus on National Health Goals display.

FOCUS ON NATIONAL HEALTH GOALS

Because sexually transmitted diseases not only cause short-term distress because of painful lesions but can also have long-term implications for fertility and future childbearing, a number of National Health Goals address them. These are:

- Reduce gonorrhea to an incidence of no more than 225 cases/100,000 people from a baseline of 300/100,000.
- Reduce primary and secondary syphilis to an incidence of no more than 10 cases/100,000 people from a baseline of 18 per 100,000.
- Reduce genital herpes from 385,000 to 142,000 first-time consultations per year.
- Reduce the incidence of pelvic inflammatory disease as measured by a reduction in hospitalizations for the condition from 311/100,000 to no more than 250/100,000 women aged 15 through 44 (DHHS, 1995).

Nurses can be instrumental in helping the nation achieve these goals by educating adolescents about effective ways to prevent STDs and recognize the signs and symptoms of these illnesses. Areas that could benefit from additional nursing research in this area include: the most effective ways to teach adolescents about safer sex practices; the reasons adolescents continue to believe that infectious diseases cannot occur to them; and strategies that would make it easier for parents to discuss this topic with adolescents.

NURSING PROCESS OVERVIEW

for Care of the Child With a Reproductive Disorder

Assessment

Assessment of reproductive health begins with the first physical examination at birth and continues at health assessments throughout childhood (see Assessing the Child for Reproductive Disorders). As with other parts of the health interview, questions regarding reproductive health and illness are generally addressed to the parents until the child is able to answer history questions reliably and independently. Once the girl has reached adolescence, a gynecologic history (Box 26-1) should be included in the health assessment. To preserve their privacy, adolescents of both genders may prefer not to be accompanied by a parent.

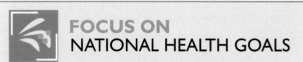

Some adolescents may visit healthcare facilities on their own for various reasons. They may be worried that they have contracted a sexually transmitted disease (STD; a disease spread by sexual relations) or that they have become pregnant, or they want to receive some form of contraception. Before they can admit their chief concern to healthcare providers, however, they may "test" the compassion of the healthcare provider by eliciting a reaction to a minor problem. Be aware that an adolescent who consults a healthcare provider with a seemingly minor concern may only be misinterpreting symptoms and is truly worried that a minor symptom is serious. On the other hand, the adolescent actually may be seeking help for another problem. Asking the adolescent, "Is there anything else that worries you? Any other way we can help you today?" may help you elicit the adolescent's primary concern (see Enhancing Communication).

A pelvic examination is unnecessary for girls who have not yet reached adolescence, but if vaginal walls need to be inspected (because of an inflammation or infection), an otoscope and ear tip can be used. Cotton-tipped applicators moistened with sterile normal saline solution can be used to take culture specimens without causing discomfort. For the adolescent girl,

ASSESSING the Child for Reproductive Disorders

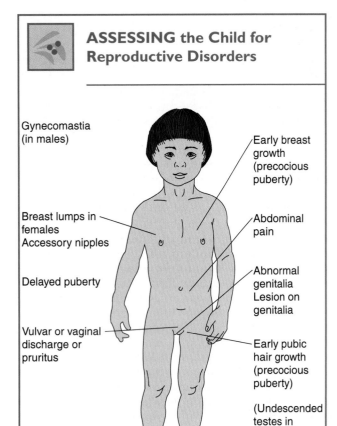

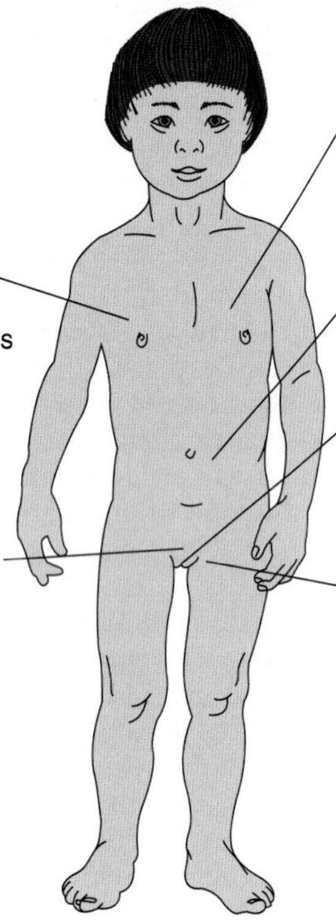

the pelvic examination becomes an important part of health assessment. Because the first pelvic examination can be frightening and embarrassing, spend time with the patient before the procedure to teach her about what is being assessed. A three-dimensional model of internal organs and some representative instruments may be more useful than a verbal description of anatomy. Let her look at and handle a speculum. A small speculum (a Graves, Hoffman, or Pederson) should be used for examining young girls. For their comfort, warm the speculum first.

Allow the adolescent to choose whether she wants a parent to remain in the room with her. Remaining beside her as a support person helps to make the examination less embarrassing. To protect her self-esteem, be sure the girl meets the person who will examine her before she is placed in a lithotomy position (see Focus on Cultural Competence).

A young adolescent may be uncomfortable in a lithotomy position and can be examined in a dorsal recumbent one instead.

Nursing Diagnosis

Selected nursing diagnoses used for children with reproductive disorders include the following:

- Pain related to vaginal infection
- Body image disturbance related to fibrocystic breasts
- Anxiety related to absence or irregularity of menstrual periods in adolescent
- Fear related to surgery on genital organs

BOX 26.1

TAKING A GYNECOLOGIC HISTORY

The nurse who is assessing an adolescent's gynecologic health history must be especially conscious of the patient's sense of modesty and need for privacy. To ensure privacy, conduct the interview without the parent or caregiver present.

Menstrual History

At what age did menarche begin?
What is the frequency and duration of menstrual periods?
What is the amount of menstrual flow? (Document by amount of pads or tampons used.)
Do you experience discomfort? (Document if first day, all days, and so forth, and action taken to relieve it.)
Do any sisters or your mother have dysmenorrhea also (endometriosis is familial)?
Do you experience premenstrual syndrome (e.g., irritability, moodiness, headache, or diarrhea) 1 or 2 days before menses?
What were the dates of your last two menstrual periods and the duration and type of flow?

Reproductive Tract History

Have you had any vaginal discharge? (Document amount and whether pad is necessary or not—include duration, frequency, description, associated symptoms, actions taken.)
Is there vaginal pruritus?
Is there any vaginal odor?
Have you had reproductive tract surgery?

Sexual History

Have you had an STD (herpes, gonorrhea, and syphilis)?
Are you currently sexually active? Heterosexually? Homosexually? Bisexually?
Is there discomfort (dyspareunia) or postcoital spotting?
Do you have any concerns (worried about frequency, position, partner's satisfaction with coitus)? Is orgasm experienced?

Contraception History

What contraceptive currently do you use? (Document length of time used, satisfaction, any problems.)
What types were used in the past?

Breast Health

Have you ever noticed any abnormality (lump, discharge, pain)?
Have you ever had breast surgery?
Have you breast-fed a child?

ENHANCING COMMUNICATION

Terry is a 16-year-old you see at a pediatric clinic. He has mild upper respiratory symptoms.

Less Effective Communication

Nurse: Terry? Doctor Jensen doesn't feel you need anything for your cold. Just drink a little extra fluid and take it easy for a couple days.
Terry: Don't I need a prescription? Some penicillin or something?
Nurse: No. Colds are caused by viruses. Penicillin isn't necessary.
Terry: I want to be sure I get over this. I'd really like an antibiotic of some kind.
Nurse: One really isn't necessary.
Terry: I have a bad cough. I don't think I mentioned that.
Nurse: Doctor Jensen listened to your chest. You don't have anything serious there.
Terry: My stomach doesn't feel very good either. Can't I have something?
Nurse: Sorry. Goodbye now.

More Effective Communication

Nurse: Terry? Doctor Jensen doesn't feel you need anything for your cold. Just drink a little extra fluid and take it easy for a couple days.
Terry: Don't I need a prescription? Some penicillin or something?
Nurse: No. Colds are caused by viruses. Penicillin isn't necessary.
Terry: I want to be sure I get over this. I'd really like an antibiotic of some kind.
Nurse: One really isn't necessary.
Terry: I have a bad cough. I don't think I mentioned that.
Nurse: Doctor Jensen listened to your chest. You don't have anything serious there.
Terry: My stomach doesn't feel very good either. Can't I have something?
Nurse: How many more symptoms do you have that you didn't mention before?
Terry: Well, I have a rash and I'm scared I might have a sex disease.

Adolescents can have difficulty discussing reproductive tract symptoms. If they have too much difficulty, they can try to obtain an antibiotic by describing respiratory or abdominal symptoms. Being alert that adolescents do this helps you to recognize a "growing" history of this type.

Outcome Identification

Identifying goals and outcomes usually stems from an assessment of the child's knowledge about the reproductive system and ways that illness can affect reproductive and sexual functioning. Educating the child about reproductive health may be one of the next areas to plan. When establishing goals with adolescents, remember that it will be difficult to meet goals requiring a wholesale change in lifestyle. It may be more effective to plan for change one step at a time.

FOCUS ON CULTURAL COMPETENCE

Different cultures have different attitudes toward reproductive disorders. Adolescents in Middle Eastern countries, for example, are extremely modest, and so are extremely uncomfortable having pelvic examinations done for reproductive disorders. Adolescents from these countries may be more comfortable if the examiner is a woman.

Implementation

Interventions for children with reproductive disorders should always include education about reproductive functioning and measures for maintaining reproductive and sexual health and preventing illness. Health education regarding the importance of testicular self-examination for adolescent males (see Focus on Nursing Research) and breast self-examination for adolescent females should be stressed at all healthcare visits (see Chapter 13). An organization helpful for referral for adolescents is:

FOCUS ON NURSING RESEARCH

Do High School Health Teachers Provide Instruction About Testicular Self-Examination?

This study compared high school health teachers' beliefs about teaching about testicular cancer and testicular self-examination with what they were actually teaching. As could be expected, those instructors who perceived testicular cancer to be a major threat were most apt to include information about it in health classes. Less than half of the respondents were providing testicular cancer instruction; information on self-examination was provided by less than one-third. Male health educators were more likely than females to teach about testicular cancer and testicular self-examination. Teachers having previous preparation in teaching the topics provided more instruction than those without such instruction.

This is an important research study for nurses because it points out how few boys (less than half) receive information on these important topics in school. It stresses the importance of nurses supplying this information during healthcare visits or health counseling.

Source: Wohl, R. E. & Kane, W. M. (1997). Teachers' beliefs concerning teaching about testicular cancer and testicular self-examination. *Journal of School Health, 67*(3), 106.

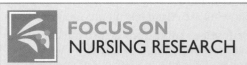

National Women's Health Network
514 10th Street
Suite 400
Washington, DC 20004

Essential nursing interventions also include supporting parents and children through difficult decisions and frightening procedures and providing close observation and empathetic counseling after surgery. Surgery for undescended testes is an example of a procedure that can be traumatic for the child, especially if performed during a developmental stage in which he views such surgery as castrating. Being certain that the child receives good preparation for surgery and reassurance that he will not be mutilated is an essential nursing intervention.

Outcome Evaluation

The responses of children to reproductive dysfunction vary both with the severity of the illness and the specific age and fears of the child. It is safe to assume, however, that children who have suffered from such an illness are at risk for a loss of self-esteem or confusion about their body image. Evaluation of goals and outcomes must include long-term evaluation of the child's coping abilities and self-image. If the child suffers from an STD, evaluation should also address the child's knowledge about avoiding STDs in the future and willingness to seek help should an infection recur. An STD infection in a young child should be investigated as the result of possible sexual abuse.

The following are examples of outcome criteria:

- Child states discomfort from vaginal infection is tolerable after beginning medication.
- Child states she is able to view self as confident despite fibrocystic breasts.
- Child states she is able to wait 6 months without worrying about not yet having a menstrual period.
- Child states he feels less fearful about pending surgery after talking with the healthcare provider.

DISORDERS CAUSED BY ALTERED REPRODUCTIVE DEVELOPMENT

Genetic sex or *biologic gender* (sex chromosome XX or XY) is determined at conception. However, development of the reproductive system, including external genitalia, occurs over two distinct periods: reproductive organs and genitalia begin to differentiate in utero by the 8th week, with growth and refinement occurring over the next several months. This period constitutes the first phase of reproductive development. The second phase occurs with specific endocrine changes that are triggered during puberty; this is a period of maturation of primary and secondary sexual characteristics.

Three disorders related to reproductive development are discussed: ambiguous genitalia, which is a rare condition with different causes and which occurs during fetal development; precocious puberty; and delayed puberty.

Ambiguous Genitalia

To understand ambiguous genitalia, it is important to understand how reproductive organs develop in utero. Although external sexual characteristics generally follow from the XX or XY chromosome, it is possible under certain circumstances for structures generally considered "male" or "female" to develop in either chromosomal gender. Usually, a diagnosis of ambiguous genitalia means that external sexual organs in the child did not follow the normal course of development, so that at birth the external sexual organs are so incompletely or abnormally formed that it is impossible to clearly determine the child's sex by simple observation. For instance, a male infant with *hypospadias* (urethral opening on the underside of the penis) and *cryptorchidism* (undescended testes) may appear more female than male on first inspection (see Chapter 25 for a discussion of hypospadias). Alternatively, a chromosomal female (XX) fetus may become "masculinized" with exposure to androgen in utero (the clitoris is so enlarged that it appears more like a penis, labia may be partially fused so it is difficult to tell them from a male perineum, or the urethra may be displaced so far forward that it is located on the clitoris); the newborn will appear to be a boy on initial inspection. Likewise, under certain conditions, a chromosomal male (XY) may become "feminized," with a lack of fusion of the labioscrotal folds and an incompletely formed penis.

The most common cause of in vitro virilization of females is *congenital adrenocortical syndrome*. The adrenal gland produces androgen instead of adequate cortisone, causing the clitoris to become the size of a typical newborn male's penis (see Chapter 27).

If testosterone was produced in utero but the müllerian duct development was not suppressed, a child may be a **hermaphrodite** (having both ovaries and testes) and, consequently, malformed external genitalia. Children with ambiguous genitalia are often termed **pseudohermaphrodites** because as infants they have some external features of both sexes, although only either ovaries or testes (or neither) are present (Diamond & Sigmundson et al, 1997).

Assessment

If there is any question about the child's gender, a karyotype test will help to establish whether the child is genetically male or female. This involves drawing a specimen of blood, allowing the white blood cells to reach a division stage, then examining them. *Laparoscopy* (introduction of a narrow laparoscope into the abdominal cavity through a half-inch incision under the umbilicus) may determine if ovaries or undescended testes are present. *Intravenous pyelography* is used to establish whether a male has a complete urinary tract. Exploratory surgery may be necessary to establish whether gonads are present.

Therapeutic Management

Once the child's true gender is determined, the extent of necessary reconstructive surgery is determined in consultation with the parents. This may involve correction of a hypospadias or cryptorchidism, removal of labial adhesions, or surgical removal of an enlarged clitoris. When removal of an enlarged clitoris is involved, the parents must consider what the absence of this organ will mean to the girl in terms of later sexual enjoyment. Parents may be well advised to delay this type of surgery until the girl can decide for herself whether she wants it done. Nonfunctioning ovaries or testes are generally removed to prevent malignancy later in life.

If an infant is chromosomally male but does not have an adequate penis, a decision to raise the child as a female might be made, although construction of an artificial penis is more likely.

NURSING DIAGNOSES AND RELATED INTERVENTIONS

When identifying goals and outcomes, be aware that parents under stress may have difficulty making long-range plans. The birth of a child with a perplexing defect produces a particularly high level of stress, hampering parents' ability to think clearly and calmly about their situation.

Nursing Diagnosis: Anxiety related to ambiguous sex of child at birth

Outcome Identification: Parents will demonstrate confidence in healthcare team and increased knowledge about child's condition and necessary care.

Outcome Criteria: Parents voice willingness to support treatment plan, including additional necessary tests, and state they are prepared to make decisions with guidance from healthcare team.

If the sex of the child is unclear, parents should be told this immediately. If told first that their child is a boy, only to be told 24 hours later that "he" is really a girl, parents can have difficulty accepting this drastic change. During this period when the baby's sex is yet to be determined, avoid calling the baby "it." Rather, say "the baby" or "your child." Explain how sexual organs form in utero and that every child has the potential to be externally female or male.

To promote bonding, help parents understand that their child is otherwise perfect (assuming this is true). As the child grows, additional counseling may be needed to help the child adjust to an abnormal appearance or function.

Precocious Puberty

The development of breast or pubic hair before age 8 years or menses before age 9 years is considered precocious sexual development (Plotnick, 1997). Often, such development is expressed as isolated breast or pubic hair growth but can proceed to complete spermatogenesis and menstrual function. Precocious puberty occurs more often in girls than in boys.

This condition is caused by the early production of gonadotropins by the pituitary gland; gonadotropins stimulate the ovaries or testes to produce sex hormones. Such stimulation can occur because of a pituitary tumor, cyst, or traumatic injury to the third ventricle next to the pituitary gland. It also can occur because of estrogen-secreting cysts or tumors of the ovary or testosterone-secreting cysts of the testes. In rare instances, it occurs because of an estrogen- or testosterone-secreting adrenal tumor. In girls, ingestion of a mother's oral contraceptives can also initiate menarche-like changes.

In children affected by precocious puberty, a tumor must be ruled out. When no physical cause, such as a tumor, is detected, the phenomenon appears to occur only because the gonadostat of the hypothalamus was triggered several years too early.

Assessment

Children have increased breast development and accelerated skeletal maturation. Girls have vaginal bleeding with little pubic or axillary hair because of still low androgen secretion. Boys have obvious genital growth. The diagnosis of early puberty is confirmed by serum analysis for estrogen or androgen; these will be at adult levels.

Therapeutic Management

A synthetic analogue to luteinizing hormone-releasing hormone (LHRH) is currently available as Factrel. Administration of this analogue desensitizes the pituitary to the child's own prematurely elevated hypothalamic LHRH. The preparation is administered subcutaneously daily. When discontinued at age 12 or 13 years, puberty progresses normally.

NURSING DIAGNOSES AND RELATED INTERVENTIONS

Nursing Diagnosis: Body image disturbance related to precocious puberty

Outcome Identification: Child will demonstrate adequate level of confidence in self and body in 3 months.

Outcome Evaluation: Child voices an understanding of what is happening and does not evidence excessive shyness or reluctance to interact with peers.

Children who develop precociously may have difficulty interacting with peers because they appear so different from other members of their group. Parents may have difficulty as well and worry about the children becoming sexually active, particularly about girls becoming pregnant (Figure 26-1).

These parents may need reassurance that upon reaching the age of normal puberty, the child will again be the same as other children; the fact that the child's sexual growth started early does not mean the genitals will be out of proportion to the rest of the body as an adult.

Parents must also understand that the child is fully fertile and able to inseminate or conceive when early puberty occurs. Oral contraceptives are not advisable for girls this young because the increased load of estrogen will hasten the closing of epiphyseal lines of long bones too early and possibly stunt their growth permanently.

Parents may need to be reminded that, although their child appears to be much older, the changes are only in sexual characteristics. Household tasks, responsibility, and expectations must be geared to the child's chronologic age, not to outward appearance.

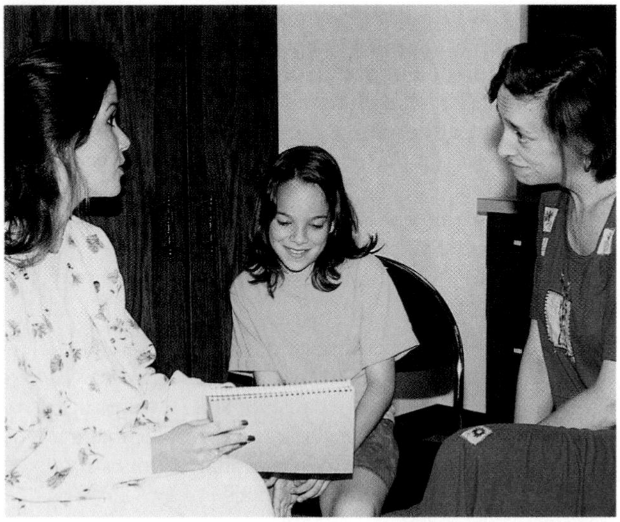

FIGURE 26.1 A child with precocious puberty. Here the nurse provides teaching and reassurance about the child's early sexual development.

Delayed Puberty

Delayed puberty is, as the name implies, the failure of pubertal changes to occur at the usual age. The family history of many children reveals a family tendency for late maturation. If so, the child needs a thorough physical examination that will disclose whether some secondary sex characteristics are present or if endocrine stimulation is beginning.

If girls have not begun to menstruate by age 17 years and pathology has been ruled out, menstrual cycles can be started by administering estrogen. Many girls worry considerably about delayed menstruation, but once reassured that development is merely delayed, they are usually willing to wait for menarche to occur on its own.

Similarly, boys who are distressed by their lack of development may receive testosterone supplements to stimulate hair and genital growth (Plotnick, 1997).

✔ **CHECKPOINT QUESTIONS**

1. Does precocious puberty occur more often in males or females?
2. Girls have until what age before they are considered to have delayed puberty?

REPRODUCTIVE DISORDERS IN MALES

Common reproductive disorders in males include structural alterations in the penis or testes such as phimosis and cryptorchidism, inflammation such as balanoposthitis, and, in adolescents, testicular cancer.

Balanoposthitis

Balanoposthitis is inflammation of the glans and prepuce of the penis. It is generally caused by poor hygiene and may accompany a urethritis or a regional dermatitis.

Assessment

The prepuce and glans become red and swollen; a purulent discharge may be present. The boy may have difficulty voiding because of crusting at the meatal opening and because acidic urine touching the denuded surface of the glans causes pain.

Therapeutic Management

Medical treatment involves local application of heat; this can be carried out with warm wet soaks or warm baths. A local antibiotic ointment may be prescribed. If *phimosis* (a tight foreskin) appears to be contributing to the condition, circumcision may be advocated after the inflammation subsides. This will prevent the condition from recurring.

Although balanoposthitis is painful, a boy may tolerate the discomfort for several days because he is too embarrassed to discuss the problem. He may think it was caused by masturbation (which can contribute to the irritation) or sexual activity, and is reluctant to seek help for fear of being criticized. He can be reassured that the problem is local and will have no long-range effect. Any discharge should be cultured to rule out gonorrhea.

Phimosis

In the normal infant, the foreskin is tight at birth and even held by adhesions. Generally, it cannot be retracted. After a few months, the adhesions should dissolve and the foreskin will become retractable. If not, the infant may have phimosis. With this, the foreskin remains so tight that it interferes with voiding, and balanoposthitis may develop because the foreskin cannot be retracted for cleaning. True phimosis is rare but can be corrected by circumcision (Dewan et al, 1996). The technique of circumcision is discussed in Chapter 5.

Cryptorchidism

Cryptorchidism is failure of one or both testes to descend from the abdominal cavity to the scrotum. The testes descend into the scrotal sac during months 7 to 9 of intrauterine life. They may descend any time up to 6 weeks after birth; rarely do they descend after that point.

The cause of undescended testes is unclear. Fibrous bands at the inguinal ring or inadequate length of spermatic vessels may prevent descent. Testes apparently descend because of stimulation by testosterone; hence, it is possible that a lower than normal level of testosterone production prevents descent. About 30% of premature infants and 3% to 4% of term infants are born with undescended testes (Roth & Gonzales, 1997).

Assessment

Early detection of undescended testes is important, because the warmth of the abdominal cavity may inhibit development of the testes and affect spermatogenesis. After puberty, sperm production deteriorates rapidly in undescended testes, and the testes may undergo a malignant change. Anchoring the testes in the scrotal sac may not prevent malignancy but will allow the boy to perform preventive measures such as testicular self-examination.

It is more common for the right testis to remain undescended than the left one. In approximately 20% of all cases, both testes remain undescended. Some children may be diagnosed with undescended testes when, in fact, poor examining technique caused the testes to retract. If the child is supine or the examining room is chilly, the scrotal sac may appear to be empty. Excessive palpation or stroking the inner thigh may also stimulate the cremasteric reflex and cause retraction. In these instances, testes descend when the child is standing or after a warm bath.

An undescended testis may be at the inguinal ring (true undescended testis) or ectopic (still in the abdomen). Laparoscopy is effective in identifying undescended testes. Because testes arise from the same germ tissue as the kidneys, the kidney function of children with ectopic testes is usually evaluated. If undescended testes and other factors (e.g., ambiguous genitals) pose questions about the child's gender, a *karyotype* may be done to determine true sex.

Therapeutic Management

Sometimes the testes descend spontaneously during the first year of life, so treatment is usually delayed until 6 to 18 months. Children may be given chorionic gonadotropin hormone to stimulate testes descent, but this therapy is successful only in approximately 20% of cases. If necessary, surgery (**orchiopexy**) by laparoscopy during the infant or toddler years will correct the condition (El-Gohary, 1997).

NURSING DIAGNOSES AND RELATED INTERVENTIONS

If an orchiopexy is scheduled, nursing goals focus on parent and child teaching, preoperative preparation, and postoperative care.

Nursing Diagnosis: Knowledge deficit related to parents' and child's inexperience with surgical procedure and postoperative treatment plan

Outcome Identification: Parents and child (if old enough) will demonstrate increased level of knowledge about surgical procedure by time of admission.

Outcome Evaluation: Parents (and child) state what will be done during surgery.

Boys who are old enough to understand need good preparation for this type of surgery. Use an anatomically correct picture to point out the exact site at which surgery will be performed. Reassure the boy that his penis itself will not be cut. The child may not voice a fear of mutilation, but you can assume that it exists, especially in preschool children.

During surgery, an internal suture may be inserted to hold the testis in place. Although the child may be discharged from the hospital the same day, his activity will be limited until approximately the second day after surgery.

Nursing Diagnosis: Body image disturbance related to change in physical appearance

Outcome Identification: Child will evidence an adequate level of self-acceptance during surgical experience.

Outcome Evaluation: Child (if verbal) states he views self as whole person and interacts with peers without excessive shyness or hesitancy.

Postoperative evaluation should ascertain that the suture line is healing well and that both testes can be palpated in the scrotum. It should also address the boy's feelings about the surgery and the changes in his body. He may need an opportunity to express his fears about mutilation or castration by playing with puppets or dolls after surgery. When he reaches puberty, he should be taught testicular self-examination to assess any early symptoms of malignancy, such as nodules or growths (see Chapter 13).

Hydrocele

When a testis descends into the scrotum in utero, it is preceded by a fold of tissue, the *processus vaginalis.* Fluid that may collect in this space (**hydrocele**) can be revealed by prenatal sonogram (Pretorius et al, 1998). At birth, the scrotum of the newborn appears enlarged. On *transillumination* (the shining of a light through the scrotal sac), the area is illuminated by the water and shines or glows (Barber, 1996). If the hydrocele is uncomplicated, the fluid will gradually be reabsorbed into the body and no treatment is necessary. The child's parents can be assured that the hydrocele is only excess fluid and that the scrotal enlargement is not due to an abnormal testis, tumor, or hernia.

A hydrocele may form later in life due to *inguinal hernia* (abdominal contents extruding into the scrotum through the inguinal ring, with accompanying fluid). If this is the case, the hernia must be repaired for the hydrocele to be reabsorbed (see Chapter 24). Injection of a drug to decrease fluid production (*sclerotherapy*) may also be effective.

Varicocele

A **varicocele** is abnormal dilation of the veins of the spermatic cord (Figure 26-2). It tends to occur most often on the left side. Identifying a varicocele is important in adolescents because, although asymptomatic, the increased heat and congestion in the testicles can lead to infertility. No treatment is necessary unless fertility becomes a concern, at which time the varicocele can be surgically removed. The patient may report some local tenderness and edema for a few days after surgery. Edema can be minimized by applying ice for the first few hours postoperatively.

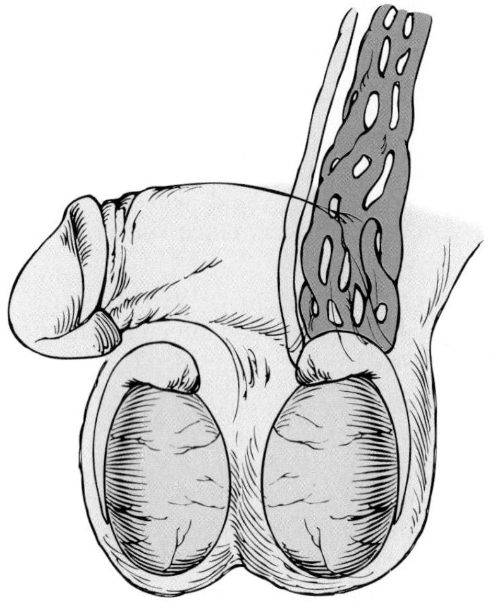

FIGURE 26.2 Identifying and correcting varicocele in adolescent males is important because the condition is associated with infertility.

Testicular Torsion

Testicular torsion (twisting of the spermatic cord) is a surgical emergency. It occurs most frequently in early adolescence, although it can be present in newborns (Elder, 1998). The boy apparently has less than normal testicular support, which allows the spermatic cord to twist. It usually results from a sports activity. The boy experiences severe scrotal pain and perhaps nausea and vomiting; the testis feels tender to palpation and edema begins to develop. If the condition is not recognized promptly (within 4 hours), irreversible change in the testes may occur from lack of circulation to the organ. Boys need to be educated about the phenomenon so that they report symptoms promptly.

Testicular Cancer

Testicular cancer is rare (only 1% of all malignancies). It usually occurs between ages 15 and 35 years, often in association with cryptorchidism. If discovered early, testicular cancer is one of the most curable cancers (O'Callaghan & Mead, 1997).

Symptoms include painless testicular enlargement and a feeling of heaviness in the scrotum. The disease metastasizes rapidly, leading to abdominal and back pain due to retroperitoneal node extension, weight loss, and general weakness. **Gynecomastia** (enlargement of the breasts) may arise from human chorionic gonadotropins (HCG) produced by the tumor. HCG and alpha-fetoprotein, which are considered tumor markers, can be detected in blood serum.

Therapy for testicular malignancy is **orchiectomy** (removal of the testis) followed by radiation or chemotherapy. A gel-filled prosthesis may be inserted for a symmetric appearance. Infertility in the opposite testis results after radiation therapy. For some patients "sperm banking," or preserving frozen sperm before the procedure, may be presented as an option for future family planning.

Teaching males to perform testicular self-examination for early detection is as important as teaching females to perform breast self-examination (see Chapter 13).

> **✔ CHECKPOINT QUESTIONS**
>
> 3. Why is it important that undescended testes be brought down into the scrotal sac before puberty?
> 4. What is the first symptom of testicular torsion?

REPRODUCTIVE DISORDERS IN FEMALES

The most frequent reproductive disorders in females involve vaginal or menstrual irregularities. Other disorders are caused by structural alterations of the reproductive organs, such as imperforate hymen, **pelvic inflammatory disease** (PID), or infections caused by STDs.

Menstrual Disorders

Because menstruation is an ongoing process throughout half of a woman's life, it affects her self-image significantly. An irregularity such as a painful cycle can exert a major influence on daily activities and should never be taken lightly; it is a health concern requiring as much time and attention as that given to other concerns.

Menstrual disorders generally fall into two categories: (1) menstruation that is painful or uncomfortable and (2) infrequent or too-frequent cycles.

Mittelschmerz

Some women may experience abdominal pain during ovulation from the release of accompanying prostaglandins. It may also be caused by a drop or two of follicular fluid or blood spilling into the abdominal cavity. This pain, called **mittelschmerz,** may range from a few sharp cramps to several hours of discomfort. It is typically felt on one side of the abdomen (near an ovary) and may be accompanied by scant vaginal spotting.

An advantage of mittelschmerz pain is that it clearly marks ovulation. If pain is felt in the right lower quadrant, it can be differentiated from appendicitis by the lack of associated symptoms (i.e., nausea, vomiting, fever, abdominal guarding, and rebound tenderness) as well as by its occurrence in the menstrual cycle. Usually mittelschmerz is of limited duration and intensity and, therefore, not a great source of discomfort.

Dysmenorrhea

Dysmenorrhea is painful menstruation. For generations, it was thought to be mainly psychological, needing no treatment other than reassurance that it was a normal phenomenon and something women should endure. Today, it is known that the pain is due to the release of prostaglandins in response to tissue destruction during the ischemic phase of the menstrual cycle (Kennedy,

1997). Prostaglandin release causes smooth muscle contraction in the uterus.

Dysmenorrhea can also be a symptom of an underlying illness such as pelvic inflammatory disease, *uterine myomas* (tumors), or *endometriosis* (abnormal formation of endometrial tissue.

Assessment. As many as 80% of adolescents have some discomfort with menstruation; in approximately 10% the discomfort seriously interferes with daily living. Dysmenorrhea is *primary* if it occurs in the absence of organic disease; it is *secondary* if it occurs as a result of organic disease. There may be a "bloating" feeling and light cramping 24 hours before menstrual flow. Pain is mainly noticed, however, when the flow begins. Colicky (sharp) pain is superimposed on a dull, nagging pain across the lower abdomen. Accompanying this is an "aching, pulling" sensation of the vulva and inner thighs. Some adolescents have mild diarrhea with the abdominal cramping. Mild breast tenderness, abdominal distention, nausea and vomiting, headache, and facial flushing may be present.

Therapeutic Management. Painful symptoms can generally be controlled by an analgesic such as acetylsalicylic acid (aspirin). Acetylsalicylic acid works well as an analgesic for dysmenorrhea because it is a mild prostaglandin inhibitor. Although adolescents are generally advised not to take aspirin because of its link to Reye's syndrome, girls may take it safely at the beginning of a menstrual period as long as they do not have additional flulike symptoms. A major breakthrough in relieving menstrual discomfort was achieved by the discovery that the anti-inflammatory drug ibuprofen (Motrin, Advil, Nuprin) is a stronger prostaglandin inhibitor and relieves more severe menstrual pain. Ibuprofen is currently available over the counter. Also effective are naproxen and bromfenac sodium (Mehlisch & Fulmer, 1997). Low-dose oral contraceptives to prevent ovulation may also be effective if pregnancy is not desired. One disadvantage of this is the possible adverse effects of long-term estrogen administration.

During the first year or two of menstruation dysmenorrhea rarely occurs, because early menstrual cycles are usually **anovulatory.** As ovulation begins, typical menstrual discomfort begins.

NURSING DIAGNOSES AND RELATED INTERVENTIONS

Nursing Diagnosis: Pain related to dysmenorrhea

Outcome Identification: Client will not experience pain above a tolerable level.

Outcome Evaluation: Client states that she has some control over pain through nonpharmacologic or pharmacologic methods.

Several nonpharmacologic solutions may help relieve dysmenorrhea. Decreasing sodium intake a few days before an expected menstrual flow by omitting salty foods such as potato chips, pretzels, and ham and other luncheon meats, and by not adding salt to foods, may help reduce "bloated" feelings. Abdominal breathing (breathing in and out slowly, allowing the abdominal wall to rise with each inhalation) may also be helpful. Applying heat to the abdomen with a heating pad or taking a hot shower or tub bath may relax muscle tension and relieve pain. Caution young girls not to apply heat to their abdomen for abdominal pain unless they are actually menstruating; if the pain results from an inflamed appendix, heat can cause rupture of the appendix and life-threatening peritonitis. Resting may help to relieve vulvar pain; abdominal massage (effleurage or light massage) may feel soothing. Adolescents who remain sexually active during their menses may discover that orgasm helps relieve pelvic engorgement and, therefore, cramping.

Menorrhagia

Menorrhagia is an abnormally heavy menstrual flow. It may occur in girls close to puberty and in women nearing menopause because of anovulatory cycles. Without ovulation and subsequent progesterone secretion, estrogen secretion continues and causes extreme proliferation of endometrium.

Assessment. It is difficult to determine when a menstrual flow is abnormally heavy, but one method is to ask the client how long it takes her to saturate a sanitary napkin or tampon. A sanitary napkin or tampon holds approximately 25 mL of fluid. Saturating a pad or tampon in less than 1 hour means the flow is heavier than usual. There is often an unusual amount of flow in clients using intrauterine devices (IUDs). With oral contraceptives the flow is often light, but may seem alarmingly heavy once the pills are discontinued. Usually, however, this is just a return of the adolescent's normal flow.

A heavy flow can indicate endometriosis (see below), a systemic disease (anemia), blood dyscrasia such as a clotting defect, or a uterine abnormality such as a myoma (fibroid) tumor. It can be a symptom of infection such as pelvic inflammatory disease or an indication of early pregnancy loss that is coincidentally occurring at the time of an expected menstrual period.

It is important to determine the cause of menorrhagia because it can lead to anemia from excessive iron loss, thus requiring iron supplements to achieve sufficient hemoglobin formation. The adolescent who is losing excessive blood because of anovulatory cycles may be administered progesterone during the luteal phase to prevent proliferative growth during this phase of the cycle; if the ability to conceive is unimportant, adolescents may be placed on a low-dose oral contraceptive, which decreases the flow.

Metrorrhagia

Metrorrhagia is bleeding between menstrual periods. This is normal in some adolescents who have spotting at the time of ovulation ("mittelstaining"). It may also occur in clients on oral contraceptives (breakthrough bleeding) for the first 3 or 4 months. Additionally, vaginal irritation from infection may cause midcycle spotting. Spotting may also represent a temporarily low level of progesterone production and endometrial sloughing (dysfunctional uterine bleeding or a luteal phase defect), a condition that tends to occur near the end of the reproductive years.

If metrorrhagia occurs for more than one menstrual cycle and the client is not on oral contraceptives, she should be referred to her primary care provider for examination, because vaginal bleeding is also an early sign of uterine carcinoma or ovarian cysts.

Endometriosis

Endometriosis is the abnormal growth of extrauterine endometrial cells, often in the cul-de-sac of the peritoneal cavity, the uterine ligaments, and the ovaries. This abnormal tissue results from excessive endometrial production and a reflux of blood and tissue through the fallopian tubes during menstrual flow. As many as 25% of women in the United States have endometriosis. It tends to occur most often in white nulliparous women, but there is also a familial tendency. Daughters of women with endometriosis may develop symptoms of dysmenorrhea early in life and may be encouraged to have children before overgrowth of the endometrium becomes so extensive that it interferes with conception.

The excessive production of endometrial tissue may be related to a deficient immunologic response. In many women, it appears to be related to excess estrogen production or a failed luteal menstrual phase. Many women with endometriosis do not ovulate or ovulate irregularly. Estrogen secretion continues through the cycle rather than becoming secondary to progesterone late in the cycle, as happens with normal ovulation. This proliferation of tissue then forces the blood back into the fallopian tubes.

Endometriosis causes dysmenorrhea when the abnormal tissue responds to estrogen and progesterone stimulation by swelling and then sloughing its layers in the same manner as the uterine lining. This causes inflammation of surrounding tissue in the abdominal cavity and an even greater release of prostaglandins. Abnormal tissue in the pelvic cul-de-sac may cause *dyspareunia* (painful coitus) because it puts pressure on the posterior vagina. Infertility may result when the fallopian tubes become immobilized and blocked by tissue implants or adhesions, preventing peristaltic motion and ova transport.

Assessment. Pelvic examination may show that the uterus is displaced by tender, fixed, palpable nodules. Nodules in the cul-de-sac or on an ovary may be palpable as well. If the endometriosis is minimal, the woman will not experience related symptoms. If the condition is moderate or extensive, she may experience dysmenorrhea or dyspareunia (Duleba, 1997).

Therapeutic Management. Treatment for endometriosis can be medical or surgical, depending on the extent of the disease. Estrogen–progesterone-based oral contraceptives may stimulate implant regression as the tissue sloughs under the influence of the progesterone. Danazol, a synthetic androgen, also helps shrink the abnormal tissue (see Drug Highlight: Danazol). Laparotomy and excision by laser surgery is the most effective measure, but because it is a highly invasive procedure, a course of conservative medical treatment may be tried first.

WHAT IF? What if an adolescent girl with endometriosis tells you that she feels strange taking a male hormone? How would you explain the action of this drug in reference to the endometriosis?

DRUG HIGHLIGHT

Danazol (Danocrine)

Class: Androgen and hormone

Action: Suppresses release of follicle stimulating hormone (FSH) and luteinizing hormone (LH) to inhibit ovulation and treat endometriosis; decreases estrogen and progesterone levels and inhibits synthesis of sex steroids to decrease nodularity, pain, and tenderness of fibrocystic breasts; and binds to steroid receptors in cells of target tissues. Danazol is also used to treat precocious puberty, gynecomastia, and menorrhagia.

Pregnancy risk category: C

Dosage: Endometriosis (begin therapy during menstruation or after evidence that patient is not pregnant): 800 mg/d, PO, in two divided doses decreasing gradually to maintain amenorrhea; for mild endometriosis, 200–400 mg, PO, in two divided doses over 3 to 6 months.

Fibrocystic breast condition (begin therapy during menstruation or after evidence that patient is not pregnant): 100–400 mg/d, PO, in two divided doses for 2 to 6 months.

Possible adverse effects: Dizziness, headache, fatigue, fluid retention, weight gain, edema, acne, oily skin or hair, mild hirsutism, decreased breast size

Nursing Implications:

- Assess for conditions that contraindicate drug therapy, including known allergy to danazol, impaired liver function, abnormal genital bleeding, pregnancy, or lactation.
- Document baseline measurements: weight, hair distribution pattern, skin color, texture and oiliness, breast condition (nodularity), vital signs, peripheral edema, emotional status, etc.
- Teach patient about possible adverse effects of therapy; for example, females should know that androgenic effects may not subside when therapy ends. Male patients should know that sperm should be tested periodically to detect changes that require discontinuing therapy. Both sexes should monitor liver function with regularly scheduled blood tests.
- Advise patients to report the following adverse effects: abnormal facial hair growth, deepening of the voice, unusual bleeding or bruising, fever, chills, sore throat, vaginal itching or irritation.

Amenorrhea

Amenorrhea, or absence of a menstrual flow, strongly suggests pregnancy but is by no means definitive because it may also result from tension, anxiety, fatigue, chronic illness, extreme dieting, or strenuous exercise. Competitive swimmers, long distance runners (50 to 75 miles weekly), and ballet dancers notice that intensive training causes their periods to become scant and irregular. This appears to be associated with their low ratio of body fat to body muscle, which leads to excessive secretion of prolactin. An elevation in prolactin causes a decrease in LHRH from the hypothalamus, followed by a decline in follicle-stimulating hormone, follicular development, and estrogen secretion. Menstrual cycles generally return to normal within 3 months of discontinuing strenuous training and conditioning.

Adolescents who wish to maintain a normal cycle while training for a sports event may take bromocriptine (Parlodel), which can reduce high prolactin levels by acting on the hypothalamus and initiating menstruation each month. Many adolescents, however, view the absence of menstrual periods as a benefit during sports training. If a menstrual flow is delayed and pregnancy is suspected, bromocriptine should be discontinued, because it is potentially teratogenic.

Amenorrhea also occurs when females diet excessively, partially as a natural defense mechanism to limit ovulation and as a means of conserving body fluid. Women with *anorexia nervosa* or *bulimia* (eating disorders described in Chapter 33) often develop amenorrhea after approximately 3 months of excessive dieting or bingeing and dieting; as in athletes, this is due to an increase in prolactin.

Premenstrual Syndrome

Premenstrual syndrome (PMS) is a condition occurring in the luteal phase of the menstrual cycle. PMS has both behavioral and physiologic symptoms. Because of the variety of possible symptoms, the incidence of PMS can be considered quite high: it has been estimated that as many as 30% of women experience some degree of PMS, a cluster of symptoms that includes anxiety, fatigue, abdominal bloating, headache, appetite disturbance, irritability, and depression (Peters, 1997). For some women, these symptoms can be incapacitating.

The cause of PMS is unknown, but it may be due to the drop in progesterone just before menses. A syndrome similar to PMS may occur in women after tubal ligation: decrease in the blood supply to the ovary apparently results in decreased luteal function and low progesterone levels. In some women, a vitamin B-complex deficiency may lead to estrogen excess, causing an abnormal ratio of estrogen to progesterone; other related causes may be poor renal clearance leading to water retention, an endometrial toxin from the presence of ischemic tissue, hypoglycemia that leads to a surge of adrenaline, and low calcium levels.

Symptoms of PMS vary from cycle to cycle and throughout life. Therapy is aimed at correcting specific symptoms.

Clients who think they have PMS should keep a diary of when symptoms occur. If they are aware of recurring patterns that indicate PMS, they will be better able to recognize the cause of their increased tension or heightened emotional reactions to everyday stressors. They should be certain their diet is high in vitamins and calcium and low in salt. Some females benefit from vaginal progesterone suppositories to increase their progesterone level. If they suspect they are pregnant, they should not use progesterone suppositories, since progesterone can harm the fetus. This syndrome needs to be studied in greater depth so that better diagnostic techniques and treatment can be developed.

Other Reproductive Disorders in Females

Imperforate Hymen

The *hymen* is a membranous ring of tissue partly obstructing the vaginal opening. An *imperforate hymen* totally occludes the vagina, preventing the escape of vaginal secretions and menstrual blood.

Before menarche, the child with an imperforate hymen generally has no symptoms. With onset, the menstrual flow is obstructed. It builds up in the vagina, causing increased pressure in the vagina and uterus and eventual abdominal pain. Palpation of the abdomen will reveal a lower abdominal mass. On vaginal examination, an intact, bulging hymen is evident.

The treatment is surgical incision or removal of the hymenal tissue. The girl may have local pain following the incision, which can be relieved by a mild analgesic and warm baths.

Careful explanation of this condition will help the girl understand that this will not interfere with sexual relations or future childbearing. Because most girls of early menstrual age have scant knowledge of anatomy, pictures of the reproductive tract will make it clear that this is a local and minor problem.

Adenosis

From 1940 to 1970, women experiencing bleeding in early pregnancy were commonly given diethylstilbestrol (DES), a nonsteroidal estrogen, to prevent spontaneous abortion. As many as 2 million women received the drug, which was later found to be ineffective and led to **adenosis** (the formation of vaginal cysts) in female offspring.

In the normal female fetus, the upper vagina, exterior cervix, and endocervix are covered with columnar epithelium in early stages. During late fetal development, these areas gradually change to squamous epithelium, except in the endocervix, where the original columnar formation remains. When estrogen was taken by the mother, however, the change in tissue was inhibited and the fetus was left with only columnar epithelium. At puberty when the squamous epithelium began to develop, it grew so rapidly that it led to adenosis and possibly vaginal carcinoma (**adenocarcinoma**).

Males born of pregnancies in which DES was administered had a possibility of developing hypoplastic testes, epididymal cysts, and alteration in sperm production as they reached maturity. The condition is very rare today because DES is no longer prescribed during pregnancy.

Toxic Shock Syndrome

Toxic shock syndrome (TSS) is an infection usually caused by toxin-producing strains of *Staphylococcus au-*

reus organisms. Organisms typically enter the body through vaginal walls damaged by the insertion of tampons at the time of a menstrual period. As many as 70% of women in the United States used tampons in 1980, the year that TSS reached its peak incidence. The incidence of disease has since fallen because women have become more cautious about heavy tampon usage (Chance, 1996).

Assessment. The symptoms of TSS appear in Empowering the Family: Preventing Toxic Shock Syndrome. Any female who develops fever with diarrhea and vomiting during a menstrual period should suspect TSS. Remember, however, a number of females have mild diarrhea as a normal accompaniment to dysmenorrhea (see Box 26-2 for symptoms of TSS).

Therapeutic Management. Women or adolescents with suspected TSS need a careful vaginal examination and removal of any tampon particles, as well as cervical and vaginal cultures for *S. aureus.* Iodine douches may reduce the number of organisms present vaginally. *S. aureus* is generally resistant to penicillin but not to penicillinase-resistant antibiotics (i.e., cephalosporins, oxacillins, or clindamycins). Intravenous fluid therapy to restore circulating fluid volume and increase blood pressure or vasopressors such as dopamine (Intropin) may be necessary to increase the blood pressure. Diuretic therapy to shift fluid back to the intravascular circulation and support of renal and cardiac failure may be necessary. Recovery occurs in 7 to 10 days; fatigue and weakness may remain for months afterward.

The rate of TSS recurrence is 28% to 64%, generally within 2 months of the first attack. Recurrence probably happens because the organism is not completely eliminated from the body.

BOX 26.2

SYMPTOMS OF TSS*

- Temperature more than 38.9°C (102°F)
- Vomiting and diarrhea
- A macular (sunburn-like) rash that desquamates on palms and soles 1 to 2 weeks after illness
- Severe hypotension (systolic pressure less than 90 mm Hg)
- Shock, leading to poor organ perfusion
- Impaired renal function with elevated blood urea nitrogen or creatinine at least twice the upper limit of normal
- Severe muscle pain or creatine phosphokinase at least twice the upper limit of normal
- Hyperemia of mucous membrane
- Impaired liver function with increased total bilirubin and increased serum glutamic-oxaloacetic transaminase at twice the upper limit of normal
- Decreased platelet count
- Central nervous system symptoms of disorientation, confusion, severe headache

* Three symptoms must be present for diagnosis.

NURSING DIAGNOSES AND RELATED INTERVENTIONS

Nursing Diagnosis: Knowledge deficit related to safe tampon use

Outcome Identification: The client will demonstrate increased knowledge of tampon use by end of health care visit.

EMPOWERING THE FAMILY:
Preventing Toxic Shock Syndrome

Although toxic shock syndrome can occur for other reasons, it most often occurs during a menstrual flow when tampons are used. Measures to help prevent the syndrome are:

- Do not use tampons.
- Use only tampons made of natural materials such as cotton, not synthetics such as cellulose or polyester; avoid high-absorbency tampons.
- Change tampons at least every 4 hours during use.
- Alternate the use of tampons with sanitary pads.
- Avoid handling the portion of the tampon that will be inserted vaginally.
- Do not use tampons near the end of a menstrual flow when excessive vaginal dryness can result from scant flow.
- Do not insert more than one tampon at a time to avoid abrasions and to keep the vaginal walls from becoming too dry.
- Avoid deodorant tampons, sanitary pads, and feminine hygiene sprays; these products can irritate the vulvar–vaginal lining.
- If fever, vomiting, or diarrhea occurs during a menstrual period, discontinue tampon use and immediately consult a healthcare provider because these are symptoms of TSS.
- Anyone who has had one episode of TSS is well advised not to use tampons again or at least not until two vaginal cultures for *Staphylococcus aureus,* the bacteria usually responsible for TSS, are negative.

Outcome Evaluation: The client states common rules such as not handling the portion of the tampon that will be inserted vaginally.

The risk of developing TSS has decreased greatly since tampon manufacturers recalled the products most likely to cause it. Educating females about menstrual hygiene and precautions for tampon use has lowered the incidence still further.

Vulvovaginitis

Vulvovaginitis is inflammation of the vulva or vagina. It is accompanied by pain, odor, pruritus, and a vaginal discharge. It may occur in a girl of any age but tends to be more frequent as the girl reaches puberty, and a change to adult *p*H and the presence of vaginal secretions make the vagina more receptive to infections. The display Empowering the Family: Tips for Relieving the Pain of Vulvitis discusses common measures to relieve discomfort.

Preschool and School-Age Children. Vaginal discharge may occur before menarche, but bleeding is rarely seen. If bleeding is present, its cause must be determined. A cystitis can cause urethral bleeding; scratching from rectal pruritus will lead to rectal bleeding. The cause of true vaginal bleeding in this early age group is generally either irritation of an inserted foreign object in the vagina, infestation of pinworms, or *vaginitis* (inflammation or infection). Sexual abuse must also be investigated as a cause of any bleeding, tenderness, or infection (see Chapter 34). Precocious puberty must also be ruled out.

Treatment for pinworm is discussed in Chapter 22. If there is a foreign body in the vagina, it should be removed. Vaginal examination is necessary first to locate the object and then to confirm that it has been fully removed. This may be difficult for girls to accept, and vaginal manipulation and stretching can be painful. A small speculum helps reduce the pain. A local antibiotic ointment or warm bath may be ordered to reduce accompanying infection and inflammation.

Sometimes daily bubble baths can cause vulvar irritation. This can be quickly remedied by discontinuing the bubble baths; irritation from such a compound can lead not only to local discomfort but to urinary tract infection as well.

A few preschool or school-age children develop a vaginitis from streptococcus or from *Escherichia coli* introduced from the anus by improper perineal care after voiding or bowel movements. A tight hymen then traps the microorganisms in the vagina and leads to infection. The girl needs to be reminded to wipe from front to back following voiding or bowel movements.

Adolescents. As a girl enters puberty, she may notice a slight vaginal discharge due to increased vaginal secretions. She can be reassured that this is normal. To keep from developing vulvar irritation, girls should wear cotton underpants rather than nylon (so moisture is absorbed better) and dry the vulva thoroughly after bathing or swimming.

Some girls may develop vulvar irritation from personal hygiene sprays or douches. These products are unnecessary. Good hygiene can be achieved by daily washing and frequent changing of tampons or pads during menstruation. This will prevent chafing or stasis of menstrual blood and help prevent irritation and excessive odor.

Pelvic Inflammatory Disease

Pelvic inflammatory disease (PID) is infection of the pelvic organs: the uterus, fallopian tubes, ovaries, and their supporting structures. The infection can extend to cause pelvic peritonitis. Although sexual transmission accounts for approximately 75% of all PIDs (gonorrheal and chlamydial or-

EMPOWERING THE FAMILY: Tips for Relieving the Pain of Vulvitis

- Wash vulva twice a day with mild, nonperfumed soap and water and pat dry. This removes secretions and decreases irritation. Wash and dry from front to back to prevent spreading rectal contamination forward.
- Take sitz baths or apply warm moist compresses three times a day to soothe area and keep it free of irritating discharge.
- After drying cleansed area, apply cornstarch for comfort and to absorb residual moisture. Avoid products such as talc, which has been associated with ovarian cancer.
- Avoid bubble bath or feminine hygiene sprays because ingredients in these products may cause local irritation or contribute to urinary tract infections.
- Take acetaminophen (Tylenol) every 4 hours. Acetaminophen is an analgesic medication that relieves pain and reduces itching, which is a mild pain sensation.
- Avoid scratching, which may increase abrasions and introduce a secondary infection. Instead, apply a cold compress to minimize itching sensation.
- Wear cotton underwear, which allows air to circulate and moisture to evaporate, rather than nylon or silk, which prevents circulation and preserves moisture.
- Sleep without underwear.
- Use an anesthetic spray or hydrocortisone cream only as prescribed.
- Carefully follow instructions provided by nurse or physician for caring for a vaginal infection; only when the infection subsides will the vulvitis clear.

ganisms are frequently responsible), infections from other causes such as *E. coli* and *Streptococcus* are beginning to occur more frequently and may be as severe.

PID begins with a cervical infection that spreads by surface invasion along the uterine endometrium and then out to the fallopian tubes and ovaries. It is most likely to occur at the end of a menstrual period, because menstrual blood provides an excellent growth medium for bacteria and there is loss of the normal barrier of cervical mucus during this time.

Assessment. As peritoneal tissue becomes inflamed and edematous, a purulent exudate forms. If the process is untreated, it enters a chronic phase and fibrotic scarring with stricture of the fallopian tubes will result. With acute PID, the adolescent notices severe pain in the lower abdomen. She may have an accompanying heavy purulent discharge. As the infection progresses, she will develop a fever. Leukocytosis and an elevated erythrocyte sedimentation rate will be present on laboratory testing. On a pelvic examination, any manipulation of the cervix causes severe pain. It may be difficult to palpate the ovaries because of tenderness and abdominal guarding. If the PID enters a chronic phase, the abdominal pain lessens but dyspareunia and dysmenorrhea may be extreme. If the ovaries are affected, intermenstrual spotting may occur. Diagnosis can be aided by sonogram and laparoscopy (Ivey, 1997).

Therapeutic Management. Therapy involves administration of analgesia for comfort plus specific antibiotics such as cefoxitin, doxycycline, or clindamycin (Barber, 1996). Limiting activity also helps relieve the pain. In some women, a pelvic abscess forms and must be drained through the cul-de-sac before healing will occur.

Women who have had one episode of PID have an increased chance of a second occurrence because the immune protection of the tubes and ovaries may be damaged. They should not have coitus with an infected partner, and they should avoid coitus during menstruation, when their protective mechanisms are lowest. Early childbearing may be recommended if they plan to have children, because extensive tubal scarring could impair fertility. It is important for adolescents to recognize the symptoms of PID and to seek early help for the best outcome.

CHECKPOINT QUESTIONS

5. Why does endometriosis lead to dysmenorrhea?
6. What condition must be ruled out in young girls with vulvovaginitis?

BREAST DISORDERS

Males have few breast disorders. Gynecomastia (enlarged breast tissue) may occur temporarily in preadolescent boys in response to a rising estrogen level. Particularly noticeable in obese males, this enlargement fades with a normal increase in testosterone production. It may also occur in teens as a result of steroid use in body building sports. If this is the cause, counseling regarding drug use is in order. Breast disorders that concern adolescent females include additional nipples, lesions such as cysts, infection, and injury.

Accessory Nipples

As the name implies, *accessory nipples* are additional breast nipples. They occur along the mammary lines (Figure 26-3). They are generally not as protuberant as true nipples; they also lack areolar pigmentation. Many girls are unaware that they have an accessory nipple, and think it is a large mole. Accessory nipples are present at birth; and parents should be told what they are so they can inform their daughters later, as some growth in accessory nipples may occur at puberty or during pregnancy in response to estrogen stimulation.

In a few instances, actual breast tissue is present beneath the accessory nipple. If so, it is subject to the same diseases as other breast tissue. If the accessory nipple or accessory breast tissue is cosmetically distressing to the adolescent, it can be removed by simple surgical excision.

WHAT IF? What if an adolescent girl has an accessory nipple with breast tissue underneath? Should she perform breast self-examination for this additional breast tissue?

Breast Hypertrophy

Breast hypertrophy is abnormal enlargement of breast tissue. In the average girl, breast development halts after puberty as soon as progesterone levels rise to mature strength. Progesterone levels remain low until menstrua-

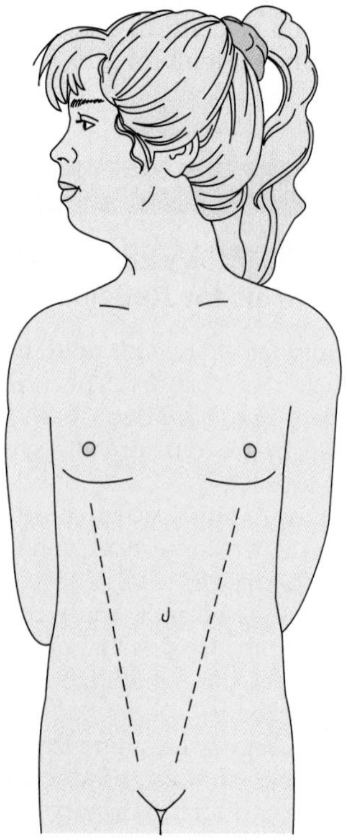

FIGURE 26.3 Nipple lines along which supernumerary nipples occur.

tion cycles are fully established. If this process is a lengthy one, breast growth may last for several years.

Breast hypertrophy can lead to both physical and emotional stress. The girl may feel pain and fatigue in the back or shoulders from attempting to maintain good posture despite the weight of heavy breast tissue. She may feel self-conscious and try to minimize her breast size by slouching and developing poor posture or rounded shoulders.

Adolescent girls with large breasts may find it difficult to adapt to such a new appearance. They may be treated as provocative sex objects and feel they should live up to this image. This can make it difficult for them to find their own identity. They may hear comments such as "I wish I had your problem" rather than receiving support and understanding from parents, peers, and healthcare providers.

If breast hypertrophy interferes with the girl's physical and emotional well-being, she can have surgical breast reduction. Adolescents need to seriously consider the consequences of this procedure before undertaking it. If a large amount of glandular tissue is removed, breast-feeding may no longer be possible. The adolescent needs to be told realistically that changing her physical appearance will reduce physical discomfort, but changing her self-concept must come from within. An adolescent with large breasts must conscientiously perform breast self-examination, because it is easier for a cancerous lesion to escape detection in large amounts of breast tissue than in a smaller breast. Pregnancy and lactation may be a particularly difficult time because breasts that are already large become even heavier with milk formation.

Breast Hypoplasia

Breast hypoplasia is less-than-average breast size. In most instances, this does not represent a decreased amount of glandular or functional breast tissue but a reduced amount of fatty tissue, which as a rule will not interfere with breast-feeding. If an adolescent feels that having small breasts interferes with self-esteem, she can have surgical augmentation to increase breast size, although currently this is not advised because the safety of breast implants remains controversial.

For augmentation, an incision is made under the breast and a silicon implant is inserted under the breast tissue next to the musculus pectoralis major. It is important for the adolescent to realize that her breast tissue is not being replaced by the implant; she still needs to do monthly breast self-examination. Because the original breast tissue is in front of the implant, she will be able to perform self-examination.

The client may notice decreased nipple sensation for approximately 1 year after the procedure. Breasts with implants in place may feel firmer than normal on palpation due to the formation of a fibrotic band or capsule around the implant.

Some women elect not to breast-feed with implants in place because a breast infection would necessitate removal of the implant. A traumatic blow to the breast, for example, from an automobile accident, requires examination by the augmentation surgeon to be certain that the implant did not rupture and cause the contents of the implant to leak into the bloodstream and cause an embolus. In addition, women with implants should have yearly examinations to guard against complications such as absorption of foreign matter into the breast tissue.

Breast Tenderness or Fullness

Many women notice a day or two of premenstrual breast fullness and tenderness each month. Some may find palpable granular or fine nodular lumps in their breasts during this time. This is a benign occurrence and part of the monthly change in hormone stimulation. For accurate assessment, breast self-examination should be done after, not before, a menstrual period. If a lump or tenderness persists, the woman should consult a healthcare provider for additional assessment and care, because the change might signal a lesion or other problem.

Fat Necrosis

If struck during a fall or other traumatic injury, breast tissue will be tender, painful, inflamed or reddened, and possibly bruised. A few days later, necrosis or disintegration may occur in the fatty layer. As the area heals, fibrotic scar tissue forms. This may leave a firm, palpable lump in the breast. It is not freely movable; it may cause skin or nipple retraction or dimpling on the skin surface. Unlike malignant breast growths, post-traumatic breast lumps tend to be well delineated (Staren & O'Neill, 1998).

It is generally recommended that such fibrotic areas be biopsied and then excised. The surgical procedure usually leaves little scarring and the woman no longer needs to worry about the lump in her breast. Although at one time breast trauma was thought to be a precipitating factor of breast carcinoma, no direct correlation between the two has been established. The association may exist because a woman who examines her breasts after an injury may find an already existing carcinoma.

Fibrocystic Breast Condition

Fibrocystic breast condition is the most common benign breast condition in women of all ages. It can occur as early as puberty when estrogen rises to adult levels. More commonly, however, it affects women between the ages of 20 and 45 years. Round, fluid-filled cysts form in the connective breast tissue (Figure 26-4). The woman is able to palpate freely movable, well-delineated breast lumps. Lumps may also be visible on the surface of the breasts (most often in the upper outer quadrant). The consistency of these lesions varies with the menstrual cycle, changing from firm and hard to soft and flexible, depending on the amount of serous fluid present. Oral contraceptives help reduce the incidence and size of cysts. The lesions tend to shrink or even disappear during pregnancy and lactation, and they totally disappear with menopause.

Fibrocystic breasts can be painful; the breasts may feel tender and "stretched," interfering with active sports and other strenuous activity. This discomfort can be relieved with a simple analgesic such as acetaminophen (Tylenol) or warm compresses. Decreasing sodium intake as well as short-term use of a mild diuretic can reduce the fluid retention just before menses.

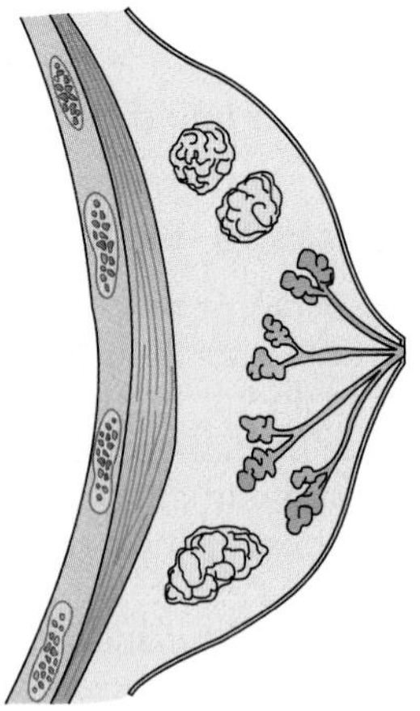

FIGURE 26.4 Round, fluid-filled cysts form in breast tissue in fibrocystic breast condition.

The formation of fibrocystic lesions may be increased in some women with the use of methylxanthines found in caffeine, theophylline, and theobromine. These women should avoid coffee, cola drinks, tea, chocolate, some toffee candy, and medications such as aspirin compound or Excedrin. Discontinuing smoking can also decrease the occurrence of fibrocystic lesions. A supplement of vitamin E may be helpful.

If these measures do not decrease the fibrocystic symptoms, cysts may be aspirated under a local anesthetic by injection of a thin sterile needle attached to a small syringe. This procedure not only reduces the size of the cyst but also provides fluid for biopsy.

Danazol (Danocrine) is a synthetic androgen that helps reduce the symptoms of fibrocystic breast condition by suppressing estrogen formation in the ovaries.

In addition to being physically distressing, fibrocystic breasts can cause women to worry that each lump may be malignant. They can be reassured that the disease itself does not lead to breast carcinoma. Breast carcinoma can occur in a woman with fibrocystic breast condition, however, and may even metastasize before she seeks health consultation, having assumed that all her breast lesions are benign. As a result, she needs more consultation than the average woman. In addition to a yearly breast examination, she needs to perform monthly breast self-examinations, and have an annual breast sonogram, which involves no x-ray exposure and can efficiently locate fluid-filled cysts.

Fibroadenoma

Fibroadenomas are tumors consisting of both fibrotic and glandular components that occur in response to estrogen stimulation. The tumors may increase in size during adolescence and during pregnancy and lactation, or when a woman takes an estrogen source such as an oral contraceptive.

Unlike fibrocystic lesions, fibroadenomas are round and well delineated, feeling firmer and more rubbery than fluid-filled cysts. Occasionally they calcify and feel extremely hard. They are typically painless, freely movable, and tend not to cause skin retraction. Like fibrocystic lesions, they do not become malignant.

Such tumors can be surgically excised so that the woman no longer has to worry about them. Because the incision is small, it leaves little scarring at the site.

✔ CHECKPOINT QUESTIONS

7. If an adolescent girl has breast augmentation, can she still breastfeed?
8. Should adolescents with fibrocystic breasts continue to do breast self-examinations?

SEXUALLY TRANSMITTED DISEASES

Sexually transmitted diseases (STDs) are those diseases spread through sexual contact. They range in severity from easily treated infections, such as trichomoniasis, to human immunodeficiency virus (HIV) which, despite advances in therapy, is life threatening.

A condom provides the best protection against STDs and should always be used in addition to washing the genitals well with soap and water, voiding immediately after coitus, and choosing sexual partners who are at low risk for infection (avoiding intravenous drug users and prostitutes). None of these practices guarantees protection, however. STD organisms are becoming more and more resistant to antibiotics (Erbelding & Quinn, 1997). Educate adolescents that little immunity develops from STDs, which means such diseases can be contracted repeatedly (Saxena & Jenkins, 1997).

Candidiasis

The candidal organism is a fungus that thrives on glycogen. As many as 40% of adult females have asymptomatic candidal vaginal infections; this rate rises even higher during pregnancy when high estrogen levels lead to glycogen levels that produce a favorable environment for fungal growth. Because oral contraceptives produce a pseudopregnancy state, pill users also have frequent vaginal candidal infections. When a woman is being treated with an antibiotic (which destroys normal vaginal flora and lets fungal organisms grow more readily), she is particularly susceptible to this infection. Incidence is also strongly associated with diabetes mellitus because hyperglycemia provides a glucose-rich environment for candidal growth.

Assessment

Because of the scant mucus production in the premenses period, symptoms may be most acute at this time. The adolescent notices vulvar reddening, burning and itching, and even bleeding from hairline fissures. The vagina sometimes shows white "patches" on the walls. The patches are adherent and cannot be scraped away without bleeding. A thick, cream cheese–like discharge can usually be observed at the vaginal introitus. The adolescent may notice pain on coitus or tampon insertion. Candidal infections may also be present at other body sites, such as the oral cavity or a moist area such as the umbilicus.

Candidal infections are diagnosed by removing a sample of discharge from the vaginal wall and placing it on a glass slide; three or four drops of a 20% potassium hydroxide (KOH) solution are then added and the mixture is protected by a coverslip. Under a microscope, typical fungal hyphae indicate the presence of *Candida* organisms (Table 26-1).

Therapeutic Management

Therapy for candidal infections includes vaginal suppositories or cream applications of antifungal preparations such as miconazole (Monistat), nystatin, and clotrimazole, usually once a day for 7 days. These are generally administered at bedtime so the drug does not drain from the vagina immediately afterward. During the day, the girl may want to wear a sanitary napkin to avoid staining from vaginal discharge. Although sexual contact is not the usual means of contracting the initial candidal infection, a reinfection cycle may occur through sexual activity. If the adolescent is sexually active, treatment of the male partner may be necessary to break the cycle. Treatment should not be interrupted until it is complete, even during a menstrual period. Because miconazole, nystatin, and clotrimazole are available without a prescription, the adolescent needs to be advised how to differentiate a candidal infection from other infections or to consult a health-care provider for assistance and treatment. (See the Nursing Care Plan: The Adolescent With Candidiasis.)

If a girl has frequent candidal infections, her urine should be tested for glucose to rule out diabetes mellitus. If she is using an oral contraceptive, she might be counseled to use another contraceptive method.

Trichomoniasis

Trichomonas vaginalis is a single-cell protozoan that is spread by coitus. Up to 25% of adult men and women have asymptomatic trichomoniasis. The incubation period is 4 to 20 days.

With a trichomonal infection, the girl will notice vaginal irritation and a frothy white or grayish-green vaginal discharge. The frothiness of the discharge is an important typical finding. The upper vagina is reddened and may have pinpoint petechiae. Extreme vulvar itching is present. By contrast, males with the same infection rarely report any symptoms.

Assessment

The infection is diagnosed by microscopic examination of vaginal discharge combined with lactated Ringer's or normal saline solution. Trichomonads typically appear as rounded, mobile structures (see Table 26-1).

Therapeutic Management

Oral metronidazole (Flagyl) eradicates trichomonal infections. However, a pregnancy test should be performed before Flagyl is prescribed, because this drug may be teratogenic. If the adolescent is pregnant, an alternative treatment is douching with a povidone-iodine (Betadine) or vinegar solution. Treatment with Flagyl and use of condoms by her sexual partner will help prevent recurrence of *Trichomonas* in both parties. Be aware that *Trichomonas* infections cause such inflammatory changes in the cervix or vagina that a Pap test taken during this time may be misinterpreted as showing abnormal tissue. Because the drug interacts with alcohol to cause acute nausea and vomiting, advise the adolescent not to drink alcoholic beverages during the course of treatment.

Bacterial Vaginosis

Bacterial vaginosis is the invasion of *Gardnerella* or *Haemophilus*. These organisms thrive in the vagina, a body area with a reduced oxygen level. The associated discharge is milk-white to gray and has a fishlike odor. Pruritus may be intense. Microscopic examination of the discharge in normal saline solution shows gram-negative rods adhering to vaginal epithelial cells, which are termed "clue cells" (see Table 26-1).

The treatment is oral metronidazole for 7 days; the woman's sexual partner should also be treated to prevent recurrence of the infection (Adger, 1997).

Chlamydia Trachomatis Infection

Chlamydia trachomatis infections are becoming increasingly common. Symptoms include a heavy grayish-white discharge and vulvar itching. The incubation period is 1 to 5 weeks. Diagnosis is made by culture of the organism. Therapy is oral doxycycline or tetracycline for 7 days. *Chlamydia* infection in a mother may cause eye infection or pneumonia in the newborn (see Chapter 14). During pregnancy, the infection is treated with erythromycin, since tetracycline is teratogenic.

Genital Warts

Genital warts are lesions caused by the human papilloma virus. They are rapidly growing structures on the vulva, vagina, or cervix. Large growths may be excised by cautery or cryotherapy, since they can become cancerous. Small growths may be removed by applying podophyllin (see Chapter 14).

Herpes Genitalis

Genital herpes is caused by the herpesvirus *hominis* type 2 (HSV-2). This is one of four similar herpes viruses: cytomegalovirus, Epstein-Barr, varicella-zoster, and herpes type 1 and type 2. Genital herpes occurs in epidemic proportions in the United States, and its incidence appears to be growing yearly. Unlike most other STDs, there is no known cure. The disease involves a lifelong process and may be a precursor to cervical cancer. The virus, spread by skin-to-skin contact, enters a break in the skin or mucous membrane. For the newborn, the virus can be systemic and even fatal (see Chapter 6).

Assessment

Herpes is diagnosed by a culture of the lesion secretion from its location on the vulva, vagina, cervix, or penis or by

(*text continues on page 822*)

TABLE 26.1 Common Vulvovaginitis Infections

CAUSATIVE AGENT	SYMPTOMS	COMMON THERAPY
Candida 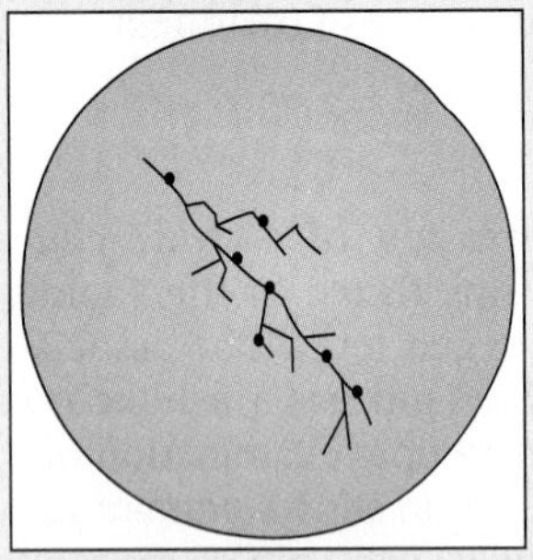	Vulvar reddening and pruritus; thick, white, cheeselike vaginal discharge	Nystatin or miconazole (Monistat) suppositories; bathing with dilute sodium bicarbonate solution may relieve pruritus
Trichomonas 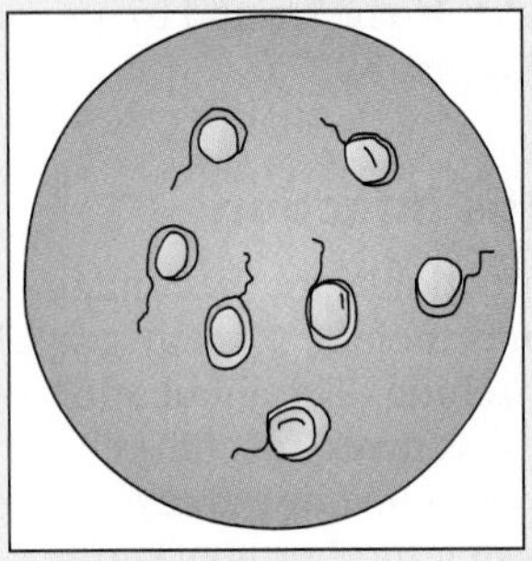	Thin, irritating frothy gray-green discharge; strong, putrid odor; itching	Metronidazole (Flagyl) orally; douching with weak vinegar solution to reduce pruritus
Herpesvirus type II	Painful pinpoint vesicles on an erythematous base with a watery vaginal discharge possible; voiding may be irritating and painful	Bathing with dilute sodium bicarbonate solution, applying lubricating jelly to lesions or an oral analgesic such as aspirin may be necessary for pain relief; topically applied acyclovir (Zovirax) helps heal lesions
Gardnerella 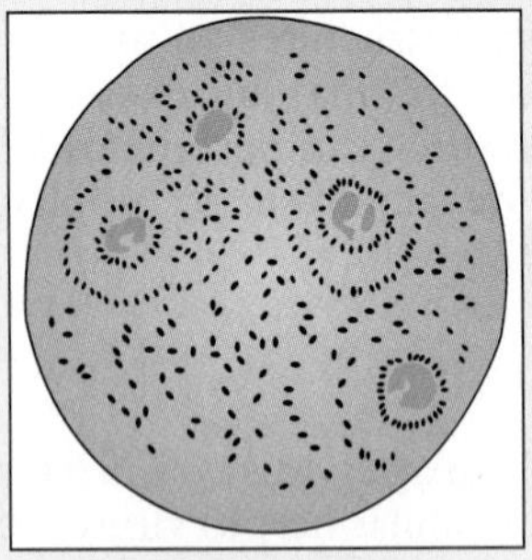	Edema and reddening of vulva, milky gray discharge, fishlike odor	Metronidazole (Flagyl) or clindamycin
Chlamydia trachomatis	Watery gray-white vaginal discharge, vulvar itching	Tetracycline or doxycycline; erythromycin during pregnancy
Neisseria gonorrhoeae	May be symptomless; may have profuse yellow-green vaginal discharge	Ceftriaxone and doxycycline; oral amoxicillin
Enterobius vermicularis (pinworm)	Rectal pruritus, especially on rising in the morning	Oral administration of an anthelmintic, such as mebendazole (Vermox)
Treponema pallidum (syphilis)	Painless ulcer on vulva or vagina	Benzathine penicillin, administered intramuscularly
Streptococcus	Vaginitis, vulvar itching; edema and reddening of vulva	Antibiotic, e.g., amoxicillin
Foreign body	Vaginal discharge; odor	Removal of foreign body during pelvic examination

Nursing Care Plan

THE ADOLESCENT WITH CANDIDIASIS

An 18-year-old female college freshman is seen at the student health center complaining of intense vaginal itching. "It started a couple of days after I started taking the antibiotic the dentist prescribed for my abscessed tooth."

Assessment: Well-proportioned female; sexual maturity stage 5. Menarche at age 12 years. Menses regular, every 29 days with moderate flow. Denies history of oral contraceptive use or other reproductive or health problems. Sexually active for approximately 1 year with same partner. "We always use a condom. You can never be too careful."

On examination, vulva reddened and excoriated. "It burns and itches terribly. It even hurts to sit. I've tried not scratching, but sometimes, I just can't help it." Thick white cheese-like discharge noted at vaginal introitus. White adherent patches noted on vaginal walls. Specimen of discharge examined and is positive for Candida. Miconazole (Monistat) vaginal cream prescribed for 7 days. "How did I get this? From my boyfriend? Does he need to be treated too?"

Nursing Diagnosis: Pain related to irritation, excoriation and pruritus associated with candidal infection

Outcome Identification: Adolescent will verbalize relief within 24 hours.

Outcome Evaluation: Adolescent identifies appropriate measures to promote comfort; reports relief of pain after use of comfort measures.

Interventions	Rationale
1. Instruct adolescent in use of miconazole cream daily at bedtime.	1. Miconazole is effective in treating candidal infections, the source of the adolescent's discomfort. Using it at bedtime improves the drug's effectiveness by preventing the cream from oozing out of the vagina.
2. Strongly urge that the adolescent refrain from scratching. Suggest use of cool compresses to perineal area.	2. Scratching exacerbates the irritation and may lead to further excoriation and possible secondary infection. Cool compresses help to minimize the itching sensation.
3. Instruct the adolescent to gently wash the perineal area at least two times per day with mild unscented soap and water and to pat rather than rub dry.	3. Frequent cleansing of the perineal area removes irritating drainage. Use of unscented mild soap prevents exposing the perineal area to additional irritants. Rubbing an area increases blood flow to the area, increasing the edema and inflammation, thus increasing the risk for further irritation and subsequent itching.
4. Recommend the use of sitz baths three to four times a day.	4. Sitz baths are soothing and help keep the area free of irritating discharge.
5. Encourage the adolescent to wear cotton underwear.	5. Cotton underwear permits air to circulate and moisture to evaporate, minimizing the risk for further irritation.
6. Recommend the use of an over-the-counter analgesic such as acetaminophen or ibuprofen.	6. Acetaminophen and ibuprofen are effective analgesics.

Nursing Diagnosis: Knowledge deficit related to cause and treatment of candidal infection

Outcome Identification: Adolescent will verbalize accurate information about candidiasis.

Outcome Evaluation: Adolescent reports contributing factors associated with development of infection; demonstrates correct technique for administering miconazole cream; reports boyfriend has an appointment within 48 hours for evaluation.

(continued)

Interventions	Rationale
1. Explore what the adolescent knows about candidal infections. Explain the possible relationship between this infection and use of antibiotics for tooth abscess.	1. Exploration provides a baseline for building teaching strategies. Antibiotics destroy the normal vaginal flora, promoting the overgrowth of fungal organisms.
2. Demonstrate the procedure for inserting miconazole cream. Have adolescent return demonstrate the procedure.	2. Demonstration aids in learning. Return demonstration helps to evaluate adolescent's understanding.
3. Advise adolescent to wear a sanitary pad during the day and reinforce the use of comfort measures.	3. Wearing a sanitary pad helps to prevent staining from vaginal discharge. Comfort measures, if used properly and consistently, aid in relieving the pain, irritation, and itching.
4. Encourage the adolescent to have her boyfriend come in for an evaluation. Urge her to avoid sexual activity until infection is resolved. If not possible, instruct her to have partner wear a condom.	4. Although sexual contact is not the usual means of contracting the initial infection, a reinfection cycle can occur with sexual activity, thus necessitating treatment of the partner. Avoidance of sexual activity and use of a condom help to minimize the risk for reinfection.
5. Recommend that the adolescent notify her dentist for a possible change in antibiotic for the abscessed tooth.	5. Some antibiotics are more prone to promoting candidal growth than others. A switch to another antibiotic may be necessary to resolve the abscess and minimize the risk for a recurrent candidal infection.
6. Instruct the adolescent in signs and symptoms of recurrent candidal infection.	6. Knowledge of these signs and symptoms allows for early recognition and prompt treatment should the infection recur.

isolation of HSV antibodies in serum. The incubation period is 3 to 14 days. On first contact, extensive primary lesions originate as a group of pinpoint vesicles on an erythematous base. Within a few days, the vesicles ulcerate and become moist, draining, open lesions. The client may have accompanying flulike symptoms with an increased temperature; vaginal lesions may cause profuse discharge. Pain is intense on contact with clothing or acidic urine.

After the primary stage that lasts approximately 1 week, lesions heal but the virus lingers in a latent form, affecting the sensory nerve ganglia. It will flare up and become an active infection during illness, PMS, fever, overexposure to sunlight, or stress. A secondary response usually produces only local lesions rather than systemic symptoms.

Therapeutic Management

Acyclovir (Zovirax) controls the virus by interfering with deoxyribonucleic acid reproduction and decreasing symptoms. The drug is available as a topical ointment. If applying this to a client, protect yourself with a finger cot or glove so that you do not contract the virus or absorb the drug. Sitz baths three times a day and applying a soothing substance such as cornstarch to reduce discomfort afterward may be helpful. An emollient (A & D Ointment) also reduces discomfort, but its moisture tends to prolong the active period of the lesions.

Because of the association with cervical cancer, any female with genital herpes should have a yearly Pap test for the rest of her life. Condoms will help prevent the spread of herpes among sexual partners.

People with herpes may have difficulty establishing sexual relationships for fear of infecting a partner. Because herpes is communicated only by direct contact, infected individuals need to inform their partner when they have any active lesions and take extra precautions to decrease the danger of spreading the virus.

Hepatitis B

Hepatitis B can be spread by semen so is considered an STD. It is discussed in Chapter 22 with other forms of hepatitis.

Gonorrhea

Gonorrhea is transmitted by *Neisseria gonorrhoeae,* a gram-positive diplococcus that thrives on columnar transitional epithelium of the mucous membrane. Symptoms begin after a 2- to 7-day incubation period, and, in males, include *urethritis* (pain on urination and frequency of urination) and a urethral discharge. Without treatment, the infection may spread to the testes, scarring the tubules and causing permanent sterility. Untreated, the infection is easily spread among sexual partners.

Although symptoms of gonorrhea in females are not as visible, there may be a slight yellowish vaginal discharge. Bartholin's glands may become inflamed and painful. If left untreated, the infection may spread to pelvic organs, most notably the fallopian tubes (PID). Tubal scarring can result in permanent sterility. In both males and females, untreated gonorrhea can lead to arthritis or heart disease from systemic involvement.

An infant may contract gonorrhea in the birth canal from its mother. This leads frequently to gonorrheal ophthalmia.

Assessment

A urine culture for gonococcal bacillus, in addition to vaginal and urethral cultures, should be done on all children with vulvovaginitis or urethral discharge. In males, a first voiding may reveal gonococci if a midstream specimen is inconclusive.

Therapeutic Management

The treatment for gonorrhea is one intramuscular injection of ceftriaxone plus oral doxycycline for 7 days (CDC, 1998). Sexual partners should receive the same treatment.

Approximately 24 hours after treatment, the gonorrhea is no longer infectious. Approximately 7 days after treatment, a client should return for a follow-up culture to verify that the disease has been completely eradicated (few people take this precaution). A sexually active client should be given a serologic test for syphilis along with the gonorrheal culture. If the dose of ceftriaxone and doxycycline has effectively eliminated the gonorrhea, no additional treatment for syphilis is necessary. Most states require that gonorrhea be reported to the health department; adolescents are asked to name sexual contacts.

NURSING DIAGNOSES AND RELATED INTERVENTIONS

Nursing Diagnosis: Anxiety related to having contracted a reportable STD

Outcome Identification: Client will demonstrate reduced anxiety by end of health care visit.

Outcome Evaluation: Client voices confidence in ability to cope with this problem and demonstrates understanding of both illness and treatment regimen.

People who seek treatment for STDs need to feel they can trust healthcare personnel and reveal information without fear of criticism. Assure the client of absolute confidentiality in naming his or her sexual contacts. Without being told who put them at risk, these people can then be notified by a health department investigator that they have been exposed to a particular STD. This vital information will help prevent further spread of the disease.

Some people are reluctant to seek treatment for gonorrhea because they have heard stories that therapy involves 10 to 15 days of intramuscular injections. Because they have no symptoms, some girls may avoid going for what they think will be extremely painful treatment. Alert them that treatment is simple. This is an insidious disease, and even though no symptoms are apparent, it can have disastrous long-term effects if left untreated.

Syphilis

Syphilis is a systemic disease caused by the spirochete *Treponema pallidum.* It is transmitted by sexual contact with a person who has an active spirochete-containing lesion; it is also reportable.

Following an incubation period of 10 to 90 days, a typical lesion appears, generally on the genitalia (penis or labia) or on the mouth, lips, or rectal area from oral-genital or genital-anal contact. The lesion (termed a *chancre*) is a deep ulcer and generally painless despite its size. Lymphadenopathy may be present but is unlikely to be noticed by the affected individual. A lesion in the vagina may not be immediately evident. Without treatment, a chancre lasts approximately 6 weeks and then fades.

Approximately 2 to 4 weeks after the chancre disappears, a generalized macular copper-colored rash appears. Unlike many other rashes, it affects the soles and the palms. A serologic test for syphilis yields a positive result at this time. There may be secondary symptoms of generalized illness such as low-grade fever and adenopathy. With or without treatment, this stage of syphilis will also fade.

The next stage is a latency period that may last from only a few years to several decades. The only indication of the disease is the serologic test, which continues to yield a positive result.

The final stage of syphilis is a destructive neurologic disease that involves major body organs such as the heart and the nervous system. Typical symptoms are blindness; paralysis; severe, crippling neurologic deformities; mental confusion; slurred speech; and lack of coordination. This third stage should be identified before it becomes fatal.

Assessment

Syphilis is diagnosed by the recognition of the various symptoms of the three stages and by serologic serum tests, usually VDRL (Venereal Disease Research Laboratory), ART (automated reagin test), RPR (rapid plasma reagin test), or FTA-ABS (fluorescent treponemal antibody absorption test).

Therapeutic Management

The therapy effectively arrests the disease at whatever stage it has reached. Benzathine penicillin G given intramuscularly in two sites is effective therapy. For the adolescent sensitive to penicillin, either oral erythromycin or tetracycline can be given for 10 to 15 days. As with gonorrhea, sexual partners are treated in the same way as the person with the active infection.

Because syphilis can be treated so easily, one would think it would be easy to eradicate. In reality, however, because the primary chancre is painless, many individuals are either unaware of it or choose to ignore it, thereby transmitting the disease to unsuspecting partners. Adolescents, in particular, need accurate information about STDs to become aware of the symptoms. They should be able to feel they can report the disease to healthcare personnel and that they can name sexual contacts without fear of being criticized. If a woman develops syphilis during pregnancy, the disease can be spread to the fetus (Rawstron et al, 1997).

Human Immunodeficiency Virus

HIV is carried by semen as well as other body fluids so is considered an STD. Invasion of the virus is discussed with other immune disorders in Chapter 21.

CHECKPOINT QUESTIONS

9. What are the typical symptoms of a candidal vaginal infection?
10. Why is gonorrhea an especially serious STD?

KEY POINTS

The cause of ambiguous genitalia is unknown but may be related to the level of testosterone produced in utero. The true sex of children is established by a karyotype of chromosomes.

Precocious puberty is the development of secondary sex characteristics before the age of 8 years. Children may be treated with a synthetic analogue of luteinizing hormone–releasing hormone to reduce development. Without effective support, such children are at high risk for body image disturbance.

Delayed puberty is the failure to develop secondary sex characteristics by the age of 17 years. Girls may be administered estrogen to promote development; boys may be administered testosterone.

Balanoposthitis (inflammation of the glans and prepuce) and phimosis (constricted foreskin) occur in boys. Phimosis can be treated with circumcision.

Cryptorchidism is failure of one or both testes to descend during intrauterine life. The condition is surgically corrected to prevent cancer from developing later in life.

Testicular cancer is rare but tends to occur in young men. Boys need to be taught testicular self-examination for early detection.

Dysmenorrhea is a menstrual disorder that occurs frequently in adolescent girls. Therapy for this is a prostaglandin inhibitor such as ibuprofen.

Untreated endometriosis (the abnormal growth of extrauterine endometrial tissue) can lead to infertility later in life. Therapy is administration of the synthetic androgen danazol or surgery to reduce the size of the abnormal tissue.

Vulvovaginitis (inflammation of the vulva and vagina) or pelvic inflammatory disease are infections that can occur in adolescents. Therapy to prevent fallopian tube scarring and infertility later in life is essential.

Conditions such as fibrocystic breasts can occur in adolescents. Adolescent girls need to learn breast self-examination to detect and monitor abnormalities that could be a sign of breast cancer.

Sexually transmitted diseases such as candidiasis, trichomoniasis, *Chlamydia trachomatis,* genital warts, herpes genitalis, gonorrhea, and syphilis are increasing in incidence in the adolescent population. An important health teaching area with children is the need to follow safer sex practices. Girls need to be taught, in addition, ways to avoid toxic shock syndrome.

When teaching about STDs, it is important to stress that they do not confer immunity and thus can be contracted more than once.

Children who are born with a reproductive tract disorder frequently adjust well when young. They may need counseling at puberty or when they become aware of the impact of their disorder on their sexual functioning or their ability to reproduce.

CRITICAL THINKING EXERCISES

1. Helen is the 15-year-old you met at the beginning of the chapter who had been diagnosed as having gonorrhea. She said she was glad she had contracted the disease early in life because now she will never get it again. What health teaching does Helen need to be better informed about her disease?
2. You care for a 15-year-old girl who has no breast development and also has not menstruated as yet. She asks you if it is time to worry. How would you counsel her?
3. A 12-year-old was born with undescended testes. He had surgery for this at age 2 years. He is concerned now that he is at high risk for testicular cancer. How would you counsel him?

REFERENCES

Adger, H. (1997). Sexually transmitted diseases. In Johnson, K.B. & Oski, F.A. *Oski's essential pediatrics*. Philadelphia: Lippincott.

Barber, N. (1996). Genitourinary disorders. In Burns, C. et al. *Pediatric primary care*. Philadelphia: Saunders.

Centers for Disease Control and Prevention. (1998). 1998 guidelines for treatment of sexually transmitted diseases. *MMWR, 47*(rr-1), 1.

Chance, T.D. (1996). Toxic shock syndrome: role of the environment, the host and the microorganism. *British Journal of Biomedical Science, 53*(4), 284.

Department of Health and Human Services. (1995). *Healthy people 2000: Midcourse review*. Washington, D.C.: DHHS.

Dewan, P.A. et al. (1996). Phimosis: is circumcision necessary? *Journal of Paediatrics and Child Health, 32*(4), 285.

Diamond, M. & Sigmundson, H.K. (1997). Management of intersexuality: guidelines for dealing with persons with ambiguous genitalia. *Archives of Pediatrics and Adolescent Medicine, 151*(10), 1046.

Duleba, A.J. (1997). Diagnosis of endometriosis. *Obstetrics and Gynecology Clinics of North America, 24*(2), 331.

Elder, J. S. (1998). Bilateral neonatal testicular torsion. *Journal of Urology, 159*(4), 1413.

El-Gohary, M.A. (1997). The role of laparoscopy in the management of impalpable testes. *Pediatric Surgery International, 12*(5), 463.

Erbelding, E. & Quinn, T.C. (1997). The impact of antimicrobial resistance on the treatment of sexually transmitted diseases. *Infectious Disease Clinics of North America, 11*(4), 889.

Ivey, J.B. (1997). The adolescent with pelvic inflammatory disease: assessment and management. *Nurse Practitioner, 22*(2), 78.

Kennedy, S. (1997). Primary dysmenorrhoea. *Lancet, 349*(9059), 1116.

Mehlisch, D.R. & Fulmer, R.I. (1997). A crossover comparison of bromfenac sodium, naproxen sodium, and placebo for relief of pain from primary dysmenorrhea. *Journal of Women's Health, 6*(1), 83.

O'Callaghan, A. & Mead, G.M. (1997). Testicular carcinoma. *Postgraduate Medical Journal, 73*(862), 481.

Peters, S. (1997). The puzzle of premenstrual syndrome: putting the pieces together. *Advance for Nurse Practitioners, 5*(10), 41.

Plotnick, L.P. (1997). Puberty and gonadal disorders. In Johnson, K.B. & Oski, F.A. *Oski's essential pediatrics*. Philadelphia: Lippincott.

Pretorius, D.H. et al. (1998). Hydroceles identified prenatally: common physiologic phenomenon? *Journal of Ultrasound in Medicine, 17*(1), 49.

Rawstron, S.A. et al. (1997). Congenital syphilis: detection of treponema pallidum in stillborns. *Clinical Infectious Diseases, 24*(1), 24.

Roth, D.R. & Gonzales, E.T. (1997). Disorders of renal development and anomalies of the collecting systems, bladder, penis and scrotum. In Johnson, K.B. & Oski, F.A. *Oski's essential pediatrics*. Philadelphia: Lippincott.

Saxena, S.B. & Jenkins, R.R. (1997). Sexually transmitted diseases in adolescents: screening and treatment. *Comprehensive Therapy, 23*(2), 108.

Staren, E. D. & O'Neill, T.P. (1998). Breast ultrasound. *Surgical Clinics of North America, 78*(2), 219.

Wohl, R.E. & Kane, W. (1997). Teachers' beliefs concerning teaching about testicular cancer and testicular self-examination. *Journal of School Health, 67*(3), 106.

SUGGESTED READINGS

Brosens, I. (1997). Diagnosis of endometriosis. *Seminars in Reproductive Endocrinology, 15*(3), 229.

Cecchi, M. Et al. (1997). Painless treatment of hydrocele. *International Urology & Nephrology, 29*(4), 457.

Hayward, C. et al. (1997). Psychiatric risk associated with early puberty in adolescent girls. *Journal of the American Academy of Child and Adolescent Psychiatry, 36*(2), 255.

Hurst, J. L. et al. (1998). Tamoxifen-induced regression of breast cysts. *Clinical Imaging, 22*(2), 95.

Kaplan, B., et al. (1997). Clinical evaluation of a new model of a transcutaneous electrical nerve stimulation device for the management of primary dysmenorrhea. *Gynecologic and Obstetric Investigation, 44*(4), 255.

Laga M. & Dallabetta, G. (1997). Sexually transmitted diseases: treating the whole syndrome. *Lancet, 350*(4S), 2528.

Martin, T.V., Anderson, K.R. & Weiss, R.M. (1997). Laparoscopic evaluation and management of a child with ambiguous genitalia, ectopic spleen and Meckel's diverticulum. *Techniques in Urology, 3*(1), 49.

Mortola, J.F. (1997). Premenstrual syndrome. *Current Therapy in Endocrinology and Metabolism, 6*, 251.

Munday, P.E. (1997). Clinical aspects of pelvic inflammatory disease. *Human Reproduction, 12*(11), 121.

Styne, D.M. (1997). New aspects in the diagnosis and treatment of pubertal disorders. *Pediatric Clinics of North America, 44*(2), 505.

Nursing Care of the Child With an Endocrine or Metabolic Disorder

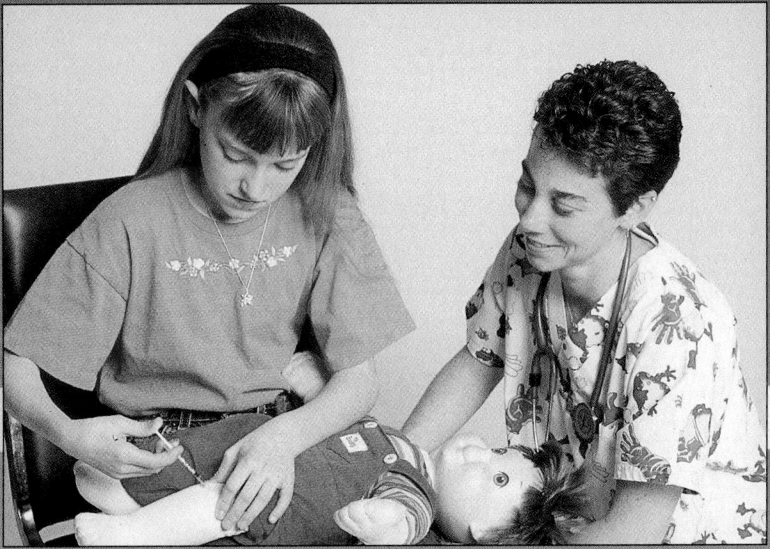

27 CHAPTER

Key Terms

- carpal spasm
- exophthalmos
- glycosuria
- hormones
- hyperfunction
- hyperglycemia
- hypofunction
- hypoglycemia
- hypothalamus
- ketoacidosis
- latent tetany
- manifest tetany
- pedal spasm
- polydipsia
- polyuria
- sella turcica
- Somogyi phenomenon

Objectives

After mastering the contents of this chapter, you should be able to:

1. Describe the different endocrine glands and their functions.
2. Assess a child with a disorder of endocrine function.
3. Formulate nursing diagnoses for the child with altered endocrine or metabolic function.
4. Develop appropriate outcomes for the child with endocrine or metabolic dysfunction.
5. Plan nursing care, for example, health teaching, for the child with altered endocrine or metabolic function.
6. Implement nursing care, for example, teaching insulin administration, for the child with an endocrine or metabolic disorder.
7. Evaluate outcomes to be certain that goals of nursing care were achieved.
8. Identify national health goals related to childhood endocrine or metabolic disorders that nurses could be instrumental in helping the nation achieve.
9. Identify areas related to care of children with endocrine or metabolic disorders that could benefit from additional nursing research.
10. Analyze ways that care of the child with altered endocrine or metabolic function can be family centered.
11. Synthesize knowledge of endocrine and metabolic dysfunctions and the nursing process to ensure quality child health nursing care.

Rob is a 16-year-old with type I diabetes. You see him in an ambulatory clinic. Rob's diabetes was diagnosed when he was 7 years old. His records indicate that his disease control has been generally good over the years, but in the last 6 months he has "forgotten" to take his insulin at least once a week. When you ask about this, he mentions that sports after school plus a weekend job, a new girlfriend, and a new car have occupied his time and interrupted what used to be a strict schedule of home-cooked meals and rigid bedtimes. Is Rob's history unusual for an adolescent? What health teaching do you think will most help him reestablish control?

In the previous chapters, you learned about growth and development of well children. In this chapter, you will add information about the dramatic changes, both physical and psychosocial, that occur when children develop an endocrine or metabolic disorder. This is important information because it builds a base for care and health teaching.

After you have studied the chapter, turn to the Critical Thinking Exercises at the end of the chapter to help sharpen your skills and test your knowledge.

The endocrine system is composed of a small group of glands that work together with the neurologic system to regulate and coordinate all body systems (Figure 27-1). The glands produce chemicals called **hormones**, which are expelled into surrounding tissue and picked up by the bloodstream where they act individually and in concert to affect various organ systems. (The word *hormone* is from the Greek *hormaein,* which means "to set in motion.") Each gland of the endocrine system has specific functions that are necessary for regulating body processes; each hormone secreted acts on a specific target (or designated) organ.

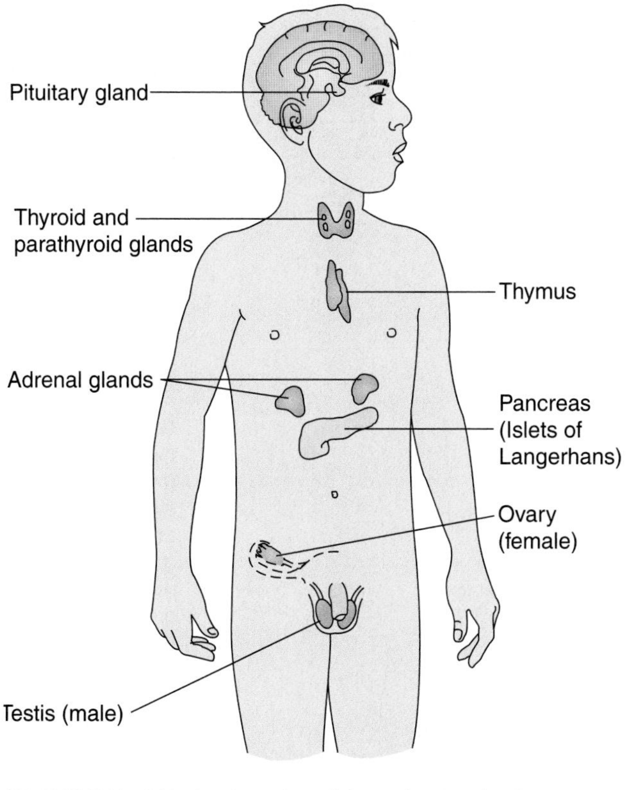

FIGURE 27.1 Location of the endocrine glands.

Dysfunction of the glands or action of the hormones results in a variety of disorders, most of which have long-term implications. Parents—and children as soon as they are old enough—need to understand these diseases to the best of their ability and to participate in the long-term plan of care. National Health Goals related to endocrine and metabolic disorders and children are presented in the Focus on National Health Goals box.

NURSING PROCESS OVERVIEW

for Care of the Child With an Endocrine or Metabolic Disorder

Assessment

Endocrine and metabolic disorders as a group commonly cause changes in normal growth or activity patterns. This is usually detected when height and weight are assessed and compared with standards for the child's age at a health visit (see Managing and Delegating Unlicensed Assistive Personnel). Obese children

FOCUS ON NATIONAL HEALTH GOALS

Diabetes mellitus is a disorder with serious consequences in both children and pregnant women. A number of National Health Goals address reducing the incidence of this disease:

- Reduce diabetes-related deaths to no more than 34/100,000 people from a baseline of 38/100,000.
- Reduce the most severe complications of diabetes, such as perinatal mortality, to 2% from a baseline of 5%, and major congenital malformations from the illness from 8% to 4%.
- Reduce diabetes to a prevalence of no more than 25 per 1000 people from a baseline of 28/1000 (DHHS, 1995).

Nurses can be instrumental in helping the nation achieve these goals by educating women about the possible effects the illness can have on pregnancy and educating children about ways to prevent the long-term effects of the illness. Nursing research could shed additional light on these goals by asking questions such as: How should women be taught that fetal anomalies from hyperglycemia occur very early in pregnancy so they must be certain to enter pregnancy in good glucose control? Long-term effects of diabetes are not noticeable in childhood, but how can children be educated to plan a healthy lifestyle to prevent these effects in adult life? How soon in life can children be expected to be responsible for glucose monitoring and insulin injection? What methods are best for encouraging children to be in charge of their own diet?

MANAGING AND DELEGATING UNLICENSED ASSISTIVE PERSONNEL

Children with endocrine or metabolic disorders are often identified first through routine height and weight measurements. Weighing babies at birth and at health visits is often done by unlicensed assistive personnel. Be certain that they understand the importance of these measurements so they do not do them carelessly. Help them learn to compare a new reading with the previous reading so they can identify a marked difference in height or weight (or a gradual trend) and can alert the primary care provider to a change in these measurements.

may have thyroid deficiencies. Short children may have pituitary difficulties. An acute loss in weight is often the first symptom of diabetes mellitus in children.

Taking a day history (asking the parent or child to describe all the child's actions on a typical day) will help you distinguish between a normally "quiet" child and one with decreased endocrine function producing inactivity and chronic fatigue in the child. (For example, the quiet child lies down after school and reads; the ill child lies down and sleeps.) Taking a day history also differentiates between a child who is merely active and one who is overly active because of hyperthyroidism. (The healthy child appears to "go constantly" but can sit through a favorite television program or a meal. The child with increased thyroid production may be unable to sit quietly at all.)

Assess dietary and elimination habits. Extreme thirst or appetite may occur with endocrine malfunction. Frequent voiding in children most often reflects a urinary tract infection but may be evidence of excessive urine excretion (polyuria), as occurs with pituitary dysfunction or diabetes mellitus.

On physical examination, the child's general appearance should be observed for excessive tiredness, scaling or dry skin, drooping eyelids or protrusion of the eyeballs (**exophthalmos**), and poor muscle tone (see Assessing the Child With an Endocrine Disorder).

Nursing Diagnoses

Nursing diagnoses relevant to children with endocrine or metabolic disorders include the following:

- Fluid volume deficit related to constant excessive loss of fluid through urination
- Risk for altered nutrition, less than body requirements related to inability to use glucose because of diabetes mellitus
- Altered body image related to abnormal height
- Health seeking behaviors related to self-administration of insulin
- Knowledge deficit related to treatment needs
- Fear related to illness outcome
- Grieving related to poor acceptance of long-term illness
- Altered family processes related to child's chronic illness

Outcome Identification and Planning

Although most endocrine and metabolic disorders have long-term implications, parents and children may find it easier to work with short-term goals at first—particularly if they are having difficulty accepting the diagnosis and the long-term nature of the disorder. Because symptoms usually are not acute, it is easy for children and parents to forget medications. Helping parents create reminder charts is an effective measure to increase therapeutic compliance.

The school situation must be carefully evaluated for any child with chronic illness. Teachers may have to be alerted to the child's health problem so they do not make excessive or inappropriate demands (e.g., insisting that the child with hyperthyroidism submit neat handwriting assignments when the child cannot do so).

Selected organizations for referral include the following:

American Diabetes Association
P.O. Box 25757
1160 Duke Street
Alexandria, VA 22314

Little People of America
7238 Piedmont Drive
Dallas, TX 75227-9324

National Tay-Sachs and Allied Disease Association
2001 Beacon Street
Brookline, MA 02146

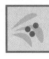

ASSESSING the Child With an Endocrine Disorder

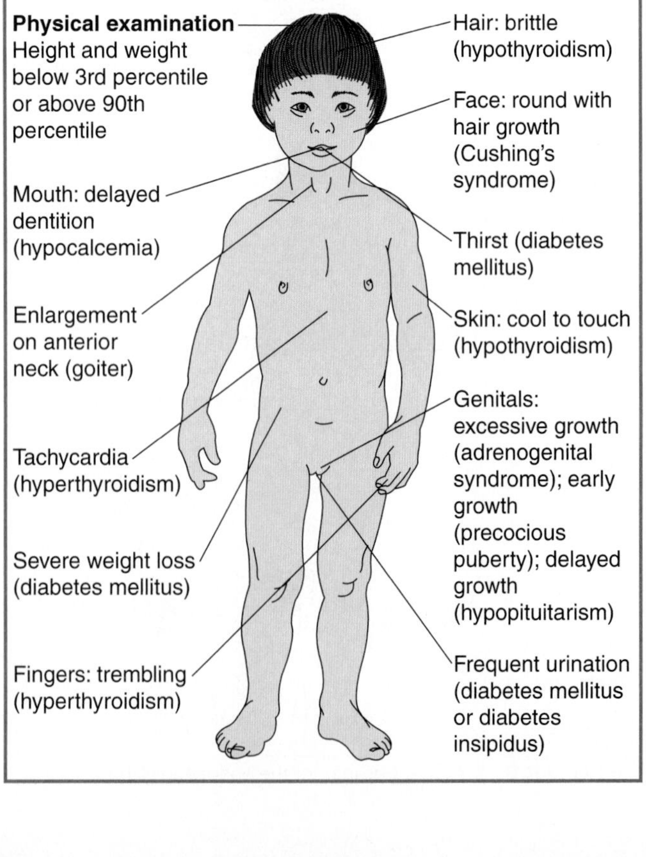

Implementation

Interventions for children with endocrine or metabolic disorders must always be carried out with the long-term aspects of care in mind. Bribing children to take a medicine, for example, is never good practice. It has no place with children who must continue to take a medication for the rest of their lives (bribery quickly becomes ineffective). As children grow older and can better understand their disorder, explanations of why they must continue to take medication need to become more detailed.

Outcome Evaluation

Children with disorders of endocrine or metabolic function need to be evaluated periodically throughout childhood; growth and activity will necessitate changes in medication dosages or schedules. These checkups provide good opportunities for health teaching to equip children to meet new situations that arise as they mature. Body appearance becomes increasingly important as children enter adolescence, for example, because being like, not unlike, their peers grows even more important. Seemingly well-adjusted school-age children may now have extreme difficulty accepting their illness. Compliance with a medication program may become erratic. Only by periodic reevaluation can these problems be identified so that health care plans can be modified and adapted to the child's needs, enabling the child and family to continue coping with a long-term illness.

The following are examples of outcome criteria:

- Child states reasons for complying with medication regimen.
- Child's blood pressure and pulse remain within normal limits for age; specific gravity of urine is between 1.003 and 1.030; skin turgor is good; child states thirst is not excessive.
- Parents demonstrate correct insulin injection technique and state they are comfortable administering an injection to their child.

THE PITUITARY GLAND

The work of the pituitary gland is directed by the **hypothalamus,** an organ that is located in the center of the brain and is the regulator of the autonomic nervous system. About 1 cm long, 1.0 to 1.5 cm wide, and 0.5 cm thick, the pituitary rests in the **sella turcica,** a depression of the sphenoid bone. It is covered by a tough membrane, which also joins the gland to the hypothalamus.

There are several distinct regions of the pituitary: the anterior lobe, or *adenohypophysis;* the posterior lobe, or *neurohypophysis;* and the intermediate lobe (*pars intermedia*), which lies between the anterior and posterior lobes. Each of these regions appears to have its own function and secretes specific hormones.

Pituitary Hormones

The regions of the pituitary gland store and release eight hormones; four of these—antidiuretic hormone (ADH), thyrotropin, corticotropin, and somatotropin—are prominently involved in childhood illnesses (Table 27-1).

DISORDERS CAUSED BY PITUITARY GLAND DYSFUNCTION

Illnesses caused by pituitary malfunction result from tumor growth of the pituitary or hypothalamus, interference with circulation to the gland, trauma, inflammation, structural abnormalities, erratic or nonfunctional feedback mechanisms, and, possibly, autoimmune responses.

Growth Hormone Deficiency

When production of human *growth hormone (GH;* somatotropin) is deficient, children remain short. Such children are well proportioned but simply miniature in size. This may result from a nonmalignant cystic tumor of embryonic origin that places pressure on the pituitary gland or from increased intracranial pressure from another cause. In most children with hypopituitarism, the cause of the defect is unknown (Plotkin, 1997).

It is difficult to predict exactly what height will be reached in the untreated child because this varies with each individual. Without treatment, however, most children will not reach a height over 3 or 4 ft.

Assessment

The child with deficient production of GH is generally normal in size and weight at birth. Within the first few years of life, however, the child begins to fall below the third percentile of height and weight on growth charts. The face appears infantile because the mandible is recessed and immature; the nose is usually small. The child's teeth may be crowded in a small jaw (and may erupt late). The child's voice may be high pitched, and there is a delayed onset of pubic, facial, and axillary hair and genital growth. History, physical findings, and a decreased level of circulating GH contribute to the diagnosis.

Evaluate the family history for traits of short stature or to detect if the main problem is constitutional delay (innocent late development). If at all possible, obtain estimates of the parents' height and siblings' height and weight during their periods of growth. Assess thoroughly the child's prenatal and birth history for suggestion of intrauterine growth retardation or severe head trauma at birth, which could have injured the pituitary gland. Assess the health history for chronic illness, such as heart, kidney, or intestinal disorders, that could contribute to the decreased level of growth. Take a 24-hour nutrition history and ask carefully about urinary and bowel function. Parents often report that their child is a "picky eater," yet the 24-hour history does not reveal a poor appetite that is extensive enough to halt growth. Be certain to assess the child's feelings about being short and the actual height.

A pituitary tumor must be ruled out as the cause of decreased GH production. Suddenly halted growth suggests a tumor; gradual failure suggests an idiopathic involvement. A history of vision loss, headache, increase in head circumference, nausea, and vomiting also suggests a pituitary tumor. The history of a child with hypopituitary dwarfism typically reveals a well child except for the abnormal lack of growth.

TABLE 27.1 Common Pituitary Hormones and Their Purposes

PITUITARY HORMONE	SOURCE AND TARGET ORGANS	ACTIONS AND EFFECTS
Antidiuretic hormone (ADH)	Secreted by the neurohypophysis Target organ: kidney	• ADH helps regulate fluid volume and urine output. It decreases urinary output by increasing water reabsorption. This increases extracellular fluid volume, resulting in a vasopressor effect (increased blood pressure). When the plasma concentration increases or overall circulating vascular volume decreases, more ADH will be released. • If blood pools in the body periphery, decreasing core body volume, ADH will be released. • Postural changes (from a lying to a standing position); exposure to high temperatures (blood shifts to peripheral structures to begin the cooling process); and positive-pressure respiration (decreased blood volume in the vena cava) stimulate ADH release. • Trauma, pain, and anxiety increase ADH release. • When ADH levels fall, little or no water is reabsorbed, and urinary output increases. • Alcohol consumption inhibits ADH secretion; as a result, urine output increases.
Corticotropin (ACTH)	Secreted by the adenohypophysis Target organ: kidneys	• ACTH stimulates the adrenal gland to produce glucocorticoid and mineralocorticoid hormones. Increased production of adrenal gland secretions decreases ACTH production and vice versa. • If a child receives synthetic ACTH or a corticosteroid, natural ACTH production is temporarily depressed. If these synthetic hormones are given for a long time, then stopped abruptly, the decreased amount of natural ACTH may not be enough to stimulate adrenal gland activity. The child will experience symptoms of adrenal insufficiency. • When discontinuing ACTH and high doses of corticosteroids, dosage decreases must be reduced gradually to protect adrenal function. The medication should never be stopped abruptly.
Somatotropin (growth hormone—GH)	Secreted by the adenohypophysis Target organ: None; acts on all body cells	• GH increases bone and cartilage growth and increases gastrointestinal absorption of calcium. If GH production is inhibited, dwarfism will occur; if GH production is excessive, gigantism or overgrowth will occur. • GH decreases catabolism of protein in cells by freeing fatty acids for energy, which in turn frees glucose for glycogen storage (GH is both protein and glucose sparing). • GH production increases when hypoglycemia occurs and during sleep. • GH is released from the adenohypophysis based on a release factor from both the hypothalamus and the liver. • The amount of GH secretion is influenced by exercise, sleep, nutrition, and thyroid and adrenal function.
Thyrotropin (TSH)	Secreted by the adenohypophysis	• TSH stimulates the thyroid gland to produce thyroid hormones (thyroxine and triiodothyronine). • Too little TSH leads to atrophy and inactivity of the thyroid gland; too much TSH causes hypertrophy (increase in size) and hyperplasia (increase in the number of cells) of the gland. • A feedback message of increased thyroid secretion lowers TSH production; decreased thyroid production increases TSH production.

A physical assessment, including a funduscopic examination and neurologic testing, should be done to detect a lesion or tumor. Blood studies for hypothyroidism, hypoadrenalism, and hypoaldosteronism are performed, because these conditions also influence growth. The wrist is examined by x-ray film to determine bone age. Epiphyseal closure of long bone is delayed with GH deficiency but is proportional to the height delay. A skull series, computed tomography (CT) scan, magnetic resonance imaging, or sonogram will be performed to detect possible enlargement of the sella turcica, which would suggest a pituitary tumor.

Normally, GH level rises after a period of sound sleep or a period of activity. If the level is low during these test periods, the hormone's response to artificial stimulation can be tested. If normal children are given a test dose of insulin, for example, they will become hypoglycemic. **Hypoglycemia** (low glucose level) stimulates the release of circulating GH. Intravenous infusion of arginine or oral administration of clonidine or propranolol will have the same effect. In children with GH deficiency, an increase in the level of GH does not occur in these instances.

These studies obviously call for careful nursing attention so that children do not become extremely hypoglycemic or refuse to cooperate with the number of blood samples and the intravenous line necessary for the studies. If the child is not concerned about being short, these studies may not seem important; it may be difficult to tolerate the pain associated with the procedures (although application of EMLA creme greatly reduces the discomfort). Use a heparin lock so that blood sampling will involve as few venipunctures as possible; provide enjoyable activities during the testing period.

Therapeutic Management

Growth hormone deficiency is treated by the administration of intramuscular human GH injection two or three times a week (Birnbacher et al, 1998) (see the Drug Highlight box). The dose is increased at puberty to mimic the normal increase at that time (Codner et al, 1997). Because the time of the dose affects the hormone's effectiveness, GH is usually given at bedtime. Fortunately, because these children have delayed epiphyseal closure, with therapy, they will still be able to grow to normal height. Some may need leuteinizing hormone-releasing hormone to delay epiphyseal closure. When human GH was in short supply, available only from cadavers, few children were able to receive treatment for their condition. Today, however, advances in recombinant DNA synthesis have made adequate amounts of synthetic GH available to all who need it. Some children, however, develop antibodies to GH, and its effect is therefore decreased. Other treatment will depend on accompanying pituitary dysfunctions. Some children may need supplements of gonadotropin or other pituitary hormones as well.

DRUG HIGHLIGHT

Somatropin (Nutropin, Humatrope)

Class: Hormone

Action: Long-term treatment of children who have growth failure from inadequate production of pituitary hormone, renal failure, and Turner's syndrome; may be used to promote healing in severe burns

Pregnancy risk category: C

Dosage: Somatropin dosage is individualized. The drug is administered by injection.

Possible adverse effects: Injection site pain, glucose intolerance, hypothyroidism, bone problems (particularly the hip), blood abnormalities, rare intracranial hypertension in first 8 weeks of therapy

Nursing Implications:

1. Advise parents that hip x-rays are performed before therapy begins. Thereafter, parents should be alert for limping or complaints of knee or hip pain, which should be reported to their primary care provider.
2. Children need periodic thyroid function tests and funduscopic examination (to detect rare intracranial hypertension).
3. Tell parents that growth hormone may interact with glucocorticoid therapy (e.g., prednisone) and interfere with the effect of the growth hormone. They should make sure that all health care practitioners know that the child is receiving growth hormone.

NURSING DIAGNOSES AND RELATED INTERVENTIONS

Nursing Diagnosis: Self-esteem disturbance related to short stature

Outcome Identification: Child will demonstrate adequate self-esteem by the end of the treatment period.

Outcome Evaluation: Child speaks positively about self; identifies friends and activities enjoyed with peers.

If a child has been consistently behind in growth since early life, parents may simply assume the child is going to be short as an adult. The parents become concerned only when the child reaches puberty and fails to develop secondary sex characteristics. When investigation reveals the child's true problem, parents may feel guilty that they did not become alarmed earlier. They may feel resentment toward health care personnel who did not alert them to the problem. Parents should be encouraged to discuss these feelings and may need support accepting their child in this new light (see the Enhancing Communication box).

Children may need some help in accepting themselves at the ultimate height they achieve, especially if this is only in the fifth percentile, not the 50th. You may need to remind parents to assign duties and responsibilities to children that match their chronologic age, not physical size, to promote their feelings of maturity and self-esteem.

Pituitary Gigantism

Overproduction of GH is generally caused by a tumor of the anterior pituitary (an adenoma). An overproduction of GH before the epiphyseal lines of the long bones have closed may cause excessive growth. Weight is excessive also, but it is proportional to height. Such excessive growth generally becomes evident at puberty when prepubertal growth is excessive. The skull circumference generally exceeds normal, and the fontanelles may close late or not close at all. *Acromegaly* (enlargement of the bones of the head and soft parts of the hands and feet) may accompany the excessive growth in stature, although acromegaly becomes more pronounced after the epiphyseal lines of the long bones close and linear growth is no longer possible. The tongue may be so enlarged and thickened that it protrudes from the mouth, giving the child a dull, apathetic appearance. X-ray films or sono-

ENHANCING COMMUNICATION

Peggy, a 10-year-old fifth grader, has been diagnosed with hypopituitarism. She is only 3 ft tall and has shown no secondary sex development as yet. The physician has prescribed injections of growth hormone three times weekly. While observing her and her mother, you notice that Peggy is wearing a dress more suitable for a first grader than a fifth grader.

Less Effective Communication

Nurse: Mrs. Stone, do you have any questions about Peggy's care?

Mrs. Stone: Not really; I think everyone is exaggerating the importance of being tall, though. Look how cute she is playing with that puzzle on that little table over there.

Nurse: She is cute, but is she happy with being so short?

Mrs. Stone: Well, her size has made her better at gymnastics than the taller girls—and tap dancing. She's won two contests—probably because she looks so much younger than she is.

Nurse: But how does she feel about her size? Have you talked to her about how she thinks she will feel about her size in the future when she's grown up?

Mrs. Stone: I can't imagine her grown up—not when she's so tiny and cute now.

Nurse: Well, you realize that the growth hormone injections that I will be teaching you to give will make her grow.

Mrs. Stone: Yes, but I hope she doesn't grow too much. I don't want to lose my baby.

Nurse: Let's go over the injection technique now so I'm sure you can give them effectively.

More Effective Communication

Nurse: Mrs. Stone, do you have any questions about Peggy's care?

Mrs. Stone: Not really; I think everyone is exaggerating the importance of being tall, though. Look how cute she is playing with that puzzle on that little table over there.

Nurse: She is cute, but is she happy with being so short?

Mrs. Stone: Well, her size has made her better at gymnastics than the taller girls—and tap dancing. She's won two contests—probably because she looks so much younger than she is.

Nurse: But how does she feel about her size? Have you talked to her about how she thinks she will feel about her size in the future when she's grown up?

Mrs. Stone: I can't imagine her grown up—not when she's so tiny and cute now.

Nurse: Well, you realize that the growth hormone injections that I will be teaching you to give will make her grow.

Mrs. Stone: Yes, but I hope she doesn't grow too much. I don't want to lose my baby.

Nurse: Well, let's talk a little bit about how Peggy's growing up makes both you and Peggy feel before we review the injection technique.

Children with hypopituitarism are often viewed as cute and petite by parents and treated as if they were the age of a child their size, not their chronologic age. When therapy to make them taller begins, some parents have difficulty accepting that growth may change not only the child's appearance, but also the parent–child relationship—that growing up means growing away toward independence. Exploring how the parents and the child feel about this may help them view the coming change as a positive and exciting new stage in their relationship. In such instances, a positive outlook on growth will help ensure adherence to and acceptance of therapy.

grams of the skull will reveal enlargement of the sella turcica. Untreated, a child may reach a height of over 8 ft.

If the cause of the increased hormone production is a tumor, surgery to remove the tumor or cryosurgery (freezing of tissue) is the primary treatment. If no tumor is present, irradiation or radioactive implants of the pituitary may be successful in reducing the GH production. Other hormones may be affected when GH secretion is halted this way, so it may be necessary in later life for the patient to receive supplemental thyroid extract, cortisol, and gonadotropin hormones.

It is difficult for a child always to be bigger and taller than playmates, and the problem continues to be very real and distressing in adulthood. These children need to be identified during regular health screening so that the cause of such excessive growth can be determined and treatment offered.

Diabetes Insipidus

Diabetes insipidus is a disease in which there is decreased release of antidiuretic hormone (ADH) by the pituitary gland. This causes less reabsorption of fluid in the kidney tubules. Urine becomes extremely dilute, and a great deal of fluid is lost from the body. Diabetes insipidus may reflect an autosomal dominant trait, or it may be transmitted by a sex-linked recessive gene; it may result from a lesion, tumor, or injury to the posterior pituitary; or it may have an unknown cause. In a rare type of diabetes insipidus, pituitary function is adequate, but the nephrons are not sensitive to ADH (a kidney etiology).

Assessment

The child with diabetes insipidus evidences excessive thirst (**polydipsia**), relieved only by drinking water, not breast milk or formula, and excessive urination (**polyuria**). The specific gravity of the urine will be low (1.001–1.005); the normal values are more often 1.010 to 1.030. Urine output may reach 4 to 10 L in a 24-hour period (the normal is 1–2 L), depending on age.

Signs and symptoms of diabetes insipidus usually present gradually. The polyuria may be noticed first as bedwetting in the toilet-trained child. Weight loss from the large loss of fluid occurs. Untreated, the child will lose such a quantity of water that dehydration and death may result.

X-ray film, CT scan, or ultrasound study of the skull will reveal whether a lesion or tumor is present. A further test is the administration of vasopressin (Pitressin). The child's urine output is measured for a baseline. Vasopressin is then administered. The drug decreases the blood pressure, alerting the kidney to retain more fluid to maintain vascular pressure. If the fault of the dilute urine is with the pituitary, not the kidney, the child's urine output will decrease.

Therapeutic Management

If a tumor is present, it is removed by surgery. If the cause is idiopathic, the condition can be controlled by the administration of desmopressin (DDAVP), an arginine vasopressin. In an emergency, this can be given intravenously. For long-term use, it is given intranasally or orally (Boulgourdjian et al, 1997). When given as an intranasal spray, it can be placed on a cotton ball and held against the mucous membrane of the nose for 3 to 5 minutes once or twice a day. Nasal irritation may result from intranasal administration; intranasal administration will not be effective if the child has an upper respiratory infection and swollen mucous membranes. Caution children that they will notice an increasing urine output just before the next dose is due.

Vasopressin is not effective if the kidney tubules are resistant to ADH. If this happens, excessive thirst can be relieved by lowering the child's intake of sodium and protein and by administering a diuretic that reduces reabsorption of sodium ions.

NURSING DIAGNOSES AND RELATED INTERVENTIONS

Nursing Diagnosis: Risk for fluid volume deficit related to constant, excessive loss of fluid through urination

Outcome Identification: Child will maintain adequate fluid volume during the illness.

Outcome Evaluation: Child's blood pressure and pulse are within normal limits for age; specific gravity of urine is between 1.003 and 1.030; skin turgor is good; child states thirst is not excessive.

Teach About Long-Term Therapy. At least one parent must learn injection technique in addition to the child if an intramuscular medication is required. Explain the difference between diabetes insipidus and diabetes mellitus, the disorder most people think of when they hear the word diabetes, so that they are not confused about differences in therapy.

Encourage Communication. Caution parents that they should always notify health care providers that the child has diabetes insipidus when seeking any type of health care. Surgery poses particular dangers because of the fluid restrictions that accompany most procedures. Encourage children to wear a MedicAlert tag identifying them as having diabetes insipidus. With the child's and parent's permission, inform school personnel that the child may need to use the bathroom frequently; help the child and family plan frequent bathroom stops and adequate fluid intake on long trips.

✔ CHECKPOINT QUESTIONS

1. Why must children be monitored closely following insulin or arginine testing for growth hormone deficiency?
2. Why may children with diabetes insipidus be reluctant to take their medication during the day at school?

THE THYROID GLAND

The thyroid gland is responsible for controlling the rate of metabolism in the body through production of the hormones thyroxine (T_4) and triiodothyronine (T_3) by the follicular cells of the thyroid.

A third hormone, thyrocalcitonin, is produced by the interstitial cells of the gland. Thyrocalcitonin is released if a high serum calcium level occurs. This hormone inhibits bone resorption, thereby slowing the rate of release of calcium from bone to plasma and a resulting lowered serum calcium level. It reflects the reverse action of parathyroid hormone, which elevates serum calcium levels.

Assessment of Thyroid Function

Radioimmunoassay of T_4 and T_3 is a specific blood study to determine how much protein-bound iodine (PBI) is present. If a child has recently taken large amounts of cough medicine containing iodide or had an iodine-based, contrast-media study, such as urography or bronchography, the PBI level may be abnormally elevated. The small amount of iodine ingested from iodized salt does not affect PBI levels.

Children who have low circulating albumin levels will have abnormally low PBI levels, because iodine is carried bound to protein. Phenytoin (Dilantin), a common anticonvulsant given to patients with recurrent seizures, may displace thyroxine from binding globulin and further contribute to these low PBI levels.

Another test of thyroid function is a radioactive iodine uptake test. The child is given an oral dose of a solution containing radioactive iodine (^{123}I). The thyroid gland "traps" this iodine, and 24 hours later, after the maximum amount has been trapped, the amount of radioactive iodine present can be determined. It is important in this type of test that the child swallow all the solution. In infants, this is generally given as a gavage feeding so that accuracy of the dose can be ensured.

An uptake of less than 10% of the test dose suggests hypothyroidism. If the child vomits after ingesting the substance, this event should be recorded and called to the attention of the laboratory; it will obviously result in a lower uptake value, because only a part of the actual dose was available for uptake. Be certain the child does not receive iodine or thyroid extract in any other form during the test time; it will compete with the uptake of the radioactive iodine and, again, the value will be falsely low.

DISORDERS OF THE THYROID GLAND

Congenital Hypothyroidism (Thyroid Dysgenesis)

Thyroid hypofunction causes reduced production of both T_4 and T_3. Congenital *hypofunction* occurs as a result of an absent or nonfunctioning thyroid gland. The condition may not be noticeable initially, because the mother's thyroid hormones maintain adequate levels in the fetus during pregnancy. The symptoms of congenital hypothyroidism become apparent, however, during the first 3 months of life in a formula-fed infant and at about 6 months in a breastfed infant. The disorder occurs in 1 in 4000 live births and about twice as often in girls as in boys (Donohoue, 1997a). Because congenital hypothyroidism causes progressive physical and cognitive impairment, early diagnosis is crucial. In most states, a screening test for hypothyroidism is mandatory at birth (using the same few drops of blood obtained for a Guthrie or phenylketonuria [PKU] test).

Assessment

Parents may report that their child sleeps excessively. The tongue becomes enlarged, causing respiratory difficulty, noisy respirations, or obstruction (Figure 27-2). The child may develop trouble feeding because of sluggishness or choking. The skin of the extremities is usually cold, and the overall body temperature may be subnormal because of slowed metabolism. A slow metabolic rate is also revealed by slow pulse and respiratory rates. Prolonged jaundice, due to the immature liver's inability to conjugate bilirubin, may be present. Anemia may increase the child's lethargy and fatigue.

The child's neck becomes short and thick. The facial expression is dull, as the result of cognitive impairment, and open-mouthed because of the child's attempts to breathe around the enlarged tongue. The extremities are short and fat, with hypotonic muscles, giving the infant a floppy, rag-doll appearance. Deep tendon reflexes are slower than normal. Generalized obesity usually occurs. Hair is brittle and dry. Dentition is delayed, or teeth may be defective when they do erupt.

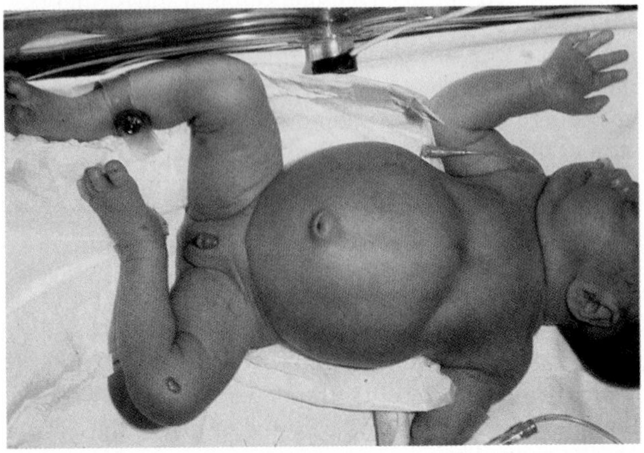

FIGURE 27.2 An infant with congenital hypothyroidism. Notice the short, thick neck and enlarged abdomen.

The hypotonia affects the intestinal tract as well, so the child has chronic constipation; the abdomen enlarges because of poor muscle tone. Many infants have an umbilical hernia. Overall, the skin is dry and perhaps scaly, and the child does not perspire. Infants will have low radioactive iodine uptake levels, low serum T_4 and T_3 levels, and elevated thyroid-stimulating factor. Blood lipids will be increased. X-ray films may reveal delayed bone growth.

Therapeutic Management

The treatment for hypothyroidism is oral administration of synthetic thyroid hormone, sodium levothyroxine. A small dose is given at first, and then the dose is gradually increased to therapeutic levels. The child will need to continue taking medication indefinitely. Supplemental vitamin D may also be given to prevent the development of rickets when, with the administration of thyroid hormone, rapid bone growth begins.

Further cognitive impairment can be prevented as soon as therapy is started, but any degree of impairment already present cannot be reversed.

Helping parents administer medication is a major nursing role. Be certain that parents know the rules for long-term medication administration with children, as described in the Empowering the Family display. Periodic monitoring of T_4 and T_3 will help to ensure an appropriate medication dosage. If the dose of thyroid hormone is not adequate, the T_4 level will remain low, and there will be few signs of clinical improvement. If the dose is too high, the T_4 level will rise, and the child will show signs of hyperthyroidism: irritability, fever, rapid pulse, and perhaps vomiting, diarrhea, and weight loss.

Thyroiditis (Hashimoto's Disease)

Thyroiditis is the most common form of acquired hypothyroidism in childhood; the age of onset is often 10 to 11 years, and there may be a family history of thyroid disease. It occurs more often in girls than in boys. The decrease in thyroid secretion is caused by the development of an autoimmune phenomenon that interferes with thyroid production. Stimulation of thyroid-stimulating hormone (TSH) from the pituitary increases when thyroid hormone production decreases in an attempt to cause the thyroid to be more effective.

Assessment

In response to TSH, there is hypertrophy of the thyroid (goiter), and body growth is impaired by lack of thyroxine. In infants, congenital goiter can lead to airway obstruction; in children, the condition leads to obesity, lethargy, and delayed sexual development.

Antithyroid antibodies are present in serum. The enlarged thyroid may become nodular in response to the oversecretion of TSH. Although in childhood, a nodular

EMPOWERING THE FAMILY: Guidelines for Successful Long-Term Medicine Administration

1. Teach children about the type and purpose of medicine they will be taking. Knowing the purpose of something maintains interest and cooperation.
2. Always be certain to anticipate obtaining prescriptions so a ready supply is on hand before vacations, summer camp, holidays.
3. Avoid bribing children to get them to take their medicine. After a time, a bribe becomes too difficult to maintain.
4. The earlier you can involve children in administering their own medication, the sooner they can achieve an independent lifestyle.
5. Be aware of the lifespan of the medicine being administered so outdated medication is not used.
6. Do not store medicine carelessly. Consider all medicine a potential poison and keep it out of the reach of small children.
7. Use a dose-reminder system such as a chart on the refrigerator, bathroom door, or school locker.
8. Plan times for medication administration that allow for a normal lifestyle (e.g., no getting up at 2 AM, or having to interrupt a school class for an injection).

thyroid is usually benign, an investigation into the possibility of thyroid malignancy must be considered. For diagnosis, children are administered radioactive iodine. If the nodes are benign, there is generally a rapid uptake of radioactive iodine ("hot nodes"). If there is no uptake ("cold nodes"), carcinoma is a much more likely diagnosis (extremely rare at this age).

Therapeutic Management

Treatment for thyroiditis is the administration of synthetic thyroid hormone (sodium levothyroxine), the same as for congenital hypothyroidism. With adequate dosage, the obesity will diminish and growth will begin again. It is important that the disease be recognized as early as possible so that there is time to stimulate growth before the epiphyseal lines close at puberty.

Hyperthyroidism (Thyrotoxicosis or Graves' Disease)

Hyperthyroidism is oversecretion of thyroid hormones by the thyroid gland. Thyrotoxicosis is the body's response to excessive production of thyroid hormones. Thyrotoxicosis in children usually occurs at the time of puberty or during adolescence and is more common in girls than in boys. Overactivity of the thyroid gland can occur from the gland being overstimulated by the thyrotropic hormone of the pituitary (TSH) due to a pituitary tumor. More frequently, hyperthyroidism and thyrotoxicosis in children are caused by an autoimmune reaction that results in production of immunoglobulin G (IgG), which stimulates the thyroid gland. An exophthalmos-producing pituitary substance causes the prominent-appearing eyes that accompany hyperthyroidism in some children.

Assessment

Graves' disease often follows a viral illness or a period of stress. Some children may have a genetic predisposition to development of the disorder. With overproduction of T_3 and T_4, children gradually experience nervousness, loss of muscle strength, and easy fatigue. Their basal metabolic rate is high; blood pressure and pulse are increased. They perspire freely. They are always hungry, and although they eat constantly, they do not gain weight and may even lose weight because of the increased basal metabolic rate. On x-ray examination, bone age will appear advanced beyond the chronologic age of the child. Unless the condition is treated, the child will not be able to reach normal adult height, because epiphyseal lines of long bones will close before normal height is attained.

The thyroid gland, which is usually not prominent in children, appears as a swelling on the anterior neck (goiter) and can be confirmed by ultrasound. When the child protrudes the tongue or extends the hands, fine tremors are noticeable. In a few children, the eye globes will be prominent (exophthalmos), giving the child a wide-eyed, staring appearance. Laboratory tests will show elevated T_4 and T_3 levels and an increased radioactive iodine uptake. TSH level will be low or absent because the thyroid is being stimulated by antibodies, not by the pituitary gland.

Therapeutic Management

Therapy consists first of a course of a beta-adrenergic blocking agent, such as propranolol, to decrease the antibody response. After this, the child is placed on an antithyroid drug, such as propylthiouracil or methimazole (Tapazole), to suppress the formation of thyroxine. While taking the drug, the child must be monitored to prevent a depressed white blood cell level (leukopenia) from occurring as a side effect. If serious leukopenia results, the drug should be discontinued until the white blood cell count returns to normal so that the patient does not contract an infection.

Because the thyroid stores considerable thyroid hormone that must be used up first, it will take about 2 weeks for these drugs to have an effect. The child will generally have to take the drug for years before the condition "burns itself out." The exophthalmos may not recede but will not become worse from the time therapy is instituted.

If the child has a toxic reaction to medical management (lowered white blood cell count) or is noncompliant about taking the medicine, radioiodine ablative therapy with ^{131}I to reduce the size of the thyroid gland can be accomplished (Foley & Charron, 1997). Surgical removal of part or almost all of the thyroid gland may be necessary in a young adult and can be completed safely (Liu et al, 1998). After both radioiodine ablative therapy and thyroidectomy, supplemental thyroid hormone therapy may be needed indefinitely.

NURSING DIAGNOSES AND RELATED INTERVENTIONS

Nursing Diagnosis: Self-esteem disturbance related to lack of coordination and presence of prominent goiter

Outcome Identification: Child will demonstrate adequate self-esteem by the end of the treatment period.

Outcome Evaluation: Child states positive traits about self and identifies friends and activities enjoyed.

Hyperthyroidism begins gradually and may become fairly involved before it is detected. Children at puberty should be suspected of having hyperthyroidism if they are losing weight or having behavior problems in school because of new hand tremors and tongue tremors that make it hard for them to write or speak. Behavior problems may also arise because of the nervousness and inability to sit still during class.

The parents need support in giving the medication or making sure that the child takes the medicine every day. Caution them not to stop medicine abruptly or a thyroxine crisis (sudden onset of symptoms) can occur. Some parents ask if their child can have surgery as a cure so that long-term administration of medicine will not be required. Help them understand that surgery will not dispel the need for medication. Instead, another kind of medicine will be needed. If a large portion of the thyroid gland is removed, it may be necessary to give medicine indefinitely to make up for the missing gland. In any event, it is preferable to try a course of medical management before resorting to surgery.

Because the onset of hyperthyroidism is gradual, children may be aware of their difficulties in school before their parents are. Increasing symptoms, for example, exophthalmos, may lead to an appearance about which the other children tease them. After therapy, these children need to be encouraged to return to activities that require fine coordination or social interaction and to think of themselves as well again.

✔ CHECKPOINT QUESTIONS

3. What is the chief (most serious) effect of congenital hypothyroidism?
4. Why are children who develop hyperthyroidism at puberty often seen as behavior problems in school?

THE ADRENAL GLAND

The two adrenal glands are located retroperitoneally just above each kidney. (Because of their location, they are also referred to as suprarenal glands.) The adrenal glands are made up of two distinct parts, which differ not only in tissue origin, but also in function. The *adrenal medulla* is a small core surrounded by the *adrenal cortex.* Although each of these parts has different functions and releases different hormones, together they protect the body against acute and chronic forms of stress.

Adrenal Hormones

The adrenal cortex produces cortisol (a glucocorticoid), androgen, and aldosterone (a mineralocorticoid)—three hormones important in childhood illness. Norepinephrine and epinephrine, hormones important for maintaining blood pressure, are produced by the adrenal medulla.

Cortisol

Cortisol is a glucocorticoid that is necessary for glucose and protein metabolism. It is released by the adrenal cortex in response to adrenocorticotropic hormone (ACTH) stimulation from the pituitary gland. ACTH is strongly influenced by biorhythm or circadian rhythms. In the hours just before and after a person awakens, ACTH reaches its highest peak. The level decreases again gradually throughout the day and night. The level of ACTH secretion also increases during periods of emotional stress, leading to increased production of cortisol. Severe trauma, major surgery, hypotension, extreme cold, and acute or chronic illness also increase production of cortisol.

Glucocorticoids are named for their ability to regulate serum glucose and protein levels. This regulation is accomplished primarily by increasing the amount of glucose formed by the liver (gluconeogenesis) and decreasing use of glucose by tissue. Free fatty acids are released from tissue stores into the plasma, making them available for energy. Protein synthesis in cells is halted, which frees up amino acids for liver production of protein. Cortisol is necessary during a time of stress to allow the body to have glucose and protein available for emergency processes.

Cortisol is also important in decreasing an inflammatory response. In the bloodstream, it causes a reduced number of eosinophils and lymphocytes while red blood cell and platelet production are increased. A drawback of this response is that the decreased number of lymphocytes may allow infection to occur.

Aldosterone

Aldosterone is secreted in response to renin-angiotensin, serum potassium, and sodium levels. Renin is released from kidney nephrons in response to a lowered blood pressure; shortly thereafter, it is converted to angiotensin II. In the presence of angiotensin II, aldosterone is released from the adrenal cortex. When angiotensin is decreased, the production of aldosterone stops. When serum potassium levels rise, aldosterone secretion increases. Lowered levels of potassium decrease aldosterone secretion. Sodium influences aldosterone by a reverse process (when sodium levels are low, aldosterone secretion increases; an increased sodium concentration inhibits aldosterone secretion).

The action of aldosterone causes salt to be retained by the body; as sodium is retained, fluid is also retained. Aldosterone plays a direct role in stabilizing blood volume and pressure because of its role in maintaining sodium balance. Infants born with an inability to produce aldosterone will quickly become dehydrated, and their lives will be in immediate danger.

Androgen

Androgen is the hormone responsible for muscular development, increase in linear size, growth of body hair, and the increase in sebaceous gland secretions that cause typical acne at puberty.

DISORDERS OF THE ADRENAL GLAND

Disorders of the adrenal gland include those related to **hypofunction**, which can lead to acute or chronic insufficiency, and those related to **hyperfunction**, which most often leads to overproduction of androgen.

Acute Adrenocortical Insufficiency

Insufficiency (hypofunction) of the adrenal gland may be either acute or chronic. In many adrenal syndromes, only one hormone is involved, and the symptoms are directly related only to that hormone. In acute adrenocortical insufficiency, the entire cortical adrenal gland function suddenly becomes insufficient. This occurs generally in association with severe overwhelming infections in which there is hemorrhagic destruction of the adrenal glands. It is seen most commonly in meningococcemia. It can occur when corticosteroid therapy, which has been maintained at high levels for long periods, is abruptly stopped.

Assessment

The symptoms of acute adrenocortical insufficiency are acute and sudden. The blood pressure drops to extremely low levels; the child appears ashen gray and may be pulseless. Temperature is elevated; dehydration and hypoglycemia are marked. Sodium and chloride blood levels will be very low, but serum potassium will be elevated, because there is usually an inverse relationship between sodium and potassium values. The child is prostrate, and convulsions may occur. Without treatment, death may occur abruptly (Donohoue, 1997b).

Therapeutic Management

Treatment involves the immediate replacement of cortisol (intravenous Solu-Cortef) and deoxycorticosterone acetate (DOCA), the synthetic equivalent of aldosterone, and intravenous 5% glucose in normal saline solution to restore blood pressure, sodium, and blood glucose levels. A vasopressor may be necessary to elevate the blood pressure (August, 1997).

Acute adrenal cortical insufficiency is a medical emergency. Although seen less often than in the past because of antibiotics that quickly halt the course of infectious disease, it is not an obsolete entity. Now that more conditions are being treated with corticosteroids, the chances that acute adrenal cortical insufficiency will occur from sudden withdrawal of steroids is actually increasing.

Adrenogenital Syndrome (Congenital Adrenal Hyperplasia)

Adrenogenital syndrome is inherited as an autosomal recessive trait. The primary defect is an inability to synthesize cortisol from its precursors. When the adrenal gland is unable to produce cortisol, the amount of pituitary adrenotropic hormone increases, stimulating the adrenal glands to improve function. Although the adrenals enlarge (hyperplasia), they still cannot produce hydrocortisone; androgen begins to be overproduced.

Assessment

The excessive androgen production masculinizes the female child or increases the size of genital organs in male infants (Figure 27-3). This process begins during fetal life, so that the female infant is born with a clitoris so enlarged it appears more like a penis. Because her labia are typically fused as well, the girl resembles a boy with undescended testes and hypospadias. Internal female organs are generally normal, although a sinus between the urethra and vagina may be present (see discussion of ambiguous genitalia in Chapter 26). If the condition is not recognized at birth and the child remains untreated, pubic and axillary hair and acne will appear precociously and a deep masculine voice will develop. At puberty there will be no breast development or menstruation.

The male child may appear normal at birth, but by 6 months of age signs of sexual precocity appear. By 3 or 4 years of age boys will have pubic hair and enlargement of the penis, scrotum, and prostate. They may have acne and a deep, mature voice. The testes do not enlarge, however, and although they are normal in size, they appear small in relation to the size of the penis. Spermatogenesis does not occur, so the child is not fertile.

Children with adrenogenital syndrome will have increased levels of testosterone in blood plasma, an important point for diagnosis. By determining the amount of other

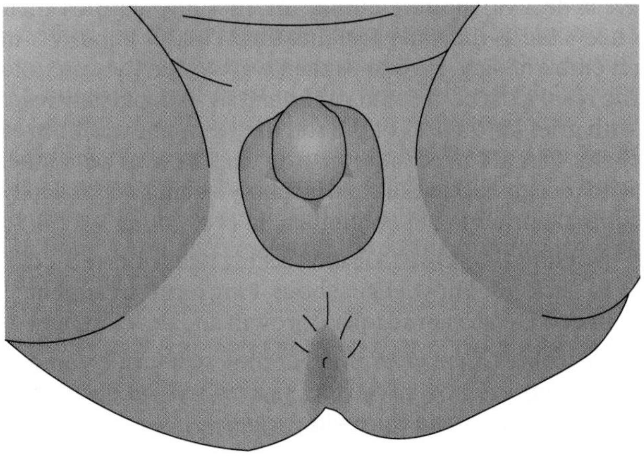

FIGURE 27.3 A female infant with adrenogenital syndrome. Note the abnormally enlarged clitoris.

Children learn quickly that if they continuously give injections in one site, scar tissue (lipohypertrophy) will form there, and no pain will be felt on injection. This is a dangerous practice, however, because insulin no longer absorbs well from this site; the child will have to increase the dose beyond what he or she actually needs for glucose metabolism, because a portion of each dose is "locked" in the tissue. Should the child then inject this larger dose of insulin into a new site, there is a potential for overdose (which would cause hypoglycemia).

Insulin should be given at room temperature. This diminishes subcutaneous atrophy and ensures its peak effectiveness. Parents may keep additional bottles in the refrigerator to increase the insulin's shelf life.

When a low-dose insulin syringe is used, the needle is so short (about 0.5 in) that children can administer insulin by bunching skin at the site and giving the injection to themselves at a 90-degree angle, a technique more closely resembling that of intramuscular than subcutaneous injection. With this technique, because the needle is so short, the insulin is deposited in the subcutaneous tissue. This technique is easier for children to learn because it takes less coordination to administer an injection at a 90-degree angle than at a 45-degree subcutaneous angle (Figure 27-6). Automatic injection devices are easy for children to use and promote early independence (Figure 27-7).

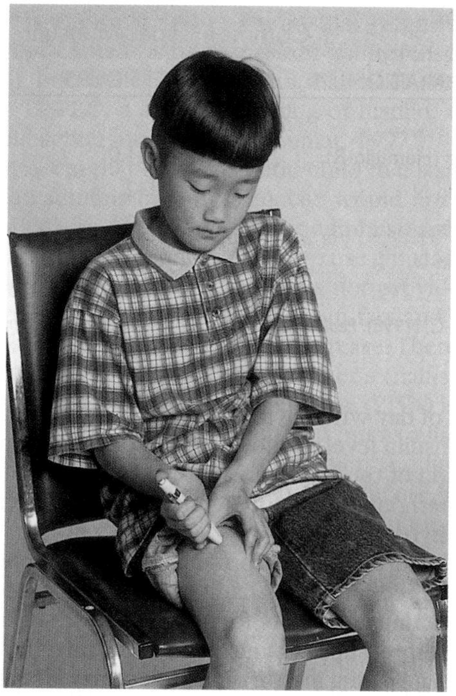

FIGURE 27.7 Injection of insulin by an automatic dispenser.

Insulin Pumps. An insulin pump is an automatic device approximately the size of a transistor radio. A syringe of regular insulin is placed in the pump chamber; a thin polyethylene tubing leads to the child's abdomen where it is implanted into the subcutaneous tissue by a small-gauge needle. Throughout the day, the pump edges the syringe barrel forward, infusing insulin at a continuous rate into the subcutaneous tissue. Before a snack or meal, the parent or child presses a button on the pump and forces a bolus of insulin forward to increase the insulin injection for managing these times of high carbohydrate intake. The site of the pump insertion is cleaned daily and covered with sterile gauze; the site is changed every 24 to 48 hours to ensure that absorption is still optimal.

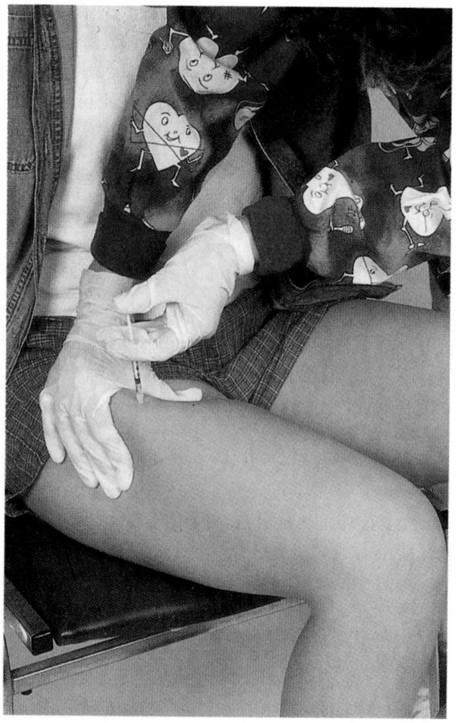

FIGURE 27.6 Insulin is usually injected at a 90-degree angle with a short needle. This angle places the insulin in the subcutaneous space.

Restrictions with pump therapy include keeping it dry; a child must remove the pump (not the syringe and tubing) while showering. The needle and syringe must be removed to bathe or swim (caution children not to leave it disconnected for over an hour or they will become hyperglycemic). A disadvantage of pump therapy is that the pump is always present. Children usually prefer to wear clothing that hides the pump's outline (it can be held against the abdomen by an over-the-shoulder sling or hung from a belt around the waist). To assess the pump's delivery of insulin, the child must do blood glucose determinations throughout the day. When pump therapy first begins, a parent must wake at 2 AM and test the child's blood glucose level because this is such a vulnerable time for hypoglycemia (the pump is delivering insulin, but the child has not eaten since bedtime).

Intranasal Insulin. In the future, insulin may be administered intranasally because it is absorbed well across mucous membranes. This will release the child from the chore of daily injections. Intranasal drug absorption is reduced, however, if the child develops a cold or allergies that cause edema of the nasal membrane. Absorption can be influenced as well by whether the insulin is applied while the child is upright or lying down at the time of administration.

Nutrition. Children with type I diabetes need to consume a diet appropriate for their age in the proportion of 50% carbohydrate, 20% protein, and 30% fat. The meal pattern should be three spaced meals with a snack in the midafternoon and evening.

Urine Testing. Urine testing has the disadvantage of not being as accurate as blood serum testing and is now used only to test for ketonuria when the child is ill or to detect nocturnal hypoglycemia. An Acetest tablet or dipstick technique may be used. Warn parents and children that Acetest tablets are poisonous. They must be kept out of the reach of smaller siblings. Acetone appearing in the urine is a sign that fat is being used for energy, which occurs with infection or when not enough food has been ingested.

Serum Monitoring. Children as young as early school age can learn the techniques of finger puncture and reading a computerized monitor. Using a spring-loaded puncture device helps minimize pain, and an automatic readout monitor, such as a Glucometer, simplifies the procedure and gives a more accurate reading than matching the shade of blood on a test strip to the colors on the test strip container (Figure 27-8). When blood is analyzed by these monitors, a whole blood value is being measured, not the serum glucose level. This means that the result will be about 15% higher than a serum determination; that is, a blood determination of 115 mg/dL equals 100 mg/dL of serum.

The "Honeymoon" Period. After the child's diagnosis has been confirmed and the blood glucose level has been initially regulated by insulin, there invariably follows a honeymoon period when only a minimal amount of insulin, or none at all, is needed for glucose regulation. Apparently, the exogenous insulin stimulates the islet cells to produce natural insulin, as if they are being reminded of their true function. Unfortunately, after a month or even up to a year, the islet cells begin to fail once again and diabetic symptoms recur. This can be upsetting to parents if they begin to believe that the child was wrongly diagnosed or that a cure has taken place. The parents and child need to be cautioned that symptoms will inevitably recur. Sometimes the child is maintained on a minimum amount of insulin during this period to keep everyone from having unrealistic expectations of a cure.

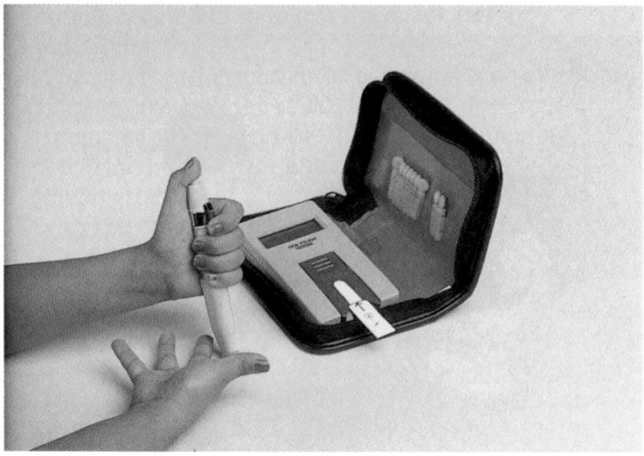

FIGURE 27.8 A child uses an automatic lancet for blood sampling (*left*). Blood glucose level will be determined by the glucometer (*right*).

Complications. Whenever children with diabetes undergo a stressful situation, either emotionally or physically, they may need increased insulin to maintain glucose homeostasis. When seen at health care facilities for periodic checkups, they should be asked not only whether they are having any difficulty with blood testing or insulin injection, but how things are at home and at school.

Interview children separately from their parents so that they can feel free to talk about anything that may be happening or going wrong. There must be cooperation between primary health care personnel and school health care personnel so that conflicts about the children's regimen do not cause problems or tensions while at school. Parents may have to meet with schoolteachers to prevent them from treating diabetic children as invalids. Sometimes children are embarrassed to have to do serum testing in school, especially in the public lavatory. It may be easier for them if they can go to the nurse's office for privacy when testing (see the Focus on Cultural Competence). Diabetic children may want to play a team sport, but the school coach may not believe a child with diabetes should play sports. Educate parents that children with well-regulated diabetes can participate in all school activities.

WHAT IF? What if your patient is a diabetic 13-year-old boy who wants to play soccer and baseball on his school teams? His parents tell you that both teams are coached by the same teacher, who thinks that diabetic children should be excluded from sports altogether. The parents prefer not to dispute the coach's decision. What information can you give the parents and the patient about diabetes and diabetes control that they can share with the coach? How can you present this information to benefit the patient and/or help change the coach's mind?

FOCUS ON CULTURAL COMPETENCE

How people view endocrine disorders can be culturally influenced. Because many of these disorders are inherited, they cluster in various populations so that there is a high incidence of the condition in family or friends or else people know nothing about the condition. In the past, because many endocrine disorders lead to changes in body appearance, particularly overgrowth or undergrowth, and because the reason for these changes was poorly understood, children with these disorders were poorly accepted. Before insulin was available for treatment of diabetes, children with the disorder did not live to adulthood. Being aware of the way that these diseases used to be viewed aids in understanding a parent's anxiety at diagnosis of these disorders and helps with nursing care planning to include reassurance and modern concepts of therapy in education.

type Ia resulted in catch-up growth. *Journal of Inherited Metabolic Disease, 20*(6), 790.

Plotnick, L. P. (1997). Growth, growth hormone and pituitary disorders. In K. B. Johnson & F. A. Oski (Eds.). *Oski's essential pediatrics*. Philadelphia: Lippincott-Raven.

Shapiro, L. J. (1997) Signs and symptoms of inborn errors of metabolism. In K. B. Johnson & F. A. Oski (Eds.). *Oski's essential pediatrics*. Philadelphia: Lippincott-Raven.

Sheth, D. P. (1997). Hypocalcemic seizures in neonates. *American Journal of Emergency Medicine, 15*(7), 638.

Taketomo, C. (1998). *Pediatric dosing handbook and formulary*. Ohio: Lexi-Comp.

Wappner, R. S., & Brandt, I. K. (1997a). Disorders of amino acid metabolism. In K. B. Johnson & F. A. Oski (Eds.). *Oski's essential pediatrics*. Philadelphia: Lippincott-Raven.

Wappner, R. S., & Brandt, I. K. (1997b). Defects in carbohydrate metabolism. In K. B. Johnson & F. A. Oski (Eds.). *Oski's essential pediatrics*. Philadelphia: Lippincott-Raven.

White, P. C. (1997). Abnormalities of aldosterone synthesis and action in children. *Current Opinion in Pediatrics, 9*(4), 424.

Wolfsdorf, J. I., & Crigler, J. F. (1997). Cornstarch regimens for nocturnal treatment of young adults with type I glycogen storage disease. *American Journal of Clinical Nutrition, 65*(5), 1507.

SUGGESTED READINGS

Allwinkle, J. (1997). The challenge of diabetes. *Community Nurse, 3*(1), 17.

Bianco, C. M. (1996). Clinical snapshot: diabetes insipidus. *American Journal of Nursing, 96*(8), 30.

Chao, T., Wang, J. R., & Hwang, B. (1997). Congenital hypothyroidism and concomitant anomalies. *Journal of Pediatric Endocrinology and Metabolism, 19*(2), 217.

Davies, P. (1996). Caring for patients with diabetes insipidus. *Nursing96, 26*(5), 62.

Grimberg, A., & Cohen, P. (1997). Optimizing growth hormone therapy in children. *Hormone Research, 48*(5), 11.

Jeffcoate, W. (1997). Probability in practice in the diagnosis of Cushing's syndrome. *Clinical Endocrinology, 47*(3), 271.

Loriaux, T. C. (1996). Endocrine assessment: Red flags for those on the front lines. *Nursing Clinics of North America, 31*(4), 695.

Ober, K. P. (1997). Work-up of endocrine abnormalities. *Hospital Medicine, 32*(10), 15.

Rusterholtz, A. (1996). Interpretation of diagnostic laboratory tests in selected endocrine disorders. *Nursing Clinics of North America, 31*(4), 715.

Shield, J. P. & Baum, J. D. (1998). Advances in childhood onset diabetes. *Archives of Disease in Childhood, 78*(4), 391.

Suevo, D. M. (1997). The infant of the diabetic mother. *Neonatal Network: Journal of Neonatal Nursing, 16*(5), 25.

Tomky, D. (1997). Diabetes: New look at an old adversary. *Nursing, 27*(11), 41.

Weissburg-Benchell, J. et al. (1995). Adolescent diabetes management and mismanagement. *Diabetes Care, 18*(2), 177.

Zadik, Z., & Zung, A. (1997). Final height after growth hormone therapy in short children: Correlation with siblings' height. *Hormone Research, 48*(6), 274.

Nursing Care of the Child With a Neurologic Disorder

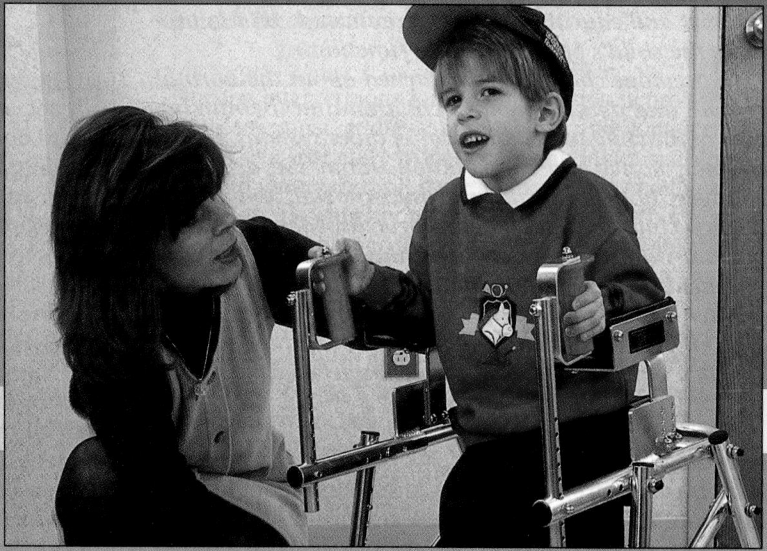

28

CHAPTER

Key Terms

- astereognosis
- automatisms
- autonomic dysreflexia
- central nervous system (CNS)
- cerebrospinal fluid (CSF)
- choreoathetosis
- choreoid
- decerebrate posturing
- decorticate posturing
- diplegia
- doll's eye reflex
- dyskinetic
- dystonic
- graphesthesia
- hemiplegia
- kinesthesia
- neuron
- paraplegia
- peripheral nervous system (PNS)
- pulse pressure
- quadriplegia
- status epilepticus
- stereognosis

Objectives

After mastering the contents of this chapter, you should be able to:

1. Describe common neurologic disorders in children.
2. Assess a child with a neurologic disorder.
3. Formulate nursing diagnoses for the child with a neurologic disorder.
4. Establish appropriate outcomes for the child with a neurologic disorder.
5. Plan nursing care for the child with a neurologic disorder.
6. Implement nursing care, such as monitoring medicine compliance, for the child with a neurologic disorder.
7. Evaluate outcomes for achievement and effectiveness of care.
8. Identify National Health Goals related to neurologic disorders and children that nurses could be instrumental in helping the nation achieve.
9. Identify areas related to care of children with neurologic disorders that could benefit from additional nursing research.
10. Analyze ways that care of the child with a neurologic disorder can be optimally family centered.
11. Integrate knowledge of neurologic disorders and the nursing process to achieve quality child health nursing care.

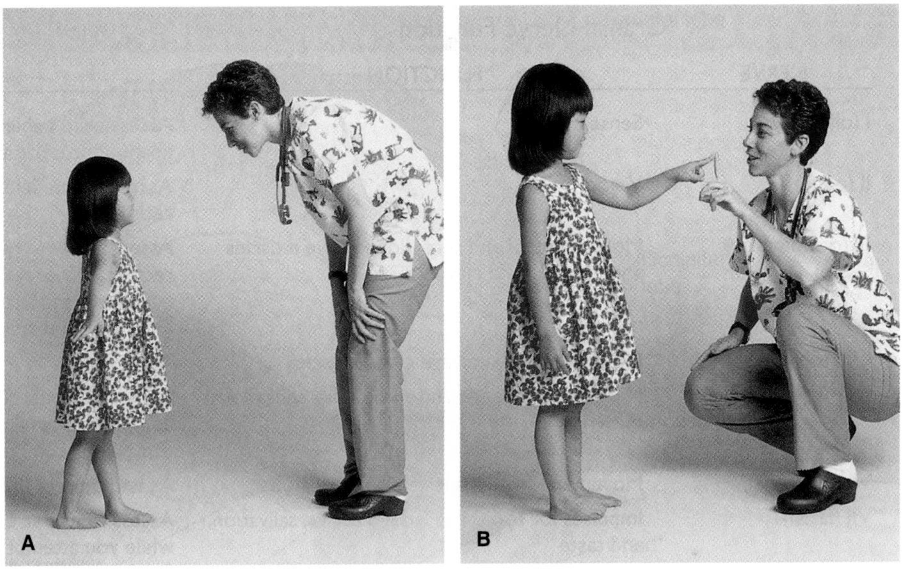

FIGURE 28.3 (A) Observing a child attempt a tandem walk. (B) Nose-to-finger test is an assessment of cerebellar function.

you touch him with an object. Light touch is tested by a wisp of cotton, deep pressure by pressure of your finger, pain by a safety pin, temperature by test tubes filled with hot or cold water. Vibration is tested by touching the child's bony prominences (iliac crest, elbows, knees) with a vibrating tuning fork. Warn the child that on pin testing, he will feel a momentary prick. Otherwise, he may be unwilling to close his eyes again for further testing.

Reflex Testing

Deep tendon reflex testing, which is part of a primary physical assessment (see Chapter 13), is also a basic part of a neurologic assessment. In newborns, reflex testing is especially important, because the infant cannot perform tasks on command to demonstrate the range of his neurologic function (see Chapter 5).

Diagnostic Testing

A variety of diagnostic tests may be ordered to provide more information should any abnormalities be detected in the health history, physical examination, or neurologic examination. Many of these tests are invasive, and it is best to try to schedule the least invasive procedures first, before the painful or more frightening procedures are done. Preparing the child and the child's family for these procedures is an important nursing responsibility. When explaining tests, take into account not only the child's chronologic age but also the child's level of cognitive functioning. Otherwise, explanations may not be well understood. Be sure also to provide an explanation that includes a description of all of the sensory experiences the child might undergo, that is, not only what will be done but also how the child might feel, or what he or she might see or hear or even smell or taste (if appropriate).

Lumbar Puncture

Lumbar puncture is the introduction of a needle into the subarachnoid space (under the arachnoid membrane) at the level of L4 or L5 to withdraw cerebrospinal fluid (CSF) for analysis. The procedure is used most frequently to diagnose hemorrhage or infection in the CNS or to diagnose an obstruction of CSF flow. Lumbar puncture is contraindicated if the needle insertion site is infected (to avoid introducing pathogens into the CSF) or if there is a suspected elevation of CSF pressure. In the latter, the increased pressure in the subarachnoid space may cause the brain stem to be drawn down into the spinal cord space, compressing the medulla and compromising the action of the cardiac and respiratory centers. EMLA cream should be applied to the puncture site 1 hour before the procedure to reduce pain.

For the procedure, the newborn is seated upright with the head bent forward (Figure 28-4*A*). The older infant or child is placed on his side on the examining table. His head is flexed forward, his knees are flexed on his abdomen, and his back is arched as much as possible. This position opens the space between the lumbar vertebrae, facilitating needle insertion (Figure 28-4*B*). Children younger than school age need to be held in this position, because they may be frightened by someone working on their back unseen; they may try to turn over or turn their head to see what is happening. It helps a school-age child or adolescent if you stand by the table facing him and gently rest your hand on the back of his head, keeping it bent forward. This helps to maintain good position without the impression of restraining him.

Children need good preparation for a lumbar puncture, because they cannot see what is happening. Let them know that the health care provider will wash their back with a solution that feels cold and that he will inject a local anesthetic that might sting like a mosquito bite. Warn them that they probably will feel pressure but not pain as the lumbar puncture needle is inserted. Remind them to remain absolutely still throughout the procedure. You might describe the position as "rolling into a ball" or "folding up like an astronaut in a small spaceship." Occasionally during a lumbar puncture, the needle will press against a dorsal nerve root and the child will experience

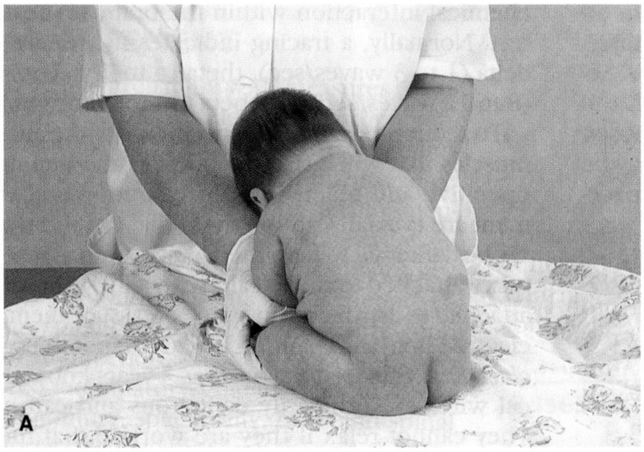

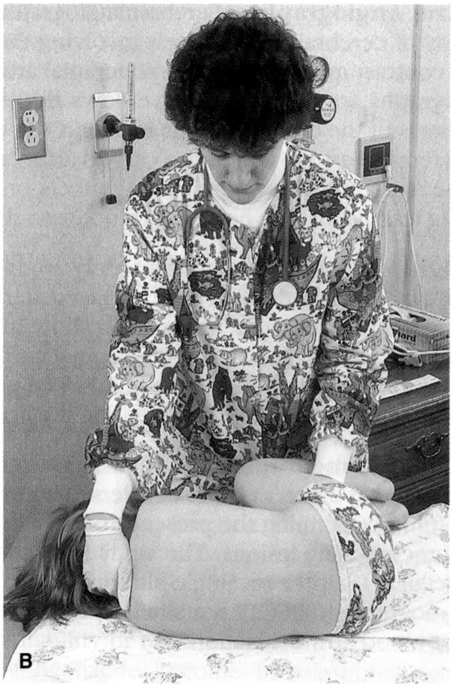

FIGURE 28.4 (**A**) Positioning an infant for a lumbar puncture. (**B**) Positioning a young child for a lumbar puncture.

a shooting pain down one leg. Reassure the child that this feeling passes quickly and does not indicate an injury.

When the insertion stylette is removed and CSF drips from the end of the needle, the procedure has been successful. An initial pressure reading is made, which varies with the child's age. To confirm that the subarachnoid space in the cord is patent with that in the skull, the examiner may ask a child who is older than 3 years to cough, or ask you to press on the child's external jugular during the procedure. Either of these measures will cause an increase of CSF pressure if fluid can flow freely through the subarachnoid space. Typically three tubes of 2 to 3 mL of CSF are collected, a closing pressure reading is taken, and the needle is withdrawn. Samples are usually sent for culture, sensitivity, glucose, and red blood cells. A *colloidal gold test* determines whether there is an alteration in the albumin–globulin ratio of CSF. An increased level of gamma-globulin is suggestive of multiple sclerosis or meningitis. The first sample obtained may contain blood or skin pathogens from the puncture, so it should not be sent for determination of blood cell content or culture. Throughout the procedure, sterile technique must be strictly observed to ensure that an uncontaminated sample of fluid is sent for culture and also to prevent introducing pathogens into the CSF.

Lumbar puncture involves at least momentary pain, so children need to be comforted afterward. The child may need to lie flat for at least 1 hour after the procedure. Drinking fluids will reduce spinal headaches that may come on as a result of the reduction in CSF volume or invasion of a small air pocket during the puncture. Lying flat helps prevent cerebral irritation caused by air rising in the subarachnoid space, and a quick intake of fluids will increase the amount of CSF in the body. Some children may have a headache despite these precautions and need an analgesic for pain relief. Post–lumbar puncture headache is seen less frequently in young children than in adults; assessing for it is important.

If a child had minimally increased CSF pressure at the time of the puncture, closely observe afterward to prevent respiratory and cardiac difficulty from medulla pressure. Take vital signs every 15 minutes for several hours. An increase in blood pressure or a decrease in pulse and respiration is an important sign of increased intracranial compression. Other important signs are a change in consciousness, pupillary changes, or decrease in motor ability.

Ventricular Tap

In infants, CSF may be obtained by a subdural tap into the ventricle through the coronal suture or anterior fontanelle. The scalp over the insertion site must be shaved or the hair clipped and the area prepared with an antiseptic. The infant's head must be held firmly while in a supine position to prevent movement during the procedure, which could cause the needle to strike and lacerate meningeal tissue.

Fluid must be removed from this site slowly rather than suddenly, to prevent a sudden shift in pressure that could cause intracranial hemorrhage. After the procedure, a pressure dressing is applied to the site, and the infant is placed in a semi-Fowler's position to prevent prolonged drainage from the puncture site. After the procedure, comfort the infant to both reduce the stress of a painful procedure and prevent him from crying excessively, an action that could increase intracranial pressure.

X-ray Film Techniques

A flat-plate skull x-ray film may be used to obtain information about increased intracranial pressure or skull defects such as fracture or craniosynostosis (premature knitting of cranial sutures). Increased intracranial pressure is suggested when skull sutures are separated. When the process is chronic, other subtle changes such as a flattening of the sella turcica or an increase in the convolutions of the inner table of the skull may be present.

Outcome Identification: Parents will verbalize accurate information about the cause and prognosis of CP by next visit.

Outcome Evaluation: Parents state they understand that cause of disease is unknown and that disease is not progressive.

It is important for parents to understand that CP is a nonprogressive disease. The brain damage that occurred during pregnancy or at birth will not recur. The child's condition may seem to grow more apparent with age, however. Motor deficits of the upper extremities, for example, may not be strikingly evident until the child attempts fine motor tasks in school. Without follow-up care, contractures from spasticity may result, further reducing existing motor function (Percy, 1997).

Caution parents also that CP is a single name for a wide variety and extent of diseases. Although another child may have such severe CP that he has no useful function in his extremities, their own child may not be affected to the same extent. Conversely, although they know someone with CP who is able to hold a full-time job, their child may not necessarily be able to do as well some day. Each child's potential must be evaluated individually.

Nursing Diagnosis: Risk for disuse syndrome related to spasticity of muscle groups

Outcome Identification: Child will achieve maximum mobility possible during childhood.

Outcome Evaluation: Child walks with a minimum of support or equipment; skin and tissue remains intact.

When caring for the child with CP, it is important to promote any function that is not already impaired and to prevent any further loss of function. Major areas to be addressed include self-care, communication, ambulation, education, safety, nutrition, parental support, and establishment of self-esteem in the child.

Learning to be ambulatory is an important part of self-care because it helps determine how independent the child can become (Strauss et al, 1998). This is difficult to achieve because of lack of muscle group coordination. Surgery to lengthen heel tendons may be needed even after the continuous use of leg braces. Other additional devices such as wheeled walkers or scooter boards also may be used (Figure 28-9). Medication to reduce spasticity has little effect, although baclofen (Lioresal) may be prescribed for some children to improve motor function. Cerebellar pacemakers may reduce spasticity in some children.

Preventing contractures is important. Formerly children were fitted with extensive braces. The weight of these braces, however, often impeded muscle movement and prevented children from learning to walk. This added to their disability. Partial leg braces, however, may be used to encourage children to bring their heels down and keep the heel cords from tightening. If leg braces are prescribed, parents may need some encouragement and support to insist that their children wear them. Remind parents that partial leg braces for stretching the heel cords should be worn for long periods during the day to be effective. Just putting them on when the child is going outside is not enough.

Passive and active muscle exercises also are important in preventing contractures. Parents can be taught to do passive exercises and to play games with the child that encourage active exercise. At health care visits, remind parents that these exercises are an important part of their child's therapy and must be done consistently each day.

Nursing Diagnosis: Risk for self-care deficit related to impaired mobility

Outcome Identification: Child will achieve independent self-care by puberty.

Outcome Evaluation: Child feeds and dresses self; manages elimination independently.

Children need to learn self-care measures such as dressing, toothbrushing, bathing, and toileting so they can gain self-esteem from accomplishing these tasks. Modifications such as straps attached to their toothbrush or feeding utensils may be necessary so they can hold it more securely. Advise parents to always supervise children during bathing. Their lack of coordination could cause them to slip underwater and drown. However, encourage the parents to allow children to scrub themselves and wash their hair. Toileting is often difficult because they do not have the muscle group coordination to achieve successful bowel evacuation. A high-roughage diet will prevent constipation and aid bowel evacuation. Voiding may be equally difficult because the child may lack sufficient voluntary muscle control.

The parents need considerable support and guidance. Helping the child with self-care activities often requires patience to allow the child to accomplish the task. Doing so, however, helps to instill confidence and self-esteem in the child.

Nursing Diagnosis: Risk for altered growth and development related to activity restriction secondary to cerebral palsy

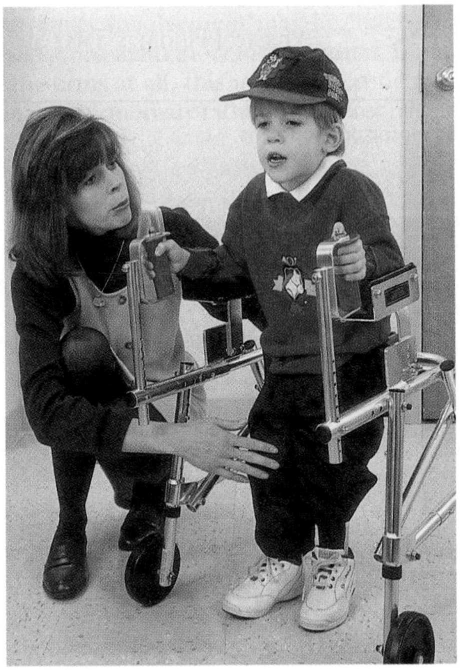

FIGURE 28.9 Wheeled walkers give a child added stability for walking and keep heel cords from shortening.

Outcome Identification: Child will demonstrate age-appropriate developmental milestones within the limits of his disease.

Outcome Evaluation: Child receives environmental stimulation; expresses interest in people and activities around him; attends school setting that is as free of restrictions as possible.

Children with CP may be unable to pursue stimulating activities and surroundings. Therefore, these things must be brought to them. Some children may need more stimulating activities than others because they have difficulty concentrating on one activity for any length of time. An activity should be neither too difficult nor too easy for the child. Choose toys and activities appropriate to the child's intellectual, developmental, and motor levels.

A preschool program is important for providing exposure to the outside world. If at all possible, school-age children with cerebral palsy should be mainstreamed so that they can be among other children. Under federal law, children with disabilities must be provided an education in the least restrictive setting possible. If they are cognitively impaired, their combined mental and motor deficits may severely limit their abilities, making school placement difficult. You may need to advocate that a child be placed in a school setting that is consistent with his or her intellectual abilities.

Nursing Diagnosis: Risk for altered nutrition, less than body requirements, related to difficulty sucking in infancy and in feeding self as older child

Outcome Identification: Child will demonstrate intake of adequate nutrients throughout childhood.

Outcome Evaluation: Child's weight will remain within 5th to 95th percentile on height–weight chart; skin turgor remains good; specific gravity of urine is 1.003 to 1.030.

Providing adequate nutrition to children with CP is often difficult. As infants, they often suck poorly because uncoordinated movements of the tongue, lips, and jaw and tongue thrusting cause them to push food out of their mouth (a retained primitive reflex). Their lip and tongue control may be poor, with weak or uncoordinated jaw muscles. Older children may have difficulty holding and controlling a spoon to bring food to their mouth. Spasticity causes children to hyperextend the head when leaning forward to take a bite, so they never feel comfortable while eating. Parents need guidance in finding a feeding pattern that works for their child. Manually controlling the jaw may help control the head, correct neck and trunk hyperextension, and stabilize the jaw and assist with feeding. If children cannot chew or swallow well, a liquid or soft diet may be necessary. Other children can handle solids and finger foods but may take longer to eat than the average child. They may need protection for their clothing and the floor. It may take longer for them to eat than the rest of the family, so people will need to wait patiently for them to finish.

A hyperactive gag reflex may cause children to vomit after feeding. Be certain that infants are positioned on their side or upright after feeding to prevent aspiration.

Nursing Diagnosis: Impaired verbal communication related to neurologic impairment

Outcome Identification: Child will achieve satisfactory communication with caregivers and significant others by school age.

Outcome Evaluation: Child can verbally make needs known to strangers and family members.

Most children with CP benefit from speech therapy, which helps them learn to speak slowly and coordinate their lips and tongue to form speech sounds. Be patient with children, and allow them to form words deliberately. If they try to hurry to please you, their speech will be much less clear, and communication will be impaired. For the child who cannot speak clearly, provide an alternative form of communication, such as flash cards or a picture board. Touch-screen computer programs are often used in school settings to aid communication.

Long-Term Care

Because CP is not always diagnosed early in infancy, parents may not learn that their child has a chronic disease until nearly 2 to 4 years later. They will need a great deal of support and education to help them cope with their grief and disappointment and care of the child.

Help parents encourage children with CP to reach their fullest potential within the limits of their disorder. Evaluations at health care visits should note not only whether the child is achieving this goal but also whether he and his family members find satisfaction and acceptance in his achievements. Listen to parents during health care visits and encourage them to discuss the difficulties of daily living, such as feeding problems. They may grieve because their child is not able to accomplish all of the major things they had wished for during pregnancy, and they may feel defeated by the day-to-day strain of caring for the child's multiple special needs.

CHECKPOINT QUESTIONS

5. What are the four types of cerebral palsy?
6. What measures should you teach the parents of a child with cerebral palsy to use to prevent contractures?

INFECTION

Nervous system tissue is as susceptible to infection as all other body tissue. Common major infections are meningitis, encephalitis, Guillain-Barré syndrome, Reye's syndrome, and botulism.

Bacterial Meningitis

Meningitis is an infection of the cerebral meninges. In the United States, it is caused most frequently by *Haemophilus influenzae* type B, *Neisseria meningitidis* (meningococcal meningitis), or group B *Streptococcus pneumoniae* in children older than age 2 months. *Diplococcus pneumoniae* (pneumococcal meningitis) as a cause occurs less frequently. In newborns, group B *Streptococcus* and *Esch-*

erichia coli are common causes of meningitis (Lebel, 1997). In children with myelomeningocele who develop meningitis, *Pseu-domonas* infection is common. Children who have had a splenectomy are particularly susceptible to meningococcal meningitis.

Meningitis occurs most often between the ages of 1 month and 5 years; half of these cases occur in children younger than 1 year old. Although the disease may occur in any month, its peak incidence appears to be in the winter.

Pathologic organisms generally are spread to the meninges from upper respiratory tract infections, by lymphatic drainage possibly through the mastoid or sinuses, or by direct introduction by a lumbar puncture or skull fracture. Once organisms enter the meningeal space, they multiply rapidly and spread throughout the CSF. Organisms invade brain tissue through meningeal folds that extend down into the brain itself. An inflammatory response may lead to a thick, fibrinous exudate that blocks CSF flow. Brain abscess or invasion of the infection into cranial nerves may result in blindness, deafness, or facial paralysis. Pus that accumulates in the narrow aqueduct of Sylvius may cause obstruction leading to hydrocephalus. Brain tissue edema puts pressure on the hypopituitary gland, causing increased production of antidiuretic hormone. This causes increased edema because the body cannot excrete adequate urine. The current routine immunization of children with *H. influenzae* vaccine has reduced the number of those who contract meningitis. Meningococcal vaccine is recommended for children older than 5 years of age who have been exposed to someone with this form of meningitis or for children who have had their spleen removed.

Assessment

The symptoms of meningitis may occur insidiously or suddenly. Children generally have 2 or 3 days of upper respiratory tract infection. They become increasingly irritable because of headaches. They may have convulsions. In some children, convulsions or shock are the first noticeable signs of illness. As the disease progresses, signs of meningeal irritability occur, as evidenced by a positive Brudzinski's and Kernig's signs (Figure 28-10). Their back may become arched and their neck hyperextended (opisthotonos). There may be cranial nerve paralysis (most typically of the third and sixth nerves, so that children are not able to follow a light through full visual fields). If open, the fontanelles are bulging and tense; if they are closed, children may develop papilledema. If the meningitis is caused by *H. influenzae,* children may develop septic arthritis. If it is caused by *N. meningitidis,* a papular or purple petechial skin rash may develop.

In the newborn, the symptoms are often vague, for example, poor sucking, weak cry, and lethargy. After this

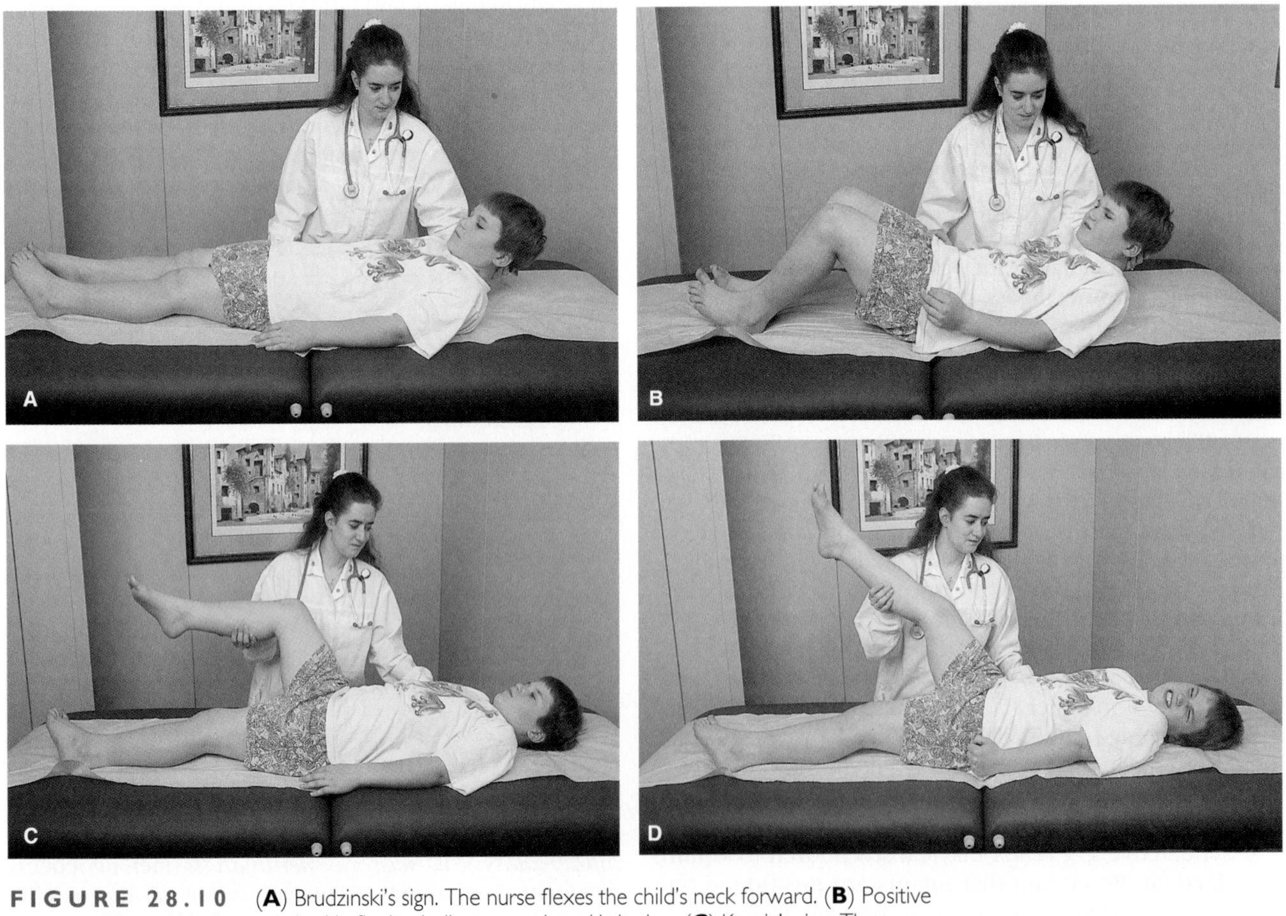

FIGURE 28.10 (**A**) Brudzinski's sign. The nurse flexes the child's neck forward. (**B**) Positive response. Bilateral hip, knee, and ankle flexion indicates meningeal irritation. (**C**) Kernig's sign. The nurse flexes the child's hip and knee, forming a 90-degree angle. (**D**) Positive response. As the leg is extended, pain, resistance, and spasm are noted, indicating meningeal irritation.

generalized beginning, sudden cardiovascular shock, convulsions, or apnea may occur. Because the infant has open fontanelles, nuchal rigidity appears late and is not as useful a sign for diagnosis as in the older child.

Meningitis is diagnosed by history and analysis of CSF obtained by lumbar puncture. A child with a febrile convulsion should be assumed to have meningitis until CSF findings prove otherwise. CSF results indicative of meningitis include an increase in white blood cell and protein levels and a lowered glucose level (bacteria have fed on the glucose). In a healthy child, the glucose level in the CSF is equal to that of the serum glucose. Because meningitis often spreads and causes septicemia, a blood culture is done as well. A fulminating (overwhelming) meningitis often leads to leukopenia. If children have had close association with someone with tuberculosis, a tuberculin skin test to rule out tuberculosis meningitis should be done. A CT scan, MRI, or ultrasound may be ordered to examine for abscesses. Typically, intracranial pressure is often over 300 mm Hg.

Therapeutic Management

Antibiotic therapy as indicated by sensitivity studies is the primary treatment measure. Usually given intravenously for rapid effect, intrathecal injections (directly into the CSF) may be necessary to reduce the infection, because the blood–brain barrier may prevent an antibiotic from passing freely into the CSF. If the organism is identified as *H. influenzae,* ampicillin generally is the drug of choice. In other instances, cefotaxime, ceftriaxone, chloramphenicol, gentamycin, or tobramycin may be used. Therapy will be continued for a minimum of 8 to 10 days. In some children, it will take a month before the CSF cell count is back to normal. A corticosteroid such as dexamethasone or the osmotic diuretic, mannitol, may be administered to reduce intracranial pressure and help prevent hearing loss, but its use is controversial.

In addition to standard precautions, children with meningitis are placed on droplet precautions for 24 hours after the start of antibiotic therapy to prevent infection transmission. Antibiotics also may be prescribed for the immediate family members of the ill child or others who were in close contact with the child.

Meningitis is always a serious disorder. It can run a rapid, fulminating, possibly fatal course, although if symptoms are recognized early enough, and if treatment is effective, the child will recover with no sequelae. For a good outcome, children must receive rapid diagnosis and treatment. Neurologic sequelae, such as learning problems, convulsions, hearing and cognitive impairment, and inability to concentrate urine, must be assessed after the infection.

NURSING DIAGNOSES AND RELATED INTERVENTIONS

When a child has meningitis, the parents may feel responsible for the illness. They knew the child had a cold, and they wonder whether they could have prevented meningitis if only they had taken him to a physician as soon as the cold symptoms started. Assure them that the symptoms of meningitis occur insidiously and that no one could have predicted the full extent of the disease from the first signs.

Encourage parents to care for the child during the illness, both to help make the child more comfortable and to help them manage their own anxiety. Teach them good infection control techniques so they can perform these tasks safely.

Nursing Diagnosis: Pain related to meningeal irritation

Outcome Identification: Child will experience a tolerable degree of pain during the course of illness.

Outcome Evaluation: Child states that pain is tolerable; shows no facial grimacing or other signs of discomfort.

For a child with meningitis, dealing with hospitalization and the numerous invasive treatments and procedures is usually difficult. If the child had a lumbar puncture on admission, his initial impression may become one of people restraining him for a painful procedure. Continuous intravenous infusions contribute to this impression. Remember that the child feels pain when his head is flexed forward and will usually be more comfortable without a pillow. Be careful not to flex the child's neck when turning or positioning him.

On admission, a child may be extremely irritable. Although he would benefit from puppet play or drawing that would help him express how he feels about so many intrusive procedures, he is too uncomfortable to play, appearing as though nothing seems to comfort him. This is the result of the disease process, and he cannot help feeling this way. Be aware of this so as not to interpret the child's withdrawal as unfriendliness and feel hurt when advances are rebuffed. Parents also need to understand that the child's behavior is because of the disease and not anything that they did or are doing. The child needs a good explanation of everything that is happening. He needs extra attention from health care personnel consistently, not just when they perform painful procedures. As the child recovers, irritability lessens and the child usually will show more interest in communicating his feelings. Promote rest for the child by keeping stimulation in his room to a minimum.

Nursing Diagnosis: Risk for altered tissue perfusion (cerebral), related to increased intracranial pressure

Outcome Identification: Child will remain free of signs and symptoms of altered cerebral tissue perfusion during course of illness.

Outcome Evaluation: Child's vital signs return to normal; child is alert and oriented; motor, cognitive, and sensory function are within acceptable parameters for the child's age; specific gravity of urine is 1.003 to 1.030.

Observe the child carefully for signs of increased intracranial pressure. Carefully monitor the rate of all intravenous infusions to prevent overhydration. Measure urine specific gravity to detect oversecretion or undersecretion of antidiuretic hormone from pituitary pressure. Measure the child's head circumference and weigh him or her daily.

Monitor hearing acuity (reduced if there is compression of the eighth cranial nerve) by asking the child a question or observing whether the infant listens to a music box or your voice.

Group B, Beta-Hemolytic Streptococcal Meningitis

A major cause of meningitis in newborns is the group B, beta-hemolytic streptococcal organism. The organism is contracted either in utero or from secretions in the birth canal at delivery. It can spread to other newborns if good handwashing technique is not used.

Group-B beta-hemolytic streptococci colonization may result in early-onset or late-onset illness. With the early-onset form, symptoms of pneumonia become apparent in the first few hours of life.

The late-onset type often leads to meningitis instead of pneumonia. At approximately the age of 2 weeks, the infant may gradually become lethargic, developing a fever and upper respiratory symptoms. The fontanelles will bulge from increased intracranial pressure. Mortality from the late-onset type is lower (15% compared to 40% in early-onset type), but neurologic consequences such as hydrocephalus may occur. Treatment is with antibiotics, such as penicillins and cephalosporins, effective against group B, beta-hemolytic streptococcal infections.

It can be difficult for parents to understand how their infant suddenly became so ill. They may need considerable support in caring for the infant who is left neurologically disabled (Lebel, 1997).

> **CHECKPOINT QUESTIONS**
>
> 7. What two signs would you use to evaluate for meningeal irritation in the child with meningitis?
> 8. For how long should the child with bacterial meningitis be placed on droplet precautions?

Encephalitis

Encephalitis is an inflammation of brain tissue and, possibly, the meninges as well. It can arise from protozoan, bacterial, fungal, or viral invasion. Enteroviruses are the most frequent cause, followed by arboviruses (togavirus). A number of encephalitis viruses, such as St Louis encephalitis and eastern equine encephalitis, are borne by mosquitoes and are seen most during the summer months. In endemic areas, mosquito repellents are strongly suggested. Encephalitis also can result from direct invasion of the CSF during lumbar puncture. It may occur as a complication of common childhood diseases, such as measles, mumps, or chickenpox. Therefore, it is crucial that children receive immunization against these childhood diseases.

Assessment

Symptoms of encephalitis may begin gradually or suddenly. These include headache, high temperature, and signs of meningeal irritation, such as nuchal rigidity (positive Brudzinski's sign and Kernig's sign). There may be symptoms of ataxia, muscle weakness or paralysis, diplopia, confusion, or irritability. The child becomes increasingly lethargic and eventually comatose.

The diagnosis is made by the history and physical assessment. Laboratory studies of CSF generally indicate an elevated leukocyte count and elevated protein and glucose levels. An EEG shows widespread cerebral involvement. A brain biopsy may be done, usually from the temporal lobe, to identify the possible virus.

Therapeutic Management

Treatment for the child with encephalitis is primarily supportive. An antipyretic is given to control fever. Take and record vital signs frequently, because brain stem involvement may affect cardiac or respiratory rates. Mechanical ventilation may be required to maintain the child's respirations during the acute phase. If the cause is viral, antibiotics will not be effective. Anticonvulsants, such as carbamazepine (Tegretol), phenobarbital, or phenytoin (Dilantin), may be prescribed for seizures. A steroid such as dexamethasone may be prescribed to decrease brain edema and intracranial pressure.

Encephalitis is always a serious diagnosis because, even though the child may recover from the initial attack, there may be residual neurologic damage, such as seizures or learning disabilities. Parents may find it hard to believe that their child is seriously ill because she only seemed tired and had a slight headache. They will find it even harder to accept a diagnosis of permanent impairment such as learning disabilities. Follow-up care after the hospitalization is important for the child's rehabilitation and to help them deal with their grief, shock, and anger. Although complete recovery is possible, parents may find themselves with a child whose health and abilities have been permanently changed.

Reye's Syndrome

Reye's syndrome is acute encephalitis with accompanying fatty infiltration of the liver, heart, lungs, pancreas, and skeletal muscle. It occurs in children from 1 to 18 years of age regardless of sex. A sibling has an increased risk of developing the disease, perhaps because of a genetic susceptibility.

The cause of Reye's syndrome is unknown, but it generally occurs after a viral infection such as varicella (chickenpox) or an upper respiratory infection. Research has identified an association between the use of acetylsalicylic acid (aspirin) and nonsteroidal anti-inflammatory agents (NSAIDs) during the viral infection with the onset of Reye's afterward. It is a perplexing disease, and its seriousness may be difficult for parents to understand when it follows such common infections. Anticipatory guidance to parents and children about avoiding the use of aspirin and NSAIDs during viral infections has led to a decrease in the incidence of Reye's syndrome (Louise, 1997).

Assessment

After seeming to recover from an initial viral illness, children may become ill again 1 to 3 weeks later, with lethargy, vomiting, agitation, anorexia, confusion, and combativeness. The vomiting may be so severe it leads to dehydration. Symptoms in adolescents may mimic those of drug intoxication such as inappropriate language, visual hallucinations, pupillary dilation, slurred speech, and staggering gait. Liver infiltration involves mitochondrial fatty droplet infiltration, enzyme abnormalities, particularly serum aspartate transaminase (AST [glutamic-oxaloacetic transaminase—SGOT]) and serum alanine transaminase (ALT [glutamic-pyruvic transaminase—SGPT]), and hypothrombinemia. Hypoglycemia will be present, and blood ammonia levels will be elevated because of poor liver function. Although CSF findings remain normal, cerebral symptoms progress from confusion to stupor to deep coma, with seizures and respiratory arrest resulting from pressure on the brain stem.

If left untreated, Reye's syndrome is rapidly fatal. Without acute respiratory support, as many as two thirds of children with the disease die within 2 or 3 days of onset. If diagnosed early and promptly treated, the child usually recovers quickly and generally without any residual neurologic effects.

Laboratory diagnosis of Reye's syndrome is confirmed by elevated ALT (SGPT) and AST (SGOT) liver function tests, elevated serum ammonia, normal direct bilirubin, delayed prothrombin time and partial thromboplastin time, decreased blood glucose, elevated blood urea nitrogen, elevated serum amylase, elevated short-chain fatty acids, and an elevated white blood count. A lumbar puncture is usually done to rule out other infection. CSF findings are normal, except for slightly elevated opening pressure. A skull CT scan or sonogram will be normal at first. Later this will show cerebral edema and decreased ventricle size. An EEG may be ordered. A liver biopsy will show fatty infiltration, establishing a definitive diagnosis. However, the child is at an increased risk for hemorrhage from the delayed prothrombin time (Louis, 1997).

Therapeutic Management

At the onset of Reye's syndrome, the child is not infectious. Therapy is directed toward supporting respiratory function, controlling hypoglycemia, and reducing brain edema. The child will be started on a 10% or 15% dextrose solution to reduce cerebral edema and to correct hypoglycemia. Mannitol or a corticosteroid also may be ordered.

Reye's syndrome is categorized by stages of involvement from 1 to 5, depending on the amount of the child's lethargy or presence of coma. In stages 1 and 2, the child responds to stimuli but may exhibit lethargy or delirium and possibly combativeness. With stages 3 through 5, the child is unresponsive to stimuli with a progressively deepening coma. Frequent neurologic assessments are necessary to evaluate the child's status and possible progression to a more serious stage of involvement. Blood sugar, electrolytes, and prothrombin level are monitored carefully. Sedating children who are combative (struggling against procedures, thrashing wildly) is controversial because it renders the neurologic evaluation invalid. On occasion, phenobarbital may be given.

If children progress to stage III involvement, fluid intake must be carefully regulated to prevent overload and increased cerebral edema. A central venous pressure line or pulmonary artery catheter may be inserted to monitor hemodynamic status. Intracranial pressure also needs to be monitored closely. An indwelling urinary catheter may be inserted to assess urine output and evaluate fluid status. A nasogastric tube may be inserted to prevent vomiting and aspiration. If the child seems in danger of respiratory arrest, an endotracheal tube and mechanical ventilation may be used to maintain $PaCO_2$ between 20 and 25 mm Hg. A low $PaCO_2$ causes cerebral vasoconstriction and lowers intracranial pressure. Pancuronium bromide may be administered to paralyze respiratory muscles, allowing for maximum ventilation. If the child awakens from coma in an intensive care unit, orient the child to the surroundings, because the child's last clear memory may be the day before becoming ill.

Guillain-Barré Syndrome

Guillain-Barré (inflammatory polyradiculoneuropathy) is a perplexing syndrome involving both motor and sensory portions of peripheral nerves. It affects both sexes and occurs most often in school-age children (Parke, 1997).

The cause of the condition is unknown, but it is suspected that the reaction is immune mediated, following upper respiratory and gastrointestinal illnesses and immunization. Inflammation of the nerve fibers apparently causes temporary demyelinization of the nerve sheaths.

Assessment

Children experience peripheral neuritis several days after the primary infection. Tendon reflexes are decreased or absent. Muscle paralysis and paresthesia (loss of sensation) begins first in the legs and then spreads to involve the arms and trunk and head. The symmetrical nature of the disorder helps to differentiate it from other types of paraplegia. Cranial nerve involvement leads to facial weakness and difficulty in swallowing. As the respiratory muscles become involved, spontaneous respirations are no longer possible. Ten percent to 20% of those who develop the syndrome will have respiratory involvement severe enough to warrant mechanical ventilation.

A significant laboratory finding is an elevated CSF protein level. An EEG may show denervation and decreased nerve conduction velocity.

Therapeutic Management

Treatment of Guillain-Barré syndrome is supportive until the process runs its course (paralysis peaks at 3 weeks, followed by gradual recovery). A course of prednisone to halt the autoimmune response may be tried, but its use is controversial. Plasmapheresis or transfusion of immune serum globulin may shorten the course of the illness.

Care of the child with Guillain-Barré includes preventing all of the effects of extreme immobility while guarding respiratory function. The child's cardiac and respiratory function must be closely monitored. An indwelling urinary catheter is usually inserted to monitor urine output. Enteral or total parenteral nutrition may be used to maintain protein and carbohydrate needs. If the child has discomfort from neuritis, adequate analgesia needs to be administered.

To prevent muscle contractures and effects of immobility, the child should have passive range-of-motion exercises every 4 hours. Turning and repositioning the child every 2 hours also is important to protect skin integrity. Providing adequate stimulation for the long weeks when the child is unable to perform any care for himself or herself is also important. Most children recover completely, without any residual effects of the syndrome, although they may continue to have minor problems such as residual weakness.

Botulism

Botulism occurs when spores of *Clostridium botulinum* colonize and produce toxins in the immature intestine. The source of the spores is generally unknown, but honey and corn syrup are frequent contaminants and should be avoided. The disease is not infectious and generally occurs in infants younger than 6 months of age.

With infant botulism, symptoms occur within a few hours of ingestion of contaminated food. Almost immediately there is generalized weakness, hypotonia, listlessness, a weak cry, and a diminished gag reflex. This is followed by a flaccid paralysis of the bulbar muscles that leads to diminished respiratory function. The organism can be cultured from stools or serum. Electromyography may be helpful to support the diagnosis.

Treatment is supportive care. The antitoxin for botulism is rarely given to infants because it is made from a horse serum base and can cause a hypersensitivity reaction; it is generally not necessary for full recovery. Infant botulism may account for some fatalities from sudden infant death syndrome (Cherington, 1998).

CHECKPOINT QUESTIONS

9. What is the most frequent cause of encephalitis?
10. What factors are associated with the development of Reye's syndrome?
11. Why is the antitoxin rarely given to infants with botulism?

PAROXYSMAL DISORDERS

A paroxysmal disorder is one that occurs suddenly and recurrently. Convulsions, headaches, and breath-holding spells are the most frequent types seen in childhood.

Recurrent Convulsions

A *convulsion* is an involuntary contraction of muscle caused by abnormal electrical brain discharges. Approximately 2% to 4% of children will have at least one convulsion by the time they reach adulthood (Glaze, 1997). These episodes are always frightening to parents and other children. Although convulsions may be idiopathic (without cause), they also can be attributed to infection, trauma, or tumor growth. Familiar or polygenic inheritance may be responsible. Fifty percent of seizures are unexplainable. They are not so much a disease as symptoms of an underlying disorder and should be investigated carefully (see Focus on Cultural Competence).

FOCUS ON CULTURAL COMPETENCE

The degree of understanding about the cause of disorders such as recurrent seizures varies in different cultures. Because the cause of recurrent seizures is often unknown (idiopathic), it has in the past been attributed to an invasion by evil spirits. Many people today still fear that recurrent seizures will lead to cognitive impairment. Adults with recurrent seizures may be refused jobs because they are viewed as undependable. Being aware of these common misconceptions helps the nurse appreciate parents' anxiety about the diagnosis of recurrent seizures. It can accentuate the need for careful planning to maintain self-esteem in the child.

The term *epilepsy* comes from a Greek word meaning "to take hold of" and refers to a person with chronic convulsions. The preferred terms now are *seizures* or *convulsions,* because epilepsy carries the stigma of cognitive impairment, behavioral disorders, institutionalization, or just unexplainable strangeness.

The types and causes of seizures vary according to the child's age. They have been classified into two major categories: partial seizures and generalized seizures (Box 28-2). With partial seizures, only one area of the brain is involved; with generalized seizures, the disturbance involves the entire brain, and loss of consciousness usually occurs. It is important that seizures be differentiated by their degree of severity so that appropriate management and drug therapy can be instituted (Carpay et al,1998).

BOX 28.2

CLASSIFICATION OF SEIZURES

Partial (Focal) Seizures

- Simple partial seizures (no altered level of consciousness)
  - Simple partial seizures with motor signs (includes Aversive, Rolandic, and Jacksonian march)
  - Simple partial seizures with sensory signs
- Complex partial (psychomotor) seizures (some impairment or alteration in level of consciousness)

Generalized Seizures

- Tonic-clonic seizures (formerly grand mal)
  - Tonic
  - Clonic
- Absence seizures (formerly petit mal)
- Atonic seizures (formerly "drop attacks")
- Myoclonic seizures
- Infantile spasms

Seizures in the Newborn Period

Seizure activity in the newborn period may be difficult to recognize because it may consist only of twitching of the head, arms, or eyes, slight cyanosis, and perhaps respiratory difficulty or apnea. Afterward, the infant may appear limp and flaccid. Whereas older children often have seizures of unknown cause, 75% of seizures in neonates have a known cause. Some possible causes include:

- Trauma and anoxia (head trauma involved with the birth process, tight maternal cervix, poor use of forceps, or placenta previa)
- Metabolic disorders (hypoglycemia [glucose level below 30 mg/100 mL in the full-term infant; 20 mg/100 mL in the preterm infant]; infants of diabetic mothers; hypocalcemia; and lack of pyridoxine [vitamin B_6])
- Neonatal infection (CNS infection or prolonged rupture of membranes before delivery)
- Kernicterus

Because of the nervous system's immaturity, EEGs in the newborn may be normal, despite extensive disease. Therefore, a noticeably abnormal EEG generally means a poor prognosis, indicating that the involvement this early in life must be severe. Because nearly 20% of all newborns have abnormal CSF values as compared with adult standards, lumbar puncture is also not too revealing. Protein is increased, and there may be a few red blood cells from rupture of subarachnoid capillaries from the pressure of birth.

A high dosage of anticonvulsant medication may be needed to control convulsions in newborns because they metabolize drugs more rapidly than older infants. In adults, for example, phenobarbital may be administered in the range of 1.5 mg per kilogram of body weight per day. In newborns, the dose might be as high as 3 to 10 mg/kg/day.

Seizures in the Infant and Toddler Periods

Seizures commonly seen in this age group are **infantile spasms,** a form of generalized seizures—"salaam" and "jackknife"—or infantile myoclonic seizures, characterized by very rapid movements of the trunk with sudden strong contractions of most of the body including flexion and adduction of the limbs. The infant suddenly slumps forward from a sitting position or falls from a standing position. These episodes may occur singly or in clusters as frequently as 100 times a day. They are most common in the first 6 months of life.

The cause is unknown, but the spasms apparently result from a failure of normal organized electrical activity in the brain. Sometimes, the seizures accompany a preexisting form of neurologic damage. Approximately 95% of these infants are cognitively impaired. In approximately 50% of those affected, there is an identifiable cause such as trauma or a metabolic disease such as phenylketonuria. In the other 50%, there may be no identifiable cause. They may follow invasion by viruses such as herpes or cytomegalovirus.

In infants whose development was previously normal, intellectual development appears to halt and even regress after seizures start. Most children with infantile spasms show high-amplitude slow waves and spikes, a chaotic discharge called *hypsarrhythmia,* on an EEG tracing.

The response to treatment with anticonvulsant therapy is poor. Parenteral adrenocorticotropic hormone (ACTH) therapy is commonly used. High-dose valproic acid or clonazapine may be used in children who do not respond to parenteral ACTH therapy. The infantile seizure phenomenon seems to "burn itself out" by 2 years of age. The associated cognitive or developmental lag remains, however, so children need follow-up planning and care.

Seizures from Poisoning or Drugs. The possibility of poisoning must be considered in all children who have a first seizure. Although poisoning is most likely in the age-group between 6 months and 3 years, it must be considered again in adolescence when drugs may be intentionally self-administered. Seizures also can be a late symptom of encephalopathy caused by lead poisoning.

Seizures in Children Older Than 3 Years of Age

More than half of children who develop recurrent seizures during school age have an idiopathic type—the cause of the seizures cannot be discovered. Fortunately, even without a clearly understood cause, medication controls these idiopathic seizures in almost all affected children. Other seizures in this age-group occur because of organic causes. They generally result from focal or diffuse brain injury that has left residual damage. The injury may have been the result of laceration of brain tissue in a car accident or fall, hemorrhage due to blood dyscrasia, infection (meningitis or encephalitis), anoxia, or toxic conditions such as lead poisoning. The possibility that a growing brain tumor is causing brain irritation also must be considered.

Complex Partial (Psychomotor) Seizures. Complex partial (psychomotor) seizures vary greatly in extent and symptoms and tend to be the most difficult to control. At one time, this type of seizure was believed to be a result of dysfunction in the temporal lobe. However, technological advances have shown that these seizures may arise from other areas of the brain also. In most children, a CT scan or MRI is normal. The child may have a slight aura, but it is rarely as definite as that seen with tonic-clonic seizures.

As an example, the seizure may begin with a sudden change in posture, such as an arm dropping suddenly to the side. Other motor, sensory, and behavior signs may include **automatisms** (complex purposeless movements, such as lip smacking, or fumbling hand movements). The child slumps to the ground, unconscious. He may have circumoral pallor. He regains consciousness in less than 5 minutes. He may be slightly drowsy afterward but does not have an actual postictal stage as in tonic-clonic seizures. The child with this type of seizure generally has a normal EEG.

Common drugs used are phenytoin (Dilantin), carbamazepine (Tegretol), valproic acid (Depakene), primidone (Mysoline), and phenobarbital (see Drug Highlight boxes). If these are not effective, surgery to remove the epileptogenic focus may be attempted.

Partial (Focal) Seizures. Parital seizures originate from a specific brain area. A typical partial seizure with motor signs begins in the fingers and spreads to the wrist, arm, and face in a clonic contraction. If the movement remains localized, there will be no loss of consciousness. When the spread is extensive, the seizure may become generalized, then impossible to differentiate from a tonic-clonic convulsion. Thus, it is important to observe children carefully as a convulsion begins. A partial seizure with sensory signs may include numbness, tingling, paresthesia, or pain originating in one area and spreading to other parts of the body. These types of seizures may be caused by something as specific as a rapidly growing brain tumor. Documenting the spread can help localize the spot where the seizure first began.

DRUG HIGHLIGHT

Phenytoin (Dilantin)

Action: Phenytoin is an anticonvulsant that stabilizes neuronal membranes and prevents hyperexcitability caused by excessive stimulation and limits the spread of seizure activity without causing general central nervous system depression

Pregnancy risk category: D

Dosage: Initially, 5 mg/kg/day in 2 to 3 equally divided doses up to a maximum of 300 mg/day with a maintenance dose of 4 to 8 mg/day.

Possible adverse effects: Nystagmus, ataxia, slurred speech, confusion, fatigue, irritability, nausea, gingival hyperplasia, liver damage, and blood dyscrasias

Nursing Implications:

- Administer the drug with food to minimize gastrointestinal upset and enhance absorption. Instruct parents to do the same.
- Advise parents to have the prescription filled each time with the same brand of drug, because differences in bioavailability have been reported.
- Obtain serum drug levels as ordered to monitor for drug's effectiveness and prevent possible toxicity. Keep in mind that the therapeutic range is 10 to 20 μg/mL.
- Monitor liver function studies and blood counts periodically.
- Inform parents about the need for follow-up laboratory tests.
- Instruct the child and parents about oral hygiene measures to prevent gum problems. Encourage frequent dental checkups.
- Suggest that the parents obtain a medical alert bracelet and have the child wear it in case of an emergency.
- Warn parents not to discontinue the drug abruptly or change the dose unless ordered by the health care provider.
- Instruct parents to notify the health care provider if the child develops nystagmus, ataxia, or diminished mental capacity. These are signs of possible toxicity.

DRUG HIGHLIGHT

Carbamazepine (Tegretol)

Action: Carbamazepine is an anticonvulsant whose exact mechanism of action is unknown. It is believed to inhibit polysynaptic responses and block post-tetanic potentiation.

Pregnancy risk category: C

Dosage: Initially in children 6 to 12 years of age, 100 mg orally bid on the first day, increased gradually in 100-mg increments at 6- to 8-hour intervals until best response is achieved, or 10 to 30 mg/kg/day in divided doses tid or qid. Not to exceed 1000 mg/day.

Possible adverse effects: Dizziness, drowsiness, behavioral changes, nausea, vomiting, gastrointestinal upset, abnormal liver function tests, bone marrow depression, rash, photosensitivity

Nursing Implications:

- Administer the drug with food to minimize gastrointestinal upset. Instruct parents to do the same.
- Obtain serum drug levels as ordered to monitor for drug's effectiveness and prevent possible toxicity. Keep in mind that the therapeutic range is 4 to 12 μg/mL.
- Monitor liver function studies and blood counts periodically.
- Inform parents about the need for follow-up laboratory tests.
- Suggest that the parents obtain a medical alert bracelet and have the child wear it in case of an emergency.
- Instruct parents and child about avoiding alcohol, sleep-inducing, or over-the-counter drugs, which could cause dangerous synergistic effects.
- Warn parents not to discontinue the drug abruptly or change the dose unless ordered by the health care provider.
- Instruct parents to notify the health care provider if the child develops bruising, bleeding, or signs of infection. These are signs of possible bone marrow depression.

Absence Seizures. Absence seizures, formerly known as *petit mal,* are classified as generalized seizures. They usually consist of a staring spell that lasts for a few seconds. A child might be reciting in class when he pauses and stares for 1 to 5 seconds before continuing the recitation; he is unaware that time has passed. Rhythmic blinking and twitching of the mouth or an extremity may accompany the staring. Absence seizures can occur up to 100 times per day. An EEG usually shows a typical 3 wave/sec spike and slow-wave discharge. Such seizures tend to occur more frequently in girls than boys. The usual age of occurrence is 6 to 7 years.

Children with absence episodes may be accused of daydreaming in school and may be referred to the school nurse for behavior problems. These children generally have normal intelligence, although if they have frequent episodes, they may be doing poorly in school because they are missing instructional content.

Absence seizures can usually be demonstrated in children by asking them to hyperventilate and count out loud. If they are susceptible to such seizures, they will breathe in and out deeply, possibly 10 times, stop and stare for 3 seconds, then continue to hyperventilate and count, unaware that they paused.

No first aid measures are necessary for absence seizures. Downplaying the importance of these episodes will help children maintain a positive self-image.

Absence seizures can be controlled by ethosuximide (Zarontin) or by valproic acid. If seizures are fully controlled by medication, children can participate in normal school activities and ride a bicycle. If seizures cannot be controlled fully, parents need to anticipate potentially hazardous situations during the child's day, such as crossing a busy street on the way to school or learning to drive. This is crucial for adolescents who are eager to get a driver's license. The tendency for developing seizures should be evaluated carefully, for the child's own safety as well as others.

Approximately one third to one half of all children with absence seizures "outgrow them" by adulthood. This does not mean that treatment is not necessary during childhood. Absence seizures usually occur independently of tonic-clonic seizures, although it is possible for children to manifest both types. Some children's seizure pattern changes from absence involvement to tonic-clonic involvement as they approach adulthood.

Tonic-Clonic Seizures. Typical tonic-clonic seizures (formerly termed *grand mal seizures*) are generalized seizures, consisting of four stages. There may be a *prodromal* period of hours or days, an *aura,* or warning, immediately before the seizure, the tonic-clonic convulsion, and finally, a postictal state. Not all four stages occur with every seizure.

The prodromal period may consist of drowsiness, dizziness, malaise, lack of coordination, or tension. Parents may observe simply that the child is "not himself." As the child reaches school age, he may be able to predict from these vague preliminary feelings when he is going to have a seizure.

The aura, or second phase, may reflect the portion of the brain in which the seizure originates. Smelling unpleasant odors (often reported as feces) denotes activity in the medial portion of the temporal lobe. Seeing flashing lights suggests the occipital area; repeated hallucinations arise from the temporal lobe; numbness of an extremity relates to the opposite parietal lobe; and a "Cheshire cat grin" is from the frontal lobe. Young children, unable to describe or understand an aura, may scream in fright or run to their parent with its onset. Note exactly what symptoms the child experiences during this time, because this may help to localize the involved brain portion.

The third phase is the tonic stage. All muscles of the body contract, and the child falls to the ground. Extremities stiffen; the face distorts. Although this phase lasts only about 20 seconds, the respiratory muscles are contracted, and the child may experience hypoxia and turn cyanotic. Contraction of the throat prevents swallowing, so saliva collects in the mouth. The child may bite his tongue when his jaws contract. As the chest muscles contract initially, air is pushed through the glottis, producing a guttural cry.

The convulsion then enters a clonic stage, in which muscles of the body rapidly contract and relax, producing quick, jerky motions. The child may blow bubbles or foamy saliva and, if he bit his tongue when his jaw spasmed shut, he may have blood in his mouth. He may be incontinent of stool and urine. This phase usually lasts about 20 to 30 seconds.

After the tonic-clonic period, the child falls into a sound sleep, called the *postictal period.* He will sleep soundly for 1 to 4 hours and will rouse only to painful stimuli during this time. When he awakens, he often experiences a severe headache. He has no memory of the seizure.

Convulsions may occur only at night. The child wakes in the morning with a bitten tongue, blood on the pillow, or a bed wet with urine. In the child with persistent bedwetting, the possibility of nocturnal seizures must be considered.

Children with this type of convulsion generally have an abnormal EEG pattern, although this is not always the case. Other family members may have similarly abnormal EEG patterns without any symptoms.

Therapy usually includes the daily administration of anticonvulsants such as phenobarbital, which has the advantage of being inexpensive (see Drug Highlight box). However, drowsiness and sleepiness may interfere with the child's ability to perform in school. Phenobarbital dosages should be tapered, never stopped suddenly, because the body becomes dependent on it. Rapid withdrawal may precipitate a convulsion.

Children with tonic-clonic convulsions also may be given phenytoin sodium (Dilantin) to control seizures. One nontoxic side effect of phenytoin is painless hypertrophy of the gums. Unless the gum hypertrophy is extensive, however, it is not sufficient reason to discontinue Dilantin. Other commonly prescribed drugs include valproic acid (Depakane) and carbamazepine (Tegretol; Glaze, 1997). Medications are usually continued until the child has been seizure free for 2 to 3 years.

Some children may be placed on a ketogenic diet. This diet is high in fat and low in protein and carbohydrate. It causes the child to have a high level of ketones, which is believed to decrease myoclonic or tonic-clonic seizure activity. Because a ketogenic diet is monotonous for children and difficult for parents to prepare, however, it is hard to maintain for very long.

WHAT IF? A child with a history of seizures controlled with phenobarbital is brought to the clinic. His mother states that he's been very sleepy, especially in school. She reported that she cut his phenobarbital dosage in half. How would you respond to this parent?

Status Epilepticus. Status epilepticus refers to a seizure that lasts continuously for more than 30 minutes or a series of seizures from which the child does not return

DRUG HIGHLIGHT

Phenobarbital

Action: Phenobarbital is a central nervous system (CNS) depressant that acts as an anticonvulsant.

Pregnancy risk category: D

Dosage: 3 to 6mg/kg/day orally or 4 to 6 mg/kg/day parenterally for 7 to 10 days until achievement of a blood level of 10 to 15 μg/mL, or 10 to 15 mg/kg/day IV or IM. In status epilepticus, 15 to 20 mg/kg IV administered over 10 to 15 minutes.

Possible adverse effects: Somnolence, sedation, confusion, ataxia, lethargy, hangover, paradoxical excitement, nausea, vomiting, constipation, diarrhea, epigastric pain, bradycardia, hypotension, syncope, hypoventilation, respiratory depression, pain or tissue necrosis at the injection site.

Nursing Implications:

- When giving parenterally, administer IV doses slowly directly into tubing or running infusion. Inject a partial dose and assess response before continuing. If giving IM, administer deeply into a large muscle.
- Monitor IV site carefully for signs of irritation or extravasation.
- Assess vital signs closely—especially pulse, blood pressure, and respiratory rate—during IV administration.
- Administer the oral form of the drug with food to minimize gastrointestinal upset. Instruct parents to do the same.
- Warn the parents and child that the drug will make the child drowsy. Advise the child to change positions slowly and sit at the edge of the bed for a few minutes before arising. Assist parents with safety measures to protect the child from injury.
- Monitor laboratory tests for liver and renal function and blood counts if the child is on long-term therapy.
- Inform parents about the possible need for follow-up laboratory tests.
- Suggest that the parents obtain a medical alert bracelet and have the child wear it in case of an emergency.
- Instruct parents and child about avoiding alcohol, sleep-inducing, or over-the-counter drugs, which could cause increased CNS depression.
- Warn parents not to discontinue the drug abruptly or change the dose unless ordered by the health care provider.
- Instruct parents to notify the health care provider if the child develops severe dizziness, weakness, or drowsiness that persists.

to his or her previous level of consciousness. This is an emergency situation requiring immediate treatment. Otherwise, permanent brain injury, exhaustion, respiratory failure, and death may occur. Intravenous diazepam (Valium) or phenobarbital followed by intravenous phenytoin halts seizures dramatically. Diazepam must be administered with extreme caution, however, because the drug is incompatible with many other drugs, and any accidental infiltration into subcutaneous tissue causes extensive tissue sloughing. Parents may administer diazepam by enema at home. Lorazepam, a long-acting benzodiazepine, also may be used in place of diazepam because it has a longer duration of action and causes less respiratory depression in children older than 2 years of age. Oxygen administration helps to relieve cyanosis.

Febrile Convulsions

Convulsions associated with high fever (102° to 104°F [38.9° to 40.0°C]) are the most common in preschool children, or between 5 months and 5 years of age, although seizures may occur as early as 3 months and as late as 7 years. There generally are no more than five to seven such episodes in the child's life. The seizure shows an active tonic-clonic pattern, which lasts 15 to 20 seconds. The EEG tracing is normal. There usually is a history of other family members having had similar convulsions.

It is unclear whether seizures are initiated by a consistently high fever or a sudden spike of temperature. The seizure subsides quickly once the fever is lowered.

Prevention of Febrile Convulsions. Because these convulsions arise with high fever, they are largely preventable. If acetaminophen is given to keep fever below 101°F (38.4°C), convulsions rarely occur. They happen most often when children develop a fever at night, when the parent is not aware of it, when the temperature is already high, or when a parent is reluctant to give acetaminophen in large enough doses to be therapeutic. Although this type of seizure can be prevented by phenobarbital, prophylactic use during an upper respiratory infection is not recommended. Phenobarbital takes 2 or 3 days to reach therapeutic blood levels. By this time, convulsions would already have occurred. In addition, phenobarbital may reduce cognitive function in children.

The child who has one febrile convulsion usually is not given further treatment, but parents should be counseled not to let the child develop a second high fever. A child who has had two or more febrile seizures may be placed on a maintenance dose of phenobarbital. Whether this prevents further seizures is unproven. For this reason, the practice is controversial. Instruct parents that every child who has a febrile seizure must be seen by a health care provider. A good rule of thumb is to assume that the child in this situation has meningitis until it is ruled out by a complete neurologic workup.

Therapeutic Management. Teach parents that after the seizure subsides, they should sponge the child with tepid water to reduce the fever quickly. Advise them not to put the child in the bathtub, however, because it would be easy for the child to slip underwater should a second seizure occur. A parent also might not be able to hold the convulsing child's head above water. Alcohol or cold water is also not advisable. Extreme cooling causes shock to an immature nervous system, and alcohol can be absorbed by the skin or the fumes inhaled in toxic amounts, compounding the child's problems. Parents should not attempt to give oral medications such as acetaminophen, because the child will be in a drowsy, or *postictal,* state after the seizure and might aspirate the medicine. If attempts to reduce the child's temperature by sponging are unsuccessful, advise parents to put a cool washcloth on the child's forehead, axillary, and groin areas and transport the child, lightly clothed, to a health care facility for immediate evaluation.

Additional treatment will depend on the underlying cause of the fever. A lumbar puncture will be performed to rule out meningitis. Antipyretic drugs to reduce the fever below seizure levels will be administered. Appropriate antibiotic therapy will be started, depending on the type of infection.

Many parents need to be assured that febrile convulsions do not lead to brain damage and that their child is almost always completely well afterward.

CHECKPOINT QUESTIONS

12. A parent describes the child's seizure as starting with a twitch in the fingers and progressing to the arm and face. What type of seizure is the parent describing?
13. How can you assess for the occurrence of absence seizures in a child?

Assessment of the Child With Seizures

A thorough pregnancy history is obtained on children with seizures. Events immediately before the seizure as well as an accurate description of the seizure itself also should be recorded. Investigate the child's overall behavior in the last few weeks. Is the child an A student who has been getting Ds lately? Has the parent noticed bedwetting? These might be possible signs of absence or nocturnal seizures.

A complete physical and neurologic examination and blood studies are necessary to rule out metabolic or infectious processes. Prepare the child for a lumbar puncture to rule out meningitis or bleeding in the CSF. A CT scan, skull x-ray film, or EEG may be done if indicated. During the EEG, the child may be stimulated with rhythm patterns or flashing lights or may be asked to hyperventilate to see whether a seizure can be provoked.

NURSING DIAGNOSES AND RELATED INTERVENTIONS

Nursing Diagnosis: Risk for injury related to tonic-clonic seizure

Outcome Identification: Child will remain free of injury during seizure.

Outcome Evaluation: Child exhibits no signs of aspiration or traumatic injury.

The child must be protected from hurting himself during a tonic-clonic convulsion (see Empowering the Family). Restraining the child's thrashing extremities is not advisable, because it is difficult for the adult and could result in injury to either person because of the amount of force needed to keep the child still. In early school-aged children, it is particularly important to avoid inserting a tongue blade because these children often have loose anterior teeth that are on the verge of falling out.

Remaining calm is also important; be aware that people are frightened by the sight of a child convulsing, because the action is so forceful and violent. It is reassuring for them to see someone calm and in control of the situation and that there is no reason to be afraid. If the child passes rapidly from one convulsion into another (status epilepticus), provide supplemental oxygen and anticonvulsant therapy to counteract this.

EMPOWERING THE FAMILY:
Safety During Seizures

- Remain calm.
- Move away furniture or any sharp object.
- Turn your child gently on his side or abdomen with his head turned to the side to prevent aspiration of unswallowed mouth secretions.
- Don't restrain him other than to keep his head turned to the side so that mouth secretions continue to drain. Restraining the child could result in injury because of the amount of force necessary.
- Do not attempt to place a stick or padded tongue blade between the child's teeth. Trying to force a tongue blade into the mouth this way could break the tongue blade or loosen teeth.
- Try to keep onlookers from crowding the area. A convulsing child is an abnormal sight and always attracts a crowd. Ask people who are only interested spectators to move away.
- Be aware that a child having this type of convulsion may have some slight cyanosis during the tonic and clonic stages, but these stages are so short that administering oxygen is not needed.
- Following any convulsion, telephone your primary care provider and notify him or her of the convulsion so arrangements for any necessary follow-up care can be made.
- If your child should pass rapidly from one convulsion into another (status epilepticus), he may need supplemental oxygen and you may need to administer diazepam. If this happens, telephone your emergency medical service number.

Nursing Diagnosis: Altered family processes related to diagnosis of long-term illness in child

Outcome Identification: Family will maintain functional system of support for each member throughout the course of the illness.

Outcome Evaluation: Child, parents, and other family members express fears and questions about disease to health care team; parents discuss ways to accommodate illness (e.g., medication schedules, school, sports activities, plans for vacation, and discipline) in their daily life.

As soon as the diagnosis of a convulsive disorder is made, parents and children need to be told that it is likely to signify a long-term disease. Although the seizures can be controlled with medication, the disease is not cured. If the child neglects her medication, seizures are apt to recur (see the Nursing Care Plan). Most children are given tablets rather than liquid medication, because the latter tends to settle at the bottom of the bottle, resulting in overdiluted or overconcentrated doses that might allow seizures to break through. Parents need instruction on planning to ensure an adequate supply of medications, especially for a trip away from home or for summer camp. Abrupt discontinuation of seizure medications (particularly phenobarbital) may result in severe seizures.

The child will need to be monitored frequently during childhood to be certain that a medication dosage is adequate. He or she will need periodic blood sampling to ascertain whether therapeutic blood levels of the medication are being maintained.

Provide parents with as much information as possible about the cause of their child's seizures. This will help them feel that they are dealing with a known disease, not an unexplainable and unpredictable illness. If the cause of the seizures is unknown, parents can be reassured that the treatment is known. Their child can be expected to respond to anticonvulsant medication as well as the child whose seizures have a known cause such as recent trauma.

Although it may be difficult, parents need to treat children with seizures as a normal member of the family. They need to know that scolding the child, asking her to do household chores, or insisting that she do her homework will not cause seizures. A few children with absence seizures can initiate them by hyperventilating and may try to manipulate those around them to gain sympathy. The few children who use this extreme form of manipulation should be referred for counseling.

Assure parents that occasional seizures in children are not harmful. Unless status epilepticus occurs and the child becomes anoxic, the chance that their child will be injured during a seizure is remote. They need to be informed so they do not worry about the child becoming cognitively impaired or heed other popular misconceptions about seizures. Although some children who have seizures are also cognitively impaired, the impairment and the seizures were caused by the same event; the seizures did not cause the impairment. At every health care visit, parents need time to ask questions about their child's care and to express any concerns they have. There are so many "scare stories" about convulsions that every parent is likely to believe some of these stories unless counseled otherwise (see Enhancing Communication).

As a rule, children with convulsions should attend regular school and participate in active sports. Many teachers are frightened of the responsibility of having a child with convulsions assigned to their classes. They need to become well informed about seizure control. Children with seizures should participate in gym classes. Being physically active tends to reduce the frequency of seizures and is healthier than being sedentary.

In many children, seizures increase at puberty. This may be the result of glandular changes or of sudden growth and the need for an increased medicine dosage. It may result in part from adolescent rebellion against prescribed medication routines. It is important to respect the adolescent's feelings and need for independence. However, assist the adolescent with channeling his feelings in a more positive manner.

All anticonvulsant medications are potentially teratogenic to a fetus. Adolescent girls must be made aware of this. They may choose to delay childbearing until later in life, when their medication can be reduced or even discontinued.

Breath-Holding

Breath-holding is a phenomenon that occurs in young children when they are stressed or angry. The child breathes in and, because he is upset, does not breathe out again or else breathes out and then does not inhale again. As brain cells become anoxic, the child becomes cyanotic and slumps to the floor, momentarily unconscious. With loss of consciousness, the child begins breathing again. Color returns to normal and he is revived. The child needs no therapy except reassurance that he is all right. Breath-holding is frightening but represents the immaturity of the child's neurologic control. This differs from a tamper tantrum in which a child deliberately attempts to hold his breath and pass out (see Chapter 9).

Headache

Headache in children younger than school age is extremely rare, although children may report "headache" in imitation of their parents. Preschoolers may have headache with a fever because of increased cerebral blood flow and intracranial pressure. As the child reaches school age, headaches may occur as a result of conditions such as eyestrain and sinusitis or possibly as serious as a brain tumor. Headache pain results from meningeal or vascular irritation. The brain itself is insensitive to pain, so a cerebral tumor may be present for a long time before meningeal irritation occurs and pain symptoms are apparent. With a brain tumor, pain becomes evident on changing body position, so a young child who reports headache after getting up should be carefully evaluated. Pain from a brain tumor is also generally occipital, so asking the child to indicate where it hurts will help determine whether there is a tumor.

Migraine Headache

Migraine headache refers to a specific type of headache that may or may not begin with an aura of visual disturbance such as diplopia or a zigzag pattern across the visual field.

Nursing Care Plan

THE CHILD WITH RECURRENT CONVULSIONS

A 12-year-old male is admitted to the acute care facility following a tonic-clonic seizure. His mother states, "He hasn't had a seizure in over a year."

Assessment: Well-proportioned male sleeping soundly on left side since admission. Seizure episode occurred approximately 1 hour ago. Vital signs within age-appropriate parameters. Reacts to painful stimuli only. Deep tendon reflexes depressed. "He was watching television this morning and then told me the light was hurting his eyes and that everything was turning orange. Suddenly he just fell to the floor and started shaking. His face became distorted and he started foaming from his mouth. Some had little specks of blood in it. I called 911 and they brought him here."

Diagnosed with seizures 3 years ago. Currently taking phenobarbital and phenytoin (Dilantin) four times a day. "Since my husband and I divorced 6 months ago, he's been taking charge of his own medicines because I went back to work full time. He's told me he hates to take them because he feels like they slow him down. Now I'm not sure if he really has been taking them like he should." Child leaves for school when mother leaves for work at 7 A.M. and takes the late bus home from school after baseball practice, getting home around 6 P.M. Mother noticed some small blood spots on the child's pillow twice in the last week. "Maybe he had a seizure during the night?"

Child is in seventh grade and is a B student. Plays on the middle school baseball team. Has a 7-year-old sister. Mother states, "They get along fairly well, except for their occasional fights."

Lumbar puncture performed; pressures within normal limits; specimens sent for cell count, glucose, and culture. Serum drug levels obtained: phenobarbital level 7 µg/mL; phenytoin level 6 µg/mL.

Nursing Diagnosis: Risk for injury related to diminished level of consciousness resulting from seizure episode

Outcome Identification: Child will remain free of injury now and during future seizures.

Outcome Evaluation: Child and parent state safety measures to prevent injury. Child exhibits no signs of aspiration or traumatic injury.

Interventions	Rationale
1. Maintain a patent airway with the child lying on his side until alert and responsive. Provide privacy and institute seizure precautions.	1. Side-lying position reduces the risk for aspiration. Privacy minimizes possible embarrassment for the child. Seizure precautions minimize the risk of injury when the child's level of consciousness is diminished and also if another seizure should occur.
2. Monitor vital signs and neurologic status every 15 minutes until the child is fully awake.	2. Frequent monitoring provides information about the extent of involvement and resolution of the seizure.
3. Observe for signs and symptoms of respiratory distress. Administer oxygen as ordered and monitor oxygen saturation levels with pulse oximetry.	3. Respiratory distress may indicate aspiration. Oxygen administration aids in preventing hypoxemia. Oxygen saturation levels provide objective evidence of tissue perfusion.
4. Provide a calm, restful environment. Minimize the child's exposure to external stimuli. Administer anticonvulsants as ordered.	4. Following a tonic-clonic seizure, a calm, restful environment is necessary to allow the child to sleep. The child's drug levels are subtherapeutic. Administering anticonvulsants reduces the risk for further seizure activity by increasing serum drug levels.

(continued)

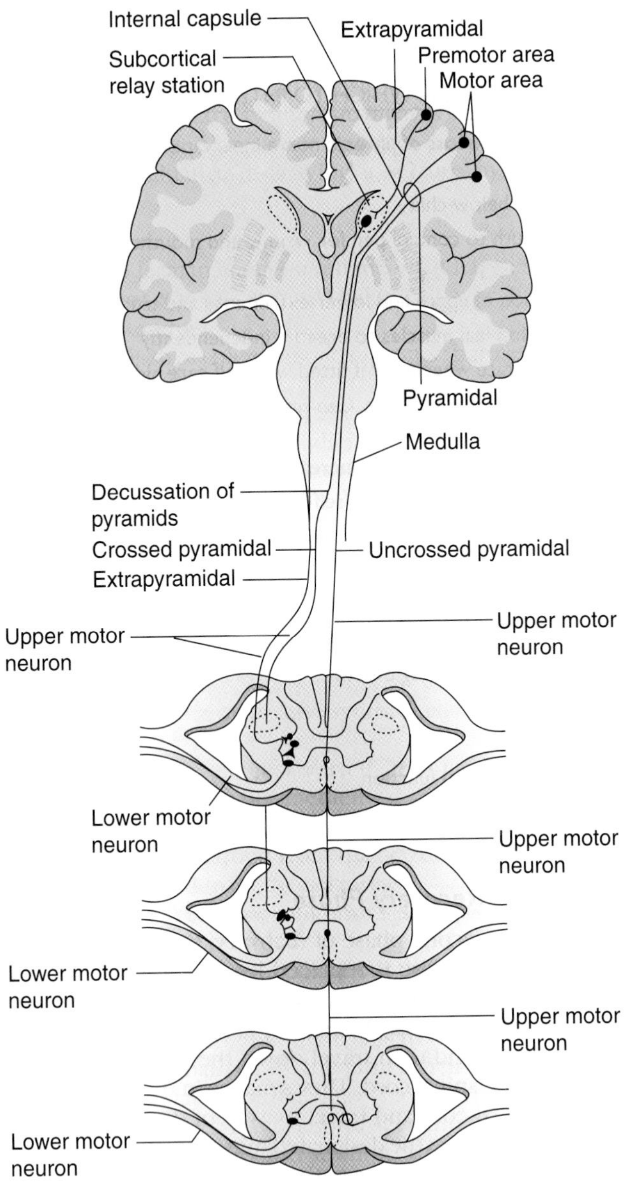

FIGURE 28.11 Diagram of motor pathways between the cerebral cortex, one of the subcortical relay stations, and lower motor neurons in the spinal cord. Decussation (crossing of fibers) means that each side of the brain controls skeletal muscles on the opposite side of the body.

remain flaccid, because lower motor neurons cannot send impulses for contraction.

During this phase, if the child's bladder is allowed to fill, the resultant sensory stimulation relayed to the damaged cord will initiate a powerful sympathetic reflex reaction (**autonomic dysreflexia**), and the child will show signs of hypertension, tachycardia, flushed face, and severe occipital headache. This is an emergency situation, and if the severe hypertension is not relieved, cerebral vascular accident can result.

Third Recovery Phase

The third phase of recovery from spinal cord injury is the final outcome, or permanent limitation of motor and sensory function. If the compression of the spinal cord is caused by edema that is then relieved, no permanent motor and sensory disability will occur.

Assessment of Spinal Cord Injury

Spinal cord injury should be suspected whenever a child has sustained a forceful trauma of any kind. The signs of spinal cord injury vary according to the level of the injury. The cervical and thoracolumbar areas of the spine are the ones most likely to sustain injury.

It is important that a child with suspected spinal cord injury not be moved until the back and head can be supported in a straight line to prevent further injury to the spinal column from twisting or bending. In the emergency department, do not attempt to move the child from the stretcher to an examining table until spinal x-ray films are done. This will reduce any unnecessary movement. When moving the child onto the x-ray table, log-roll him gently so that additional injury does not result. If resuscitation is necessary, maintain the head in a neutral position; do not hyperextend it. To keep the neck immobilized, do not remove a child's football or motorcycle helmet or neck brace.

The child will need a thorough neurologic assessment to determine the level of injury. Help maintain spinal immobilization during procedures.

WHAT IF? You are caring for the child with a spinal cord injury and he suddenly develops hypertension, tachycardia, diaphoresis, and headache. What would you initially assess for? How would you intervene?

TABLE 28.6 Characteristics of Upper and Lower Motor Nerve Lesions After Spinal Shock Phase

FINDING	UPPER MOTOR LESION	LOWER MOTOR LESION
Spasticity	Present	Absent (flaccidity present)
Clonus	Present, increased	Absent
Tendon reflexes	Increased	Absent
Babinski reflex	Present	Absent
Reflexes below level of lesion	Present	Absent
Reflex at level of lesion	Absent	Absent
Atrophy of muscles	Absent or present only to slight degree	Present (muscle fasciculations may be present)

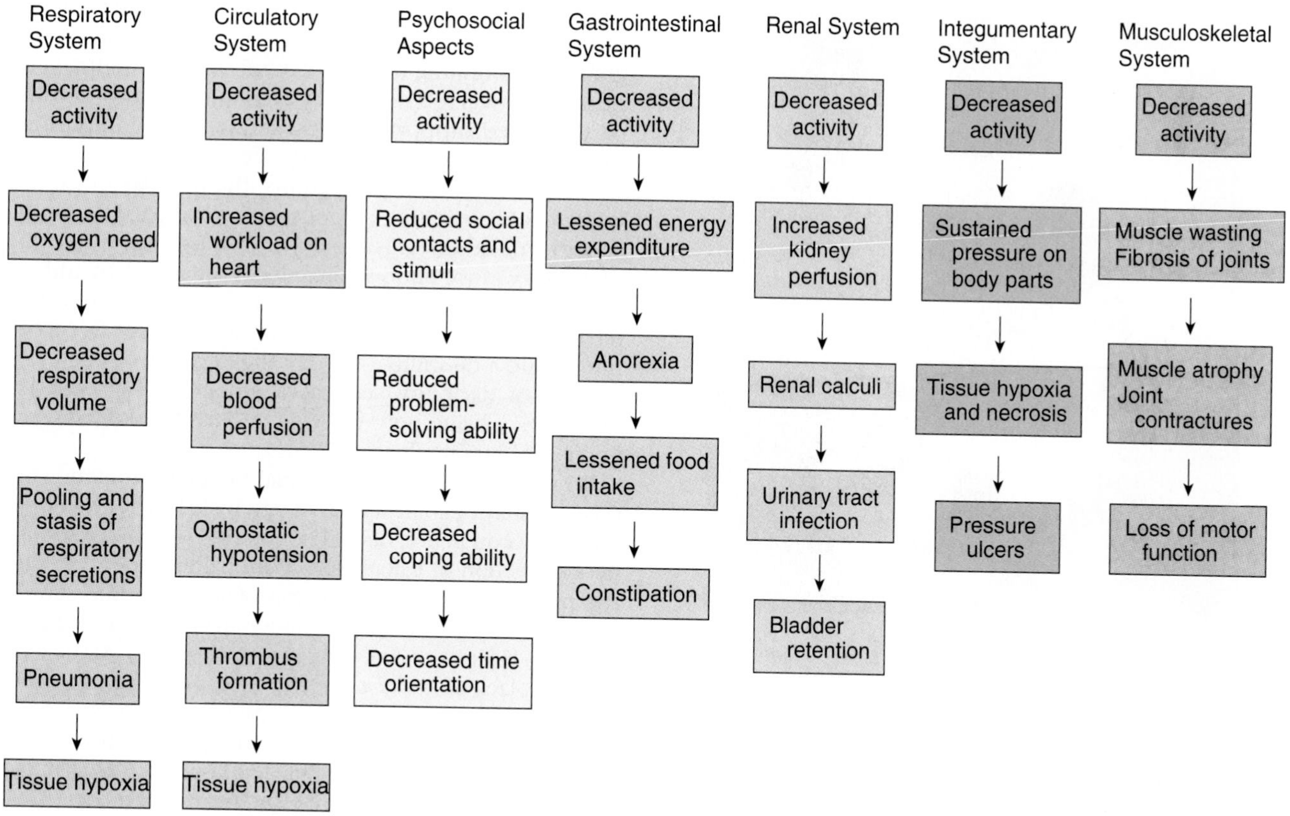

FIGURE 28.12 Effects of immobilization.

NURSING DIAGNOSES AND RELATED INTERVENTIONS

During the first phase of recovery, the child's major problems are those resulting from almost complete immobility: pressure sores on bony prominences; loss of appetite and subsequent poor nutrition from depression or being in the supine position; urinary calculi from excessive calcium loss; atrophy of flaccid muscle groups; and urinary retention and bladder infection. These effects of immobility are shown in Figure 28-12.

Nursing Diagnosis: Impaired physical mobility related to effects of spinal cord injury

Outcome Identification: Child will achieve the optimal level of mobility possible after injury.

Outcome Evaluation: Child demonstrates movement of all extremities with a minimum of artificial support and equipment; participates in exercise program within limitations; exhibits ability to move about environment within limitations.

Children may be placed in cervical traction with Crutchfield tongs and a traction belt (Figure 28-13) or by halo traction (see Chapter 30). Having tongs inserted into the skull is a very frightening procedure for children. They are afraid that the tongs will burrow into their skull and strike their brain. Children need someone they know and trust to help them lie still during the procedure. To relieve edema at the injury site and prevent further injury, corticosteroids may be administered.

To promote circulation and prevent loss of calcium that results from inactivity, full range-of-motion exercises must be done approximately three times per day. These are time consuming but important in maintaining joint function.

During the second phase of recovery, when spasticity of muscle groups occurs, preventing contractures becomes an important nursing responsibility. Specialized splints, boots, or even hightop sneakers may be used to prevent footdrop (Figure 28-14). A muscle relaxant, such as diazepam, may be ordered to prevent painful muscle spasm. Holding legs and arms at the joints helps reduce the spasms. If children have upper extremity mobility but will be left with lower extremity paralysis, exercises to strengthen the upper ex-

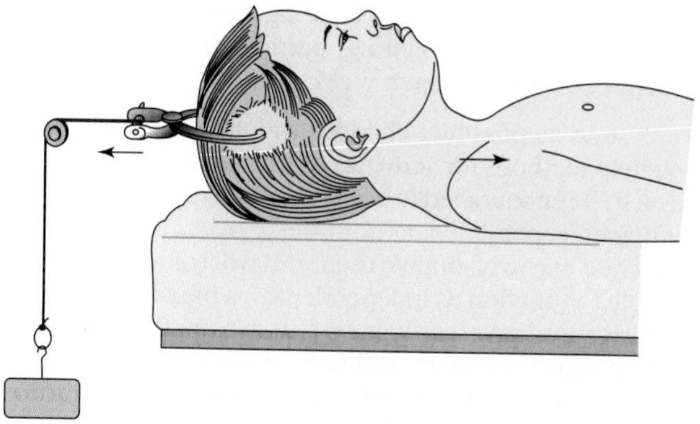

FIGURE 28.13 Crutchfield tongs used to create spinal traction.

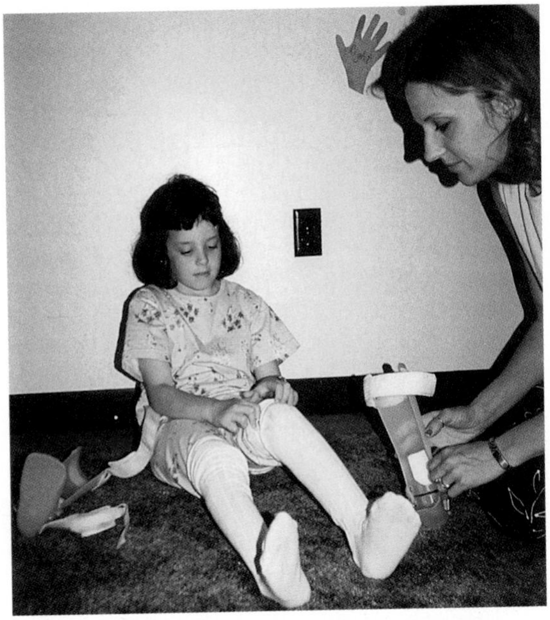

FIGURE 28.14 Specialized splints are used for a child with a low spinal cord injury to prevent contractures and foot drop. Here the physical therapist prepares to apply the splint to the child's leg.

tremity muscle groups will be started. Strengthening the arms will help children be able to lift themselves from bed to wheelchair or raise themselves with a trapeze over the bed when changing positions.

One major problem of ambulation after spinal cord injury is helping a child's body readjust to a vertical position after being maintained in the supine position for so long. When the child is raised, blood tends to pool in dilated blood vessels below the level of the lesion. This pooling of blood results in a pseudohypovolemia and hypotension, and the child may faint. Gradually increasing the angle of the bed will help the child become acclimated to the upright position without experiencing vascular pooling.

Nursing Diagnosis: Self-care deficit related to spinal cord injury

Outcome Identification: Child will demonstrate ability to perform as many activities of daily living as possible within his level of functioning.

Outcome Evaluation: Child states intention of taking over self-care; practices using equipment for eating, bathing, and toileting; participates in one new aspect of self-care each week.

As soon as possible, children should be introduced to self-help methods for activities of daily living. Most parents need to be encouraged to allow the child to become as self-sufficient as possible and not to take over complete care. The child may well outlive them and will some day need to be able to function as independently as possible.

With autonomic nervous system dysfunction, the child will be unable to sweat and will become hyperthermic if covered too warmly; if not covered warmly enough, the capillaries will dilate, and he will lose considerable heat into the environment. If the room temperature cools at night, be careful to dress the child appropriately for sleeping.

Specific measures for bowel evacuation may be necessary, depending on the level of the injury. A bowel program incorporating the use of stool softeners, suppositories, and bowel retraining may be required. The child and parents need support and instructions in accomplishing this task and gaining independence.

For some children and parents, the first day of using a wheelchair is exciting (proof they can be partially ambulatory). For others, it is the day they must face the reality that they cannot undo the results of the accident and are faced with a lifelong disability. For some parents who have nearly overcome their grief and almost accepted their child's disability, the day they are introduced to a symbol of disability such as a wheelchair or long-leg braces may bring new grieving and a sense of loss (see Focus on Nursing Research).

When the child reaches sexual maturity, limitations in this area may become apparent. If a male has had an upper motor neuron injury, he will not be able to achieve spontaneous erection or ejaculation. With manual stimulation of the penis, however (stimulation of lower motor neuron function), he may be able to achieve an erection and engage in coitus. Ejaculation and fertility remain limited. At the time of injury, lack of lower extremity motor control may seem the greatest loss. In adolescence, loss of normal sexual function may become even more disturbing. With most spinal cord injuries, a female is not able to experience orgasm but is nonetheless able to conceive and bear children.

The limitations caused by a spinal cord injury will become especially evident to the child (and the parents) when choosing a vocation and selecting an appropriate school program (children cannot be denied normal

FOCUS ON NURSING RESEARCH

What Is the Quality of Life in Patients With Spinal Cord Injury?

Three groups of spinal cord–injured patients—those who had sustained a pediatric spinal cord injury, a second group newly injured and a third group with chronic adult injury—were interviewed as to their health-related quality of life. Patients with pediatric spinal cord injury assigned the lowest importance to moving; they scored lower on the importance of working capability. The quality-of-life scores of patients who had sustained their injury in childhood were significantly higher than those of the newly injured patients or chronic adult patients.

This study is important to nurses because it stresses the long time span that is needed for many children to adjust to a devastating injury. It stresses how important it is to offer psychological support to children and families undergoing this type of crisis.

Kannisto, M., Merikanto, J., Alaranta, H., Hokkanen, H., & Sintonen, H. (1998). Comparison of health-related quality of life in three subgroups of spinal cord injury patients. *Spinal Cord, 36*(3), 193.

schooling by federal law in the United States, even with a severe physical disability).

Counseling and rehabilitation are crucial aspects to achieve an optimal level of functioning and independence.

Nursing Diagnosis: Risk for impaired gas exchange related to spinal cord injury

Outcome Identification: Child will achieve optimum respiratory function possible.

Outcome Evaluation: Respiratory rate is within acceptable parameters; lungs clear; airway patent.

If the cervical level of the cord is involved, the child will need ventilatory assistance. He may be intubated at first, but orotracheal or nasotracheal intubation is only a temporary measure to maintain a patent airway. A tracheostomy may be done for long-term airway management and to prevent sloughing of pharyngeal tissue from the pressure of the intubation tube. If this is required, the parents will need instruction about caring for the tracheostomy and working with a mechanical ventilator. A phrenic nerve pacemaker may be used to stimulate the diaphragm to contract and initiate respirations. If the child has a thoracic level injury, rare because the rib cage gives extra strength to thoracic vertebrae, the child will be able to breathe on her own but will have reduced vital capacity. Periodic positive-pressure breathing treatments may be necessary to encourage increased lung filling. Be careful when positioning the child to prevent compromising chest movement with equipment or other restricting objects. Other respiratory care measures, such as suctioning and chest physiotherapy, are also important.

Nursing Diagnosis: Risk for altered skin integrity related to immobility

Outcome Identification: Child's skin will remain intact.

Outcome Evaluation: Child's skin remains clean, dry, and intact without signs of erythema or ulceration.

To prevent skin breakdown, the child should be turned about every 2 hours (always be sure to log-roll or maintain immobilization with a striker frame or Circo-Electric bed). The use of an alternating-pressure mattress may be helpful. With loss of sensation in body parts, the child is unable to report skin irritation from a wrinkled sheet or wet clothing. If incontinent, the bedding must be changed immediately to prevent skin breakdown. Once children begin to be ambulatory, their legs and buttocks should be checked regularly to prevent pressure ulcers from developing from sitting in a wheelchair or using leg braces (Harding-Okimoto, 1997).

Nursing Diagnosis: Risk for altered urinary elimination related to spinal cord injury

Outcome Identification: Child will demonstrate ability to eliminate urine within limits of injury.

Outcome Evaluation: Child's urine output is adequate for intake; Child identifies measures to assist with voiding; demonstrates procedure for self-catheterization.

To prevent urinary retention during the first phase of recovery, a Foley catheter will be inserted, or the bladder can be emptied by periodic suprapubic aspiration, catheterization, or Credé maneuver (pressing on the bladder to evacuate it). Second-stage spasticity causes periodic reflex emptying. This rarely empties the bladder completely, however, so the same problems of stasis and infection continue. Encouraging a child to drink cranberry juice will help acidify the urine and limit bacterial growth. To live independently, the child will need to learn self-catheterization to empty the bladder.

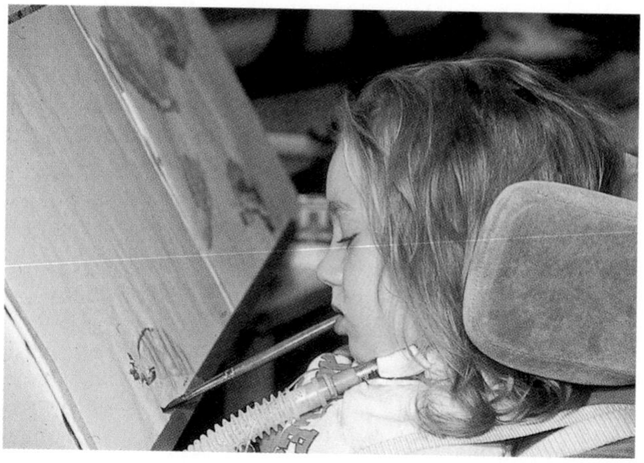

FIGURE 28.15 A 6-year-old girl with a cervical spine injury adapts to her disability by using her mouth to hold a paintbrush and participate in age-appropriate activities.

Nursing Diagnosis: Anticipatory grieving related to loss of function secondary to spinal cord injury

Outcome Identification: Child and parents will express their grief regarding spinal cord injury during recovery period.

Outcome Evaluation: Child and parents openly discuss their feelings about injury and its effect on their lives.

The second recovery phase is the time for parents and children to begin thinking about what this degree of disability will mean to them and to face its full extent. Children and parents typically react to the initial diagnosis with grief. They may still be in denial or shock when the second phase begins. With no sudden miracle cure in sight, they may begin to move through stages of anger, bargaining, depression, and then acceptance (the accident happened; we must go on from this point). They need assistance and support to work through these feelings. Both the parents and the child may need counseling to reach acceptance. Incorporation of a rehabilitation program can help in maximizing the child's potential despite the limitations imposed by the injury (Figure 28-15).

CHECKPOINT QUESTIONS

16. During which recovery phase would you expect to observe loss of autonomic nervous system function?
17. Why does spastic paralysis occur in a child with spinal cord injury?
18. Which area of the spinal cord is most likely to sustain an injury in a child?

KEY POINTS

Nerve cells are unique in that they do not regenerate if damaged. This makes neurologic disease a long-term type of illness. Parents and children alike need support from health care providers to cope with problems that continue to occur over a long period. Many neurologic disorders cause problems with balance. Be certain that children are capable of ambulating safely before allowing them out of bed without assistance. Some children need to wear a helmet to protect the head from trauma if they should fall.

Increased intracranial pressure arises from an increase in the CSF volume or from blood accumulation, cerebral edema, or space-occupying lesions. Neurologic changes such as increased temperature and blood pressure and decreased pulse and respirations that occur with this are subtle. Always compare assessments with previous levels to detect that a consistent, although minor, change is occurring.

Cerebral palsy is a nonprogressive disorder of upper motor neurons. The exact cause is generally unknown, but the condition is associated with anoxia before, during, or shortly after birth. Four major types are identified: spastic (there is excessive tone in the voluntary muscles), dyskinetic or athetoid (abnormal involuntary movement), atonic (decreased muscle tone), and mixed (symptoms of both spasticity and athetoid movements are present).

Meningitis is infection of the cerebral meninges. It is caused most frequently by bacterial invasion. Children need follow-up afterward to monitor for hearing acuity and undersecretion of antidiuretic hormone.

Encephalitis is inflammation of brain tissue. This is always a serious diagnosis, because the child may be left with residual neurologic damage such as seizures or learning disabilities.

Reye's syndrome is acute encephalitis with accompanying fatty infiltration of the liver, heart, and lungs associated with the use of aspirin and NSAIDs in children with a viral infection. Its incidence is declining.

Guillain-Barré syndrome is inflammation of motor and sensory nerves. The reaction may be immune mediated, after an upper respiratory illness. Temporary demyelinization of the nerve sheaths occurs with loss of function.

Botulism occurs when spores of *Clostridium botulinum* produce toxins in the intestine. Because honey and corn syrup may be sources of the organism, they should not be given to infants.

Recurrent convulsions are involuntary contractions of muscle caused by abnormal electrical brain discharges. Common types seen in children are infantile spasms, partial (focal), absence, and tonic-clonic. Seizures may occur from fever in children younger than 7 years of age. Therapy is administration of anticonvulsant drugs.

Spinal cord injury is occurring at increased rates in children from sports and motor vehicle accidents. Children pass through a first, second, and third recovery phase after the injury.

CRITICAL THINKING EXERCISES

1. Tasha is the 2-year-old newly diagnosed with cerebral palsy you met at the beginning of the chapter. Her parents are concerned about long-term problems. Would you encourage them to concentrate on these or on more short-term concerns?
2. A 2-year-old diagnosed with bacterial meningitis has severe neck pain when she is moved. Her mother asks you not to worry so much about intake and output so her daughter can rest. How would you answer her mother? Suppose you call the child's name and she does not answer you? Why is this a particular cause of concern with a child with meningitis?
3. A high school senior who is your neighbor tells you that he thinks he has the flu and that he took some aspirin for it. When you tell him it is not wise for children to take aspirin for flulike symptoms, he tells you that advice is "just for babies." How would you respond and how would you pursue the matter with him?
4. A spinal cord injury can cause severe disability in adolescents. If you were designing a program to teach measures to prevent spinal cord injury, what topics would you include in your presentation?

REFERENCES

Carpay, H. A. et al. (1998). Epilepsy in childhood: an audit of clinical practice. *Archives of Neurology, 55*(5), 668.

Cherington, M. (1998). Clinical spectrum of botulism. *Muscle and Nerve, 21*(6), 701.

Department of Health and Human Services. (1995). *Healthy people 2000: midcourse review.* Washington, D.C.: DHHS.

Fishman, M. A. (1997). Evaluation of the child with neurologic disease. In Johnson, K. B. & Oski, F. A. *Oski's essential pediatrics*. Philadelphia: Lippincott-Raven.

Glaze, D. G. (1997). Status epilepticus. In Johnson, K. B. & Oski, F. A. *Oski's essential pediatrics.* Philadelphia: Lippincott-Raven.

Gorman, C. et al. (1998). Alterations in self-perceptions following childhood onset of spinal cord injury. *Spinal Cord, 36*(3), 181.

Harding-Okimoto, M. B. (1997). Pressure ulcers, self-concept and body image in spinal cord injury patients. *SCI Nursing, 14*(4), 111.

Kannisto, M., Merikanto, J., Alaranta, H., Hokkanen, H., & Sintonen, H. (1998). Comparison of health-related quality of life in three subgroups of spinal cord injury patients. *Spinal Cord, 36*(3), 193.

Kornberg, A. J. & Prensky, A. L. (1997). Cerebral vascular disease in childhood. In Johnson, K. B. & Oski, F. A. *Oski's essential pediatrics*. Philadelphia: Lippincott-Raven.

Lebel, M. H. (1997). Meningitis. In Johnson, K. B. & Oski, F. A. *Oski's essential pediatrics*. Philadelphia: Lippincott-Raven.

Louise, P. T. (1997). Reye's syndrome. In Johnson, K. B. & Oski, F. A. *Oski's essential pediatrics*. Philadelphia: Lippincott-Raven

Metsahonkala, L. et al. (1998). Social environment and headache in 8- to 9-year old children: a follow-up study. *Headache, 38*(3), 222.

Parke, J. T. (1997). Peripheral neuropathy. In Johnson, K. B. & Oski, F. A. *Oski's essential pediatrics.* Philadelphia: Lippincott-Raven.

Percy, A. K. (1997). Static encephalopathy. In Johnson, K. B. & Oski, F. A. *Oski's essential pediatrics.* Philadelphia: Lippincott-Raven.

Pinto-Martin, J. A. et al. (1998). Short interpregnancy interval and the risk of disabling cerebral palsy in a low birth weight population. *Journal of Pediatrics, 132*(5), 818.

Poyhonen, M., et al. (1997). Risk of malignancy and death in neurofibromatosis. *Archives of Pathology and Laboratory Medicine, 121*(2), 139.

Riccardi, V. M. (1997). Phakomatoses and other neurocutaneous syndromes. In Johnson, K. B. & Oski, F. A. *Oski's esential pediatrics.* Philadelphia: Lippincott-Raven.

Rosman, N. P. (1997). Acute head trauma. In Johnson, K. B. & Oski, F. A. *Oski's essential pediatrics*. Philadelphia: Lippincott-Raven.

Schoenen, J. (1997). Acute migraine therapy: the newer drugs. *Current Opinion in Neurology, 10*(3), 237.

Strauss, D. J. et al. (1998). Life expectancy of children with cerebral palsy. *Pediatric Neurology, 18*(2), 143.

Wood, N. W. (1998). Diagnosing Friedreich's ataxia. *Archives of Disease in Childhood, 78*(3), 204.

SUGGESTED READINGS

Cantu, R. C. (1998). Epilepsy and athletics. *Clinics in Sports Medicine, 17*(1), 61.

Celano, R. T. (1998). Diagnosing pediatric epilepsy: an update for the primary care clinician. *Nurse Practitioner 23*(3), 69.

De Lorenzo, R. A. (1997). Demystifying the neurological examination. *Journal of Emergency Medical Services, 22*(9), 68.

De Michele, G. et al. (1998). Determinants of onset age in Friedreich's ataxia. *Journal of Neurology, 245*(3), 166.

Edwards-Beckett, J. & King, H. (1996). The impact of spinal pathology on bowel control in children. *Rehabilitation Nursing, 21*(6), 292.

Hope, M. E. & Kailis, S. G. (1998). Medication usage in a spinal cord injured population. *Spinal Cord, 36*(3), 161.

Kelly, M. T. & Hays, T. L. (1997). Implementing the ketogenic diet. *Topics in Clinical Nutrition, 13*(1), 53.

Reid, D. E. et al. (1997). Central nervous system perfusion and metabolism abnormalities in Sturge-Weber syndrome. *Journal of Child Neurology, 12*(3), 218.

Simmons, B. (1997). What do you think? What practical strategies can nurses utilize to assess, treat, and prevent urinary tract infections among persons with SCI/D? *SCI Nursing, 14*(4), 129.

Telatar, M. et al. (1998). Ataxia-telangiectasia: identification and detection of founder-effect mutations in the ATM gene in ethnic populations. *American Journal of Human Genetics, 62*(1), 86.

Ward, M. R. (1997). Reye's syndrome: an update. *Nurse Practitioner, 22*(12), 45.

Nursing Care of the Child With a Disorder of the Eyes or Ears

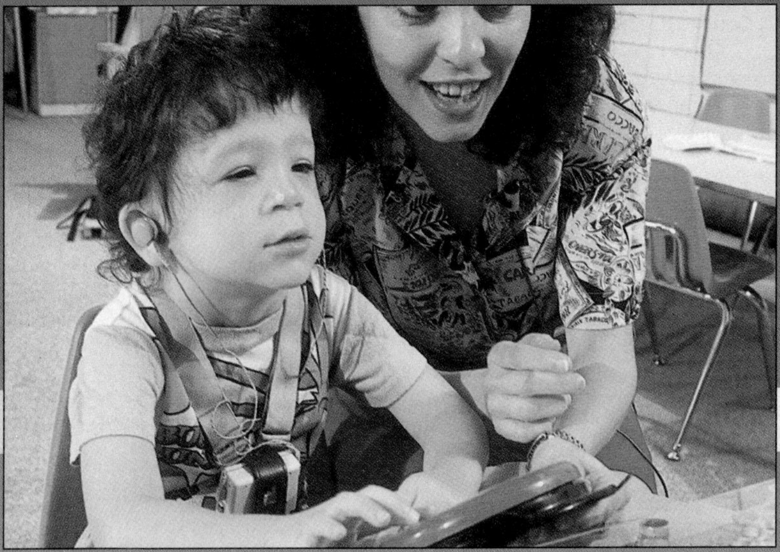

29

CHAPTER

Key Terms

- accommodation
- amblyopia
- astigmatism
- cones
- convergence
- diplopia
- enucleation
- extraocular muscles
- fovea centralis
- goniotomy
- hyperopia
- light refraction
- myopia
- myringotomy
- nystagmus
- orthoptics
- ptosis
- rods
- stereopsis
- strabismus
- tympanocentesis

Objectives

After mastering the contents of this chapter, you should be able to:

1. Describe the structure and function of the eyes and ears and disorders of these organs that affect children.
2. Assess the child who has a disorder of vision or hearing.
3. Formulate nursing diagnoses related to the child with a disorder of vision or hearing.
4. Establish appropriate outcomes for the child with a disorder of vision or hearing.
5. Plan nursing interventions for the child with a disorder of vision or hearing.
6. Implement nursing care to meet the specific needs of the child who has a disorder of the eyes or ears.
7. Evaluate outcomes for achievement and effectiveness of care.
8. Identify National Health Goals related to vision and hearing disorders of children that nurses could be instrumental in helping the nation achieve.
9. Identify areas related to care of children with vision or hearing disorders that could benefit from additional nursing research.
10. Use critical thinking to analyze ways that nursing care of children with a dysfunction of vision or hearing could be more family centered.
11. Integrate knowledge of childhood disorders of the eyes or ears with the nursing process to achieve quality child health nursing care.

Carla Vander, a 4-year-old child, is brought to the clinic for evaluation. Her mother states, "I think she has another ear infection. She's had a fever for 2 days and says that her ear hurts. This is just like what happened 2 weeks ago when she had an ear infection. Why does this keep happening?" How would you answer Ms. Vander? What information does she need to know about ear infections?

In previous chapters, you learned about growth and development of well children. In this chapter, you'll add information about the changes, physical and psychosocial, that occur when a child develops a disorder of vision or hearing. This is important information because it builds a base for care and health teaching.

After you've studied this chapter, turn to the Critical Thinking Exercises at the end of the chapter to help sharpen your skills and test your knowledge.

Impairment of the eyes or ears always poses a threat to normal growth and development, because so much of how a child learns about the world is achieved through these sensory organs. Infants first learn how to interact with others by watching their parents' faces. They learn to speak by listening to words spoken to them. They continue to depend on sensory input for stimulation throughout life.

Eye and ear disorders may be transitory. However, they always have the potential for becoming long-term illnesses if they permanently affect vision and hearing. This is an area in which health promotion, illness prevention, and health rehabilitation are important aspects of nursing care. Because of the importance of vision and hearing, National Health Goals have been established. Those related to vision and hearing disorders in children are shown in the Focus on National Health Goals.

FOCUS ON NATIONAL HEALTH GOALS

Adequate vision and hearing ability are necessary for normal growth and development; three National Health Goals address goals in these areas:

- Reduce acute middle ear infections among children aged 4 and younger, as measured by days of restricted activity or school absenteeism, to no more than 105 days per 100 children from a baseline of 131 days per 100 children.
- Reduce significant hearing impairment to a prevalence of no more than 82/1000 people from a baseline of 88.9/1000.
- Reduce significant visual impairment to a prevalence of no more than 30/1000 people from a baseline of 34.5/1000 (DHHS, 1995).

Nurses can be instrumental in helping the nation achieve these goals by screening for vision and hearing at all well child assessments, paying particular attention to those children who have been cared for in neonatal intensive care units. Nursing research questions that might yield helpful information include: Can infants who are prone to hearing and vision disorders be better identified before discharge from a neonatal intensive unit? What are effective techniques for teaching adolescents to avoid excessive sound levels, such as those associated with loud music? What are effective ways to teach school-age children to avoid eye injury?

NURSING PROCESS OVERVIEW

for Health Promotion of Vision and Hearing

Assessment

All newborns should be assessed for their ability to focus on or see an examiner's face and to follow an object from the periphery to midline. Observe the infant closely to ensure that the newborn's interest is evoked by sight, not sound. Newborn vision can be further tested by optokinetic nystagmus testing (the infant is shown alternating black and white stripes), visual-evoked potential testing (similar but checkerboard-appearing pictures are shown), and forced-choice preferential looking testing (the infant is shown a pattern and a plain picture; the seeing child focuses on the pattern; Traboulsi & Maumenee, 1994).

Assessing newborn infants for hearing loss is an equally important part of newborn care. Newborns should quiet to the sound of a soothing voice. (For this you need to stay out of sight so you are certain the infant is not quieting to your face.) Newborns should startle or attune to a loud noise made near them. Instruments for testing newborn hearing are being developed that will provide for better documentation of the newborn's ability to respond to a noise.

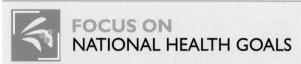

Children should be assessed for vision problems and hearing loss by history throughout childhood. (Is a parent or teacher concerned about vision? Does a parent worry that a child may not be hearing well? Is a child having any difficulty in school?) Vision should also be assessed by inspection: Do the child's eyes follow a moving light into all six fields of vision? Is a red reflex present? Do the child's eyes appear to be in straight alignment? Both vision and hearing acuity should be checked periodically. Children also should be assessed for their ability to speak clearly and age appropriately, because language is influenced by hearing. Detailed vision and hearing assessment is discussed in Chapter 13 with other aspects of physical assessment. (See Assessing the Child for Signs and Symptoms of Vision or Hearing Disorders.)

Nursing Diagnosis

Health promotion in regard to safety measures for eye and ear health is a major responsibility of the nurse. Related nursing diagnoses include the following:

- Health-seeking behaviors related to prevention of trauma to eyes or ears
- Knowledge deficit related to importance of early diagnosis and treatment of ear infection

Nursing diagnoses for the child with vision or hearing impairment should focus on the child and

ASSESSING the Child for Signs and Symptoms of Vision or Hearing Disorders

History

Chief concern: Are symptoms of vision or hearing difficulty present—blurriness of vision, squinting, turning head, leaning toward speaker, ignoring instructions?

Past health history: Has child had any exposure to loud noises? Eye trauma? Ear infection?

Family medical history: Do any family members have a hearing disorder? What is the vision level of parents?

Physical assessment

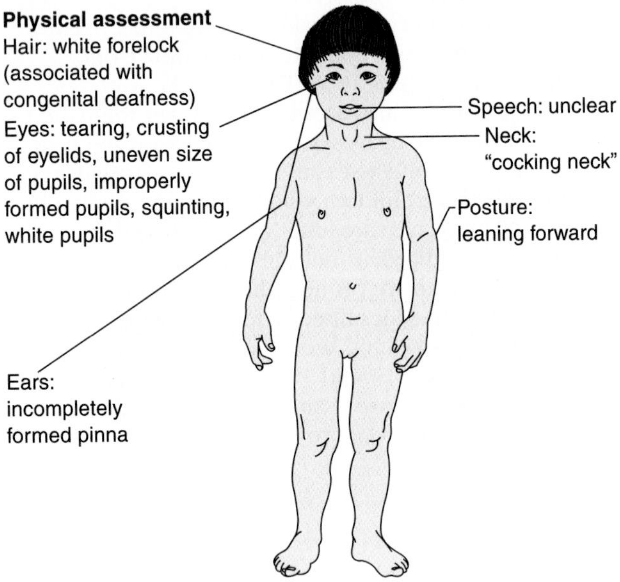

parents' responses to loss of sight or hearing, not on the deficit itself (Carpenito, 1997). Such nursing diagnoses might include:

- Self-care deficit related to impaired visual acuity
- Risk for injury related to hearing loss
- Risk for altered self-esteem related to long-term vision deficit
- Impaired verbal communication related to congenital hearing deficit
- Social isolation related to effects of hearing loss
- Dysfunctional grieving related to child's loss of sight
- Family coping, potential for growth, related to child's traumatic injury and subsequent loss of vision in one eye

Outcome Identification and Planning

Be certain that outcomes established are realistic and address areas in which you can have some impact. By listening attentively to parents' concerns and providing useful anticipatory guidance, you can help to increase the child's ability to function effectively. Because many eye and ear disorders cause pain, helping parents reduce pain is a major nursing responsibility. Outcomes should always address preventive aspects of care in all areas of daily living.

When parents learn that a child has a vision or hearing impairment, they generally need help in planning for schooling and activities such as toilet-training and self-care. You need to discuss with these parents the importance of talking to and touching their infant; of teaching her how to communicate and learn about the world around her through touch as well as through her other functioning senses.

Children with sensory impairment benefit from very early preschool education programs. They are exposed to interesting and stimulating tasks when their sense of initiative is strongest and so they can accomplish learning tasks despite their disability. It may be difficult for parents to relinquish their children to such programs during the day, especially at such an early age. It takes careful planning to enable parents to accept this separation.

Parents of children with hearing impairments may need to be encouraged to talk to their children, even in infancy. Although the infant may not be able to hear what the parents are saying, observing facial expressions and spontaneous body movements that accompany verbal speech will help him or her learn important aspects of communication. The older child may not be able to hear her mother say, "I'm so proud of you," but she can see the happiness on her mother's face.

Implementation

Nursing interventions for the child with a disorder of the eye or ear range from providing anticipatory guidance and teaching children and parents measures to promote eye and ear health to preparing a child for surgery. Nursing interventions also include helping a child and parents adjust to aids that will improve hearing, speech, or sight. Referrals to organizations that can provide information and support to parents of children with vision or hearing impairment can be particularly useful, especially when the impairment will be long term. Some of the organizations concerned with sensory impairment include the following:

Alexander Graham Bell Association for the Deaf
3417 Volta Place NW
Washington, DC 20007

American Foundation for the Blind
15 West 16th Street
New York, NY 10011

American Speech-Language-Hearing Association
10801 Rockville Pike
Rockville, MD 20852

National Association for the Visually Handicapped
22 West 21st Street
New York, NY 10010

National Federation of the Blind
1800 Johnson Street
Baltimore, MD 21230

Recording for the Blind
20 Roszel Road
Princeton, NJ 08540

Outcome Evaluation

As stated before, a disorder of the eyes or ears can turn from an acute, one-time illness into a chronic and developmentally debilitating condition if steps are not taken to treat the initial problem quickly and completely. Even the most rigorous preventive care and attention, however, cannot avert the occurrence of some serious disorders affecting vision and hearing. Nursing care must then focus on helping the child and parents adjust to this condition and making sure that the child receives the stimulation needed to grow and develop on a normal continuum.

Continuous follow-up is essential, too. Self-esteem is an important factor to be evaluated. Does the child see herself as well or ill; as a person able to do things or as helpless? Plans to promote self-esteem may have to be devised. Some parents may require help with their own feelings of worth. (Feeling inferior to other parents is common in parents of children with disabilities.) They may need help in letting go as children begin school. The growth of parents in allowing their child to be independent is just as important to evaluate as the child's own progress toward independence.

The following are examples of outcome criteria:

- Parent voices importance of giving full 10-day supply of antibiotic to child for otitis media therapy.
- Parents state concrete plans for enrolling child in preschool program.
- Child wears corrective lenses for major portion of each day.
- Child demonstrates methods to communicate effectively with health care providers.

HEALTH PROMOTION AND RISK MANAGEMENT

All children should be screened routinely for vision and hearing problems. A history and physical examination performed at each health maintenance visit can provide important clues to possible problems and need for further evaluation. Pay special attention to any questions or concerns voiced by the parents at these visits. As the child grows older and attends school, often the school nurse assumes a major responsibility for vision and hearing testing. General guidelines for evaluation are shown in Table 29-1.

Providing anticipatory guidance to parents about safety measures to prevent accidental injury is another major nursing responsibility. Empowering the Family summarizes safety measures for preventing eye injuries and hearing loss in children.

In addition to safety measures, parents need instruction about measures to prevent eye and ear infections, which may lead to long-term problems. Promoting compliance with treatments, specifically for otitis media, is essential because this disorder is a common cause of impaired hearing in children.

If the child has a vision or hearing impairment, safety measures take on even greater importance. Assist the parents with measures to adapt the child's environment to meet his needs while promoting growth and development and independence as much as possible. Supplement verbal explanations with tactile and visual aids as appropriate and allow the child to use drawings, writing, or gestures to respond and communicate. Encourage the use of specialized devices such as a talking picture board if the child is hearing impaired with limited speech. Provide ample time for interaction and incorporate the use of therapeutic play (see Managing and Delegating Unlicensed Assistive Personnel). Children with vision or hearing impairments need to attend regular classrooms in school, if possible, so that they have contact with seeing and hearing children (Giangreco et al, 1998). School nurses need to advocate for such placements.

VISION

Vision occurs because light rays reflect from an object through the corneas, aqueous humors, lenses, and vitre-

TABLE 29.1 Health Promotion Guidelines

AGE	VISION ASSESSMENT PARAMETERS	HEARING ASSESSMENT PARAMETERS
Infant	Ability to follow objects Corneal reflex Ability to turn to light stimuli	Startle reflex (at birth) Ability to track sounds (3 to 6 months) Ability to recognize sounds (6 to 8 months) Ability to locate sounds (8 to 12 months)
Toddler	Corneal light reflex Cover test Smooth ocular movements Hand–eye coordination	Ability to react to soft sounds (whispers) Ability to track source of sounds Ability to form a noun–verb sentence by 2 years Ability to follow simple directions
Preschooler	Corneal light reflex Cover test Snellen E chart (or modification)	Awareness of pitch and tone Pure tone audiometry (starting at age 4 years) Understandable language with increasing vocabulary
School age	Visual acuity testing every 1 to 2 years	Pure tone audiometry at ages 6, 8, and 11 years
Adolescent	Visual acuity testing every 1 to 2 years	Pure tone audiometry at ages 14 and 18 years

Children with either vision or hearing impairment need special preparation and orientation for a hospital or ambulatory health visit so they can fully understand what is going to happen during the visit.

Help children with vision impairment work through new experiences by letting them feel equipment as much as possible. Guide their hands through the steps of a new procedure you are teaching them.

Otitis media (middle ear infection) is a common childhood illness. Children need therapy with antibiotics to correct this. With serous otitis media, some children have myringotomy tubes placed to relieve pressure and supply air access to the middle ear.

Use photos, drawings, or demonstration with hearing-impaired children to help them learn new skills. Contact a signing interpreter as appropriate to be certain that children understand instructions.

CRITICAL THINKING EXERCISES

1. Carla is the 4-year-old with an ear infection you met at the beginning of the chapter. What information would be important to ascertain from her mother about the Carla's previous ear infection? How would you counsel this parent about preventing future episodes?
2. A 4-year-old boy is going to have eye surgery. What special steps do you want to take to prepare him for this surgery? Is he old enough to appreciate the importance of seeing?
3. A 14-year-old who is profoundly hearing-impaired from developing meningitis as a preschooler uses sign language to communicate. How could you communicate effectively with him while he's hospitalized? What are his rights as a patient in regard to having an interpreter provided for him?
4. You are going to teach a first-grade class on ways to prevent eye and hearing injuries. What would you include in your class? How would your teaching plan be different if the class was for 16-year-olds?

REFERENCES

Bachmann, K. R., & Arvedson, J. C. (1998). Early Identification and intervention for children who are hearing impaired. *Pediatrics in Review, 19*(5), 155.

Bance, M. L. et al. (1998). Vestibular stimulation by multichannel cochlear implants. *Laryngoscope, 108*(2), 291.

Behl, D. D., Akers, J. F., Boyce, G. C., & Taylor, M. J. (1996). Do mothers interact differently with children who are visually impaired? *Journal of Visual Impairment and Blindness, 90*(6), 501.

Carpenito, L. J. (1997). *Nursing diagnosis: application to clinical practice* (7th ed.). Philadelphia: Lippincott.

Department of Health and Human Services. (1995). *Healthy people 2000: midcourse review.* Washington, DC: DHHS.

Giangreco, M. F. et al. (1998). Impact of planning for support services on students who are deaf-blind. *Journal of Visual Impairment and Blindness, 92*(1), 18.

Kline, M. W. (1997a). Otitis externa. In Johnson, K. B. & Oski, F. A. *Oski's essential pediatrics.* Philadelphia: Lippincott-Raven.

Kline, M. W. (1997b). Otitis media. In Johnson, K. B. & Oski, F. A. *Oski's essential pediatrics.* Philadelphia: Lippincott-Raven.

Leguire, L. E. et al. (1995). Levodopa/carbidopa treatment for amblyopia in older children. *Journal of Pediatric Ophthalmology and Strabismus, 32*(3), 143.

Lennerstrand, G., et al. (1998). Treatment of strabismus and nystagmus with botulinum toxin type A: an evaluation of effects and complications. *Acta Ophthalmologica Scandinavica, 76*(1), 27.

Litt, M. et al. (1998). Autosomal dominant congenital cataract associated with a missense mutation in the human alpha cystalllin gene CRYAA. *Human Molecular Genetics, 7*(3), 471.

Mandal, A. K. et al. (1998). Surgical results of combined trabeculotomy-trabeculectomy for developmental glaucoma. *Ophthalmology, 105*(6), 974.

Morrow, G. L., & Abbott, R. L. (1998). Conjunctivitis. *American Family Physician, 57*(4), 735.

Pulido, J. S. et al. (1997). Perforating BB gun injuries of the globe. *Ophthalmic Surgery and Lasers, 28*(8), 625.

Strachan, D. P., & Cook, D. G. (1998). Health effects of passive smoking: parental smoking, middle ear disease and adenotonsillectomy in children. *Thorax, 53*(1), 50.

Traboulsi, E. I., & Maumenee, I. H. (1997). Eye problems. In Johnson, K. B. & Oski, F. A. *Oski's essential pediatrics.* Philadelphia: Lippincott-Raven.

SUGGESTED READINGS

Brown, S. & Story, I. (1998). A new approach to visual acuity screening for pre-school children. *Ophthalmic Epidemiology, 5*(1), 21.

Daly, K. A. et al. (1997). Knowledge and attitudes about otitis media risk: implications for prevention. *Pediatrics, 100*(6), 931.

Daw, N. W. (1998). Critical periods and amblyopia. *Archives of Ophthalmology, 116*(4), 502.

Dote-Kwan, J. et al. (1997). Impact of early experiences on the development of young children with visual impairments revisited. *Journal of Visual Impairment and Blindness, 91*(2), 131.

Gonococcal conjunctivitis outbreak. (1998). *Communicable Diseases Intelligence, 22*(3), 39.

Tully, S. B. (1998). The right angle: otitis media and infant feeding position. *Advance for Nurse Practitioners. 6*(4), 44.

Weber, C. M., & Eichenbaum, J. W. (1997). Acute red eye: differentiating viral conjunctivitis from other, less common causes. *Postgraduate Medicine, 101*(55), 185.

Weinstock, V. M. et al. (1998). Screening for childhood strabismus by primary care physicians. *Canadian Family Physician, 44*(2), 337.

Wheeler, L., & Griffin, H. C. (1997). A movement-based approach to language development in children who are deaf-blind. *American Annals of the Deaf, 142*(5), 387.

Yetman, R. J., & Coody, D. K. (1997). Conjunctivitis: a practice guideline. *Journal of Pediatric Health Care, 11*(5), 238.

Nursing Care of the Child With a Musculoskeletal Disorder

30

CHAPTER

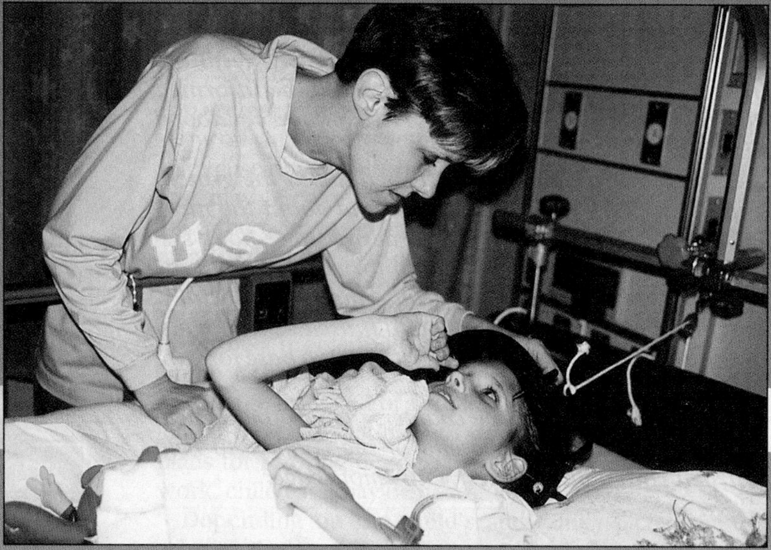

Key Terms

- apposition
- arthroscopy
- cartilage
- diaphysis
- epiphyseal plate
- epiphysis
- fracture
- long bones
- malleoli
- metaphysis
- myopathy
- periosteum
- petaling
- remodeling
- resorption
- sequestrum
- smooth muscle
- striated muscle
- traction

Objectives

After mastering the contents of this chapter, you should be able to:

1. Describe common musculoskeletal disorders in children.
2. Assess the child with a musculoskeletal disorder.
3. Formulate nursing diagnoses related to the child with a musculoskeletal disorder.
4. Establish appropriate outcomes for the child with a musculoskeletal disorder.
5. Plan nursing care, such as age-appropriate diversional activities, for the child with a musculoskeletal disorder.
6. Implement nursing care for the child with a musculoskeletal disorder.
7. Evaluate outcomes for achievement and effectiveness of care.
8. Identify National Health Goals related to musculoskeletal disorders and children that nurses can be instrumental in helping the nation to achieve.
9. Identify areas related to care of the child with a musculoskeletal disorder that could benefit from additional nursing research.
10. Use critical thinking to analyze ways that care of the child immobilized by a cast or traction can be more family centered.
11. Integrate knowledge of musculoskeletal disorders with nursing process to achieve quality child health nursing care.

Outcome Evaluation

Children with musculoskeletal disorders invariably need follow-up care after discharge from an ambulatory visit or inpatient care, because bone healing is a slow process. Parents may ask to have x-rays taken frequently to evaluate healing progress. They may need to be reminded that x-rays are never taken on children unless there is a documented need for them (excessive radiation is possibly associated with the development of leukemia in children).

Both parents and children may need support at reevaluation visits when learning that a cast or brace must stay on longer or that they must continue exercises. Praise for their management thus far is an effective intervention for helping parents realize that they can cope with the situation in the future.

During reevaluation visits, spend time assessing the child's body image and self-esteem. Does the child view himself or herself as a well person with, for example, a right leg shorter than the left leg, or as a deformed person who is inferior to others? Success of treatment is incomplete if a child's self-concept is impacted.

Some examples of outcomes may include the following:

- Child states he or she feels no pain or numbness in extremity.
- Child demonstrates allowable weight-bearing activities with casted lower extremity.
- Parents accurately state child's care needs to be met both in and out of the hospital.
- Child states positive aspects of self; participates in activities; establishes friendships with peers.

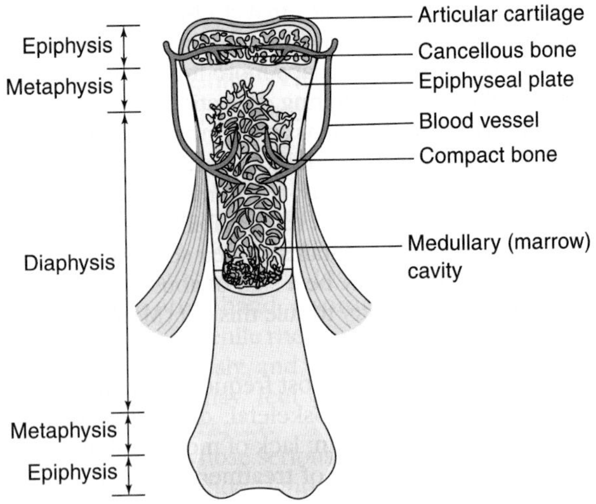

FIGURE 30.1 Structure of a bone.

THE MUSCULOSKELETAL SYSTEM

Bones and Bone Growth

Bones are generally classified by their shape as long, short, flat, or irregular. **Long bones** are the bones of the extremities, including the fingers and toes, in which most childhood bone disorders are found. The short bones are the bones found in the ankle and wrist. Flat bones are found in the skull, ribs, scapula, and clavicle. Irregular bones are found in the vertebrae, the pelvis, and the facial bones of the skull.

Long bones are composed of a long central shaft (the **diaphysis**), a rounded end portion (the **epiphysis**), and a thin area between them (the **metaphysis**) (Figure 30-1). Increase in the length of long bones occurs at the cartilage segment (the **epiphyseal plate**). As **cartilage** (connective tissue) cells grow away from the shaft, they are replaced by bone, thereby increasing bone length. Injury to this area in a growing child is always potentially serious, because it may halt growth, stimulate abnormal growth, or cause irregular or erratic growth. The central shafts of long bones are covered by an outer sensitive layer of **periosteum**. Bone width increases by growth at the inner surface of the periosteum. Injury to the periosteum, such as may occur with osteomyelitis, can also threaten bone growth.

Although it is easy to think of bones as rigid, solid structures, they are, in fact, living tissue, for which nutrients for growth must be supplied. Calcium, one of the main components of bone, is an important element for bone formation, **remodeling** (new bone tissue replacing old bone tissue), and **resorption** (bone breakdown). These processes are influenced by parathyroid hormone, calcitonin, vitamin D, other minerals, nutrients, and enzymes. "Bone age" can be determined by an x-ray of the wrists that shows the ossification level of bones. The inner core of long bones is filled whereas yellow and red marrow, which is responsible for red blood cell, white blood cell, and adipose cell formation. Red marrow is primarily involved with red blood cell production, while yellow marrow is chiefly involved with adipose cell formation. The blood supply to bones is abundant so that the marrow can actively supply enough red blood cells for the body. As with other tissues, if the blood supply is cut off, bone cells die.

The bones of children tend to be more resilient than the bones of adults. This means that accidents that might result in severe breaks to adult bones are apt to result in lesser breaks or only torsional twists in children. Bones tend to heal more quickly in children than in adults; therefore, children usually are incapacitated for a shorter time following an injury.

Muscle

The skeletal muscular system is composed of one type of muscle, called **striated muscle,** which is the predominant muscle in the body (differentiated from **smooth muscle**, which is responsible for, among other things, gastrointestinal peristalsis). Activation of skeletal muscle occurs with innervation from a motor nerve and is under voluntary control. **Myopathy**, or disease of the muscular system, can be inherited (as in muscular dystrophy) or acquired (as in myasthenia gravis).

ASSESSMENT OF MUSCULOSKELETAL FUNCTION

In addition to the history and physical examination, diagnostic tests frequently are ordered for children with musculoskeletal dysfunction. These may include x-rays and bone scans, bone and muscle biopsy, electromyography, and arthroscopy. Ultrasound and magnetic resonance studies may reveal soft-tissue disease.

X-ray

Because bones are opaque, they outline well on x-ray. Bone x-rays provide information about a specific bone, groups of bones, or a joint. They can also provide information abut soft-tissue structure, swelling, or calcification. However, other tests are indicated to confirm problems with cartilage, tendons, and ligaments.

Bone Scan

A bone scan is a study of the uptake of intravenously injected radioactive substances by the bone. The distribution and concentration of the substance are evaluated to determine the problem. For example, areas of increased metabolic activity will cause the substance to concentrate in that area. A bone scan provides information of very early bone disease and healing, often before it is visible in x-rays.

Electromyography

Electromyography studies the electrical activity of skeletal muscle and nerve conduction. It can determine the location and cause of several disorders, such as myasthenia gravis and muscular dystrophy and lower motor neuron and peripheral nerve disorders.

For the test, needle electrodes are inserted into muscle masses; the electrical activity of the muscle at rest and in motion is detected by audioamplification and recorded on an oscilloscope. Normally, resting muscle is quiet. If defects, such as fasciculations, are present, abnormal noises or oscilloscope spikes will be observed.

Although the needle electrodes are small, the test may be frightening for children because they are pricked by needles. They need support from someone they know during the procedure. Before and after the procedrue, provide opportunities for therapeutic play so that they can express their anxiety and feelings.

Muscle or Bone Biopsy

A muscle or bone biopsy involves removal of a tissue sample for examination of its microscopic structure. It can provide evidence about infection, malignant bone growth, inflammation, or atrophy of the area. Either type may be done during surgery or as an ambulatory procedure.

Muscle biopsy is generally done under a local anesthetic, but if children cannot cooperate, it may be done under a general anesthetic. Caution children that they will feel the initial prick of an anesthetizing needle; as the actual biopsy needle enters the muscle mass, they will feel an additional momentary pain. They can be assured that the amount of tissue taken from them is no larger than the inner bore of the biopsy needle or the lead in a pencil.

Arthroscopy

Arthroscopy involves direct visualization of a joint with a fiberoptic instrument. It is usually done under local anesthesia in an ambulatory care setting. Arthroscopy allows a joint, most commonly the knee, but also the hip, shoulder, elbow, or wrist, to be examined without a large incision. It is most commonly used to diagnose athletic injuries and to differentiate between acute and chronic joint disorders.

HEALTH PROMOTION AND RISK MANAGEMENT

Health promotion focuses on thorough assessment at all health maintenance visits. The child's ability to achieve developmental milestones, specifically gross and fine motor abilities, provides important information about his or her musculoskeletal function. In addition, the ability to get around directly influences a child's exploration of the environment and exposure to stimuli. If this is impaired, it also can interfere with his or her growth and development. Screening, such as for scoliosis in the prepubescent child and adolescent, is also an important health promotion measure.

Safety is paramount for any child to prevent injury. Anticipatory guidance for parents is essential to minimize the risk of injury, specifically to the extremities, in all aspects of every day life. As the child grows and becomes active in sports, parental and child education takes on an even greater role.

Nutrition education is important to ensure adequate calcium intake necessary for bone growth and healing. However, if the child requires bedrest, calcium intake should be moderated to reduce the risk of renal calculi.

If the child experiences a musculoskeletal disorder, education helps to prevent complications, maximize the child's ability to function, and minimize the risk of residual impaired physical mobility. Parents and children need instruction about all aspects of treatment and follow-up, for example, caring for the child requiring a cast, traction, brace, or drug therapy, such as antibiotics for osteomyelitis or nonsteroidal anti-inflammatory drugs (NSAIDs) for JRA. Teaching provides a basis for enhancing compliance, maximizing the effectiveness of treatment, and minimizing the possible long-term risk for problems.

✓ **CHECKPOINT QUESTIONS**

1. At what part of the long bone does an increase in bone length occur?
2. What diagnostic test involves inserting needle electrodes into the child's muscles?

THERAPEUTIC MANAGEMENT OF MUSCULOSKELETAL DISORDERS IN CHILDREN

Various methods may be used as therapy for a child with a musculoskeletal disorder. These may include casts, traction, distraction, and open reduction. Amputation is discussed in Chapter 32.

Casting

Casts may be used in the treatment of a variety of musculoskeletal system disorders—from simple fractures in the extremities to correction of congenital structural bone disorders (see Chapter 18 for a discussion of the latter).

Cast Application

Casts are created from either plaster of paris or synthetic material, such as fiberglass. Fiberglass is an attractive material to use for children's casts because it is light, comes in colors, and is water resistant. A special waterproof liner can be used, allowing the cast to be immersed in water. Unfortunately, it is more expensive and may not be practical for casts that need frequent changing.

Children need an explanation of what to expect with casting. To maintain alignment of body parts, a physician gently exerts a pull on the body part (manual traction) being casted during cast application. If a large body cast is being applied, children may be positioned on a special cast table with traction apparatus at the chin and pelvis. These tables are stark, steel tables and may resemble torture racks children have seen in horror movies. Allow someone to accompany them to the cast room to hold their hand or talk to them during the application. Most children (and adults) are unaware that traditional casts are formed from strips of gauze impregnated with the casting material. The normal curiosity of children as they watch a cast grow and mold to their body part makes casting a pleasant procedure. Some children look forward to having a cast put in place. It may be a badge of courage, a conversation piece, or an "autograph book."

Before the cast is applied, a tube of stockinette is stretched over the area, and a soft cotton sheet is placed over bony prominences. This stockinette is pulled up and over the raw edges of the cast as it is applied to form a smooth, padded surface (Figure 30-2). Caution children that when wet strips of plaster of paris are first applied, they feel cool. Almost immediately, the strips begin to generate heat as evaporation begins, and body parts feel warm. If the cast is a full-body cast, children may become uncomfortably warm with perspiration possibly running from their forehead. Assure them that this feeling of warmth is transient and is never enough to cause a burn.

A plaster cast takes from 10 to 72 hours to dry depending on its size. Fiberglass casts usually dry within 5 to 30 minutes. When moving a child in a wet cast, always use open palms to move the cast. Fingers indent the cast and may cause pressure points that could result in pressure ulcers under the cast. Support the cast on soft pillows also to avoid indenting the cast. Avoid covering a cast with clothing or bedclothes so that it dries as rapidly as possible (Figure 30-3). If a plaster cast has been applied, turn children about every 2 hours to allow the underside of the cast to dry. The use of heaters or fans to dry the cast is not advised because they can cause uneven drying and heat can cause a burn under the cast.

A window may be placed in a cast if an infection is suspected. It also may be used with an open fracture to permit observation and care of the wound site. If the child has a body or hip spica cast, windowing may prevent uncomfortable abdominal distention.

NURSING DIAGNOSES AND RELATED INTERVENTIONS

Nursing Diagnosis: Risk for altered peripheral tissue perfusion related to pressure from cast

Outcome Identification: Child will exhibit signs and symptoms of adequate tissue perfusion during the time the cast is in place.

Outcome Evaluation: Child states he or she feels no pain or numbness in extremity; distal nail bed blanches

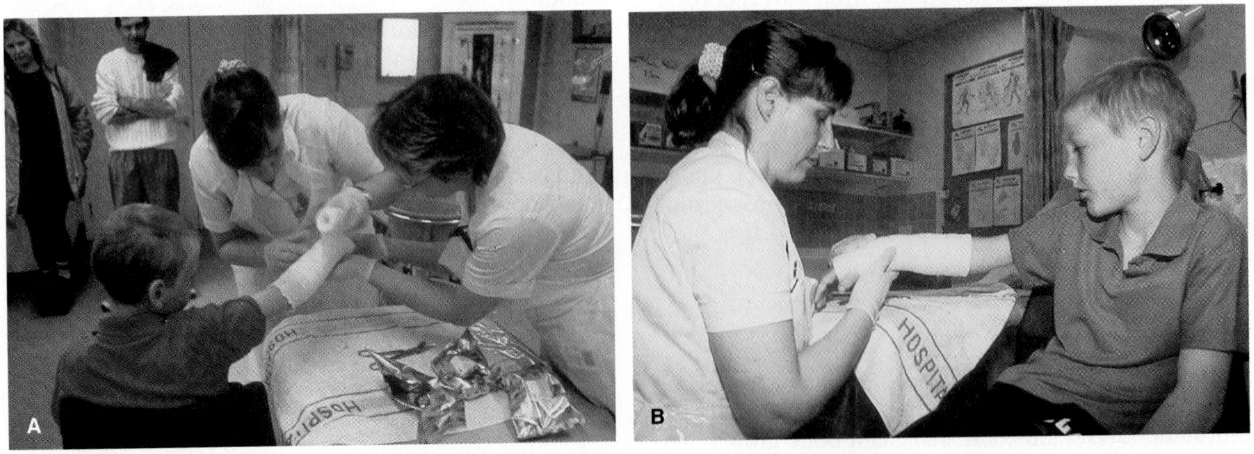

FIGURE 30.2 Cast application. (**A**) A fiberglass cast is applied to a young boy's arm over a stockinette already in place. (**B**) While applying the finishing touches to the young boy's cast, the nurse assesses the extremity.

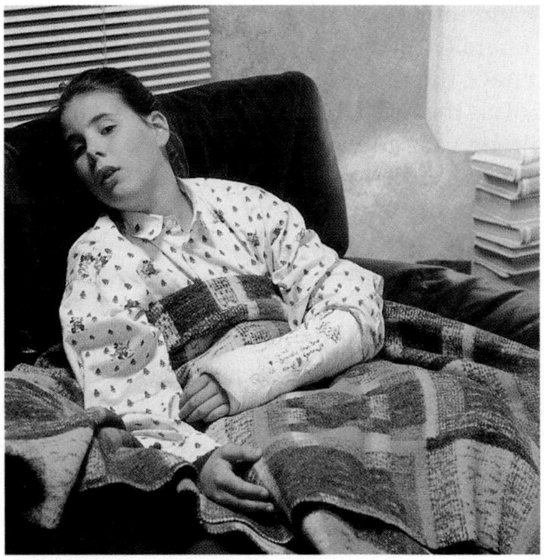

FIGURE 30.3 A young girl with her left arm in a plaster cast lies quietly on the sofa.

and refills in less than 5 seconds; pedal pulses are palpable; area surrounding cast is warm and pink.

If an extremity has been casted, keep it elevated to prevent edema in the part. Check circulation frequently, such as every 15 minutes during the first hour, hourly for the first 24 hours, and then every 4 hours thereafter. Assess for color, warmth, presence of pedal pulses, and sensations of numbness or tingling. Signs of impaired neurovascular function include pallor (including blueness or coldness of a distal part), pulselessness, pain in the casted part, or paresthesia, such as numbness or tingling in the part as if it were "asleep." (Children younger than 6 or 7 years have difficulty describing this feeling; however, they may whine or cry with the discomfort of the sensation.) Edema that does not improve with elevation is also an important sign. Any of these symptoms requires immediate attention, because neurovascular impairment can lead to nerve ischemia and destruction, possibly causing permanent paralysis of an extremity.

Nursing Diagnosis: Risk for impaired tissue integrity related to pressure from cast

Outcome Identification: Child's skin will remain intact during time cast is in place.

Outcome Evaluation: Child reports no pain under cast; cast remains dry and free of stains; skin surrounding cast edges is clean, dry, and free of erythema or irritation.

When a cast is dry, edges that are not smooth or covered by a fold of stockinet must be smoothed by applying adhesive tape strips to prevent skin irritation. This is termed **petaling** (Figure 30-4). If a cast surrounds the genital area, cover the cast with plastic to prevent urine from impregnating it, or cover the edges of the cast surrounding the genital area with plastic or waterproof material. Placing an infant on a Bradford frame while the cast is in place may help urine and feces to drain away from the cast. Pin diapers so that they do not cover areas of the cast not protected by the plastic covering; otherwise, a soaked diaper will wet the cast. Instead, fold the diaper so that it fits a smaller area. In some children, a sanitary pad absorbs urine well and keeps the cast dry. Plastic pants should not be used over a cast because they tend to hold the moisture and urine, preventing drying. Using a urine collecting device often is ineffective, because the tape required to keep it in place for a long time may cause skin irritation.

Keeping children in a semi-Fowler's position by using pillows or raising the head of the bed helps to direct urine and feces downward and prevents soaking of the back of a body cast. Because a cast is heavy, an infant tends to slip down a great deal, so he or she needs frequent repositioning to remain in the raised position.

Prevention is of the utmost importance. Once urine has penetrated a cast, there is no way to remove it. A urine-soaked cast becomes very malodorous. Not only is the odor unappealing, but it may mask the odor of a pressure sore under the cast. Heavy soaking tends to weaken the cast, causing loss of support.

Make certain that when children are being fed or are feeding themselves, they have a bib or a cover over the top edge of a cast so that crumbs and fluid are not spilled inside. Toys should be chosen carefully for the same reason. A piece of food inside a cast will mold and macerate the skin; a small part of a toy dropped inside a cast can cause irritation and a pressure ulcer.

If a child spills food on a cast or the cast becomes soiled, it can be cleaned with a damp cloth. Scouring powder without a chlorine base (such as Bon Ami) may be used. Using chlorine-based scouring powder causes the plaster to deteriorate and weaken.

Nursing Diagnosis: Parental health-seeking behaviors related to care of child with cast at home.

Outcome Identification: Parents will demonstrate ability to care for child following cast application.

Outcome Evaluation: Parents state plans for adapting home environment and lifestyle to accommodate

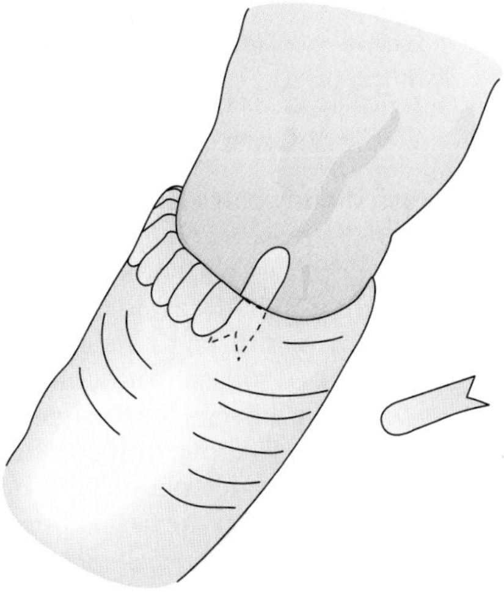

FIGURE 30.4 Technique for petaling a cast with adhesive tape. This smooths the rough edges and prevents irritation of the child's skin.

child with cast; parents demonstrate measures to check neurovascular status.

If the child has an upper extremity cast, be sure parents understand how to position the extremity properly, such as with a sling. If the cast is on a lower extremity, instruct the child and parents in the amount of weight bearing allowed to the affected extremity and in the use of crutches, if prescribed.

Handling a child in a large cast is a major task for parents. For many, it may seem so overwhelming that they do not see how they will be able to care for the child at home. Assure them that the child is quite comfortable in the cast, despite its awkward, constricting appearance. Allow them to observe you moving the child and positioning him or her before they attempt these maneuvers themselves. Be sure to caution them that if an abduction bar is used with a cast, it must never be used as a handle for lifting the cast. Such use can break the bar from the cast or weaken its support.

A body cast is heavy, so caution parents to use good body mechanics (lift with the thighs, not the back) when turning or positioning the child. Be sure to act as a role model for this. Be certain that parents have had adequate handling and positioning practice before a child goes home so that they can care for a child confidently. If a cast is bulky, parents often appreciate suggestions on ways to help move the child from room to room, such as using a toy wagon with a flat board on top or using a skateboard for the child to propel himself or herself. It is important to point out that all children thrive on being touched. Children in a large body cast need their head and arms stroked (or any areas of the body that are not covered by a cast). Demonstrate how even a child in a large hip spica cast can be held, cuddled, and supported for feeding. Otherwise, parents may tend to neglect this aspect of care.

Many children complain of itching inside a cast at about the end of the first week. If the area is immediately under the edge of the cast, the itching is probably the result of dry skin caused by the drying effect of the plaster. Reaching a hand under the edge of the cast and massaging the area generally relieves the itching. Applying hand lotion may relieve the dryness. If the area is unreachable, blowing cool air through the cast with a fan, a hair dryer set on cool air, or a vacuum cleaner attachment may relieve the uncomfortable feeling. Caution the child and parents not to use implements such as a coat hanger or knitting needle to scratch the area. These can injure the skin, causing infection under a cast (see Empowering the Family: Cast Care at Home).

Transporting the child in the car, particularly fitting a bulky cast into an infant car seat, can be a major problem. Before a child is discharged, give parents a telephone number to call if they have any questions about their child's care or condition.

Cast Removal

Most casts remain in place for 4 to 8 weeks and are then removed, using an electric cast cutter with a rapidly vibrating, circular disk (Figure 30-5). The disk makes a very loud noise as it cuts through the cast material and also generates heat. To the child, the disk appears capable of cutting through not only the plaster but an arm or leg as well. The person removing the cast generally demonstrates that the disk does not cut skin by touching a thumb to the edge of it. Not all children are totally convinced by the demonstration, however, and may require additional support while the disk moves from one end of a cast to the other, such as saying, "It's all right to cry; I know this looks scary" or by holding your hands over the child's ears to lessen the noise.

The skin of the child's extremity looks macerated and dirty after the cast is removed; a good bath usually washes away most of this. If an arm has been casted in flexion, the elbow may feel stiff and even sore as the child is asked to extend it for the first time. Children often use extremities with caution after a cast has been removed. Therefore, advise parents to allow the child to begin using the extremity again at his or her own pace. As children naturally play

EMPOWERING THE FAMILY: Cast Care at Home

- Keep the casted body part elevated on a pillow for the first day to decrease swelling.
- Avoid touching the cast with other than your palm (no fingers) until it is dry to avoid denting it.
- Observe the body part distal to the cast for swelling or blueness, and ask your child to move the part about every 4 hours for the first 24 hours; if he or she is unable to move or if swelling, blueness, or pain is present, telephone your health care provider (this could mean the cast is pressing on a nerve or constricting a blood vessel).
- Monitor strenuous activities, such as roughhousing, while the cast is in place; urge usual activities so your child remains active.
- Ask your child to think through how wearing a cast will change his or her day, such as making it difficult to eat in a cafeteria at school or carry books to classes, and brainstorm how to solve these problems.
- Be certain your child knows not to put anything inside the cast. If itching occurs inside the cast, blowing some cool air into it from a hair dryer can be comforting.
- Be certain your child keeps the cast dry (cover with a plastic bag to shower); no swimming is allowed.
- Be certain to keep your return appointment for follow-up care. Because children grow so rapidly, they can outgrow a cast rapidly. This could put pressure on nerves and lead to permanent disability.

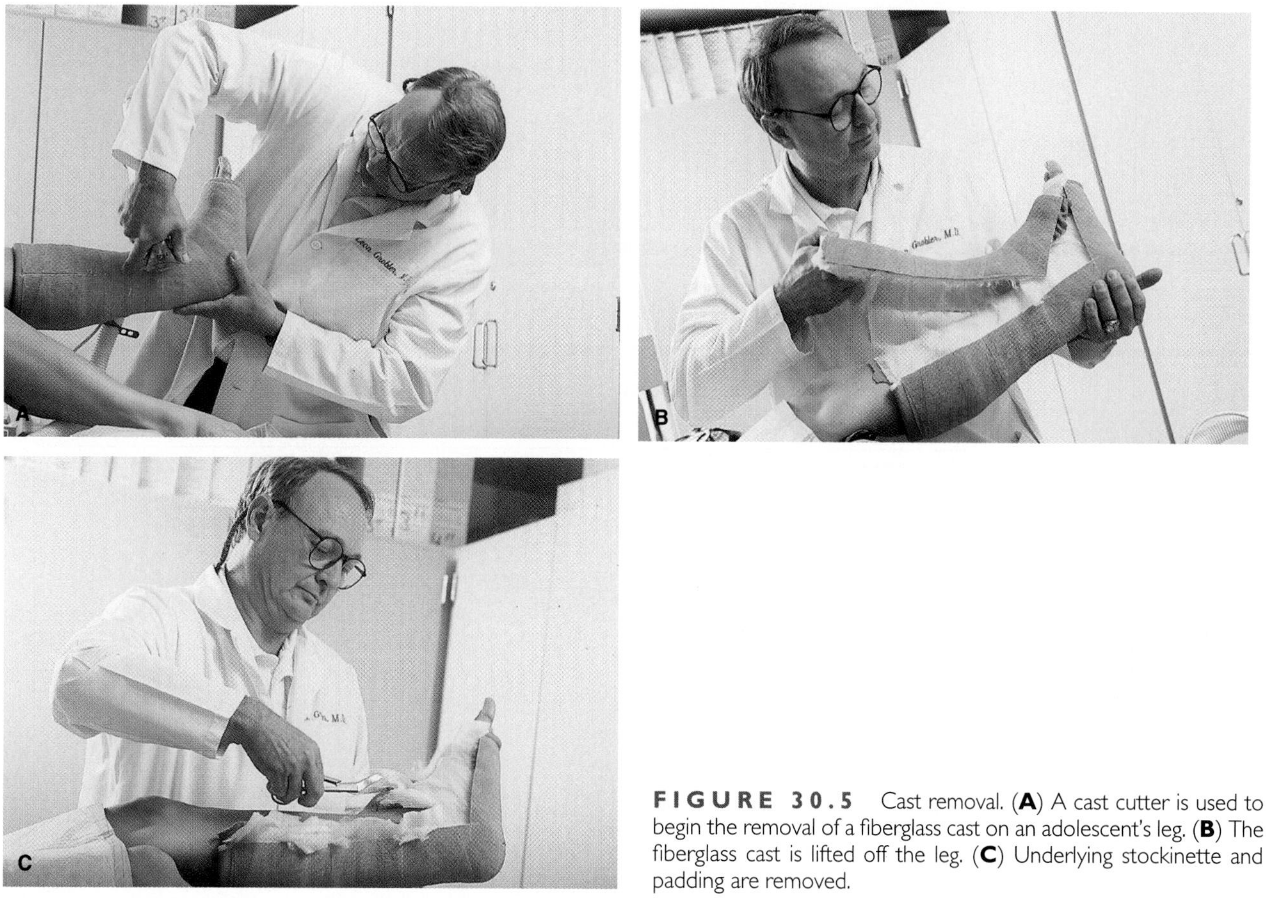

FIGURE 30.5 Cast removal. (**A**) A cast cutter is used to begin the removal of a fiberglass cast on an adolescent's leg. (**B**) The fiberglass cast is lifted off the leg. (**C**) Underlying stockinette and padding are removed.

and reach for objects, they gradually forget to favor the arm or leg, and full function then returns. Once healing has taken place, the extremity is as strong as it was before the fracture. The child does not need to continue to favor the extremity to protect it from a second fracture.

Crutches

Crutches are prescribed for children for one of three reasons: to keep weight off one or both legs, to support weakened legs, or to maintain balance. Usually, a physical therapist measures crutch length and gives beginning instruction in crutch walking. Be familiar with measuring and supervising crutch walking to offer emotional support to children as they learn and to assess progress at follow-up visits.

Fit and Adjustment

If crutches are properly fitted, there should be a space of 1 to 1½ in between the axilla crutch pad and the child's axilla. When the child stands upright and places his hands on the handrests of the crutches, the elbows should flex about 20 degrees. This degree of flexion ensures that when the child bears weight on the crutch, the body weight will be borne by the arm, not the axilla. Pressure of a crutch against the axilla could lead to compression and damage of the brachial nerve plexus crossing the axilla, resulting in permanent nerve palsy. Teach children not to rest with the crutch pad pressing on the axilla but always to support their weight at the hand grip.

Always assess the tips of crutches to see that the rubber tip is intact and not worn through. The tip prevents the crutch from slipping when it is in place. Be certain that the child is walking with the crutches placed about 6 in to the side of foot. This distance furnishes a wide, balanced base for support.

Explore with children any problems crutches may cause with their daily activities. If they carry books to school, for example, they may prefer to wear a backpack until they are free of crutches so they can leave their hands free for the handrests. Caution parents to clear articles, such as throw rugs and small footstools, out of the paths at home. If there are small children at home, the parents will need to keep the traffic areas free of toys to prevent an accident.

Crutch Walking

Two main crutch-walking patterns are used (Figure 30-6). A two-point gait is used when a child needs support for weakened muscles or balance but may bear weight on both lower extremities. The child places the right crutch and left foot forward, then left crutch and right foot forward, and so on. Using the crutch opposite a foot provides a wider base of support than using the crutch next to the foot. Caution children to take small steps until they feel confident.

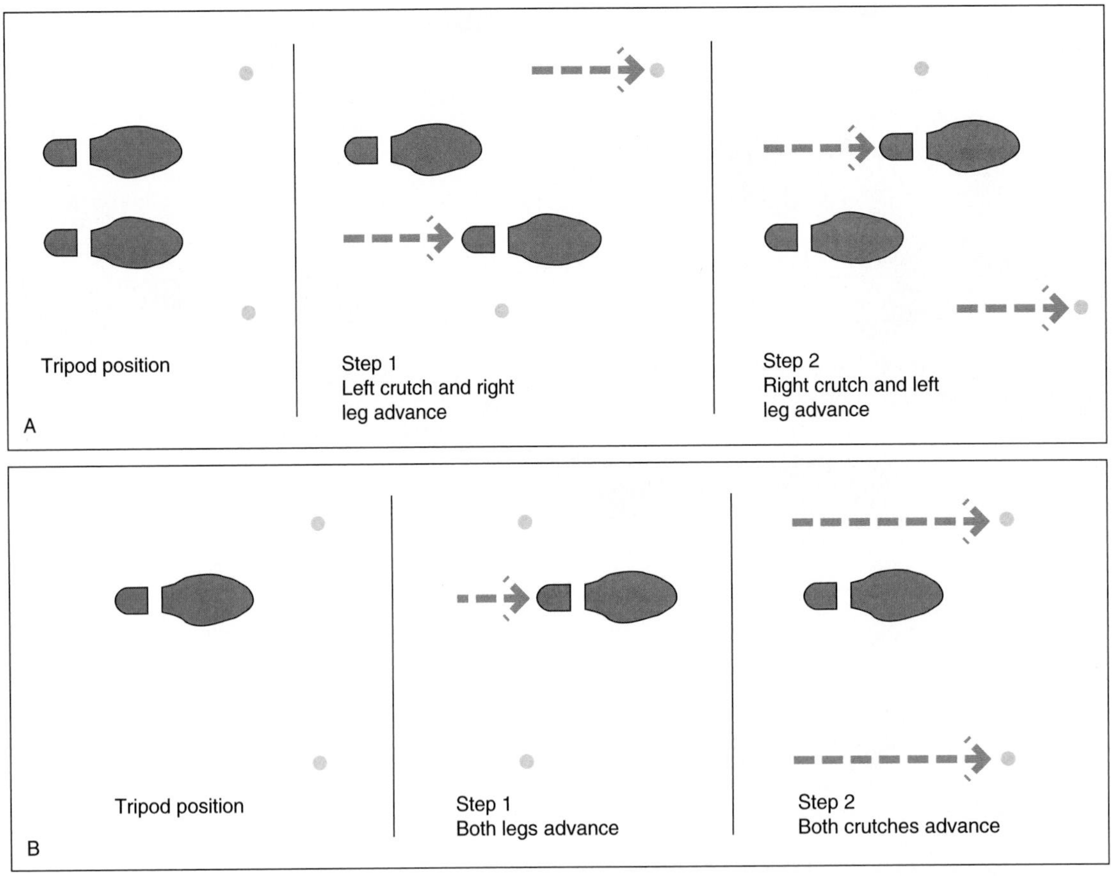

FIGURE 30.6 Crutch-walking patterns. (**A**) Two-point gait. (**B**) Swing-through gait.

A three-point swing-through gait is used when no weight bearing is allowed on one foot. For this, the crutches are both brought forward. The weight of the body is shifted forward as both legs are swung through the crutches. The child bears weight on the unaffected (good) leg and moves the crutches forward again. It takes strong arm support to bear full weight on crutches this way. Be certain the child is bearing weight on the hands and not the axillae when swinging through. Some children use a swing-through gait rather recklessly and need to be advised to slow their pace to a safer one.

To walk downstairs using a swing-through gait, children place the crutches on the lower step, then swing the unaffected (good) foot forward and down to that step. To go upstairs, they place their unaffected (good) foot on the elevated step, then raise the crutches onto the step and lift themselves up. To help children remember this pattern, a saying—"angels" (the good foot) go up; "devils" (the bad foot with the crutches) go down—is traditionally used.

A third type of crutch walking, the four-point gait, may be used. However, this method requires the ability to move both legs separately and bear weight on each leg.

Traction

Traction, used to reduce dislocations and immobilize fractures, involves pulling on a body part in one direction against a counterpull exerted in the opposite direction. Although still necessary for some conditions, its use is declining. In straight (running) traction, a child's body weight serves as the counterpull. In suspended or balanced traction, the body part is suspended by a sling, and the counterpull and primary pull are accomplished by pulleys and weights. Skin traction (in which skin provides the counterpull) or skeletal traction (in which bone provides the counterpull) may be used. Skin traction is used when only minimal traction is necessary; the child's skin must be in good condition for this procedure. Skeletal traction is used when a longer period of traction or greater strength of traction pull is needed. Types of traction are illustrated in Figure 30-7. Use of traction in the home allows the child to interact with family members and should be encouraged (Draper & Scott, 1998).

Skin Traction

Bryant's traction, used for fractured femurs in younger children (younger than 2 years), is an example of skin traction (Figure 30-8). It also may be used in preparation for surgical repair of congenital developmental defects, such as developmental hip dysplasia (see Chapter 18). This type of traction is being used less frequently because the elevation of the extremities causes blood to pool at the hips. This and the possible tourniquet effect of the traction strips, bandages, and traction itself increase the risk for possible vasospasm and avascular necrosis.

Buck's extension is an example of skin traction used for immobilizing lower extremity fractures in older children.

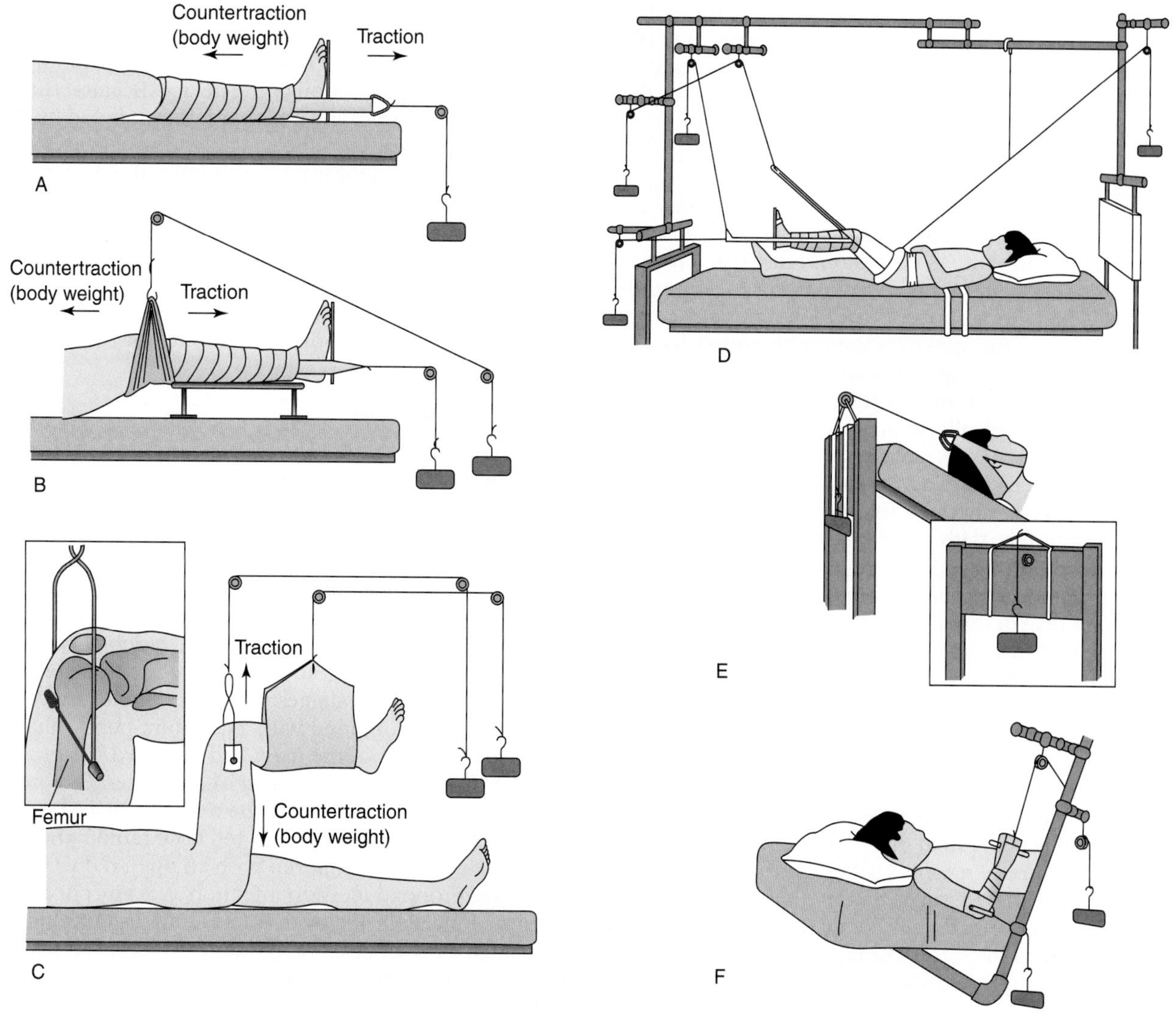

FIGURE 30.7 Types of traction. (**A**) Buck's extension. (**B**) Russell. (**C**) 90-degree. (**D**) Balanced suspension. (**E**) Cervical skin traction. (**F**) Dunlop's traction (skeletal).

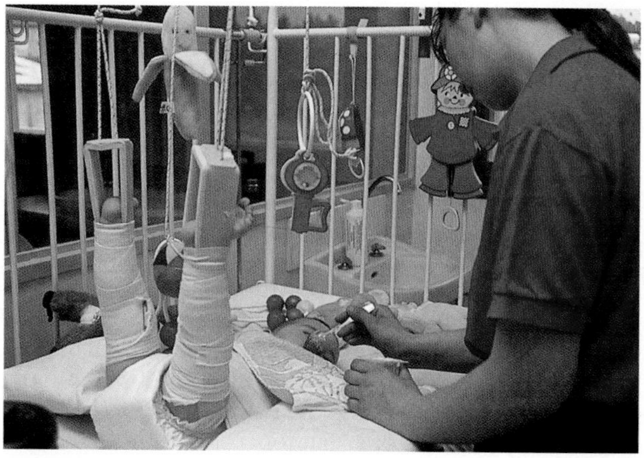

FIGURE 30.8 An infant in Bryant's traction. Here, the father feeds the infant while the infant is maintained in traction.

Dunlop's traction is used to immobilize the upper extremity. (This can be skin traction or skeletal traction if a wire or pin is used to immobilize.) Cervical skin traction may be used to decrease muscle spasms in the back. This type of traction uses a halter-type device attached to weights (McCarthy, 1998). With this type of traction, the head of the bed is elevated to provide some countertraction.

Skeletal Traction

Skeletal traction involves the use of a pin, such as a Steinmann pin, or wire, such as a Kirschner wire, passed through the skin into the end of a long bone. The pin or wire can be inserted in an emergency department under local anesthesia if the child can hold absolutely still, but usually it is done under general anesthesia in the operating room. With skeletal traction, ropes strung over pulleys and attached to weights exert a pull on the extremity at the pin site. Cotton gauze squares usually are placed around the ends of the pin on the outside. Be sure to observe the pin sites daily for drainage. Odorous or excessive drainage or erythema may be a sign of infection at the pin site. (See the Nursing Care Plan: The Child in Skeletal Traction.)

Traction-Related Care

Children in traction need to be assessed carefully for neurovascular impairment, as do children in casts. The extremity in traction should be checked every 15 minutes during the first hour, hourly for 24 hours, and every 4 hours thereafter for signs of pallor (or blueness), lack of warmth (coldness), tingling, absent peripheral pulse, edema, or pain. Traction can lead to hypertension because the head typically is positioned lower than the lower extremities. Assess once a day for this.

Be careful when changing the child's bed linens or carrying out nursing functions that you do not move the weights or interfere with the traction. Provide good skin care on the child's back, elbows, and heels, which may become irritated. A trapeze suspended over the bed provides a great deal of mobility and assists children in using a bedpan and positioning themselves in bed.

Being in traction is not as dramatic for children as being placed in a cast. There is nothing for people to autograph. There is an unspoken feeling from other children that "if what you have is really serious, you'd have a cast." Explain to children why this type of treatment is best for them. Keep them informed of x-ray reports, for example, "The fracture is being held in just the right position; the bone is beginning to reform." Although they cannot see progress, they can be assured that it is happening.

Children need to maintain contact with their school friends through cards, letters, or tape-recorded messages. If hospitalized, their bed should be located so that they can see unit activities. Whether at home or in the hospital, allow frequent visitors of their own age to help maintain peer relationships.

Children in traction are generally not "ill" children. They feel well except for the leg or arm being held in correct position. Therefore, they have the energy and need the stimulation of well children. Keeping them occupied and exposed to activities appropriate to their age group is a major part of nursing care (Figure 30-9).

Distraction

Distraction involves the use of an external device to separate opposing bones, thus encouraging new bone growth. It can be used to lengthen the bone when one limb is shorter than the other. It also can be used to immobilize fractures or correct defects when the bone is rotated or angled.

A device such as the Ilizarov external fixator is used to achieve distraction (Figure 30-10). It consists of wires that are inserted through the bone. The wires are attached to either full or half rings, which are secured to telescoping rods. If used for bone lengthening, each day the rods are adjusted approximately 1 mm to stimulate bone growth until the desired length is achieved. The device remains in place until consolidation is complete and there is no pain, limp, or edema. At this time, the bone is healed and can bear weight.

The child and parents need thorough preparation for the surgery and application of the device. Because the device is external, large, and awkward, they need to be prepared for its appearance and the reactions of others to it. Provide suggestions for ways to minimize the device's appearance, such as wide-legged pants with adjustable closures. Parents also need instructions about adjusting the telescoping rods, if ordered; providing care to the wire insertion sites; assessing for signs and symptoms of infection; and instituting activity restrictions. Follow-up care is essential to ensure the optimal outcome for the child.

Open Reduction

Open reduction is a surgical technique used to align and repair bone. If there is a spinal fracture or both bones of a forearm or lower leg are fractured, open reduction may be necessary to stabilize the bones. Internal fixation, such as the use of rods or screws, is rarely used with children except in those with scoliosis.

Once an open reduction is completed, the area is generally casted to provide support. Invariably, serosanguineous fluid oozes from an open-reduction site. Any stain on the cast that suggests oozing from a surgical incision should be outlined with a ballpoint pen so that an increase in the size of the mark can be noted. Do not use a magic marker for this, because the fluid tends to penetrate through the cast. Noting the time you make the pen mark on the cast allows you to tell how rapidly the spot is increasing in size. Children with an open-reduction incision are prone to incision infection as is any child after a surgical incision. Be aware of systemic symptoms (increased pulse, increased temperature, lethargy) and local signs (edema, pain, tingling, blueness or coolness of the distal extremity) of infection.

> ✔ **CHECKPOINT QUESTIONS**
>
> 3. Why might a window be used with a cast?
> 4. When using crutches, where should the child bear the weight?

DISORDERS OF BONE DEVELOPMENT

Flat Feet (Pes Planus)

The term *flat feet* refers to relaxation of the longitudinal arch of the foot. Many parents worry that their children have this problem. Only rarely, however, does this occur. Parents become concerned because, normally, a newborn's foot is flatter and proportionately wider than an adult's. A transverse arch rarely is visible. A longitudinal arch may not be present until a child has been walking for months. Parents notice that when their child walks in the sand or makes wet tracks on the bathroom floor, he or she makes an impression of a "flat foot."

Evaluate children's feet for this by having them stand on tiptoe. In this position, a longitudinal arch should be visible. If they can stand on their heels with the soles of

Nursing Care Plan

THE CHILD IN SKELETAL TRACTION

A 10-year-old male with a fracture of the left femur was placed in skeletal traction 2 days ago. He is scheduled to remain hospitalized for the next 2 weeks.

Assessment: 10-year-old male admitted with fracture of left femur after being struck by a car while riding his bicycle. Placed in balanced suspension traction with pin placed in distal portion of femur. Skin around pin insertion site slightly reddened. Small amount of serosanguinous drainage observed oozing from pin site. Traction weights attached and hanging freely.

Left lower extremity pale, pink, and warm with pedal pulses present. Capillary refill of 3 seconds. Able to wiggle toes on command. States he does not feel numbness or tingling. Right lower extremity findings within normal limits. Vital signs within age-acceptable parameters. States he has some pain, rating it a 4 on a numerical scale of 1 to 10 (no pain to severe pain). Relieved with codeine and acetaminophen as ordered. Abdomen soft, nontender; bowel sounds active but slow. Bowel movement 2 days ago. Voiding clear yellow urine in adequate amounts.

During morning assessment, child states, "I'm so bored. I have to stay like this for 2 whole weeks? I'll go stir crazy." Child enjoys playing baseball with friends and video games.

Nursing Diagnosis: Diversional activity deficit related to immobilization and hospitalization secondary to skeletal traction

Outcome Identification: Child will participate in age-appropriate activities during hospitalization.

Outcome Evaluation: Child reports fewer feelings of boredom; communicates with friends on telephone and during visits; participates in activities offered.

Interventions	Rationale
1. Discuss typical interests, hobbies, and activities that the child likes and dislikes.	1. Ascertaining likes and dislikes provides a foundation on which to build future suggestions.
2. Work with the child to plan nursing care that allows time for rest and activities. Involve the child in care as appropriate.	2. Active participation lessens the feelings of boredom and passivity, enhancing the feelings of control, autonomy, and individualism.
3. Provide age-appropriate play items, such as video games, arts and craft supplies, and music, within easy access to the child. Use therapeutic play.	3. Play enhances a child's mental, emotional, and social well-being. Therapeutic play aids in ventilating feelings and anxiety.
4. Encourage the parents to bring in favorite items from home. Provide time for the child and parents to verbalize their feelings.	4. Items with personal meaning help to foster a sense of familiarity, promoting interest and stimulation. Verbalizing feelings aids in reducing frustration and anxiety.
5. Move the child to a room with another child of the same age, sex, and physical capabilities. Change the position of the child's bed in the room and transport the child in bed out of the room periodically.	5. Interaction between children with similar characteristics promotes socialization, fostering growth and development. Changing the bed's position or transporting the child in bed out of the room alters sensory stimuli and prevents monotony.
6. Encourage the child to telephone friends as appropriate. Urge the parents to have the child's friends visit.	6. Contact with peers is essential to maintain relationships and promote growth and development.

(continued)

Nursing Diagnosis: Risk for peripheral neurovascular dysfunction related to the effects of the fracture and use of skeletal traction

Outcome Identification: Child will remain free of signs and symptoms of neurovascular compromise.

Outcome Evaluation: Child's extremities pink, warm, dry, with palpable pedal pulses and capillary refill of 3 seconds or less bilaterally. Child denies any numbness or tingling in extremity.

Interventions	Rationale
1. Assess neurovascular status of left lower extremity, including temperature, color, pedal pulse, edema, and capillary refill at least every 4 hours or more often as indicated. Compare findings with unaffected extremity.	1. Changes in neurovascular function often begin with minor changes. Frequent assessment allows for early detection and prompt intervention should any problems occur. Comparing the affected with the unaffected extremity provides a basis for evaluation.
2. Monitor the child's ability to move his toes and detect sensation in the left lower extremity.	2. Ability to move toes and detect sensations indicate intact motor and sensory function.
3. Maintain traction with left leg in proper alignment.	3. Proper positioning with intact traction promotes adequate bone healing and circulation.
4. Instruct the child to report any numbness, tingling, increased pain, or feelings of coldness.	4. Symptoms such as these indicate decreased blood supply to nerve or muscle tissue.

Nursing Diagnosis: Risk for infection related to open wound at pin insertion site

Outcome Identification: Child will remain free of signs and symptoms of infection.

Outcome Evaluation: Pin site is clean and dry without purulent drainage. Temperature within age-appropriate parameters.

Interventions	Rationale
1. Assess vital signs, especially temperature, every 4 hours or more often as indicated.	1. Vital signs, especially temperature, are reliable indicators of infection.
2. Inspect pin insertion site at least every 8 hours for signs of redness, swelling, irritation, or drainage. Obtain culture of pin site as ordered.	2. The skin provides the first line of defense against infection; insertion of pin disrupts this defense, providing an entrance for microorganisms. Frequent monitoring of the pin insertion site allows for early detection of problems and prompt intervention should any signs be noted.
3. Perform pin site care according to the institution's policy. Adhere to standard precautions and use aseptic technique.	3. Pin site care helps keep the area clean, minimizing the risk for infection. Standard precautions and aseptic technique minimize the risk for infection transmission.
4. Provide a well-balanced diet with adequate protein and calories. Limit calcium intake as ordered.	4. Adequate nutrition is essential for overall body function. Calories and protein are needed for tissue repair. Calcium intake is necessary for bone healing. Too much calcium, however, increases the risk for renal calculi development from immobility.
5. Anticipate antibiotic administration based on culture reports.	5. Antibiotic therapy specific to the organism involved is necessary to treat the infection, should one occur.

Nursing Diagnosis: Risk for disuse syndrome related to prolonged bedrest and immobilization secondary to skeletal traction

Outcome Identification: Child remains free of any signs and symptoms of complications of immobility.

Outcome Evaluation: Child's skin integrity remains intact; lungs clear to auscultation. Child voids in adequate amounts; has a bowel movement at least every other day; maintains range of motion of unaffected extremities; exhibits signs of adequate peripheral blood flow.

(continued)

Interventions	Rationale
1. Assess skin surfaces at least every 8 hours for signs of redness, irritation, or pressure. Provide frequent skin care measures, padding bony prominences and using pressure-reducing devices as appropriate. Encourage frequent position changes within the limits of traction, and urge child to use over-bed trapeze bar to shift body weight.	1. Frequent position changes, skin care measures, and pressure-reducing devices reduce the risk for skin breakdown. Use of the over-bed trapeze allows the child to participate in care and activities.
2. Assess respiratory status at least every 4 hours; auscultate lungs for adventitious sounds. Encourage coughing, deep breathing, and use of incentive spirometer at least every 2 hours.	2. Immobilization leads to stasis of respiratory sections, decreased chest expansion, and shallow respirations. Adventitious breath sounds are abnormal, indicating compromised respiratory function. Coughing, deep breathing, and incentive spirometry help to clear the airway, expand the lungs, and mobilize secretions for expectoration.
3. Assess urine elimination. Monitor intake and output. Encourage fluid intake of at least 2 L per day with limited calcium intake.	3. Immobilization leads to urinary stasis and increases the risk for urinary calculi (from bone demineralization). Increased fluid intake helps to promote urine excretion. Limiting calcium intake reduces the risk for renal calculi.
4. Assess bowel sounds and elimination patterns. Institute a diet high in fiber and ensure adequate fluid intake. Allow child to use fracture pan in bed for elimination. Anticipate the need for a bowel program if no bowel movement in 3 days.	4. Immobilization leads to decreased peristalsis. High-fiber foods and adequate fluid intake promote peristalsis and enhance bowel elimination. A fracture pan may be helpful in allowing the child to assume the normal anatomic position for defecating without interfering with the traction. Additional assistance such as with a bowel program may be necessary for effective bowel elimination.
5. Have the child perform active range-of-motion exercises to unaffected extremities as appropriate. Encourage use of isometric exercises to the affected leg.	5. Exercise helps to maintain muscle strength and tone and prevent contractures.
6. Anticipate the need for antiembolism stockings or intermittent compression devices for the unaffected leg.	6. Immobility results in venous stasis. Antiembolism stockings or intermittent compression devices promote venous return.
7. Monitor vital signs and laboratory test results, such as serum calcium levels, coagulation studies, and white blood cell counts.	7. Vital signs are important indicators of overall body function. Immobility results in bone demineralization, which may lead to hypercalcemia. Increased serum calcium levels increase blood coagulability, which, when coupled with venous stasis, increases the child's risk for thrombosis. White blood cell count provides information about the possibility of infection.
8. Allow the child to participate in planning and to do as much as possible in all aspects of care. Vary the routine and physical environment whenever possible.	8. Participation in care activities promotes feelings of control and self-esteem. Varying the routine and environment reduces monotony of the situation and provides stimulation.

the feet off the ground, the feet probably are normal. Examine the ankle joint to be certain a full range of motion is present to demonstrate that the Achilles' tendon is not shortened. Tarsal and metatarsal joints should normally show a full range of motion.

Some children experience foot pain at the end of the day. This probably occurs not from lack of a longitudinal arch, but from poor arch development. The arch can be strengthened and the pain usually can be eliminated if the child walks on tiptoe for 5 to 10 minutes daily or practices picking up marbles with the toes. For an older child, standing pigeon toed (toes pointed in) and throwing the weight forward onto the lateral aspect of the feet tends to strengthen arches.

Teach parents that children do not need a hightop or rigid shoe for foot development. Shoes with strong foot support may actually prevent the arch from forming adequately and should be avoided (Cappello & Song, 1998).

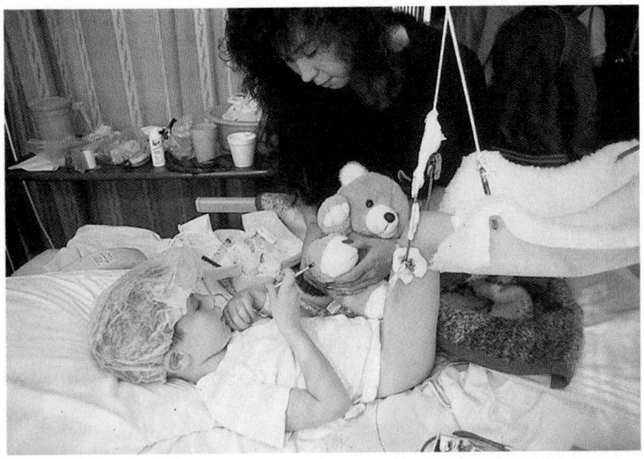

FIGURE 30.9 A child in skeletal traction engages in play.

Bowlegs (Genu Varum)

Genu varum is the lateral bowing of the tibia. If present, the **malleoli** (rounded prominence on either side of the ankles) of the ankles are touching and the medial surface of the knees is over 2 in (5 cm) apart (Figure 30-11*A*).

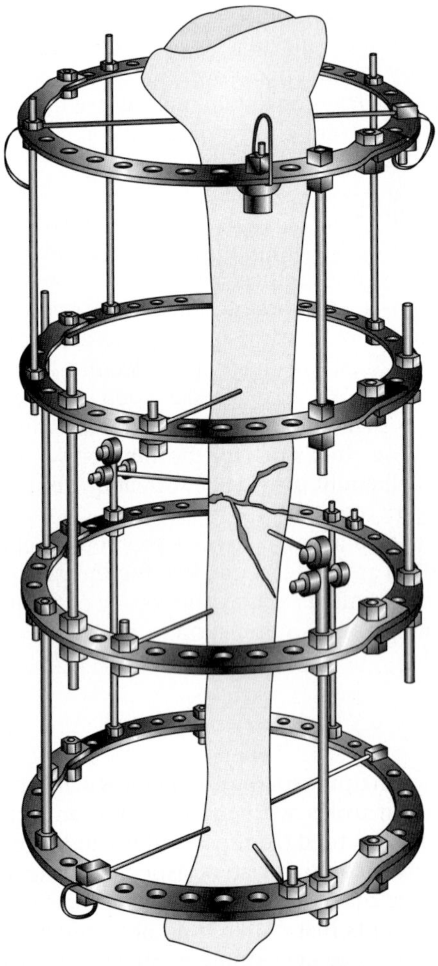

FIGURE 30.10 Ilizarov device in place to treat comminuted fracture.

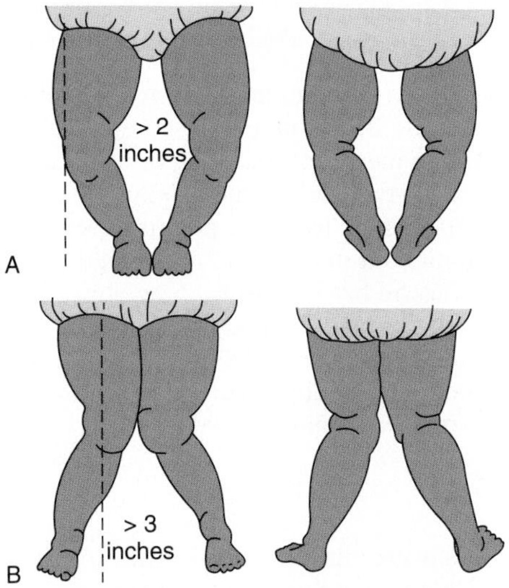

FIGURE 30.11 (**A**) Genu varum. (**B**) Genu valgum.

Children may develop this condition as part of normal development, but it is seen most commonly in 2-year-olds. Record the extent of the bowing at health maintenance visits by approximating the medial malleoli of the ankles and measuring the distance between the patellas (knees) for changes.

Genu varum gradually corrects itself by about 3 years of age and at the latest by school age. If the problem is becoming rapidly worse or persists beyond this time, children need referral to an orthopedist for further evaluation.

Blount's Disease (Tibia Vara)

Blount's disease is retardation of growth of the epiphyseal line on the medial side of the proximal tibia (inside of the knee), resulting in bowed legs. Unlike the normal developmental aspect of genu varum, however, Blount's disease is a serious disturbance in bone growth that requires treatment.

Because it is not possible to rule out Blount's disease by appearance alone, almost all children with bowed legs have an initial x-ray. With Blount's disease, the medial aspect of the proximal tibia will show a sharp, beaklike appearance on x-ray.

Bracing or osteotomy may be necessary to correct this deformity or prevent it from becoming more severe. Explain to the parents why their child requires treatment or surgery when another child on the block with a similar appearance (developmental genu varum) is expected to outgrow the problem.

Knock Knees (Genu Valgum)

Genu valgum or knock knee, appears as the opposite of genu varum. The medial surfaces of the knees touch, and the medial surfaces of the ankle malleoli are separated by more than 3 in (7.5 cm) (see Figure 30-11*B*).

This is seen most commonly in children 3 to 4 years old. No treatment is necessary for genu valgum. The problem tends to correct itself as the child grows. By school age, few children continue to have the problem. Those children who do, or those in whom the abnormality is becoming more pronounced, need a referral to an orthopedist for further evaluation. The severity of the deformity should be measured at regular health maintenance visits by approximating the medial aspects of the knees and measuring the distance between the medial malleoli of the ankles.

Toeing-In

Toeing-in (pigeon toe) in children may occur as a result of foot, tibial, femoral, or hip displacement. Assess for this when a parent describes a child as "always falling over her feet" or "awkward."

Metatarsus adductus is turning in of the forefoot. The heel is in good alignment; only the forefoot is turned in. This may develop or become more pronounced in infants who sleep prone with feet adducted or older children who watch television by kneeling, resting on their feet, and turning their feet in. If the child stood on a copying machine and made a print, the turning in of the foot would be well demonstrated.

Most instances of metatarsus adductus resolve without therapy. Those that persist beyond 1 year can be corrected by passive stretching exercises. Wearing shoes on the opposite feet may help some infants. Wearing a Denis Browne splint at night may be necessary. A Denis Browne splint consists of a pair of shoes connected by a metal or plastic rod. The shoes are positioned to keep the foot in the correct alignment and are then held firmly to the rod by metal or plastic plates.

A few infants with extremely rigid, incorrect foot posture may require casts rather than splints for correction. Early detection is important. Treatment for metatarsus adductus is most effective if it is begun before an infant walks. With early treatment, the prognosis is excellent.

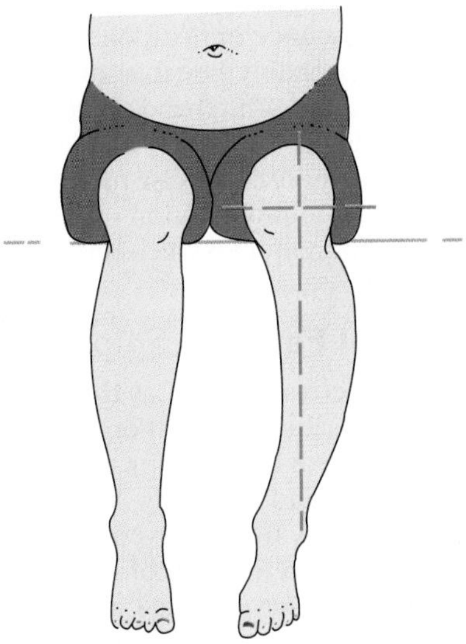

FIGURE 30.12 Toeing-in caused by inward tibial torsion. In good alignment, a line drawn from the anterosuperior iliac crest through the patella should intersect the second toe.

Inward tibial torsion also may be evidenced as toeing-in. This condition is diagnosed when a line drawn from the anterior superior iliac crest through the center of the patella intersects the fourth or fifth toe (or a position even more lateral) (Figure 30-12). Ordinarily, such a line should intersect the second toe.

Tibial torsion, a normal developmental finding, usually improving as the tibia grows, needs no treatment. Parents will need a good explanation of why no treatment is necessary. Reassure them at periodic health maintenance visits that patience and time will correct tibial torsion.

Inward femoral torsion can be detected if you have a child lie supine and attempt to rotate his or her leg internally and then externally at the hip. Normally, internal rotation is about 30 degrees, and outward rotation is about 90 degrees. With inward femoral torsion, the degree of internal rotation is closer to 90 degrees. In some children, the femur rotates so far that the patellar bones face each other. As with tibial torsion, no treatment is necessary. Inward femoral rotation will not correct itself, but a compensating tibial torsion will develop and make feet appear straight (Sponseller, 1997).

A fourth cause of toeing-in may be improper hip placement or hip dysplasia, a problem that is very serious and needs early therapy for correction (see Chapter 18).

Limps

Observation of a child's gait is part of the health assessment at any health maintenance visit. Gait is a variable characteristic; however, limping is never normal. Although it may reflect a simple problem (a recently stubbed toe), it may also reflect serious bone or muscle involvement, such as with osteomyelitis or cerebral palsy.

History is important in determining the cause of the limp. When children have pain in the lower extremities, they protect their extremities by limping—stepping gingerly and quickly on an affected leg. Although children may seem to be favoring an ankle or a knee, ask them specifically what hurts. They may be favoring a hip. Because a hip hurts, they may be walking gingerly on the leg and causing pain in a knee.

The lower extremities need careful, thoughtful examination, including inspection, measurement of leg length, range of motion, palpation, and a neurologic examination. X-ray or bone scan may be necessary to rule out a pathologic process (Fordham et al, 1998).

Growing Pains

Listen to parents carefully when they state that their child has "growing pains." What they are reporting may be symptoms indicative of rheumatic fever or JRA rather than a simple, transient phenomenon. Growing pains occur most frequently in the muscle of the calf, never in a joint. Children wake at night because of the pain. Such cramping generally is associated with a day of vigorous activity or wearing new shoes with a heel of a different height than before. Children with genu varum (bowlegs) tend to have more of such pain than other children. Growing pains should be evaluated seriously at health maintenance visits to detect possible symptoms of disease.

WHAT IF? The parents of a child report that their child has been waking up at night because of pain in the calf. How would you evaluate this child further?

Osteogenesis Imperfecta

Osteogenesis imperfecta is characterized by the formation of pathologic fractures (Ablin, 1998). It occurs in two main forms: a severe form that is recognized at birth (osteogenesis imperfecta congenita) and a form that occurs later in life (osteogenesis imperfecta tarda).

Children with the congenital form are born with countless fractures. They develop many more fractures during childhood. This condition appears to be inherited as a *recessive trait.* Children with the late-occurring form may have associated deafness, dental deformities, and an unusual blueness of the sclera because of poor connective tissue formation. This disorder is inherited as a *dominant trait.* X-ray reveals a particular ribbon-like or mosaic pattern in bones, which aids in diagnosis.

In both instances, the major clinical manifestation is a tendency to fracture easily due to poor collagen formation. In some children, their bones are so fragile, fracture results not only from trauma, such as a fall, but from simple walking. It can occur from the force of birth.

As the child grows older, the multiple breaks tend to cause limb and spinal column deformities, interfering with alignment or growth. Growth hormone may be administered to stimulate growth. Calcitonin aids bone healing. Biphosphonates may be prescribed to increase bone mass. Children need to be protected from trauma, fractures need to be aligned and casted, and children need to be educated about a lifestyle that is productive yet minimizes the risk of trauma. Lightweight leg braces or intermedullary rods may be effective in strengthening bones.

Always be careful when caring for a child with this disorder. Be sure to raise side rails on cribs or beds. Keep floors dry and remove objects that could cause falls. Always lift children gently and avoid lifting them by a single arm or leg.

Legg-Calvé-Perthes Disease (Coxa Plana)

Legg-Calvé-Perthes disease is avascular necrosis of the proximal femoral epiphysis. This occurs more often in boys than girls and has a peak age of incidence between 4 and 8 years of age (Sponseller, 1997). It usually occurs unilaterally but may occur bilaterally.

The affected child notices pain in the hip joint accompanied by spasm and limited motion. X-ray studies are used to distinguish between Legg-Calvé-Perthes disease and a simple synovitis (inflammation of the hip joint), which begins with the same symptoms. X-ray changes may not be apparent when a child is first seen but appear after about 3 weeks. For this reason, most children seen for a synovitis of the hip joint are asked to return in 3 weeks for a repeat x-ray.

Legg-Calvé-Perthes disease passes through four stages. First is the synovitis stage, or period of painful inflammation. Following this is a necrotic stage, during which bone in the femur head becomes smaller and shows increased density on x-ray. This stage lasts 6 to 12 months. A third stage is a fragmentation stage. Resorption of dead bone occurs over a 1- to 2-year period. The fourth stage, a reconstruction stage, marks final healing with deposition of new bone occurring.

Treatment for Legg-Calvé-Perthes disease focuses on keeping the head of the femur within the acetabulum to act as a mold to preserve the shape of the femoral head and maintain range of motion.

Initially, rest is used to reduce inflammation and restore motion. To keep the head of the femur correctly positioned within the acetabulum, "containment" devices, such as abduction braces, casts, or leather harness slings, or weight-bearing devices, such as abduction ambulation braces or casts (after bedrest and traction), may be used.

A reconstructive surgery technique (an osteotomy to center the femur head in the acetabulum followed by cast application) also may be used. This technique returns the child to normal activity within 3 to 4 months.

Parents and children need thorough education about treatment and care because a majority of it occurs on an outpatient basis. Be sure parents understand the need for a containment device. Without the apparatus, the femur head tends to remold in a mushroom shape. This makes the hip unstable thereafter. Because the shape does not conform well to the acetabulum, degenerative changes may occur later in life, leading to chronic pain, reduced mobility of the hip joint, and possible permanent disability.

It may be difficult for children to accept the extended treatment period involved with this disorder. Be certain that parents and children understand the long-term consequences. In addition, the parents may need assistance with devising appropriate activities for the child during treatment because of the device and limited weight bearing allowed.

Osgood-Schlatter Disease

Osgood-Schlatter disease is thickening and enlargement of the tibial tuberosity resulting from microtrauma. Children notice pain and swelling over the tibia tubercle. The pain is aggravated by running and squatting. This tends to occur in early adolescence or preadolescence in children who are athletic, probably because of rapid growth at these times (Kaeding & Whitehead, 1998).

Therapy depends on the extent of the bone changes. Limiting strenuous physical exercise may be all that is necessary. Occasionally, immobilization of a leg in a walking cast or immobilizer for about 6 weeks may be required.

Slipped Capital Femoral Epiphysis

Slipped epiphysis (coxa vera) is, as the name implies, a slipping of the femur head in relation to the neck of the femur at the epiphyseal line. The proximal femoral head displaces posteriorly and inferiorly. The cartilage covering the femur head may be destroyed by necrosis, resulting in permanent loss of motion of the femur head. An avascular necrosis similar to Legg-Calvé-Perthes disease may occur. With both complications, surgical reconstruction of the hip joint will be necessary.

This disorder occurs most frequently in preadolescence. It is twice as frequent in African Americans as other races and twice as frequent in boys as in girls. It is more common in obese or rapidly growing children. This suggests that it occurs due to the influence of growth hormone and excessive weight bearing in the preadolescent child.

The onset of symptoms is gradual. On inspection, children often will be observed limping and holding their leg externally rotated to relieve stress and pain in the hip joint. They may complain first of pain in their knee, because favoring the hip joint puts abnormal stress on the knee. On physical examination, internal rotation of the hip is difficult and painful. X-ray will reveal the slipped epiphysis at the femur head (Loder, 1998).

Early detection is important because correction is easiest if it is attempted before the condition has progressed to epiphyseal destruction. Surgery with pinning or external fixation, such as with skeletal traction, is used to stabilize the femur head. Following surgery, the child may have activity restrictions or be confined to bed. Because it is most common in preadolescence, these children need continued support. Help them to understand the potential seriousness of the condition. Although they may not like being restricted or confined in this way, supportive communication and education can help them accept this as necessary to maintain good healing and function of the hip joint. Encourage frequent visits and telephone calls with friends to provide optimal growth and development.

Although this condition usually is unilateral, about 30% of affected children later develop the same condition in the opposite hip. All children with a slipped epiphysis, therefore, need follow-up care, with careful attention to the condition of the opposite hip (Sponseller, 1997).

✔ CHECKPOINT QUESTIONS

5. Are bowed legs common in 15-month-olds?
6. Should you prepare a child with Legg-Calvé-Perthes disease for a short or long period of therapy?

INFECTIOUS AND INFLAMMATORY DISORDERS OF THE BONES AND JOINTS

Osteomyelitis

Osteomyelitis is infection of the bone. It is most often caused by *Staphylococcus aureus* in older children and *Haemophilus influenzae* in younger children and is carried to the bone site by septicemia (blood infection). It may follow extensive impetigo, burns, or something as simple as a furuncle (skin abscess). Children with sickle cell anemia have a special susceptibility to *Salmonella* invasion in long bones (Sponseller, 1997). It also may occur directly from outside invasion from a penetrating wound, open fracture, or contamination during surgery.

Osteomyelitis begins typically as a metaphysis infection because the blood supply is sluggish in that portion of the bone. An abscess forms, spreading along the shaft of the bone under the periosteum, possibly extending to and penetrating the bone marrow. Sinuses may form between the marrow and the periosteum or between the infected bone and the skin above. If the epiphyseal plate is infected, altered bone growth may result.

Assessment

Osteomyelitis generally begins with acute symptoms. Children show systemic malaise, fever, and irritability. They may have sharp pain at the bone metaphysis. By the second day, the area of skin over the infected bone will feel warm to the touch; edema will be present. Edema reduces the blood supply to vast expanses of bone, causing death of bone tissue. This dead bone tissue appears dense on x-ray. It is called **sequestrum.**

Blood studies will reveal an increased white blood cell count, C-reactive protein, and sedimentation rate, and the blood culture generally is positive. X-ray may not reveal bone changes (formation of sequestrum) until 5 to 10 days after the beginning of the infection. Computed tomography may demonstrate early stage bone changes. Some children with osteomyelitis are not seen at health care facilities as soon as they should be, because parents account for the pain as "growing pain." Children with systemic symptoms, such as fever, malaise, and joint pain, must be evaluated carefully so that developing osteomyelitis, if present, can be detected early.

Therapeutic Management

Medical treatment involves limitation of weight bearing on the affected part, bedrest, immobilization, and administration of an antibiotic as indicated by the blood culture. Generally, the antibiotic is administered intravenously. This therapy is usually initiated in the hospital and then continued at home, often using an intermittent infusion device or peripherally inserted central catheter. Intravenous (IV) antibiotic therapy may continue for 3 to 6 weeks and orally for 2 weeks thereafter, depending on the duration of symptoms, response to treatment, and sensitivity of the organism.

If there is pus formation under the periosteum, it may be aspirated using a technique similar to bone marrow aspiration. Following the procedure, a tube may be inserted into the area for instillation of an antibiotic solution. A drainage tube may be inserted and attached to suction to evacuate the subperiosteum area.

NURSING DIAGNOSES AND RELATED INTERVENTIONS

Nursing Diagnosis: Parental health-seeking behaviors related to care of the child with osteomyelitis

Outcome Identification: Parents understand child's care needs within 24 hours.

Outcome Evaluation: Parents accurately identify child's care needs to be met in the hospital and at home; parents demonstrate procedure for IV antibiotic administration.

When planning for the child with osteomyelitis, be certain that the long-term immobilization necessary for care will be considered. Parents may need to make major changes in their lifestyle for the child remaining in a hospital or to give care at home for an extended length of time.

Parents have many questions when osteomyelitis is diagnosed because at first, the defect does not show on x-ray. They may be startled to hear their physician talking about 6 weeks of home care. They may be suspicious, anxious, and afraid that hospitalization and administration of IV antibiotics are really unnecessary. At the point that the x-ray reveals the process, often they will become more supportive and understanding of the care given to their child.

Handle the extremity gently when giving care because the child has pain. Demonstrate to the parents how to do this. Provide instructions to the parents about good food sources of calcium and protein for bone healing. If the child had surgery and drainage tubes in place, institute infection-control precautions because the drain evacuates infected material.

When the child is discharged, be sure to instruct the parents about follow-up antibiotic care at home. Ensure that parents understand the importance of giving medication even though the child's symptoms may have completely disappeared. Review with them measures to care for the IV site and antibiotic adminstration. Also review the signs and symptoms of infection, measures for wound care and infection control, and possible adverse effects of antibiotic treatment. A referral for home care follow-up is important to ensure continued support and education.

If osteomyelitis is not entirely eradicated with the initial treatment, it will return and result in a chronic infectious process with open, draining sinuses and bone deformity in years to come. Growth plates can be destroyed, leading to shortening of an extremity (Wall, 1998).

Synovitis

Synovitis, an acute, nonpurulent inflammation of the synovial membrane of a joint, occurs most commonly in the hip joint in children. The peak age of incidence is between 2 and 10 years. Children notice pain in their groin, the lower portion of the thigh or knee, or the buttocks. Pain is intense and most noticeable in the morning when they first awaken. Children may wake at night or in the morning, crying from the pain of turning over. Pain again becomes worse later in the day when children become tired.

Aside from the localized pain, children feel well except that they generally hold the joint flexed in a position of comfort. On physical examination, range-of-motion exercises will cause pain. An x-ray may reveal capsular swelling at the involved joint.

The treatment of synovitis is bedrest until muscle spasm from pain has passed. With some children, flexion contractures occur, requiring countertraction in addition to bedrest.

In most children, 3 days of bedrest will reduce the synovitis. However, some children may need 10 to 14 days. Synovitis must be differentiated from septic arthritis restricted to one joint. With septic arthritis, the child tends to be systemically ill, and blood studies will reveal an increased white blood cell count.

It is important that children and parents understand that synovitis is a simple inflammation process that will heal without sequelae. Bedrest is important for this recovery, however, and must be enforced.

Apophysitis

Adolescents who are growing rapidly are prone to apophysitis, or inflammation of the epiphysis of a heel bone. The heel feels tender, and pain on walking may be acute.

Pain generally can be relieved by adding a lift to the heel of the adolescent's shoe, reducing the tension on the heel cord. When pain has subsided, adolescents need to practice exercises to stretch the heel cord. This can be accomplished by having an adolescent stand on a slanting board, which elevates the foot and toes above the level of the heel, for 20 minutes about three times a day.

Apophysitis is an annoying condition, particularly for adolescents who feel a need to excel in sports to win peer approval. They need assurance that although this annoying pain may persist for months, it is not a serious disorder. It helps to put the slant board by the telephone or somewhere where they will be reminded of it daily. Many adolescents feel that they are too busy and do not have the time for such an exercise three times a day unless they can combine it with another activity, such as talking on the telephone or watching television.

✔ CHECKPOINT QUESTIONS

7. What organism typically causes osteomyelitis in the older child?
8. Where does synovitis most commonly occur?

DISORDERS OF SKELETAL STRUCTURE

Scoliosis: Functional (Postural)

Scoliosis is a lateral (sideways) curvature of the spine. It may involve all or only a portion of the spinal column. It may be functional (a curve caused by a secondary problem) or structural (a primary deformity).

Functional scoliosis occurs as a compensatory mechanism in children who have unequal leg lengths and sometimes in children with ocular refractive errors that cause them constantly to tilt their head sideways. The pelvic tilt caused by unequal leg length or the neck tilt results in a spinal deviation (necessary for the child to stand upright). The curve that occurs in functional scoliosis tends to be a C-shaped curve, in contrast to that in structural scoliosis, which tends to be S-shaped (composed of two separate curves). There is little change in the shape of vertebrae on x-ray with functional curves.

To rectify functional scoliosis, the difficulty causing the spinal curvature must be corrected. A lift inserted in one shoe will correct unequal leg length (leg length is measured from the anterior iliac spine to the bottom of the medial malleolus). Correcting ocular refractive errors will improve problems caused by head tilt. In addition, children must be reminded to maintain good posture during everyday activities. Walking with a book on the head for 10 minutes, three times a day or hanging by the hands from a door frame (chinning themselves) stretches the back and is often helpful. Sit-ups and push-ups are good exercises. Swimming also is good exercise, because the reaching involved stretches the spine.

Parents and children need to be assured that functional scoliosis is a disorder that can be corrected. Children need to be aware of this to prevent problems with self-esteem and body image. Reinforce the need for good posture and exercise with the child and parents. Caution parents about nagging children of this age to do exercises or maintain good posture. Puberty is an age of rebellion and exertion of independence. Children may choose to ignore the parents' requests. Be open with them, helping them to understand the need for treatment. Let them know that you understand that children of their age feel they do not have to do everything their parents want them to do. Help them to find alternative, more positive ways to exert their independence.

Scoliosis: Structural

Structural scoliosis is idiopathic, permanent curvature of the spine accompanied by damage to the vertebrae. The spine assumes a primary lateral curvature. To allow children to hold their head level, a compensatory second curve develops, giving the spine an S-shaped appearance (Figure 30-13). The primary curve is often a right thoracic convexity. As the original curve becomes severe, rotation and angulation of vertebrae occur. The thoracic rib cage will rotate to become very protuberant on the convex curve. Vertebral growth may halt because of extreme pressure changes (Sarwark & Kramer, 1998).

A family history of curvature of the spine is found in up to 70% of children with scoliosis, although no specific inheritance pattern has been documented. It is five times more common in girls than boys with a peak incidence age of 8 to 15 years. As long as children are growing, the spinal curves will become more severe. This is why the symptoms become most marked at prepuberty, a time of rapid growth.

Assessment

All children older than 10 years should be assessed for scoliosis at all health assessment visits.

Often, the condition develops insidiously and may be very prominent before it is noticed, because of the preadolescent's and adolescent's need for privacy. A parent might notice when doing laundry that the daughter's bra straps are adjusted to unequal lengths. The parents might notice that the girl finds it difficult to buy jeans that fit correctly because of uneven iliac crests. They might notice that the girl's skirts or dresses hang unevenly. The diagnosis of structural scoliosis is made on physical examination by asking the child to bend forward (Cole et al, 1998) (see Nursing Procedure 13-2).

X-rays and photographs help to estimate the extent of the deformity and serve as a baseline description. Children's bone age is established by x-ray of the wrists. If children have a vertebral rotation causing rib imbalance, pulmonary function studies and a chest x-ray may be done to provide further baseline information. If bone growth is complete or nearly complete, little more deformity will result, so no correction may be necessary. On the other hand, if children have 1 to 2 years of bone growth remaining, some correction most likely will be undertaken.

Therapeutic Management

If the spinal curve is less than 20 degrees, no therapy is usually required except for close observation until the child reaches about 18 years of age.

If the curve is greater than 20 degrees, treatment may be a conservative, nonsurgical approach using braces or trac-

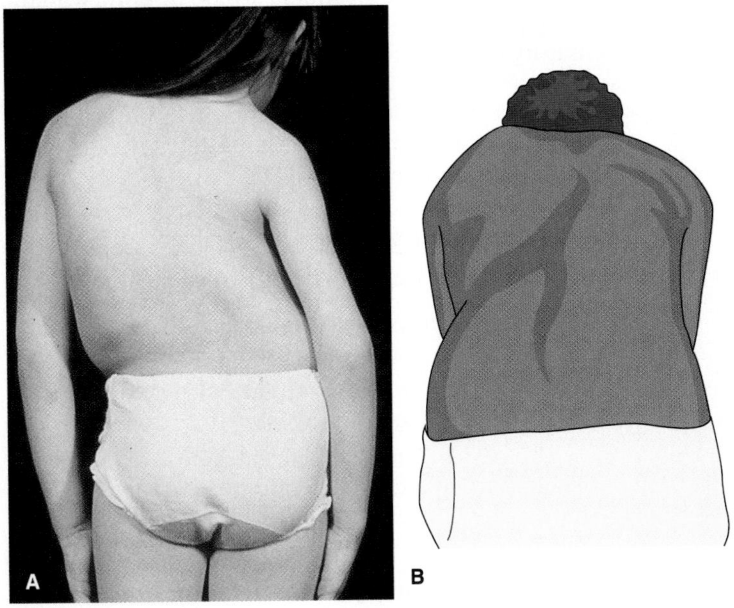

FIGURE 30.13 Assessing scoliosis. (**A**) Child with scoliosis (standing). (**B**) Child with scoliosis (bending over).

tion, surgery, or a combination of both. Regardless of the type of treatment chosen, the child must be prepared for it to be long term. The goal of both surgery and mechanical bracing is to maintain spinal stability and prevent further progression of the deformity until bone growth is complete.

During prepuberty and adolescence, children are very concerned about body image and are very impatient with scoliosis correction, often wanting their problem corrected immediately. They need a great deal of support at health care visits to help them cope with the time needed for correction.

Electrical stimulation may be used for mild to moderate curvatures. Leads are applied with a lubricant along the convexity of the spinal curve. Low pulsating current from a battery is applied for 6 to 8 hours a night while the child sleeps. This is believed to cause the muscles to contract at regular and frequent intervals, possibly helping to straighten the spine. Its effectiveness needs to be more fully evaluated (Allington et al, 1996).

Bracing. If the curve is greater than 20 degrees but less than 40 degrees and the child is still skeletally immature, bracing may be used. The Milwaukee brace was the first type used for this purpose. Other names are the Wilmington, Boston, or Charleston brace; they are used to improve spine alignment. A Milwaukee brace is a torso brace consisting of an anterior rod, two posterior rods, leather pads, and a plastic torso piece. A ring with a padded throat mold encircles the neck. Milwaukee braces are made individually for each child according to his or her specific dimensions. A Boston brace is a prefabricated plastic shell (customized to the child) that fits under the child's arms. Children may find the Boston brace more cosmetically acceptable because it can be hidden under loose clothing. Other bracing devices, such as the thoracic-lumbar-sacral orthosis, also may be used (Figure 30-14).

Children and parents need thorough instructions on how to apply the brace. Marking the strap holes to be used can help ensure that the child always uses the correct holes. Frequent follow-up health care visits are necessary to check the fit of the device, making sure that it fits snugly without rubbing on body prominences, such as the iliac crests. Caution children and parents to notify the health care provider if rubbing occurs. Caution them not to loosen straps to decrease the discomfort. This makes the brace fit loosely, and it will not exert adequate compression and traction this way.

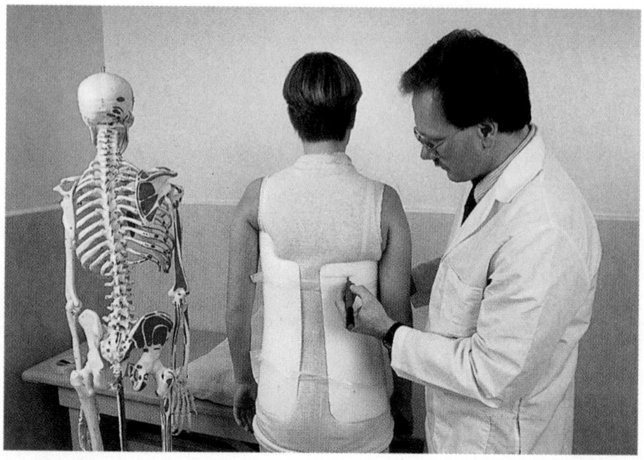

FIGURE 30.14 A teenage girl is fitted with a thoracic-lumbar-sacral orthotic device for treatment of scoliosis.

During the first couple of weeks they wear the brace, children may notice slight muscle aches resulting from the new alignment. If neck and pelvic traction were applied beforehand, this aching may be minimized. A mild analgesic will decrease the discomfort in most children. Rest also provides considerable relief. Children need to be cautioned not to remove the brace during this time because removing it will compound the problem of discomfort by prolonging the period of adjustment.

Typically, the device is worn for a majority of hours during the day, depending on the curvature, the child's age, and any underlying problems associated with the curvature. For example, a Milwaukee brace usually is worn 23 hours a day, 7 days a week for maximum correction. It is worn over a tee shirt to prevent the leather and plastic pads from touching skin surfaces. Leather tends to deteriorate when exposed to sweat, and skin excoriation may occur with long exposure to leather or plastic. Children can remove the brace once a day to bathe or shower. In addition, children may be able to remove it for an hour every day while they swim because this strengthens muscles. If the hour is for swimming, children must be certain to spend the hour actively swimming.

In addition to wearing the brace, exercises done several times a day are usually prescribed:

- To increase pelvic tilt (by standing against a wall and pushing the small of their back [lumbar area] toward the wall)
- For lateral strengthening (by standing straight and moving their body away from the major pad of the brace)
- To correct thoracic lordosis (by standing as tall as they can and pushing back against the posterior bars of the brace with their posterior chest)

These exercises may be taught to children before the brace is applied, but they should always be done with the brace in place after it is fitted. The brace checks the compensatory curve of the spine; without the brace in place, such exercises may increase the spinal deformity by increasing the extent of the minor curve. How long bracing should be used before spinal fusion surgery is scheduled is becoming controversial.

NURSING DIAGNOSES AND RELATED INTERVENTIONS

Nursing Diagnosis: Self-esteem disturbance related to obviousness of the brace used for scoliosis

Outcome Identification: Child will demonstrate positive self-concept by 1 week.

Outcome Evaluation: Child states positive aspects of self; participates in activities; establishes friendships with peers.

It may be easier for children to accept Milwaukee braces today than it once was because the braces are more compact and because teenage clothing tends to be more casual and looser. Even though choosing clothes is easier than it once was, it may still be a major problem for some children. They need time at health care visits to voice concerns about their appearance. Encourage children to voice what it feels like to have to wear a brace of this size constantly. Help them to concentrate on things they can do, such as having a friend over or going to the movies, rather than those they cannot do because of the brace (play basketball, make the track team). If appropriate, another type may be used, which is smaller and less obvious (see Enhancing Communication).

Encourage children in Milwaukee braces to be as active as possible. They may comment at first that they feel awkward or "so much taller" that they are afraid they will fall. The only way to get comfortable with this feeling is to walk and get used to the new sensation of actually being a little taller. Braces may be awkward at school if chairs are attached to desks. Advocate for the child with the school nurse for seating arrangements that are comfortable.

Friends typically ask questions about what happened to a child. The sooner children expose themselves wearing a brace to friends and family, the sooner these questions will cease. The brace is adjusted about every 3 months to accomplish more alignment. Children may need more frequent visits than this, however, to be able to express the problems they are having with social and school adjustment. However, do not underestimate an adolescent's ability to adjust to new situations. Children can see by looking in a mirror that their spine is curved, and they want this corrected. Often, they will endure discomfort if they have hope that they will emerge at the end of the correction period without an obvious physical deformity (see Focus on Cultural Competence).

Parents must be firm about insisting that the child wear the brace continuously to experience the maximum benefits. If bracing does not work, children must have spinal alignment and fusion surgery. Be certain that children do not think spinal surgery is a simple, quick procedure, similar to an appendectomy, and therefore preferable to bracing. If children think this, they may avoid wearing the brace, hoping that surgery will then be prescribed. However, do not depict surgery as horrible. In some children, the scoliosis continues to worsen despite good bracing, and surgery will be necessary.

The brace typically is worn until the child's spinal growth stops (about 14½ years in girls, 16½ years in boys), as demonstrated by spinal x-ray. Bracing is not discontinued abruptly, however. When this point is reached, children are weaned from it gradually because some demineralization of vertebrae may have occurred during the long period of bracing. Gradual resumption of activity allows remineralization and continued spinal support. They may continue to wear the brace at night for a prolonged period (1–2 years).

Halo Traction. Traction is the use of opposing forces to straighten and reduce spinal curves. Halo traction is achieved using a ring of metal (a halo) held in place by about four stainless steel pins inserted into the skull bones. Countertraction is applied by pins inserted into the distal fe-

FOCUS ON CULTURAL COMPETENCE

The way that parents or a child react to the diagnosis of a musculoskeletal disorder can be culturally influenced. In a culture in which beauty and looking similar to others are important values, being asked to wear a Milwaukee or halo brace would be very hard to accept. Because an adolescent culture is often one that respects athletics, beauty, and conformity, adolescence may be a very difficult time for a child to maintain body image and self-esteem when a musculoskeletal disorder is present.

ENHANCING COMMUNICATION

Stacey is a 13-year-old who was diagnosed with structural scoliosis after a routine screening at school. She is being fitted with a Milwaukee brace.

Less Effective Communication

Stacey: Look at this thing; it's so ugly!
Nurse: It is awkward, but it's not too bad.
Stacey: You don't have to wear it. All my friends are going to laugh at me now!
Nurse: You need to wear this brace to help correct your spine.
Stacey: I know, but . . . I'm going to look like such a freak!
Nurse: You need to wear it. Otherwise your spine will be deformed.
Stacey: I know. I know.

More Effective Communication

Stacey: Look at this thing; it's so ugly!
Nurse: It is awkward, but it's not too bad.
Stacey: You don't have to wear it. All my friends are going to laugh at me now!
Nurse: You need to wear this brace to help correct your spine.
Stacey: I know, but . . . I'm going to look like such a freak!
Nurse: You'll feel like a freak?
Stacey: Yeah, how can I go to school? What can I wear?
Nurse: There are ways to try and make this brace look less obvious.
Stacey: Really? How?
Nurse: Let's talk about this. Now, what do you usually like to wear to school?

In the first scenario, the nurse focuses on stressing the need for wearing the brace but fails to identify and acknowledge the adolescent's concerns about how she will look. In the second scenario, the nurse picks up on the adolescent's clues about body image and self-esteem and works with her to develop possible strategies to enhance these areas and promote compliance with wearing the brace.

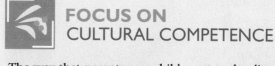

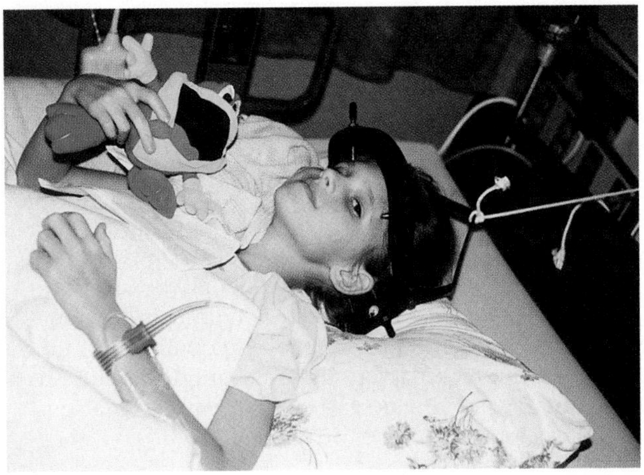

FIGURE 30.15 A 9-year-old girl in halo traction.

murs or iliac crests (Figure 30-15). A halo traction apparatus is a bulky apparatus that looks frightening. Children have some real fear that when the pins are inserted into their skull (done under general anesthesia), the pins will slip and penetrate their brain. They may worry that the apparatus will be so heavy that it will strain or break their neck.

Halo traction is generally used when children have respiratory involvement, cervical instability, a high thoracic deformity, or decreased vital capacity from severe spinal curvature and rotation. Children need to see photographs of the apparatus or talk to children who have the apparatus in place before having it applied. They need time to express their feelings about being placed in such a cumbersome device. Children may react to the apparatus with nausea, diarrhea, or chronic sadness until they see that they can adjust to it. Orientation must be as thorough for the parents as it is for the child. Parents may show symptoms of nausea like the child's for the first few days after the application of such traction. They are generally too unsure of themselves to care for the child during the first week, so they need support to parent during this time.

Careful explanations about the child's care before it is given will help reduce anxiety. Stressing positive aspects, such as what the child can do, and explaining that the traction will help the spinal curvature may encourage children to accept such extreme traction (see Focus on Nursing Research).

For the first 24 hours after applying the apparatus, children generally experience pain at the pin insertion sites. A generalized headache may occur, requiring analgesia. Accepting halo traction is difficult, even without this pain. Offer adequate analgesia for comfort (Olson, 1996).

Children in halo traction need frequent shampoos to keep the pin sites clean. Crusting around the pin sites can be reduced by cleaning the pin insertion sites daily with half-strength hydrogen peroxide or other appropriate solution. Encourage children to be as self-sufficient as possible. Be certain that parents or children have a telephone number they can call for help or if they have questions once the child returns home.

When optimal spinal correction has been achieved, halo traction equipment is removed easily. The pin sites in the skull heal within a week without obvious scarring.

FOCUS ON NURSING RESEARCH

Does Scoliosis Have a Significant Psychological Impact on Adolescents?

For this study, 685 adolescents with scoliosis in Minnesota, 12 to 18 years of age, were identified from the overall school-age population of 75,000 (a prevalence of 1.97%). They were matched with control subjects who did not have scoliosis. Information was collected by a self-administered questionnaire, the Adolescent Health Survey, which investigated such areas as peer relations, body image, and health-compromising behaviors such as suicidal thought and alcohol consumption. Results showed that students with scoliosis had significantly more thoughts about suicide and worried more about body development and peer interactions than their peers without scoliosis.

This is an important study for nurses because nurses are often the people who spend the most time with adolescents with scoliosis in health care settings and therefore have the most opportunity to assess them for how they are adjusting to this potentially devastating event in their life.

Payne, W. K., Ogilvie, J. W., Resnick, M. D., Kane, R. I., Transfeldt, E. F. & Blum, R. W. (1997). Does scoliosis have a psychological impact and does gender make a difference? *Spine, 22*(12), 1380.

Surgical Intervention: Spinal Instrumentation. Surgical correction is generally necessary when the degree of curvature is greater than 40 degrees. Instruments, such as rods, screws, and wires, are placed next to the spinal column to provide firm reduction of the curvature; the spine is then fused in the corrected position. Bone from the iliac crests may be used to strengthen the fusion procedure.

Preoperative Nursing Care. Prior to spinal instrumentation, extensive x-rays will be taken to plan the exact location of the rods. Introduce children to deep-breathing exercises and incentive spirometry before surgery to increase lung function postoperatively. Deep-breathing exercises are particularly important in children whose scoliosis has caused chronically reduced lung capacity.

Children need a good explanation of what they can expect after surgery. This surgery involves bone destruction, so they can expect to have pain. It is a major operation, so they can expect to feel tired and "not themselves" for a number of days. Teaching young adolescents about these events helps them to adjust to the postoperative period. They appreciate being treated like adults. Be aware, however, that early adolescents are not adults, and although they seem eager to breathe deeply and cooperate with routines before surgery, these requests may be overwhelming for them postoperatively, and their behavior may not be nearly as adult as they anticipate. Intrathecal anesthesia offers a great deal of pain relief. Allowing children to use a patient-controlled analgesia system offers both pain relief and a feeling of control.

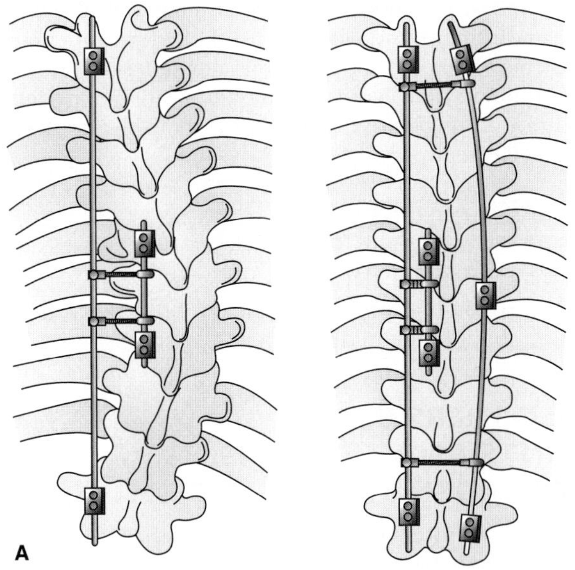

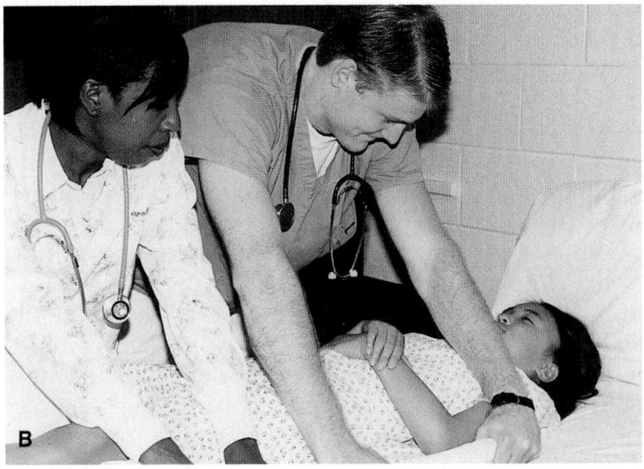

FIGURE 30.16 (**A**) Cotrel-Dubousset rods to correct scoliosis. A short distraction rod is linked to a longer one to correct the major curve. A convex rod is then applied. (**B**) Preparing to log roll. Two nurses use a draw-sheet to roll the child in one coordinated movement to the side-lying position.

The type of rods used depends on the degree of spinal curvature and the age of the child. Harrington rods were the first such rods manufactured, so the surgery is frequently referred to as Harrington rod placement, even though newer types of rods are now more commonly used. Luque rods and Wisconsin segmental spinal instrumentation use a segmental approach. Cotrel-Dubousset rods also are commonly used. These are attached to the vertebrae using hooks or screws (Figure 30-16*A*).

Postoperative Care. Following surgery, the child's bed must not be gatched, because once rods are in place and the spinal fusion has been done, the back must not be bent. Tape the gatch of the bed in place or unplug electric controls so that the bed cannot be raised by accident by a parent or by uninformed auxiliary personnel (see Managing and Delegating Unlicensed Assistive Personnel). In some instances, a child may receive postoperative care on a Stryker frame. If so, introduce a frame preoperatively. A nasogastric tube generally is inserted prior to surgery to prevent abdominal distention; major surgery may cause paralytic ileus and lack of bowel tone.

When the child returns from surgery, he or she must lie flat and must be log-rolled (always by two people) to a side-lying position every 2 hours to enhance respiratory status unless segmented rods were used (see Figure 30-16*B*). Perform neurovascular assessment of lower-extremity function every hour for the first 24 hours. Feel the lower extremities for warmth. Ask the child if he or she can feel you touch a foot. Ask the child to wiggle his or her toes. Neurologic dysfunction may result from bleeding or compression caused by a bone particle dislodged during the spinal fusion. Vital signs must be recorded carefully. Circulatory pressure changes resulting from realignment of the chest cage and reduced rotation of the spine may result in circulatory impairment. There is usually extensive blood loss during spinal fusion surgery. A drainage system, such as a Hemovac, may be inserted next to the incision to evacuate any accumulating drainage. The procedure itself or the blood loss may cause shock.

The child will have nothing by mouth until bowel sounds return. An indwelling urinary catheter is generally in place because voiding may be difficult due to the horizontal position that must be maintained and the edema at the lower spinal cord innervation points.

Even though the parents have been prepared for the fact that spinal fusion is major surgery, they may be shocked by the child's appearance after surgery. They may be afraid to touch the child to provide comfort. They may be unaware that although their child may be 14 or 15 years old, he or she would probably enjoy being touched now because of feeling so ill and frightened.

Gradually, pain is reduced, and the child can take fluids and then solids. Because of the need to maintain a dependent position following surgery, there may be a rapid release of calcium from bones. Calcium intake should,

MANAGING AND DELEGATING UNLICENSED ASSISTIVE PERSONNEL

Unlicensed assistive personnel may be assigned to care for children following scoliosis surgery. Be certain they understand that the child has had rods inserted next to the spine, so they cannot bend the back. Alert them that such surgery causes a high level of pain so they are responsive to children's requests for additional analgesia.

Unlicensed assistive personnel are also often assigned to help with the application or removal of casts in emergency departments or with the long-term care of children with chronic orthopedic disorders. Be certain they understand that cast applicaton must be followed by instructions on cast care and ways the child can take active measures to accommodate the cast to his or her life style.

Be certain they realize that most children with an orthopedic disorder do not feel ill; therefore, they need activities provided for them to occupy their time. If they are oriented to view this as a part of care, unlicensed assistive personnel can be instrumental in providing this type of activity.

therefore, be moderate at first rather than extensive to prevent renal calculi.

After 2 to 4 days, the child is allowed out of bed to sit up. He or she may feel very dizzy at first and must get used to sitting by attempting it for short periods at a time. Some children will have a body cast applied before hospital discharge to help ensure spinal fusion. Activity will be allowed gradually.

Instrumentation rods are left in place permanently unless they cause irritation later. Removing the rods is as extensive a procedure as inserting them. The average child will never be aware that they are in place. However, they must always be conscious of good posture (never slumping in chairs; stooping, not bending, to pick up objects from the floor). Extremely active gymnastics or trampoline work is contraindicated. The rods do not interfere with other sports or, although ovaries receive significant doses of radiation, with childbearing in girls.

Children may be afraid to move or behave normally following spinal fusion, because they have been in some type of restraining device for such a long time. They need time to readjust to the freedom of normal body movement. They may need to be reassured frequently that with the spinal fusion, their problem finally is corrected. No further curvature can occur after this point, so it is safe for them to be without support.

Correction of scoliosis may have taken years. Following surgery, children need an opportunity to talk at health care assessments about how they feel to be free of this problem. If the correction was not as complete as the child wished (children with severe scoliosis cannot expect 100% correction), they need time to talk about their disappointment and to adjust to their new appearance. They may feel that they have missed adolescence or "the best time of their lives." Emphasize positive experiences and point out positive attributes to help the adolescent gain self-esteem.

CHECKPOINT QUESTIONS

9. What are the two types of scoliosis?
10. Following spinal instrumentation surgery, how should the child be moved?

DISORDERS OF THE JOINTS AND TENDONS: COLLAGEN-VASCULAR DISEASE

Collagen is protein composed of bundles of fibers forming the connective tissue of the tendons, ligaments, and bones. Because this tissue is found throughout the body, collagen diseases are systemic. They also tend to be long term.

Juvenile Rheumatoid Arthritis

Juvenile rheumatoid arthritis (JRA) primarily involves the joints of the body, although it also affects blood vessels and other connective tissue. To be classified as JRA, symptoms must begin before 16 years of age and last longer than 3 months. The peak incidence occurs at two times in childhood: 1 to 3 years and 8 to 12 years. The cause of

TABLE 30.1 Comparing Different Types of Juvenile Rheumatoid Arthritis

CHARACTERISTIC	POLYARTHRITIS	PAUCIARTICULAR	SYSTEMIC ONSET
Number of joints involved	Five or more	Four or less	Any number
Joints affected	Usually small joints of fingers and hands Also possibly weight-bearing joints Often same joint on both sides of body	Usually large joints, such as knees, ankle, or elbow Usually particular joint on one side of body	Any joint
Sex affected	More girls than boys	More girls than boys (most common type)	Boys and girls equally
Body temperature	Low-grade fever	Low-grade fever	High spiking fever lasting for weeks or months
Other symptoms	Stiffness and minimal joint swelling, leading to limited motion Rheumatoid nodules or bumps on elbow or other body area receiving pressure from chairs, shoes, or other object (+)Rheumatoid factor (in approximately 20% of cases) (+)ANA titer (possible) Elevated white blood cell count, complement, and sedimentation rate	Iridocyclitis (eye inflammation) Painless joint swelling with little redness (+)ANA titer (possible) (+)HLA antigen (possible in boys)	Macular rash on chest, thighs Inflammation of heart and lungs Anemia Enlarged lymph nodes, liver, and spleen Rarely +rheumatoid factor and ANA titer Elevated white blood cell count

JRA is unknown, although it is probably an autoimmune process in which the child has developed circulating antibodies (immunoglobulins) against his or her own body cells. This is revealed by an antinuclear antibody level. T lymphocytes may also be involved in the process. A genetic predisposition may increase the risk in some people. JRA can occur in children as young as 6 months of age. It is slightly more common in girls than boys. Acute changes rarely continue past 19 years.

Three separate types of JRA exist. Major distinctions of these types are outlined in Table 30-1. Types differ mainly by the type of joint affected and the severity of systemic effects.

Assessment

Children with systemic JRA are often admitted to a hospital for diagnosis of their persistent fever and rash because these may be present before joint involvement is present. When arthritis is diagnosed, parents may be surprised, believing that arthritis is a disease of older adults only. Regardless of the type of JRA, assess children for signs and symptoms of the disease and for the effect their disease is having on self-care. (Do they need help eating, dressing, ambulating, or toileting?) Assess also the child's and parents' understanding of the illness and planned therapy. Children and parents typically bear the major responsibility for carrying out therapy at home.

Children with pauciarticular arthritis need to be screened every 6 months for uveitis (inflammation of the iris, ciliary body, and choroid membrane of the eye), because severe uveitis can lead to blindness (Boone et al, 1998).

Therapeutic Management

Because JRA is a long-term illness, therapy includes a balanced program of exercise, rest, and medication administration.

Exercise. To preserve muscle and joint function, a set program of physical activities to strengthen muscles and put joints through a full range of motion should be instituted. To reduce joint destruction, however, activities that place excessive strain on joints should be avoided. Running, jumping, prolonged walking, and kicking should be avoided if active lower extremity synovitis is present. School-age children can cooperate to avoid these activities. Parents of preschool children need to create interesting alternative activities so that the child avoids these motions.

Extremes of immobilization should also be avoided. To prevent this, children need to perform full range-of-motion exercises twice every day. It is best if these exercises can be incorporated into a dance routine or a game, such as "Simon says." This will make the exercise a family participation time to be anticipated rather than a dull routine that must be followed. Swimming and tricycle or bicycle riding are excellent activities to encourage because these provide smooth joint action. Encourage children to do as much self-care as they can because the natural motions of activities such as dressing and brushing teeth exercise joints.

Children should attend school if possible. Active children tend to show fewer contractures and less decalcification of bones than do inactive children. Children with JRA fatigue easily, however, and may need a shortened school day. If a school day is to be shortened, it is often better if the starting time is moved to midmorning. This allows the child time for a warm bath in the morning before school, which reduces the pain and increases movement of involved joints, and for rest after taking medications to minimize the inflammation. An activity such as sitting on a toilet may be uncomfortable if hip and knee joints are painful. An elevated toilet seat may be helpful because it reduces bending. Children may be unable to dress themselves independently because they cannot manage buttons or zippers with painful finger joints. Modifying these activities not only helps children feel good about themselves, but increases their overall level of activity.

Acutely inflamed joints should be rested passively and actively during the period of acute inflammation (Figure 30-17). To maintain muscle strength during this time, children may perform isometric exercises (exercises that do not change the length of muscles). Support inflamed joints in good body alignment, positioning large joints with pillows for support. To further prevent contractures, encourage children to sleep prone.

Heat Application. Heat reduces pain and inflammation in joints and increases comfort and motion. Heat can be applied by the use of warm water soaks for 20 to 30 minutes. Scheduling a hot bath on arising can help to eliminate stiff joints and make a child feel well enough to begin to function for the morning. Paraffin soaks can be useful for wrist and finger inflammation.

Splinting. Splinting is used to immobilize a joint in good body alignment. These are worn continuously during periods of active inflammation, even during sleep. If splints are removed, joints tend to assume a flexed, more comfortable position, possibly resulting in a contracture. Splints should not be worn once inflammation has subsided because the splint can actually cause a contracture and deformity with extended use.

Nutrition. Children with JRA, as with almost all chronic diseases, eat poorly because of anorexia, joint pain, and fatigue. Help parents plan mealtimes for "best times" of the day to overcome these problems.

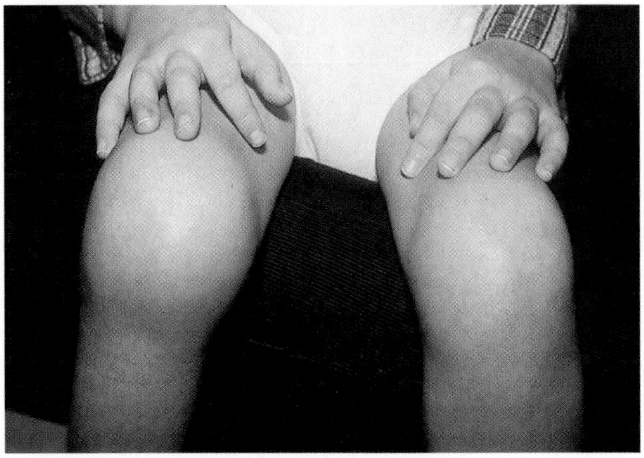

FIGURE 30.17 The knees of a child with juvenile rheumatoid arthritis. Note the degree of joint enlargement and swelling.

Medication. The NSAIDs are the drugs of choice for children with JRA. Those approved for use in children 12 years and older include tolmetin (Tolectin), naproxen, and ibuprofen. NSAIDs taken one to four times a day are used to control pain and inflammation, thereby reducing joint swelling, joint discomfort, and morning stiffness. They may contribute to improvement in malaise and irritability. NSAIDs must be taken for at least 6 to 8 weeks to ensure effectiveness.

Aspirin also may be used because it is both analgesic and anti-inflammatory. This is given in large doses three to four times a day. Educate parents that aspirin and NSAIDs may cause gastrointestinal upset and bleeding. Advise parents to give the medications with food. For example, have the child drink a glass of milk first. Most parents think of aspirin or NSAIDs as a drug to give children only when they have pain. Teach that they should continue to give it even if the child has no noticeable pain at the time of administration. Its anti-inflammatory action is important in preventing pain.

Slow-acting anti-inflammatory drugs (SAARDs), also called disease-modifying antirheumatic drugs, are used when NSAIDs have been ineffective. In contrast to the immediate pain relief or anti-inflammatory effect, these drugs modify the natural progress of the disease over weeks to months. Examples include gold salts, penicillamine, and hydroxychloroquinine.

Cytotoxic drugs, such as cyclophosphamide, azathioprine, chlorambucil, and methotrexate, may be used in children who have severely debilitating disease that has not responded to NSAIDs or SAARDs.

Steroids, such as prednisone, may be added to the drug therapy if the disease is severe or life threatening or is an incapacitating systemic disease that has not responded to other anti-inflammatory agents. Although they are the most potent anti-inflammatory drugs, they are avoided if at all possible because of the numerous adverse effects. When they are prescribed, usually the lowest possible dose given for the shortest time is the rule.

WHAT IF? A child with JRA states, "The school nurse told our class never to take aspirin because it causes Reye's syndrome." How would you respond?

NURSING DIAGNOSES AND RELATED INTERVENTIONS

Nursing Diagnosis: Knowledge deficit related to care necessary to control disease symptoms

Outcome Identification: Parents and child will demonstrate increased knowledge of care regimen within 1 week.

Outcome Evaluation: Parents and child follow instructions regarding exercise and medication.

Parents and children need to understand the necessity of taking an active role in therapy. Help them plan exercise and medication programs around school and other activities. Children with JRA are irritable and fatigue easily, which may interfere with the plans. Assist them with writing schedules that allow for a balance of rest periods with exercise to maximize the possibility of success.

Children with JRA need ongoing follow-up care to evaluate the disease and how they view themselves. Assist them with measures that allow them to view themselves as well again following such a long period of pain and illness. Children who are left with joint contractures may require soft-tissue surgery, such as contracture release, tendon reconstruction, and synovectomy, or orthopedic surgery, such as equalization of leg length and orthoplasty, at a later date. Surgery may be delayed until growth is complete so further growth will not influence the outcome.

About half of children with JRA will recover without joint deformity (Flato et al, 1998). One third will continue to have the disease into adulthood. About one sixth will be left with severe, crippling deformities after several years. Children need a great deal of support to perform exercises, wear splints, and take daily medication as prescribed. They need time set aside at health care visits to talk about how it feels to discover that the joints of the hands are gradually becoming more and more useless. Provide hope for recovery. Children may have difficulty following a therapy regimen if they see nothing ahead except complete disability.

✔ CHECKPOINT QUESTIONS

11. Does bracing for scoliosis always prevent the need for spinal surgery?
12. What type of drugs are the drugs of choice for treating JRA?

DISORDERS OF THE SKELETAL MUSCLES

Myasthenia Gravis

For nerve conduction to cause muscles to contract effectively, a neurotransmitter, acetylcholine, must be released at synaptic junctions. Myasthenia gravis is an interference in this process, leading to symptoms of progressive muscle weakness. The fault may be the impaired synthesis or storage of acetylcholine, insufficient acetylcholine release, blockage of acetylcholine factor present at motor end plates, or opposition of acetylcholine by an antiacetylcholine factor. The defect is probably a motor end plate insufficiency (a decreased number of acetylcholine receptors present). This probably occurs from an autoimmune process (autoantibodies may block receptor sites for acetylcholine) (Herrmann et al, 1998). There is some evidence of an inherited tendency. The thymus gland is usually enlarged in people with the condition, suggesting that thymopoietin may be overproduced, leading to neuromuscular blockage.

Assessment

If a mother has myasthenia gravis, an infant may evidence transient disease symptoms at birth from transfer of antibodies. The newborn is "floppy," sucks poorly, and has weak respiratory effort. Ptosis (drooping eyelids) may be present. The symptoms disappear within 2 to 4 weeks, but if not recognized when they occur, they may prove fatal because of respiratory difficulty.

If myasthenia gravis does not occur in the newborn period, the onset generally is delayed until the child is about 10 years old. The condition occurs more frequently in girls than boys (about 5:1). The child begins to notice symptoms of blurred or double vision (diplopia). Ptosis is present because of weakness of the extraocular muscles. Symptoms grow more intense as facial, neck, jaw, swallowing, and intercostal muscles become affected. There is extreme fatigue, becoming more noticeable as the day progresses. Symptoms increase with emotional stress, fatigue, menstruation, respiratory infections, and alcohol intake. In the most severe form, all muscles, including those of respiration, become paralyzed.

Obtaining an accurate history is important in diagnosis. On physical examination, children are asked to perform repetitive movements. If you ask a child to look upward and hold that position, he or she will gradually demonstrate ptosis. Most children will have myography performed to document the poor muscle function. Chest x-ray and a computed tomography scan demonstrate an enlarged thymus gland. Administration of edrophonium (Tensilon), which prolongs the action of acetylcholine and therefore increases muscle strength, renews exhausted muscles in a few minutes. If this occurs, the diagnosis is positive for myasthenia gravis.

Therapeutic Management

Myasthenia gravis is treated by the administration of anticholinesterase drugs, such as neostigmine (Prostigmin), which prolong acetylcholine action (see Drug Highlight). The dose of these agents must be individually determined. If toxicity occurs, it is similar to the symptoms of the original disease. Atropine is the antidote for an overdose of anticholinesterase drugs and should be available when the dosage is first being determined. In some children, prednisone may be added to their medication regimen to decrease the amount of anticholinesterase medication required. In some children, plasmapheresis to remove immune complexes from the bloodstream is effective in reducing symptoms. Excision of the thymus gland is rarely performed in children younger than 12 years because there is an increased risk of children developing neoplastic growths without a thymus gland.

Teach parents and children that symptoms become worse under stress. Parents will need to prepare children well for new experiences (menstruation, high school, a parental divorce, surgery) to minimize stress. Help children plan their day to include rest periods, possibly advocating for a special school schedule that allows for this. If chewing and swallowing are difficult, ensure a rest period before meals. Children may need to eat a soft diet and learn to eat slowly and cautiously to avoid choking and aspiration. Scheduling medication administration for about an hour before mealtime is often helpful. If symptoms of muscle weakness suddenly become very severe, children should be seen at a health care facility, because paralysis of intercostal muscles may lead to respiratory arrest.

DRUG HIGHLIGHT

Neostigmine (Prostigmin)

Action: Neostigmine is an antimyesthenic agent that increases the concentration of acetylcholine, prolonging and exaggerating its effects and facilitating neuromuscular transmission.

Pregnancy risk category: C

Dosage: Orally, 2 mg/kg daily in divided doses every 3 to 4 hours or 0.01 to 0.04 mg/kg per dose intramuscularly, intravenously, or subcutaneously every 2 to 3 hours as needed

Possible adverse effects: Salivation, dysphagia, nausea, vomiting, increased peristalsis, abdominal cramps, cardiac arrhythmias, increased respiratory secretions, urinary frequency, miosis, and diaphoresis

Nursing Implications:

- If ordered intravenously, administer the drug slowly directly into a vein or into the tubing's injection port of an intravenous infusion.
- Assess the child for increased muscle weakness, indicating possible cholinergic crisis. Keep atropine sulfate readily available as the antidote.
- If given orally, administer the drug with food or milk to minimize gastrointestinal upset. Instruct parents to administer the drug exactly as prescribed.
- Anticipate administering larger portions of the divided doses approximately one-half hour before times of greater fatigue.
- Review possible adverse effects with parents and child. Advise parents to watch for signs of excessive salivation, emesis, or frequent urination and to notify the health care provider if any occurs.
- Encourage parents to control the child's environmental temperature as much as possible to prevent diaphoresis from too hot or too humid an environment.
- Inform parents that an increase in muscle weakness may be related to drug overdose or exacerbation of the disease. Urge them to report any signs of increased weakness to the health care provider.

Dermatomyositis

Dermatomyositis involves degeneration of skeletal muscle fibers. The cause of the disorder is unknown. Symptoms generally begin insidiously with muscle weakness. Children are unable to perform tasks that they could manage previously, such as competing in gym classes, lifting objects, or climbing onto a high stool. Muscle pain is infrequent. Skin symptoms are present (swollen upper eyelids, a confluent rash on the cheeks that increases to become telangiectatic and scaling). Subcutaneous calcifications may appear, making the skin feel unusually firm. Muscle breakdown causes creatinine to appear in the urine. A muscle biopsy will reveal lack of electrical activity in muscle fibers. It is more common in girls, occurring between the ages of 5 and 14 years. Approximately 20% of children with this disorder have JRA.

Corticosteroids improve muscle strength. Immune globulins may also be helpful. Children who survive beyond the first year after diagnosis have a good prognosis for prolonged remissions. Unfortunately, many adults with dermatomyositis develop neoplastic complications.

Muscular Dystrophy

Muscular dystrophy is progressive degeneration of skeletal muscles, apparently from lack of a protein necessary for muscle contraction. It is a group of disorders that leads to gradual degeneration of muscle fibers. All the disorders are inherited.

Types

Congenital Muscular Dystrophy. Congenital muscular dystrophy is inherited as an autosomal recessive trait. The disease process begins in utero. The infant may be born with severe myotonia; muscle degeneration may make respiratory muscle movement difficult. Diagnosis is by serum enzyme analysis and muscle biopsy. Most of these infants die before they are 1 year old because they cannot sustain respiratory function.

Facioscapulohumeral Muscular Dystrophy. Facioscapulohumeral muscular dystrophy is inherited as a dominant trait, carried on the number 4 chromosome. Symptoms begin after the child is 10 years old. The predominant symptom is facial weakness. The child is unable to wrinkle his or her forehead and cannot whistle. Serum enzyme analysis and muscle biopsy are used in diagnosis. The symptoms generally progress so slowly that a normal lifespan is possible.

Pseudohypertrophic Muscular Dystrophy (Duchenne's Disease). Duchenne's disease, the most common form of muscular dystrophy, is inherited as a sex-linked recessive trait. Therefore, it occurs only in boys.

Assessment

Children generally have a history of meeting motor milestones, such as sitting, walking, and standing, later than the average infant. At about 3 years old, symptoms become acute and obvious. It is difficult to lift the young child with this condition by placing your hands under the axillae. The child seems to slip through your hands because of the lax shoulder muscles. In contrast, calf muscles are hypertrophied (measure larger than normal) because the muscles become so degenerated that they are replaced by fat and connective tissue (DeVivo & DiMauro, 1997).

Children have a waddling gait and have difficulty climbing stairs. They can rise from the floor only by rolling onto their stomachs, then pushing themselves to their knees. To stand, they press their hands against their ankles, knees, and thighs (they "walk up their front"); this is Gower's sign. They may walk on their toes, which leads to the development of a short heel cord. Speech and swallowing become difficult. Many boys with this type of muscular dystrophy show delays in meeting developmental milestones.

As the disease progresses, the muscle weakness becomes more pronounced. Scoliosis of the spine and fractures of long bones may occur from abnormal muscle tension and lack of muscle support. By junior high school age, most boys are confined to a wheelchair, unable to walk independently. Tachycardia occurs as heart muscle weakens and enlarges. Pneumonia develops easily as the child's cough reflex becomes weak and ineffective. Death from heart failure may occur at about 20 years.

The diagnosis is based on the history and physical findings, muscle biopsy showing fibrous degeneration and fatty deposits, electromyography showing a decrease in amplitude and duration of motor unit potentials, and an elevated level of serum creatine phosphokinase.

Therapeutic Management

Boys with muscular dystrophy should be encouraged to remain ambulatory for as long as possible. Help the child and family plan a program of active and passive daily range-of-motion exercises. Splinting and bracing may be necessary to maintain lower extremity stability and avoid contractures. If children become overweight, remaining ambulatory becomes more difficult for them. Encourage a low-calorie, high-protein diet to avoid this. To prevent constipation, encourage a high-fiber and high-fluid diet. Advocate for a stool softener if necessary.

Because the disease is progressive, assist the child and family with achieving the optimal level of activity within the child's limitations. Provide support and education to assist them with coping. Help children and parents locate a parent support group. Organizations such as the Muscular Dystrophy Association can be helpful in supplying information about the disease and support through the long period of illness.

✔ CHECKPOINT QUESTIONS

13. What is the underlying pathophysiologic problem associated with myasthenia gravis?
14. What is the most common form of muscular dystrophy?

INJURIES OF THE EXTREMITIES

Finger Injuries

It is not uncommon for a child to sustain a finger injury from a slammed car door. This injury, which causes a crushing blow to the tip of the finger, is excruciatingly painful. The fingernail may be lacerated and detached. As blood accumulates under an attached fingernail, pain continues to increase. An incision under the distal end of the nail or a stab wound through the attached nail helps to relieve pain. Fingernails often are lost following these injuries, but they grow back readily with little scarring. Reassure parents that although fingernails may be lost, the cosmetic effect will invariably not be a problem.

Parents may feel embarrassed and guilty when they bring in a child for this type of injury. The accident usually occurred because they closed a door without looking for the child's finger. They appreciate how much this hurts and are angry with themselves for being so careless. Reassure parents that this is a common childhood injury.

The fingertip will be x-rayed to make certain that the tip of the distal phalanx is not broken. The rule, "If the child can bend it, it's not broken," does not apply to this injury, because the fracture is often distal to the last phalangeal joint. Any open wound is cleaned well. If the distal phalanx is fractured, a splint should be applied to the finger. A follow-up visit is necessary to ensure that healing has occurred.

Bicycle-Spoke Injuries

Children who ride in child bicycle seats or over the back wheel of a bicycle can catch a foot or ankle between the spoke and the frame of the bicycle, resulting in a crushing, lacerating injury that quickly becomes edematous. Children can also injure their fingers in bicycle spokes. An x-ray is needed to rule out a fracture.

The wound usually is contaminated with spoke grease and needs cleaning with an appropriate antiseptic. It may be necessary to soak the area first with a solution of lidocaine, a local anesthetic, because of the amount of pain present. Sutures and a splint may be necessary. If it is a foot injury, the child may need to limit weight bearing by using crutches.

Soft-tissue injuries are painful. Edema and ecchymosis are extensive. Elevating the body part by propping it on pillows helps to reduce pain and edema. Such a major tissue injury may take up to 6 weeks to heal. Advise parents of this at the time of the injury. Otherwise, they may worry that the child's injury is not healing.

Fractures

A **fracture** is a break in the continuity or structure of bone. Because children experience falls during their growth years, fractures of long bones are common childhood injuries. Many fractures in early childhood are the greenstick variety (one side of a bone is broken; the other is only bent) because of the high resilience of immature bone. These fractures cause minimal pain, swelling, or deformity, the usual hallmarks of fracture. The various types of fractures are described in Table 30-2. Fractures in children tend to be different than in adults because of the following:

- Bone in childhood is fairly porous (allowing bone to bend rather than break).
- The periosteum is thick (causes greenstick fractures).
- Epiphyseal lines may cushion a blow so bone does not break.
- Healing is rapid as a result of overall increased bone growth.

Many fractures in children occur at the epiphyseal line. These are always serious fractures because bone growth occurs at this point. Damage to the area may lead to complications of bone growth (undergrowth, overgrowth, or uneven growth, resulting in angulation). If a child is involved in an accident that causes severe trauma, such as an automobile accident, compound (open) fractures may result. These are always serious injuries because the severed bone may lacerate nerves or blood vessels. The open wound may become infected, and correction will most likely involve a surgery with the risks of anesthesia.

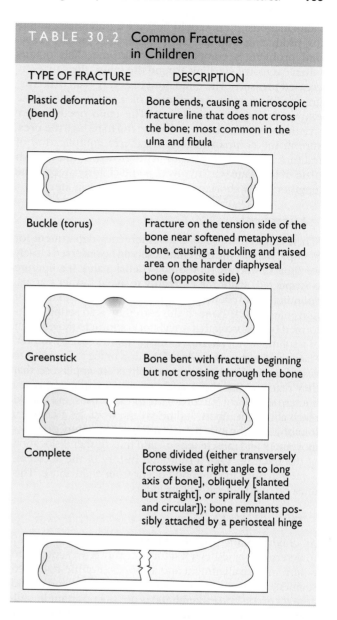

TABLE 30.2 Common Fractures in Children

TYPE OF FRACTURE	DESCRIPTION
Plastic deformation (bend)	Bone bends, causing a microscopic fracture line that does not cross the bone; most common in the ulna and fibula
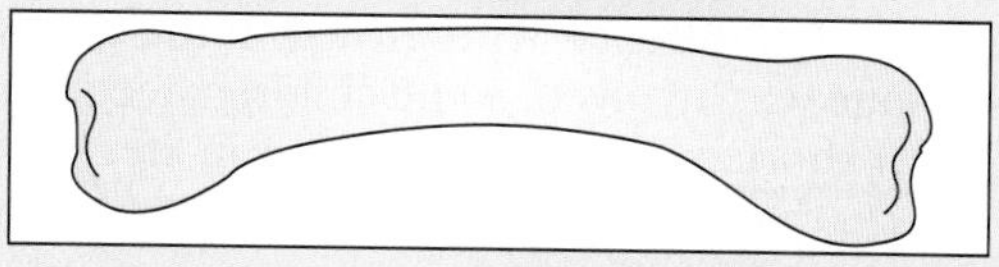	
Buckle (torus)	Fracture on the tension side of the bone near softened metaphyseal bone, causing a buckling and raised area on the harder diaphyseal bone (opposite side)
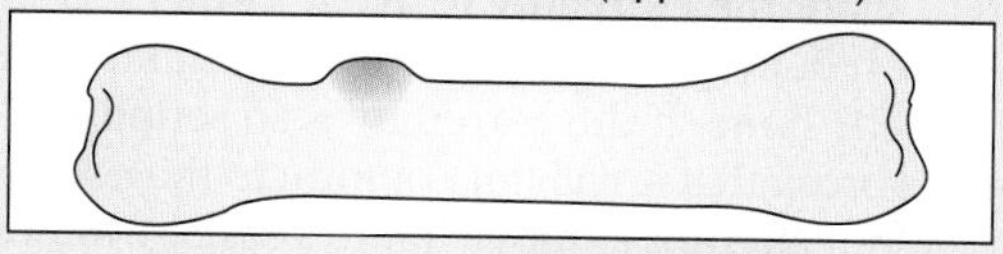	
Greenstick	Bone bent with fracture beginning but not crossing through the bone
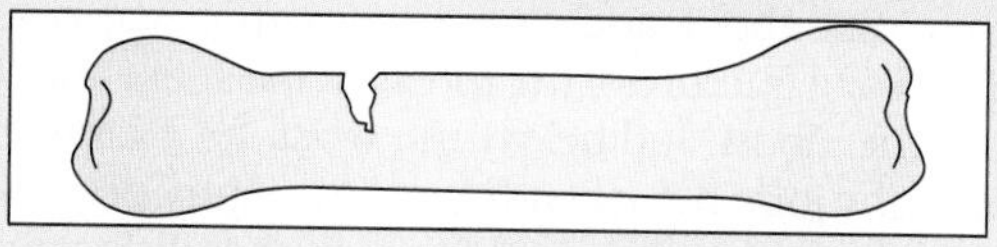	
Complete	Bone divided (either transversely [crosswise at right angle to long axis of bone], obliquely [slanted but straight], or spirally [slanted and circular]); bone remnants possibly attached by a periosteal hinge
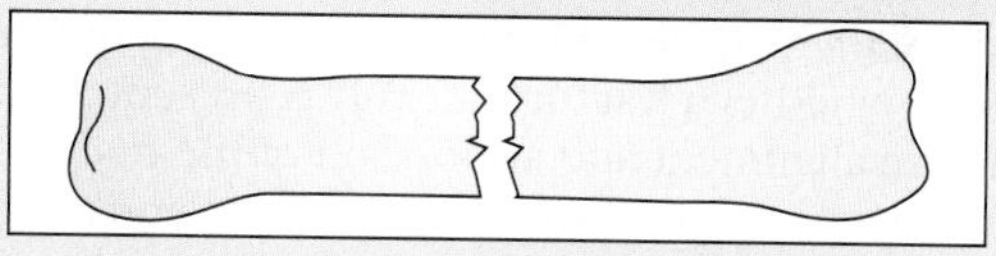	

If a fall is from a high distance or caused by a violent force, such as a speeding automobile, breaks may be complex or the formation may be compounded (the bone pierces the skin) or comminuted (the parts of the bone are fragmented).

Fractures heal relatively slowly compared with other body injuries. Immediately following a fracture, a hematoma forms at the site of the break; over the next several days, this is infiltrated by capillaries to lay down granulation tissue. Over the next several weeks, osteoblasts invade the new tissue, and calcium is deposited (termed *callus*) to form new bone. When callus formation is extensive (enough for movement at the fracture site to be impossible), clinical healing or clinical union has occurred. Complete healing does not occur until all the temporary callus formation has been replaced by mature bone cells and the bone has once more regained its normal shape and contour.

A number of complications may occur following traumatic fractures. One is fat embolus or the release of fat from the broken bone into the bloodstream. This can travel to the brain and cause symptoms of confusion or hallucinations. It also could become a pulmonary embolus, producing dyspnea, tachycardia, and cyanosis. A second problem is compartment syndrome. This occurs when excessive swelling around the injury site causes increased pressure. The child notices severe pain that is aggravated by passive stretching. Color and warmth of the extremity may remain normal. The child needs a constricting device such as a cast removed to reduce the pressure in the compartment. A long-term complication of fracture may be interference with growth if the growth plate of the bone was involved. Some children need bone lengthening or shortening procedures later in life.

Assessment

When children are seen in an emergency department for multiple trauma, the extremities should be observed closely for signs of fracture (deformity, edema, pain). If a fracture is suspected, splint the extremity to avoid further trauma. Splinting also reduces pain, because it prevents further movement of the bone. If the extremity is so seriously deformed by the break that it will not conform to the contour of a splint, do not attempt to move it into a splint position. Place sandbags on the sides of the arm or leg to immobilize it, and leave it in that position. Splints are applied so that they reach a joint above and a joint below the suspected fracture site. (For a fracture of the forearm, the splint should reach above the elbow and below the wrist, for example.) Immobilizing the joint below and above the injury prevents movement and muscle tension and thus further dislocation of the fracture. Take a thorough history of the accident. Some fractures in childhood occur from child abuse. This must be ruled out with all accidents.

Therapeutic Management

All children with a suspected fracture will need an x-ray to determine whether a fracture actually is present and to determine the alignment and apposition of the fractured segments of bone. **Apposition** (the amount of end-to-end contact of the bone fragments) is not as important in children as in adults. Bayonet or side-to-side apposition may be established or left in children up to 10 to 12 years old, because as the child grows and remodeling occurs, the bone will develop with normal contour and length. Side-to-side apposition results in a rapid, strong union and actually is the preferred position in some fractures.

If skin has been broken, children may need tetanus immunization. A hematocrit determination to estimate blood loss and cross-matching for replacement therapy may be necessary. An IV line is generally established to provide a route for fluid or blood replacement or for administration of an IV antibiotic to reduce the possibility of infection through the open wound.

All children with fractures are in some pain. Generally, they are frightened not only from the pain, the appearance of the fracture, and their inability to use the extremity, but also from the frightening situation that led to the fracture (a fall, an automobile accident). Spend time comforting and helping children to realize that they are now safe and will not be injured further. If they can relax enough to lie still and not move the fractured extremity, pain will decrease. When children have a compound fracture, they are as frightened at the sight of blood as they are of the deformity and pain. However, assure children and parents that unless the bone has been crushed, the bone fragments can be brought back into line. After this, the bone will heal with the same strength as before.

Forearm Fractures

Because a child often falls on an outstretched arm, fractures of the forearm are common. In children, most fractures of the forearm involve the distal third; a smaller number of such accidents occur in the middle or proximal third. The injury may involve a fracture of the radius, a fracture of both the radius and ulna, or a displacement of the epiphyseal plate of the radius. In young children, the injury usually is a greenstick fracture. Sometimes greenstick fractures are broken completely before casting to prevent the bone's resuming its "bent" position within the cast. Refer to this as "straightening" the bone, rather than "breaking" the bone. If a greenstick fracture is slight so that the degree of angulation is not great, it may not be reduced or brought into a straight line. As callus is formed and the bone remodels itself, it will naturally straighten into good alignment.

If the fracture is complete and overriding is excessive, traction to the fingers may be used as a part of the cast. This "banjo" traction is cumbersome and limits the child's use of that hand. With almost all casts, the hand is covered up to the first phalangeal knuckle to prevent the child from moving the hand excessively and damaging the edge of the cast, which will loosen it and put the arm into poor alignment.

Volkmann's Ischemic Contracture

When an arm is flexed and put into a cast, the radial artery and nerve may be compressed at the elbow, causing nerve injury or severe impairment of circulation. If the fracture is in the proximal third of the radius, the child generally is admitted to the hospital for 24 hours so that signs of circulatory or nerve impairment can be observed carefully.

If symptoms of compression are present but not detected within 6 hours, Volkmann's contracture and possible permanent damage to the arm will result. The arm is left permanently flexed at the elbow. The wrist is hyperextended, and the fingers assume a flexed, clawlike, useless position. If a child is going to be discharged following application of a cast, inform parents about the symptoms of compression so that its development can be detected. If a child is admitted to the hospital for 24 hours, the radial pulse (if palpable at the edge of the cast) should be taken hourly along with checks for coldness, blanching, and color for the first 8 hours. In some instances, the cast will be applied incompletely for 24 hours, the elbow portion just being splinted and wrapped with elastic bandages. After 24 hours, when edema has subsided and the chance of compression is less, the rest of the arm is casted.

Elbow Fractures

If a child falls and stops the fall with a hand, the elbow may hyperextend, transmitting the force of the blow to the distal humerus and causing a supracondylar fracture of the humerus. The fracture of the humerus is reduced and stabilized with an arm cast, a splint, or traction, depending on the position of the fracture. Although the fracture may be minor, the child is usually admitted to the hospital for overnight observation to prevent possible Volkmann's contracture. Elevate the cast on pillows or suspend the hand by a strip of gauze or traction apparatus to reduce edema.

Explain to parents why the child needs to be hospitalized so that they can keep the accident in perspective. The child is not being admitted because this is a serious fracture that will take an unusually long time to heal but because of the possibility of an immediate complication. If there is no indication of a complication within 24 to 48 hours and the arm can be casted, the child will be discharged.

Epiphyseal Separations of the Radius

When children break a fall with an outstretched arm, they may cause a separation of the epiphysis of the distal radius. When this occurs, the wrist must be casted to restabilize the epiphysis. Although epiphyseal injuries are always serious because injury to an epiphysis may cause growth disturbances, distal radial injury rarely causes serious sequelae in children. Advise parents that it is important to keep appointments for follow-up visits, however, so growth disturbances can be detected early and correction started. Stapling the epiphysis may be done to arrest abnormal growth if it occurs. Stimulation of the epiphyseal line may increase growth if growth retardation occurs (Rettig, 1998).

Clavicle Fractures

When young children fall and catch themselves with an outstretched arm, the force of the blow may be transmitted to the clavicle, causing fracture of the clavicle rather than of the arm. Clavicles also may be fractured during birth.

Swelling is often present at the site of the break. The child refuses to use the arm, and it hangs at the side. In the newborn, a Moro reflex is demonstrated only on the unaffected side. Newborns are treated by having the arm on that side immobilized against the chest. Following x-ray diagnosis, an older child is placed in a figure-eight splint of stockinet placed over the shoulders and under the armpits keeping the arm adducted and flexed across the chest. This is left in place for about 3 weeks. The child should keep it dry—no swimming or showering during this time. The parent often needs to tighten it every morning to keep it firmly in place. These stockinet wraps tend to get soiled in 3 weeks. Parents are usually apologetic about the appearance of the stockinet when they return for a repeat x-ray after 3 weeks; they are worried that the soiled appearance of the splint reflects the quality of their housekeeping or child care. Assure them that the soiled splint proves that they followed instructions well and left the splint in place for 3 weeks.

Parents may need reassurance that this splint is adequate therapy. They may ask, "The bone is broken, after all—why is my child not being placed in a cast?" Acknowledge their concern with a statement such as, "Most people think that when there is a broken bone, a cast is needed, but this is an exception." Doing so allows parents to voice their concern and receive further assurance.

Fracture of the Femur

Children who are involved in automobile accidents or who fall from considerable heights and land on their feet may suffer a fractured femur. Child abuse should be considered in an infant who sustains a fractured femur because there are few normal instances when this could occur in an infant.

Even if these fractures are closed so the skin is not broken, blood loss may be extensive because of the size of the bone broken. As the child lies on the examining table in the emergency department, the child holds the leg externally rotated; the thigh may appear abnormally short or deformed. Often the child is in a great deal of pain, possibly with signs of shock from pain and blood loss. Children are always frightened from the force of the accident that caused such a severe injury.

Fractured femurs usually cannot be casted immediately because strong tendon spasm causes poor alignment and overriding of the femur segments. Therefore, alignment must be initiated first by traction.

For a child younger than 2 years old, Bryant's traction is used (see Figure 30-8). For the older child with a fractured femur, skeletal traction with a pin through the distal femur is used. When muscle spasm has been reduced enough to allow close approximation of the bone edges and callus formation is good (7–14 days), the child is removed from traction and placed in a hip spica cast. A young child will remain in a cast for an additional 3 to 4 weeks. In older children, healing of a fractured femur requires an extended time. In a child who is 12 years old, firm union of the bone fragments will take about 12 weeks. Help the child and family identify ways for the child to continue school work and contact with friends if he or she is unable to attend school because of the large cast during this time.

Dislocation of the Radial Head

If a small child is lifted by one hand, as happens when a parent pulls on one arm to lift the child over a curb or up a step, the head of the radius may escape the ligament surrounding it and become dislocated (nursemaid's elbow). The child holds the arm flexed at the elbow with the forearm held pronated. The child winces with pain when the radial head is palpated.

A simple dislocation of the radial head can be reduced by a physician, using gentle pressure on the radial head while the arm is flexed and supinated. Relief of pain is immediate, and the child begins to use the arm again.

Assure parents that this is a common injury in small children. Parents feel guilty because they caused this dislocation. They rarely need to be cautioned that lifting a child in this manner is not wise. Be aware, however, that a dislocation of the radial head can occur from extremely rough handling as is seen in child abuse. Investigate the circumstances of the injury very closely.

Athletic Injuries

Knee Injuries

Participation in sports, such as football, skiing, or track, can cause knee injuries in children. As football increases in popularity with young children, knee injuries are occurring more frequently. These injuries generally involve the ligaments (the medial, lateral, posterior, or cruciate ligaments [figure-eight ligaments that stabilize the knee]) surrounding the knee. Following the injury, the child has severe pain in the knee with localized edema. An x-ray will be taken to rule out fracture (Landry, 1997).

If the injury is mild (only a few torn fibers), bedrest with ice applied to the knee is often the only therapy needed. Local infiltration of an anesthetic may be necessary to minimize pain. After 24 hours, heat is applied to the leg to hasten healing.

If the injury is more severe, the knee joint may fill with fluid. The child will need bedrest and ice applied to the joint. The abnormal synovial fluid will be aspirated, and a compression dressing will be applied to discourage accumulation of further fluid. After 24 hours, heat treatments will be started to hasten healing.

If the injury is severe, a cast may be applied for complete immobilization. It takes as long for a severe ligament injury to heal as it does for a bone fracture, so the cast will remain in place for about 8 weeks. Arthroscopy may be done to visualize and surgically repair the knee ligaments. Arthroscopic surgery makes repair of ligaments or cartilage a minor procedure and limits the necessity for immobilization and a cast.

A severe twisting motion to the knee may cause a dislocation of the kneecap (it moves to the posterior surface of the knee). The knee appears deformed, and the child is in acute pain. Immediate treatment for a dislocated kneecap is to slide it again to the front of the knee. Following this, the child will usually have to use a leg immobilizer for 1 week. If the problem is chronic or occurs frequently, surgery to strengthen the ligaments may be necessary.

Throwing Injuries

Throwing places repeated stress on the upper extremity, particularly the elbow joint. The injury tends to occur during the forward motion of the arm or the follow-through. Children are unable to extend their elbow completely because of minute tears and fibrous contractures in the muscle. They notice pain and tenderness and loss of complete elbow extension for 24 to 48 hours after the injury. Resting the arm and applying ice packs for 15 to 20 minutes three times a day relieves the pain. An antiinflammatory agent may be helpful. A limited number of cortisone injections into the elbow musculature may be helpful. Exercises to strengthen flexor muscles help to prevent this type of injury.

"Little Leaguer's elbow" is epiphysitis of the medial epicondylar epiphysis. Throwing curve balls and breaking pitches increases the stress in this area because of the forceful flexion and pronation required. An x-ray of the elbow may reveal increased growth, separation, and fragmentation of the medial epicondylar epiphysis. This injury may occur in as many as 95% of Little League pitchers between the ages of 9 and 14.

Children generally need extra protection against injury until the epiphyseal growth centers at the elbow have fused at 14 to 17 years of age. Children who participate in Little League sports need time for proper warm-up. They should be encouraged to refrain from throwing curve balls or breaking pitches and should be limited to pitching about six innings per week with a 3-day rest between games. Treatment for Little Leaguer's elbow is rest and immobilization until pain, tenderness, and limitation of movement have passed. If the injury is not treated adequately, permanent damage to the epiphyseal line and elbow deformity can occur.

Strains and Sprains

A strain is a muscle-tendon injury. A sprain is a ligament injury. Strained or sprained ankles are common but difficult childhood injuries. The joint is painful and swollen. They are typical injuries that occur with in-line skating (Jerosch et al, 1998).When the x-ray reveals no fracture, the child may feel as though someone has said that the injury is not serious but "just a sprain." He or she finds the extension of the swelling and pain baffling. Some children may be accused by parents of "putting on" pain, because the injury is "only a sprain."

Help the child and parents to understand that strains and sprains are truly painful. Because a cast is not used and an ankle is not immobilized completely, strains and sprains are often more painful than fractures, which are casted.

If the injury is recent, an ice pack should be applied for approximately 20 minutes at a time to reduce edema at the site. An elastic bandage may be applied for firm support. The child may be given crutches to limit weight bearing for the next 3 or 4 days. Make certain that the parents of the child understand how the elastic bandage is applied so that it can be rewrapped if it loosens and that the child is using the crutches properly before being discharged from the emergency department.

KEY POINTS

Bone and muscle disorders tend to be long-term disorders. Help children and their families to think about how the disorder will affect tasks of daily living to help the child better adjust to a cast or brace. Help children plan self-diversional activities as necessary so they continue to grow developmentally while confined to a cast or traction.

As a rule, if a bone is broken, children need additional calcium in their diet to aid bone healing. If they are on strict bedrest, however, this should only be a moderate addition to their diet to prevent renal calculi from forming.

Many children have casts applied to allow broken bones to heal. If broken bones are not easily aligned, children are placed in traction.

Developmental disorders that occur in children are flat feet (pronation), genu varum (bowlegs), and genu valgum (knock knees). The majority of these disorders are corrected naturally by normal growth.

Slipped epiphysis is slipping of the femur head in relation to the neck of the femur at the epiphyseal line. It occurs most frequently in obese or rapidly growing boys.

Osteomyelitis is infection of the bone. It can result in extensive destruction of the bone. Antibiotic therapy is necessary to combat the infection.

Scoliosis is a lateral curvature of the spine. It is treated by bracing or surgery.

Juvenile rheumatoid arthritis occurs in a number of different forms: polyarthritis, pauciarticular, and systemic onset. Therapy is exercise, heat application, splinting, and administration of medications, such as NSAIDs, methotrexate, or aspirin.

Myasthenia gravis can occur in a transient form at birth from transfer of antibodies from a mother with the illness or as a primary form later in childhood. Therapy is administration of anticholinesterase drugs, such as neostigmine (Prostigmin), that prolong acetylcholine action.

Muscular dystrophy is the inherited progressive degeneration of skeletal muscles. Different types that can occur are congenital, facioscapulohumeral, and pseudohypertrophic. Children and parents need long-term support throughout this long-term illness.

A fracture or bruise of soft tissue could have resulted from any trauma, including child abuse. Be certain to secure a detailed history of an injury to be certain that the history is consistent with the degree of injury.

Volkmann's ischemic contracture is a complication that occurs when an arm is casted in a bent position and a radial artery and nerve are compressed at the elbow. Frequent assessments of finger color and warmth are safeguards to prevent this from occurring.

CRITICAL THINKING EXERCISES

1. Jeffrey is the 10-year-old with osteomyelitis that you met at the beginning of the chapter. How would you explain what has happened to Jeffrey's mother? Develop a teaching plan to addresss this issue.
2. A 14-year-old wears a Milwaukee brace 23 hours a day for scoliosis. During the last month, she turned down an invitation to the high school prom and has dropped out of the high school band and the one after-school club to which she belonged. She tells you she is dropping activities to have more "time to study." Would you be concerned about her?
3. Your patient is a 3-year-old with JRA. You notice when he returns for a follow-up visit to the arthritis clinic that the inflammation in his joints is worse than at his last visit. He has a great deal of pain. His mother tells you she has been giving him acetaminophen instead of aspirin for therapy because her primary doctor said not to give aspirin to children younger than 18 years. How would you explain these contradictory instructions? Why do children with JRA receive aspirin?
4. A parent has three athletically inclined boys in grade school. She is concerned with guiding them into sports that will be safe for them during their growing years. What advice would you give her?

REFERENCES

Ablin, D. S. (1998). Osteogenesis imperfecta: a review. *Canadian Association of Radiologists Journal, 49*(2), 110.

Allington, N. J., & Bowen, J. R. (1996). Adolescent idiopathic scoliosis: treatment with the Wilmington Brace. *Journal of Bone and Joint Surgery, 78*(7), 1056.

Boone, M. I. et al. (1998). Screening for uveitis in juvenile rheumatoid arthritis. *Journal of Pediatric Ophthalmology and Strabismus, 35*(1), 41.

Cappello, T., & Song, K. M. (1998). Determining treatment of flatfoot in children. *Current Opinion in Pediatrics, 10*(1), 77.

Cote, P. et al. (1998) A study of the diagnostic accuracy and reliability of the Scoliometer and Adam's forward bend test. *Spine, 23*(7), 796.

Department of Health and Human Services. (1995). *Healthy people 2000: midcourse review.* Washington, DC: DHHS.

DeVivo, D. C., & DiMauro, S. (1997). Hereditary and acquired types of myopathy. In Johnson, K. B. & Oski, F. A. *Oski's essential pediatrics.* Philadelphia: Lippincott-Raven.

Draper, P. & Scott, F. (1998). Using traction. *Nursing Times, 94*(12), 31.

Flato, B. et al. (1998). Outcome and predictive factors in juvenile rheumatoid arthritis and juvenile spondyloarthropathy. *Journal of Rheumatology, 25*(2), 366.

Fordham, L. et al. (1998). Pediatric imaging perspective: acute limp. *Journal of Pediatrics, 132*(5), 906.

Hermann, D. N. et al. (1998). Juvenile myasthenia gravis: treatment with immune globulin and thymectomy. *Pediatric Neurology, 18*(1), 63.

Jerosch, J. et al. (1998). Injury pattern and acceptance of passive and active injury prophylaxis for inline skating. *Knee Surgery, Sports Traumatology, Arthroscopy, 6*(1), 44.

Kaeding, C. C., & Whitehead, R. (1998). Musculoskeletal injuries in adolescents. *Primary Care: Clinics in Office Practice, 25*(1), 211.

Landry, G. L. (1997). Sports medicine. In Johnson, K. B. & Oski, F. A. *Oski's essential pediatrics* Philadelphia: Lippincott-Raven.

Loder, RT. (1998). Slipped capital femoral epiphysis. *American Family Physician, 57*(9), 2135.

McCarthy, L. (1998). Safe handling of patients on cervical traction. *Nursing Times, 94*(14) 57.

Monk, M. (1998). Interviewing suspected victims of child maltreatment in the emergency department. *Journal of Emergency Nursing, 24*(1), 31.

Olson, R. S. (1996). Halo skeletal traction pin site care: toward developing a standard of care. *Rehabilitation Nursing, 21*(5), 243.

Payne, W. K., Ogilvie, J. W., Resnick, M. D., Kane, R. I. Transfeldt, E. F., & Blum, R. W. (1997). Does scoliosis have a psychological impact and does gender make a difference? *Spine, 22*(12), 1380.

Rettig, A. C. (1998). Elbow, forearm and wrist injuries in the athlete. *Sports Medicine, 25*(2), 115.

Sarwark, J. F. & Kramer, A. (1998). Pediatric spinal deformity. *Current Opinion in Pediatrics 10*(1), 82.

Sponseller, P. D. (1997). Bone, joint and muscle problems. In Johnson, K. B. & Oski, F. A. *Oski's essential pediatrics.* Philadelphia: Lippincott-Raven.

Wall, E. J. (1998). Childhood osteomyelitis and septic arthritis. *Current Opinion in Pediatrics, 10*(1), 73.

SUGGESTED READINGS

Bridwell, K. H. (1997). Spinal instrumentation in the management of adolescent scoliosis. *Clinical Orthopaedics and Related Research, 6*(335), 64.

Giannini, S. (1998). Operative treatment of the flatfoot: why and how. *Foot and Ankle International, 19*(1), 52.

Hergenroeder, A. C. (1998). Prevention of sports injuries. *Pediatrics, 101*(6), 1057.

Lindner, A. et al (1997). Outcome in juvenile-onset myasthenia gravis: a retrospective study with long-term follow-up of 79 patients. *Journal of Neurology, 244*(8), 515.

Lipp, E. J. (1998). Athletic physeal injury in children and adolescents. *Orthopaedic Nursing, 17*(2), 17.

Murray, D. J. et al. (1997). Transfusion management in pediatric and adolescent scoliosis surgery: efficacy of autologous blood. *Spine, 22*(23), 2735.

Myers, A., & Sickles, T. (1998). Preparticipation sports examination. *Primary Care: Clinics in Office Practice, 25*(1), 225.

Weinstein, S. L. (1997). Natural history and treatment outcomes of childhood hip disorders. *Clinical Orthopaedics and Related Research, 6*(344), 227.

Williams, C. J. et al. (1997). Hypercalcaemia in osteogenesis imperfecta treated with pamidronate. *Archives of Disease in Childhood, 76*(2), 169.

Zionts, L. E., & Shean, C. J. (1998). Brace treatment of early infantile tibia vara. *Journal of Pediatric Orthopedics, 18*(1), 102.

Nursing Care of the Child With a Traumatic Injury

31

CHAPTER

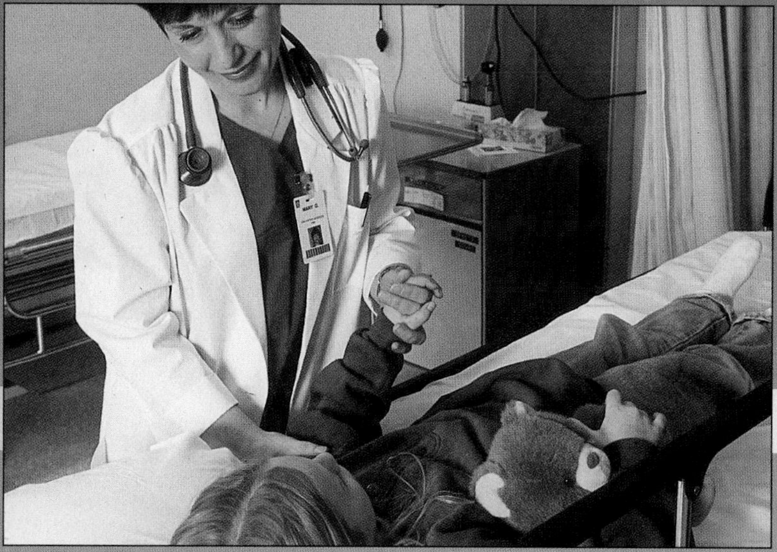

Key Terms

- allografting
- autografting
- bougie
- contrecoup injury
- débridement
- drowning
- escharotomy
- heterografts
- homografting
- near drowning
- otorrhea
- plumbism
- postural vertigo
- rhinorrhea
- stupor

Objectives

After mastering the contents of this chapter, you should be able to:

1. Describe the causes and consequences of common accidents and injuries in childhood and measures to prevent them.
2. Assess a child injured from an accident.
3. Formulate nursing diagnoses related to the injured child.
4. Establish appropriate outcomes for the injured child.
5. Plan nursing care related to the injured child.
6. Implement nursing care for the child with an injury.
7. Evaluate outcomes for achievement and effectiveness of care.
8. Identify National Health Goals related to children and trauma that nurses can be instrumental in helping the nation to achieve.
9. Identify areas related to care of children with traumatic injuries that could benefit from additional nursing research.
10. Use critical thinking to analyze ways that accidents and injuries can be prevented in childhood.
11. Integrate knowledge of injuries in childhood with nursing process to achieve quality child health nursing care.

Jason, a 4-year-old, is seen in the emergency room following an automobile accident. He is lethargic and stuporous, with the only visible signs of trauma being an area of the middle forehead that is red and edematous. Vital signs reveal the following: temperature, 99.4°F (37.5°C); respirations, 18; pulse, 62; and blood pressure, 110/62. His left pupil is more dilated than his right; it reacts sluggishly to light. His Glasgow Coma score is 8. "I'm sure he's not injured badly. He was wearing his seat belt," his mother tells you. You are the triage nurse. Would you rate Jason as a child to be seen immediately, or could he be given second priority?

In previous chapters, you learned about the growth and development of well children and care of the child with a disorder of other body systems. In this chapter, you'll add information about the characteristic changes, both physically and psychosocially, that occur when children experience a traumatic injury. This is important information because it provides a base for care and health teaching.

After you've studied the chapter, turn to the Critical Thinking Exercises at the end of the chapter to help sharpen your skills and test your knowledge.

Accidents cause more deaths in the 1- to 4-year age group than the next six most prevalent diseases combined. In the 15- to 24-year age group, they cause more deaths than all other combined causes. If accidents could be prevented, a major cause of childhood morbidity and mortality would be eliminated. Accident reduction is certainly a realistic goal. However, total elimination may not be possible, because many children believe that accidents will not happen to them and do not take sensible precautions against them. Some parents lead children into accidents by overestimating their development and giving them responsibility beyond their capabilities.

Family stress plays a large role in childhood poisoning accidents. In a classic study, Sobel (1970) compared the home environments of children who had poisoned themselves with those of matched children with no poisoning history. This study looked at the availability of poisons and the presence of stress in the house. The results showed that both types of houses had poisons available. The families in which poisonings occurred, however, had more stress factors, such as illness of the mother, marital discord, or illness in another family member. Eliminating accidents in children, therefore, is not a simple procedure, because it involves reducing family stress as well. National Health Goals related to children and trauma are shown in the Focus on National Health Goals box.

The frequency of different types of accidents varies according to age group (Table 31-1). Because the anatomy and physiology of children are different from those of adults, they are affected by accidents differently than adults.

NURSING PROCESS OVERVIEW

for Care of the Child With a Traumatic Injury

Assessment

When children are seen at health care facilities because of accidents, neither they nor their parents may be at their best because of the stress of the situation. They may be apprehensive and frightened not only about what *has* happened, but also about what could have happened. Children often feel guilty and are afraid that they will be scolded or punished. Their parents may feel equally guilty; for example, they may

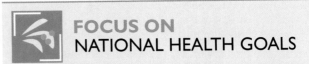

FOCUS ON NATIONAL HEALTH GOALS

A number of National Health Goals are concerned with trauma and children:

- Reduce homicides to no more than 3.1/100,000 in children aged 3 and younger and 1.4/100,000 in persons aged 15–34 from baselines of 3.9 and 1.7/100,000, respectively.
- Reduce assault injuries among people aged 12 and older to no more than 10/1000 people from a baseline of 11.1/1000.
- Reduce by 20% the incidence of weapons-carrying by adolescents aged 14 through 17.
- Reduce residential fire deaths to no more than 3.3 per 100,000 children aged 4 and younger from a baseline of 4.4/100,000.
- Reduce drowning deaths to no more than 2.3/100,000 children aged 4 and younger from a baseline of 4.2/100,000.
- Increase to at least 50% the proportion of primary care providers who routinely provide age-appropriate counseling on safety precautions to prevent unintentional injury (DHHS, 1995).

Nurses can be instrumental in helping the nation achieve these goals by being primary care providers who provide counseling on safety precautions to parents and children. Additional nursing research would be helpful in areas such as the following: what are effective ways to communicate safety information to parents at well child visits when time is at a premium; what ways should safety teaching given after an accident to prevent a further accident be different from that given as primary prevention; and is there an association between children setting fires and their exposure to fire experiences with fireplaces or candles?

TABLE 31.1 Most Frequent Accidents in Children by Age Group

AGE (y)	TYPE OF ACCIDENT
0–1	Falls, inhalation of foreign objects, poisoning, burns, drowning
1–4	Falls, drowning, motor vehicles, poisoning, burns
5–9	Motor vehicles, bicycle accidents, drowning, burns, firearms
10–14	Motor vehicles, drowning, burns, firearms, falls, bicycle accidents
15–18	Motor vehicles, drowning, falls, firearms

feel that if they were really "good" parents, they would have been watching more closely. They may feel defensive because they are worried about being criticized. People under stress do not hear well and may not perceive correctly the information given to them. Information they receive in the emergency department may be grossly misinterpreted or not heard at all.

Children are likely to be in pain. They are frightened not just from the pain of the injury, but also from the circumstance of the injury. Children count on their parents to keep them safe, yet they have been hurt. The trust is broken momentarily. How can they be safe here if their parents no longer are protecting them?

Assess children's conditions quickly when they are first seen. They may be seriously hurt and not cry because they are in shock. They may be hemorrhaging, but if they are bleeding internally, blood may not be evident. Because the emergency department nurse is often the first person who sees a child after an injury, be ready to make a preliminary assessment of the extent of the child's injuries before a physician arrives. Accidents become fatal when lung, heart, or brain function becomes inadequate. These three body systems, therefore, must be evaluated first. Table 31-2 lists signs and symptoms to assess to determine the respiratory, cardiovascular, and neurologic status of an injured child.

TABLE 31.2 Important Assessments on Initial Examination of an Injured Child

BODY SYSTEM	ASSESSMENT
Respiratory system	Quality of respirations
	Rate of respirations
	Sound of obstruction (wheezing, stridor, retractions, coughing?)
	Color (cyanotic?)
	Oxygen hunger (restlessness, inability to lie flat?)
Cardiovascular system	Color (pallor from hemorrhage or cardiovascular collapse?)
	Gross bleeding
	Pulse rate (increases with hemorrhage)
	Blood pressure (decreases with hemorrhage)
	Feeling of apprehension from altered vascular pressure
Nervous system	Level of consciousness (child answers questions coherently?; infant attunes to parent's voice?)
	Pupils (equal and reacting to light?)
	Bumps or bruises on head or spinal column
	Loss of motion or sensory function in a body part

While you conduct a preliminary assessment of a child's major body systems, take a brief history of the accident. What happened? How long ago did it happen? What have the parents done? If the child fell, how far did he or she fall? On what body part did the child land? (A head injury is more likely to be serious than an ankle injury, although a child may be in more pain and have more obvious symptoms with the lesser injury.) Ask parents what they think are a child's major injuries. Children may complain about one body part at first, but then a small cut elsewhere begins to bleed, and they focus on the minor bleeding as their major injury. If parents say, "At first, he acted as if his stomach hurt," this may be the first suggestion that he has a splenic rupture.

It is often difficult to evaluate children in an emergency department, because they are so frightened that they cannot stop crying to report which body parts are painful or to indicate which parts should be assessed first. A few minutes spent attempting to calm children and get them past this initial fright is time well spent unless symptoms of major body system disturbances require that you direct your immediate efforts elsewhere. Parents need frequent explanations of care given or planned, because as long as they are worried and tense, children cannot be calmed easily.

A proportion of traumatic injuries in children result from child abuse. Ask yourself if this could be a possibility (see Chapter 34).

Nursing Diagnosis

The nursing diagnosis used most frequently with injured children is Pain. Depending on the particular injury, a number of other nursing diagnoses are relevant, as are those that relate to the suffering that parents experience when their child is injured. Examples of possible nursing diagnoses include the following:

- Ineffective airway clearance related to burned esophageal tissue
- Impaired mobility related to severe burn injury
- Body image disturbance related to change in physical appearance with thermal burns
- Parental fear related to outcome after head injury in child
- Altered family processes related to child's accident
- Anxiety related to apprehension and lack of knowledge regarding medical treatment of child

Outcome Identification and Planning

Parents in an emergency department are rarely ready for long-term planning. They have great difficulty in coming up with answers even to the most straightforward questions. Establishing outcomes is often difficult with injured children because both they and their parents are too frightened to plan. Long-term planning may have to be delayed until the immediate concern of the injury has passed.

On discharge from the emergency department, parents need printed instructions about the child's care at home and whom to call if they have questions about care or progress. They also need an appointment (or the number to call for a return appointment) for follow-up care. If the child is admitted to the hospital from the emergency department, it is helpful if the nurse who cared for the child in the emergency department can accompany him or her to the hospital unit. The first people who care for a child after an injury become very important to the child and parents. Parents have difficulty letting them go and accepting new caregivers. A transition period, a "passing on of care," helps a parent to accept the child's new caregivers as being as dependable and trustworthy as the emergency department staff.

Implementation

The extent of a child's injury depends on the injuring agent, the part of the body injured, and often the immediate care, including both physical and psychological management.

The diameter of the airway in children is smaller than in adults, so an injury to this body area almost always will result in a greater danger of airway closure than in adults. This could happen from the child inhaling a substance, such as water, that directly obstructs the airway or from inhaling toxic fumes that cause inflammation along the lining of the airway, resulting in obstruction. A blow to the neck can result in edema of surrounding tissues, pushing the airway closed.

Most injuries involve some blood loss. Fortunately, a child's circulatory system is capable of rapid compensation for blood loss by vasoconstriction. Because the total volume of blood in a child is reduced, however, blood loss in children is always potentially serious.

Often, large portions of the child's body must be exposed to view so that care can be easily given. This means that rapid cooling can occur. Because of the large body surface area of children in relation to weight, always be conscious of body temperature and take active measures to decrease cooling by keeping the child covered as much as possible during examination times.

Parental consent must be obtained for treatment procedures even in an emergency, except for life-saving actions, such as cardiopulmonary resuscitation procedures. In these instances, action can and should be taken to save the child's life with or without parental permission (it is assumed that parents would consent to life-saving procedures). Delaying emergency procedures until parents can be located may result in permanent disability or death. Standard precautions are maintained in emergency situations, the same as at any other time.

A part of nursing intervention in an emergency department should be helping parents to understand why an injury happened and helping the parents plan ways to make their house or community safe for children.

Outcome Evaluation

After an injury, children need follow-up care to be certain that the immediate interventions were adequate and that healing is taking place. Evaluation visits are also the time to determine if the child's environment has been changed and is safer now than at the time of the accident (if applicable). At that time, parents may have been too anxious to hear health supervision information. Now, with the accident behind them, they are ready for such information and prepared to make changes.

When an injury could not have been anticipated, parents appreciate hearing one more time that such an accident could not have been avoided and that they are good parents. This helps them maintain adequate self-esteem to continue to function well as parents.

Examples of outcome criteria follow:

- Child is able to swallow fluids without distress following esophageal burns.
- Child states pain is at tolerable level within half hour.
- Child has full range of motion in hand following thermal injury.

HEALTH PROMOTION AND RISK MANAGEMENT

Nurses in every care setting have the unique opportunity among health care professionals to provide child and family teaching concerning the prevention of accidents. Even in the acute care setting when an accident has already occurred, nurses can provide invaluable instruction to families about safeguarding their children against future accidents. In the community setting, nurses have a greater opportunity for assessment of the unique threats present in particular environments, for example, lead-based paint in older homes, the presence of kerosene heaters in a home, and the risk of drowning in a home that has a swimming pool. Nurses, therefore, need to be knowledgeable about the interventions to be used and the measures to prevent injury. Instructing families in prevention requires a broad awareness of older and more modern threats in the environment.

Poisoning is frequently the cause of serious injuries in children younger than 6 years. Common household agents are often the cause. Since the Poison Prevention Packaging Act of 1970, potentially hazardous products are sold in child-resistant containers. Passage of this Act initiated a decrease in the incidence of childhood poisonings.

The home environment may still contain products that may be hazardous and poisonous to children if handled improperly. Plants, cosmetics, and cleaning products, although harmless to adults, may be considerably dangerous to children if ingested or absorbed through the skin. Parents must be made aware of these dangers and taught strategies for maintaining a safe home environment. This includes knowledge of basic first aid.

Measures for a safe home environment include child-resistant locks on low cabinets where household products are stored and moving plants to a higher surface or removing them from the home until the child is older. In addition, parents should anticipate that an accident may occur. Even in the safest environment, a child can be injured. Along with knowledge of basic first aid, the phone number of the local poison control center should be posted by the phone. Parents should also have an emergency first aid kit and syrup of ipecac on hand (see Drug Highlight box later in the chapter).

CHECKPOINT QUESTIONS

1. What types of accidents are the most common in children between the ages of 5 and 9 years?
2. What legislation has contributed to a decrease in the number of childhood poisonings?

HEAD TRAUMA

Children receive head injuries when they are involved in multiple trauma accidents, such as automobile accidents. Falls from swing sets, porches, and bunk beds also cause many head injuries. Sometimes children are struck on the head by an object, such as a baseball, rock, or hockey puck, or fall from a bicycle (see the Focus on Nursing Research).

Head injuries are serious not only because they cause an immediate life threat to the child, but also because a number of complications may follow. With a depressed skull fracture, the incidence of recurrent seizures after the injury is as high as 30% to 60%. Recurrent seizures occur primarily in children who were unconscious for longer than 24 hours or who had convulsions during the acute phase of illness (Rosman, 1997). Many of these children show focal abnormalities on an electroencephalogram (EEG). A number of children with seizure involvement will have a normal EEG, however, so by itself, EEG is of limited value in predicting post-traumatic seizures.

Some children experience memory deficits or minor personality changes after head injury. Symptoms such as headache, irritability, and **postural vertigo** (sensation of faintness or an inability to maintain normal balance—also known as posttrauma syndrome) also may occur. Behavioral manifestations may include aggressiveness or poor school performance (Cattelani et al, 1998). It often is difficult to determine whether these symptoms are organic or the result of being treated differently than usual by anxious parents.

FOCUS ON NURSING RESEARCH

How Can Iron Burns to the Hand Be Better Prevented?

Burns from irons can be serious in children in that they result in both functional and cosmetic deformities. For this study, the charts of 82 pediatric patients who had had iron burns to the hand were reviewed. Results showed that most injuries occurred in low-income, single-parent, single-child households. They tended to occur most commonly in male children under 2 year of age. Although most burns were minor partial-thickness and treated in the outpatient setting with no adverse effects, 15% of children experienced full-thickness burns that required grafting. Ten percent of children developed complications such as hypertrophic scarring and scar contracture. The researchers recommend that parents be better educated about the consequences that can result from leaving a child unattended in the presence of a hot iron.

This is an important study for nurses as nurses are the people most apt to discuss household safety measures with parents. Cautioning them that iron burns can leave significant impairment in a child could help to reduce the incidence of this common childhood injury.

Brown, R. L., Greenhalgh, D. G., & Warden, G. D. (1997). Burn prevention forum: iron burns to the hand in the young pediatric patient: a problem in prevention. *Journal of Burn Care and Rehabilitation, 18*(3), 279.

Immediate Assessment

All children with head trauma need an assessment of neurologic function as soon as they are seen and at frequent intervals to detect increased intracranial pressure. Increasing pressure will put stress on the respiratory, cardiac, and temperature centers, causing dysfunction in these areas. With increased pressure, the pupils become slow or unable to react immediately. Level of consciousness and motor ability decrease, pulse rate decreases, respiratory rate decreases, and temperature and pulse pressure increase.

Assess vital signs to detect changes in these areas, and observe children's pupils to be certain that they are equal and react to light. Assess children's level of consciousness and motor function. Stabilize the neck with a brace until cervical trauma has been ruled out.

Immediate Management

After a head injury, brain edema is likely because fluid rushes into the inflamed and bruised area. A central venous line and arterial line may be inserted. Intracranial pressure monitoring may be begun (see Chapter 28). A CT scan or magnetic resonance imaging (MRI) will be ordered to determine areas of edema or bleeding. An attempt may be made to decrease brain edema by intravenous administration of a hypertonic solution, such as mannitol. This will increase intravascular pressure and shift edema fluid back into the blood vessels. Steroids such as dexamethasone may be added to decrease inflammation and edema. Keeping the hand elevated about 30 degrees, intubation, and hyperventilation (keeping the PCO_2 below 25 mm Hg) are also effective in reducing intracranial pressure (Kochanek et al, 1997).

NURSING DIAGNOSES AND RELATED INTERVENTIONS

Nursing Diagnosis: Risk for fluid volume excess related to administration of hypertonic solution

Outcome Identification: Child will remain free of effects of increased fluid load during the course of treatment.

Outcome Evaluation: The child's respiratory rate remains between 16 to 24 per minute; specific gravity of urine is between 1.003 and 1.030; pulse remains between 60 to 100 beats per minute; blood pressure will remain consistent for age group; lungs are clear to auscultation.

When hypertonic solutions are being infused into children, assess vital signs frequently to be certain that the fluid load being called into the intravascular system does not overtax it. This fluid must be excreted by the kidneys to keep the vascular system from being overloaded. Keep accurate intake and output records, and test the specific gravity of urine to detect the development of pituitary compression and resultant overproduction or underproduction of antidiuretic hormone from the posterior pituitary.

Nursing Diagnosis: Risk for altered growth and development related to late sequelae of head injury

Outcome Identification: Child will maintain normal function following head trauma.

Outcome Evaluation: Child shows no evidence of any alteration in thought processes, seizure activity, or memory at follow-up visits. Cognitive and physical development are appropriate for age.

Helping care for the child with a head injury may be difficult for parents because they are so worried. Offer information on the child's progress as it is available to you. Urge parents to help care for the child to increase their sense of control.

It is important during the acute phase of illness that parents be informed about the dangers of trauma. If they ask about the possibility that personality changes or seizures will develop later in life, their questions should be answered truthfully. At the same time, don't give unnecessary warnings about observing the child carefully in the months to come. Head injuries by themselves are worrisome enough to parents and children without adding to their burden.

Skull Fracture

A skull fracture is a crack in the bone of the skull. It is important that skull fractures be recognized in children, because associated cerebral injury often occurs under the fracture. Many skull fractures are simple linear types, most often involving the parietal bones. In some children, the skull does not fracture, but the suture lines separate. This occurs more commonly in the lambdoid suture line; a coronal suture separation is rarer and, if present, indicates severe trauma (Figure 31-1).

Assessment

If the base of the skull is fractured, children generally have orbital or postauricular ecchymosis. They may have **rhinorrhea** or **otorrhea** (clear fluid draining from the nose or ear). This is escaping cerebrospinal fluid—a serious finding, because it means the child's central nervous system is open to infection. Nasal discharge may be tested with a glucose reagent strip if there is doubt about the source of the drainage. Cerebrospinal fluid will be positive for glucose, whereas the clear, watery drainage of an upper respiratory tract infection will not.

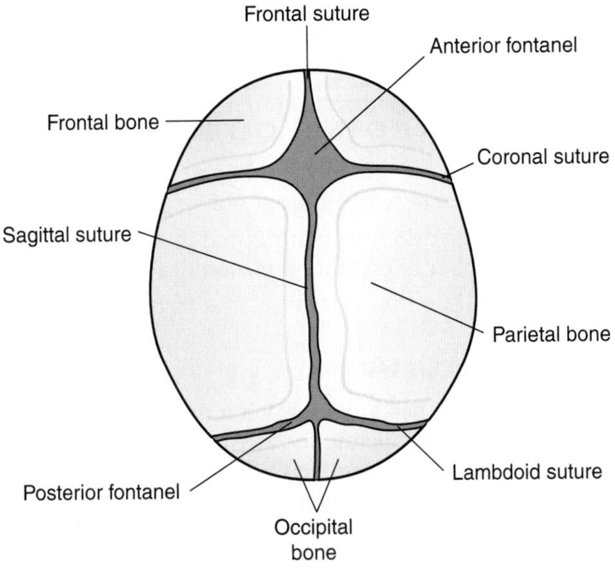

FIGURE 31.1 Location of sutures.

Skull fractures are confirmed by skull x-ray. Take a careful history of the accident so that the strength of the blow to the head can be judged. Shock rarely occurs with an isolated head injury. If children are in shock, bleeding points other than the head injury should be investigated.

If a skull fracture is linear with no underlying pathology, no treatment except observation and prescription of an analgesic is necessary. In about 3 weeks, children need a repeat x-ray to confirm that healing has taken place. Parents can be assured that a second x-ray this soon is not harmful but necessary.

If a fracture is depressed (a bone fragment is pressing inward) or compounded (bone is broken into pieces), surgery will be necessary. Cranial surgery is discussed in Chapter 28.

Therapeutic Management

If cerebrospinal fluid is draining from the nose, children will be hospitalized. Keep them in a semi-Fowler's position so fluid drains out, not inward, to reduce the possibility of introducing infection. Make certain that they do not attempt to hold their nose or pack their nostrils with something to halt the drainage. Because coughing and sneezing may allow air to enter the meningeal space, coughing may be suppressed by medication. If the drainage is excoriating to the upper lip, coat the space with petrolatum. Children may be placed on a prophylactic antibiotic to reduce the risk for meningitis. If the drainage does not stop within a few days, surgery will be necessary to repair the fracture and reduce the danger of meningitis. Air that enters intracranial spaces generally is absorbed rapidly. If x-rays at 72 hours still show air in the cerebral spaces, it implies that a skull defect remains. Surgery may be indicated to close the defect.

Potential Complications

A long-term complication of even a linear fracture may be a *leptomeningeal cyst.* This results from projection of the arachnoid membrane into the fracture site. With the interfering tissue, bone cannot heal and actually erodes so that the fracture site becomes progressively larger, not smaller. This will be evident on a follow-up x-ray. It may be suspected if a child develops focal seizures or symptoms of increased intracranial pressure. The defect may be palpated on the skull as an underlying indentation. Surgical resection will be necessary to remove the cyst.

Subdural Hematoma

Subdural hematoma is venous bleeding into the space between the dura and arachnoid membrane (Figure 31-2*A*). It occurs when head trauma lacerates minute veins in this area. The collection of blood generally is bilateral.

Subdural hematomas tend to occur in infants more than older children. Symptoms may occur within 3 days of trauma or as late as 20 days. Infants generally have symptoms of increased intracranial pressure. Seizures, vomiting, hyperirritability, and enlargement of the head may occur. Anemia from the substantial blood loss is a prominent sign. Angiocardiography or sonogram will reveal the extent of the hematoma.

In infants, accumulated subdural blood may be removed by a subdural puncture through the lateral aspect of a patent anterior fontanelle. The procedure is similar to a lumbar puncture. Infants must be held extremely still during the procedure so that they do not move and cause the aspiration needle to be inserted incorrectly. Half of the success of subdural puncture depends on the ability of the person to hold the child still.

Subdural punctures may have to be repeated daily to empty the subdural space. When the space is empty, it will be occluded by expanding brain tissue. If the space has not been occluded after 2 weeks of daily punctures, active bleeding is still present, and surgery generally is necessary to reduce the space and halt bleeding.

In older children, surgery generally is necessary because the anterior fontanelle is closed, and the space cannot be reached by puncture.

Epidural Hematoma

Epidural hematoma is bleeding into the space between the dura and the skull (Figure 31-2*B*). This happens when head trauma is severe. Subdural hemorrhage is generally venous bleeding, but epidural hemorrhage is usually a result of rupture of the middle meningeal artery and is therefore arterial bleeding. It usually is intense and causes rapid brain compression.

At the time of the injury, children are usually momentarily unconscious. They then regain consciousness and, to the untrained eye, appear to be well for minutes or hours. Then signs of cortical compression—vomiting, loss of consciousness, headache, convulsions, or hemiparesis (paralysis on one side)—are observed. On physical examination, unequal dilatation or constriction of the pupils may be pres-ent. Decorticate posturing (see Chapter 28) may be seen, indicating that there is extreme pressure on upper cortical centers. If the pressure is allowed to continue unchecked, cortical compression may be so

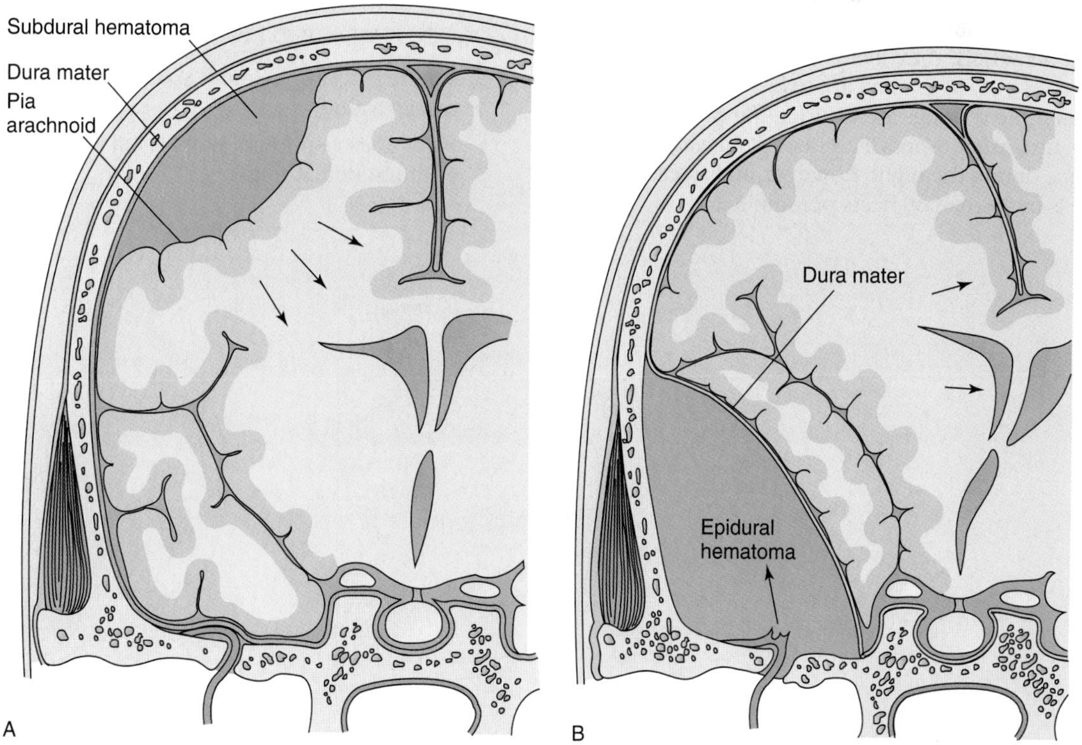

FIGURE 31.2 (**A**) Subdural hematoma. The dark area in the upper left area of the drawing is the hematoma. Note the shift of structures. (**B**) Epidural hematoma. The dark area in the lower left area of the drawing is the hematoma. Note the broken blood vessel and the shift of midline structures.

great that brain stem, respiratory, or cardiovascular function is impaired.

As a rule, the closer to the time of the injury that symptoms of compression occur, the more extreme the amount of blood loss. The treatment is surgical removal of the accumulated blood and cauterization or ligation of the torn artery. The earlier the process is recognized and treated, the lesser the chance of residual damage from extreme pressure or anoxia to a brain portion.

Concussion

Concussion is defined as a head injury from a hard, jarring shock. Concussion may occur on the side of the skull that was struck (a *coup injury*) or on the opposite side of the brain (a **contrecoup injury;** Figure 31-3). As the brain recoils from the force of the blow and strikes the posterior surface of the skull, this second injury occurs. Children have at least a transient loss of consciousness at the time of the injury. They may vomit and may show irritability after regaining consciousness. They may have a convulsion within minutes of the trauma. They typically have no memory (amnesia) of the events leading up to the injury or of the injury itself. For some children, being asked questions about the accident is extremely upsetting because they do not remember anything that happened and feel a frightening loss of control. The child requires a skull x-ray to rule out skull fracture and observation for 24 hours to rule out severe brain trauma, edema, or laceration. The child usually can be observed at home by the parents, who are instructed to rouse him or her every 1 to 2 hours to check the level of consciousness (Roddy et al, 1998).

To be certain that children are alert, they should be asked to name a familiar object, such as a favorite toy, or to name the color of some object shown to them. Telling parents their name or where they live is equally revealing. Occasionally, parents are instructed not to keep waking children because multiple wakings are disorienting and can be confused with unconsciousness. Parents should wake the child at least once during the night, however, and assess that the pulse rate is more than 60 beats per minute.

Give parents the telephone number to call if they have any questions about their child's care. Advise them to call if their child's behavior changes in any way that makes them suspicious. Many parents will need to set an alarm clock to wake themselves during the night to assess their child's status. There is an old belief that if children fall asleep following a head injury, they will die in their sleep; thus, some parents may keep shaking children awake or make them walk continuously. Be certain they understand that it is all right for children to sleep, but they must wake them at least once to assess their status. (See the Nursing Care Plan: A Child With a Concussion.)

WHAT IF? In the emergency room, parents state that their 5-year-old daughter has been vomiting and is lethargic after being hit by a baseball bat during a playground game. She keeps saying she wasn't hit. "Why won't she tell us the truth?" her father asks you. How would you answer him?

Contusion

A brain contusion occurs when there is tearing or laceration of brain tissue (Figure 31-4). The symptoms are the same as for concussion except they are more severe. In addition, there are specific symptoms related to the lacerated brain area (focal seizure, eye deviation, loss of speech). Surgery may be necessary to halt bleeding. The child's prognosis depends on the extent of the injury and effectiveness of therapy.

CHECKPOINT QUESTIONS

3. Where is a simple linear skull fracture most commonly found?
4. How does a subdural hematoma differ from an epidural hematoma?

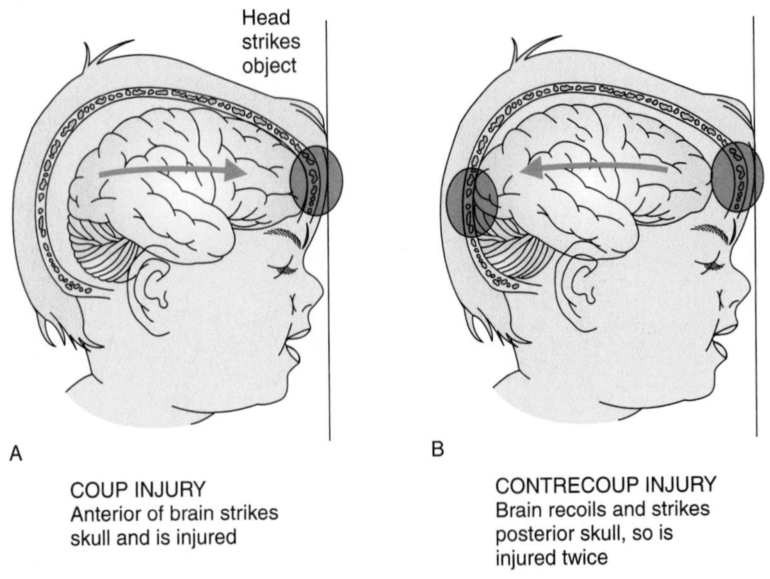
Head
strikes
object
A
COUP INJURY
Anterior of brain strikes
skull and is injured
B
CONTRECOUP INJURY
Brain recoils and strikes
posterior skull, so is
injured twice

FIGURE 31.3 Etiology of (**A**) coup and (**B**) contrecoup injuries.

Nursing Care Plan

THE CHILD WITH A CONCUSSION

A 3½-year-old child clutching her teddy bear is brought to the emergency department by her parents. Her parents state that she was playing on the swings in the backyard, when she fell off, hitting her head on the metal support. "She was out for a minute or two."

Assessment: 3½-year-old female visibly upset and crying. Height and weight at 75th percentile for age. Child unable to report or recall anything about the incident. "We should have been watching her more closely. We just turned our backs for one minute. What kind of parents are we?"

Alert and oriented. Able to name teddy bear brought in with her. Pupils equal, round, reactive to light and accommodation bilaterally. 1.5-cm raised area noted on left parietal area. Skin intact without evidence of bleeding. Child cries when area touched. Negative otorrhea or rhinorrhea. Small 2-cm abrasion noted on right knee; 3-cm abrasion noted on right hand. No other injuries noted. Able to move all extremities through range of motion.

Vital signs: Temperature: 98.2°F (36.8°C); pulse: 128; respirations: 32; blood pressure 110/70. A diagnosis of concussion is made and child is to be discharged home to parents.

Nursing Diagnosis: Risk for injury related to effects of concussion

Outcome Identification: Child will remain free of signs and symptoms of injury following concussion.

Outcome Evaluation: Child remains alert and oriented; easily arousable. Pupils equal, round, react to light and accommodation; vital signs within age-acceptable parameters; exhibits no signs or symptoms of neurologic dysfunction.

Interventions	Rationale
1. Assess the child's vital signs, level of consciousness, and neurologic function initially, and then every ½ hour or according to institution's policy until discharge.	1. Assessment provides a baseline for evaluation. Changes in vital signs, level of consciousness, or neurologic function indicate a worsening of the child's condition and possibly increasing intracranial pressure.
2. Orient the child to her surroundings and explain what has happened. Offer explanations about any treatments or procedures that are to come.	2. Children often have no memory of events leading up to or at the time of the injury. Orientation and explanation help to minimize the child's fear of the unknown and of her situation.
3. Obtain a skull x-ray and other diagnostic tests as ordered, such as CT scan or MRI.	3. Skull x-ray rules out a possible skull fracture secondary to the trauma. CT scan or MRI helps determine any areas of bleeding or edema if present.
4. Institute measures to calm the child. Speak slowly and softly and minimize distractions. Encourage the parents to hold and stroke the child.	4. Crying increases intracranial pressure. Involving the parents provides them with a concrete activity, helping to provide some sense of control over the situation.
5. Instruct the parents to observe the child for the next 24 hours for changes. Advise them to rouse the child approximately every 2 hours during daytime hours and at least once during the night, asking the child to name a familiar object, color, or something she's been shown or to state her name or where she is.	5. Observation is necessary to rule out the possibility of severe brain trauma, edema, or laceration. Waking the child every 2 hours provides time for assessing the child's level of consciousness.
6. Warn parents not to awaken the child too frequently.	6. Multiple frequent waking can be disorienting to the child and be confused with unconsciousness.

(continued)

Interventions	Rationale
7. Review the signs and symptoms of increased intracranial pressure or decreased neurologic function with the parents. Give them a telephone number to call if they have any questions or notice any behavior changes that are suspicious.	7. Understanding of what to look for allows the parents to be comfortable with caring for the child at home. Availability of contact, if necessary, provides the parents with a sense of reassurance and support.
8. Recommend that the parents call their primary health care provider for an appointment once they are at home.	8. Appointment with the child's health care provider allows for additional follow-up.

Nursing Diagnosis: Situational low self-esteem related to feelings of guilt about the child's accident

Outcome Identification: Parents will express positive feelings about themselves as parents.

Outcome Evaluation: Parents state the impact of the child's accident on their view of themselves as parents; identify steps taken after child's fall; participate actively in child's care; report some degree of control over the situation.

Interventions	Rationale
1. Attempt to identify the meaning and effect of the child's accident on the parents.	1. Identification of the meaning and effect of the child's accident assists in determining the degree of impact of the situation on the parents.
2. Encourage the parents to express their feelings about themselves as parents and their role in the child's accident.	2. Sharing of feelings permits a safe outlet for emotions and also aids in highlighting the parents' awareness of the possible impact on their self-esteem.
3. Review and reinforce positive actions as parents. Point out positive behaviors related to maintaining the child's safety and prompt action when the accident happened.	3. Positive actions and behaviors provide a foundation for rebuilding self-esteem.
4. Clarify any misconceptions that the parents may have. Reinforce with them that even with the most constant supervision, it is not always possible to prevent all accidents.	4. Understanding that accidents can happen even with the best of supervision helps to alleviate possible feelings of guilt and anxiety.
5. Assist the parents with participating in the child's care during hospitalization and after discharge. Reinforce previous instructions about observing the child.	5. Ability to perform one's role promotes self-esteem; active participation enhances feelings of control.
6. Reinforce with the parents about calling the institution with any questions.	6. Awareness of additional support helps to reduce feelings of anxiety.

Coma

Coma (unconsciousness from which children cannot be roused) or **stupor** (grogginess from which children can be roused) may be present in children following severe head trauma. Coma and stupor are both symptoms of underlying disorders; a history of the injury must be obtained so that treatment can be directed specifically toward the cause.

Obtain a history to determine the circumstances immediately prior to the time the child became comatose. Assess children in coma carefully and completely so that the cause of the decreased consciousness can quickly be determined.

Assessment

Although head injury is most likely to be the underlying cause of coma or seizure, metabolic disturbances, such as diabetes mellitus, dehydration, severe hemorrhage, or drug ingestion, also must be considered as possible causes. Vital signs often provide good clues. A child with increased intracranial pressure will show a decreased pulse rate, decreased respiratory rate, and increased blood pressure. Diabetes leads to increased respirations. Hemorrhage leads to an increased pulse rate and a decreased blood pressure. Drug ingestion may lead to increased or decreased measurements, depending on the drug ingested.

Undress children completely so that all body parts can be inspected. Irregular breathing, such as hyperventilation, may occur from medullary pressure from brain injury. If bulbar (brain stem) compression is present, children cannot swallow effectively or safely. Turn them on the side to prevent aspiration. Count respirations and pulse and measure blood pressure to establish baseline values. Observe the eyes for signs of increased intracra-

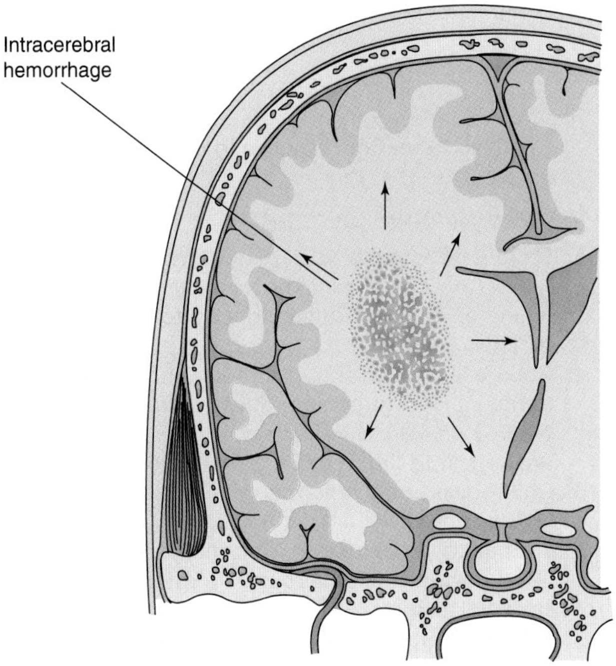

FIGURE 31.4 Intracerebral hemorrhage. The central large dark area represents the hemorrhage. Note the midline shift.

nial pressure. If both pupils are dilated, irreversible brain stem damage is suggested, although such a finding may be present with poisoning from an atropine-like drug. Pinpoint pupils suggest barbiturate or opiate intoxication. One pupil dilated more than the other suggests third cranial nerve damage. The eye may be deviated downward and laterally as well. This may be caused by a tentorial tear (the membrane between the cerebellum and cerebrum) and herniation of the temporal lobe into the torn membrane. This situation requires immediate surgery to correct temporal compression.

The retina of the eye should be examined for papilledema. If increased pressure is longstanding (more than 24–48 hours), papilledema will be present. If the increased pressure is of a shorter duration, papilledema may not be present. Lack of a doll's eye reflex suggests that compression of the oculomotor nerves (third, fourth, or sixth) or the brain stem is involved. Observe for posturing, such as decerebrate posturing, which suggests cerebral compression and dysfunction.

Coma is usually graded according to a standard scale so changes can be evaluated accurately. Figure 31-5 shows the Glasgow Coma Scale, a commonly used evaluation system. Because this system was devised to be an adult assessment scale, it must be modified for use with children; such a modification is shown in Box 31-1.

A score of 3 to 8 suggests severe trauma (less than 5 carries a very severe prognosis); a score of 9 to 12, moderate trauma; and 13 to 15, slight trauma. Many laboratory studies are helpful in determining the cause of coma. Blood glucose, blood electrolytes, blood urea nitrogen (BUN), liver function tests, blood gas studies, lumbar puncture, and toxicology tests may be ordered to rule out possible causes, such as bacterial meningitis or hemorrhage.

Therapeutic Management

If children are unconscious for more than a transient period, they generally are admitted to the hospital for observation. Place children who are comatose on their side to reduce the risk of aspiration. Oral suctioning to remove

Glasgow Coma Scale			A.M.		P.M.						A.M.				
Assessment	Reaction	Score	8	10	12	2	4	6	8	10	12	2	4	6	8
Eye Opening	Spontaneously	4	X						X	X	X	X	X		
Response	To speech	3		X				X							
	To pain	2			X	X	X								
	No response	1													
Motor Response	Obeys verbal command	6	X						X	X	X	X	X		
	Localizes pain	5		X	X										
	Flexion withdrawal	4				X		X							
	Flexion	3					X								
	Extension	2													
	No response	1													
Verbal Response	Oriented x3	5	X						X	X	X	X	X		
	Conversation confused	4		X				X							
	Inappropriate speech	3			X										
	Incomprehensible sounds	2				X	X								
	No response	1													

FIGURE 31.5 Glasgow Coma Scale scoring for a child. A score of 3 to 8 denotes severe trauma; 9 to 12, moderate trauma; 13 to 15, slight trauma. Notice the gradual improvement from coma in this example.

BOX 31.1

SCORING FOR GLASGOW COMA SCALE

Eye Opening

4. Child opens his or her eyes spontaneously when you approach.
3. Child opens his or her eyes in response to speech (spoken or shouted).
2. Child opens his or her eyes only in response to painful stimuli, such as pressure on a nail bed.
1. Child does not open his or her eyes in response to painful stimuli.

Motor Response

6. Child can obey a simple command such as "hand me a toy" (infant smiles or attunes).
5. Child moves an extremity to locate a painful stimuli applied to the head or trunk and attempts to remove the source.
4. Child attempts to withdraw from the source of pain.
3. Child flexes his or her arms at the elbows and wrists in response to painful stimuli to the nail beds (decorticate rigidity).
2. Child extends his or her arms (straightens the elbows) in response to painful stimuli (cerebrate rigidity).
1. Child has no motor response to pain on any extremity.

Verbal Response

5. Child is oriented to time, place, and person (child over age 4 years knows name, date, and where he or she is; infant appears to recognize parent).
4. Child is able to converse, although not oriented to time, place, or person (does not know who or where he or she is; infant says words but does not appear to differentiate parents from others).
3. Child speaks only in words or phrases that make little or no sense ("I want frazzle no"; infant's vocabulary is less than it is normally).
2. Child responds with incomprehensible sounds, such as groans.
1. Child does not respond verbally at all.

Source: Modified from Teasdale, G., & Bennett, B. (1974). Assessment of coma and impaired consciousness: A practical scale. *Lancet, 2,* 81.

mucus from their mouths and pharynx may be necessary. If children have acute signs of respiratory difficulty, endotracheal intubation or tracheostomy may be necessary to ensure respiratory function.

An intravenous route is established so that when specific measures are determined (blood replacement, electrolyte replacement, fluid replacement), a route for immediate administration will be available. Blood will be drawn for a complete blood count, electrolyte determination, toxicology tests, and cross-matching. If the cause of the coma is unknown, a lumbar puncture and EEG may be done. Skull x-rays, CT scan, or MRI may be taken.

Lumbar puncture has little value at first in predicting the severity of a head injury, because any degree of cerebral contusion generally leads to an increased cerebrospinal fluid pressure. Lumbar punctures cannot be done with increased intracranial pressure; brain stem compression can result. Obtain children's vital signs and assess neurologic status, such as state of consciousness and the ability of pupils to react to light, every 15 to 20 minutes. Accurately and carefully record this information so that a picture of gradual change will become apparent.

A child's prognosis following coma depends on the initial cause of the coma. If the increased intracranial pressure can be relieved before any permanent brain damage results, the effects of the coma will be transient. Prognosis is always guarded, however, because coma in itself reflects a major health problem to children.

NURSING DIAGNOSES AND RELATED INTERVENTIONS

Care of the child in coma is directed toward maintaining body function in an optimum state until the child reawakens.

Nursing Diagnosis: Risk for ineffective airway clearance related to brain stem pressure

Outcome Identification: Child's airway will remain unobstructed during course of illness.

Outcome Evaluation: Child's respiratory rate is between 16 and 20 breaths per minute; there are no retractions or signs of obstruction.

Some children who are comatose will require endotracheal intubation or tracheostomy to ensure an open airway. Some will be placed on mechanical ventilation. Maintaining the $PaCO_2$ level below 30 mm Hg may help reduce cerebral edema. Oxygen may be prescribed if arterial blood gases reveal poor oxygenation of body cells (PaO_2 below 55 mm Hg). Endotracheal tubes are replaced with a tracheostomy after 3 or 4 days to prevent necrosis of the pharynx from pressure of the tube.

Nursing Diagnosis: Risk for impaired skin integrity related to lack of mobility

Outcome Identification: Skin will remain intact during the period of coma.

Outcome Evaluation: No areas of broken or irritated skin are present.

Bathe children who are comatose daily to stimulate skin circulation. Include the hair as part of the bath about every 3 days. Change position at least every 2 hours to prevent pressure ulcer formation and development of hydrostatic pneumonia from pooled secretions. When turning, assess skin for reddened points. Keep linen dry and free from wrinkles. Perform passive range-of-motion exercises to maintain muscle tone and prevent contractures. Be certain that exercises are thorough, not merely including a few motions. Without thoroughness, this type of exercise does not prevent contractures and wastes nursing time. Using sheepskin, an egg carton, or an alternating pressure or water mattress also can be important in decreasing pressure to the skin.

Nursing Diagnosis: Risk for altered nutrition, less than body requirements related to inability to take oral food or fluid

Outcome Identification: Child will remain well nourished during period of coma.

Outcome Evaluation: Child's skin turgor is normal; weight remains within acceptable percentile; hourly urine output remains over 1 mL/kg/hr.

Children who are unconscious cannot be fed orally or they might aspirate. Nutrition, therefore, must be maintained by nasogastric feedings, gastrostomy tube, intravenous fluid, or total parenteral nutrition. Intravenous fluid is only a short-term answer because adequate protein and fat cannot be supplied solely by this route. Nasogastric or gastrostomy feedings are effective. Always aspirate the tube for stomach contents before giving a feeding to check tube placement and assess gastric residual amounts. Always return any amount of stomach residue aspirated because if this is discarded each time, the child will lose a large amount of stomach acid, possibly leading to alkalosis. Check whether the amount of the feeding should be reduced by the amount of fluid remaining in the stomach before feeding the full amount of prescribed formula.

Give mouth care at least twice daily with clear water and a padded tongue blade. Coat lips with petrolatum to prevent drying and cracking. If the child's eyes tend to dry, close them to prevent corneal ulceration. Artificial tears (methylcellulose) may be prescribed to keep eyes from drying. Gauze patches over eyes will keep them closed and moist.

✔ CHECKPOINT QUESTIONS

5. What is the most common underlying cause of a coma in a child?
6. A child has a Glasgow Coma score of 10. What does this indicate?

ABDOMINAL TRAUMA

When children are brought to a health care facility after suffering a multiple-injury trauma, several medical specialists may be required: a neurosurgeon for consultation about a head injury; an orthopedic physician for consultation about a fractured extremity; and a thoracic surgeon to intubate or investigate lung trauma. The nurse may serve the important function as the person who is best able to observe a total child and recognize subtle signs of abdominal trauma.

Assessment

Abdominal trauma can result from any object striking the abdomen. In young children, abdominal trauma is generally nonpenetrating and occurs from a direct blow to the abdomen from an object such as a baseball bat or an automobile dashboard. All children who have multiple trauma, such as from automobile accidents, need observation for abdominal injury. Monitor vital signs frequently until they are stable. Hypotension (under 80 mm Hg systolic pressure in older children; under 60 mm Hg in infants) generally suggests hemorrhage, which may be hidden abdominal bleeding. In addition, children may have increasing pallor and rapid respirations. If internal bleeding is present, blood pressure will show little improvement when intravenous fluid is administered.

When abdominal trauma is suspected, a nasogastric tube is passed and stomach contents aspirated to be checked visually for blood and to test for occult blood. Attach the tube to low suction if the presence of blood is established. An indwelling urinary (Foley) catheter is also inserted to examine urine for blood and to evaluate urine output. This may indicate accompanying kidney or bladder trauma. If the urine contains blood, an emergency intravenous pyelogram may be ordered. Be aware that having nasogastric tubes or catheters passed is always frightening for children (unsure of their anatomy, they have no clear idea where the tubes are going). Following an accident, when they are already frightened, they need a great deal of support to accept this (see Enhancing Communication).

An abdominal x-ray may be ordered to rule out a fractured pelvis, a condition that could contribute to blood loss. Air under the diaphragm on the x-ray suggests gastric or intestinal rupture and escape of air from these organs into the peritoneal cavity. Free fluid in the abdomen, shown on x-ray when children are turned on their side, suggests leakage of bowel fluid or splenic rupture and pooling of blood. If the x-ray does not suggest the source of the fluid, an abdominal paracentesis may be done. This procedure is very frightening to children not only because it is intrusive, but also because children's abdomens are likely to be tender. Parents may be so frightened by the sight of the procedure that they are unable to remain with a child while this is done. A nurse, therefore, needs to be present to offer support (Figure 31-6).

For a paracentesis, children are placed in a sitting or side-lying position; their abdomen is cleaned with an antiseptic and covered with a sterile drape. Caution children that they will feel a pinprick as a local anesthetic is inserted into their abdominal wall and feel pressure as the paracentesis needle is inserted. Appreciate children's concern. It is almost impossible for them to lie still while the procedure is being done. Comments such as "Don't cry; be a good boy" are not therapeutic. "It's all right to cry; I know this is scary" is much more comforting and achieves better results, because it lets children know that you understand what you are asking of them.

ENHANCING COMMUNICATION

Danny, a 6-year-old boy with multiple trauma, comes into the emergency room with his father. He is being assessed for abdominal injuries.

Less Effective Communication

Mr. Varton: Why are you looking at his belly? He didn't hurt that.

Nurse: We need to investigate his entire body just to make sure that there aren't any problems. He's had major trauma. He needs to have a central intravenous line and indwelling urinary catheter inserted and a CT scan to rule out any problems.

Mr. Varton: Are you sure? I don't want to put him through any more. He's already in so much pain and he's so upset. I'm just not sure about all this stuff. What if something else goes wrong?

Nurse: If you don't consent to these tests and treatments, we cannot take care of your child.

Mr. Varton: He needs help. Do what you have to. But I'm still not sure.

More Effective Communication

Mr. Varton: Why are you looking at his belly? He didn't hurt that.

Nurse: We need to investigate his entire body just to make sure that there aren't any problems. He's had major trauma. He needs to have a central intravenous line and indwelling urinary catheter inserted and a CT scan to rule out any problems.

Mr. Varton: Are you sure? I don't want to put him through any more.

Nurse: By consenting to these tests, we will be better able to care for your child.

Mr. Varton: He's already in so much pain and he's so upset. I'm just not sure about all this stuff. What if something else goes wrong?

Nurse: This must be very difficult for you to see your child in such pain. Can you tell me how you're feeling or what you're afraid of?

Mr. Varton: I'm really not sure. I'm just so scared that he might die.

Nurse: That's understandable. Let me explain a little more about what we're doing and why these things are necessary. Maybe I can help to calm some of those fears.

In the first scenario, the nurse focuses on obtaining the parent's consent but fails to recognize the fear and apprehension in the parent. In the second scenario, the nurse recognizes and attends to the fears of the parent, helping to establish a sense of support and trust.

It is often difficult for parents to appreciate the seriousness of abdominal trauma, because the signs are not as dramatic or obvious as those of fractured extremities or lacerations. They may ask why an x-ray is necessary. When children are asked to turn on the x-ray table so that an abdominal fluid level can be revealed, they may perceive this as unnecessary manipulation of an injured child. Some parents may not bring a child to an emergency department immediately following abdominal trauma, because they are unaware that serious injury can result to this part of the body. Without frightening them, explain that an injury need not be obvious at first glance to be serious and need care.

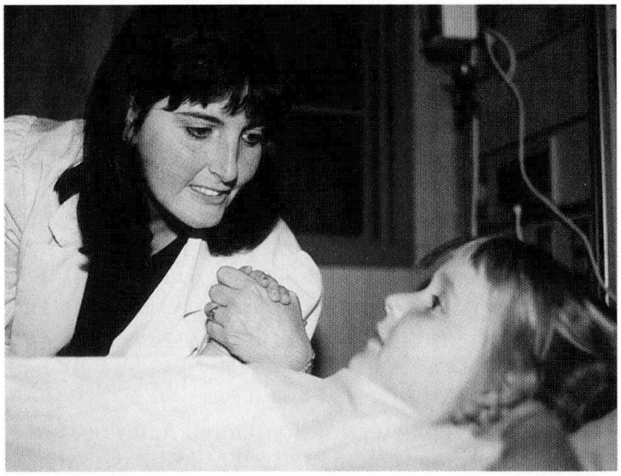

FIGURE 31.6 Prior to a paracentesis, the nurse provides support to the child to help alleviate her fears.

NURSING DIAGNOSES AND RELATED INTERVENTIONS

Nursing Diagnosis: Pain related to abdominal injury

Outcome Identification: Child will experience a tolerable level of pain during period of recovery.

Outcome Evaluation: Child states that level of pain is tolerable; child does not grimace when thinks he or she is not being observed.

Most children with abdominal trauma have pain because they are not routinely administered an analgesic following abdominal trauma so the location of the pain can help to identify which organs may be injured. If parents did not recognize that the child was injured, guilt and fear compound the problem. Goal setting is usually concerned with the immediate diagnostic procedures or surgery that is anticipated. Interventions differ according to the specific injury present.

Splenic Rupture

The spleen is the most frequently injured organ in abdominal trauma because in children this is usually palpable under the lower rib. Children with splenic injury will have tenderness in the left upper quadrant. They notice this especially on deep inspiration, when the diaphragm moves down and touches the spleen. They may hold their left shoulder elevated to keep the diaphragm raised on the left side to keep this from happening. Occasionally, children will notice radiated left shoulder pain when they lie in a supine position (Kehr's sign). An abdominal x-ray will show little about the spleen itself but perhaps will reveal a broken rib over the spleen, suggesting the extent of the trauma to that area. Fluid in the abdomen will suggest bleeding from some source. Obtaining blood on abdominal paracentesis strongly suggests splenic rupture.

An intravenous line is started immediately for fluid replacement and an intravenous pyelogram will be done to rule out damage to the left kidney, which, because of its location in that area, probably also suffered trauma. A complete blood count is done to estimate the extent of the blood loss. Blood is typed and cross-matched so blood for replacement can then be readied if necessary. Children will be admitted to a hospital unit for observation if the blood loss from rupture appears mild. If severe, immediate surgery will be performed. Partial or total splenectomy may be necessary to halt bleeding and save their life.

After a splenectomy, children are very susceptible to infection, particularly pneumococci infections. Therefore, most children are immunized with pneumococci vaccine to prevent this.

Liver Rupture

Children with liver rupture or laceration usually have severe abdominal pain, most marked on inspiration when the diaphragm descends and touches the liver. They show symptoms of blood loss, including tachycardia, hypotension, anxiety, and pallor. Their hematocrit will be low or falling. Such children need to be prepared for immediate surgery, because the liver is a highly vascular organ, and blood loss from it is acute and damaging.

Occasionally, a communication between an artery and a bile duct occurs at the time of trauma. With this, symptoms are not immediate, but gastrointestinal (GI) bleeding, such as hematemesis, or melena may occur in a few days. The child may have colicky upper abdominal pain that may be relieved by emesis. Liver studies, such as a liver arteriogram, will be necessary to reveal the extent of the problem.

Following both liver and spleen surgery, children need careful observation for return of bowel function, assessment for the possibility that peritonitis may develop, and careful reintroduction of oral nutrition.

DENTAL TRAUMA

Injuries to teeth occur most often from falls in which children strike their upper front incisors and from blows to the face by objects such as baseball bats or hockey sticks. They are always potentially serious because they can lead to aspiration or malalignment of future teeth. When a tooth is knocked out, parents should rinse the tooth in water and replace it in the child's mouth or drop the tooth in a salt solution or milk and bring it to the emergency department with them. If permanent teeth that have been knocked out recently are washed with saline in the emergency department and replaced, there is a good chance that they will reimplant successfully. Some dentists advocate immersing the tooth in an antiseptic and then an antibiotic solution before replacing it. If a tooth is replaced, it generally is wired into place to hold it in good alignment. Children receive a course of oral antibiotics, such as penicillin, to prevent infection. They must eat only soft food until the tooth has firmly adhered.

If a blow to a child's teeth was extensive, an x-ray may be taken to rule out a mandibular or maxillary fracture. If a portion of a tooth cannot be located, the possibility of aspiration must be considered and confirmed or ruled out by a chest x-ray. In young children, often a tooth is not knocked out but is pushed back up into the gum. These teeth gradually regrow, and although they may darken in color, they usually are healthy. If the affected tooth is a deciduous tooth, the permanent tooth is rarely injured even though it is already formed in the gum. At the appropriate time, the permanent tooth will erupt normally.

✔ **CHECKPOINT QUESTIONS**

7. What does air under the diaphragm on abdominal x-ray suggest?
8. Which organ is most frequently injured in the child with abdominal trauma?

NEAR DROWNING

Drowning is defined as death due to suffocation from submersion in liquid. Inhaled water fills and therefore blocks the exchange of oxygen in the alveoli. More than 3500 children die from drowning annually. The term **near drowning** is used to describe the child with a submersion injury who requires emergency treatment and who survives the first 24 hours postinjury.

Drowning accidents occur most frequently in the summer months, when more children are swimming and boating. Toddlers and preschool-age children who cannot swim are the most frequent victims of drowning and near-drowning accidents, although children (and adults) of all ages and swimming abilities are at risk. Small children may fall into neighborhood swimming pools or adolescents may take dares to swim farther than their ability or swim under the influence of alcohol, which impairs their decision-making ability and their physical coordination.

Pathophysiology of Drowning

If children hyperventilate prior to swimming underwater, excess carbon dioxide is blown off; during an extended period of underwater swimming, carbon dioxide levels rise, but not adequately to cause children to experience distress. This results in decreased oxygen levels with drowsiness and listlessness (children drown without struggling or realizing their danger).

When children first inhale water, they cough violently from the irritation of the water in their nose and throat. If children cannot get their head out of water at that point, water will enter the larynx. The larynx will go into spasm, preventing any air from entering the trachea, and asphyxia will result. If children are ventilated at this point, treatment generally is very effective because there is little water in the lungs. The condition more closely simulates asphyxia that occurs with croup or when a foreign body, such as a nut, lodges in the larynx and stops air flow.

If treatment is not given at this point, the larynx relaxes from the asphyxia and water enters the lungs. Children can no longer exchange oxygen, because the alveoli fill with water. Hypoxia deepens, and cardiac arrest occurs.

Additional changes that occur when water enters the lungs depend on whether the water is fresh or salt. The osmotic pressure of the hypertonic salt solution in salt water causes fluid to diffuse from the bloodstream and enter the alveoli, increasing the amount of fluid in the lung tissue. Tachycardia and decreased blood pressure from hypovolemia will result. Blood viscosity increases (increased hematocrit level). The presence of pulmonary edema will cause increased hypoxia. In fresh water, which is hypotonic, fluid in the lungs is absorbed into the bloodstream. This may lead to hemolysis of red blood cells, a dilution of plasma, and possible hypervolemia with tachycardia and increased blood pressure. If the release of potassium from destroyed red blood cells is great enough with fresh-water drowning, cardiac arrhythmias may occur. In both instances, loss of surfactant from the lung alveoli, caused by introduction of water, will cause alveolar collapse.

Very young children display a mammalian diving reflex when they plunge under cold water. Immediately, a lifesaving bradycardia and shunting of blood away from the periphery of their body to their brain and heart occurs. This is triggered when water is 70°F (21°C) or less and their face is submerged first. Children have fully recovered after being submerged up to 40 minutes in water that is very cold (0°C–15°C; 32°F–60°F).

Emergency Management

When children are pulled from the water following drowning, mouth-to-mouth resuscitation should be started at once. If cardiac arrest has occurred with the hypoxia, simultaneous measures to initiate cardiac action must be taken. The techniques of cardiopulmonary resuscitation for infants and children are discussed in Chapter 40.

Assuming that cardiopulmonary resuscitation is effective, children need follow-up care at a health care facility, because they are certain to be acidotic from accumulated CO_2 and hypoxic (from lack of oxygen because of the water in the alveoli).

Follow-up care aims to increase children's oxygen and carbon dioxide exchange capacity, using the lung areas that are not filled with water. Children are intubated with a cuffed intratracheal tube; mechanical ventilation with positive end-expiratory pressure may be necessary to force air into the alveoli. Because children swallow water, vomiting usually occurs as the child is revived. The cuff of the intratracheal tube prevents vomitus from being aspirated. Children are given 100% oxygen so that as much space as possible in the available lung alveoli can be used. Generally, either isoproterenol, albuterol, or racemic epinephrine is administered by aerosol to prevent bronchospasm and, again, to allow children to make maximum use of the oxygen administered. Intravenous aminophylline may also be used to open the airways. If a child aspirated salt water, plasma may be administered to replace protein loss into the lungs and prevent hypovolemia.

If the child's body temperature is very low, gradual warming (not using a warming blanket) is advised so metabolism need does not rise sharply before alveolar space is ready to accommodate this. Extracorporeal membrane oxygenation may be used. A nasogastric tube is placed to compress the stomach, prevent vomiting, and free up breathing space (Hutchison, 1997).

Unfortunately, neurologic damage occurs in as many as 21% of near-drowning incidents. If the child is awake or only lethargic at the scene of the accident and immediately afterward in the hospital, the prognosis is greatly improved over that of the child who is comatose.

NURSING DIAGNOSES AND RELATED INTERVENTIONS

Nursing Diagnosis: Risk for infection related to foreign substance in respiratory tract

Outcome Identification: Child will remain free of signs and symptoms of infection following near drowning.

Outcome Evaluation: Child's temperature remains below 37.0°C orally; rales are absent on lung auscultation; respiratory rate is within age-acceptable parameters.

Children may be placed on a prophylactic antibiotic to prevent pneumonia and additional airway interference (Ender & Dolan, 1997). Assess vital signs and auscultate lung sounds for adventitious sounds, such as rales (also called crackles) or fine rhonchi. Turning the child every 2 hours if on bedrest and encouraging deep breathing and incentive spirometry every hour help to aerate the lungs fully and prevent the accumulation of fluid, which promote infection.

Nursing Diagnosis: Fear related to near-drowning experience

Outcome Identification: Child will demonstrate that he or she can manage this degree of fear.

Outcome Evaluation: Child discusses fears; child states that he or she understands that although frightening, the experience is over, and he or she is now safe.

Children must be admitted to the hospital for observation and monitoring of blood gases until water from the alveoli is absorbed and they once again can ventilate effectively on their own. Children may wake at night while in the hospital from a nightmare that they are drowning. Frequently reassure them that they are now safe and definitely out of the water. Near drowning is a thoroughly frightening experience. Children need to verbalize this fright. They will need support from parents before they engage in an activity such as swimming again after such a frightening experience.

✔ CHECKPOINT QUESTIONS

9. What do very young children display when they plunge into cold water?
10. What is the rationale for prophylactic antibiotic therapy after a near-drowning episode?

POISONING

Poisoning occurs most commonly between the ages of 2 and 3 years and in children of all socioeconomic groups. Common agents in childhood poisoning include soaps, detergents or cleaners, and plants. It can occur from over-the-counter drugs, such as vitamins, iron compounds, aspirin, or acetaminophen, or prescription drugs, such as antidepressants. Poisoning is entirely preventable. Parents must be educated regarding the high risk for poisoning and strategies for maintaining a home environment that is safe for children of all ages. Be aware that when poisoning occurs in an older child, it may be a suicide attempt (Harrington et al, 1998).

NURSING DIAGNOSES AND RELATED INTERVENTIONS

Nursing Diagnosis: Risk for injury related to maturational age of child and presence of poisons

Outcome Identification: Child will not ingest a poison during childhood.

Outcome Evaluation: Parents identify poisonous and toxic items in the home and describe how they are stored safely; parents state local poison control center number; parents describe measures to seek help immediately if poisoning occurs.

Emergency Management of Poisoning at Home

Teach parents that if they discover that a child has swallowed a poison, they should immediately call the emergency poison control center number in their community. Information they need to provide includes the following:

- Child's name, telephone number, address, weight, and age
- How long ago the poisoning occurred
- The route of poisoning (oral, inhaled, sprayed on skin)
- How much of the poison the child took (This may be difficult for parents to judge if they do not know how much was in the bottle. If they just answer, "a whole bottle," ask them to read from the bottle how much that is.)
- If the poison was in pill form, whether there are pills scattered under a chair or if they are all missing and presumed swallowed
- What was swallowed; if the name of a medicine is not known, what it was prescribed for and a description of it (color, size, shape of pills).
- The child's present condition (sleepy, hyperactive, comatose)

If one child has swallowed a poison, parents must investigate whether other children have also poisoned themselves. A preschooler often gives a younger sibling some of the "candy" he or she has been eating. Ask if parents have transportation to the health care facility or if they need an ambulance.

Parents should keep a bottle of syrup of ipecac (an emetic) with their emergency first aid supplies (see Drug Highlight). Before they administer this emetic, however, they should call a poison control center to make certain that vomiting is desirable. Unless the poison was a caustic, corrosive, or a hydrocarbon, vomiting is the most effective way to remove the poison from the body—more effective even than lavage. In 90% of children, vomiting will occur within 20 minutes of being given ipecac. If vomiting does not occur in 20 to 30 minutes, another dose of ipecac can be given. Parents should, however, begin transport to a health care facility for follow-up treatment as soon as the first dose of ipecac is given.

If parents do not have ipecac in the house, making children vomit by placing a finger in the back of the throat (gagging them) is effective. Ask parents to bring any vomited material to the health care facility with them so it can be analyzed for content.

> **DRUG HIGHLIGHT**
>
> **Syrup of Ipecac**
>
> *Action:* Syrup of ipecac is an emetic agent used in the treatment of drug overdose and poisoning. It produces vomiting by locally irritating the gastrointestinal mucosa and stimulating the brain's chemotrigger receptor zone for vomiting.
>
> *Pregnancy risk category:* C
>
> *Dosage:* For children <1 year: 5 to 10 mL orally followed by 1 cup (200 mL) of water or clear fluid. For children >1 year: 15 mL orally followed by 2 to 3 glasses of water or clear fluid. Dosage may be repeated if vomiting does not occur within 20 minutes.
>
> *Possible adverse effects:* Mild CNS depression, nausea, diarrhea.
>
> *Nursing Implications:*
> - Make sure vomiting is the desired implementation for the poison ingested. Use activated charcoal if vomiting of ipecac does not occur or if ipecac overdose occurs.
> - If the child doesn't vomit within 30 minutes of the repeated dose, prepare for gastric lavage.
> - Administer the drug to a conscious child only. Always administer ipecac before using activated charcoal; charcoal will inactivate the ipecac.
> - Instruct parents to keep this drug readily available in the home in case of accidental poisoning. Advise them to call the local poison control center for instructions.
> - If vomiting is indicated for poisoning, tell parents to administer the drug as soon as possible after poisoning.
> - Urge the parents to bring the child to the emergency department as quickly as possible.
> - Teach parents about the possible sources of poisons in the home and how to minimize the risk of poisoning.

Emergency Management of Poisoning at the Health Care Facility

Although not done routinely, if a child has ingested a potentially fatal dose, further removal of the poison may be carried out by gastric lavage (Vale, 1997). When performing lavage, always place the first specimen returned in a separate specimen container or emesis basin to save for a toxicology analysis. Later specimens are often too dilute for an analysis (Nursing Procedure 31-1).

After lavage, activated charcoal may be administered, either through the lavage tube or orally. Activated charcoal is supplied as a fine black powder that is mixed with water for administration. It combines with the poison and inactivates it. As the charcoal is excreted through the bowel over the next 3 days, stools will appear black. Never administer activated charcoal before ipecac because it will inactivate the ipecac. Never administer it if acetylcysteine (Mucomyst; the specific antidote for acetaminophen poisoning) will be used, because charcoal inactivates acetylcysteine.

Another way to speed removal of a poison from the body is to administer a saline cathartic. Saline cathartics are harsh laxatives and should be used with caution in young children. Severe dehydration and electrolyte imbalance could occur.

Always follow emergency measures with an education program to prevent poisoning from happening again. Specific measures for each age group are discussed in previous chapters with problems and concerns of the age group.

Salicylate Poisoning

About 25% of childhood poisonings are salicylate (aspirin) poisonings, although this percentage is decreasing because of safety packaging and less use of aspirin for childhood fever.

NURSING PROCEDURE 31.1: GASTRIC LAVAGE

Purpose

To dilute and remove toxic contents from the stomach

Procedure	**Principle**
1. Wash your hands; identify child; explain the procedure.	1. Handwashing prevents spread of microorganisms. Explanations encourage client compliance and cooperation.
2. Assess child for current status; analyze appropriateness of procedure.	2. If child is vomiting, stomach lavage may be unnecessary. Lavage should not be begun if the ingested substance was a flammable liquid or caustic until an antidote is administered.
3. Organize supplies, including nasogastric (NG) tube, normal saline, basin, tape, asepto or barrel syringe with catheter tip.	3. Organization speeds emergency care and enhances effectiveness.
4. Restrain child as necessary. Pass NG tube into stomach using usual technique, then position child on side with head slightly elevated. Aspirate all stomach contents possible.	4. Aspirating before diluting stomach contents allows you to secure a sample of contents for laboratory analysis. Positioning on side reduces possibility of aspiration if child vomits.
5. Remove plunger from syringe; attach barrel to NG tube, and elevate about 12 in over the child's stomach level. Pour a designated amount of irrigating solution into syringe; allow it to flow into the stomach by gravity.	5. Proper technique allows procedure to be carried out efficiently. Proper positioning allows fluid to be instilled by gravity. Don't force irrigating solution into the stomach because this might force the poison into the small intestine or cause vomiting with aspiration.
6. Remove the syringe and lower the end of the NG tube. Allow the stomach contents to drain by gravity into the basin. If necessary, attach syringe and apply gentle suction. Note the amount and color of the drainage.	6. Aspiration can injure the stomach lining if the catheter rests against the stomach wall. Notify the child's physician if the return fluid is bloody because it suggests a caustic poison.
7. Repeat the procedure until the stomach contents return clear (about 10 times).	7. It is important to remove as much of the toxic contents as possible.
8. Remove the NG tube. Position the child comfortably on the side.	8. Keeping the child on the side helps prevent aspiration if further vomiting occurs.
9. Record the type and amount of irrigating solution used and the child's reaction to the procedure.	9. Evaluation allows determination of whether procedure has been successful. Documentation allows further follow-up based on previous results.
10. Plan health teaching, such as safe rules for household poisons.	10. Health teaching is important to prevent future accidents.

Assessment

An overdose of salicylate causes a myriad of metabolic consequences, including increased metabolic rate, interference with the use of carbohydrate, decreased prothrombin production, and stimulation of the respiratory center of the brain, causing hyperventilation (hyperpnea and tachypnea). Hyperventilation leads to respiratory alkalosis as excessive amounts of carbon dioxide are "blown off." Because of the increased metabolic rate and an inability to use carbohydrates, the body begins to use protein and fat sources for energy. This causes the initial alkalosis to be quickly replaced by metabolic acidosis. The increased metabolism will also lead to a high fever and dehydration. Within 2 hours of ingestion, children have marked tachycardia, tachypnea, and perhaps hypoglycemia. They may have fever, vomiting, and diarrhea. They may have central nervous system signs, such as restlessness, stupor, convulsions, or coma. Because salicylate also interferes with the formation of prothrombin, areas of purpura may appear on the child's skin. Irritation to the gastric lining may lead to stomach ulcer. Tinnitus (ringing in the ears), a specific toxic effect of salicylate overdose, may occur.

Symptoms increase in severity, depending on the amount of aspirin ingested (Table 31-3). Symptoms begin when children ingest 150 to 200 mg of salicylate per kilogram of body weight. The peak blood level is reached within 2 to 3 hours of ingestion.

A simple test for detecting salicylate poisoning is to test a urine specimen with a strip of Phenistix. If there is salicylate secretion in the urine, the strip will turn brownish purple. Phenistix may also be used as a quick test of blood serum. If the strip turns tan when a blood sample is placed on it, the serum salicylate level is less than 70 mg/100 mL; if purple, the serum level is more than 70 mg/100 mL.

Therapeutic Management

With salicylate poisoning, parents should administer syrup of ipecac to induce vomiting. If a child has not vomited by the time he or she is seen at a health care facility, a repeat dose of ipecac or gastric lavage will be initiated.

TABLE 31.3 Levels of Salicylate Poisoning

DOSE INGESTED (mg/kg)	SYMPTOMS
<150	None
150–300	Mild to moderate hyperpnea, lethargy and excitability, metabolic acidosis that can be compensated
300–500	Severe tachypnea and hyperventilation; possible convulsions; uncompensated metabolic acidosis; pyrexia
>500	Coma, uncompensated metabolic acidosis; convulsions, severe pyrexia

Next, implementations to support metabolic and respiratory function and encourage salicylate elimination are initiated. If the serum salicylate level is more than 50 mg/100 mL, children usually are admitted to a health care facility for observation. Offer fluid orally to dilute the poison and prevent dehydration. If children will not drink, intravenous fluid may be administered. Administering sodium bicarbonate to create an alkaline urine (pH over 8) aids salicylate excretion. With some children, hemodialysis may be necessary to remove the salicylate load and maintain normal potassium levels (potassium is exchanged for H^+—hydrogen ion—in urine so it reaches high levels).

Continue to monitor vital signs every 2 to 4 hours. Test urine for pH. Even though the child's temperature is elevated, a method of decreasing temperature (administering aspirin) is obviously contraindicated following aspirin intoxication. Dress children lightly and sponge with tepid water or use a cooling blanket. Test stool for occult blood to see if gastric irritation from aspirin is occurring. Observe especially for signs of hypoglycemia (coma, profuse sweating, disorientation) or metabolic acidosis (rapid, deep breathing; disorientation). Serum blood glucose levels may be ordered periodically based on clinical signs of hypoglycemia.

The prognosis of the child with salicylate poisoning depends on the amount of salicylate ingested and the speed with which treatment was begun. Some parents do not call for aid immediately after aspirin poisoning, because they do not think of aspirin as a harmful drug. They may think that the dose was too small to cause a problem. In addition, they may feel guilty because they realize they were careless about putting the bottle of medicine away after use.

Assurance that the child is excreting the salicylate would include the following: positive Phenistix test; a urine pH above 8; respiratory and cardiac rates and temperature level returning to normal; no progression of ecchymotic or petechial areas; and return of a normal serum glucose level.

NURSING DIAGNOSES AND RELATED INTERVENTIONS

Nursing Diagnosis: Self-esteem disturbance related to child's poisoning

Outcome Identification: Parents demonstrate confidence in their ability to provide safe care for the child (and other family members) within 24 hours.

Outcome Evaluation: Parents state guidelines for continued assessment of child at home; parents state ways they can improve "childproofing."

After the child is stabilized, take some time to talk to parents about how they feel about this event. Remember that poisoning tends to happen in homes where there is stress. If stress was already present, how has this poisoning added to it?

Before children are discharged from a health care facility, be certain parents are comfortable with any further assessment measures they will need to continue at home, such as temperature taking and urging a high fluid intake. Talk to the parents about childproofing their home.

Acetaminophen Poisoning

Parents are now using acetaminophen (Tylenol) as a substitute for aspirin to treat childhood fevers. In many homes, it is now more available than aspirin. Told that acetaminophen is safer than aspirin, parents may not be as careful about putting this substance away as they were with aspirin. If their child swallows acetaminophen, they may delay bringing him or her for help, thinking it is a harmless drug.

Acetaminophen in large doses is not an innocent drug. It can cause extreme liver destruction. Immediately after ingestion, the child will experience anorexia, nausea, and vomiting. Soon, serum aspartate transaminase (AST [SGOT]) and serum alanine transaminase (ALT [SGPT]) liver enzymes become elevated. The liver may be tender. Liver toxicity occurs with an acetaminophen load greater than 200 μg/mL by 4 hours and 50 μg/mL by 12 hours.

Syrup of ipecac is administered to induce vomiting. This can be followed by acetylcysteine every 4 hours for 72 hours orally. This agent prevents hepatotoxicity by binding with the breakdown product of acetaminophen so it will not bind to liver cells (Mariscalco, 1997). Acetylcysteine, unfortunately, has an offensive odor and taste. Administer it in a carbonated beverage to help the child swallow it. In small children, it is administered directly into the nasogastric tube following lavage to avoid this difficulty. If the child is admitted to the hospital for observation, continue to observe for jaundice and tenderness over the liver; assess ALT and AST levels.

Caustic Poisoning

Ingestion of a strong alkali, such as lye, often contained in toilet bowl cleaners or hair care products, may cause burns and tissue necrosis in the mouth, esophagus, and stomach.

Assessment

After a caustic ingestion, the child has immediate pain in the mouth and throat and drools saliva from an inability to swallow. The mouth turns white immediately from the burn. Later, the mouth turns brown as edema and ulceration occur. There may be such marked edema of the lips and mouth that it is difficult to examine them. The child may immediately vomit blood, mucus, and necrotic tissue. The loss of blood from the denuded, burned surface may lead to systemic signs of tachycardia, tachypnea, pallor, and hypotension.

A chest x-ray is ordered to determine if pulmonary involvement has occurred from any aspirated poison or an esophageal perforation has allowed poison to seep into the mediastinum. An esophagoscopy under anesthesia may be done to assess the esophagus. This may be omitted because there is a possibility an esophagoscope might perforate the burned esophagus. After 2 weeks, a barium swallow may be done to reveal the final extent of the esophageal burns.

Therapeutic Management

Parents should always call a poison control center to ask for advice on how to proceed. *With caustic poisoning, vomiting should not be induced, because the corrosive substance will burn as it comes up just as it did going down.* Diluting the poison with milk or water is a good emergency measure. Parents should not waste time trying to get children to swallow anything, however. They should immediately take them to a health care facility for treatment.

There is a high possibility that pharyngeal edema will be severe enough to obstruct children's airway by even 20 minutes after the burn. Intubation may be necessary to provide a clear airway.

To detect respiratory interference, assess vital signs closely, especially respiratory rate. In infants, increasing restlessness is an important accompanying sign of this. Assess children for the degree of pain involved. A strong analgesic may need to be ordered and administered to achieve pain relief.

NURSING DIAGNOSES AND RELATED INTERVENTIONS

Nursing Diagnosis: Risk for ineffective airway clearance related to burns of esophagus and mouth

Outcome Identification: Child will maintain adequate respiratory function.

Outcome Evaluation: Child's respiration rate will remain within 16 to 20 breaths per minute.

Starting therapy immediately with a steroid such as dexamethasone (Decadron) and continuing it for about 4 weeks will reduce the chance of permanent esophageal scarring. Children may be placed on a prophylactic antibiotic to reduce the possibility of infection and additional inflammation in the denuded mouth and esophageal area.

Children who respond well to steroid therapy will recover with no important sequelae. Children who do not receive steroid therapy for some reason may have scarring of the esophagus, resulting in complete obstruction. To correct complete obstruction, repeated surgical procedures are necessary. Sometimes transplantation of intestinal tissue or a synthetic graft is required to replace stenosed esophageal tissue. If partial obstruction is present, a string is passed through the nose and esophagus and exited through a gastrostomy opening to form a continuous loop. **Bougies** (flexible, cylindrical, metal instruments) are tied to the string and pulled through the esophagus to dilate it and increase the lumen size. This may be done as often as once or twice a week up to 1 year following the burn.

Nursing Diagnosis: Risk for altered nutrition, less than body requirements related to esophageal stricture from burn scarring

Outcome Identification: Child will ingest an adequate intake for age following ingestion.

Outcome Evaluation: Child's diet meets recommended daily allowance requirements for age.

Oral intake commonly will be a problem for the first week because of soreness in the child's mouth. Observe children carefully the first time they drink to observe for signs that an esophageal perforation has occurred (coughing, choking, cyanosis). Intravenous fluid may be needed as a supplement. If a child is totally unable to swallow, gastrostomy feedings or total parenteral nutrition may be necessary. When children are able to take food, they should begin with a liquid diet. Liquid passing through the burned and scarring esophagus tends to maintain esophageal patency, so it is therapeutic for the burn and nutritious for the child.

Hydrocarbon Ingestion

Hydrocarbons are substances contained in products such as kerosene and furniture polish. Because these substances are volatile, fumes rise from them, and their major effect is respiratory irritation (see Chapter 19).

CHECKPOINT QUESTIONS

11. When is vomiting contraindicated with poisoning in a child?
12. What is the antidote for acetaminophen poisoning?

Iron Poisoning

Iron is frequently swallowed by small children because it is an ingredient in vitamin preparations, particularly pregnancy vitamins. When it is ingested, it is corrosive to the gastric mucosa, and the symptoms of iron ingestion reflect this irritation. The immediate effects of iron toxicity are nausea and vomiting, diarrhea, and abdominal pain. After 6 hours, these symptoms fade, and the child's condition appears to improve. By this time, however, hemorrhagic necrosis of the lining of the GI tract has occurred. By 12 hours, melena (blood in stool) and hematemesis (blood in emesis) will be present. Lethargy and coma, cyanosis, and vasomotor collapse also may occur. Coagulation defects may occur; hepatic injury also can result. Shock from an increase in peripheral vascular resistance and decreased cardiac output can occur. Long-term effects can be gastric scarring from fibrotic tissue formation.

Assessment

It is difficult to estimate the amount of iron a child has swallowed, because parents can only guess at the number of pills in the bottle, and the amount of elemental iron in compounds varies. Serum iron and iron-binding concentration should be measured. A level of more than 500 μg/100 mL serum iron is a significant level. A toxic dose is 20 to 30 mg/kg of body weight; 60 to 180 mg/kg is a potentially lethal amount (Fortenberry & Mariscalco, 1997).

Therapeutic Management

Having children vomit by taking syrup of ipecac helps to remove any iron not yet absorbed. This may be followed by gastric lavage with a bicarbonate solution to convert the remaining ferrous iron to a less absorbable carbonate compound. A cathartic may be given to help a child pass enteric-coated iron pills. Activated charcoal has no effect.

A child who has ingested a potentially toxic dose (40–60 mg/kg of body weight of elemental iron) is admitted to the hospital for therapy with a chelating agent, such as intravenous or intramuscular deferoxamine. Chelating agents combine with metal and allow metal to be excreted from the body. Deferoxamine causes urine to turn orange as iron is excreted. An exchange transfusion is another way that excess iron can be removed from the body. An upper GI series and liver studies will be done 1 week after ingestion to screen for long-term effects. The hope is that the iron load was removed from the stomach in time so that not all of it was absorbed.

Assist with emergency measures, such as gastric lavage, and administer chelating agents as ordered. Test any stool passed for the next 3 days for occult blood to assess for stomach irritation and subsequent GI bleeding. Be certain that parents understand the importance of follow-up studies if any of these are prescribed.

NURSING DIAGNOSES AND RELATED INTERVENTIONS

Nursing Diagnosis: Parental knowledge deficit related to the danger of iron as a poison

Outcome Identification: Parents will acknowledge that iron is a dangerous substance to children in toxic dosages following the ingestion.

Outcome Evaluation: Parents state ways they have safeguarded their child from iron exposure.

Iron poisoning occurs frequently because parents do not think of iron pills or vitamins containing iron as real medicine. As mentioned, poisoning tends to happen when a family is under stress. Pregnancy in the mother is a form of stress, and almost all pregnant women take iron compounds. The 9 months of pregnancy are therefore a likely time for iron poisoning to occur in an older sibling. When you instruct parents to use an iron supplement for themselves or their children, stress that overdoses can be fatal to small children. Teach them to think of iron as they would any other medicine and keep it out of the reach of small children.

WHAT IF? A 3-year-old girl is seen in the emergency room after ingesting prenatal vitamins. What test would you use to detect gastric bleeding from iron ingestion?

Lead Poisoning

Lead in the body interferes with red blood cell function by blocking the incorporation of iron into the protoporphyrin compound that makes up the heme portion of hemoglobin

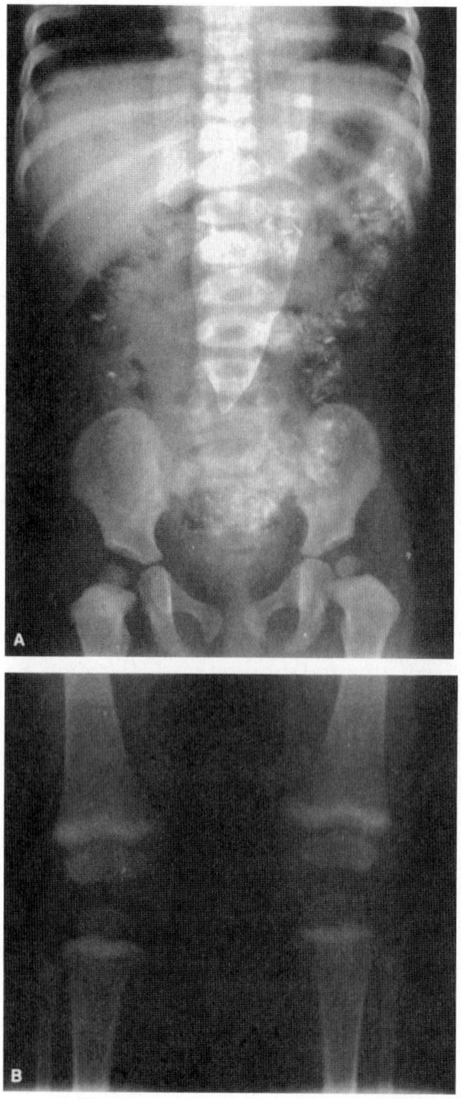

FIGURE 31.7 (**A**) Ingested paint chips (white crescents) in the intestinal tract. (**B**) A radiograph of the long bones of a child with chronic lead ingestion showing the characteristic "lead line" or white marking at the epiphyseal line.

in red blood cells. This leads to a hypochromic, microcytic anemia. Kidney destruction may occur, causing excess excretion of amino acids, glucose, and phosphates in the urine. The most serious effects are lead encephalitis or inflammation of brain cells from the toxic lead content. Lead poisoning (**plumbism**), like all forms of poisoning in children, tends to occur most often in the toddler and preschool child. Sources of lead poisoning are described in Chapter 9, along with guidelines for its prevention.

Assessment

The usual source of ingested lead is from paint chips or paint dust. Paint tastes sweet, and a child will pick chips up off the floor or off the walls over and over again. If a crib rail is painted with lead paint, a child will ingest it as he or she teethes on the rail. Chewing on window sills is also common. In fishing communities, swallowing lead sinkers can be a common source. Restoring an older home saturates the air with lead dust. In such homes, lead plumbing may con-taminate the drinking water.

All children who live in housing built before 1950 should be screened for lead poisoning yearly (AAP, 1998). The most widely used method of screening for lead levels is the blood lead determination. Unfortunately, this test requires using atomic absorption spectrophotometry, which is a costly procedure that is not available in all communities. Free eryth-rocyte protoporphyrin tests are a simple screening procedure, involving only a finger stick. Because protoporphyrin is blocked from entering heme by lead, it will be elevated in lead poisoning.

Many children with fairly high blood lead levels are asymptomatic. Others show insidious symptoms of anorexia and abdominal pain from the presence of lead in the stomach. One of the major effects of excessive lead levels is encephalopathy. The child usually has beginning symptoms of lethargy, impulsiveness, and learning difficulties. As the child's blood level of lead increases, severe encephalopathy with seizures and permanent neurologic damage will result.

Basophilic stippling (an odd striation of basophils) may be apparent on a blood smear. An x-ray of the abdomen may reveal paint chips in the intestinal tract (Figure 31-7*A*). "Lead lines" (areas of increased density) may be present near the epiphyseal line of long bones (see Figure 31-7*B*). The thickness of the line shows the length of time lead ingestion has been occurring. Damage to the kidney nephrons from the presence of lead leads to proteinuria, ketonuria, and glycosuria. Cerebrospinal fluid may have an increased protein level. Lead poisoning is usually said to be present when the child has two successive blood lead levels greater than 10 μg/dL. A classification of levels of lead poisoning is shown in Table 31-4.

Therapeutic Management

A child with a blood lead level between 10 and 14 μg/dL needs to be rescreened to confirm the level. If the lead level is 15 or above, the child needs active interventions to prevent further lead exposure. All children with lead levels over 25 μg/100 mL require treatment. A major part of treatment is removing the child from the environment containing the lead source or removing the source of lead

TABLE 31.4 Classification of Lead Poisoning Risk

CLASS	BLOOD LEVEL CONCENTRATION (μg/dL)
Class I (low risk)	Lead under 9
Class IIa (rescreen)	Lead 10–14
Class IIb (moderate risk)	Lead 15–19
Class III (high risk)	Lead 20–44
Class IV (urgent risk)	Lead 45–69
Class V (urgent risk)	Lead greater than 70

(Centers for Disease Control. [1991]. *Preventing lead poisoning in young children.* Washington, DC: U.S. Department of Health and Human Services, Public Health Service.)

from the child's environment. Removing the lead source may be difficult. If the family lives in a rented apartment, the landlord may be legally obligated to remove the lead. Simple repainting or wallpapering does not remove a source of peeling paint adequately. After some months, the new paint will begin to peel because of the defective paint underneath. The walls must be covered by paneling or masonite. Plastic-covered contact paper can be used temporarily and is less expensive than paneling.

Until such repairs are made, children may be removed from the home. Children with blood lead levels of greater than 30 μg/100 mL may be admitted to the hospital for chelating therapy with agents such as dimercaprol (BAL) or edetate calcium disodium (CaEDTA), one of the most commonly used chelating agents (see Drug Highlight).

Chelating agents remove the lead from soft tissue and bone (although not from red blood cells) and eliminate it in the urine. Injections of EDTA, which must be given intramuscularly into a large muscle mass, are painful and may be combined with 0.5 mL of procaine. EDTA also removes calcium from the body; therefore, serum calcium must be measured periodically to determine whether it is at a safe level. Intake and output must be measured for assurance that kidney function is adequate to handle the lead being excreted. BUN, serum creatinine, and protein in urine may also be assessed. If kidney function is no adequate, EDTA may lead to nephrotoxicity or kidney damage.

DRUG HIGHLIGHT

Edetate Calcium Disodium (EDTA)

Action: EDTA is an antidote agent that is used to pull heavy metals, such as lead, from soft tissue and bone, forming a soluble compound that can be eliminated in the urine.

Pregnancy risk category: C

Dosage: 35 mg/kg IM bid (for a total of approximately 75 mg/kg/d). In mild cases, divide total daily dose every 8 to 12 hours for 3 to 5 days. Give a second course after a rest period of 4 days or more.

Possible adverse effects: Nausea, vomiting, diarrhea, electrolyte imbalance

Nursing Implications:

- Monitor pupillary reflexes, orientation, urinalysis, and serum BUN and electrolytes. Ensure adequate renal function prior to administration.
- Apply EMLA cream to injection site prior to administration to decrease pain associated with injection. Anticipate use of procaine hydrochloride added to syringe as ordered to minimize pain.
- Administer IM deep into a large muscle mass to help minimize pain.
- Encourage fluid intake to facilitate excretion of compound. Monitor intake and output and urine-specific gravity.
- Keep patient supine for a short period due to possible postural hypotension.

BAL has the advantage of removing lead from red blood cells, but because of severe toxicity, it is only used with children who have severe forms of lead intoxication. Penicillamine (Cuprimine) is another drug used for lead poisoning. It is given orally following BAL or EDTA. Weekly complete blood count and renal and liver function tests accompany the administration of penicillamine. It may be given for as long as 3 to 6 months.

NURSING DIAGNOSES AND RELATED INTERVENTIONS

Planning can be difficult when parents are upset by their child's exposure to lead. They may experience a loss of self-esteem and sense of powerlessness when realizing that their financial circumstances or lifestyle has hurt their child.

Nursing Diagnosis: Knowledge deficit related to the dangers of lead ingestion

Outcome Identification: Parents will acknowledge the danger of lead ingestion to their child and potential sources of lead in their environment.

Outcome Evaluation: Parents state ways they have safeguarded their child against further lead ingestion; parents identify measures to reduce lead in the environment.

Teach parents about the risk of lead poisoning. Teach them to keep toddlers away from windowsills and other common sources of lead paint. Placing the television or an overstuffed chair against the windowsill may be effective as a temporary measure. As a rule, children's cribs should be placed about 3 ft away from walls in older homes to reduce the risk of children picking at loose wallpaper when they first wake in the morning or before they fall asleep at night (plaster, which contains lead, clings to the wallpaper).

All children with elevated lead levels need careful follow-up care to determine the seriousness of their condition and to ensure that they are kept from a lead source. Because children who recover from symptomatic lead poisoning have a high incidence of permanent neurologic damage, all children with elevated blood lead levels need appropriate follow-up care to evaluate development and intelligence.

Insecticide Poisoning

Children can be poisoned by insecticides by accidental ingestion or through skin or respiratory tract contact when playing in an area that has recently been sprayed with one. Long-term exposure may result from exposure to a parent's clothing if he or she comes home covered with insecticide spray. Once thought to be only a rural problem, the increase in the use of lawn sprays by commercial companies now makes this a suburban problem as well.

Many insecticides have an organophosphate base that leads to an accumulation of acetylcholine at neuromuscular junctions. Within a few minutes to 2 hours of exposure, children develop nausea and vomiting, diarrhea, excessive salivation, weakness of respiratory muscles, confusion, depressed reflexes, and possibly seizures.

If insecticide is swallowed, vomiting should be induced by syrup of ipecac or gastric lavage. Activated charcoal may be helpful in neutralizing any poison remaining. If clothing is contaminated, it should be removed and the child's skin and hair washed. To prevent contacting the insecticide yourself, wear gloves while giving such a bath.

Intravenous atropine is an effective antidote to reverse symptoms. Pralidoxime also may be effective.

Plant Poisoning

Plant poisoning (ingestion of a growing plant) occurs because parents do not think of plants as being poisonous. Common plants to which children may be exposed and the effects when they are ingested are shown in Empowering the Family.

Recreational Drug Poisoning

Adolescents and even grade-school children are brought to health care facilities by parents or friends because of a drug overdose or a "bad trip" caused by an unusual reaction or the effect of an unfortunate combination of drugs.

Children are often extremely disoriented following this form of ingestion. They may be having hallucinations. Obtaining a history may be difficult because children may have no idea what they took except that it was a red or a yellow capsule. They may know but may be reluctant to name a drug if it was obtained illegally.

Assessment

Even though the child may not appear to hear well or may not seem coherent, try to elicit a history from him or her. Avoid shouting or aggravating, with the knowledge that children who are having a paranoid reaction will be unable to cope rationally with this approach. If friends accompany an ill child, point out that your role is not that of a law enforcer. Your role is to help the child, and you cannot do that effectively unless the drug is identified. Approaching a child's friends this way is more likely to result in their naming the drug. If a child is brought in by parents who have no idea what drug could possibly have been taken, ask them to have someone at home check the child's bedroom for drugs (provided the child became ill while at home).

Try to determine whether the ingestion was an accident (a child was unaware that two drugs would react this way or took a wrong dose) or whether a child was actually attempting suicide. In the first instance, children will need counseling about drug use or about which drugs do not mix. If the incident was an attempted suicide, children will need observation and counseling toward more effective coping mechanisms in self-care. All poisonings or drug ingestions in children older than 7 years of age should be considered potential suicides until established otherwise.

Blood should be drawn for electrolyte levels and a toxicology screen. If a child is vomiting, save vomitus for analysis also.

Therapeutic Management

Children need supportive measures for their specific symptoms, including oxygen administration; electrolyte replacement (particularly if there is accompanying nausea and vomiting); and perhaps intravenous fluid administration in an attempt to dilute the drug.

Children who have swallowed a recreational drug need immediate treatment followed by empathetic investigation into the events leading to the poisoning. This potentially lethal ingestion may act as a turning point in the child's life, possibly alerting the child and family to the fact of a drug problem and the need for help. Factors such as reduction of fear and anxiety, increased coping mechanisms, knowledge of the effects of drug use, and availability of referral sources for a drug problem are important areas to address.

EMPOWERING THE FAMILY: **Identifying Poisonous Plants**

A number of common plants that can lead to poisoning in children, and the symptoms they produce, include the following:

English ivy	Nausea, vomiting, excess salivation, diarrhea, abdominal pain
Holly (berries)	Vomiting, diarrhea, abdominal pain
Hydrangea	Nausea, vomiting, muscular weakness, convulsions, dyspnea
Lily of the valley	Vomiting, abdominal pain, diarrhea, cardiac disturbances
Mistletoe	Vomiting, diarrhea, bradycardia
Morning glory (seeds)	Nausea, diarrhea, hallucinations
Philodendron	Swelling of the tongue, lips, irritation of mouth
Poinsettia	Nausea, vomiting
Rhubarb (leaves)	Irritant action on gastrointestinal tract
Rhododendron	Nausea, vomiting, abdominal pain, convulsions, limb paralysis

CHECKPOINT QUESTIONS

13. What type of agent is used for treating lead toxicity?
14. How might a child be poisoned by insecticides?

FOREIGN BODY OBSTRUCTION

Foreign bodies can become lodged in the throat or other body openings, causing stasis of secretions and infection. Direct obstruction or laceration of the mucous membrane may also result, with serious consequences.

Whether a foreign substance is inhaled or embedded elsewhere, nursing interventions will focus first on comforting the child and aiding in the substance's removal and then on teaching the child and parents ways to avoid such occurrences in the future.

Foreign Bodies in the Ear

Any child with a history of draining exudate from the ear canal needs an otoscopic examination to establish the reason for the drainage. In toddlers and preschoolers, the drainage often is the result of a foreign body in the ear canal. The object might be a small piece of a toy, a piece of paper, a transistor battery, or food, such as a peanut.

Removing foreign bodies from the ear is difficult because children are afraid that the instrument used will hurt them, so they have difficulty lying still for the procedure. If there is reason to think that the tympanic membrane is intact, irrigating the object from the ear canal with a syringe and normal saline may be possible. This should not be done if the object is a substance, such as a peanut, that will swell when wet. If it is possible that the tympanic membrane is ruptured, the ear canal must not be irrigated or fluid will be forced into the middle ear, possibly introducing infection (otitis media).

Often, it is better to wait for an otolaryngologist to care for the child, because trauma to the ear canal in an attempt to remove a foreign body will increase the edema and make removal even more difficult.

Foreign Bodies in the Nose

Foreign objects stuffed into the nose eventually cause inflammation and purulent discharge from the nares. The odor accompanying such impaction is often the first sign noticed by a parent. Objects pushed into the nose generally can be removed with forceps. A local antibiotic might be necessary after removal if ulceration resulted from the local irritation.

Foreign Bodies in the Esophagus

Children tend not to chew food well and to swallow portions that are too big to pass safely through the esophagus. Candy, such as Lifesavers, are common objects caught in the esophagus. Intense pain at the site where the object is lodged will result. If it is an object that will dissolve, such as a Lifesaver or a piece of digestible meat, offer the child fluid to drink to help flush the object into the stomach. Even after the object dissolves or passes into the stomach, children will feel transient pain at the original site of the obstruction.

An object that is a part of a toy or a chicken bone (other objects frequently swallowed) that will not dissolve and should not be passed is removed by esophagoscopy. Small coins, such as pennies and dimes, generally pass by themselves without difficulty.

Parents (or children themselves if adolescents) should observe stools over the next several days to determine when the coin passes through the GI tract (this takes about 48 hours). Without frightening them, caution parents to observe for signs of bowel perforation or obstruction, such as vomiting or abdominal pain, until an object has passed. If there is any doubt, an x-ray taken 3 days to a week after ingestion will establish whether the object has been evacuated from the body.

WHAT IF? What if you received a call from your neighbor stating that her 2-year-old son swallowed a quarter? Would you reassure her that this size coin passes readily, or would you recommend she see her primary care provider?

Subcutaneous Objects

Children receive many wood splinters in hands and feet. These usually are removed easily by a probing needle and tweezers following cleaning with an antiseptic solution. If the penetrating object is metal, such as a sewing needle or nail, its presence can be detected by x-ray. If the object is one that would have been in contact with soil, such as a rusty nail, the child needs tetanus prophylaxis following extraction of the object.

TRAUMA RELATED TO ENVIRONMENTAL EXPOSURE

Frostbite

Frostbite is tissue injury caused by freezing cold. Cells at the site actually die. Cold exposure leads to peripheral vasoconstriction, so oxygen supply is cut off to surrounding cells. In children, the body parts involved are usually the fingers or toes.

Assessment

The affected part appears white or erythematous with edema and feels numb. Degrees of frostbite are summarized in Table 31-5. Explore the cause of frostbite by careful history taking. It occurs most frequently in children who are skiing or snowmobiling for long periods. If parents fail to provide adequate clothing because they underestimated the degree of cold outside, the possibility of neglect or child abuse must be ruled out as a cause. Frostbite also can occur from inhalant abuse (Kurbat & Pollack, 1998).

TABLE 31.5 Degrees of Frostbite

DEGREE	DESCRIPTION
First	Mild freezing of epidermis; appears erythematous with edema
Second	Partial- or full-thickness injury; appears erythematous with blisters and pain occurring after rewarming
Third	Full thickness (epidermis, dermis, and subcutaneous tissue); appears white
Fourth	Complete necrosis with gangrene and possible ultimate loss of body part

Therapeutic Management

Always warm frostbitten areas gradually. Sudden warming will increase the metabolism rate of cells. Without adequate blood flow to the area because of still-present vasoconstriction, additional damage will occur.

NURSING DIAGNOSES AND RELATED INTERVENTIONS

Nursing Diagnosis: Pain related to frostbite damage to cells

Outcome Identification: Child will experience a minimum amount of pain following injury.

Outcome Evaluation: Child states that pain is controlled at a tolerable level.

As soon as warming begins, the area becomes painful from cells that are injured, but not destroyed, registering their anoxic state. Children need an analgesic for pain. The pain is usually extreme. Do not underestimate its extent. Epidural anesthesia can be used if the feet are involved (Punja et al, 1998).

During the next few days after severe frostbite, necrosis of destroyed tissue will occur, and affected tissue will slough away. Apply a dressing as necessary to avoid secondary bacterial contamination of a necrotic injury site. Assess body temperature conscientiously to detect early symptoms of infection.

✔ CHECKPOINT QUESTIONS

15. If a child swallowed a chicken bone, how would the child be treated?
16. What results if a frostbitten area is warmed too quickly?

BITES

Mammalian Bites

Dog bites account for approximately 90% of all bites inflicted on humans, and children and adolescents are involved in one third to one half of reported incidents. Cat bites, wild animal bites, and human bites also constitute a threat, although less common to children. All of these bites can cause abrasions, puncture wounds, lacerations, and crushing injuries related to the size of the animal and location of the bite. The biggest concerns associated with animal bites are the possibility of long-term scarring and disfigurement and the possibility of infection, especially rabies, from the presence of microorganisms in the animal's mouth. This latter subject is discussed in Chapter 22.

Snakebite

Most fatal snakebites (envenomation) in the United States are copperhead (found in Eastern and Southern states) and rattlesnake bites (found in almost every state). A few bites occur from cottonmouth moccasins or coral snakes (both found in Southeastern states). The effect of rattlesnake, copperhead, and cottonmouth bites is to cause a failure of the blood coagulation system (Bond & Burkhart, 1998). Intracranial hemorrhage is the cause of death. Coral snakes are known for the small coral, yellow, and black rings encircling their body. Fortunately, they are shy and seldom bite. The effect of venom injected through the bite of these snakes is to cause neuromuscular paralysis.

Assessment

Snakebites tend to occur during the warm months of the year, from April to October. Reaction to a poisonous snakebite is almost immediate. A white wheal forms at the site, showing the puncture marks, accompanied by excruciating pain at the site. Purplish erythema and edema begin to extend rapidly from the site.

By the time children are seen at a health care facility, sanguineous fluid may ooze from the bite. Systemic symptoms, such as dizziness, vomiting, perspiration, and weakness, may be present. Because snake venom interferes with blood coagulation, children may have hematemesis or bleeding from the nose, intestines, or bladder from subcutaneous or internal hemorrhage. The pupils may be dilated, showing the potent effect on cerebral centers. If children are not treated, convulsions, coma, and death may result.

Emergency Management at the Scene

At the scene of a snakebite, apply a cold compress to the bite in the hope of slowing the spread of the venom and to reduce the formation of edema. Urge the child to lie quietly to slow circulation. Keep the bitten extremity dependent, again to slow venous circulation. Commercial snakebite kits have rubber suction cups in them for suctioning out venom. These should be used. Excising the bite with a knife and sucking out the venom orally (often shown in old western movies) is of questionable value and contradicts rules of standard precautions. If the person administering the treatment has open mouth lesions, such as carious teeth, the procedure may be dangerous to that person (venom is not dangerous when swallowed, only when absorbed through open lesions). Excising the bite also may lead to secondary infection and if done too vigorously, may injure tendon or muscle. No time should be wasted before children are taken to a health care facility for treatment.

Emergency Management at the Health Facility

In the emergency facility, ask the child or a person who was with him or her to describe the snake. In areas where snakebites are frequent, keep available photographs of the venomous snakes in the area. Even a preschooler may be able to identify the snake by pointing to a photograph. Specific antivenin will be administered. Because rattlesnakes, copperheads, and cottonmouth moccasins are all one type of snake (pit vipers), one form of antivenin acts against all of these bites. Specific antivenin is prepared for coral snake or cobra bites and is kept at most zoos. If the child receives antivenin promptly after a bite, the prognosis for full recovery is good. Tetanus prophylaxis is instituted if the child's immunization status is unknown or if it has been more than 10 years since a tetanus immunization was given.

Antivenin contains a horse-serum base. Therefore, before the serum is injected intramuscularly or intravenously, a skin test is first performed to prevent a possible anaphylactic reaction to the serum. If the serum is given intramuscularly, it should not be injected into an edematous body part because medication is absorbed poorly from edematous areas. Giving antivenin in the limb opposite the bitten limb will be just as effective as administering it into the bitten limb.

NURSING DIAGNOSES AND RELATED INTERVENTIONS

Nursing Diagnosis: Fear related to seriousness of child's condition

Outcome Identification: Parents and child will demonstrate ability to keep fear within manageable limits.

Outcome Evaluation: Parents and child voice that they are able to cope with the degree of fear present.

Children with snakebites are extremely frightened. Their parents who have seen old cowboy movies showing the agony of snakebite also are thoroughly frightened. Children need a great deal of support from health care personnel because parents may be too frightened to offer the support.

As a final care measure, teach children safety rules for avoiding snakebites:

- Looking for snakes before stepping into underbrush
- Not lifting up rocks without looking at what could be under them
- Listening for the telltale sound of a rattlesnake
- Being aware that snakes sun on rocks
- Knowing the markings of poisonous snakes

BURN TRAUMA

A burn is injury to body tissue caused by excessive heat. They commonly occur in children of all ages after infancy. They are the second cause of accidental injury in children 1 to 4 years of age and the third cause in children 5 to 14 years. Toddlers are often burned by turning pans of scalding water over on themselves or by biting into electrical cords. Older children are more apt to suffer burns from flames when they move too close to a campfire, heater, or fireplace or if they play with matches. Some burns (particularly scalding) are symptoms of child abuse (Bennett & Gamelli, 1998). As many as 50% of burns could be prevented with improved parent and child education.

With a thermal burn, tissue damage occurs when heat is greater than 104°F (40°C). Any thermal burn tends to be more serious in children than in adults because the same size burn covers a larger surface of a child's body.

Assessment

When children are brought to a health care facility with a thermal injury, the first questions must be, "What is the extent of the burn? What is the depth of the burn? Where is the burn?" Burns are classified according to the criteria of the American Burn Association as major, moderate, or minor burns. These classifications are shown in Table 31-6. It is important that along with the size and depth, the location of the burn is assessed. Face and throat burns are particularly hazardous because there may be unseen burns in the respiratory tract. Resulting edema will lead to respiratory tract obstruction. Hand burns are also hazardous, because if the fingers and thumb are not positioned properly during healing, adhesions will inhibit full range of motion in the future. Burns of the feet and genitalia often become secondarily infected if the child is sent home after only initial treatment. Genital burns are also hazardous because edema of the urinary meatus may prevent a child from voiding.

With adults, a "rule of nine" is a quick method of estimating the extent of a burn. Each upper extremity represents 9% of body surface; each lower extremity represents two 9s, or 18%, and the head and neck represent 9%. Because the body proportions of children are different from those of adults, this rule does not always apply and is misleading in the very young child. Data for determining the extent of burns in children are shown in Figure 31-8.

Depth of Burn

Assessing the depth of burns is not always easy. Descriptions of tissue at different burn depths appear in Table 31-7

TABLE 31.6 Classification of Burns

CLASSIFICATION	DESCRIPTION
Minor	First-degree burn or second degree <10% of body surface or third degree <2% of body surface; no area of the face, feet, hands, or genitalia burned
Moderate	Second-degree burn between 10% and 20% or on the face, hands, feet, or genitalia or third-degree burn <10% body surface or if smoke inhalation has occurred
Severe	Second-degree burn >20% body surface or third-degree burn >10% body surface

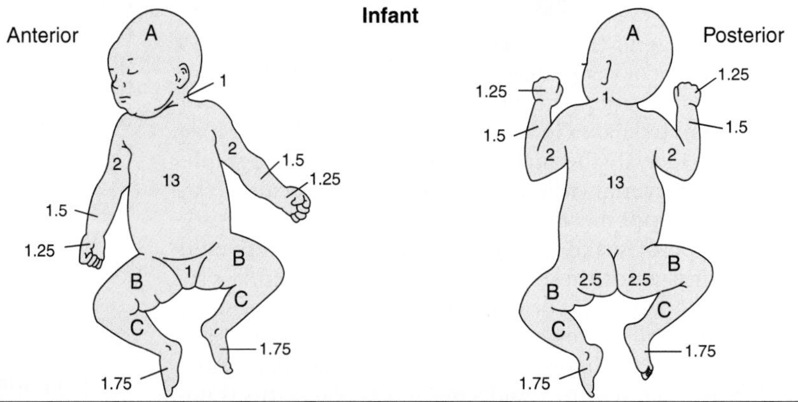

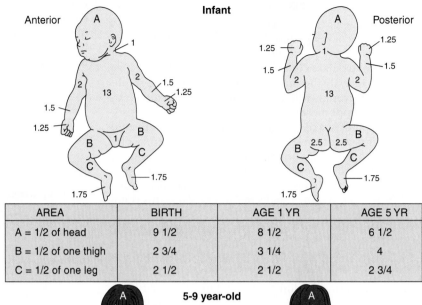

AREA	BIRTH	AGE 1 YR	AGE 5 YR
A = 1/2 of head	9 1/2	8 1/2	6 1/2
B = 1/2 of one thigh	2 3/4	3 1/4	4
C = 1/2 of one leg	2 1/2	2 1/2	2 3/4

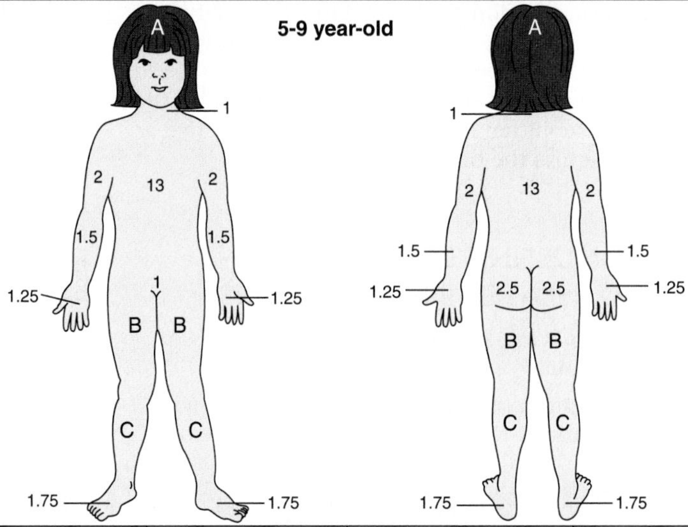

AREA	AGE 10 YR	AGE 15 YR	ADULT
A = 1/2 of head	5 1/2	4 1/2	3 1/2
B = 1/2 of one thigh	4 1/2	4 1/2	4 3/4
C = 1/2 of one leg	3	3 1/4	3 1/2

FIGURE 31.8 Determination of extent of burns in children.

and are illustrated in Figure 31-9. *Partial-thickness* burns include first- and second-degree burns. A first-degree burn involves only the superficial epidermis. The area appears erythematous. It is painful to touch and blanches on pressure (Figure 31-10*A*). Scalds and sunburn are examples of first-degree burns. Such burns heal by simple regeneration and take only 1 to 10 days to heal.

A second-degree burn involves the entire epidermis. Sweat glands and hair follicles are left intact. The area appears very erythematous, blistered, and moist from exudate. It is extremely painful. Scalds can cause second-degree burns (see Figure 31-10*B*). Such burns heal by regeneration of tissue but take 2 to 6 weeks to heal.

A third-degree burn is a full-thickness burn involving both skin layers, epidermis and dermis. It may also involve adipose tissue, fascia, muscle, and bone. The burn appears either white or black (Figure 31-11). Because the nerves, sweat glands, and hair follicles have been burned, third-degree burns are not painful. Flames lead to third-degree burns. Such burns cannot heal by regeneration because underlying layers of skin are destroyed. Skin grafting is usually necessary, and healing will take months. Scar tissue will remain at the healed site.

When estimating the depth of a burn, use the appearance of the burn and the sensitivity of the area to pain as criteria. Many burns are compound, involving first-, second-, and third-degree burns. There may be a central white area that is insensitive to pain (third degree), surrounded by an area of erythematous blisters (second degree), surrounded by another area that is erythematous only (first degree).

Undress children with burns completely so that the entire body can be inspected. A first-degree burn is painful, whereas a third-degree burn is not. Therefore, a child may be crying from a superficial burn that is obvious on the arm, although the condition needing the most immediate

TABLE 31.7 Characteristics of Burns

SEVERITY	DEPTH OF TISSUE INVOLVED	APPEARANCE	EXAMPLE
First degree (partial thickness)	Epidermis	Erythematous, dry, painful	Sunburn
Second degree (partial thickness)	Epidermis Portion of dermis	Blistered, erythematous to white	Scalds
Third degree (full thickness)	Entire skin, including nerves and blood vessels in skin	Leathery; black or white; not sensitive to pain (nerve endings destroyed)	Flame

attention is a third-degree burn on the chest, which is covered by a jacket.

Ask what caused the burn, because different materials cause different degrees of burn. Hot water, for example, causes scalding, a generally lesser degree of burn than is caused by flaming clothing. Ask where the fire happened. Fires in closed spaces are apt to cause more respiratory involvement than fires in open areas.

Ask if the child has any secondary health problem. In the anxiety over the present burn, parents forget to report important facts, for example, that the child has diabetes or is allergic to a common drug. Following a fire, parents often pick up the burned child and bring him or her to a health care facility, leaving other children unprotected at home. Ask about other children and where they are. Parents may have burned hands from putting out the fire on the child's clothes and need equal care, but in their anxiety about the child's condition, they do not mention this. Ask who put out the fire. Were any other family members or close friends hurt? Does anyone else need care?

✔ CHECKPOINT QUESTIONS

17. What layer(s) of skin is (are) involved with a second-degree burn?
18. What would be absent in a child with a third-degree burn?

Emergency Management

Mild (First-Degree) Burns

Although first-degree partial-thickness burns are the simplest type of burn, they involve pain and death of skin cells, so they must be treated seriously. Cleanse the area with an antiseptic. Apply an analgesic, antibiotic ointment and a gauze bandage to prevent infection. Do not break any blisters that are present because this invites infection. Broken blisters may be débrided (cut away) to remove possible necrotic tissue. The child should return in 2 days to have the

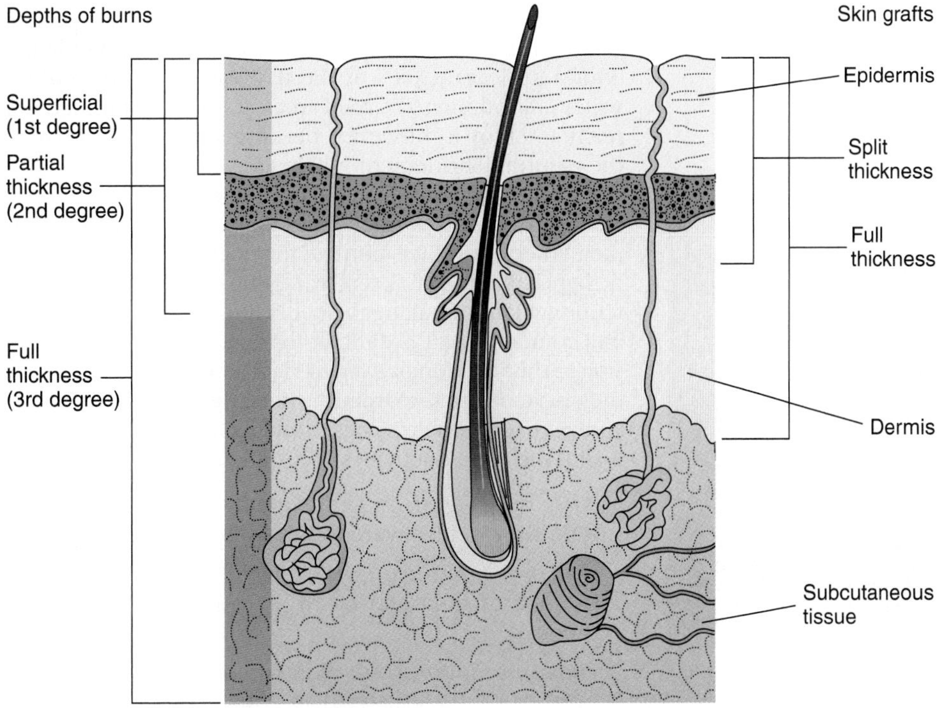

FIGURE 31.9 Depths of burns.

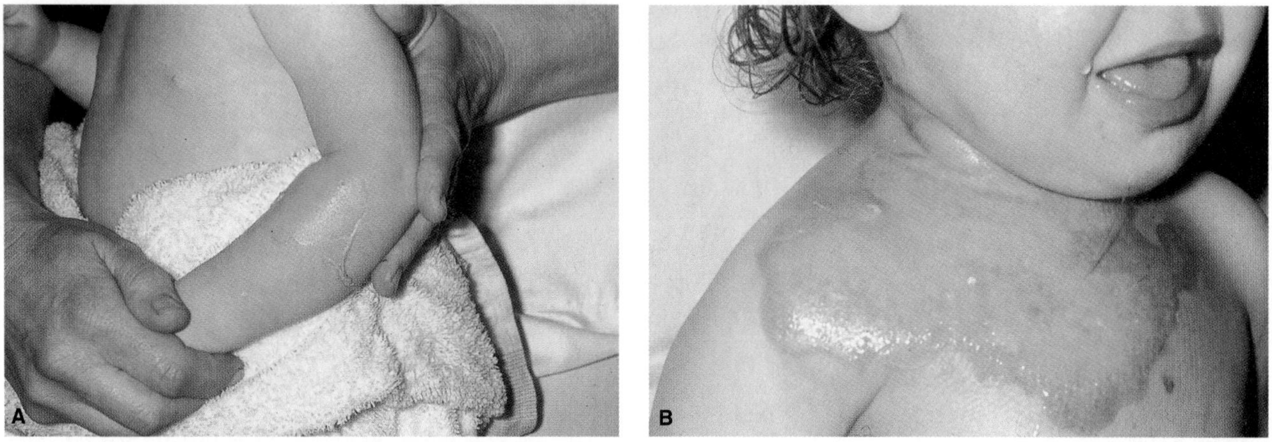

FIGURE 31.10 Partial-thickness burns. (**A**) An infant with a first-degree burn on the arm and chest caused by scalding with hot water. (**B**) A toddler with a second-degree burn caused by scalding. The area appears severely reddened and moist with some blistering.

area inspected for a secondary infection and to have the dressing changed. Caution parents to keep the dressing dry (no swimming or getting the area wet while bathing for 1 week). A first-degree burn heals in about that time.

Moderate and Severe Burns

The child with a moderate or severe burn is severely injured and needs swift, sure care to survive the injury without a disability caused by scarring, infection, or contracture.

NURSING DIAGNOSES AND RELATED INTERVENTIONS

Nursing Diagnosis: Pain related to trauma to body cells

Outcome Identification: Child will experience the minimum amount of pain possible (be certain that goal established is realistic; you cannot eliminate *all* pain).

Outcome Evaluation: Child states that pain is at a tolerable level.

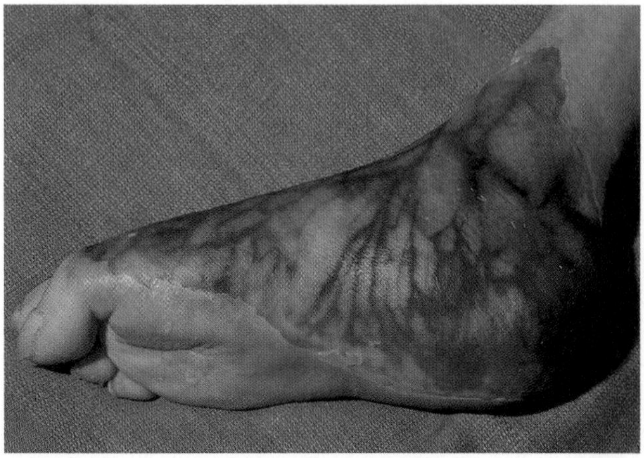

FIGURE 31.11 Full-thickness (third-degree) burn of the foot. Notice the layers of skin involved with this type of burn.

Children who have smoke inhalation may be unconscious from brain anoxia immediately following a burn. Most children, however, are awake and very aware of the pain and treatments involved, so they need immediate care to relieve this. After the first week following a major burn, some children develop symptoms of delirium, seizures, and coma that result from toxic breakdown of damaged cells and sensory deprivation, isolation, and lack of sleep. Nursing care aimed at reducing unnecessary stimuli helps to prevent these late symptoms from occurring.

A child needs an analgesic to relieve pain and to help prevent shock. Morphine sulfate is commonly given. It can be given intramuscularly, but because circulation is impaired in children with shock, intravenous administration is most effective. Attempt to premedicate prior to performing any burn care.

Daily débridement that follows emergency care is a painful procedure. Whirlpool treatment, which precedes the débridement, may at first be painful but quickly becomes a pleasant part of the day, because the swirling water is soothing to burned areas. It is difficult for a child really to enjoy it, however, because as soon as it is over, the painful débridement will begin.

For most of every day, children may be required to remain in awkward positions to keep joints overextended. If their anterior throat is burned, for example, their head will be hyperextended to keep scar tissue that forms on the anterior neck from pulling their chin down against their chest in a contracture. It is difficult for children to watch television in this position or even to view activities on the unit. If they have burns at extremity joints, they may have splints applied over burn dressings to maintain joints in extension. Again, this makes activities very difficult for them.

Nursing Diagnosis: Fluid volume deficit related to fluid shifts with severe thermal burn

Outcome Identification: Child will maintain normal balance of fluid and electrolytes during period of therapy.

Outcome Evaluation: Skin turgor is good; hourly urine output is greater than 1 mL/kg, with specific gravity between 1.003 and 1.030; vital signs are within acceptable parameters.

Immediately following a severe burn, the child's circulatory system becomes hypovolemic, due to the loss of plasma through the burn site. In addition, a great deal of fluid is sequestered in edematous tissue at the site. The outpouring of plasma, caused by increased permeability of capillaries (or damage to capillaries), is most marked during the first 6 hours after a burn. It continues to some extent for the first 24 hours. To replace this, the child may have intravenous albumin ordered (12.5 g/L of intravenous fluid).

Accompanying the hypovolemia will be a marked reduction in cardiac output. Part of this decrease apparently results from a primary response of the myocardium to the shock of thermal injury. Even with relatively minor burns, vital signs must be followed closely so that this reaction can be detected. The child may be severely anemic because of injury to red blood cells by heat and loss at the wound site, and he or she may have severe electrolyte abnormalities as a result of fluid shifts (Table 31-8). The large amount of sodium lost with the edematous burn fluid and the release of potassium from damaged cells leads to an immediate hyponatremia and hyperkalemia.

In response to injury, the adrenal gland releases epinephrine and norepinephrine. This may lead to compensatory hypertension. Monitor blood pressure closely. Both aldosterone and antidiuretic hormone levels rise in an attempt to conserve fluid.

Lactated Ringer's solution is the commercially available solution most compatible with extracellular fluid. It is one of the first fluids usually begun for fluid replacement, although normal saline may be used. The child may also need plasma replacement and additional fluid, such as 5% dextrose in water. Potassium must not be administered immediately after a burn because kidney function must first be evaluated. Intravenous fluid is generally administered by the most convenient vein that can be entered so that morphine sulfate can be administered to relieve pain. A more stable fluid line may then be inserted. The amount of fluid necessary is calculated carefully, based on predicted insensible fluid loss and loss due to the burn. A common formula used to calculate fluid needed is:

$$\frac{2000\ \text{mL/m}^2\ \text{of body surface}}{24\ \text{h}} + \frac{5000\ \text{mL/m}^2\ \text{of body surface burned}}{24\ \text{h}}$$

This fluid is administered rapidly for the first 8 hours (half of the 24-hour load), then more slowly for the next 16 hours (the second half). It is important that it be continued beyond the time of increased capillary permeability (at least the first 24 hours). The administration site, therefore, must be safeguarded carefully so that it does not become infiltrated. A central venous pressure or pulmonary artery catheter may be inserted to determine hemodynamic and fluid volume status (Carrougher, 1997).

About 48 hours after the burn, the extracellular fluid at the burn site begins to be reabsorbed into the bloodstream. The edema begins to subside; the child will have diuresis and lose weight. The heart rate will increase because of temporary hypervolemia. The hematocrit level will be low because red blood cells will be diluted. The child will need frequent electrolyte levels evaluated to determine the effectiveness of fluid balance during this period. Potassium supplements may be necessary to maintain normal heart function, because although potassium is released into serum from destroyed cells, it is rapidly excreted by the kidneys. If the child needs continued electrolyte replacement at this time, the rate of flow of fluid must be monitored carefully so that the blood volume does not exceed the child's tolerance. The child may need packed red blood cells to maintain an adequate hemoglobin level.

Nursing Diagnosis: Risk for altered tissue perfusion related to cardiovascular adjustments following thermal injury

Outcome Identification: Child's cardiovascular system will satisfactorily adjust to fluid shifts during therapy.

Outcome Evaluation: Child's vital signs stay within normal limits; hourly urine output remains greater than 1 mL/kg.

Take height, weight, and vital signs on admission, and continue to take vital signs every 15 minutes until they are stable. The pulse, blood pressure, and central venous pressure should be recorded hourly until the child passes the immediate danger of shock. Another important period occurs 48 hours after the injury when fluid is returning to the bloodstream. Make certain to evaluate vital signs and urine output carefully. Gradual changes may be as informative as sudden changes.

A complete blood count, blood typing and cross-matching, electrolyte and BUN determinations, and blood gas studies to ascertain blood levels of oxygen and carbon dioxide are also important.

Nursing Diagnosis: Risk for altered breathing patterns related to edema from thermal injury

Outcome Identification: Child will maintain respiratory function during course of illness.

Outcome Evaluation: Child's respiratory rate stays within 16 to 20 breaths per minute; lung auscultation reveals no rales.

TABLE 31.8 Fluid Shifts After Thermal Injury

FLUID SHIFTS IN FIRST 24 HOURS	REMOBILIZATION OF FLUID AFTER 48 HOURS
Burn ↓	Edematous tissue surrounding burn area ↓
Increased capillary permeability ↓	Intravascular compartment ↓
Hypoproteinemia	
Hyponatremia	Hypervolemia
Hyperkalemia	Hypernatremia
Hypovolemia	Hypokalemia

If the child breathed in smoke from a fire, the injury from the smoke inhalation can be more serious than the skin surface burns. Smoke coming from a fire is at the temperature of the fire. Breathing this in is therefore the same as exposing the upper respiratory tract to open fire. In addition, toxic substances and soot given off from fire may be extremely irritating to the respiratory tract (Schweich, 1997). Carbon monoxide is absorbed from smoke. This enters red blood cells in place of oxygen, shutting off oxygen supply to body cells. Smoke inhalation leads to loss of consciousness. Edema fluid will pass into the injured bronchioles and trachea, causing pulmonary edema or obstruction. This leads to dyspnea and stridor. The edema may be so extensive that it reduces lung function substantially. About a week after the smoke inhalation, the possible development of pneumonia because of denuded tracheal and bronchial tract areas becomes a major problem. That inhalation of smoke or flame from a fire can be more serious than the skin burns the child suffers may be difficult for parents to understand. They are relieved if they learn that the child has suffered only smoke inhalation. They need an explanation of the physiologic consequences that can result from pulmonary injury.

Obtain a history to assess if the fire occurred in a closed space, such as a garage. Assess for burns of the face, neck, or chest, which means fire was near the nose and respiratory tract. Assess the quality of the child's voice (will be hoarse if the throat is irritated from smoke). The respiratory rate of all burned children should be monitored carefully, because the respiratory rate increases with respiratory obstruction. The child may become restless and thrash because of lack of oxygen. Measurement of blood gases will demonstrate the degree of hypoxia present from carbon monoxide intoxication. Administering 100% oxygen is the best therapy for displacing carbon monoxide and providing adequate oxygenation to body cells. The child may need endotracheal intubation or tracheostomy with assisted ventilation. Intubation is best because this child is at a much higher risk for pneumonia than the average child with a tracheostomy.

Symptoms of smoke inhalation may not occur immediately but only after 8 to 24 hours. A chest x-ray taken at this time will reveal collecting edematous fluid and decreased aeration. Continue to assess the child's temperature every 4 hours for the first week after the injury to detect lung infection. The cause of fever may relate to infection in the burn area. If the burn occurred in a closed area so that the child inhaled smoke, pneumonia must also be considered as a possible reason for increasing temperature. Bronchodilators and antibiotics may be prescribed. High-frequency ventilation may be helpful to keep alveoli functioning. Some children need ECMO support (Pierre et al, 1998).

Nursing Diagnosis: Risk for altered urinary elimination related to thermal trauma

Outcome Identification: Child will not experience decreased urine output during course of illness.

Outcome Evaluation: Child's urine output will be greater than 1 mL/kg of body weight per hour.

Because the child's blood volume decreases immediately following a burn, renal function is threatened by kidney ischemia just when renal function is needed to rid the body of breakdown products from burned cells. If the child is burned over 10% of his or her body surface, urinary output may decrease immediately. Blood volume must be maintained by intravenous fluid administration to establish good urinary output once more. Urine output should be 1 mL/kg of body weight per hour. The specific gravity of urine also should be monitored to determine whether the kidneys can concentrate urine to conserve body fluid (failing kidneys lose this ability rapidly). In the days following the burn, because products of necrotic tissue and toxic substances must be evacuated by the kidney, kidney function may fail again. There are also increases in antidiuretic hormone and aldosterone. Diuresis occurs at 48 hours.

An indwelling urinary (Foley) catheter should be inserted and an immediate urine specimen obtained for analysis. A specific gravity determination performed immediately in the emergency department is helpful. Observing urinary output is a major nursing responsibility.

Hourly urine output less than 1 mL/kg suggests renal insufficiency. Free hemoglobin from destroyed red blood cells can plug kidney tubules and lead to kidney failure (acute tubular necrosis). When this is occurring, urine color will be red to black from the hemoglobin present. A diuretic such as mannitol may be administered to flush this from the kidneys. If effective, urine returns to its usual straw color.

Nursing Diagnosis: Risk for altered nutrition, less than body requirements, related to thermal trauma

Outcome Identification: Child will ingest adequate nutrients for increased metabolic needs during therapy.

Outcome Evaluation: Child's weight remains within normal age-appropriate growth percentiles; skin turgor remains normal; urine-specific gravity remains between 1.003 and 1.030.

The metabolic rate increases in children following burns as their body begins to pool its resources to adjust to the insult. If the child does not receive enough calories in intravenous fluid, he or she will begin to use protein. This is particularly dangerous because the child needs protein now for burn healing, and he or she will become acidotic (Hildreth, 1997).

A nasogastric tube may be inserted and attached to low suction as prophylactic therapy to prevent aspiration of vomitus. The tube must remain in place until bowel sounds are detected. This usually occurs within 24 hours but may take as long as 72 hours in severely burned children. The suction from a nasogastric tube may be tinged with blood (coffee-ground fluid) due to bleeding caused by stomach vessel congestion. This drainage must be observed closely for a change to fresh bleeding, which can be caused by an ulcer (Curling's ulcer). This type of ulcer results from stress. It is prevented by administering a histamine-2 receptor antagonist, such as cimetidine (Tagamet), in an attempt to reduce gastric acidity and ulcer formation.

If a bleeding ulcer occurs, gastric lavage with iced saline may be necessary. Blood for transfusion should be readily available, because the blood loss from a GI ulcer can be rapid and severe.

When children have burns over more than 30% of the body surface, paralytic ileus may occur. If this happens, within hours of the burn, symptoms of intestinal obstruction, such as vomiting, abdominal distention, and colicky pain, will appear.

Children with severe burns usually have nothing by mouth for 24 hours because of the danger of paralytic ileus. After this, most burned children are able to eat, and oral feedings are begun as soon as possible. To supply adequate calories for increased metabolic needs and spare protein for repairing cells, the diet is high in calories and protein (1800 cal/m^2/24 hours plus 22 cal/m^2 of burned area per 24 hours). Children may also need vitamin (particularly B and C) and iron supplements. High-protein drinks may be necessary in between meals to ensure an adequate protein intake.

Because adequate nutrition is important, it may be necessary to supplement the child's diet with intravenous or parenteral nutrition solutions or nasogastric tube feeding. As additional methods of stimulating interest in eating, encourage school-age children to help add intake and output columns and help the dietitian add a calorie-count list or keep track of their own daily weight (taken at the same time each day in the same clothing). It may be helpful to make contracts with older children for a good nutritional intake.

Nursing Diagnosis: Risk for injury related to effects of burn, denuded skin surfaces, and lowered resistance to infection with thermal injury

Outcome Identification: Child will not develop an infection during time of denuded tissue.

Outcome Evaluation: Child's temperature remains at 98.6°F (37°C); skin areas surrounding burned areas show no signs of erythema or warmth.

There appears to be some defect in the ability of neutrophils to phagocytize bacteria following thermal injury, and formation of immunoglobulin G antibodies apparently fails. For these reasons, the child has reduced protection against infection. *Staphylococcus aureus* and streptococci are the gram-positive organisms and *Pseudomonas aeruginosa* is the gram-negative organism most likely to invade burn tissue. Children are usually prescribed parenteral penicillin to prevent β-hemolytic streptococcal infection and tetanus toxoid to prevent tetanus.

Bacteria penetrate the burn eschar readily, offering no protection from infection. However, it does offer protection from fluid loss. Fortunately, granulation tissue, which forms under the eschar 3 to 4 weeks after the burn, is resistant to bacterial invasion.

Because the child has lost the integumentary defense against infection, prophylactic treatment is important to prevent infection. Antibiotics are not very effective in controlling burn-wound infection, probably because the burned and constricted capillaries around the burn site cannot carry the antibiotic to the area. Equipment used with the child must therefore be sterile. Personnel caring for the severely burned child should wear caps, masks, gowns, and gloves, even for emergency care. Children are placed on a sterile sheet on the examining table. Nose, throat, and wound cultures may be done.

Even though their burns may be covered by gauze dressings, children need additional protection from possible infection until adequate granulation tissue has formed to serve as a barrier against massive infection. Cultures of the burned area are taken about every third day so that invading organisms can be identified and specific therapy planned. Helping children maintain their self-esteem and keeping them from withdrawing from social contacts is one of the most difficult nursing roles when caring for a burned child during the isolation period.

Because third-degree burns heal with fibrous scarring, contracture of the joint may occur if the burn is over a movable body part (Figure 31-12). Joints are positioned carefully, often overextended, so that if some contracture occurs, the joint will eventually remain in good position. Extremities are elevated to decrease edema and tissue

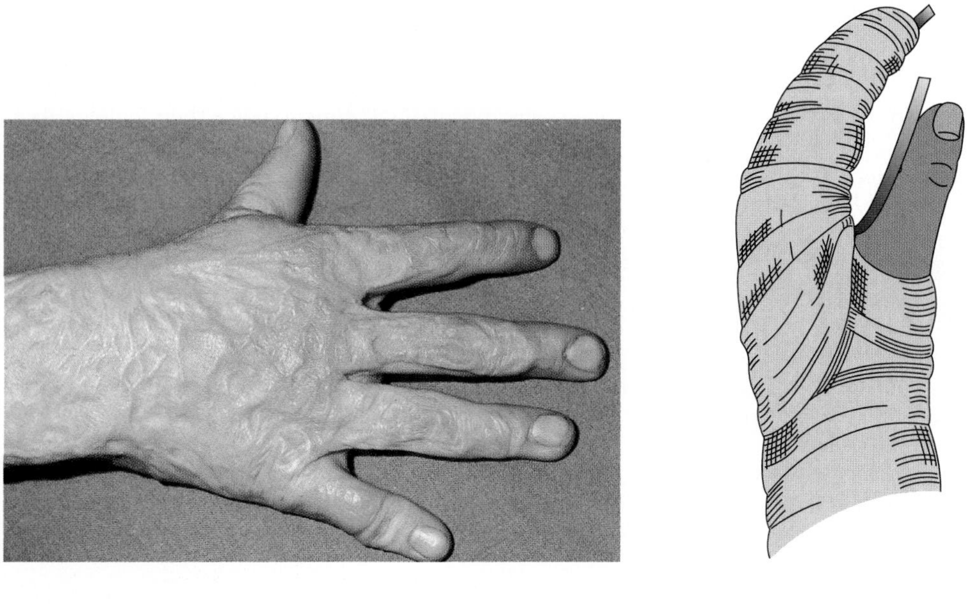

FIGURE 31.12 A child's hand scarred from third-degree burns. Note the proper extension and alignment of the hand and fingers, which were maintained by the use of splints during healing.

pressure. The overextension positions are difficult to maintain because they become uncomfortable for the child. Be certain to understand the need for these positions so that you can reinforce their importance.

Therapy for Severe Burns

Once the child has been given immediate care and is thoroughly assessed to determine the effects of the injury on all body systems, planning for burn treatment can begin.

Second- and third-degree burns may receive open treatment, leaving the burned area exposed to the air, or a closed method, covering the burned area with an antibacterial cream and many layers of gauze. These two methods are compared in Table 31-9. As a rule, burn dressings are applied loosely in the first 24 hours to prevent interfering with circulation as edema forms. Be certain not to allow two burned body surfaces, such as the sides of fingers or the back of the ears and the scalp, to touch, because as healing takes place, a webbing forms between these surfaces. Do not use adhesive tape. It is painful to remove and can leave excoriated areas providing additional entry for infection. Netting is useful to use to hold dressings in place because it expands easily and needs no additional tape.

Topical Therapy

Silver sulfadiazine (Silvadene) is the drug of choice for burn therapy to limit infection at the burn site. It is applied as a paste to the burn, and the area is covered with a few layers of mesh gauze. Silver sulfadiazine is an effective agent against gram-negative and gram-positive organisms and secondary infectious agents, such as *Candida.* It is soothing when applied and tends to keep the burn eschar soft, making débridement easier. It does not penetrate the eschar well, which is its one drawback.

Antiseptic solutions, such a povidone-iodine (Betadine), may be used to inhibit bacterial and fungal growth. Unfortunately, iodine stings as it is applied and stains skin and clothing brown. Dressings must be kept continually wet to keep them from clinging to and disrupting the healing tissue. An occlusive dressing with topical antibiotic therapy may be used.

Pseudomonas is a pathogen commonly found in burn wounds. If it is detected in cultures, gentamicin (Garamycin) cream may be applied. If a topical cream is not effective against invading organisms in the deeper tissue under the eschar, daily injections of specific antibiotics to the deeper layers of the burned area may be necessary. A rise in C-reactive protein serum level may first reveal infection in burns (Neely et al, 1998).

If a burned area cannot be readily dressed, such as the female genitalia, it can be left exposed. The danger of this method is the potential invasion of pathogens.

Escharotomy

An eschar is the tough, leathery scab that forms over moderately or severely burned areas. Fluid accumulates rapidly under eschars, putting pressure on underlying blood vessels and nerves. If an extremity or the trunk has been burned so both anterior and posterior surfaces have eschar formation, this may form a tight band around the extremity or trunk, cutting off circulation to the distal body portions. Distal parts feel cool to the touch and appear pale. The child notices tingling or numbness. Pulses are difficult to palpate and capillary refill is slow (more than 5 seconds). To alleviate this problem, an **escharotomy** (cut into the eschar) is performed. Some bleeding following escharotomy will occur. Packing the wound and applying pressure usually relieves this.

Débridement

Débridement is the removal of necrotic tissue from a burned area. Débridement reduces the possibility of infection because it reduces the tissue present for microorganisms to thrive. Children usually have 20 minutes of hydrotherapy before débridement to soften and loosen eschar, which can then be gently snipped away with forceps and scissors. Débridement is painful, and some bleeding occurs with it. Premedicate the child with a prescribed analgesic, and help the child use a distraction technique during the procedure to reduce the level of pain. Transcutaneous electrical nerve stimulation therapy may be helpful to reduce the pain of débridement. Praise any degree of cooperation. Plan an enjoyable activity afterward.

Children need to have a "helping" person with them, to hold their hand, to stroke their head, and to offer some verbal comfort: "It's all right to cry; we know that hurts. We don't like to do this, but it's one of the things that makes burns heal" (Figure 31-13). Nursing personnel need a great deal of talk time to voice their feelings about assisting with or doing débridement procedures. Be careful in serving as the "helping" person that you do not pro-

TABLE 31.9 Comparing Open and Closed Burn Therapy

METHOD	DESCRIPTION	ADVANTAGES	DISADVANTAGES
Open	Burn is exposed to air; used for superficial burns or body parts that are prone to infection, such as perineum	Allows frequent inspection of site; allows child to follow healing process	Requires strict isolation to prevent infection; area may scrape and bleed easily and impede healing
Closed	Burn is covered with nonadherent gauze; used for moderate and severe burns	Better protection from injury; easier to turn and position child; allows child more freedom to play	Dressing changes are painful; possibility of infection may increase because of dark, moist environment

ject yourself as the healer and the comforter and a fellow nurse as the hurter, or "bad guy." It helps if people alternate this chore so that on alternate days, each serves as the protector and the comforter. Research has found that when children are given some control over the process of débridement (e.g., piercing blisters), they are much better able to cope with the procedure and much less likely to suffer from depression later.

If eschar tissue is débrided in this manner day after day, granulation tissue forms underneath. When a full bed of granulation tissue is present (about 2 weeks after the injury) the area is ready for skin grafting. In some burn centers, this waiting period is avoided by immediate surgical excision of eschar and placement of skin grafts. Another trend in débridement is the use of Travase, an enzyme that can dissolve tissue.

Grafting

Homografting (also called **allografting**) is the placement of skin (sterilized and frozen) from cadavers or a donor on the cleaned burn site. These grafts do not grow but provide a protective covering for the area. In small children, **heterografts** (also called *xenografts*) from other sources, such as porcine (pig) skin, may be used. **Autografting** is a process in which a layer of skin of both epidermis and a part of the dermis (called a *split-thickness graft*) is removed from a distal, unburned portion of the child's body and placed at the prepared burn site, where it will grow and replace the burned skin. Postage stamp-sized grafts of split-thickness skin are often used. Larger areas require mesh grafts (a strip of partial thickness skin that is slit at intervals so that it can be stretched to cover a larger area) (Figure 31-14). The advantage of grafting is that it reduces fluid and electrolyte loss, pain, and the chance of infection.

Following the grafting procedure, the area is covered by a bulky dressing. So that the growth of the newly adhering cells will not be disrupted, this should not be removed or changed. The donor site on the child's body

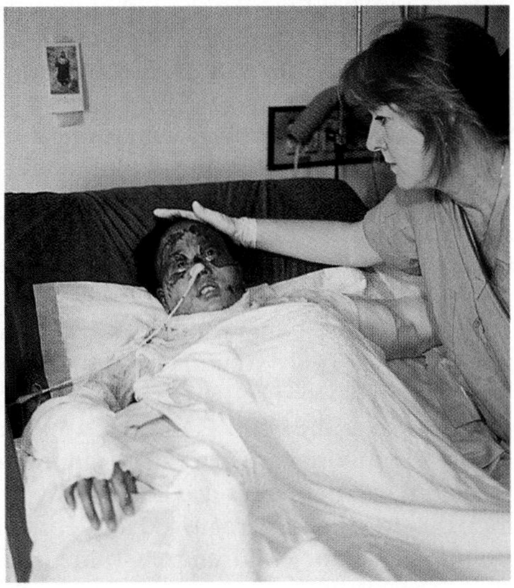

FIGURE 31.13 The nurse provides comfort and support to the child during débridement.

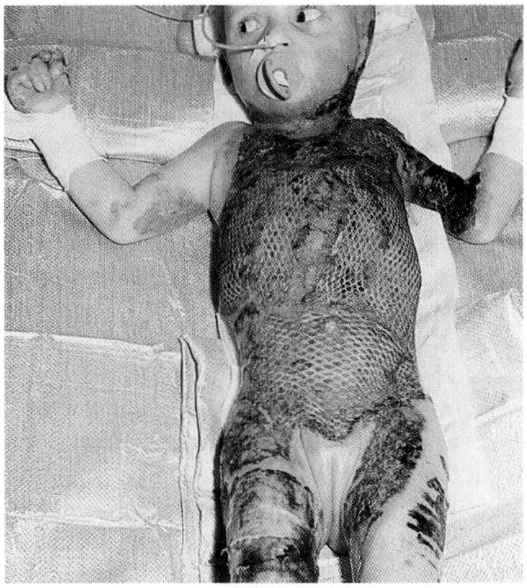

FIGURE 31.14 Mesh grafting is necessary to cover large areas of the body in this young child with third-degree burns.

(often the anterior thigh or buttocks) is also covered by a gauze dressing. Both donor and graft dressings should be observed for fluid drainage and odor. Observe the child to see if he or she has pain at either site, which might indicate infection. The child's temperature should be taken every 4 hours. A rise in systemic temperature may be the first indication that there is infection at the graft or donor site. Autograft sites can be reused every 7 to 10 days, so any one site can provide a great deal of skin for grafting.

NURSING DIAGNOSES AND RELATED INTERVENTIONS

Nursing Diagnosis: Social isolation related to infection control precautions necessary to control spread of microorganisms

Outcome Identification: Child will demonstrate that he or she is able to cope with degree of restriction necessary during course of illness.

Outcome Evaluation: Child states that he or she understands the reason for infection control precautions; child accepts it as a necessary part of therapy.

Infection control measures involved in the care of children with major burns is more than just placing the child in a private room. Aseptic technique and appropriate barriers are necessary to reduce the risk of exposing the child to infection. Health care facilities differ in their policies for preventing infection for the child with a burn. Check your agency's policy. In some agencies, all the people who come into the room wear gowns, masks, caps, and sterile gloves. The child is doubly isolated: by distance and by strangers who never touch him or her directly.

It is easy for children with burns (who were told not to play with matches or go too close to the fireplace) to interpret these precautions as punishment. Make every effort to make their environment as warm and comforting as possible, despite the isolation procedures. Place children's beds so that they can see as much unit activity as possible. Decorate walls in front of them with cards they receive or with a changing gallery of pictures drawn by staff members of things in which the children appear interested.

Children need to be able to discuss their feelings about being kept in a room by themselves. A question such as, "It's hard to understand a lot of things about a hospital; do you understand why your bed is in this special room?" gives children a chance to express their feelings.

Encourage parents to participate in the child's care as much as possible, even with wearing the gowns, gloves, and masks (depending on agency policy). Parents often do not ask to do these things spontaneously when their children are severely burned. They are in a state of grief. They do not react in a normal manner. They may believe the bulky dressings make it impossible for them to hold the child. Actually, the closed bulky dressings on the wound make it *possible* for the child to be held. If it is not possible for children to be held, help parents to see that stroking a child's face or touching a hand (even with gloves in place) gives the child a feeling of still being loved.

Nursing Diagnosis: Altered family processes related to the effects of severe burns in family member

Outcome Identification: The family will remain intact and functional during the period of rehabilitation.

Outcome Evaluation: Family voices that they are able to cope effectively with the degree of stress to which they are subjected; family demonstrates positive coping mechanisms.

Children with severe burns always have a difficult hospitalization because it involves pain, restrictions, and (at some point) awareness of the disfigurement that accompanies major burns.

Some parents grieve so deeply over the child's condition or are so concerned with other upsetting factors in their lives (many burns happen because of situational crises in the family) that their interaction with the child seems to falter or proves very difficult for them. They may avoid visiting because the sound of the child's crying when they leave is more than they can endure. At the same time, they may have lost their home and possessions to fire. They may need help in establishing priorities. It may be important that they wait at home one morning for an insurance inspector to make an estimate on damage caused by the fire to their house or furniture. Other tasks, such as shopping or housecleaning, could possibly be done by relatives or neighbors, leaving them time to visit the child.

Nursing Diagnosis: Diversional activity deficit related to restricted mobility following severe burn

Outcome Identification: Child remains interested in age-appropriate activities during rehabilitation.

Outcome Evaluation: Child expresses interest in obtaining school homework; child communicates with friends and relatives via telephone or letters.

Remember that although children's chest, abdomen, and hands may be burned, they do not stop thinking. They need stimulation in their environment. A television set is good for passing time but should not be the child's main communication with the outside world. Listening to favorite tapes, having stories read to him or her, talking about what is going on at home or what the child normally does at school, and doing schoolwork are important, too.

Toys and play material are important. Make certain to visit the child just to talk to him or her or come to play a game at times other than procedures or treatment times. The child may be hospitalized for a long time. He or she needs to view the nursing staff as friends and caregivers. Frequent visits convey to a child that he or she is not alone and that others are aware of important needs.

Nursing Diagnosis: Body image disturbance related to changes in physical appearance with thermal injury

Outcome Identification: Child will maintain self-esteem during rehabilitation period.

Outcome Evaluation: Child expresses fears about physical appearance; demonstrates desire to resume age-appropriate activities.

Children with burns are often forced to become extremely dependent on the nursing staff due to the position in which they must lie and because of bulky dressings that cover their arms or hands and prevent them from feeding themselves. They respond to this forced dependence at first with gratitude. They are hurt, and someone is taking care of them. After a period, however, the response may become less healthy. The young school-age child or preschooler may revert to bedwetting or baby talk. Older children respond by becoming openly aggressive to counteract their feelings of helplessness. They attempt to reestablish independence in the ways that they can, often by refusing to eat or to lie in a position that is best for them. Although good nutrition is vitally important for rapid healing, it may suffer because of children's need to assert their independence. Make certain when caring for burned children to allow independent decision making whenever possible. Children must take their 10 o'clock medicine, but they can choose the fluid they want to swallow after it. They must be fed meals because of the bulky dressings over their hands, but they can decide which food they will be fed first. They must have their dressings changed, but they can choose the story you will read them afterward.

Be careful not to give choices when there really are none to give. Inappropriate questions include, "Can I change your dressing now?" "Do you want dinner now?" "Will you swallow this pill?"

Immediately after a severe burn, children (if they are old enough to understand), parents, and probably the hospital staff are most concerned with whether or not they will live. When body systems have stabilized and it seems appropriate to assure parents that the child will live, thoughts turn to the child's cosmetic appearance. At first, it is easy for children and parents to ignore this problem because the burned areas are covered by dressings. Even when the dressings are removed for débridement or whirlpool, it is easy for children to assume that the appearance of the burned area is only temporary and the area will eventually heal and have a good appearance. They have probably never seen anyone with a scar from a second- or third-degree burn and have no reason to worry about it (Figure 31-15).

When children see others on the unit with burn scars, they begin to realize what healing will look like. Depending on the extent and the site of the burn, parents and children will have varying degrees of difficulty accepting this. They may lose confidence in the health care personnel.

Parents and children need time to talk about their feelings. A girl may be extremely concerned if her chest is burned because she is worried that breast tissue will not develop (a very real concern, depending on the extent of the burn). Her parents may be most concerned because they can see that although a blouse can cover her chest, her right hand will not have full function. Do not assume that your biggest concern is the same as the child's and parents' biggest concern. A father who dreamed his son would be a great track star may be most concerned about a leg scar; the child may be most concerned about a facial burn.

Children watch you as you care for them to see if you find them unattractive. As dressings are removed, children may expose parts of their body seemingly inappropriately, to see if you are shocked or revolted by them. It is easy to think that you will not react this way, but for everyone, the first sight of a severe burn is a shock and it is difficult not to react accordingly. Imagining how the child feels, realizing that this mutilated skin is his or hers, helps health care providers maintain a professional attitude (see Managing and Delegating Unlicensed Assistive Personnel).

Returning to school is difficult for children who have been hospitalized or receiving home care for a long time. Their old friends have new friends, so they may feel cut out of school activities. They look different if they have burn scars. The appearance of scar formation can be improved by the application of pressure dressings that the child wears 24 hours a day. If the child has facial burns, facing friends with a compression bandage in place may be difficult. They need a great deal of support from health care personnel to be able to endure this. Some children may need referral for formal counseling. Some parents may need formal counseling also to help them accept the child's changed appearance.

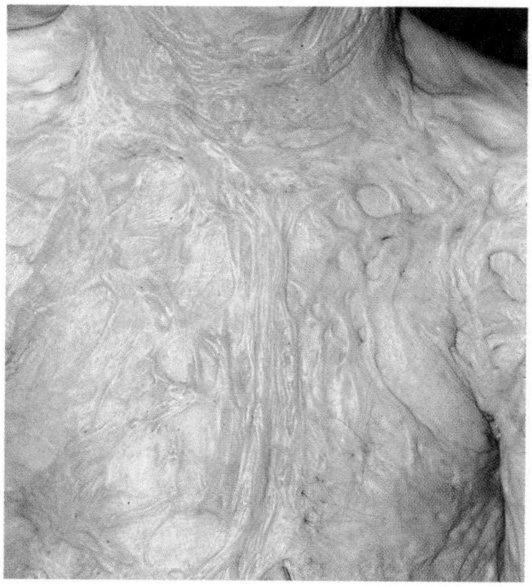

FIGURE 31.15 Extensive scarring on the chest of a 9-year-old boy with third-degree burns. The child and his family will need much support to help them deal with his appearance.

MANAGING AND DELEGATING UNLICENSED ASSISTIVE PERSONNEL

Unlicensed assistive personnel are often assigned to take vital signs in primary care or emergency rooms. This means they may be the first contact persons for families with an injured child. It is often a first reaction in people on seeing a child who has been injured to try and establish blame for the injury and then lecture on safety. Help unlicensed assistive personnel to react first to the child's needs (comfort, pain relief, airway) and secondarily to discovering the cause of the injury. This helps ensure that the child's needs are met and encourages parent cooperation, necessary for obtaining a factual history and planning for long-term care.

Be certain also that they understand that how burn tissue first looks is not how it will look eventually. This helps them to support the child through the many therapies necessary.

Electrical Burns of the Mouth

If children put the prongs of a plugged-in extension cord into their mouth or chew on an electric cord, their mouth will be burned severely (Zubair & Besner, 1997). Electrical current from the plug is conducted for a distance through the skin and underlying tissue so a tissue area much larger than where the prongs or cord actually touched is involved.

Tissue will be destroyed at the entry site, leaving an angry-looking ulcer. If blood vessels were burned, active bleeding will be present. The immediate treatment for electrical burns is to unplug the electric cord and control bleeding. Pressure applied to the site with gauze will usually control this. Most children are admitted to a hospital for at least 24 hours of observation following electrical burns of the mouth because edema in the mouth may lead to airway obstruction.

Clean the wound about four times a day with an antiseptic solution, such as half-strength hydrogen peroxide, to reduce the possibility of infection (a real danger in this area because bacteria are always present in the mouth).

Eating will be a problem for children because their mouth is so sore. They may be able to drink fluids from a cup best. Bland fluids, such as artificial fruit drinks, flat ginger ale, or milk products, are best.

Electrical burns of the mouth turn black as local tissue necrosis begins. They will heal with white, fibrous scar tissue, possibly causing a deformity of the lip and cheeks with healing. This can be minimized by the use of a mouth appliance, which helps maintain lip contour. Some children may have difficulty with speech sounds because of resulting lip scarring. They need follow-up care by a plastic surgeon to restore their lip contour and function again. Obviously, you need to review with parents the importance of not leaving "live" electrical cords where young children can reach them.

KEY POINTS

Children need total body assessment following a traumatic injury, because they may be unable to describe other injuries besides a primary one they may have suffered. Be aware that some trauma in children occurs from child abuse. Screen for this by history and physical examination. Be certain that aseptic technique is maintained when caring for trauma victims so that the child does not develop an additional unnecessary infection.

Head injuries are always potentially serious in children. Skull fractures, subdural hematoma, epidural hematomas, concussion, and contusions can occur. Coma (unconsciousness from which children cannot be roused) may be present in children following severe head trauma.

Abdominal trauma resulting in splenic or liver rupture may occur in connection with multiple trauma.

Near drowning can occur from salt or fresh water. The physiologic basis for complications following drowning differs as to whether the water was fresh or salt water.

Common substances children swallow that result in poisoning include acetaminophen (Tylenol) and salicylic acid (aspirin). Teach parents to keep the number of the local poison control center next to their telephone and always to call first before administering an antidote for poisoning.

Lead poisoning most frequently occurs from the ingestion of lead chips from older housing. Preventing this is a major nursing responsibility.

Burns are divided into three types—first, second, and third degree—depending on the depth of the burn. Burns produce systemic body reactions and require long-term nursing care.

CRITICAL THINKING EXERCISES

1. Jason is the 4-year-old you met at the beginning of the chapter. He is admitted to the hospital confused and lethargic. What are the immediate nursing considerations? Why is frequent neurologic assessment necessary? What are the signs of deterioration and improvement of this child's status?
2. A 3-year-old seen in the emergency room for acetaminophen poisoning. Her father tells you they normally lock all medicine away carefully. His wife left acetaminophen on the counter because she was suffering from a headache. Would you want to discuss the necessity of poisoning prevention with these parents, or should they have learned from this experience that their actions were not safe?
3. A 10-year-old has third-degree burns on her legs from lighting a fire to burn leaves. She will probably have a lengthy hospitalization and may need skin grafts to improve healing. What precautions does this child need to prevent infection until healing is complete?

REFERENCES

American Academy of Pediatrics. Committee on Environmental Health (1998). Screening for elevated blood lead levels. *Pediatrics, 101*(6), 1072.

Bennett, B., & Gamelli, R. (1998). Profile of an abused burned child. *Journal of Burn Care and Rehabilitation, 19*(1.1), 88.

Bond, R. G., & Burkhart, K. K. (1998). Thrombocytopenia following timber rattlesnake envenomation. *Annals of Emergency Medicine, 30*(1), 40.

Brown, R. L., Greenhalgh, D. G., & Warden, G. D. (1997). Burn prevention forum: iron burns to the hand in the young pediatric patient: a problem in prevention. *Journal of Burn Care and Rehabilitation, 18*(3), 279.

Carrougher, G. J. (1997). Management of fluid and electrolyte balance in thermal injuries: implications for perioperative nursing practice. *Seminars in Perioperative Nursing, 6*(4), 201.

Cattelani, R. et al. (1998). Traumatic brain injury in childhood: intellectual, behavioral and social outcome into adulthood. *Brain Injury, 12*(4), 283.

Department of Health and Human Services. (1995). *Healthy people 2000: midcourse review.* Washington, D.C.: DHHS.

Ender, P. T., & Dolan, M. J. (1997). Pneumonia associated with near-drowning. *Clinical Infectous Diseases, 25*(4), 896.

Fortenberry, J. D., & Mariscalco, M. M. (1997). Poisoning. In Johnson, K. B. & Oski, F. A. *Oski's essential pediatrics.* Philadelphia: Lippincott-Raven.

Harrington, R. et al. (1998). Randomized trial of a home-based family intervention for children who have deliberately poisoned themselves. *Journal of the American Academy of Child and Adolescent Psychiatry, 37*(5), 512.

Hildreth, M. (1997). Pediatric nutrition therapy: nutrition therapy for the pediatric burn patient. *Topics in Clinical Nutrition, 12*(4), 6.

Hutchison, J. S. (1997). Near-drowning. In Singh, N. C. *Manual of pediatric critical care.* Philadelphia: Saunders.

Kochanek, P. M. et al. (1997). Severe traumatic brain injury in children. In Singh, N. C. *Manual of pediatric critical care.* Philadelphia: Saunders.

Kurbat, R. S., & Pollack, C. V. Jr. (1998). Facial injury and airway threat from inhalant abuse: a case report. *Journal of Emergency Medicine, 16*(2), 167.

Mariscalco, M. M. (1997). Acetaminophen overdose. In Johnson, K. B. & Oski, F. A. *Oski's essential pediatrics.* Philadelphia: Lippincott-Raven.

Neely, A. N. et al. (1998). Efficacy of a rise in C-reactive protein serum levels as an early indicator of sepsis in burned children. *Journal of Burn Care and Rehabilitation. 19*(2), 102.

Pierre, E. J. et al. (1998). Extracorporeal membrane oxygenation in the treatment of respiratory failure: pediatric patients with burns. *Journal of Burn Care and Rehabilitation, 19*(2), 131.

Punja, K., et al. (1998). Continuous infusion of epidural morphine in frostbite. *Journal of Burn Care and Rehabilitation, 19*(2), 142.

Roddy, S. P. et al. (1998). Minimal head trauma in children revisited: is routine hospitalization required? *Pediatrics, 101*(4.1), 575.

Rosman, N. P. (1997). Acute head trauma. In Johnson, K. B. & Oski, F. A. *Oski's essential pediatrics.* Philadelphia: Lippincott-Raven.

Schweich, P. J. (1997). Emergency medicine except poisoning. In Johnson, K. B. & Oski, F. A. *Oski's essential pediatrics.* Philadelphia: Lippincott-Raven.

Sobel, R. (1970). The psychiatric implications of accidental poisonings in childhood. *Pediatric Clinics of North America, 17*(5), 653.

Vale, J. A. (1998). Position statement: gastric lavage. *Journal of Toxicology-Clinical Toxicology, 35*(7), 711.

Zubair, M., & Besner, G. E. (1997). Pediatric electrical burns: management strategies. *Burns, 22*(5), 413.

SUGGESTED READINGS

Blakeney, P., et al. (1998). Long-term psychosocial adaptation of children who survive burns involving 80% or greater total body surface area. *Journal of Trauma, 44*(4), 625.

Cortiella, J., & Marvin J. A. (1997). Management of the pediatric burn patient. *Nursing Clinics of North America, 32*(2), 311.

Deer, P. J. (1997). Elapid envenomation: a medical emergency. *Journal of Emergency Nursing, 23*(6), 574.

Knestrick, J., & Milstead, JA. (1998). Public policy and child lead poisoning: implementation of Title X. *Pediatric Nursing, 24*(1), 37.

Rabban, J. T. et al. (1997). Mechanisms of pediatric electrical injury: new implications for product safety and injury prevention. *Archives of Pediatrics and Adolescent Medicine, 151*(7), 696.

Shafi, S. et al. (1998). Impact of bicycle helmet safety legislation on children admitted to a regional pediatric trauma center. *Journal of Pediatric Surgery, 33*(2), 317.

Sheridan, R. et al. (1998). Treatment of the seriously burned infant. *Journal of Burn Care and Rehabilitation, 19*(2), 115.

Strohecker, B., & Parulski, C. J. (1997). Frostbite injuries of the hand. *Plastic Surgical Nursing, 17*(4), 212.

Suominen, P. K. et al. (1997). Does water temperature affect outcome of nearly drowned children? *Resuscitation, 35*(2), 111.

Vernon, D. D., & Gleich, M. C. (1997). Poisoning and drug overdose. *Critical Care Clinics, 13*(3), 647.

Nursing Care of the Child With Cancer

32
CHAPTER

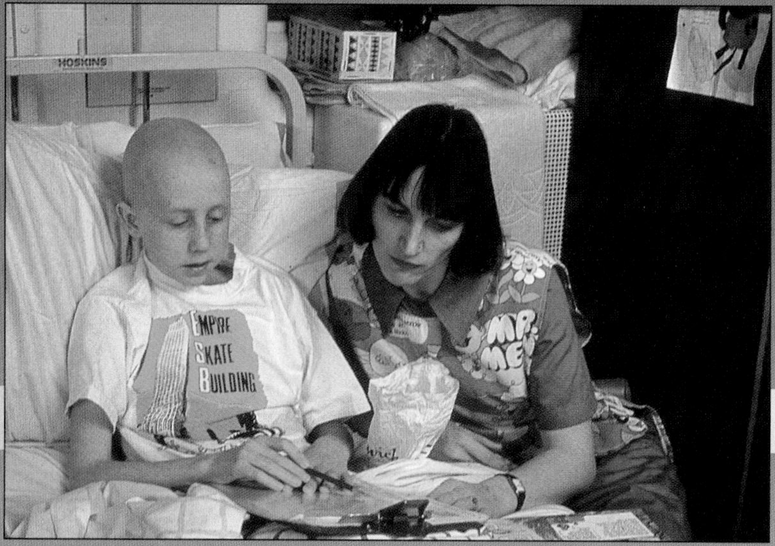

Key Terms

- biopsy
- chemotherapeutic agent
- Ewing's sarcoma
- leukemia
- lymphoma
- metastasis
- neoplasm
- neuroblastoma
- oncogenic virus
- osteogenic sarcoma
- rhabdomyosarcoma
- sarcoma
- tumor staging

Objectives

After mastering the contents of this chapter, you should be able to:

1. Define terms related to tumor growth, such as neoplasm, benign, malignant, sarcoma, and carcinoma, and describe normal cell growth and theories that explain how cells are altered to become cancerous in children.
2. Assess the child with a cancerous process, such as a rhabdomyosarcoma, neuroblastoma, Wilms' tumor, and leukemia.
3. Formulate nursing diagnoses related to the child with cancer.
4. Establish appropriate outcomes for the child with cancer.
5. Plan nursing care specific to the child with cancer.
6. Implement nursing care for the child undergoing cancer therapy.
7. Evaluate outcome criteria to be certain that nursing care goals were achieved.
8. Identify National Health Goals related to the care of the child with cancer that nurses can be instrumental in helping the nation to achieve.
9. Identify areas related to care of children with cancer that could benefit from additional nursing research.
10. Use critical thinking to propose ways that nursing care for the child with cancer can be more family centered.
11. Integrate knowledge of abnormal cell growth in children with the nursing process to achieve quality child health nursing care.

Geri is a 6-year-old you meet at a health maintenance organization clinic. He is there for a well-child checkup. His mother tells you that Geri wakes up every morning with a headache and then vomits. Immediately after that, he is fine. The problem began just after he started a new school in the fall, so she is certain it is related to this. His teacher has suggested that Geri needs an eye examination because he cocks his head to see the chalkboard. You notice that he has lost weight. "What do I do for school phobia?" his mother asks you.

Is his mother describing school phobia? What additional questions would you want to ask her to see if this is something more serious?

In previous chapters, you learned about the growth and development of well children. In this chapter, you'll add information about the dramatic changes, both physical and psychosocial, that occur when children develop cancer. This is important information because it forms a base for care and health teaching.

After you've studied the chapter, turn to the Critical Thinking Exercises at the end of the chapter to help sharpen your skills and test your knowledge.

The terms *malignant* and *cancerous* describe cells growing and proliferating in a disorderly, chaotic fashion. In adults, cancer usually occurs in the form of a solid tumor (abnormal growth). In children, the most frequent type of cancer is that of an immature blood cell overgrowth, or leukemia.

Many parents assume that the diagnosis of cancer means that the child's life will be very limited. Because of the giant strides in cancer research and treatment over the last 20 years, however, the prognosis for children with cancer improves daily. To help parents and children adjust to this illness, nursing support is necessary from the time of diagnosis throughout the long-term therapy required. National Health Goals related to cancer and children are shown in the Focus on National Health Goals box.

NURSING PROCESS OVERVIEW

for Care of the Child With Cancer

Assessment

The symptoms of cancer in children are often insidious and hard to define. Weight loss, headaches, or pain at a particular body site can often be explained away by other factors. Weight loss, however, is a common symptom of cancer. A child's height and weight should be plotted and analyzed at every health care visit. Although pain and swelling could be attributed to injury, be sure to refer children with swelling of major joints to the primary health care provider for further assessment so that bone tumors will not go undetected. See Assessing the Child with Cancer Signs.

Nursing Diagnosis

Selected nursing diagnoses established for the child with cancer address specific symptoms caused by the cancer, side effects of the cancer treatment process, or coping abilities of the child and family.

- Pain related to neoplastic process in bone
- Altered nutrition, less than body requirements, related to cancer
- Risk for infection related to immunosuppressive effects of chemotherapy
- Body image disturbance related to loss of hair following radiation treatment
- Ineffective family coping, compromised, related to long-term chemotherapy program

Outcome Identification and Planning

When a neoplasm is first diagnosed in their child, parents may be able to deal only with short-term goals and plans. They may concentrate on learning about the effect or toxic properties of a particular chemotherapeutic drug given their child, or they may ask how long the child's surgical incision will be. Dealing with such specifics helps them to control their anxiety. It prevents them from dealing with the overall picture or prognosis: that their child has a potentially lethal condition.

The family of the cancer patient needs support beginning with the diagnosis. When planning, sit down with parents and discuss the treatment protocol. Explain measures they will need to take to make their child more comfortable during therapy (e.g., not forcing food if the child is nauseated, playing games or reading stories while intravenous fluid is administered).

FOCUS ON NATIONAL HEALTH GOALS

A number of National Health Goals concern cancer prevention and children:

- Reduce rise in cancer deaths to achieve a rate of no more than 130/100,000 people.
- Increase to at least 60% the proportion of people of all ages who limit sun exposure, use sunscreens and protective clothing when exposed to sunlight, and avoid artificial sources of ultraviolet light (e.g., sun lamps, tanning booths) (DHHS, 1995).

Nurses can be instrumental in helping the nation achieve these goals by careful history taking at health assessments to reveal the symptoms of cancer, because these are often subtle in children, and active teaching to stimulate self-screening measures, such as breast and testicular examination and measures to avoid excessive sun exposure.

Areas that could benefit from additional nursing research are effective ways to teach young clients about the dangers of tanning booths or excessive sun exposure; reasons adolescents give for avoiding self-examination; and reasons parents give for delaying health care consultation after discovering an abnormal growth, unexplainable bruising, or weight loss.

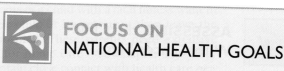

x-ray, sonography, magnetic resonance imaging, blood analysis, and biopsy.

Biopsy

A **biopsy** is the surgical removal of tissue cells for laboratory analysis. Most children with a possible diagnosis of cancer will have a biopsy performed with their initial diagnosis. Although biopsies are classified as minor surgery and usually done on an ambulatory basis, do not treat them lightly. They carry a definite surgical risk if general anesthesia is used. Moreover, they are an anxiety-producing procedure for the parents and the child. Up to this point, parents can convince themselves that the child has something innocent. A biopsy clouds this hope because the word biopsy implies that cancer is at least a possibility. For this reason, parents and children need thorough preparation for the biopsy procedure and the care the child will need following the procedure. Anxious parents do not "hear" well and may need to have postoperative instructions repeated thoroughly at a later time. Bone marrow aspiration is a frequent type of biopsy used with children. Although this can be done with local anesthesia, it is equally frightening (see Chapter 23).

Staging

Tumor staging is a procedure by which a malignant tumor's extent and progress are determined. Knowing the stage of the tumor helps the health care team design an effective treatment program, establish an accurate prognosis, and evaluate the progress or regression of the disease. In general staging, stage I refers to a tumor that can be completely removed surgically. Stage II refers to a tumor that cannot be completely removed surgically. Stages III and IV designate tumors that have extended beyond the original site or have spread systemically (**metastasis**). There are various staging systems, but one of the most common is known as the TNM system, which describes the tumor's size (T), its presence in the lymph nodes (N), and its metastasis (M) or spread to other organs, if any. A TNM system is most applicable to carcinomas. Because most childhood tumors are sarcomas (derived from connective tissue), the system is not as applicable to children as to adults.

✔ **CHECKPOINT QUESTIONS**

1. What does it mean when a tumor has metastasized?
2. What does stage II disease imply?

OVERVIEW OF CANCER TREATMENT MEASURES USED WITH CHILDREN

The treatment of a child with cancer centers on devising ways to kill the growth of the abnormal cells while protecting normal surrounding cells. This is done by a combination of surgery, radiation, chemotherapy, bone marrow transplant, and general health measures. Bone marrow transplant is discussed in Chapter 23 with common blood disorders.

Radiation Therapy

Radiation therapy changes the DNA component of a cell nucleus to a point where the cell cannot replicate DNA material and so cannot divide and grow further. Radiation is not effective on cells that have a low oxygen content (a proportion of cells in every tumor mass), nor is it effective at the time of cell division (mitosis). Radiation schedules therefore are designed so that therapy occurs over 1 to 6 weeks so that cells that are not in a susceptible stage on one day will be in a susceptible stage on another. Tumors that require such a massive dose of radiation that normal tissue through which the radiation must pass to penetrate the tumor would be destroyed in the process are said to be radioresistant.

Immediate Side Effects

Radiation has systemic and localized effects. Radiation sickness (anorexia, nausea, vomiting) is the most frequently encountered systemic effect. This occurs if the gastrointestinal tract is radiated. It also can occur to a lesser degree from the release of toxic substances from destroyed tumor cells. The child may need to receive an antiemetic before each procedure to counter nausea and vomiting. Extreme fatigue is also very common.

Long-Term Side Effects

The long-term side effects of radiation are becoming more apparent as increasing numbers of children who have had intense radiation survive. Because radiation damages all cells in its path to some extent, any body tissue can be affected (Lombardi et al, 1998).

Bone. Asymmetric growth of bones, easy fracturing, scoliosis, kyphosis, or spinal shortening can occur. Bones are most vulnerable during times of rapid growth, such as the first year of life or during a prepubertal growth spurt. Scoliosis and kyphosis can be avoided if an entire vertebra is radiated rather than one side or the other; this means that a larger area of bone may be radiated than formerly so that both sides of the vertebra are in the radiation path.

Hormone. Radiation to the head can result in long-term thyroid, hypothalamic, and pituitary gland dysfunction. This may result in growth hormone deficiency or hypothalamic-pituitary stimulation to the thyroid gland. Children's growth and thyroid function should be evaluated every 6 months for the next 3 years to detect these changes. Both hypothyroidism and hypopituitary growth failure can be treated with hormone replacement in coming years. Radiation to ovaries or testes can result in infertility. In girls, normal estrogen production may lag or fail, preventing secondary sexual changes from developing. In boys, testosterone production rarely fails. However, pretreatment sperm banking may be advocated for a boy past puberty before he undergoes radiation to the testes.

Nervous System. Long-term effects of radiation to the nervous system are demyelination and necrosis of the white matter of the brain. This can result in symptoms of lethargy, sleepiness, and seizures. Effects on the gray matter can result in learning disabilities. There may be abnormal electroencephalograph tracings; the child may have low-intensity headaches, cataracts, salivary gland damage, and a chronic change in or loss of taste.

Lungs. Radiation to the lungs may result in a chronic pneumonitis and pulmonary fibrosis or thickening. Heart effects may be pericardial thickening and reduced heart expandability. Radiation to the gastrointestinal system can result in chronic malabsorption from changes in intestinal villi. Hepatic fibrosis can result in reduced liver function. Radiation to the kidney and bladder can result in nephritis and chronic cystitis.

The possibility of these long-term effects of radiation should be explained to parents when radiation is initially discussed as a part of obtaining informed consent. At the early stage of diagnosis, however, parents rarely are concerned with these long-term effects. Their thoughts are understandably filled with such short-term goals as the achievement of a remission or destruction of the tumor.

NURSING DIAGNOSES AND RELATED INTERVENTIONS

Nursing Diagnosis: Parental and child anxiety related to radiation procedure

Outcome Identification: Parents demonstrate reduced anxiety about radiation by time of therapy.

Outcome Evaluation: Parents voice that they understand necessity of therapy and can help support child during therapy.

Before Treatment. The points where radiation therapy will be directed are marked on the child's skin, usually in indelible ink. As a rule, no cream or lotion should be applied to radiation areas until the treatment series is complete. If creams contain any metal, they may distort or interfere with the entrance of radiation. If the head will be irradiated, a dental consult may be suggested. This is because radiation therapy will slow healing if a tooth extraction is necessary.

During Treatment. Most children have had prior x-rays taken at the point that radiation therapy is begun and so are not frightened by the procedure. However, because the procedure requires them to lie still for about 20 minutes on an uncomfortable table, in a room away from personnel or their parents, they do not particularly like the procedure. Assure parents and the child that during the treatment, just as there is no sensation from x-ray exposure, the child will experience no sensation from radiation exposure. Infants are usually prescribed a sedative before therapy to ensure that they lie still during the procedure. To make this approach effective, keep the child fairly active early in the day and introduce calming activities after the sedative is administered. The child will be sleepy and may fall asleep during radiation. An older child may want to plan an activity to think about during radiation, such as selecting 10 people to take on a camping trip (and why) or choosing 10 places to visit next year and so forth.

After Treatment. If the head area is involved in therapy, alopecia (hair loss) may result. Moreover, radiation may reduce salivary gland function, leading to a constantly dry mouth. Tooth growth may be halted due to root atrophy. Radiation to bone marrow may depress white blood cell and platelet production. Children undergoing radiation therapy need their leukocyte and platelet counts monitored periodically to be certain that these remain adequate during the course of therapy. Teaching points for parents to maintain skin integrity are summarized in Empowering the Family.

Chemotherapy

A **chemotherapeutic agent** is one that is capable of destroying malignant cells. In most instances, several chemotherapeutic agents are used to cause multiple damage to cells and thereby increase the chances that cells will no longer be able to reproduce. Like radiation, chemotherapy is scheduled over a period of time so that all cells can eventually be destroyed (cells undergoing meiosis and therefore not susceptible to the chemotherapeutic agent on one day will be susceptible on the next).

Types of Chemotherapeutic Agents

Several categories of chemotherapeutic agents are available. Typically, all agents that need mixing are prepared under a hood to prevent airborne drug residue. When administering such agents, wear gloves and wash your hands well afterward to prevent skin exposure and absorption of the drug.

Alkylating Agents. Alkylating agents interfere with DNA synthesis. They are cell cycle specific; that is, they are most effective against cells in the G1 and S phases of growth. Alkylating agents commonly used with children are cyclophosphamide (Cytoxan) and chlorambucil (Leukeran).

Antimetabolites. Antimetabolites are drugs that so closely resemble natural products that a cell incorporates them into its structure. They are not the natural product, however, so the cell cannot function or replicate with them in its structure and will die. They act only in the S (synthesis) phase of the cell cycle. Methotrexate (Folex PFS), a folic acid antagonist, is an example.

Plant Alkaloids. Plant alkaloids interfere with cell mitosis (M phase). Two commonly used plant alkaloids are vincristine (Oncovin) and vinblastine (Velban).

Antibiotics. A number of antibiotics are effective in destroying malignant cells by impairing DNA synthesis. These are not cell cycle specific, which means the agents can be effective at any cell phase (resting or dividing). Dactinomycin (Cosmegan) and doxorubicin (Adriamcin) are examples.

Nitrosoureas. The action of the nitrosoureas is similar to that of the antibiotics in that these agents interfere with DNA synthesis. Nitrosoureas are not used extensively in chemotherapy with children except in brain tumor therapy because these drugs cross the blood-brain barrier.

EMPOWERING THE FAMILY: Caring for the Child Receiving Radiation Therapy

In addition to preventing infection (see the Nursing Procedure for a Child With Neutropenia), parents need to take some special actions to meet the needs of a child undergoing radiation therapy. The following interventions are designed to promote therapeutic benefits and minimize adverse effects.

Maintain Skin Integrity, Prevent Breakdown
- Expose irradiated area to air but not direct heat or sunlight.
- Avoid lengthy soaks in bath water or swimming pools.
- Use mild shampoo on hair and rinse gently with water. Air dry or pat excess moisture gently. Avoid rough towels and hair dryers.
- Encourage loose clothing, particularly at waist, wrists, and neckline.
- Supply soft toothbrush to protect gums and oral mucous membranes. Keep dry mouth moist by offering frequent sips of water—particularly if radiation decreases salivary gland secretions.
- Because some skin preparations are drying and because some interfere with radiation, do not apply creams or lotions unless prescribed.

Enhance Nutrition
- To promote retention of nutrients, administer antiemetics as prescribed.
- Encourage high-calorie meals when child is least likely to be nauseated. Praise the child's efforts to eat. Strive for peaceful and pleasant meal and snack times.
- Provide foods identified by child as special favorites. Serve easy-to-swallow foods at tolerable temperatures.

Promote Hydration
- Reduce fresh fruit and vegetables rich in cellulose, and eliminate apple juice from child's diet because these may contribute to diarrhea and subsequent fluid loss.
- If diarrhea occurs, administer antidiarrheal medication as prescribed.
- Monitor hydration status, and administer intravenous fluid replacement as prescribed.

Encourage Activity But Prevent Fatigue
- Provide adequate rest periods. Schedule activities to avoid waking child frequently at night.
- Structure the child's activities to be stimulating but not physically tiring.
- Recommend mild activity that does not stress bones that may be weakened by radiation and therefore easily fractured.

Provide Instruction and Distraction
- Prepare the child for the effects of radiation therapy, particularly hair loss. Some comfort measures may include wearing a wig or special cap, introducing play things, such as dolls without hair, and stressing that people like people for themselves, not their appearance.
- Arrange a tour of the radiation department. As possible, let the child play act and become familiar with the equipment. Provide ample time to answer questions.
- If the child needs to be sedated before radiation, encourage active games before the procedure and quiet games afterward.
- Help the child devise "mind games" to play during the procedure, for example listing 10 friends to take camping, 10 activities to do, or 10 favorite games to play.

Enzymes. Body cells need a ready supply of L-asparagine (an essential amino acid) to grow. L-Asparaginase, a chemotherapeutic agent, is an enzyme that converts L-asparagine into L-aspartic acid, thereby making L-asparagine unavailable for leukemia cell growth.

Steroids. The addition of a corticosteroid (most frequently prednisone) binds to DNA to inhibit mitosis in cells and probably RNA synthesis, preventing the formation of new cells.

Immunotherapy. Immunotherapy is the stimulation of the body's immune system to attempt destruction of foreign or malignant cells. The administration of bacille Calmette-Guérin vaccine (the vaccine for tuberculosis) is an example of this type of therapy. The tuberculin antigen stimulates the immune system to identify and destroy an antigen in hopes that the system "recognizes" that foreign tumor cells are also present and acts against them as well. Interferon is an antiviral agent that prevents growth of viruses; stimulation of interferon or interferon therapy may be used to attempt to halt malignant cell growth.

Active immunotherapy can be attempted by the injection of tumor cells taken from the child (or a child with a similar tumor type). Passive immunotherapy using serum from children with a like type of cancer is a possibility.

Although the theory of immunotherapy is sound, results have been disappointing. The immune system may be so altered by the malignant process that it cannot respond when stimulated. It is also possible that the immune response to malignant cells is so different from the response to invading microorganisms that immunotherapy is unable to stimulate it.

Chemotherapy Protocols

Chemotherapy is scheduled for children at set times and days and by different predetermined routes. At first, children may remain in the hospital for a few days of treatment; later, they must be brought in on a specific day for therapy, or parents administer it at home. Parents learn about the child's treatment protocol so that they know which drug the child will be receiving each day and on which day the drugs must be administered. Knowing the protocol and specific drug therapy helps parents begin to prepare the child for it, such as increasing fiber in the child's diet for a few days prior to the beginning of a constipation-causing drug like vincristine. An example of such a protocol is shown in Table 32-2. Chemotherapy for acute lymphocytic leukemia (ALL; the most common cancer in children) is given first in a remission phase (6 weeks), next in a sanctuary or prophylactic phase (8 weeks), and finally, in a maintenance phase (18–36 months).

While children are receiving chemotherapy, they should not be given aspirin, but acetaminophen can be used to relieve a headache or to reduce fever. Aspirin may interfere with blood coagulation, a problem already present due to lowered thrombocyte levels, and may increase the child's susceptibility to Reye's syndrome. A parent who wants to give the child vitamins should be certain that the vitamin preparation does not contain folic acid. Administration of folic acid will interfere with the effectiveness of methotrexate, a folic acid antagonist.

Live virus vaccines should not be given. The child's immune mechanism is so deficient that these vaccines could cause widespread viral disease. The child is particularly susceptible to infections and should be kept away from people with known infections. Zoster immune globulin will be needed if the child is exposed to chickenpox.

Side Effects and Toxic Reactions

All chemotherapeutic agents have side effects and toxic effects. Table 32-3 lists commonly used chemotherapeutic agents, the specific side effects, and potential toxic reactions for each agent. Malnutrition, nausea and vomiting, hair loss, stomatitis, constipation, diarrhea, cushingoid effects, and susceptibility to infection are side effects common to almost all of these agents. Nursing diagnoses and related interventions associated with these side effects are described below.

If an intravenous infusion of a chemotherapeutic agent that is a vesicant infiltrates into the subcutaneous tissue, there is apt to be extensive tissue sloughing and damage. Intravenous infusions of chemotherapeutic vesicants must be watched very carefully to prevent this process, known as extravasation, from happening. The infusion should be discontinued if extravasation occurs. Then, an ice pack applied to the site will induce vasoconstriction and prevent further spread of the toxic solution. Hyaluronidase injected into the site may speed absorption. Following this, warm compresses will hasten absorption and clearance of the solution from subcutaneous tissue.

NURSING DIAGNOSES AND RELATED INTERVENTIONS

Nursing Diagnosis: Altered nutrition, less than body requirements, related to nausea, vomiting, or anorexia resulting from chemotherapy

Outcome Identification: Child will take in adequate nutrients for needs during therapy period.

Outcome Evaluation: Child is able to eat frequent, small meals; calorie intake is adequate for age and size.

It is easy for the child with cancer to become malnourished. The fast-growing malignant cells take more than their share of nutrients from normal cells. Nausea and vomiting from chemotherapy make it difficult for the child to maintain an adequate oral intake. If stomatitis occurs as a result of chemotherapy, eating becomes difficult due to mouth pain. Not only is the oral cavity affected, but also the stomach and intestines, in which like ulcers develop to interfere with absorption. Changes in fatty acid metabolism may alter the responsiveness of body cells to insulin metabolism. Unable to use glucose effectively, cells cannot function at an optimum level. This may account for the sense of fatigue that children with cancer frequently report. Anorexia may occur from a factor produced by the tumor that acts directly on the center for hunger in the hypothalamus, reducing appetite and altering taste perception. Cyclophosphamide, a commonly used chemotherapeutic agent, is associated with taste changes. For many children, foods taste very bitter; foods are not described as sweet until they are very sweet. Because of these taste changes, foods the child used to enjoy

TABLE 32.2 Sample Protocol for Treating Acute Lymphocytic Leukemia

	REMISSION PHASE						SANCTUARY PHASE							
Day	1	8	15	22	29	36	43	50	57	64	71	78	85	92
Week	1	2	3	4	5	6	7	8	9	10	11	12	13	14
	V	V	V	V	L	L	M			M		V	M	
			M	M			M'+			M'+			M'+	
	P	P	P	P	P	P								

V = vincristine; P = prednisone; M = intrathecal methotrexate; L = L-asparaginase; M′ = methotrexate IV; + = leucovorin.

TABLE 32.3 Commonly Used Chemotherapeutic Agents

DRUG	CLASSIFICATION	METHOD OF ADMINISTRATION	SIDE EFFECTS AND TOXIC RESPONSES	SPECIAL CONSIDERATIONS
Asparaginase (Elspar)	Enzyme; deprives leukemic cells of asparagine, leading to cell death	IV	Anorexia, weight loss, nausea, vomiting, hepatotoxicity, central nervous system toxicity, anaphylactic reaction	Stay with child for first hour of infusion; take vital signs q15 min for first hour to detect anaphylactic reaction.
Carmustine (BCNU) (BiCNU)	Nitrosourea compound; crosses blood-brain barrier	IV	Nausea, vomiting, bone marrow depression (after 3–4 wk), hepatotoxicity	Child may notice burning sensation along vein during administration due to alcohol diluent.
Chlorambucil (Leukeran)	Nitrogen mustard derivative	Oral	Bone marrow depression	Monitoring of white blood cell count is necessary.
Cisplatin (Platinol)	Reacts with and injures cell nucleus	IV	Bone marrow depression, nephrotoxicity (renal dysfunction), nausea, vomiting, loss of taste, tinnitus, high-frequency hearing loss	Infusion bottle must be covered with aluminum foil to keep out light, or decomposition will result.
Cyclophosphamide (Cytoxan)	Alkylating agent (nitrogen mustard derivative)	IV, oral	Bone marrow depression, anorexia, nausea, vomiting, stomatitis, alopecia, cystitis, (hemorrhagic) hepatotoxicity	Encourage fluids; maintain IV line to limit bladder irritation; test urine for blood and specific gravity.
Cytosine arabinoside (Ara-C)	Antimetabolite (pyrimidine analog)	IV, SC, intrathecal	Nausea, vomiting, bone marrow depression, stomatitis, alopecia, photosensitivity	Child may need to wear sunglasses in bright light.
Dacarbazine (DTIC)	Alkylating agent	IV	Bone marrow depression	Extravasation causes severe tissue damage.
Dactinomycin (Cosmegan)	Antibiotic; inhibits DNA synthesis	IV	Nausea, vomiting, bone marrow depression, stomatitis	Causes tissue inflammation if it extravasates into tissue.
Daunorubicin (Cerubidine)	Antibiotic; vesicant	IV	Alopecia, bone marrow depression	Extravasation causes severe tissue damage.
Doxorubicin (Adriamycin)	Antibiotic; inhibits DNA synthesis; vesicant	IV	Nausea, vomiting, bone marrow depression, alopecia, stomatitis, possible heart toxicity	Urine may turn red; take pulse for full minute to detect arrhythmia; tissue necrosis occurs if extravasated.
Lomustine (CCNU) (CeeNu)	Alkylating agent (nitrosourea compound)	Oral	Nausea, vomiting in 6 h, bone marrow depression (after 3–4 wk)	Should be taken on an empty stomach for best absorption.
Mercaptopurine (Purinethol)	Antimetabolite (purine analog)	Oral	Bone marrow depression, nausea, vomiting, stomatitis, hepatotoxicity	Allopurinol delays the degradation of mercaptopurine and thus increases toxicity; question order if both are to be administered.
Methotrexate (Methotrexate)	Antimetabolite	Oral, IV, intrathecal	Stomatitis, bone marrow depression, nausea, vomiting, alopecia, hepatotoxicity, nephrotoxicity at high dosage	Decreased effect if administered with salicylates; often followed by leucovorin to decrease toxicity to normal cells.
Prednisone (Prednisone)	Corticosteroid; suppresses lymphocyte production	Oral	Weight gain, cushingoid facies, depressed systemic response to infection	Child needs support to accept changed appearance.

(continued)

TABLE 32.3 Commonly Used Chemotherapeutic Agents *(Continued)*

DRUG	CLASSIFICATION	METHOD OF ADMINISTRATION	SIDE EFFECTS AND TOXIC RESPONSES	SPECIAL CONSIDERATIONS
Procarbazine (Matulane)	Interferes with DNA and RNA synthesis	Oral	Nausea, vomiting, bone marrow depression	May cause blurriness of vision; avoid foods with high tyramine content.
Thioguanine	Antimetabolite	Oral	Bone marrow suppression	Monitoring of hepatic function tests is necessary.
Vinblastine (Velban)	Plant alkaloid; vesicant	IV	Alopecia, anorexia, bone marrow depression, nausea, vomiting, constipation	Tissue necrosis occurs if infiltrated.
Vincristine (Oncovin)	Plant alkaloid; vesicant	IV	Constipation, alopecia, joint and muscle pain, muscle weakness	Paresthesia of fingers and toes, footdrop may occur; may need stool softener; tissue necrosis occurs if infiltrated.
Additional Agents				
Allopurinol (Allopurinol, Lopurin, Zyloprim)	Prevents formation of uric acid from destroyed cells	IV, oral	Nausea, vomiting	
Bacillus Calmette-Guerin (BCG) vaccine*	Stimulates immune system	Intradermal	Local inflammation	
Leucovorin (citrovorum)	Folinic acid given to neutralize the toxicity of methotrexate	IV, IM, oral		
Interferon	Antiviral agent	IV, intrathecal	Fever	
Filgrastin	Granulocyte colony-stimulating factor	IV	Nausea, vomiting	Increases leukocyte count.

IV = intravenous; IM = intramuscular; SC = subcutaneous.
* Otherwise used to vaccinate against tuberculosis.

no longer taste good. Unwilling to try new foods, the child decreases oral intake.

To counteract these taste changes, you may need to suggest different foods or methods of food preparation or include a dietitian as a major health team member. Chicken, for example, often tastes less bitter than beef or pork. Sprinkling brown sugar on cereal gives a different sweet taste than plain sugar. Many children believe that sugar is bad for them so are reluctant to use a lot of it to make foods taste good. Assure them that eating is the most important thing to think about now. Carefully cleaning teeth after eating will preserve teeth even if a great deal of sugar is eaten. However, do not recommend honey as a sweetener. Botulism organisms may grow in honey, and the immunosuppressed child has little resistance to these.

Make mealtime a pleasant time; serve food that is appetizing in flavor, texture, color, and temperature. Allow the child to make choices whenever possible. Assess what are favorite foods, and urge the nutritionist (in the hospital) or parents (at home) to supply these (Figure 32-2).

A small meal that can be finished is more satisfying than a large meal half finished. Urge parents to make snack foods nutritious (e.g., a malted milkshake rather than a cola beverage). Additional good advice is to plan larger meals to be eaten early in the day before chemotherapy begins and when the child is less likely to be nauseated.

Nursing Diagnosis: Risk for fluid volume deficit related to nausea and vomiting resulting from chemotherapy

Outcome Identification: Child will remain adequately hydrated during therapy.

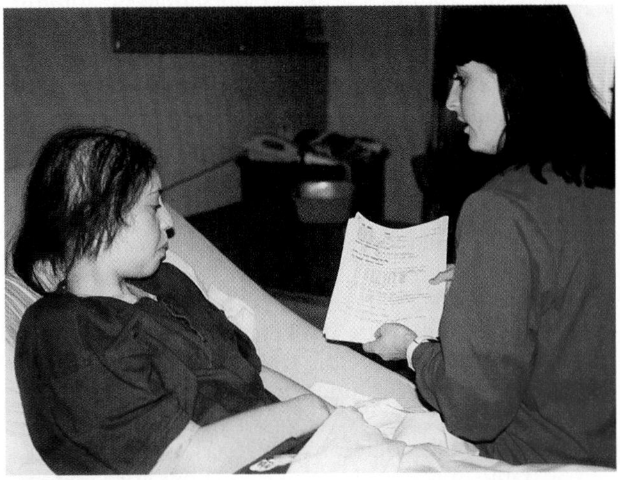

FIGURE 32.2 Children receiving radiation or chemotherapy often have reduced appetites. Here a nurse discusses nutrition and food choices with a 15-year-old with leukemia.

Outcome Evaluation: Skin turgor is good; mucous membranes are moist; vomiting does not occur more than once a day.

Nausea and vomiting are common side effects of chemotherapy because the cells lining the stomach are fast growing and so are irritated by drugs. Nausea and vomiting can often be prevented by administering an antiemetic, such as hydroxyzine (Atarax), ondansetron (Zofran), or dolasetron mesylate, before chemotherapy and at 4-hour intervals during the course of therapy. These drugs effectively prevent nausea and vomiting in children but will not necessarily relieve it once it is present. It is necessary, therefore, to give these medications prophylactically or before chemotherapy begins. For more information, see the Drug Highlight.

Antiemetic suppositories, such as trimethobenzamide (Tigan), are of limited help and not normally used with children. Many children have intense reactions to prochlorperazine (Compazine), so it also is not often administered to them.

Do not encourage children to eat if they are nauseated. Encourage them to take clear fluids, however, because this helps prevent uric acid buildup in the kidneys from the malignant cells being destroyed. If children are vomiting or cannot take even clear fluid, intravenous hydration therapy may be necessary. With a drug such as cyclophosphamide, known to cause cystitis when fluid intake is reduced, an intravenous line for adequate fluid intake must be started.

DRUG HIGHLIGHT

Dolasetron Mesylate

Drug class: Antiemetic

Action: An antiemetic used to prevent chemotherapy-induced nausea and vomiting in adults and children older than 2 years

Dosage: About 1.8 mg/kg up to a maximum of 100 mg of dolasetron may be administered 30 minutes before chemotherapy intravenously as a single dose or orally in the same amount 60 minutes before chemotherapy.

Possible adverse effects: Undesired cardiac effects may result from this drug, which should be administered with caution in patients in whom prolonged cardiac conduction interval may develop. This includes patients with hypokalemia or hypomagnesemia, those taking diuretic drugs, those with congenital QT syndrome, those on antiarrhythmic therapy, and those on high-dose anthracycline therapy.

Nursing Implications:

- Monitor patient's cardiovascular, fluid, and electrolyte status.
- For oral palatability, drug may be mixed with apple or apple-grape juice and kept at room temperature for up to 2 hours before use.
- Store vials of IV solution at room temperature and protect from light.
- Note that after dilution of IV dolasetron, injection is stable in normal lighting conditions at room temperature for 24 hours and under refrigeration for 48 hours.

WHAT IF? What if a parent tells you that she does not want her child to have an antiemetic drug before chemotherapy because she sees the nausea and vomiting as proof that the chemotherapy is working? Would you give the drug?

Nursing Diagnosis: Risk for body image disturbance related to changes in physical appearance caused by chemotherapy

Outcome Identification: Child will accept side effects affecting appearance as temporary, inevitable components of treatment within 1 week.

Outcome Evaluation: Child discusses feelings about appearance changes with nurse and parents; states that although he or she does not like them, they do not alter him or her in any other way.

Alopecia. *Alopecia,* or hair loss, is a side effect that occurs with almost all chemotherapeutic drugs because hair cells are fast-growing and easily killed. Even when forewarned that such a consequence is likely, most children and parents are surprised at the suddenness of the hair loss (entire curls may fall out at a time; the child can be totally bald in 2 to 3 days). Even so, hair loss is often a greater problem for the parents than the child. Coping mechanisms may be enhanced by wearing a wig or a scarf, playing and identifying with a doll without hair, and being reminded that those who love the child love the whole person not just the packaging (Figure 32-3). It may be possible to reduce the amount of alopecia by placing ice packs on the scalp during chemotherapy. This prevents a large uptake of drug by hair follicles. However, do not use an ice cap for children who have leukemia, because it may prevent destruction of leukemic cells near hair follicles.

Cushingoid Appearance. In children on long-term corticosteroid (prednisone) therapy, typical "moon face,"

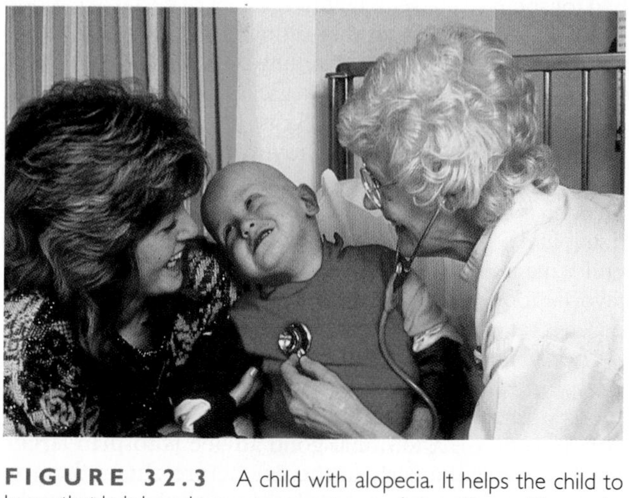

FIGURE 32.3 A child with alopecia. It helps the child to know that hair loss does not prevent warm interactions with people.

red cheeks, and increased body hair will develop. Like the loss of body hair, a cushingoid appearance may be devastating to children, the final insult in light of all the other things happening to them. Assurance that appearance will revert to normal when they are no longer on therapy may help, as will telling them that people care more about the kind of person they are than how they look.

Nursing Diagnosis: Altered oral mucous membrane related to effects of chemotherapy

Outcome Identification: Child will remain free of severe discomfort from stomatitis during course of chemotherapy.

Outcome Evaluation: Child states that mouth discomfort is at tolerable level; no signs of ulceration are present.

Stomatitis, or ulcers of the gumline and mucous membranes of the mouth, often occurs with antimetabolic drugs. The child may need a soft or light diet for comfort. Brushing the teeth with a soft swab rather than a brush or having the child just rinse the mouth with half-strength hydrogen peroxide and water is helpful. Viscous lidocaine (Xylocaine) may be prescribed to be swabbed on individual lesions for comfort. Lidocaine can cause paralysis of the gag reflex if it is swallowed, so it must be swabbed on individual lesions, *not* used for rinsing out the mouth as it is in adults. (Children younger than 8 years are likely to rinse and swallow.) Measures to reduce stomatitis are summarized in Empowering the Family.

Because mucous membrane ulcers may occur throughout the gastrointestinal tract, children on antimetabolic therapy should not have rectal temperatures taken to avoid aggravation or perforation of rectal ulcers.

Nursing Diagnosis: Risk for altered patterns of bowel elimination related to effects of chemotherapeutic agents

Outcome Identification: Child will remain free of constipation or diarrhea during course of treatment.

Outcome Evaluation: Child maintains usual pattern of bowel elimination; child reports (and parent confirms) no existence of hard or watery stools.

Constipation. Some chemotherapeutic agents, particularly vincristine, cause constipation. Children are placed on a stool softener, such as docusate sodium (Colace), to prevent hard stools from exacerbating rectal ulcers. The frequency of bowel movements should be recorded so that constipation is recognized early in its course. Additional measures for dealing with constipation include increasing the intake of fluids and dietary roughage.

Diarrhea. Diarrhea may occur from effects on the absorptive surfaces of the intestine. Keep careful records of the number and consistency of bowel movements in children receiving chemotherapy. If diarrhea is present, intravenous fluid will usually be administered to supplement fluid loss; an antidiarrheal agent may be prescribed for older children. Be certain to change diapers frequently in infants to prevent excoriation of the skin from the acid stool content. Diarrhea is frightening for children because of the loss of control they experience. Offer support and comfort for this annoying side effect of their primary therapy.

Nursing Diagnosis: Risk for diversional activity deficit related to neuropathy resulting from chemotherapy

Outcome Identification: Child will maintain usual activity level during therapy.

Outcome Evaluation: Child identifies activities in which he or she can participate that do not require fine motor skills while neuropathy is present.

Vincristine therapy will result in various neurologic symptoms, such as weakness, tingling, and numbing of the extremities, and sometimes an inability to walk. These symptoms subside when the medication is discontinued. Children may be unable to hold a pen or pencil or maneuver small parts of toys because their fingers are so affected. Think of games they can accomplish until the numbness in the hands fades. Children on bedrest may develop foot drop with vincristine. In some cases, physical therapy may be needed along with special braces or boots to prevent foot drop.

Nursing Diagnosis: Risk for infection related to therapy-induced depression of immune system

EMPOWERING THE FAMILY: Tips for Relieving the Discomfort of Stomatitis

- Oral hygiene should be seen as good and fun. Use a soft toothbrush to keep the number of germs in the mouth to a minimum and hopefully prevent infection. Another way to promote oral hygiene is to make up a game about mouth care that the whole family can play.
- Serve soft foods like mashed potatoes and pudding, rather than hard ones, such as toast crusts or crunchy cereal, to avoid further abrasions to tender gumlines.
- Encourage your child to rinse his mouth with lukewarm water three times a day (half strength H_2O_2 may be prescribed) both for comfort and to encourage healing.
- Provide nonacidic foods, such as gelatin instead of orange juice, which can sting if sores are present.
- Encourage your child to drink as much fluid as possible because this helps to keep lips from cracking.
- Keep lips well lubricated with vaseline or a commercial product. This also prevents cracking.

Outcome Identification: Child will remain free of an infection during treatment period.

Outcome Evaluation: Child's temperature remains below 98.6°F (37.0°C); no areas of erythema or drainage are found on the skin.

Children with cancer are very susceptible to infection not only because their immune system is depressed by chemotherapy, but also because they develop a degree of malnutrition that decreases the effectiveness of macrophage and phagocytosis function. A malignant process in the body decreases the body's overall ability to recognize foreign invaders and respond with the usual efficient rejection process. Frequent insertion of intravenous devices, the development of dry and cracking mucous membranes, and ulcer formation throughout the gastrointestinal tract provide ready sites for the entrance of microorganisms.

Although infection is occurring, it may be difficult to recognize because the usual response does not occur. Such common findings as local erythema, swelling, systemic fever, and swollen lymph glands may not be present or may be reduced in contrast to the degree of infection present.

Fortunately, administration of colony-stimulating factors can help the body quickly begin replacing damaged white blood cells (Nemunaitis, 1997). Even with this, bacterial infections are common. Gram-negative bacteria, such as *Escherichia coli, Pseudomonas aeruginosa*, and *Klebsiella pneumoniae*, and gram-positive bacteria, such as *Staphylococcus aureus* and streptococci, are common organisms involved in infections. Viral infections, such as varicella (chickenpox), varicella zoster (shingles), herpes simplex, viral hepatitis, and cytomegalovirus, are common invaders. Viral infections may occur because of the inability of children to produce interferon.

When bacterial infections are treated with antibiotics, overgrowth of fungal infections may occur. Candidiasis or Aspergillosis are common fungal invaders. When children are treated with immunosuppressive drugs, protozoal infections, such as *Pneumocystis carinii* pneumonia (normally a very rare pneumonia), may occur.

When infection is discovered in children with cancer, the causative agent is identified by culture. Specific antibiotics are then prescribed. The most important role in caring for children with cancer is preventing infection (see Nursing Procedure 32-1). This display identifies interventions to reduce the possibility of infection in the child with neutropenia (lowered white blood cell count).

Bone Marrow Transplantation

Transplanting bone marrow that was previously harvested from a child with cancer or transplanting marrow from a well person to a child with cancer has become a frequently used treatment for children. This can allow higher doses of chemotherapy and radiation to be used because, in the event of severe bone marrow depression, the child can have healthy marrow restored. Immune cells in the transplanted marrow may actually help to kill remaining cancer cells in the child's circulation.

If the child's own marrow is used, this is autologous transfusion. Bone marrow may be donated by someone who is histocompatible (immune compatible) with the child. This is an allogeneic transplant. A *syngeneic* transplant is one between twins.

Prior to transplant, the child receives a chemotherapy agent, such as cyclophosphamide, and total-body irradiation to kill as many marrow cells as possible, suppress the child's immune response to the transplanted tissue, and create space in the bone marrow to allow the newly transplanted cells a place to grow.

Bone marrow is removed from the child and treated to reduce the number of abnormal cells present (called purging) or removed from the donor in the operating room, under anesthesia, by the use of repeated punctures at the iliac crest. It is then processed and transfused into the child intravenously. The new marrow migrates to the bone marrow in about 3 weeks. Until this time, the child is at extreme risk for infection. Everyone coming in contact with the child must wash their hands well, and reverse isolation may be maintained. Transfusion of blood products may be necessary to maintain functional blood components until the transplanted marrow begins to function (see Managing and Delegating Unlicensed Assistive Personnel).

Not all medical centers perform bone marrow transplants, so a family may have to travel a distance for the therapy. Complications of bone marrow transplant are discussed in Chapter 23, because this technique is used with children with blood dyscrasias as well. Previously used only with children with leukemia, it is now being used in children with other cancers, such as neuroblastoma and Hodgkin's disease.

Pain Assessment

Because growing tumors displace cells, causing anoxia to those cells, pain is a common symptom experienced by children with cancer.

✔ CHECKPOINT QUESTIONS

3. Why does chemotherapy cause nausea and vomiting?
4. What are two common side effects of vincristine?

THE LEUKEMIAS

Acute Lymphocytic Leukemia

Leukemia is the distorted and uncontrolled proliferation of white blood cells (leukocytes). It is the most frequently occurring type of cancer in children. Because the abnormally proliferating cells are so immature, they may be identifiable only at the immature, or "blast" or "stem," cell stage.

The most frequent type of leukemia in children, acute lymphocytic leukemia (ALL) accounts for one third of all instances. The malignant cell involved is the lymphoblast, which is an immature lymphocyte. With the rapid prolif-

NURSING PROCEDURE 32.1: PREVENTING INFECTION IN THE HOSPITALIZED CHILD WITH NEUTROPENIA

Plan	Principle
1. Arrange for the child to occupy a private room with laminar airflow. The room should be recently cleaned and suitable for reverse isolation. Be sure to explain the rules of the room to the family and patient; for example, visitors may need to wear masks and clean gowns.	1. The patient and family need to know that rooms with laminar airflow take old "dirty air" out of the room. Requiring visitors and staff entering the room to wear masks and gowns help to protect the child (who cannot fight infection normally) from potentially dangerous microorganisms.
2. While caring for a child with neutropenia, avoid caring for patients with infections, such as bronchiolitis, diarrhea, or meningitis.	2. This precaution reduces possibility for disease spread.
3. Wash hands frequently: before child care; after handling potentially contaminated containers (e.g., tissues, diapers, other containers of body secretions or fluids); and when leaving the child's room.	3. Handwashing is the most effective safeguard against spreading infection.
4. Screen and prohibit visitors who have signs of infection (e.g., runny nose, oral herpes, rashes); who have been exposed to a communicable disease, such as chickenpox; or who have recently been vaccinated.	4. Selecting "safe" visitors prevents communication of potential infection to patient with neutropenia.
5. Keep child's immediate surroundings free of plants, fresh fruit and vegetables, flowers, goldfish, and other pets.	5. Prohibiting items that may harbor mold spores, salmonella, and other organisms helps keep immediate environment free of infecting organisms.
6. Keep child clean. Assist with daily body and oral hygiene. Wash skin with mild soap and water. Clean mouth with soft brush, disposable sponge, or cotton-tipped applicator and water rinses.	6. Personal hygiene and mouth care rid surfaces of microorganisms and preserve integrity of the skin and mucous membranes. Moisturizing ointments prevent skin breakdown.
7. Inspect mouth daily for breaks in the tissue, bleeding, or white patches, suggesting oral monilial (thrush) infection. As appropriate, apply a moisturizing and protective barrier, such as KY Jelly, to the lips.	7. Regular mouth inspection helps detect infection or the opportunity for infection early. Applying gel to lips promotes skin integrity so that infection cannot enter.
8. Take temperature and pulse and respiratory rates every 4 hours. Avoid taking rectal temperatures and administer acetaminophen (not aspirin) as prescribed.	8. Rectal temperature assessment may puncture rectal mucosa and provide entry for microorganisms. Aspirin is avoided to prevent Reye's syndrome and possible bleeding.
9. Provide gentle skin care, as prescribed, using nonirritating and nondrying lotions and nonallergenic tape on patient's skin. At the same time, inspect skin surfaces that may become entrances for infection, such as pressure points on the elbows and heels, IV and IM sites, venous access devices, diaper area, and other injection sites.	9. Careful skin care and inspection helps preserve skin integrity and prevent skin breakdown.
10. Clean injection sites well with alcohol or povidone-iodine solution. Also, change IV tubing, access sites, and dressings according to institutional protocol, usually every 24 to 48 hours.	10. Regular cleaning and changing procedures ensure the least growth of bacteria and other infective organisms.
11. Provide stool softeners, if needed, to promote smooth bowel movement.	11. Stool softeners keep hard stools from tearing rectal mucosa.
12. Arrange for patient to receive high-calorie, high-protein foods and food supplements as needed.	12. A diet rich in protein, vitamins, and minerals promotes the immune system.

(continued)

Plan	Principle
13. Assess for respiratory infection every 8 hours: auscultate chest sounds; listen for cough and throat clearing; inspect throat for redness and nasal passage for discharge. Institute measures to keep patient active and moving, such as playing games, such as "Simon Says," that encourage deep breathing.	13. These measures detect early infection and promote mobility. Movement and repositioning helps prevent infection by mobilizing static secretions that act as a growth medium for bacteria, viruses, and fungi.
14. Assess for possible genitourinary infections. Inspect color, clarity, and concentration of urine. Test pH (alkalinity suggests bacteria) and check frequency. Avoid catheterizing the patient; secure urine for testing by clean-catch method. Promote increased fluid intake. Advise female patients to wipe from front to back after voiding or defecating. If patient is menstruating, sanitary napkins should be used rather than tampons.	14. These measures help prevent and/or detect early infection. Increasing fluid intake helps move static urine so that microorganisms cannot colonize and replicate.
15. Administer and monitor granulocyte transfusions as prescribed.	15. Granulocytes are infection-fighting blood cells.
16. Do not administer any vaccine made with a live virus.	16. A child with neutropenia is susceptible to viral infection, which would be introduced by vaccine.

eration of lymphocytes, the production of red blood cells and platelets falls, and invasion of body organs by the rapidly increasing white blood cell elements begins (Mahoney, 1997a).

The highest incidence of ALL is in children between 2 and 6 years. The prognosis in children younger than 2 years or older than 10 years at the time of first occurrence is not as good as in those between 2 and 10 years. The prognosis in children who have more than 20,000 white blood cells per millimeter or who have more than 10% L2 cells (see classification of cells below) in bone marrow at the time of diagnosis is not as good as in those with a lower white blood cell count and fewer L2 cells at first diagnosis. The incidence of ALL is slightly higher in boys than girls, and the disease is seen more often in white children than in children of other races.

MANAGING AND DELEGATING UNLICENSED ASSISTIVE PERSONNEL

Unlicensed assistive personnel who may be assigned to care for children with cancer during hospital stays need to be made aware of major strides made in children's cancer therapy so that they can appreciate that most children with cancer (especially leukemia) have a favorable prognosis.

Be certain also that unlicensed personnel understand that children who are receiving chemotherapy or who have had bone marrow transplants are highly susceptible to infection. This helps them take responsibility for not spreading infection (washing hands well, not caring for an immunosuppressed child if they have an upper respiratory or herpes simplex infection, and the like).

Although it can be shown that leukemia in mice and cats is of viral origin, the cause of leukemia in children is unknown. Radiation, exposure to chemicals, or genetic factors may have some influence on the occurrence. Children with Down syndrome or Fanconi's syndrome are more likely to develop leukemia than are other children. It occurs more often in identical twins than in children who are only siblings. Bone irradiation may be implicated, so children should be submitted to as few x-rays as possible, including x-rays while in utero. Whether proximity to high-power lines is a cause is debatable (Li et al, 1998).

Assessment

The first symptoms in children usually are pallor, low-grade fever, and lethargy (symptoms of anemia caused by decreased red blood cell production). A child may have petechiae and bleeding from oral mucous membranes and may bruise easily because of low thrombocyte count. As the spleen and liver begin to enlarge from infiltration, abdominal pain, vomiting, and anorexia will occur. As abnormal lymphocytes begin to invade the bone periosteum, the child experiences bone and joint pain. Central nervous system invasion will lead to symptoms such as headache or unsteady gait.

Physical assessment will reveal painless generalized adenopathy, especially of the submaxillary or cervical nodes. Laboratory studies will reveal a variable leukocyte count. In some children, the leukocyte count is normal or even slightly decreased but includes blast (very immature) cells; in other children, there is a marked leukocytosis of the blast cells. The platelet count and hematocrit will be low, but the red blood cells present will be normocytic and normochromic (of normal size and color).

A bone marrow aspiration is done to identify the type of white blood cell involved or the type of leukemia. If there are more than 25% blast cells present, a leukemia diagnosis is established. In children, bone marrow is aspirated at the iliac crest rather than the sternum both because this is less frightening and because it yields more marrow. X-rays of the long bones may reveal lesions caused by the invasion of abnormal cells. A lumbar puncture may show evidence of blast cells in the cerebrospinal fluid (CSF).

Therapeutic Management

About 90% of children with an initial good prognosis will have long-term survival. If a child experiences a relapse, the chances of long-term survival become greatly reduced. Although remission can be reinduced, the length of each subsequent remission tends to be shorter and less effective.

Disease Classification and Prognosis. Leukemia is classified to define subgroups of cells and to predict the usual response to treatment. Lymphoblasts are classified as L1, L2, and L3, based on cell size, amount of cytoplasm present, shape of nucleus, and presence of nucleoli. A second classification system distinguishes cells as T or B. Blasts with T-cell characteristics clump or form rosettes when exposed to sheep erythrocytes and are described as being E positive. A third classification method includes the use of monoclonal antibodies that bind to antigens related to leukemic cells.

Blasts with B-cell characteristics can be recognized by the presence of immunoglobulin and antigen-antibody receptors on their surfaces. Most children with ALL have null-cell disease, or cells that are neither T nor B cell. An antigen found with null-cell ALL has been named CALLA. Approximately 40% of children with ALL are CALLA positive. This finding is associated with a good prognosis. About 15% to 20% of children have T-cell involvement; prognosis with this type is poor. B-cell incidence is extremely rare (only a 5% incidence) and has a very poor prognosis. In contrast, a subtype termed *pre-B-cell ALL* has a good prognosis.

Cure as Goal. The goal of therapy for leukemia is complete cure, based on the use of chemotherapeutic agents. A chemotherapy program is aimed at, first, achieving a complete remission or absence of leukemia cells (induction phase); second, preventing leukemia cells from invading or growing in the central nervous system (sanctuary phase); and third, maintaining the original remission (maintenance phase).

Chemotherapy in children is often administered by means of a Broviac (double-lumen catheter) into a subclavian vein. This can be clamped and "trapped" or kept open by a slow intravenous infusion so that the child can be ambulatory between treatments.

Drugs frequently used to initiate a remission are vincristine, prednisone, and L-asparaginase. Doxorubicin or daunorubicin may be used also. These are given over about a 1-month period. As many as 95% of children with ALL achieve remission with chemotherapy (a bone marrow aspiration shows fewer than 5% blasts in bone marrow). Because so many cells are destroyed by chemotherapy, a high level of uric acid is excreted during chemotherapy, which can lead to plugging of kidney glomeruli and loss of kidney function. To prevent this, a drug such as allopurinol to reduce formation of uric acid is administered with chemotherapy. Keeping a child well hydrated also helps maintain safe uric acid excretion.

Because many chemotherapy drugs do not cross the blood-brain barrier in effective concentrations, leukemic cells in the central nervous system continue to flourish even with chemotherapy. A combination of intrathecal drug administration (injection of drugs into the CSF by lumbar puncture), such as methotrexate, dexamethasone, cytarabine, and ara-C is next instituted to eradicate this source of leukemic cells (called a ***prophylaxis*** or ***sanctuary phase*** because no "sanctuary" is given to malignant cells). Cranial radiation, once used extensively for this purpose, is less used today than previously because over the long-term, minimal learning disorders may result.

Maintenance and Monitoring. The purpose of maintenance chemotherapy is to eliminate residual leukemic cells so that the child's immune system can complete the eradication. Standard maintenance therapy includes a combination of methotrexate and 6-mercaptopurine, vincristine, prednisone, and ara-C. This is given for up to 2 to 3 years. A drug such as leucovorin is usually given following systemic methotrexate to neutralize its action and protect normal cells from the effect of the drug. During the maintenance phase, the child's blood values must be monitored monthly. If there is serious bone marrow depression, medication levels may be reduced or a transfusion may be necessary.

If a bone marrow study during the maintenance phase shows that leukemic cells are again evident, a new induction phase will be started, followed by a new prophylaxis and maintenance phase. Children who are free of disease for 4 years are considered cured, and their maintenance therapy can then be stopped. Bone marrow transplantation or immunotherapy may be used with children who do not respond well to standard therapy. Newer drugs are constantly being researched to use for relapse therapy. Help parents evaluate the use of nonapproved drugs (see Enhancing Communication).

Complications

Throughout therapy, the nurse, family, and other members of the health care team need to be alert for complications of therapy. Among these problems are central nervous system, renal, and reproductive system problems.

Central Nervous System Involvement. If central nervous system involvement occurs, it can be severe and intense and can include blindness, hydrocephalus, and recurrent convulsions. The meninges and the sixth and seventh cranial nerves are the structures most often affected. With meningeal involvement, the child will have nuchal rigidity, headache, irritability, and perhaps vomiting and papilledema. A lumbar puncture will reveal the presence of blast cells in the CSF. Symptoms can be relieved by intrathecal injections of methotrexate, but check that children are not given oral or intravenous methotrexate at the same time, because some of the dose of intrathecal

ENHANCING COMMUNICATION

Len, a 10-year-old, was diagnosed with leukemia 3 months ago. His mother brings him into the emergency room because of a severe nose bleed. While you are putting pressure on his nose, you notice that both of Len's arms are covered with fresh ecchymotic bruises.

Less Effective Communication

Nurse: Is Len still having chemotherapy, Mrs. Miller?
Mrs. Miller: No. He's in remission.
Nurse: Is he taking anything that would lower his platelet count or clotting factors?
Mrs. Miller: All he takes is asparagus powder we get from Mexico.
Nurse: Why are you getting that from Mexico and not the clinic here?
Mrs. Miller: It's a new treatment and not legal here—even though it cured him.
Nurse: If he's cured, why do you think he has so many new black and blue marks?
Mrs. Miller: I don't want to think about that.
Nurse: Well, let's focus right now on getting this bleeding stopped.

More Effective Communication

Nurse: Is Len still having chemotherapy, Mrs. Miller?
Mrs. Miller: No. He's in remission.
Nurse: Is he taking anything that would lower his platelet count or clotting factors?
Mrs. Miller: All he takes is asparagus powder we get from Mexico.
Nurse: Why are you getting that from Mexico and not the clinic here?
Mrs. Miller: It's a new treatment and not legal here—even though it cured him.
Nurse: If he's cured, why do you think he has so many new black and blue marks?
Mrs. Miller: I don't want to think about that.
Nurse: Well, let's get this nose bleed stopped. Then we can take a minute to talk about what they might mean and decide what to do about them.

Of all the diseases known, there is no other disease with as many "false cures" as cancer. It is important when talking with parents to see if they are using any of these unproved methods. Some of them do no harm, so parents can continue to give them along with proven therapies. Others, however, actually interfere with the action of a chemotherapy drug and are contraindicated. In the above scenario, the parent has chosen an unproved regimen. Ignoring that this choice may be an unhelpful one and denying a potential recurrence of cancer or other problem will not be therapeutic in the long term.

methotrexate is absorbed systemically, which could lead to a toxic reaction. Inserting Silicon tubing into a cerebral ventricle and threading it under the scalp (an Ommaya reservoir) provides easy access to the CSF for sampling or injection without the need for lumbar punctures (Figure 32-4).

Renal Involvement. Kidney involvement, resulting from invasion of leukemia cells, is a serious complication. The kidneys may enlarge, and their function will be impaired. If uric acid levels rise as a result of the breakdown of leukemic cells during chemotherapy, plugging of renal tubules with uric acid crystals and kidney failure may result. Renal involvement may limit the use of chemotherapeutic agents, because they cannot be excreted effectively due to the kidney damage.

Testicular Invasion. In boys, leukemic cells tend to invade the testes. Unless this problem is specifically addressed, these cells will not be destroyed by chemotherapy and so may grow and proliferate again once chemotherapy is halted. In most boys, therefore, the testes will be radiated to destroy this sanctuary site for cells. This will unfortunately lead to sterilization later in life. If a boy is past puberty and is forming sperm, sperm banking might be suggested prior to chemotherapy and radiation so that he will have sperm for reproduction later in life.

NURSING DIAGNOSES AND RELATED INTERVENTIONS

Nursing Diagnosis: Risk for infection related to nonfunctioning white blood cells and immunosuppressive therapy

Outcome Identification: Child will remain free of an infection during course of therapy.

Outcome Evaluation: Child's temperature will remain below 98.6°F (37.0°C); no areas of erythema or drainage are present on skin.

Prevent Infection. Because the number of functioning white blood cells is reduced and the drugs used for treatment are immunosuppressive, children with leukemia are extremely prone to infection during chemotherapy. Most deaths in children result from infections, such as septicemia, pneumonia, or meningitis. *Pseudomonas* is commonly an invading organism.

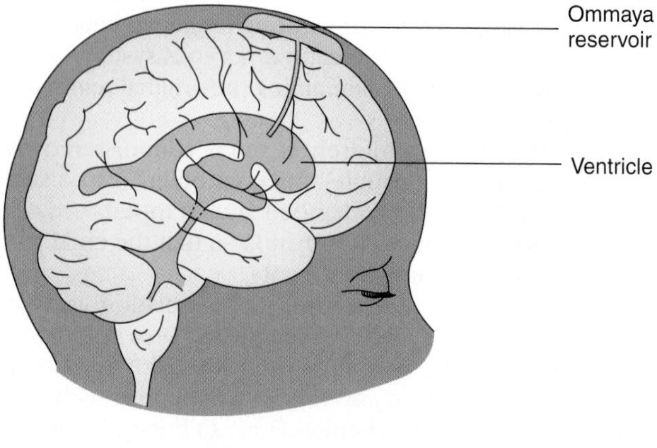

FIGURE 32.4 An Ommaya reservoir. Medication injected into the reservoir flows down to the ventricle and enters the cerebrospinal fluid.

While children are receiving care at home, parents must learn to observe them carefully and promptly report any indication of infection, such as low-grade fever or behavior that does not seem typical of the child. The sooner the symptoms are reported, the sooner anti-infective therapy can begin.

To increase the functioning leukocyte count, leukocytes may be transfused. Symptoms of fever and chills from leukocyte transfusion tend to be more common than with red blood cell transfusion. This is not a true transfusion reaction and generally not a reason to stop the transfusion.

Children may be placed on prophylactic antibiotics to reduce the possibility of infection. Parents may be advised to limit visitors, especially anyone with an infection, until the child's functioning white blood count improves.

Nursing Diagnosis: Risk for fluid volume deficit related to increased chance of hemorrhage from poor platelet production

Outcome Identification: Child will maintain an adequate fluid volume during course of therapy.

Outcome Evaluation: No evidence of hemorrhage is present (no epistaxis, hematuria, hematemesis); pulse rate and blood pressure remain normal for age group.

Prevent Blood Loss. Because the platelet count is low due to poor platelet production and the effect of chemotherapy, children with leukemia are extremely prone to massive hemorrhage. Epistaxis (nose bleed) is the most common kind of bleeding; gastrointestinal, renal, or central nervous system bleeding also may occur.

Digital pressure is usually effective in stopping epistaxis. The application of Gelfoam soaked in topical thrombin may be necessary. In some children, postnasal packing is necessary. Children may need a transfusion to replace the lost blood volume. Platelet-rich plasma or a concentrated preparation of platelets will be ordered to improve the platelet count. Unfortunately, the lifespan of transfused platelets is short (1–3 days), so frequent platelet transfusion may be necessary.

Because children with leukemia have blood samples drawn frequently, receive transfusions, and have chemotherapeutic drugs given intravenously, they need the opportunity for therapeutic play with needles and syringes or intravenous tubing so that they can work through some feelings about these intrusive, hurtful procedures. Advocate for heparin traps or subclavian lines that minimize the number of venipunctures.

Following an intramuscular injection or the removal of an intravenous needle, compress the injection site securely to prevent bleeding. If the sites for intravenous infusion become obscured by large ecchymotic areas, the child's chances of remission through chemotherapy are reduced.

Nursing Diagnosis: Pain related to invasion of leukocytes

Outcome Identification: Child will experience a tolerable degree of pain during course of illness.

Outcome Evaluation: Child states that pain is tolerable (if infant, not crying).

Manage Pain. Children with acute leukemia experience pain because of the vast number of white blood cells that invade the periosteum of the bones. Handle these children gently to keep pain to a minimum. Assess pain using a standard scale for accuracy. Reposition them frequently because they tend to remain in a position of maximum comfort if they hurt. Placing a sheepskin underneath them helps to reduce skin irritation caused by always resting in the same position.

Nursing Diagnosis: Altered health maintenance related to long-term therapy for leukemia

Outcome Identification: Child and parents demonstrate understanding of long-term health maintenance needs by hospital discharge.

Outcome Evaluation: Parents and child state importance of regular health maintenance visits; child continues chemotherapy regimen at home and keeps all ambulatory appointments.

Support the Family. During the maintenance phase of therapy, children can be allowed normal activity and should attend regular school. Parents need to report promptly any sign of infection so that antibiotic therapy can be started early. Because chickenpox can be fatal to a child who is immunosuppressed, the school should be asked to notify the child's parents if any other child in the school develops chickenpox so that appropriate immune protection can be given. Many children with leukemia are immunized by the vaccine against chickenpox.

Evaluation of children at a follow-up visit should include not only the state of blood formation, but also whether they are making forward-thinking plans or think of themselves as well children again.

Parents continue to need a great deal of support during the maintenance phase of therapy. They live from day to day, hoping that the remission will not end; they need a great deal of support if a relapse does occur. Parents who are told that their child has a heart defect that is not correctable know from the beginning that their child will die. In contrast, parents of the child with leukemia constantly hope that a remission is permanent, that their child will be one who is cured. In a sense, the child dies many times—at diagnosis and again if a relapse occurs. If death does occur, the reality of what has happened may be extremely difficult for the parents to accept. They may return to the hospital for visits weeks or months after the child's death in an effort to accept reality and work through their grief. The Nursing Care Plan summarizes care for the child with leukemia.

Acute Myelogenous Leukemia

If leukemia is acute but does not involve a lymphocytic type, it is categorized as nonlymphoid leukemia (non-ALL, or ANLL). About 25% of childhood leukemia is this type.

Acute myelogenous leukemia (AML) accounts for about 20% of all childhood leukemia. The frequency of the disorder increases in late adolescence. In its chronic form, it is the most common type of leukemia in adulthood.

Myelogenous leukemia is overproliferation of granulocytes. Granulocytes grow so rapidly that they often are forced out into the bloodstream still in the blast stage.

Nursing Care Plan

THE CHILD WITH LEUKEMIA RECEIVING MAINTENANCE CHEMOTHERAPY

A 6-year-old male with ALL is brought to the outpatient clinic for administration of maintenance chemotherapy. His father states, "He's been having trouble eating lately and I've noticed some clumps of hair on his pillow when he gets up in the morning."

Assessment: 6-year-old male diagnosed with ALL approximately 10 weeks ago. Completed induction phase of chemotherapy with some reports of nausea and vomiting; controlled with antiemetics. Weight maintained within 1 to 2 pounds of baseline weight.

Child appears pale. Weight decreased 5 pounds in last 2 weeks. "He's been having trouble keeping food down." Skin turgor sluggish. Oral mucous membranes red and irritated.Two ulcers noted on inner aspect of left cheek at gum line. "It hurts to eat."

Child's scalp is totally bald. Child states, "I'm so ugly. I look like an old man." Laboratory test results decreased from previous levels but within acceptable parameters.

Nursing Diagnosis: Altered nutrition, less than body requirements, related to inadequate intake, secondary irritation and pain of mucosal ulceration and increased vomiting

Outcome Identification: Child will demonstrate an adequate intake of nutrients to return to baseline weight.

Outcome Evaluation: Child exhibits a 1- to 2-pound weight gain by next visit; states oral ulcers are healing and no further ulcers have developed; reports food intake is increasing with decreasing episodes of vomiting. Child and father verbalize measures to control vomiting and relieve ulceration.

Interventions	Rationale
1. Administer ordered antiemetic approximately 30 minutes before initiating chemotherapy and at prescribed intervals during therapy. Instruct parent to continue antiemetic therapy at home as ordered.	1. Antiemetics administered prior to chemotherapy help to prevent nausea and vomiting from developing. Continued therapy helps to control any nausea or vomiting that does develop.
2. If the child experiences nausea, encourage him to take clear fluids until feeling has passed.	2. Taking clear fluids helps to minimize irritation of the gastrointestinal tract and decreases the risk for vomiting.
3. When the child is comfortable, question him about his food likes and dislikes. Obtain a dietary recall from the child and his father.	3. Ascertaining likes and dislikes provides a baseline for future suggestions for food choices that would be followed. A dietary recall provides information about the child's current intake and aids in planning appropriate suggestions for nutritional intake.
4. Encourage the parent to offer food early in the day before chemotherapy. Suggest frequent high-calorie snacks, such as fortified breakfast foods, milk shakes, and high-energy snack bars. Enlist the aid of the dietician.	4. Eating prior to chemotherapy enhances nutrition because the child is less likely to be nauseated at this time. Frequent high-calorie snacks provides additional calories needed without the additional expenditure of energy to eat a large meal. Assistance from the dietician ensures nutritionally sound food choices.
5. Allow child to select items from a list of appropriate foods. Develop a simple contract with the child for including appropriate food choices. Praise the child for choices and eating behavior.	5. Contracting and providing the child with choices promotes active participation and feelings of control, thus enhancing the chances for success. Praising offers positive reinforcement.

(continued)

Interventions	Rationale
6. Encourage the child to eat small, frequent meals and to eat when hungry, even if it is not mealtime.	6. Small, frequent meals decrease the amount of energy expended for eating and also minimize the risk for abdominal distention, which may exacerbate the child's nausea and vomiting.
7. Instruct the parent and child in ways to enhance the taste, protein, and caloric content of food, such as adding brown sugar, eggs, or wheat germ.	7. Chemotherapy can alter the taste of foods. Increased calorie and protein intake is necessary to meet the child's increased metabolic needs.
8. Advise parent to offer nonacidic and soft, bland, moist foods, such as mashed potatoes, puddings, milk shakes, and cooked cereals rather than foods such as toast, cold cereal, and orange juice. Assist the parent with ways to make mealtime pleasant.	8. Soft, bland, moist, and nonacidic foods minimize irritation to the child's already ulcerated mucosa. Making mealtime pleasant may help to stimulate the child's appetite.
9. Instruct child and parent in oral care and advise using a soft toothbrush or swabs to cleanse teeth. Encourage the use of warm water rinses and saline mouthwashes frequently. Teach the parent about the use of topical anesthetic application to the ulcers as appropriate.	9. Good oral care is essential to prevent further ulceration. It also helps to soothe the already ulcerated tissue. Topical anesthetics may help decrease the discomfort of the ulcers.
10. Encourage the child to drink as much fluid as possible.	10. Adequate fluid intake helps to keep mucous membranes moist and minimizes the risk of possible dehydration.
11. Reinforce with the parent the need to monitor the child's intake and output and to weigh the child twice a week at the same time each day, with the same scale, and with the child wearing similar clothing.	11. Intake and output and weight are valuable indicators of fluid balance and nutritional status if done consistently in the same manner each time. Since weight fluctuates from day to day, weighing the child twice a week rather than daily helps to deemphasize the problems, minimizing the risk for frustration.
12. Instruct the parent to keep a written record of the child's intake, weight, episodes of nausea and vomiting, and relief measures. Encourage the parent to involve the child with record keeping.	12. A written record provides objective evidence for evaluating the effectiveness of the plan and allows for feedback and further teaching. Involving the child in a concrete activity promotes active participation, helping to enhance feelings of self-esteem and control.
13. Urge the parent to contact the clinic if the child develops further ulcerations or experiences continued weight loss or an increase in nausea and vomiting.	13. Continued nausea and vomiting, weight loss, or development of more ulcers requires further evaluation and follow-up to minimize the risk of additional problems for the child.

Nursing Diagnosis: Body image disturbance related to hair loss secondary to the effects of chemotherapy

Outcome Identification: Child will verbalize positive feelings about himself.

Outcome Evaluation: Child states impact of hair loss on appearance and feelings; verbalizes measures to cope with hair loss; reports continued participation in age-appropriate activities.

Interventions	Rationale
1. Assess the child's understanding of hair loss and its cause. Review the structure and function of the hair and development of hair loss.	1. Obtaining a baseline knowledge assessment provides a foundation on which to build future teaching strategies. Reviewing and clarifying aids in learning and strengthening understanding.
2. Attempt to identify the meaning of his appearance and hair loss.	2. Identifying the meaning assists in determining the degree of its possible impact on the child.
3. Encourage the child to express feelings and thoughts about self, appearance, and hair loss. Incorporate the use of therapeutic play.	3. Sharing of feelings and concerns permits a safe outlet for emotions and also aids in highlighting the child's awareness of possible impact on body image. Therapeutic play allows the child to express his feelings.

(continued)

4. Reinforce with the child that hair is lost by breaking off at the skin surface. Remind child that the hair will grow back because the root is not damaged.	4. Reinforcement aids in clarifying any misconceptions, helping the child to understand that hair loss is temporary.
5. Assist the child with suggestions, such as the use of colorful caps, to minimize the appearance of the hair loss.	5. Minimizing the appearance of the hair loss may help the child cope better with the event and possibly enhance feelings of self-esteem and normalcy.
6. Include a few of the child's close friends as appropriate in discussion and suggestions.	6. Including the child's friends in these measures helps to decrease the child's feelings of being different and alone.

The overproliferation of granulocytes limits the production of red blood cells and platelets.

Assessment

Children with AML have the same symptoms as those with ALL. Because they do not have mature granulocytes, they are susceptible to infection and may have had many recent upper respiratory infections.

Therapeutic Management

The diagnosis is established by bone marrow aspiration and biopsy. Cells are typed (M1 to M6) to establish prognosis. Following diagnosis, chemotherapy to effect remission will begin. Doxorubicin and cytosine arabinoside are two drugs commonly used for therapy. It may take 1 to 2 months to reach a full remission.

During the maintenance phase, additional chemotherapeutic agents in common use are cyclophosphamide, 6-thioguanine, and methyl-GAG. Maintenance therapy is continued indefinitely.

Remission is more difficult to achieve in children with ANLL than in those with ALL; if one is achieved, it may be brief (Steuber, 1997). Bone marrow transplantation may be attempted following the initial remission to ensure new growth of normal granulocytes.

✔ CHECKPOINT QUESTIONS

5. What are the first signs commonly seen in the child with leukemia?
6. If a child has central nervous system involvement with leukemia, how will methotrexate be administered?

THE LYMPHOMAS

Hodgkin's Disease

Lymphomas are malignancies of the lymph or reticuloendothelial system; they are categorized as Hodgkin's or non-Hodgkin's lymphomas. Although Hodgkin's disease is better known, non-Hodgkin's lymphomas are more common in children (about 60% non-Hodgkin's to 40% Hodgkin's).

With Hodgkin's disease, there is a proliferation of lymphocytes and special *Reed-Sternberg cells* (large, multinucleated cells that are probably nonfunctioning monocyte-macrophage cells). Although Hodgkin's cells are capable of DNA synthesis and mitotic division, they are abnormal in that they lack both B- and T-lymphocyte surface markers and cannot produce immunoglobulins.

As with all neoplastic diseases, the etiology of Hodgkin's disease is unknown. It occurs more often in boys than in girls. It is rarely seen in children younger than 7 years. The incidence increases greatly during adolescence and young adulthood (McClain, 1997).

It occurs more frequently in children with rheumatoid arthritis or systemic lupus erythematosus, supporting the theory that the disease is associated with an abnormal immune response. Children who take phenytoin sodium (Dilantin) for long periods may develop a lymphoid hyperplasia that mimics Hodgkin's disease. In some children, there is an abnormal distribution of human leukocyte antigens to suggest that the disease may be inherited. Metastasis is through lymphatic channels. Late in the disease, spread to lung, liver, and bone marrow occurs.

Assessment

Symptoms of Hodgkin's disease usually begin with only one painless, enlarged, rubbery-feeling lymph node, usually a cervical node. Other nodes then become involved, along with the liver, spleen, bone marrow, and eventually the central nervous system. The child usually has accompanying symptoms of anorexia, malaise, and loss of weight. Fever may be present. The sedimentation rate will be elevated; anemia is usually present from reduced red blood cell survival and poor iron use. Serum copper is elevated; the white blood cell count is usually normal.

Hodgkin's disease is confirmed by biopsy of the lymph nodes and of the liver. Further studies (bone marrow, liver function, chest and abdominal computed tomography [CT] scan, lymphangiogram, and abdominal biopsy) are done to classify the clinical stage of the disorder. Chest x-ray reveals enlarged mediastinal nodes; the abdominal CT will reveal enlarged lymph nodes of the abdomen.

A lymphangiogram is performed by injecting dye into the hand or foot. This allows visualization of the lymphatic system. A catheter is inserted into a lymph vessel, and radiopaque dye is added as in angiography. Lymphatic channels can be visualized on x-ray films. The lymph system does not eradicate opaque dye readily; in some children, lymph chains will still be outlined on x-ray films for up to 1 year. The original dye injected into the skin to visualize the lymph vessels stains the skin a bluish green. This dye will remain as a skin stain for about 1 year. Nodes opacified from lymphangiogram dye can be used as markers of disease progress on plain, flat-plate x-ray films for 6 to 12 months.

Therapeutic Management

Four subcategories of Hodgkin's disease can be documented: lymphocyte predominant, nodular sclerosing, mixed cellularity, and lymphocyte depletion. The most frequently occurring types in children are nodular sclerosing and lymphocyte predominant. The prognosis is best for the child with the lymphocyte-predominant type and worst for the child with the lymphocyte-depletion type.

The disease is staged according to regional involvement (Table 32-4). Such staging may be determined by a laparotomy with partial or total splenectomy and liver, multiple lymph node, and bone marrow biopsy. In girls, ovaries can be repositioned at the time of laparotomy to minimize the effect of radiation on them.

Treatment depends on the clinical stage of the disease at the time of diagnosis. Children in stages I or II receive radiation therapy to all lymph nodes above the diaphragm. These stages of disease are curable in about 90% of children. Children with stage III receive radiation therapy to the groin and retroperitoneum as well as to areas above the diaphragm. Removal of the spleen at the time of laparotomy prevents the need for extensive radiation to this area. Chemotherapy may be begun. Children with stage IV disease are generally treated by a 6-month course of chemotherapy. Common treatment agents are mechlorethamine (nitrogen mustard), vincristine (Oncovin), procarbazine, and prednisone. This treatment protocol is commonly called MOPP therapy. Other drugs used are doxorubicin (Adriamycin), bleomycin, vinblastine, and dacarbazine (ABVD therapy) (Mulnar et al., 1997). If total splenectomy was done, the child will have a lifelong susceptibility to bacterial infection, most often *Pneumococcus.* Children who have had their spleens removed generally are placed on prophylactic antibiotic therapy, such as penicillin, daily for 1 to 2 years to prevent them from contracting infections. They should receive pneumococcal vaccine prior to spleen removal.

TABLE 32.4 Stages of Hodgkin's Disease

STAGE	EXTENT OF DISEASE
I	Disease affects single lymph node or single extralymphatic organ or site.
II	Disease affects two or more lymph node regions on the same side of the diaphragm, or there is localized involvement of an extralymphatic organ or site.
III	Disease affects lymph node regions on both sides of the diaphragm, or there is localized involvement of an extralymphatic organ or site.
IV	There is diffuse or disseminated involvement of extralymphatic organs with or without associated lymph node involvement.

Children should be followed conscientiously for symptoms of Hodgkin's disease relapse during adult life. A relapse is often retreatable, using a chemotherapy course different from that used initially. Adolescents with stages I and II who receive both radiation and chemotherapy have a 90% chance of a 5-year survival; this is as high as 80% in stage III. Those with stage IV and V disease, unfortunately, have a limited survival rate (25%–50%).

Long-term effects of complete radiation may be retarded bone growth, scoliosis, hypothyroidism, and nephritis. A secondary tumor may occur in as many as 10% to 12% of children from the extensive radiation. In boys, aspermia may be a complication of MOPP therapy. Girls who have their ovaries repositioned prior to radiation may have no detrimental effect on ovaries from the therapy. Newer regimens of an ABVD protocol may be used to reduce these late toxicity problems.

NURSING DIAGNOSES AND RELATED INTERVENTIONS

The nursing diagnoses most often used with Hodgkin's disease address the child's impaired immune defenses and risk for infection, fear and feelings about the diagnosis, or changed body image (particularly in the adolescent). Both the parents and the child need opportunities to express their feelings about the unfairness of this disease.

Nursing Diagnosis: Risk for powerlessness related to constant possibility of disease recurrence

Outcome Identification: Child will maintain positive attitude about self and ability of health care team to manage illness should a relapse occur.

Outcome Evaluation: Child states that he or she feels healthy during remission; participates in school and extracurricular activities; and voices confidence in health care team to treat symptoms if they recur.

The course of treatment for Hodgkin's disease is long. Some adolescents, in whom the disease is most prevalent, live from day to day wondering if symptoms will recur.

Adolescents should attend regular school during periods of remission so that they can lead as normal a life as possible. They should be told as much as they want to know about the disease. Some adolescents want to know exactly what stage they are in; others prefer not to be told so that they can continue to believe that a cure will be possible. Both adolescents and their parents need continued support from health care personnel during the long course of the disease.

Non-Hodgkin's Lymphoma

Non-Hodgkin's lymphomas are malignant disorders of the lymphocytes. They involve stem cells and lymphocytes in varying degrees of differentiation. In the pediatric population, diffuse lymphoblastic, undifferentiated, and large-cell lymphomas are commonly seen. Unlike Hodgkin's disease, spread is through the bloodstream rather than directly by lymph flow, so it is unpredictable. Metastatic spread to the central nervous system tends to occur early in the disease. The most common age of occurrence is 5 to 15 years; non-Hodgkin's lymphomas occur slightly more often in boys than in girls.

The cause of non-Hodgkin's lymphomas may be an oncogenic virus. This occurs with increased frequency in children with agammaglobulinemia and acquired immunodeficiency syndrome or who are receiving long-term immunosuppressive therapy, such as would be given following an organ transplant. Such states may reduce the body's ability to recognize and destroy oncogenic viruses or malignant cells. These lymphomas can be divided into two groups: diffuse lymphoblastic lymphomas and diffuse, undifferentiated lymphomas. Cells can be classified as T-cell, B-cell, non-T, or non-B type; the prognosis for recovery is best if cells are non-T or non-B and worst if cells are B-cell type.

Assessment

Non-Hodgkin's lymphomas of the lymphoblastic type involve the lymph glands of the neck and chest most commonly, although axillary, abdominal, or inguinal nodes may be the first involved. If mediastinal lymph glands are swollen, the child may have a cough or chest "tightness." If mediastinal nodes press on the veins returning blood from the head, edema of the face may result. Diffuse, undifferentiated types present most commonly with an abdominal mass. If abdominal nodes are involved, the child notices abdominal pain; he or she may have diarrhea or constipation, and a mass may be palpable on examination. To establish the diagnosis, biopsy of the affected lymph nodes and bone marrow is performed. It is often difficult to distinguish between undifferentiated lymphoma cells and acute lymphoblastic leukemia. This can be established by bone marrow analysis (if a bone marrow biopsy shows more than 25% blasts, the diagnosis is acute leukemia). Areas of metastases are identified by chest x-ray; lymphangiogram; gallium, liver-spleen, and CT scans; and bone marrow aspiration.

Therapeutic Management

Non-Hodgkin's lymphomas are treated by radiation of lymph nodes and by systemic chemotherapy. The initial phase of therapy is an induction phase (a time during which the child is put into remission, or no tumor can be detected by clinical means), followed by a maintenance phase up to 2 years long. Common drugs used are cyclophosphamide, vincristine, methotrexate, and prednisone (COMP therapy) and a multiple-agent program that includes cytosine arabinoside, cyclophosphamide, daunorubicin, vincristine, prednisone, BCNU, L-asparaginase, thioguanine, hydroxyurea, and methotrexate. Intrathecal chemotherapy may be included in the therapy because of the tendency for non-Hodgkin's lymphoma metastasis to the central nervous system. Because the breakdown of cells is so rapid with chemotherapy, hyperkalemia, hyperphosphate serum levels, and hypocalcemia must be carefully assessed. A granulocyte colony-stimulating factor is given to prevent neutropenia.

Autologous bone marrow transfusion (bone marrow removed at diagnosis before the disease has spread to the marrow and then replaced at a point that blood components are destroyed by chemotherapy) allows more aggressive chemotherapy to be used than formerly.

Between 80% and 90% of children with non-Hodgkin's lymphoma with minimal symptoms will achieve remission. In a few children, the disorder may transform to ALL.

Burkitt's Lymphoma

Burkitt's lymphoma (a non-Hodgkin's lymphoma) is a specifically named but rare form of cancer in the United States; it is generally seen in Africa. When this lymphoma does occur, however, it tends to affect children. Children 2 to 14 years old have the highest incidence; the peak age of incidence is 7 years.

There is an association between Burkitt's lymphoma and Epstein-Barr virus, which causes infectious mononucleosis, in that the virus is present at the same time as Burkitt's lymphoma.

The first indication of disease is a detectable mass, which is usually painless unless it blocks some body system. Common primary sites are the submaxillary lymph nodes or those of the abdomen.

A Burkitt's lymphoma is a rapidly growing tumor; the cell mass may double in size in 24 hours. Surgery is used to remove the primary tumor. This is followed by chemotherapy; cyclophosphamide, methotrexate, doxorubicin, vincristine, and prednisone are commonly used agents. To prevent central nervous system involvement, intrathecal methotrexate may be given.

Because Burkitt's lymphomas are such rapidly growing tumors, they respond dramatically to chemotherapy (the cells are almost always in a susceptible state). Tissue breakdown may be so voluminous that the uric acid level of the urine may cause renal tubule plugging unless the child is kept very well hydrated and a drug such as allopurinol is administered concurrently (McClain, 1997).

✔ CHECKPOINT QUESTIONS

7. At what age is Hodgkin's disease most likely to develop in a child?
8. What is usually the first sign of Hodgkin's disease?

NEOPLASMS OF THE BRAIN

Brain tumor is the second most common form of cancer in children and the most common solid tumor form. Tumors tend to occur between 1 and 10 years of age, with 5 years being the peak incidence. In children, brain tumors tend to occur at the midline in the brain stem or cerebellum located beneath the tentorial membrane; in contrast, they usually are lateral and above the tentorial membrane in adults. This makes them particularly difficult to remove in children without damaging normal brain tissue (Mahoney, 1997b).

Assessment

Children with brain tumor will have symptoms of increased intracranial pressure: headache, vision changes, vomiting, and an enlarging head circumference from compression of cerebral fluid drainage. Lethargy, projectile vomiting, and coma are late signs.

The headache associated with brain tumor tends to be intermittent because of pressure changes related to position and the ability of the cranium to expand to some degree and temporarily relieve the associated pressure. Headache tends to occur on arising in the morning. It becomes intense on straining, such as occurs with coughing or bowel movements. A parent may report these symptoms in the young child as an increasingly irritable child who is constipated because of reluctance to strain to pass stool. With some tumors, the pain is occipital. This is an important finding because this is an unusual location for a headache from any other cause.

Vomiting, like headache, tends to occur on arising. The child is not usually nauseated and so will eat immediately afterward, unlike the child who vomits because of gastrointestinal distress. The vomiting pattern occurs morning after morning. It will eventually become projectile after a long time, but projectile vomiting does not present as an initial symptom. Vomiting in this pattern may be discounted by parents as school phobia (reluctance to attend school) because the children are able to eat again immediately and seem to recover about a half hour after they are out of bed (at the same time the school bus leaves).

Eye changes that occur are usually diplopia due to sixth cranial nerve involvement or strabismus due to suppression of vision in one eye. Children with strabismus may tend to tilt their head to the side or partially close one eye when viewing objects to compensate for the suppression and strabismus. The child may develop a torticollis (wry neck) or ptosis (lag of the eyelid). Papilledema (swelling of the optic nerve) may be evident on funduscopic examination.

Apart from these generalized symptoms of increased intracranial pressure, a growing tumor will produce specific localized signs, such as nystagmus (constant movement on horizontal movement of the eye), cranial nerve paralysis, or visual field defects. Tumors of the cerebellum tend to cause a definite head tilt due to vision suppression. As the tumor growth continues, symptoms of ataxia, personality change (emotional lability, irritability), and seizures may occur.

Four to six months may pass from the time of initial symptoms until symptoms become localized enough to arouse suspicion of a brain tumor. When this suspicion arises, the child needs a thorough neurologic examination; skull films, a bone scan, sonogram or magnetic resonance imaging, cerebral angiography, or a CT scan will be done as needed. Myelography may be done to identify tumors that have seeded into the spinal column. Nuclear magnetic resonance scanning may detect small tumors even earlier than a CT scan reveals them. Lumbar puncture must be done cautiously or the release of CSF may cause the brain stem (under pressure from the tumor) to herniate into the spinal cord and interfere with respiratory and cardiac function.

Therapeutic Management

Therapy for brain tumors includes a combination of surgery, radiotherapy, and chemotherapy, depending on the location and extent of the tumor. Most tumors cannot be completely removed in children, so radiotherapy and chemotherapy measures become increasingly important. Radiation therapy may be intense because if tumor tissue is not rapidly proliferating, cells are not easily destroyed. Chemotherapy is limited in that many chemotherapeutic agents do not cross the blood–brain barrier (Armstrong & Gilbert, 1996). Lomustine (CCNU) and vincristine are two drugs used. Administration of the drug directly into the ventricular system by a reservoir (Ommaya) may increase drug effectiveness.

The diagnosis of brain tumor is always a serious one in children (O'Hanlon-Nichols, 1996). It is important to observe closely the child admitted for a possible diagnosis of brain tumor so that signs of increased intracranial pressure or new localizing signs are detected as they occur. Record pulse rate, blood pressure, and respiration rate with extreme accuracy so that subtle changes become apparent. Note and document episodes of irritability, drowsiness, speech difficulty, and eye involvement. Statements such as, "Child says he sees two forks when I show him one" or "Child is unable to see objects held in her left field of vision" are much more meaningful to a neurosurgeon than "Child has difficulty seeing." Describe completely any seizure activity observed, particularly the beginning movements of the seizure, because these may help to localize the point of maximum brain pressure. Side rails should be in place for protection if a seizure occurs when a child is in bed.

Preoperative Care

Before surgery, the child may receive a stool softener to prevent straining when moving bowels. Such straining can cause increased intracranial pressure. Usually no preoperative enema is given, because expelling an enema will increase intracranial pressure.

Also before surgery, a portion of the child's head is shaved. Prepare the child for this in a positive way. Emphasize that hair grows back very rapidly (Figure 32-5).

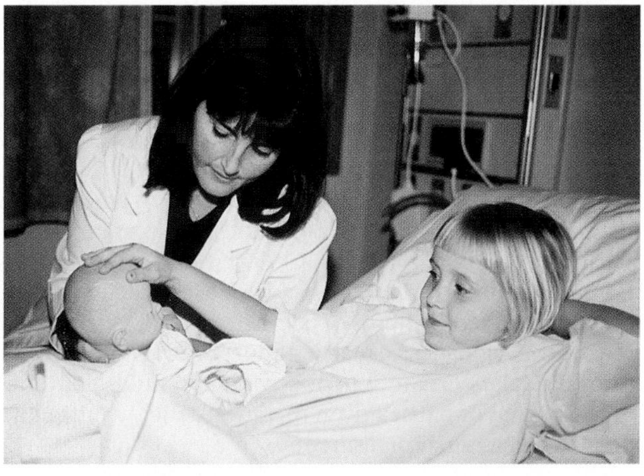

FIGURE 32.5 A nurse uses a doll to help prepare a child for shaving her head for brain surgery.

If the child will go to an intensive care unit for the first few days after surgery, a preoperative visit to meet the ICU staff should be made. Laser surgery techniques simplify a postoperative course.

Postoperative Care

After surgery, position the child as the surgeon prescribes. The position depends on the location of the tumor and the extent of surgery, but generally the child is positioned on the side opposite the incision. The bed remains flat or only slightly elevated. Do not lower the head of the bed because this tends to increase intracranial pressure from accumulation of increased blood in the area. Note carefully how much movement of the child's neck is allowed. If surgery was in the low occipital area, the surgeon may want the child to be moved as though the head and neck were a single body part. A neck brace or cast can be applied to stabilize the head and neck.

The child can be expected to be comatose or extremely lethargic for a number of days after surgery due to brain irritation and edema. In addition, the child may be on a ventilator. Unless ventilated, comatose children need to be positioned on their side so that oral secretions drain from the mouth to prevent aspiration. Many children have such extreme facial edema that their eyelids do not close completely or nasal breathing is impaired. Saline irrigation, eye drops, or eye dressings (with the eyes carefully closed under the dressings) may be ordered to keep the cornea from drying and ulcerating. Cool compresses over the eyes may help to reduce edema. Assess carefully the rate of pulse and respiration, pupillary size and ability to react to light, muscle strength (by asking the child to squeeze your hands), and level of consciousness (by asking the child his or her name or giving a simple instruction to follow).

Vital signs are taken frequently, about every 15 minutes, until they are stable and there is no apparent increase in intracranial pressure. The child's temperature may be either elevated or decreased because of the effect of the edema on the hypothalamus. Measures to reduce hyperthermia (sponging, antipyretics given by gavage or rectal administration because of lethargy or coma, or a hypothermia blanket) may be necessary to reduce the elevated temperature to below 38.4°C (101°F).

As the cerebral edema subsides and children begin to regain consciousness, they may need to be restrained to stop them from touching their head dressing or intravenous line. They should have as few restraints in place as possible, however, because if they fight restraints, intracranial pressure will increase.

The rate at which intravenous fluid is given must be regulated carefully; an increase in the infusion rate will increase intracranial pressure. Children may receive solutions of mannitol or hypertonic dextrose to aid in freeing the cerebral hemispheres of edematous fluid. As children regain consciousness, small amounts of oral fluid may be started. Make certain, when introducing fluid, that children are free of nausea from the anesthetic; vomiting increases intracranial pressure.

Observe head dressings carefully for drainage. A wet dressing is no longer a sterile dressing, because pathologic organisms may filter through its folds to reach the meninges and cause meningitis. Place a sterile towel under a wet dressing or reinforce the dressing with sterile compresses. Report signs of drainage, and estimate the extent of the seepage so that you can tell later whether seepage has increased.

Children regaining consciousness after brain surgery generally are confused as to time and place; they may have difficulty performing simple tasks they could do easily before. Help the child gradually regain independence in self-care.

Following discharge from the hospital, the child should be allowed as near-normal activity as possible. A football helmet may be necessary to protect his or her head if a section of skull was removed or is not yet firmly knit. When the bulky head dressing is removed, the child may become aware of baldness for the first time. Children need support to return to school because some children will treat them differently now, having heard from their parents that they are dying or "had to have their head fixed." Parents should make the school administration aware of what has happened to the child; the school nurse should be encouraged to take an active role in helping the child readjust to school after a considerably long absence.

Late effects may occur in children who survive a malignant brain tumor. Long-term neurologic and pituitary dysfunction and intellectual retardation are not unusual in survivors of pediatric brain tumor, especially if they were treated with high doses of cranial radiation at a very young age.

NURSING DIAGNOSES AND RELATED INTERVENTIONS

Nursing Diagnosis: Fear related to diagnosis of brain tumor

Outcome Identification: Parents and child will demonstrate ability to cope with the level of fear present by 1 week.

Outcome Evaluation: Parents and child continue to maintain function as a family, visit in hospital, and plan appropriately for discharge.

Parents of children with brain tumors generally are not prepared for their child's diagnosis. They bring the child to a health care facility because of insidious symptoms—vomiting, headache, strabismus. They may think that the child has a mild gastrointestinal upset or needs eyeglasses. They are shocked to learn that such benign symptoms are signs of a condition that may well kill their child. They are so upset at the time of the initial diagnosis that they cannot think of questions to ask. In the hours or days following the diagnosis, they have a great need to talk to people familiar with the care of children with brain tumors and to ask questions of the neurosurgeon.

Most parents want to hear a definite statement about prognosis—for example, "All the tumor can be removed; your child will be as good as new" or "Your child's chances are one in four of surviving surgery (or of having permanent effects)." Because the type of tumor, its exact location, and its extent are not fully known until the surgery, these predictions cannot be made with more than an informed guess. Parents can be assured that it is normal in these instances for a surgeon not to make much of a guess. Otherwise, they may interpret a surgeon's unwillingness to give them definite figures as incompetence or lack of interest. Parents need to be assured that earlier diagnosis would not have made a difference in the outcome. This makes it possible for them to live with themselves afterward and not be overwhelmed by the guilt that would come if they thought they could have prevented a bad outcome. Symptoms of brain tumor *are* insidious, and the average parent cannot be expected to recognize them as important.

Help parents understand that because of the importance of brain tissue, brain surgery is never minor surgery. Inform them how their child will appear following surgery: They will have a large, bulky head dressing; be drowsy or unresponsive; and have possible facial edema. Still, parents who are well prepared this way are likely to be shocked at the actual sight of their child. Following surgery, review with them once more that the child has a bulky dressing and is unconscious before you take them to the child's room.

Some parents may not "hear" the full extent of their child's diagnosis before surgery. They cannot believe that the surgeon will not be able to remove the entire tumor and cure their child. After surgery, when they are told that the entire tumor could not be removed, a very genuine grief reaction occurs. They are unable to sit and hold the child's hand, read to the child, and talk to him or her, because their minds have jumped ahead to the time when the child will die. The child may have difficulty relating to them because they are no longer acting like the parents he or she knew before but more like two strangers. When this happens, parents need a great deal of support from the time a child is first seen until the surgery, through discharge and readmissions, to the last hospital admission, when the child finally dies.

Children as young as 5 years old are aware that the head and the brain are important parts of the body. They are very aware of the feeling tone they detect in the words of parents and health care personnel. Because they undergo a number of diagnostic studies, followed by surgery and prolonged radiation therapy, they need opportunities to express their feelings about intrusive procedures through play with puppets or hospital equipment. Remember that when a patient becomes unconscious, hearing is often the last sense lost. Although children do not appear to respond to you following surgery, they may be able to hear what is said.

Types of Brain Tumors

Common sites for brain tumors in children are shown in Figure 32-6. Among the most common brain tumors are cerebellar astrocytomas, medulloblastomas, ependymomas, brain stem tumors, cerebral tumors, optic nerve tumors, and craniopharyngiomas (Table 32-5).

> **CHECKPOINT QUESTIONS**
>
> 9. Why may parents dismiss the vomiting that occurs with increased cranial pressure from tumors as unimportant?
> 10. Why may children be prescribed a stool softener prior to surgery for a brain tumor?

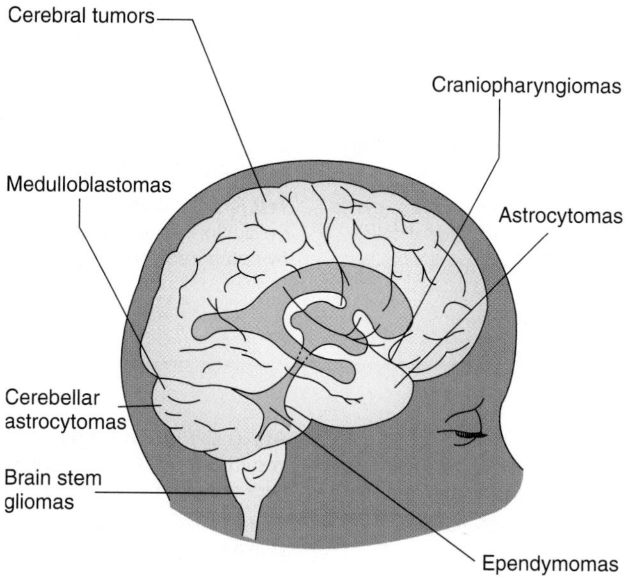

FIGURE 32.6 Common sites for brain tumors in children.

SARCOMAS

Tumors derived from connective tissue, such as bone and cartilage, muscle, blood vessels, or lymphoid tissue, are called **sarcomas.** They are the second most frequently occurring neoplasms in adolescents (only lymphomas occur more frequently). Bone tumor may arise during adolescence because rapid bone growth is occurring at this time. Because girls have a puberty growth spurt earlier than boys, bone tumors tend to occur slightly earlier in girls than boys (13 compared with 14 or 15 years of age). The two most frequently occurring types are osteogenic sarcoma and Ewing's sarcoma (Figure 32-7).

Osteogenic Sarcoma

An **osteogenic sarcoma** is a malignant tumor of long bone involving rapidly growing bone tissue (mesenchymal-matrix forming cells). It tends to occur more commonly in boys than girls. The most common sites of occurrence are the distal femur (40%–50%), proximal tibia (20%), and proximal humerus (10%–15%). Osteogenic sarcoma can occur in children who have had radiation for other malignancies as a later life effect. Children with retinoblastoma have a higher incidence than normal of osteosarcoma, as if a hereditary influence may be present. Osteosarcomas can be induced by viruses in animals.

Metastasis occurs early because of the high vascularity present in bones (Fletcher, 1997). Metastasis to the lungs is the most common site; as many as 25% of adolescents have lung metastasis already at the time of initial diagnosis. If this is present, the adolescent usually has a chronic cough, dyspnea, chest pain, and leg pain (if the tumor originates in the leg). Other common sites of metastasis are brain and other bone tissue.

TABLE 32.5 Types of Brain Tumors

TYPE	SIGNS AND SYMPTOMS	TREATMENT AND RELATED NURSING CONSIDERATIONS
Cerebellar Astrocytomas Account for about ¼ of all brain tumors in children Benign, slow growing, cystic (overgrowth of glial cells) Four grades from I (most benign) to IV (most malignant) Peak age: 5–8 y	Ataxia, head tilt, and nystagmus from increased intracranial pressure (ICP); papilledema *Test findings:* cranial suture lines separated on skull x-ray; tumor location confirmed by computed tomography (CT) scan	*Surgical removal and radiation to dissolve remaining tumor capsule* Recognize that outlook for recovery is better if tumor affects only one hemisphere and does not invade brain stem; the survival rate is about 90%. Explain to patient and family that aftereffects of surgery may be ataxia and tremor resulting from edema. Measure head circumference daily because hydrocephalus may result from postsurgical meningeal inflammation and swelling.
Medulloblastomas Fast growing, malignant, sensitive to radiation therapy Mostly in cerebellum More common in boys Peak age: 3–5 y	Ataxia and fourth-ventricle compression resulting from ICP and leading to hydrocephalus *Test findings:* The fourth-ventricle compression and tumor site and size revealed by CT scan	*Surgery, then radiation of head and spinal cord to discourage disease spread to CSF; also, intrathecal chemotherapy with lomustine (CCNU), vincristine, or methotrexate* Understand that because tumor is usually large by time of diagnosis, it may be difficult to remove fully; the survival rate is about 40%. Advise family that object of radiation and medication is to prevent spread of disease to cerebrospinal fluid (CSF). As prescribed, administer intrathecal medications through Ommaya reservoir access device in scalp instead of by lumbar puncture.
Ependymomas Arise from the floor of the fourth ventricle Grow with intermediate speed Highly sensitive to radiation therapy Occur equally in boys and girls Peak age 2–6 y	Obstructive hydrocephalus with ICP reflected by head tilt, ataxia, nystagmus, and vomiting (vomiting center is just under the fourth ventricle) *Test findings:* Ventricular obstruction on CT scan	*Surgery, then radiation of entire central nervous system to discourage metastasis to CSF. Also, chemotherapy with nitrosureas to treat recurrent symptoms* Inform caregivers that postsurgical radiation may be needed to manage disease process. Ependymomas are difficult to separate completely from the ventricle (chances that tumor will not recur are about 50%).
Brain Stem Tumors Glioma (tumor of the brain's support tissue) Almost exclusive to children Tumor located low in brain	Insidious onset: first signs, paralysis of the 5th, 6th, 7th, 9th, and 10th cranial nerves Ataxia, horizontal nystagmus, hemiparesis, and a positive Babinski reflex (toes flare upward when sole is stimulated) *Definitive sign:* paralysis of conjugate gaze (eyes unable to work together) *Test findings:* Upward displacement of the fourth ventricle (from tumor growth) on CT scan	*Radiation to reduce tumor, then chemotherapy (e.g., intrathecal methotrexate)* Discuss what to expect during radiation therapy. Excision of brain stem tumors is generally not attempted because the brain stem contains the respiratory and cardiac centers. Support patient and family because relapses are common and usually occur in about 6 months; survival is limited.
Cerebral Tumors Most tumors of the cerebral hemisphere are astrocytomas Peak incidence: school-age children	Headache and vomiting, motor weakness, or spasticity *Test findings:* Space-occupying lesion in the cerebral hemisphere on x-ray; EEG, brain scans with radioisotopes, cerebral angiography, or CT scan to identify tumor location	*Surgery and radiation* Teach and answer questions about therapeutic plan. Complete tumor removal by surgery is difficult because many essential brain parts, such as the motor and sensory areas, may be involved. The chance for full recovery after surgery and radiation is encouraging.
Optic Nerve Tumors Almost exclusive to children, particularly those around 2 y Tend to be astrocytomas	Commonly, exophthalmos, nystagmus, and strabismus (caused by diminished visual acuity) *Test findings:* Optic atrophy on funduscopy; reveals mass encroaching on third ventricle on skull x-ray or CT scan	*Surgical removal of the tumor and, possibly, radiation therapy* Prepare child and family for vision loss because the optic nerve is removed with the tumor.

(continued)

TABLE 32.5 Types of Brain Tumors *(Continued)*

TYPE	SIGNS AND SYMPTOMS	TREATMENT AND RELATED NURSING CONSIDERATIONS
Craniopharyngiomas Benign tumor located near the upper surface of the pituitary gland in the sella turcica Occur mostly in school-age children	Signs of intracranial pressure from tumor compressing the foramen of Monro and blocking CSF flow Visual field defects Growth retardation and sexual immaturity from diminished pituitary activity Excessive urine output (diabetes insipidus) from decreased secretion of antidiuretic hormone Hypothermia or hyperthermia from diminished hypothalamic function *Test findings:* Tumor detected on skull x-ray, CT scan, or magnetic resonance imaging	*Surgery with corticosteroid and hormonal therapy* Administer corticosteroids before and after surgery as prescribed to correct deficits in cortisone production that occur because of decreased pituitary stimulation to the adrenal glands. As brain edema subsides, these symptoms diminish. Anticipate symptoms of diabetes insipidus during the immediate postoperative period. In some children, corticosteroid and thyroid therapy and therapy for diabetes insipidus may have to be continued permanently. Inform the patient and family that hormonal therapy may be necessary at puberty to induce secondary sex changes and that human growth hormone may be necessary to achieve normal growth.

Assessment

Children with osteogenic sarcoma are often taller than average, indicating rapid bone growth. They notice pain and swelling at the tumor site. Often they report a history of recent trauma to the site (they fell playing basketball and bumped their knee) and attribute pain in the knee to this injury for some time. All adolescents with extremity pain and swelling, particularly near the knee, should be referred for evaluation because of the possibility that a malignant process may be at work. It is important that both adolescents and their parents understand that trauma did not cause the process; it merely called attention to the leg or arm where a malignant process was at work. This prevents adolescents from thinking they caused the tumor.

The area may be inflamed and feel warm, because tumors are highly vascular and therefore call increased blood into the area. As the tumor invades and weakens bone tissue, a pathologic fracture of the bone can occur.

For diagnosis, a biopsy is done of the area under suspicion. Because osteo cells produce alkaline phosphatase, rapidly growing bone cells will raise the serum level of this markedly, so serum analysis for alkaline phosphatase will be obtained. To see if metastasis is present, a complete blood count, urinalysis, chest x-ray, chest CT scan, and bone scans will be done. Caution children not to bear weight on an affected appendage while waiting for tests or surgery. The bone may be so weakened by the growing tumor that weight bearing may cause a fracture at the tumor site.

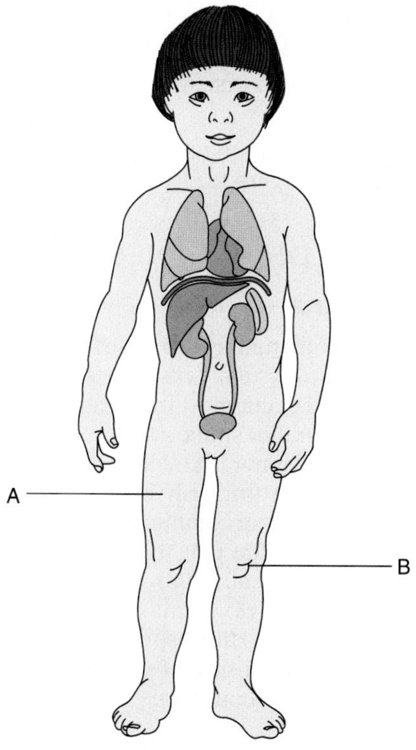

FIGURE 32.7 (**A**) The diaphysis (midshaft) is one of the most frequent sites of Ewing's sarcoma. (**B**) The epiphysis of a bone is a common site of osteogenic sarcoma.

Therapeutic Management

If the tumor is in the leg and the tumor is small at the time of diagnosis and if the child has reached adult height, the single bone involved may be surgically removed and replaced with an internally placed bone or metal prosthesis. This will preserve the child's leg. If the tumor is extensive at the time of diagnosis, the leg may be amputated at the joint above the tumor (this usually involves a total hip amputation). If the cancer has spread to the lung, metastases can usually be removed by thoracotomy.

An adolescent may have chemotherapy to shrink the tumor before surgery. Parents may be very concerned with the surgery delay and need an explanation that with bone tumor, this is an accepted and helpful intervention before surgery. Common treatment drugs include methotrexate and doxorubicin (Bruland & Pihl, 1997).

Only a few years ago, a diagnosis of osteogenic sarcoma was ominous; only a few children survived into adulthood.

Today, 60% to 65% of adolescents in whom the diagnosis is made early and who are treated rigorously can be cured.

NURSING DIAGNOSES AND RELATED INTERVENTIONS

Diagnosis of malignant bone tumor is a shock to both parents and children. The symptoms begin so insidiously that the diagnosis seems unreal. Parents can be assured that any delay in seeking treatment would not have had a marked effect on the chances for a cure. Neither the adolescent nor the parents could have been expected to seek medical attention any earlier. This is important preparation because guilt-ridden parents cannot function effectively to help a child through this extensive an illness.

Be certain that goals established are realistic. It is not realistic, for example, for adolescents to accept amputation with understanding. The highest goal you might be able to achieve is that they realize amputation is necessary to save their life.

Nursing Diagnosis: Risk for injury related to surgery and leg prosthesis

Outcome Identification: Adolescent will maintain good neurologic and circulatory function following surgery.

Outcome Evaluation: Extremity distal to surgical incision remains warm; capillary filling is under 5 seconds; adolescent reports no tingling or numbness in distal extremity.

The major danger of surgery for excising osteosarcoma and placing a prosthesis (limb salvage surgery) is that the swelling that occurs during surgery or immediately afterward can disrupt neurologic or circulatory function. Therefore, position and handle the leg carefully to present further disruption. Assess frequently for signs that the neurologic and circulatory systems are intact distal to the surgery (toes are warm and pink; capillary filling is under 5 seconds; the client reports no numbness or tingling).

Adolescents who had pain in the leg before surgery may continue to feel this pain even though the involved bone has been removed. This is known as phantom pain, and it occurs because nerve tracts continue to report pain for a period after the pain has been relieved. Although you might think that phantom limb pain could be simply explained away, this is not true. The pain is very real. The adolescent may need an analgesic to control it.

Ewing's Sarcoma

Ewing's sarcoma is a malignant tumor occurring most often in the bone marrow of the diaphyseal area (midshaft) of long bones. It spreads longitudinally through the bone (see Figure 32-7). Ewing's sarcoma occurs primarily in young adolescents and older school-age children; it is slightly more common in boys than girls. It almost never occurs in African Americans. Metastasis is usually present at the time of diagnosis; the lungs and bones are the most common sites for this. Eventually, central nervous system and lymph node sites become involved.

Assessment

Most children have had pain at the site of the tumor for some time before seeing a physician. At first, the pain is intermittent, and the child attributes it to an injury (a friend punched her leg; she bumped it against a footstool). Finally, the pain becomes constant and so severe that the child cannot sleep at night. Because of this delay, at the time of the diagnosis, multiple areas of involvement are often found.

X-ray will reveal an unusual "onion skin" reaction (fine lines disclosed on the x-ray film) surrounding the invading tumor cells. A bone scan, bone marrow aspiration and biopsy, CT scan of the lungs, and intravenous pyelogram will probably be done to determine if metastasis to the lung, bone, kidney, or lymph nodes is present. A biopsy of the tumor site will be done for a definite diagnosis. During tests, the child should not bear weight on the affected extremity because this may cause a pathologic fracture at the site.

Therapeutic Management

With Ewing's sarcoma, therapy will be a combination of surgery to remove the primary tumor, radiation, and chemotherapy. Drugs often used are vincristine, actinomycin D, cyclophosphamide, and doxorubicin. High-dose radiation to the entire involved bone may be scheduled.

About 50% of children achieve a 5-year survival rate; older children have a better survival rate than younger children. Caution adolescents to continue to be careful about stress on a leg that has received extensive radiation (no football, no weight lifting with pressure on that leg) because it may not be as strong as normal.

CHECKPOINT QUESTIONS

11. What is the usual first symptom of osteosarcoma?
12. What is a precaution to review with children waiting for surgery for Ewing's sarcoma?

OTHER CHILDHOOD NEOPLASMS

Neuroblastoma

Neuroblastomas are tumors that arise from the cells of the sympathetic nervous system; cells are very undifferentiated, highly invasive, and occur most frequently in the abdomen near the adrenal gland or spinal ganglia. They are the most common abdominal tumor in childhood (Abramson, 1997). Neuroblastoma occurs primarily in infants and preschool children; it is slightly more common in boys than girls. They may occur so early in life that they are detected by fetal sonogram (Yamagiwa et al, 1998). There may be an association between the development of neuroblastomas and fetal alcohol syndrome, Hirschsprung's disease, and neurofibromatosis. Common sites of metastasis are bone marrow, liver, and subcutaneous tissue.

Assessment

The growing tumor is most often discovered on abdominal palpation as an abdominal mass. The general symptoms of weight loss and anorexia may be present. Pressure on the adrenal gland from the tumor may cause excessive sweating, flushed face, and hypertension. Abdominal pain and constipation may be present. Compression on the spinal nerves or invasion into the intervertebral foramina may cause loss of motor function in lower extremities.

If the primary lesion is in the upper chest, children will have dyspnea; swallowing may be difficult, and neck and facial edema may occur from compression on the vena cava. If liver metastasis is present, children may have jaundice. If metastasis to the skin has occurred, blue or purplish nodules (prominent raised areas) on arms or legs may be seen.

The extent of the tumor and any metastases present are identified by an intravenous pyelogram (a mass growing on the adrenal gland just above the kidney will demonstrate kidney compression); an arteriogram (neuroblastomas are vascular tumors and incorporate veins and arteries into their structure as they grow); a sonogram or CT scan of the chest, abdomen, and pelvis; gallium bone scan; and bone marrow aspiration and biopsy. If an adrenal tumor is present, it will stimulate production of adrenal gland hormones or catecholamines. A urine sample will be tested for the presence of catecholamines or vanillyl-mandelic acid and homovanillic acid (the breakdown products of catecholamines). If children with stage IV disease have a high level of serum ferritin and the enzyme neuron-specific enolase, they have a poorer prognosis than those with low levels.

A biopsy of the tumor site will be planned so the tumor can be definitely identified and staged (Table 32-6).

Therapeutic Management

If the tumor is localized, therapy will consist of surgical removal of the primary tumor, followed by radiation therapy. Chemotherapy has not shown any added benefit for children with stage I and stage II disease. With stage III involvement, both radiation and chemotherapy are begun. A "second look" surgical procedure may be scheduled within several months to determine the effectiveness of treatment and to attempt the possible removal of further tumor. The use of aggressive chemotherapy followed by bone marrow transplantation to restore functioning bone marrow has promise in children with neuroblastoma (Dreyer & Fernbach, 1997). Immunotherapy is also a possibility.

Therapy for stage IV disease is combination chemotherapy: cyclophosphamide, vincristine, cisplatin, doxorubicin, and etoposide are frequently used. Stage IV-s disease is a unique form because it has a very high rate of spontaneous regression (about 80%). This occurs because the tumor either spontaneously degenerates or undergoes differentiation to normal tissue.

Children with stage I and stage II disease have a 5-year survival rate as high as 90%. Most children, unfortunately, are usually at a stage IV level at the time of diagnosis, so prognosis is guarded (less than 10%). Although most children have a positive initial response to therapy, recurrence is common within the first year. The prognosis in children younger than 2 years is better than that in children older than 2 years.

TABLE 32.6 Staging Neuroblastoma

STAGE	EXTENT OF DISEASE
I	Tumor is well encapsulated and completely removed by surgery.
II	Tumor cannot be completely removed by surgery or disease extends to lymph nodes.
III	Tumor extends beyond the midline; regional lymph nodes may be involved bilaterally.
IV	Distant metastases; bone, eyes, or liver is involved.

Rhabdomyosarcoma

A **rhabdomyosarcoma** is a tumor of striated muscle. It arises from the embryonic mesenchyme tissue that forms muscle, connective, and vascular tissue. The peak age of incidence of these tumors is 2 to 6 years; a second peak occurrence is during puberty. Common sites of occurrence are the eye orbit, paranasal sinuses, uterus, prostate, bladder, retroperitoneum, arms, or legs. Central nervous system invasion occurs from direct tumor extension. This results in cranial nerve palsy, nuchal rigidity, bradycardia, or bradypnea (due to brain stem compromise). Distant metastasis most commonly occurs in lungs, bone, or the bone marrow. Rhabdomyosarcomas are associated with low socioeconomic level, implying an environmental role may play a part in causing it (Hurwitz, 1997).

Assessment

The symptoms relate to the site of the tumor (Table 32-7). A biopsy specimen of the tumor is taken and examined

TABLE 32.7 Common Sites and Symptoms of Rhabdomyosarcoma

SITE OF TUMOR	SYMPTOMS
Orbit	Proptosis (extruding eye); visible and palpable conjunctival or eyelid mass
Neck	Hoarseness, dysphagia; visible and palpable mass in neck
Nasopharynx	Airway obstruction, epistaxis, dysphagia, visible mass in nasal or nasopharyngeal passages
Paranasal sinuses	Swelling, pain, nasal discharge, epistaxis
Middle ear	Pain, chronic otitis media, hearing loss, facial nerve palsy, mass protruding into external ear canal
Bladder and prostate	Dysuria, urinary retention, hematuria, constipation, palpable lower abdominal mass
Vagina	Mass protruding from uterus or cervix into vagina, abnormal vaginal bleeding
Trunk, extremities	Visible and palpable soft-tissue mass
Testicles	Visible and palpable soft-tissue mass

for tissue identification. Metastasis is ruled out by bone scan, chest x-ray, CT scan, and bone marrow aspiration.

Therapeutic Management

The primary treatment is surgical removal of the tumor, followed by radiation and chemotherapy. Because a large area of the body may be irradiated, the white blood cell count must be monitored closely. A number of chemotherapeutic drugs are effective, including vincristine, dactinomycin, cyclophosphamide, doxorubicin, and cisplatin. The child receives chemotherapy every 3 or 4 weeks for 18 to 24 months. If central nervous system extension has occurred, intrathecal chemotherapy may be included in the regimen.

A child's prognosis depends on the size of the tumor and whether metastasis was present at the time of initial diagnosis. If all the tumor can be removed and no lymph node metastasis has occurred, the chances are as high as 80% that the tumor will not recur. If some of the tumor has to be left because of its size or location, the chance of recurrence rises to about 50%. If metastasis to the lungs or bone was present at the time of the initial diagnosis, the prognosis is poor (about 20% of children with this have long-term survival). In children who do survive, long-term complications, such as cataract formation, bone neoplasm, gastrointestinal stricture, and hemorrhagic cystitis, may occur from the extensive radiation used in the primary therapy.

Wilms' Tumor

Wilms' tumor (nephroblastoma) is a malignant tumor that rises from the metanephric mesoderm cells of the upper pole of the kidney (Friar, 1995). It accounts for 20% of solid tumors in childhood; there is no increased incidence for sex or race. It occurs in association with congenital anomalies, such as aniridia (lack of color in the iris), cryptorchidism, hypospadias, pseudohermaphroditism, cystic kidneys, hemangioma, and talipes disorders. There is a tendency for bilateral involvement to occur in siblings as if an autosomal dominant inheritance pattern may be present. Metastatic spread is most often to the lungs, regional lymph nodes, liver, bone, and eventually, brain by the bloodstream. The maturity of cells (the more differentiated cells are) makes a difference in prognosis. If cells are mostly differentiated epithelial cells, the prognosis is best; if most are undifferentiated stromal cells, it is worst.

Assessment

A Wilms' tumor is usually discovered early in life (6 months to 5 years; peak at 3 to 4 years), although it apparently arises from an embryonic structure present in the child before birth. Wilms' tumors distort the kidney anteriorly so that the tumor is felt as a firm, nontender, abdominal mass. Parents sometimes are aware that their infant has a mass in the abdomen but bring him or her to a physician thinking that it is hard stool from chronic constipation. Fathers often discover the tumor when they toss a baby in the air, catch him or her by the abdomen, and feel the abdominal mass. Parents often report that the mass seemed to appear overnight. This actually can happen because tumors can hemorrhage into themselves, doubling their size in a matter of hours. Wilms' tumor may present with hematuria, and a low-grade fever may be noted. Although hypertension may also occur from excessive renin production, blood pressure is not taken routinely in children of this age, so the tumor is rarely discovered by this method. The child may be anemic from lack of erythropoietin formation.

An intravenous pyelogram will reveal a mass displacing normal kidney structure. A CT scan or sonogram will reveal any points of metastasis. Kidney function studies, such as glomerular filtration rate or blood urea nitrogen, will be done to assess function of the kidneys prior to surgery. Little time, however, can be allotted for preoperative testing, because these tumors metastasize rapidly as a result of the large blood supply of kidneys and adrenal glands.

It is important that the child's abdomen not be palpated any more than is necessary for diagnosis, because handling appears to aid metastasis. Place a sign reading "No abdominal palpation" over the child's crib to prevent this.

Therapeutic Management

Wilms' tumors are staged according to the criteria of the National Wilms' Tumor Study Group (Table 32-8) to predict therapy and prognosis. The tumor will be removed by nephrectomy (excision of the affected kidney). This is generally followed immediately by radiation therapy (omitted in stage I tumors) and chemotherapy with dactinomycin, doxorubicin, or vincristine. The chemotherapy may be given at varying intervals for as long as 15 months. A second surgical procedure may be scheduled after 2 or 3 months to remove any remaining tumor.

If tumor involvement is bilateral, the operative decisions obviously become more complex. If tumors are small, they can both be removed, leaving functioning kidney cells intact. Only the kidney with the larger tumor may be removed. Tumors may be treated initially with radiation to shrink their size and then with surgery in about 3 months to remove any remaining tumor from kidneys.

Complications can occur from Wilms' tumor therapy. Both small bowel obstruction from fibrotic scarring and hepatic damage can occur from radiation to the lesion. Nephritis in the kidney can occur. In girls, radiation to ovaries may result in sterility. Radiation to lungs may re-

TABLE 32.8 Staging Wilms' Tumor

STAGE	DESCRIPTION
I	Tumor confined to the kidney and completely removed surgically
II	Tumor extending beyond the kidney but completely removed surgically
III	Regional spread of disease beyond the kidney with residual abdominal disease postoperatively
IV	Metastases to lung, liver, bone, distant lymph nodes, or other distant sites
V	Bilateral disease

sult in interstitial pneumonia. Effects on bones can be scoliosis and hypoplasia of the ilium and lower rib cage, and epiphyseal radiation can lead to different growth rates in the two femurs. The extent of radiation may lead to the development of a second tumor. About 15% of children who survive Wilms' tumor develop a soft-tissue sarcoma, bone tumor, or leukemia in 5 to 25 years.

About 90% of children who had no metastatic spread survive for at least 5 years. In most protocols, if there is no recurrence in 2 years, the child is considered cured.

WHAT IF? What if a father tells you that he discovered a Wilms' tumor in his son when he tossed him in the air and caught him, but his mother tells you that she thinks the father caused the tumor by his rough-housing? What would you want to discuss with the parents?

Retinoblastoma

Retinoblastoma is a malignant tumor of the retina of the eye (Shields et al., 1996). A rare tumor, it accounts for only 1% to 3% of childhood malignancies. A small number (about 10%) develop because of an inherited autosomal dominant pattern. An alteration of chromosome 13 is present. Parents who have one child with retinoblastoma have about a 4% chance of having a second child with a similar tumor. If two or more children have the tumor, the parents are probably carriers, and it can be predicted that up to 50% of their children will be affected. Because of the dominant pattern of inheritance, a person who survives retinoblastoma has a 90% chance of having a child with a tumor. Parents who may be carriers, or the parent who has survived the disease, need genetic counseling so they are aware of the risk to their children. Because the 5-year survival rate for children with retinoblastoma is good (at least 90%), this will become a very important counseling role in the future (Servodidio & Abramson, 1996).

Retinoblastoma occurs most often, however, as spontaneous development, not the inherited type. Children with the inherited type tend to develop bilateral disease; those with the spontaneous type may or may not have the tumor in both eyes.

Assessment

Retinoblastoma occurs early in life, from about 6 weeks of age through the preschool period. It occurs equally in boys and girls, and there is no preference for either the right or left eye. One tumor or many individual tumors may be present. They are located on the retina or in the vitreous fluid or extend backward into the choroid, the optic nerve, and the subarachnoid space.

On examination, the child's pupil appears white (the red reflex is absent) or is described as a typical "cat's eye." The child will develop strabismus as the eye becomes nonfunctional. This tumor metastasizes readily along the course of the optic nerve to the subarachnoid space and brain; it quickly involves the second eye. Metastasis to distant body sites, such as the bone marrow and liver, occurs because of the rich blood supply to the brain.

Children with a family history should be examined at least three times yearly until they reach 5 years of age. When a tumor is suspected, an examination under general anesthesia or conscious sedation is scheduled because children this age do not comply well with eye examinations. CT scanning and sonography may be ordered to detect intraocular calcification or the presence of tumor. The possibility of distant metastasis is explored by lumbar puncture, liver and skeletal survey, and bone-marrow biopsy.

Therapeutic Management

Retinoblastomas are serious tumors affecting the retina of the eye. If the tumor is very small at the time of diagnosis, it may be treated with cryosurgery (freezing the tumor to destroy local cells). This will preserve partial vision in the eye. Photocoagulation to destroy the blood vessels supplying the tumor may be used. Localized radioactive applicators or plaques sutured to the sclera over the tumor may be used. Such plaques remain in place for 4 to 7 days. If the tumor is large, the eye will be enucleated (Boyd-Monk & Augsburger, 1997). The child may receive radiation treatment and chemotherapy (nitrogen mustard, vincristine, and cyclophosphamide are common drugs used) as well if the tumor has metastasized.

After enucleation surgery, the child has a large pressure dressing applied to the empty socket. Observe for bleeding on the dressing and assess vital signs conscientiously. Young children may need to be restrained if someone cannot be with them constantly to keep them from tugging at the dressing and removing it. After about 48 hours, the pressure dressing is removed (usually by the surgeon), and a small eye patch is applied. Irrigation of the empty socket with normal saline solution or application of an antibiotic ointment may be prescribed with future dressing changes.

An eye prosthesis is fitted about 3 weeks after surgery. Prostheses in children do not need to be removed and cleaned daily, and in children this young, leaving the prosthesis in place prevents the child from playing with it (an interesting, colorful, round ball).

As discussed earlier, the long-term survival rate for children with retinoblastoma is as high as 90%. Evaluation of the child following retinoblastoma must include not only whether metastasis can be detected, but whether the child is adjusting to the loss of sight in one or both eyes. Children who do not have binocular vision this early in life generally do not have difficulty adjusting to this. They notice it most as a school-ager when they are unable to compete in sports that require three-dimensional sight, such as baseball. They may be restricted from obtaining a driver's license. If radiation was used for therapy, cataracts may develop several years later. Any radiation therapy has the risk of leading to the development of leukemia later in life. The high incidence of osteogenic and soft-tissue sarcomas that occur may not be related to therapy as much as to a tendency for tumor growth.

NURSING DIAGNOSES AND RELATED INTERVENTIONS

Nursing Diagnosis: Decisional conflict related to approval of eye removal to save child's life

Outcome Identification: Parents and child will feel comfortable about decision regarding surgery postoperatively.

Outcome Evaluation: Parents and child state that they can accept removal of eye to save child's life.

With the diagnosis of retinoblastoma, parents are asked to make a most difficult decision. To save their child's life, they must agree to the removal of an eye. Even following this procedure, the second eye may become involved or distant metastasis may occur.

Parents need support in the decision they make. If there is metastasis at a later date, they may feel guilty that they agreed to enucleation, thinking they have put the child through the surgery for nothing. They may feel guilty that they did not notice that the child's eye was abnormal before metastasis occurred. They may have noticed that the eye was abnormal but thought nothing more than that the child needed glasses and delayed seeking health care. Be certain that parents understand fully what surgery will entail (i.e., loss of the eye). Provide time for discussion to help them work through this very emotional time in their life.

CHECKPOINT QUESTIONS

13. What is an important nursing responsibility for the child waiting for surgery for Wilms' tumor?
14. What is a common finding in the child with retinoblastoma?

KEY POINTS

Radiation is an important treatment modality in cancer therapy. Immediate side effects are anorexia, nausea, vomiting, and hair loss if radiation is to the head. Long-term effects may be growth retardation or learning disabilities.

A chemotherapeutic agent is one capable of destroying malignant cells. Common side effects are the same as for radiation therapy. Help children to use time during chemotherapy in constructive ways, such as imagining a game, to keep them mentally stimulated yet quiet.

Be aware of the need to use gloves and mix preparations under a hood when preparing chemotherapy drugs to protect yourself from adverse effects of the medication.

Leukemia is the distorted and uncontrolled proliferation of white blood cells and is the most frequently occurring type of cancer in children. About 90% of children with an initially good prognosis now have long-term survival.

Hodgkin's disease and non-Hodgkin's lymphomas are malignancies of the lymphatic system. Hodgkin's disease occurs most often in adolescents; the initial symptom is often one painless, enlarged lymph node. Therapy is radiation and chemotherapy.

Brain tumors are the most common solid tumors to occur in childhood. Beginning symptoms are usually those of increased intracranial pressure. Therapy may include a combination of surgery followed by radiation and chemotherapy.

Bone tumors occur in two main forms: osteogenic sarcoma and Ewing's sarcoma. These tumors tend to be fast growing because of the ready blood supply to bone. Therapy is surgery followed by radiation and chemotherapy.

Neuroblastomas are tumors that arise from the cells of the sympathetic nervous system. They are the most common abdominal tumor in childhood. Therapy is surgery, radiation, and chemotherapy.

Rhabdomyosarcomas are tumors of striated muscle. The peak age of incidence is 2 to 6 years. Therapy is surgery and chemotherapy.

Wilms' tumor (nephroblastoma) is a malignancy that arises from the metanephric mesoderm cells of the kidney. It is usually discovered early in life. Therapy is surgery followed by radiation and chemotherapy.

Retinoblastoma is a malignant tumor of the retina of the eye. It may be inherited as an autosomal dominant pattern. Therapy is radiation, chemotherapy, and possibly enucleation.

After a diagnosis of cancer, parents and children need help to change their thinking from an older concept of cancer as being an always painful, fatal disease to a newer concept of it as a condition for which there is therapy and hope.

Because the therapy for cancer involves so many return hospitalizations and so much parental concern, the siblings of children with cancer may begin to feel left out of family activities. Remind parents to incorporate the entire family in activities when possible to help them grow as a family during the course of therapy.

Skin cancer is a type of malignancy that begins in childhood. Cautioning children about sensible sun exposure can be an important health promotion role for nurses.

CRITICAL THINKING EXERCISES

1. Geri is the 6-year-old you met at the beginning of the chapter. His mother told you that he wakes up every morning with a headache and then vomits. She says this began just after school started, so she is certain it is related to school. The school nurse has suggested that Geri have an eye examination. What are some additional questions you would want to ask to see if you should pursue this problem further?

2. A 2-year-old is going to be receiving chemotherapy following surgery for a neuroblastoma. How would you prepare the child for this? What activities would you propose to keep the child occupied while an intravenous solution is infusing?
3. An adolescent has been diagnosed as having Hodgkin's disease. How would you explain this disease to him? He is active in a school sports program and works part-time in a supermarket. How will you answer if he asks if these activities should be stopped?

REFERENCES

Abramson, S. J. (1997). Adrenal neoplasmas in children. *Radiologic Clinics of North America, 35*(6), 1415.

Armstrong, T. S., & Gilbert, M. R. (1996). Glial neoplasms: Classification, treatment, and pathways for the future. *Oncology Nursing Forum, 23*(4), 615.

Boyd-Monk, H., & Augsburger, J. J. (1997). Treatment of primary intraocular cancers: retinoblastoma and uveal malignant melanoma. *Journal of Ophthalmic Nursing and Technology, 16*(4), 183.

Bruland, O. S., & Pihl, A. (1997). On the current management of osteosarcoma. *European Journal of Cancer, 33*(11), 1725.

Department of Health and Human Services. (1995). *Healthy people 2000: midcourse review*. Washington, DC: DHHS.

Dreyer, Z. E., & Fernbach, D. J. (1997). Neuroblastoma. In K. B. Johnson & F. A. Oski (Eds.). *Oski's essential pediatrics*. Philadelphia: Lippincott-Raven.

Fletcher, B. D. (1997). Imaging pediatric bone sarcomas: diagnosis and treatment-related issues. *Radiologic Clinics of North America, 35*(6), 1477.

Friar, M. B. (1995). Wilms' tumor and neuroblastoma. *Images, 14*(1), 5.

Hockenberry-Eaton, M., Manteuffel, B., & Botomley, S. (1997). Development of two instruments examining stress and adjustment in children with cancer. *Journal of Pediatric Oncology Nursing, 14*(3), 178.

Hurwitz, R. L. (1997). Soft tissue sarcomas. In K. B. Johnson & F. A. Oski (Eds.). *Oski's essential pediatrics*. Philadelphia: Lippincott-Raven.

Li, C. Y. et al. (1998). Risk of leukemia in children living near high-voltage transmission lines. *Journal of Occupational and Environmental Medicine, 40*(2),144.

Lombardi, F. et al. (1998). The evolving role of radiation therapy in the optimal multimodality treatment of childhood cancer. *Tumori, 84*(2), 270.

Mahoney, D. H. (1997a). Acute lymphoblastic leukemia in childhood. In K. B. Johnson & F. A. Oski (Eds.). *Oski's essential pediatrics*. Philadelphia: Lippincott-Raven.

Mahoney, D. H. (1997b). Malignant brain tumors. In K. B. Johnson & F. A. Oski (Eds.). *Oski's essential pediatrics*. Philadelphia: Lippincott-Raven.

McClain, K. L. (1997). Hodgkin's disease. In K. B. Johnson & F. A. Oski (Eds.). *Oski's essential pediatrics*. Philadelphia: Lippincott-Raven.

Mulnar, Z. et al. (1997). ABVD chemotherapy of Hodgkin's disease. *Neoplasma, 44*(4), 263.

Nemunaitis, J. (1997). A comparative review of colony-stimulating factors. *Drugs, 54*(5), 709.

O'Hanlon-Nichols, T. (1996). Clinical snapshot: Intracranial tumors. *American Journal of Nursing, 96*(4), 38.

Servodidio, C. A., & Abramson, D. H. (1996). Genetic teaching for the retinoblastoma patient. *Insight, 21*(4), 120.

Shields, C. L. et al. (1996). New treatment modalities for retinoblastoma. *Current Opinion in Ophthalmology, 7*(3), 20.

Steuber, C. P. (1997). Acute myeloid leukemia. In K. B. Johnson & F. A. Oski (Eds.). *Oski's essential pediatrics*. Philadelphia: Lippincott-Raven.

Yamagiwa, I. et al. (1998). Prenatally detected cystic neuroblastoma. *Pediatric Surgery International, 13*(2), 215.

SUGGESTED READINGS

Baer, M. R. (1998). Assessment of minimal residual disease in patients with acute leukemia. *Current Opinion in Oncology, 10*(1), 17.

Evans, A. E. et al. (1998). Hodgkin disease? *Medical and Pediatric Oncology, 30*(4), 252.

Kaneko, M. et al. (1997). Is extensive surgery required for treatment of advanced neuroblastoma? *Journal of Pediatric Surgery, 32*(11), 1616.

Kline, N. E. (1996). Neuro-oncology patients and nursing research issues. *Journal of Pediatric Oncology Nursing, 13*(1), 40.

Kopecky, E. A. et al. (1997). Review of a home-based palliative care program for children with malignant and non-malignant diseases. *Journal of Palliative Care, 13*(4), 28.

Kramarova, E., & Stiller, C. A. (1996). The international classification of childhood cancer. *International Journal of Cancer, 68*(6), 759.

Pui, C. H. (1995). Medical progress: childhood leukemia. *New England Journal of Medicine, 332*(24), 1618.

Snyder, C. L., & Stocker, J. (1997). Confronting a tempest: acute leukemia. *Nursing, 27*(2), 32.

Woodgate, R., & McClement, S. (1998). Symptom distress in children with cancer. *Journal of Pediatric Oncology Nursing, 15*(1), 3.

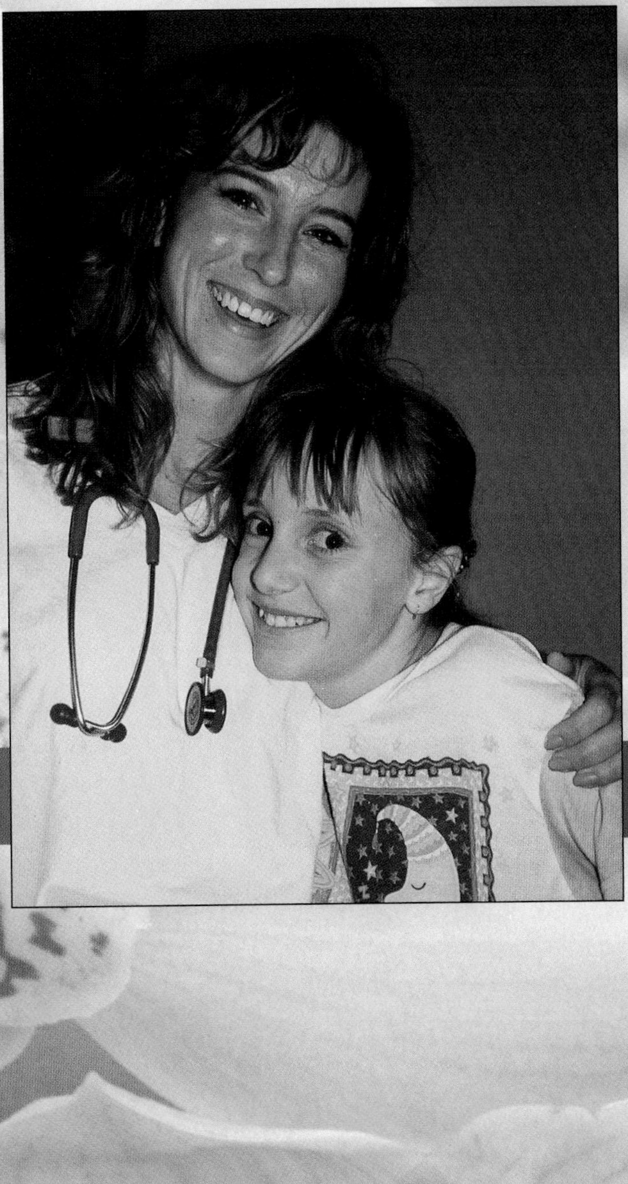

UNIT

5

The Nursing Role in Restoring and Maintaining the Health of Children and Families With Mental Health Disorders

Nursing Care of the Child With a Cognitive or Mental Health Disorder

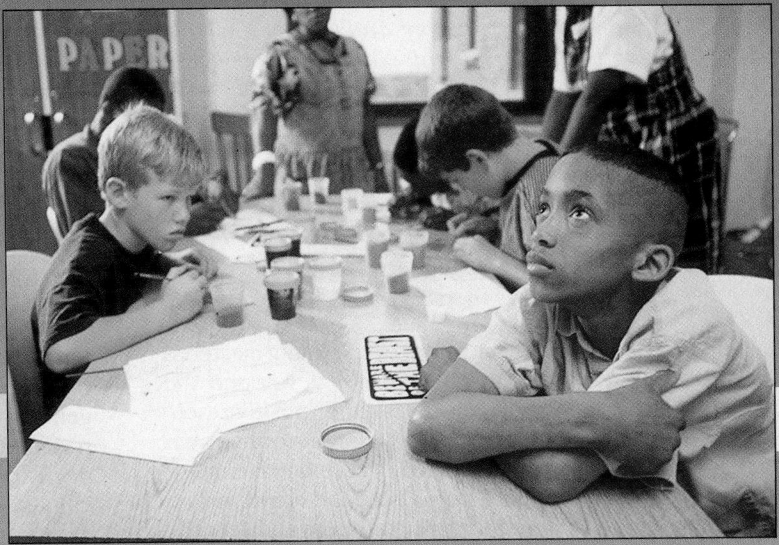

33

CHAPTER

Key Terms

- anhedonia
- binge eating
- catatonia
- choreiform movements
- complex vocal tics
- coprolalia
- dyslexia
- echolalia
- expressed emotion
- flat affect
- graphesthesia
- hyperactivity
- labile mood
- motor tics
- palilalia
- purging
- school phobia
- stereognosis
- vocal tics

Objectives

After mastering the contents of this chapter, you should be able to:

1. Describe common cognitive and mental health disorders in children.
2. Assess a child for a cognitive or mental health disorder.
3. Formulate nursing diagnoses related to the cognitive or mental health disorders of childhood.
4. Establish appropriate outcomes for the child with a cognitive or mental health disorder.
5. Plan nursing care for the child with a cognitive or mental health disorder.
6. Implement nursing care for the child with a cognitive or mental health disorder.
7. Evaluate outcomes for achievement and effectiveness of care.
8. Identify National Health Goals related to cognitive or mental health disorders that nurses can be instrumental in helping the nation to achieve.
9. Identify areas related to cognitive or mental health that could benefit from additional nursing research.
10. Analyze ways that care of the child with a cognitive or mental health disorder can be more family centered.
11. Integrate knowledge of childhood cognitive and mental health disorders and nursing process to achieve quality child health nursing care.

Todd, a second grader, is brought to the clinic by his parents. He was diagnosed with attention deficit hyperactivity disorder approximately 6 months ago. During the visit, Todd is observed to color; run to the window; run over to the door, open and close it; and then move pamphlets in the information rack. His parents feel that they are at their "wits' end" because his attention span is so short and his behavior so disruptive. How can you help?

In previous chapters you learned about the growth and development of well children and care of the child with physiologic disorders. In this chapter, you will add information about the dramatic changes that occur when children develop a cognitive or mental health disorder. This is important information because it builds a base for care and health teaching.

After you have studied the chapter, turn to the Critical Thinking Exercises at the end of the chapter to sharpen your skills and test your knowledge.

A child who is mentally healthy has successfully mastered the tasks of each developmental phase, developed the ability to trust adults, and possesses a positive self-concept and sense of contentment within his or her own limits. How is this state of health achieved and maintained? Perhaps the most important factor is a good emotional relationship with parents and a sense of safety and security in the home environment. Promoting healthy family functioning during healthcare visits, providing anticipatory guidance for parents about developmental milestones and needs, and listening carefully to clients–the children *and* the parents–are all important in fostering both the physical and mental health of children.

Mental health also implies that a child is able to use adaptive coping mechanisms appropriately to meet the normal stressors of life. Often, it is these stressors that provide the growth-producing challenges in life or help a child achieve the tasks of each developmental phase, for instance, establishing a sense of trust or independence. (This is one of the reasons why providing age-appropriate stimulation is an essential nursing responsibility.) Some stressors in life, however, go beyond what is considered "the norm." Acute illness and hospitalization are examples of increased stress. Chronic illness may provide an even greater stress, as the acute phase fades into recognition of long-term disability or an ultimately fatal prognosis. Nurses must be able to recognize the effects of illness and hospitalization on children and their families and also be able to provide interventions to prevent maladaptive coping mechanisms. Being aware of the potential emotional responses a child might have to a particular illness and implications for family functioning are essential to this ability.

Actual mental illness may develop during childhood. Children suffer from the same mental health disorders that affect the adult population, such as depression or schizophrenia. In addition, a number of disorders begin in childhood or adolescence and affect only children. Autism is an example of such a disorder. Some problems, such as separation anxiety, may consist of behavior that is considered normal at one stage of development (infancy) but pathologic at another (adolescence). Current research attributes some of these disorders to genetic vulnerability, others to disruption in family life, temperament, or inadequate parent–child bonding and attachment difficulties. Children with mental illness, whatever the cause, must be evaluated and treated by specialists in the mental health field as early in their disease process as possible. It is often the child health nurse who is first aware of such problems and thus may be instrumental, through appropriate referrals, in helping the child and family adjust to the disorder.

Cognitive and mental health disorders are addressed by the National Health Goals (see the Focus on National Health Goals box).

NURSING PROCESS OVERVIEW

for the Care of the Child With Cognitive or Mental Illness

Assessment

Both a child's personality and mental growth potential are influenced by a number of factors, including genetic makeup, cultural background, family environment, and community resources. All of these need to be taken into account when assessing a child's cognitive and mental health and well being. Assess children for emotional as well as physical

FOCUS ON NATIONAL HEALTH GOALS

Cognitive and mental health disorders in children produce major costs to a nation, as well as to individual families, because they have the potential to reduce the earning power and contribution of future citizens. Two National Health Goals directly address this:

- Reduce to less than 10% the prevalence of mental disorders among children and adolescents from a baseline of 12%.
- Reduce the prevalence of serious mental retardation in school-aged children to no more than 2/1000 children from a baseline of 2.7/1000 (DHHS, 1995).

Nurses can be instrumental in helping the nation achieve these goals by educating parents to seek prenatal care so low birth weight can be reduced, educating about ways to reduce stress in families, and identifying children in school and health care agency settings who demonstrate a high level of stress as well as other symptoms of mental illness. Additional nursing research is needed for the following questions: What are the questions that best reveal mental stress at children's health maintenance visits? Can nurses identify adolescents who are high risk for eating disorders? What support measures are most helpful to families of a child with mental illness or cognitive impairment?

problems at regular health maintenance visits. When an emotional problem has been identified or is suspected, a detailed history should be obtained of the presenting problem, presumed reason for appearance of the problem, relevant past history, child's school and social history, child's developmental history, and family history and current pattern of family functioning.

Table 33-1 lists some helpful observational data for assessing these areas.

Nursing Diagnosis

Nursing diagnoses established for ill children often address the response of children and their families to their condition or treatment. Examples of these include:

- Anxiety related to surgical experience
- Diversional activity deficit related to lack of appropriate play materials for hospitalized child
- Fear related to potential loss of independence secondary to traumatic injury
- Self-esteem disturbance related to disfiguring scars following accident
- Impaired social interactions related to hearing deficit
- Powerlessness related to loss of independence and control in hospital environment
- Decisional conflict related to lack of relevant information
- Hopelessness related to prolonged caretaking responsibilities for chronically ill child
- Ineffective family coping: compromised, related to overwhelming number of stressors placed on family at one time

Additional nursing diagnoses are appropriate when a problem of cognitive or mental health is present. Examples of these may include:

- Risk for violence, self-directed related to impulsivity
- Impaired social interaction related to short attention span and distractibility
- Altered family processes related to inability of child to follow instructions
- Altered thought processes related to the effects of schizophrenia
- Impaired verbal communication related to depression and withdrawn behavior
- Altered health maintenance related to inattention to food or hygiene needs
- Self-esteem disturbance related to lack of successful coping strategies
- Sleep pattern disturbance related to hallucinations
- Social isolation related to low self-esteem
- Ineffective family coping: compromised, related to chronic psychiatric illness in child

Outcome Identification and Planning

Although the diagnosis of a mental health disorder or a referral to a child guidance or psychiatric clinic does not carry the stigma it once did, many parents still believe that such a referral is a mark of inadequacy or a sign of failure for themselves as parents.

TABLE 33.1 Guidelines for the Mental Health Interview of the Child

Observational Data	
General appearance	Height, weight, grooming and hygiene, nutrition, physical health, distinguishing features (deformities, tics), maturity level
Motor behaviors	Fine and gross, balance, bizarre motor activity
Speech and language	Receptive, expressive, content, tone, and articulation
Affect	Range of emotion, predominant emotion (depressed, angry, anxious, happy, irritable, labile), emotional reactions to process and/or content of interview (appropriate, inappropriate)
Thought process	Estimated intellectual level via language and knowledge base (organization and thought content), orientation (to person, place, time), perceptual distortions (hallucinations, illusions, tangentiality, obsessions, delusions), attention span, learning disabilities
Ability to relate to evaluator	Eye contact, attitude toward interviewer (negative, positive, shy, suspicious, withdrawn, friendly, self-centered)
Behaviors displayed during interview	Impulsivity, aggression, inhibition, distractibility, low frustration tolerance, ability to have fun, sense of humor, creativity
Interactional Data	
Interpersonal relationships	Attitudes toward and perceptions of family, siblings, and peers, transitional objects,* pets; social skills with peers, best friend; relationships with family, siblings, and peers; conflicts; behavior problems; adjustment to changes in routine or new situations
Self-concept and image	Self-appraisal (does child like self?), comparison of self with others (sibling, peers), what does child like most about self? what would he or she like to change about self? sense of pride in accomplishments, sex role, and gender identity
Conscience	Sense of right and wrong, acceptance of guilt, ability to accept limits in the evaluation, judgment

* Inanimate objects invested with ability to allay anxiety and tension in lieu of human relationships, especially the mother–child relationship.

(Gary, F., & Kavanagh, C. K. [1991]. *Psychiatric mental health nursing.* Philadelphia: J.B. Lippincott; with permission.)

Help parents to see that this type of referral is no different from one to a cardiologist or orthopedist.

Parents can be assured that everyone recognizes the many pressures and stresses on children today that cannot be controlled or guarded against completely. Many parents find it reassuring to be told that their contact with a child guidance clinic, psychologist, or psychiatrist will be kept confidential. They also feel reassured by knowing that the healthcare personnel making the referral will continue to offer episodic or health maintenance care—that they are not being "transferred out" but asked to seek additional help only in this one area.

Implementation

Often what parents and children need most when a cognitive or mental health disorder is present is an empathetic but uninvolved person to listen to their story objectively and to provide support for them as they try to resolve and manage the situation to a satisfactory conclusion. Recognizing when you are the person best able to serve this function requires professional judgment. Serving in this capacity can be important and provide a source of personal satisfaction.

Additionally, outside organizations may be a source of support and education for the family. Organizations that might be helpful for referral include the following:

Anorexia Nervosa and Related Eating Disorders
P.O. Box 5102
Eugene, OR 97405

Autism Society of America
8601 Georgia Avenue
Suite 503
Silver Spring, MD 20910

Tourette Syndrome Association
42-40 Bell Boulevard
Bayside, NY 11361

Parents of Children with Down Syndrome
c/o Montgomery County Association for Retarded Citizens
11600 Nebel Street
Rockville, MD 20852

Toughlove International
P.O. Box 1069
Doylestown, PA 18901

Outcome Evaluation

Children who have had a cognitve or mental health disorder need ongoing evaluation by healthcare personnel at healthcare visits to determine if the circumstances that led to the problem have truly been corrected or, because they were only superficially changed, are apt to resurface. On the whole, if the circumstances surrounding the child remain the same, the child's problem may return or be manifested later in another way.

Examples of outcome criteria that might be established include:

- Child does not injure himself during the coming month.
- Parents state they are able to cope with child's disruptive behavior since prescription of antipsychotic drug.
- Child ingests a minimum of 500 calories daily with no binge eating.

HEALTH PROMOTION AND RISK MANAGEMENT

Nurses play a key role in assessing and promoting the mental health of children and their families. A working knowledge of the typical growth and development of a child provides the basis for assessment of a child's behavior. The knowledge also helps in developing appropriate educational strategies for parents so that they can better identify problems early on. Like adults, children and adolescents are exposed to stress; however, they cope with these stresses differently. Nurses can help parents better understand how children respond to and cope with stress, also aiding in early identification should problems arise. Acting as educator, facilitator, and advocate, nurses can assist children and families to identify their needs and implement measures to meet them (see Managing and Delegating Unlicensed Assistive Personnel).

Various risk factors have been associated with an increased risk for mental health disorders in children. These include:

- Trauma or neglect
- Difficult temperament
- Attachment problems
- Experience of major losses
- Negative sibling relationships
- Medical problems and illnesses
- Exposure to high-risk activities, such as drug abuse
- Poverty and homelessness
- Parental substance abuse

A thorough assessment of the child and family can provide clues to the existence of possible risk factors and initiation of strategies to reduce their impact.

If a child develops a cognitive or mental health disorder, nurses act as advocates for referrals to support services and early intervention programs, thus helping to minimize the overall effects of the disorder on the child and family.

MANAGING AND DELEGATING UNLICENSED ASSISTIVE PERSONNEL

Unlicensed assistive personnel are often assigned to care for children who need "routine care." Be certain that unlicensed assistive personnel are aware that although care may be termed "routine," there is no such thing as routine care. Each child is unique, with unique needs. Understanding this, unlicensed assistive personnel can help identify children who appear to be having more than the usual difficulty accepting an illness or undergoing a procedure so the child can receive necessary support to help modify a stress level.

CLASSIFICATION OF MENTAL DISORDERS

For many years, psychopathology in children was not classified according to a standard system; as a result, conditions were not clearly defined or described. Today, after several revisions, the American Psychiatric Association's *Diagnostic and Statistical Manual of Mental Disorders—Revised* (DSM-IV-R) (1994) provides a standardized classification system that can be used by all members of the mental health care team. Major categories of disorders that have been devised are shown in Table 33-2.

DEVELOPMENTAL DISORDERS

Developmental disorders, although not related by etiology, typically share a common feature in that there is a delay in one or more areas of development. These areas include attention, cognition, language, affect, and social and moral behavior. In addition, a delay in one area may interfere with development in another area. Developmental disorders include cognitive impairment; pervasive developmental disorders; and specific developmental disorders such as learning disabilities (reading, mathematics, disorders of written expression, and learning disorders not otherwise specified), motor skills disorders (developmental coordination disorder), and communication disorders (expressive language disorder, mixed receptive-expressive disorder, phonological disorder, and stuttering). Cognitive impairment and pervasive developmental disorders are discussed in more detail below.

Mental Retardation

The DSM-IV defines cognitive impairment on the basis of two criteria: significantly subaverage general intellectual functioning—an intelligence quotient (IQ) of 70 or below—and concurrent deficits in adaptive functioning in at least 2 major areas (APA, 1994). For infants, because available intelligence tests do not yield numerical values, a clinical judgment of significant subaverage intellectual function must be made.

TABLE 33.2 Disorders Usually First Diagnosed in Infancy, Childhood, or Adolescence

Developmental Disorders

- Mental Retardation
  - Mild Mental Retardation
  - Moderate Mental Retardation
  - Severe Mental Retardation
  - Profound Mental Retardation
  - Mental Retardation, Severity Unspecified
- Learning Disorders
  - Reading Disorder
  - Mathematics Disorder
  - Disorder of Written Expression
- Motor Skills Disorders
  - Developmental Coordination Disorder
- Communication Disorders
  - Expressive Language Disorder
  - Mixed Receptive-Expressive Language Disorder
  - Phonological Disorder
  - Stuttering
  - Communication Disorder Not Otherwise Specified
- Pervasive Developmental Disorders
  - Autistic Disorder
  - Rett's Disorder
  - Childhood Disintegrative Disorder
  - Asperger's Disorder
  - Pervasive Developmental Disorder Not Otherwise Specified

Disruptive Behaviors Disorders

- Attention Deficit/Hyperactivity Disorder
  - Combined Type
  - Predominantly Inattentive Type
  - Predominantly Hyperactive-Impulsive Type
  - Attention-Deficit/Hyperactivity Disorder Not Otherwise Specified
- Conduct Disorder
- Oppositional Defiant Disorder
- Disruptive Behavior Disorder Not Otherwise Specified

Feeding and Eating Disorders of Infancy or Early Childhood

- Pica
- Rumination Disorder
- Feeding and Eating Disorders of Infancy or Early Childhood Not Otherwise Specified

Tic Disorders

- Tourette's Disorder
- Chronic Motor or Vocal Tic Disorder
- Transient Tic Disorder
- Tic Disorder Not Otherwise Specified

Elimination Disorders

- Encopresis
  - With Constipation and Overflow Incontinence
  - Without Constipation and Overflow Incontinence
- Enuresis (Not Due to a General Medical Condition)

Other Disorders of Infancy, Childhood, and Adolescence

- Separation Anxiety Disorder
- Selective Mutism
- Reactive Attachment Disorder of Infancy or Early Childhood
- Stereotypic Movement Disorder
- Disorder of Infancy, Childhood and Adolescence Not Otherwise Specified

American Psychiatric Association. (1994). *Diagnostic and statistical manual of mental disorders* (4th ed.). Washington, D.C.: American Psychiatric Association.

Approximately 2% of children in the United States are cognitively challenged. This is not the result of a single cause, but conditions such as genetic abnormalities (e.g., fragile X syndrome and Down syndrome [trisomy 21]) and metabolic disorders (e.g., phenylketonuria). In addition, an interplay of several genes with environmental factors (polyfactorial causes) has been identified as a possible cause for some cases (Box 33-1).

Children with cognitive impairment are seen in healthcare settings for diagnosis, and they come to health settings throughout their lives for the same reasons as other children—for well-child care at ambulatory health maintenance visits; for treatment of lacerations or poisoning in emergency departments; or for treatment of illnesses such as pneumonia or appendicitis in in-service units. For these reasons, child health nurses need to be skilled in meeting the needs of cognitively challenged children.

Classification

It is unfair to categorize children only according to the results of intelligence tests, because children do not always perform well in testing situations. Commonly, cognitive impairment is classified as mild, moderate, severe, or profound according to IQ. The level of 70 was chosen as the upper limit of cognitive impairment because most children with IQs below this are so limited in their functioning that they require special services, protection, and schooling. IQ tests are considered to have an error of measurement of about 5 points. Therefore, many children with an IQ of 75 are included in special schooling programs.

Mild Mental Retardation. About 80% to 90% of children who are cognitively challenged fall into this category. In this group, a child's IQ is between 70 and 50. The category is equivalent to the educational category "educable." During early years, these children learn social and communication skills and are often not distinguishable from average children. They are able to learn academic skills up to about the sixth-grade level. As adults, they can usually achieve social and vocational skills adequate for minimum self-support. They need guidance and assistance when faced with new situations or unusual stress.

Moderate Mental Retardation. Children in this category have an IQ between 55 and 35. About 10% of cognitively challenged children fall into this category. It is equivalent to the educational category of "trainable." During preschool years, these children learn to talk and communicate but they have only poor awareness of social conventions. They can learn some vocational skills during adolescence or young adulthood and to take care of themselves with moderate supervision. They are unlikely to progress beyond the second-grade level in academic subjects. As adults, they may be able to contribute to their own support by performing unskilled or semiskilled work under close supervision in a sheltered workshop setting. They may learn to travel alone to familiar places. They need supervision and guidance when in stressful settings.

Severe Mental Retardation. Children in this group have an IQ between 40 and 20. About 4% of cognitively challenged children fall into this category. During the preschool period, these children develop only minimal speech and little or no communicative speech. They usually have accompanying poor motor development. During school years, they may learn to talk and can be trained in basic hygiene and dressing skills. As adults, they may be able to perform simple work tasks under close supervision but as a group do not profit from vocational training. They need constant supervision for safety.

Profound Mental Retardation. The IQ of this group of children is below 20. Less than 1% of cognitively challenged children fall into this group. During the preschool period, these children show only minimal capacity for sensorimotor functioning. They need a highly structured environment and a constant level of help and supervision. Some children respond to training in minimal self-care, such as toothbrushing, but only very limited self-care is possible.

BOX 33.1

COMMON CAUSES OF COGNITIVE IMPAIRMENT

Chromosomal abnormalities such as Down syndrome and fragile X syndrome
Infection *in utero* such as rubella or cytomegalic inclusion disease
Anoxia at birth such as from umbilical cord compression
Fetal alcohol syndrome
Inherited metabolic disorders such as phenylketonuria
Head trauma
Lead poisoning
Hypothyroidism
Brain malformations such as anencephaly
Prematurity
Infection such as measles encephalitis

Assessment

Assessment for cognitive impairment is done by history taking and IQ testing. Early assessment is key and should be done as soon as parents become aware that their child is experiencing problems with development. Doing so helps to prevent them from developing unrealistic expectations of the child or punishing a child for doing things that he or she doesn't understand not to do. Assessment also allows parents to look at the things the child can do and to see where they can be of most help.

Intelligence is routinely measured with standardized tests, notably the Wechsler Intelligence Scale for Children (WISC) or the Stanford-Binet. Adaptive behavioral functioning, which may vary in different environments, is judged according to several methods, including standardized instruments for assessing social maturity and adaptive skills. A composite picture of life functioning is drawn from multiple sources.

Parents may react to the diagnosis of cognitive impairment in the same way as parents who have been told that their child has a chronic or fatal illness—with a grief reaction. This may be manifested as disbelief, anger, or extreme sorrow. The grief may become chronic, always present, always waiting to strike a parent especially hard at times when the child would have reached milestones in his or her life, such as the first day of school or high school graduation. Work with the family in developing plans that are realistic. A child cannot achieve more than an individual disability will allow, but you can help parents better accept the outcome (see the Focus on Cultural Competence box).

CHECKPOINT QUESTIONS

1. What are the four major categories of cognitive impairment?
2. What level of development would you expect to see in a child who is cognitively challenged with an IQ of 45?

Therapeutic Management

To aid in planning, parents need a realistic prognosis for a child. This may be difficult to offer in early life, because infant intelligence tests are not accurate and more sophisticated tests are difficult to administer until the preschool years. Prediction based on these early tests involves some subjective input so a child's potential may be over- or underrated by them. Once parents have a realistic expectation based on the best judgement possible, however, they are ready, with guidance, to help children achieve their full potential.

NURSING DIAGNOSES AND RELATED INTERVENTIONS

Nursing Diagnosis: Health-seeking behaviors related to increasing knowledge of care needs of the cognitively challenged child

FOCUS ON CULTURAL COMPETENCE

Mental health disorders and cognitive impairment have always been perplexing to people, and so there is a history of poor acceptance of children with such disorders (Geissler, 1994). In ancient civilizations, physicians bored holes in children's heads to let out what they perceived to be evil spirits; modern television programs or movies still show distorted perceptions of how people with cognitive impairment or mental illness behave. These misperceptions make it difficult for parents to accept these diagnoses. Taking time to talk with them about modern management of mental health disorders and the ways that children with cognitive impairment can be integrated into a family can be a major intervention in helping families adjust to and grow with these disorders.

Outcome identification: Parents will demonstrate understanding of the needs of their child and care options before making any decisions.

Outcome Evaluation: Parents identify their particular options; identify child's care needs; demonstrate measures to care for child.

Parents of children with cognitive impairment have a number of important decisions to make concerning care of their child.

Institutional Care Versus Home Care. At one time, if a child was born with a syndrome such as Down syndrome, parents were advised to place the child in an institution immediately. Today, very few institutions of this type are available. Parents are encouraged to keep children at home and maintain a home and school environment for them as near normal as possible. This plan has definite advantages for children who are mildly or moderately delayed. The give-and-take of a home environment improves their ability to relate to other people. Because a small group of people cares for them, stimulation and their desire to achieve is increased.

When children are severely delayed, keeping them at home becomes a more difficult task. If both parents work to earn an adequate family income, the responsibility for constant supervision of the child is on babysitters or older children in the family. Obtaining babysitters may be difficult, further compounding the problem. Day care and/or schooling outside the home may make home care more feasible.

Parents shoulder a great deal of responsibility to provide constant watchful care, especially for the child with problems affecting judgment. This responsibility increases as both the child and the parents grow older. The parents' freedom to go on vacation or have an adult life apart from the child is restricted. They may spend so much time with the child that other children in the family feel left out, unloved, or burdensome.

If parents are unable to care for a child at home, a suitable foster home placement may be possible to offer the child the advantage of a family setting. Halfway houses or group homes (6 to 12 children living in a home with assigned counselors) provide a care setting with a home atmosphere and community experiences.

Before giving advice to any family about where a child should be raised, consider the individual circumstances of the family. Every family has its own coping mechanisms, and individual parents may be at different stages of coping, especially in the first year after the birth of a child with a severe disability. Be certain to consider the feelings of each family member and how adequately they are coping.

Health Maintenance Needs. Children with cognitive impairment need the same health maintenance supervision as other children. At healthcare visits, parents may need reinforcement and review of precautions against accidents. Remind them to treat children according to their intellectual age, not their chronologic age. All 2-year-olds would turn on the burners of the stove to see the flame if they could reach them. Most do not, however, because they cannot reach them. The mother of a 6-year-old who thinks as a 2-year-old must be exceedingly careful; her child can reach the same dangerous areas as any 6-year-old but, unfortunately, may explore and touch them with a 2-year-old's judgment.

Illness. It may be more difficult to detect illness in a child with cognitive impairment because he or she may not be able to describe the problem. For example, a child experiencing pain may respond to it by generalized crying, like an infant. Parents must observe them closely for symptoms such as tugging at an ear, refusing to swallow food, rapid breathing, or limping, because these will help to localize discomfort. When they call healthcare personnel, parents may be apologetic about their lack of ability to judge the child. Help parents to become advocates for their child. They know their child better than anyone else. The parents may not know exactly what is wrong, but they do know that something is wrong. Reasure parents that they have done the correct thing by calling to check out the problem.

When children with cognitive impairment are seen in an emergency department or an ambulatory setting for care, they need simple explanations of what will happen. The average 6-year-old sees you with a thermometer in your hand and thinks, "She's going to take my temperature." Your explanation that you are going to do that only confirms what the child has already guessed. A child who is cognitively challenged may be unable to make this association between the thermometer and what you are going to do. Your explanation, therefore, is the first introduction to the event. Make certain that it is adequate.

When children are admitted to the hospital, nursing care must meet the needs of their intellectual age, not their chronologic one. For example, whether safety precautions such as side rails or possibly restraints will be necessary must be judged according to intellectual age. The explanations and preparation for procedures also must be geared to intellectual age (see the Nursing Care Plan: A Hospitalized Adolescent With Cognitive Impairment).

When children are discharged from a hospital, parents need careful explanations of signs and symptoms to look for to ensure continued good health in the child. Remember that such signs may be more difficult to elicit, depending on the degree of the child's cognitive delay. Be sure parents have a telephone number they can call to seek further information or advice if they are unsure of their own observations in the period immediately after discharge.

Education. Most children who are cognitively impaired do well in preschool programs, possibly giving them a head start in learning to socialize with peers and to develop fine and gross motor coordination. These programs also offer parents some free time during the week to do things *they* wish to do.

The school chosen for the child depends on the degree of intellectual delay and on the school situations available in the community. Children should be included in regular classes as much as possible (Figure 33-1). This offers children a great deal of stimulation and helps them reach their best potential. It also helps them learn to work and socialize with people, something they will need to do for the rest of their lives. Advocating for school placement of a child in an inclusive program may be necessary. By federal law, children have the right to the least restrictive environment possible. Children with cognitive impairment need instructions on bus safety and on locating the correct bus for the trip home from school. If they walk to school, they need appropriate supervision to ensure safety when crossing streets.

Nursing Diagnosis: Altered growth and development related to cognitive impairment

Outcome Identification: Child will reach and maintain optimum level of functioning possible.

Outcome Evaluation: Child is able to perform self care within limits of disorder; exhibits feelings of satisfaction with accomplishments.

Self-Care Activities. Children who are cognitively challenged need to learn the maximum amount of self-care possible. Doing so provides them with a sense of control and accomplishment. Assess carefully whether children need special aids to achieve such skills as brushing teeth, combing hair, taking a bath, and eating. Even after children learn how to perform these skills, they may need continued reminders to do them because they are unaware of the reason for or importance of the skill. If you do these skills for children, such as during a period of hospitalization, they can forget how to perform them and will need to be retaught after they return home (see the Empowering the Family box.)

Play. Children with intellectual delays enjoy play like any child. Guide parents to choose toys that are appropriate for their child's developmental, not chronologic, age. Toys that cover a wide age range, such as music boxes or tape players, are good choices. Because children with cognitive impairment may be older and stronger than the age stated for that toy, toys that are developmentally correct still may not be appropriate because they break too easily to be safe.

Social Relationships. The ability to communicate may be delayed in children who are cognitively challenged because the ability to develop language is often delayed. Speech therapy may be necessary to help them articulate correct sounds. Talking picture boards (boards with pictures on them, available commercially or made by parents) to which children can point if they want something can help speed communication.

Teaching early social behavior, such as saying "thank you" and "excuse me," shaking hands, and taking turns, is important to help children relate to other children and adults. Cognitively impaired children imitate this type of behavior the same as other children. Providing good role models is an effective way of teaching social behavior.

Encourage parents to enroll children in preschool programs to help them learn to be comfortable with other children at the earliest time possible. Many programs enroll children as early as 1 year of age to begin education. As a school-age child, participating in organized groups such as Girl Scouts or Special Olympics is an important way to learn to interact with others and feel successful.

Preparation for Adulthood. As children with cognitive impairment reach adolescence, they benefit from orientation to sexual responsibility, the same as all children.

Nursing Care Plan

THE HOSPITALIZED ADOLESCENT WITH COGNITIVE IMPAIRMENT

A 14-year-old female with moderate cognitive impairment is admitted to the hospital for knee surgery. Following surgery, the child will be placed in a long leg cast and remain hospitalized for approximately 4 days.

Assessment: 14-year-old, slightly overweight adolescent with an IQ of approximately 50. Sexual maturity rating: 3. Developmental age estimated at approximately 3 years. Child observed holding favorite doll tightly. Mother states, "She talks to her about what she wants to do." Some difficulty interacting and talking with others. "She often repeats herself, asking 'What's your name?' 'What do you like to do?'" Able to feed self and use bathroom independently. Able to wash and dress self with supervision. Mother says, "She gets upset and cries easily if her routine changes." Attends special education classes at a local school. Mother planning to stay with child around the clock throughout the hospital stay.

Nursing Diagnosis: Self-care deficit (bathing/hygiene, dressing, toileting) related to application of cast and effects of hospitalization on daily routine

Outcome Identification: Child will maintain level of self care achieved prior to hospitalization.

Outcome Evaluation: Child continues to feed self independently; verbalizes need to use bathroom and assists with toileting activities; participates in bathing and dressing activities with supervision.

Interventions	Rationale
1. Assess the child's daily routine at home.	1. Obtaining information about the usual routine helps in providing suggestions for modifying the hospital routine.
2. Modify care activities as much as possible to simulate the child's daily routine.	2. Maintaining as nearly normal a routine as possible minimizes the amount of stress to which the child is exposed and helps her adjust to hospitalization.
3. With each activity or procedure, offer simple, single explanations and instructions. Include the child's doll in these explanations.	3. Simple, single instructions are necessary to help the child understand what is happening. A child with cognitive impairment may be unable to associate a particular action with its meaning. Including the child's doll is therapeutic and may help to increase the child's understanding.
4. Encourage the mother to bring in personal care items from home, such as pajamas, toothbrush, and hair brush or comb.	4. Using the child's own personal care items helps to promote a more familiar, routine environment for self care.
5. Break down each aspect of self care into simple steps. Allow the child ample time to complete each step. Praise the child for accomplishments and provide help as necessary.	5. Breaking down a task into steps prevents overwhelming the child. Allowing ample time for task completion and praising for accomplishments helps to promote independence and foster self-confidence. Providing help as needed assists in minimizing the possible feelings of frustration, stress, and ultimately failure.
6. Instruct the child to use the call bell when she needs to use the bathroom. Arrange for a bedside commode, if appropriate, and assist as necessary, such as with transferring on and off the commode.	6. Because of cast placement, the child needs assistance with toileting. A bedside commode, similar in appearance to a toilet, may be less frightening for the child to use than a bedpan.

(continued)

Nursing Diagnosis: Risk for injury related to impaired cognitive function and immobilization from cast application

Outcome Identification: Child will remain free of injury during hospitalization.

Outcome Evaluation: Child and mother use call bell when assistance is necessary. Child exhibits no signs or symptoms of injury. Mother informs staff when she is leaving the child's room.

Interventions	Rationale
1. Institute developmentally appropriate safety measures, such as raised side rails, for the child.	1. Although the child is chronologically an adolescent, she is developmentally a 3 year old.
2. Instruct the child and mother in the use of the call bell and keep the call bell within easy reach of both.	2. A call bell provides a ready access for help should it be needed.
3. Make frequent visits to the child's room and check on the child.	3. Frequent visits provide support and help to ensure safety.
4. Advise the child's mother to inform the staff about any plans to leave the child's room.	4. Knowledge that the child is alone allows for staff supervision to minimize the risk for injury.
5. Assess the neurovascular status of the affected extremity at least every 4 hours.	5. A cast can interfere with circulatory and neurologic functioning of the affected leg, placing the child at risk for injury.
6. Institute measures to prevent complications related to immobility.	6. Immobility can adversely affect any body system. Preventive measures reduce the risk of their occurrence.

Nursing Diagnosis: Diversional activity deficit related to changes in routine and separation from school and family secondary to hospitalization

Outcome Identification: Child will participate in developmentally age-appropriate activities while hospitalized.

Outcome Evaluation: Child participates in activities; demonstrates interest in staff and other children.

Interventions	Rationale
1. Explore with the mother and child the types of activities and interests that the child likes and dislikes.	1. Ascertaining likes and dislikes provides a basis for planning future suggestions.
2. Work with the mother and child to plan nursing care that allows time for rest and activities. Have the child participate in care based on the child's developmental level.	2. Active participation according to the child's developmental level minimizes feelings of boredom and enhances feelings of control and self-confidence. Expectations above the child's level promote failure.
3. Encourage the mother to bring in some of the child's favorite toys from home.	3. Items that are familiar provide stimulation and promote feelings of comfort and interest.
4. Contact the play therapist for assistance.	4. The play therapist can provide suggestions and support for developmentally appropriate activities.
5. Place the child in a room with another child who is school aged.	5. A school-aged child is younger chronologically but older developmentally. Such a roommate can provide social stimulation and act as a role model.
6. Include the child in play room activities and transport the child to the play room when possible.	6. Including the child in play room activities provides stimulation and offers opportunities for social interaction.
7. Encourage the mother to have family members and friends visit often.	7. Contact with family members and friends is essential to maintain relationships and foster growth and development, providing familiarity and additional support for the child and mother.

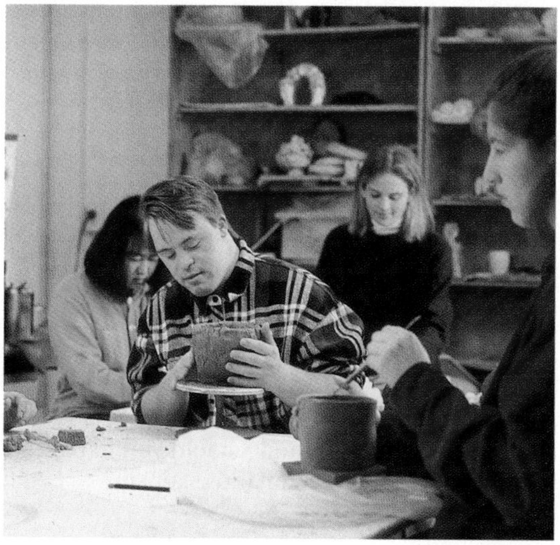

FIGURE 33.1 A teenage boy with Down syndrome participates in a high school art class.

Girls can understand a simple explanation of menstruation and necessary menstrual hygiene. Both boys and girls need explanations of how pregnancy occurs and the measures they need to take to prevent this. Help them understand socially acceptable sexual activities.

If a girl is going to use a contraceptive and lives with a responsible adult, she can be given an oral contraceptive daily by that adult. Other longer-acting contraceptives, such as Depo Provera and Norplant, are now available. Sterilization is not usually recommended because it is difficult for a cognitively impaired adolescent to understand fully the implications of this (so consent is not fully informed). If pregnancy should occur, an adolescent who is cognitively challenged can be counseled but not forced to have an abortion. If the adolescent decides to continue the pregnancy, assist her through the pregnancy.

WHAT IF? A 15-year-old female who is mildly cognitively impaired comes to the clinic for a routine checkup with her mother. During your conversation, the girl asks you if she should have a baby. How would you respond?

Pervasive Developmental Disorders: Infantile Autism

Infantile autism is a category of pervasive developmental disorders that is marked by serious distortions in psychological functioning. There may be deficits in language, perceptual, and motor development; defective reality testing; and an inability to function in social settings. There is a lack of responsiveness to other people, gross impairment in communication skills, and bizarre responses to various aspects of the environment, all developing within the first 30 months of age (APA, 1994). It is a rare condition, occurring in only 2 to 10 children out of 10,000. It occurs more often in boys than in girls.

The cause of the disorder is unknown, but it is believed to be a result of multiple factors, including genetics, perinatal complications and perhaps problems with biochemical substances in the body (Happe & Frith, 1996). As many as 50% of children with the disorder are also cognitively impaired.

Assessment

Common symptoms of autism are summarized in Box 33-2. Because of the lack of responsiveness to people that is part of the syndrome, normal attachment behavior does not develop. Infants fail to cuddle or make eye contact or exhibit facial unresponsiveness. They do not reach to be picked up. They are unable to play cooperatively or make friendships. Parents may first bring a child to a healthcare facility thinking he or she is deaf because of this.

EMPOWERING THE FAMILY:
Teaching Guidelines for the Cognitively Challenged Child

- Teach one step at a time. Short-term memory is often possible, whereas long-term memory is not. This means a child can only learn one step of a skill at a time (remembering three consecutive steps is long-term memory).
- Introduce motivators for learning such as generous praise. Learning is not rewarding all by itself when intelligence is impaired.
- Reduce the number of extra stimuli present. With too many stimuli present, a child cannot focus attention on the task to learn (or realize that the task is more important than surrounding stimuli).
- Demonstrate the skill to be learned. Seeing a skill performed is generally better than just hearing it explained.
- Keep things simple. Cognitively impaired children may have difficulty with learning principles or abstractions. They may be able to learn to wash their hands, for example, but not why they should wash them (other than it pleases you).
- Give praise accordingly. Remember that accomplishing even the most simple skill may be very difficult. Learning to tie shoes may take the same effort as another child spends learning mathematics. Learning to cross streets safely may be equivalent to earning a high school diploma.

The impairment in communication is shown in both verbal and nonverbal skills. Language may be totally absent. If a child does speak, grammatical structure may be impaired (the use of "you" when "I" is intended is common). There is inability to name objects (nominal aphasia) and abnormal speech melody, such as question-like rises at the end of statements. **Echolalia** (repetitive words or phrases spoken by others) and concrete interpretation also may be present.

Bizarre responses to the environment include intense reactions to minor changes in the environment (screaming if a toybox is moved across the room) and attachment to odd objects (always carrying a string or a shoe). Autistic children often persist in repetitive hand movements. Rocking and rhythmic body movements are often observed. They are intensely preoccupied by objects that move, such as a fan, the swirling water in the toilet bowl, or a spinning top. Music often holds a special interest for them. Hitting, head banging, and biting also may be present.

In contrast to these mannerisms, long-term memory may be excellent. Autistic children may be able to recall dates and spoken words from conversations that took place years before. This excellent memory previously led to the belief that most of these children have normal intelligence. Actually only about 25% of them have an IQ above 70 (APA, 1994). Intelligence testing is difficult, however, because they do not respond well to test situations and they score poorly on verbal parts of these tests. Tasks requiring manipulative or visual skills or immediate memory may be performed at above-normal levels.

Children with autism have a **labile mood** (e.g., crying occurs suddenly followed immediately by giggling or laughing). They may react with overresponsiveness to sensory stimuli, such as light or sound, but then be unaware of a major event in the room, such as the sounding of a fire alarm.

Therapeutic Management

Autism is a perplexing condition. Parents need a great deal of support so that they do not reject the child because he or she seems to be rejecting them. Behavior modification therapy may be effective in controlling some of the bizarre mannerisms that accompany autism, but because the basic cause of the disorder is not known, therapy will not always succeed (Weeks & Laver-Bradbury, 1997).

BOX 33.2

COMMON SYMPTOMS IN THE CHILD WITH AUTISM

Social isolation, abnormal social interaction
Stereotyped behaviors
Resistance to any change in routine
Abnormal responses to sensory stimuli
Insensitivity to pain
Inappropriate emotional expressions
Disturbances of movement
Poor development of speech, impaired communication
Specific, limited intellectual problems

As children mature, they develop greater awareness of and attachment to parents and other familiar adults. A day care program can help to promote social awareness. Some children may eventually reach a point where they can become passively involved in loosely structured play groups. Some children may be able to lead independent lives, although social ineptness and awkwardness may remain, especially if accompanied by cognitive impairment.

✔ CHECKPOINT QUESTIONS

3. What areas are important to address for the child who is cognitively challenged to reach his optimal level of functioning?
4. What assessment findings would you expect to find with a child with infantile autism?

Specific Developmental Disorders

Specific developmental disorders may be characterized by the more narrowed area of development involved with the delay. Typically, these include learning disorders, communication disorders, and motor skills disorders.

Learning disorders, although the degree may vary, generally involve a discrepancy between actual achievement and what is expected based on the person's age and intelligence. Learning disorders may be verbal—involving reading, such as **dyslexia** (reading disability)—or nonverbal (e.g., a delay in learning mathematics).

Communication disorders involve speech (motor aspect) or language (formulation and comprehension of verbal communication) problems. Categories include expressive disorder, mixed receptive-expressive disorder, phonologic disorder, and stuttering. Motor skills disorders, as the name implies, involve problems with motor coordination.

DISRUPTIVE BEHAVIOR DISORDERS

The disruptive behavior disorders include attention deficit hyperactivity disorder (ADHD); attention-deficit disorder, predominantly inattentive or predominantly hyperactive-impusive type; and the conduct disorders. These disorders may begin with behavior problems that are not so different from what most families experience; thus, parents may be unaware of the need for intervention. By the time they seek help, they may already be extremely distressed about the unmanageability of their child.

It is important that these disorders be diagnosed as early as possible, before the child's behavior leads to a deteriorating level of self-esteem and compromised social skills and complications in family functioning develop. The home environment may be the most important factor in determining whether the disorder turns into a more complicated psychopathologic process or whether it can be channelled into purposeful, productive activity.

Attention Deficit Hyperactivity Disorder

One of the most controversial childhood mental health disorders, ADHD is estimated to occur in about 6% of school-age children in the U.S. Boys are affected more frequently than girls. The possible causes of ADHD, as well as the reliability of symptoms for establishing its diagnosis and treatment methods, have been under debate for the last 50 years. It may well be that ADHD serves as an umbrella diagnosis for a variety of behavioral-attention problems with a variety of causes. ADHD occurs more frequently among some families than in the general population, indicating a possible genetic etiologic component. ADHD has also been associated with situational anxiety, abuse, and neglect and may be one component in the development of a psychiatric illness such as schizophrenia. Both drug and behavior-modification treatment methods have been used with success, which may support the theory of varying causes.

The disorder is characterized by three major behaviors: inattention, impulsiveness, and hyperactivity. Children with ADHD are unable to complete tasks effectively because of inattention or impulsivity. They are easily distracted and often may not seem to listen. They act before they think and have difficulty with such tasks as awaiting turns in games. They exhibit excessive or exaggerated muscular activity, such as excessive climbing onto objects, constant fidgeting, and aimless or haphazard running. They may shift excessively from one activity to another.

Assessment

The disorder is diagnosable by 36 months of age, although it is often difficult to identify the disorder until later, when the child is asked to sit still in school for longer periods. Diagnosis is made on the basis of history and neurologic assessment. When the disorder is first suspected, a thorough initial history to reveal the extent of the problem should be recorded. Some children have enough control in a one-to-one situation that the behavior is not apparent in these settings. A child whom parents report as hyperactive, therefore, may not be hyperactive in an ambulatory healthcare setting.

The history is especially important in evaluating the extent of the problem. The pregnancy and birth history, the child's ability to meet developmental milestones, and a typical day for the child should be reviewed carefully. The term **hyperactivity,** or excess movement, is commonly carelessly used to describe any active child. Have the parent give an exact description of what the child is unable to do, such as sitting still long enough to finish a full meal or running to the window 10 times in 15 minutes, to document that hyperactivity truly exists.

Assess for activity that is not only excessive but also disorganized. Children with ADHD may not be able to sit still long enough to eat a meal or finish a school project. In school, they move from the back of the room to the front of the room, to the window, to the teacher's desk, to their own desk. They perform repetitive activities such as pencil tapping, arm swinging, and finger tapping. They may leave a project they are working on or a television program they are watching intently to run to the window or open the refrigerator door, unaware of why they are running. This is driven or compulsive behavior.

Variability is another important symptom. Everyone has days when they perform at their peak and days when performance is less than optimum. In children with ADHA, behavior may be so variable that they have good and bad *moments.* This type of variability causes children to lose track of systems and methods, not just answers, so school performance may falter. When asked to add, for example, a child might add 4 and 3 correctly and 5 and 4 correctly, but then lose track of the system and add 2 and 3 as 23 or 32.

A high level of impulsiveness may cause children to make statements without thinking, to touch objects they have just been told not to touch, or to speak or act before they have time to think about what they want to say or do. When angered, they may shout or strike out before they can be offered an explanation. They may be unable to wait in line for a drink of water—their impulsiveness tells them that they must have their drink immediately.

Usually, children can filter out stimuli that are not important to them at that moment. Children with ADHD seem to have an "all-or-none" reaction to stimuli. They may block out all incoming stimuli and as a result, do not hear their parents or a teacher calling them. They may be disciplined at school for something such as not answering a fire drill (unaware that a bell was ringing and that children around them were moving toward the exit). At other times they may be unable to suppress any incoming stimuli. They mean to concentrate on a desk assignment in school, but outside the window they hear a bird singing; next to them they smell a girl's perfume; they feel their watch on their wrist—so they cannot concentrate on the problem at hand. This may be reported by parents or teachers as an exceedingly short attention span.

Children with ADHD may also have difficulty with concepts such as *right* and *left, before* and *after, in front of, in back of, yesterday,* and *tomorrow,* because these concepts call for sequencing. If children cannot tell the difference between left and right, they can have difficulty forming common letters such as *b* and *d,* which vary only in the direction of the bottom loop. They can have difficulty with common tasks such as washing their hands, because they never know which way to turn a faucet. Turning door knobs and keys, tying shoe laces, and screwing on bottle caps are all complex tasks for a child who has difficulty with sequencing or space perception. They may show awkward motor movements and cannot work all muscles gracefully in proper sequence. These children may reach beyond an object, possibly spilling a glass of milk at the table at every meal.

Long after the average child is speaking in fluent sentences, children with ADHD may have difficulty using conjunctions or prepositions correctly (sequencing of words). They may have difficulty learning to read. To read words of more than one syllable, they must sound the first syllable, then retain that sound in their mind while they sound the second. If they have difficulty retaining the first syllable long enough to connect it with the second, they cannot construct the word. Similarly, they can have difficulty with arithmetic, because they may be unable to retain the sum of two numbers long enough to add the sum of a third. Spelling may be equally difficult. Not only are they unable to sequence the letters in a word correctly, but they also cannot retain memory rules such as "i before e" to help them.

Children with ADHD do not have a deficit in intelligence, although they may seem to because of their impulsive behavior. They may be unaware that their behavior is upsetting to family, friends, and teachers and thus are not anxious about their inability to conform to society's rules.

These children often show many "soft" neurologic signs, such as inability to use a pencil or scissors well. A thorough neurologic examination often is difficult because their attention span is so short. On such an exam they often have difficulty performing tests such as a finger-to-nose test or rapid hand movements, such as touching one finger after another with their thumb. They tend to show "mirroring" with this movement (the second hand imitates what the first hand attempts to do). Cerebellar difficulty may be evidenced further by inability to perform a tandem walk or a heel-to-shin test. They may be able to identify one touch but not two simultaneous touches on their body. They may not show the normal responses of **graphesthesia** (ability to recognize a shape that has been traced on the skin) or **stereognosis** (ability to recognize an object by touch). When asked to stand with arms outstretched, **choreiform movements** (aimless movements) and rising of the fingers are often present. More definite neurologic signs, such as a unilateral Babinski reflex or strabismus, may also be present. Testing through the use of games may be necessary, so that their attention is maintained long enough to complete the assessment.

IQ testing is used to document the child's intelligence. The WISC, the test most often chosen, consists of two portions: a verbal scale and a performance scale. The child is given three final scores: verbal IQ, performance IQ, and combination or full-scale IQ. The child with perceptual and motor deficits tends to do poorly on the performance scale but average or better on the verbal scale. Children with language difficulty typically do poorly on the verbal scale but average or above on the performance scale. Children with ADHD show a "scatter" pattern on both performance and verbal portions, doing well on some portions and poorly on others.

Children who have difficulty filtering out stimuli do poorly on group-administered intelligence tests because they are too distracted by those around them. These children, therefore, should take IQ tests individually. Neurologic examinations also should be performed in rooms free of distractions such as attractive toys.

Children with ADHD are often referred to a healthcare facility because they have had difficulty in school. Parents may have been assured on previous occasions that although their child had difficulty settling down to tasks, this was because he was "all boy" or "every child is different." They may need time to accept that their child has a condition that interferes with learning. Active listening is essential. This is a difficult situation that may have persisted for a long time. The parents may be unaware themselves of the strain this has produced until they start to describe it.

✔ CHECKPOINT QUESTONS

5. What are the three major characteristics of ADHD?
6. What is the underlying problem associated with difficulty of concepts such as before and after?

Therapeutic Management

A variety of treatment methods are used, often in combination, in the management of ADHD.

Environment. It is important that a stable learning environment be constructed for children with ADHD. This may include special instruction, free from the distractions of an entire class. Parents may have difficulty accepting the fact that their child needs special schooling (the intelligence test, after all, said that he or she was above average). They may need help in seeing that the condition interferes with intellectual functioning and that a special program must be constructed for the child to succeed.

Parents having difficulty at home with discipline and management often appreciate some support and advice. Encourage them to be fair but firm and set consistent limits. Although every child has a right to an opinion, many decisions that the average child enjoys making for himself or herself must be made for this child. "Do you want to wear your red or your blue shirt today?" is less effective than "Here is your blue shirt to wear today."

Children who are easily distracted have difficulty completing chores or picking up their toys. They can be assigned age-appropriate chores with the understanding that a parent must give many reminders to them to get the job completed. Teach parents to give instructions slowly and make certain that they have the child's attention before beginning instructions. Breaking down a chore into several steps may help (get the toybox is one step; pick up toys is a second). This helps to avoid confrontation that may arise later if children do not hear or do not process what is said to them.

All children like to participate in dinner conversation or discussions about their day. Children with ADHD often have difficulty telling a story or repeating a joke told to them (a sequencing problem). Suggest parents help them by asking questions such as "Why?" "Where?" or "Who?" to reach the point of the story. Also encourage parents to be certain that when they correct behavior, their anger is about something the child has deliberately done wrong, not about some incident that happened because of the child's inability to sequence, filter, or integrate concepts. Punishment should follow an offense quickly because a child quickly forgets what he or she did. As with all children, parents should make certain the child understands that the parent is angry at the behavior, not the child. Children with ADHD commonly develop poor self-esteem because although they are intelligent, they cannot succeed. Help parents to build, not hinder, the development of self-esteem at every stage possible.

Medication. A number of medications are helpful in controlling the excessive activity of the child with ADHD and lengthening the attention span or decreasing the distractibility so that he or she can function in a normal classroom. Dextroamphetamine (Dexedrine) was the first drug used for this purpose.

More recently, methylphenidate hydrochloride (Ritalin) or pemoline (Cylert) have been prescribed for this disorder (see the Drug Highlight box). These drugs have side effects of insomnia and anorexia, so the child must

DRUG HIGHLIGHT

Methylphenidate Hydrochloride (Ritalin)

Action: Methylphenidate is a central nervous system stimulant that appears to act paradoxically in children with ADHD.

Pregnancy risk category: C

Dosage: Initially, 5 mg orally before breakfast and lunch, gradually increasing the dosage in 5- to 10-mg increments weekly, not to exceed 60 mg/day.

Possible adverse reactions: Nervousness, insomnia, anorexia, nausea, abdominal pain, pulse rate changes, hyper- or hypotension, tachycardia, leukopenia, anemia, and growth suppression.

Nursing Implications:

- Administer the drug exactly as prescribed and instruct parents in same. Instruct parents to have child swallow timed-release tablets whole and to refrain from chewing or crushing them.
- Instruct the parents to administer the drug before 6 PM to prevent interference with sleep.
- Advise the parents and child to avoid over-the-counter drugs, such as cold remedies and cough syrups, which may contain alcohol.
- Obtain baseline vital signs and monitor on follow-up visits for changes.
- Arrange for follow-up laboratory tests, including complete blood count for children on long-term therapy.
- Assess child's growth on subsequent visits for possible growth suppression.
- Anticipate need to interrupt therapy periodically to evaluate need for continuation of drug.

be closely observed. The insomnia may be relieved by administering the drug early in the day. Children receiving the drugs for long periods need careful height and weight assessment to evaluate for possible growth suppression and also to determine that long-term anorexia is not causing weight loss (St. Dennis & Synoground, 1996). Periodically, the dosage may be interrupted—a "Ritalin vacation"—to determine if continued therapy is needed.

Diet. Dietary treatment of ADHD has been proposed but not substantiated in research. The Feingold diet (omitting salicylates and food dyes) became popular in the 1980s, but studies of this treatment have yielded contradictory findings. It has been found that food-dye restriction might be helpful for a small subgroup of children with ADHD (Ward, 1997). Megavitamin treatments have also proved ineffective and possibly dangerous.

Family Support. Parents of a child with ADHD often need frequent healthcare visits while their child is growing up. A responsive, listening ear is crucial to their ability to handle the challenge of raising a child with these symptoms. Any parent can grow short tempered and irritable at times with a child who does not seem to hear them or follow what they say. They may need reminders at intervals that their child does not act this way on purpose. Help them to understand that because of a very complex and as yet ill-understood syndrome, the behavior is the best their child can achieve.

Attention-deficit disorder is a common childhood condition. Research has shown that some children with ADHD continue to experience problems with impulsivity and inattention (although hyperactivity may be less overt) into adulthood. Many parents of children with ADHD have similar symptoms of restlessness, impulsivity, and high activity, although these may not pose the same problems as in childhood (when the child is expected to sit at a desk for 6 to 8 hours a day). Adults may find careers that allow them to cope with these behaviors better than "sitting at a desk job."

Conduct Disorders

Conduct disorders represent the most common psychiatric diagnosis of children and adolescents. The essential feature of these disorders is a repetitive and persistent pattern of violations of personal rights or societal rules, such as disobedience, stealing, fighting, destruction of property, fire setting, and early sexual behavior (APA, 1994).

Children may show aggressive behavior by purse snatching, mugging, or robbery with confrontation, or in less overt ways by persistent truancy, lying, or vandalism. Many teenage runaways may fall into this category.

Often these children fail to demonstrate a normal degree of affection, empathy, or ability to bond with others. They may have few meaningful peer relationships. Egocentrism is strong; they manipulate others for favors without any effort to return them. Feelings of guilt or remorse appear to be lacking. Unless there is an obvious immediate advantage, they do not extend themselves to others.

Conduct disorders are seen more frequently in males than in females, particularly when property or violent crimes are involved; however, the prevalence of conduct disorders in girls is increasing, possibly reducing the male predominance over time. A number of etiologic factors have been described for this disorder, including genetic predisposition, neurologic deficit correlates, and sociologic factors related to poverty and cultural disadvantage. In addition, the home environment is frequently characterized by rejection, frustration, and harsh and inconsistent discipline. Parents may have marital conflicts or substance abuse problems or children may have had a series of step-parents or foster parents.

Therapy for children with conduct disorders focuses on modifying the home environment and training in social and problem-solving skills. Social skills training teaches the child to recognize how his or her behavior affects others. Problem-solving skills training teaches the child to generate alternative solutions to a situation, sharpen thinking about the consequences of choices, and evaluate his or her response. Parental training is also important, but this may be difficult because parents are under stress already. Learning improved parenting skills to cope with a child exhibiting acting-out behavior is difficult. Removing the child from the home to a structured day-care environment may be necessary. Unfortunately, the child may interpret this as more rejection, further compounding the problem. Any new environment that is created must be consistent and loving, not institutional, to be effective. If hospitalized, children with conduct disorder can be very disruptive.

Teaching parents behavior therapy (rewarding positive behavior) can also be effective. TOUGHLOVE is a national organization that can be helpful to some parents as a support group. The mainstay of the organization's philosophy is to set basic rules that children must follow or else move out of the parents' home. Critics of the method caution that although this approach may be effective in making children display acceptable behavior, it may not actually change the behavior (just drive it underground).

Numerous medications such as haloperidol, carbamazepine, propranolol, and lithium carbonate have been used to treat aggressive behavior. Research has shown that haloperidol has been most effective in children and adolescents.

✔ CHECKPOINT QUESTIONS

7. What medication is most frequently used to treat ADHD?
8. What methods are used as therapy for conduct disorders?

ANXIETY DISORDERS OF CHILDHOOD OR ADOLESCENCE

Because anxiety is considered a normal part of certain phases of development (e.g., stranger anxiety of the 6- to 8-month old, separation anxiety in the toddler, fear of mutilation and the dark in the preschooler, and performance anxiety of the school-ager or adolescent), genuine anxiety disorders in children may often be overlooked. When left untreated, children may cope with fear by becoming overdependent on others for support or by turning away from the problem and withdrawing into themselves. This can leave a child socially immature and unable to achieve in school.The DSM-IV indentifies separation anxiety disorder as an anxiety disorder in children. **School phobia** is a common finding with anxiety disorder. In this instance, the child refuses to go to school; instead, he or she stays home with the primary attachment person (see Chapter 11).

Separation Anxiety

Separation anxiety, a normal phase of development in the toddler (see Chapter 9), is considered a disorder when an older child shows excessive anxiety about separation or the possibility of separation from those to whom the child is attached. Children may worry when apart from parents that they will have an accident or become ill. They may have difficulty falling asleep at night or insist on sleeping with parents or just outside their parents' bedroom door. They may experience acute distress, frequent nightmares about separation, and reluctance and refusal to separate. Repeated reports of physical symptoms when separated or when separation is anticipated are also possible. Such a degree of anxiety can be incapacitating to children; it may prevent them from visiting at friend's houses, enjoying a camp experience, or enjoying school.

Separation anxiety tends to run in families and occurs slightly more frequently in girls than in boys. Unresolved internal conflicts, uncertainty about one's caregiver, and parent-induced anxious attachment are psychodynamic factors attributed to this disorder. Temperament is also considered a contributing factor.

Treatment for separation anxiety includes individual counseling sessions combined with antidepressant medication. In addition, family therapy may be helpful in allowing the family to gain greater insight into the dynamics of the problem and the child to gain more confidence in his or her ability to function independently.

EATING DISORDERS

Pica

Children who eat nonfood substances such as dirt, clay, paint chips, crayons, yarn, or paper are said to have pica. *Pica* is the Latin word for magpie (a bird that will eat anything). Although this disorder is rarely diagnosed, it may be common. Its primary danger lies in the possibility of accidental poisoning. Other complications include constipation, gastrointestinal malabsorption, fecal impaction, and intestinal obstruction. In children, this disorder is seen predominantly between the ages of 1 and 6, although it may be present into adolescence. Often it is not diagnosed until the child presents with a pica-induced complication, such as lead poisoning (see Chapter 31).

The condition may occur as a reaction to stress. There is an increased incidence of pica in children with cognitive impairment, possibly because of their inability to distinguish edible from inedible substances. It is highly associated with iron deficiency anemia; it occurs at a high incidence in pregnant teenage girls. With these children, correcting the anemia also corrects the pica. Keeping the child safe from ingesting inedible substances is a major nursing responsibility (LeBlanc et al, 1997) (see the Focus on Nursing Research).

Rumination Disorder of Infancy

The term *rumination* comes from the Latin word for "chewing the cud" (as cattle do). Rumination is the act of regurgitating and reswallowing previously ingested food. It is a rare disorder that generally affects infants between the ages of 3 to 12 months. It is seen most often in children who are cognitively challenged. Both organic and environmental theories have been explored to explain this disorder. In some children, the existence of gastroesophageal reflux disorder has been implicated. It has also been postulated that rumination is a form of self-stimulation by the infant, similar to head banging and body rocking. It may be related to an understimulating environment, but attempts to implicate the role of the primary caregiver in causing this disorder have failed. Most infants with rumination disorder seem happy and well cared for.

A parent may report that a child is constantly "spitting up" or vomiting or smells sour. Children can lose a great deal of fluid and electrolytes through this process and may show signs of failure to thrive. (Failure to thrive as a distinct problem is discussed in Chapter 34.) Distracting

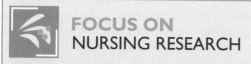

FOCUS ON NURSING RESEARCH

If Children With Pica Eat Soil, Could They Ingest a Lethal Dose of Toxic Substances?

Although paint is the usual substance eaten by children with pica, some children ingest substantial amounts of soil as a manifestation of pica. The EPA assumes that the average child ingests no more than 200 mg soil/day (from soil on hands or toys). For this study, it was assumed that a child with pica might eat up to 50 gm of soil daily. Soil samples of this size were analyzed for toxic contaminants. The researchers concluded that if this large a dose of soil were eaten, children could ingest a contaminant dose approximating or exceeding the acute human lethal dose recommended by the EPA.

This is an important study for nurses because nurses are often the people who obtain health histories in ambulatory settings. It stresses the importance of asking a broad question such as "Does your child ever eat nonedible substances," not merely asking if a child has ever been seen eating chipped paint.

Calabrese, E. J., Stanek, E. J., James, R. C., & Roberts, S. M. (1997). Soil ingestion: a concern for acute toxicity in children. *Environmental Health Perspectives, 105*(12), 1354.

infants by holding, rocking, and talking to them tends to decrease rumination. Thickening formula with cereal occasionally is effective because this is more difficult to regurgitate. When the problem is severe, hospitalization may be necessary to provide an alternative feeding environment for the child. Attachment between the child and parent may be at risk because of the anxiety the parents suffer from their infant's constant regurgitation of food and lack of growth. Parents need support, reassurance, and education to help them reestablish this bond.

✔ CHECKPOINT QUESTIONS

9. Is separation anxiety seen more frequently in boys or girls?
10. What type of anemia is strongly associated with pica?

Anorexia Nervosa

Anorexia nervosa is a disorder characterized by preoccupation with food and body weight, creating a feeling of revulsion to food to the point of excessive weight loss (APA, 1994). Characteristics include:

- Fear of loss of control
- Intense fear of gaining weight or becoming fat
- Severely distorted body image
- Refusal to acknowledge seriousness of weight loss
- Low self-esteem (George, 1997)

Anorexia nervosa occurs most often in girls (95%), usually at puberty or during adolescence, between 13 and 20 years of age. It is more common among sisters and daughters of mothers who also had the disorder.

The DSM-IV categorizes anorexia into two types:

- Restricting—weight is controlled by restricting food intake or with excessive exercise
- **Binge eating/purging**—episodes of uncontrollable intake of large amounts of food over a specified period of time (binge eating) following by self-induced vomiting or the use of laxatives, enemas, or diuretics (purging)

The specific cause of anorexia nervosa is unknown, but most theories have focused on psychodynamic views of the disorder as a phobic-avoidance response to food resulting from the sexual and social tensions generated by the physical changes associated with puberty. Anorexia nervosa tends to occur in girls who are described by their parents as perfectionist, "model children." They may be overvalued by both parents. Parents are fairly demanding and controlling (see Box 33-3). Girls who develop this disorder tend to have a poor self-image (they cannot live up to their parents' expectations). By excessive dieting, girls are able to feel a sense of control over their own body.

Anorexia nervosa often occurs in girls who were mildly overweight before the onset of the illness. Some girls seem reluctant to grow up or mature physically. Lack of nutrition causes delayed psychosexual development. With a lean, nearly starved appearance, they do not appear as sexually developed or as old as they are. Some girls may be worried that they are pregnant, and the starvation may be an unconscious attempt to abort the pregnancy. In some girls, a period of stress or an unpleasant sexual encounter may have occurred prior to the anorexia nervosa. They may be attempting subconsciously to prevent further such sexual encounters.

Assessment

Girls with anorexia nervosa have an intense fear of becoming obese, perceive food as revolting and nauseating, and refuse to eat or else vomit food immediately after eating. They often state that they "feel fat" when they are ac-

BOX 33.3

FAMILY CHARACTERISTICS OF CHILDREN WITH ANOREXIA

- Lacking clear boundaries between generations (enmeshment)
- Oversensitivity of family to experiencing emotions and reactions of other family members
- Avoidance of conflict (maintenance of harmony) and overprotectiveness
- Rigid, unchanging patterns of relating to one another

Marshall, L. (1998). Eating disorders. In M. Boyd and M. Nihart. *Psychiatric nursing: Contemporary practice.* Philadelphia: Lippincott-Raven.

ENHANCING COMMUNICATION

Brenda is a 15-year-old female who is diagnosed with anorexia nervosa. She is 5 feet, 8 inches tall and weighs 95 pounds.

Less Effective Communication

Nurse: Let's talk about your weight, Brenda.
Brenda: I'm fat. Look at this belly of mine.
Nurse: You need to eat at least three good meals a day.
Brenda: I do. I eat a lot.
Nurse: You should have a healthy breakfast. After all, it is the most important meal of the day.
Brenda: I eat huge breakfasts. I'm just so active, I don't gain weight.

More Effective Communication

Nurse: Let's talk about your weight, Brenda.
Brenda: I'm fat. Look at me.
Nurse: You feel fat?
Brenda: Yes, just look at me.
Nurse: Tell me what you eat for a typical breakfast.
Brenda: A lot. I pig out for breakfast.
Nurse: What did you eat this morning?
Brenda: A quarter piece of toast.
Nurse: Tell me more about what it is that you eat.

In the first scenario the nurse is intent on getting the client to eat. In the second scenario the nurse is attempting to obtain more information about the client, her image of herself, and her diet.

tually as much as 25% below normal weight. Refusal to eat may be accompanied by the use of laxatives or diuretics and extensive exercising to further lose weight. Girls may ingest ipecac to induce vomiting. These measures lead eventually to excessive weight loss, acidosis or alkalosis, dependent edema, hypotension, hypothermia, bradycardia, and lanugo formation (fine, neonatal-like hair). Compulsive mannerisms such as handwashing may develop. If the process is allowed to continue without therapy, it can lead to starvation and death. The use of ipecac can be exceptionally damaging and possibly cardiotoxic. The mortality rate for the illness is between 1% and 15%.

Therapeutic Management

By the time most children are seen at healthcare facilities, they are often already extremely underweight, pale, and lethargic. Amenorrhea is the most common physical symptom. Often the child's parents have tried various methods of getting the child to eat, such as threatening, coaxing, and punishing; as a result, parent–child relationships may be strained. Parents may feel guilty for insisting their child lose weight if the girl was once overweight.

Planning and outcome identification need to be realistic. A girl who grows nauseated just looking at food cannot quickly begin to ingest a large amount of it. When caring for children with anorexia nervosa remember that, although the condition began as a psychosocial problem, by the time a girl is seen for care, starvation and its effects are a second important component. Typically, oral foods are withheld and intravenous fluid therapy is initiated for at least 2 or 3 days. Total parenteral nutrition may be necessary to supply fat and protein. Girls generally accept total parenteral nutrition well because they view it as medicine, not as food. Enteral feedings may also be accepted and used to restore weight.

Numerous strategies may be used. Initially, physical complications associated with the disorder need to be treated. In addition, establishing trust and effective communication are crucial to help the child resolve interpersonal issues (see Enhancing Communication Box). Other therapeutic interventions include:

- Medications such as antidepressants, for example, fluoxetine (Prozac)
- Identification of emotional triggers
- Self monitoring (awareness training)
- Education

Gradual weight gain is recommended. Rapid gain of weight is not desirable because a girl may again begin dieting to reduce this weight gain. Weighing her once a week is better than every day to reduce her concentration on weight. Box 33-4 describes common strategies for assisting family and friends to help the child with anorexia.

Children who have had anorexia nervosa need continued follow-up after weight is regained to be certain that they do not revert to their former dieting pattern (Figure 33-2). Counseling continues for 2 to 3 years to be certain that self-image is maintained. With counseling, most girls will achieve full recovery.

BOX 33.4

WHAT FAMILY MEMBERS AND FRIENDS CAN DO TO HELP THOSE WITH EATING DISORDERS

- Tell the person you are concerned, that you care and would like to help. Suggest that the person seek professional help.
- If the person refuses to seek help, encourage reaching out to an adult such as a teacher, school nurse, or counselor.
- Do not discuss weight, the number of calories being consumed, or particular eating habits. Try to talk about things other than food, weight, counting calories, or exercise.
- Avoid making comments about the person's appearance. Concern about weight loss may be interpreted as a compliment; comments about weight gain may be interpreted as criticism.
- Offer support but keep in mind that ultimately, the responsibility and decision for accepting help and to change is with the person.
- Read and educate yourself about these disorders.

Marshall, L. (1998). Eating disorders. In M. Boyd and M. Nihart. *Psychiatric nursing: Contemporary practice.* Philadelphia: Lippincott-Raven.

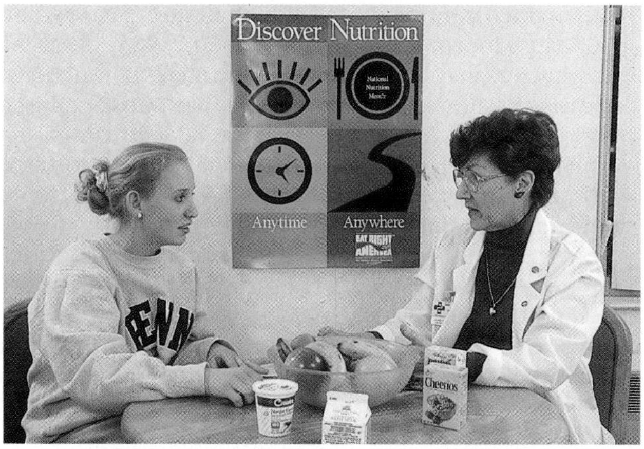

FIGURE 33.2 This anorexic teen, who is in the later stages of treatment, continues to meet with the counselor to discuss her food choices, exercise program, and overall well-being.

> WHAT IF? During a routine health maintenance visit, you notice that a teenage girl has lost 20 pounds in the last 6 months. Her mother states, "She's the perfect daughter, always getting straight A's in school." How would you respond?

Bulimia Nervosa

Bulimia refers to recurrent and episodic binge eating and purging, accompanied by an awareness that the eating pattern is abnormal but not being able to stop. A period of depression or guilt usually follows the period of bingeing. Like anorexia nervosa, bulimia typically is seen in adolescence or early adult life and predominantly in girls. The disorder may last for months or years. Periods of normal eating may be interspersed, or the girl may constantly move from bingeing to fasting. Food consumed during a binge often has a high-caloric content and a texture that facilitates rapid eating. It may be eaten secretly, such as late at night or in the privacy of a bedroom. Following ingestion of this food, the girl notices abdominal pain; she vomits to decrease the physical pain of abdominal distention and to improve self-concept (she feels more in control).

Children with bulimia may abuse purgatives, laxatives, and diuretics to aid in weight control. The combination of frequent vomiting and the use of these drugs can result in serious physical complications, notably electrolyte abnormalities, which can ultimately lead to changes as severe as cardiac arrest. People with bulimia may also have severe erosion of their teeth because of the constant exposure to acidic gastrointestinal juices from vomiting. Esophageal tears may also result.

Like adolescents with anorexia nervosa, these girls exhibit great concern about their weight and overall body image and appearance. In contrast with anorexia, most girls with bulimia are only slightly underweight and so may be discounted as merely slim unless a thorough history is obtained. As with anorexia nervosa, counseling is aimed at increasing the girl's self-esteem and sense of control (Walsh & Devlin, 1998).

> ✔ **CHECKPOINT QUESTIONS**
>
> 11. Does anorexia nervosa also occur in boys?
> 12. How does bulimia differ from anorexia nervosa?

TIC DISORDERS

Tic disorders are abnormalities of semi-involuntary movement thought to result from dysfunction in the basal ganglia. *Tics* are rapid, repetitive muscle movements, such as rapid eye blinking or facial twitching. They generally become more pronounced during periods of stress and usually diminish in sleep. **Motor tics** include eye blinking, neck jerking, and facial grimacing. Simple **vocal tics** include coughing, throat clearing, snorting, and barking. Complex motor tics include facial gestures, grooming behaviors, jumping, touching, and smelling objects (Lechman et al, 1997).

Children are most prone to these disorders between the ages of 9 and 13. They occur more frequently in boys than in girls and tend to be familial. The tic disorders are subclassified into Tourette's syndrome, chronic motor or vocal tic disorder, and transient tic disorder. Treatment generally focuses on reducing areas of stress in a child's life. Pointing out the mannerism to the child is not usually helpful and may intensify the manifestations. Behavior modification may be successful in curing a particular tic. If the stress is not removed, however, a child may substitute another nervous mechanism for the original tic.

Tourette's Syndrome

Tourette's syndrome is an inherited disorder in which the child suffers from a syndrome of motor and phonic vocal tics (Jankovic, 1997). **Complex vocal tics** include the repeated use of words or phrases out of context—specifically, **coprolalia** (use of socially unacceptable words, usually obscenities), **palilalia** (repeating one's own words), and echolalia. Some children with this syndrome have nonspecific electroencephalographic abnormalities and soft neurologic signs. Typically, the age of onset is around 7 years, with motor tics generally occurring before vocal tics. Although tics can be suppressed for brief periods, the syndrome lasts a lifetime. It occurs three times more frequently in boys than in girls. Often there is some other form of tic in other family members. Children with Tourette's syndrome can develop low self-esteem because of coprolalia before the syndrome is fully diagnosed. This syndrome responds to administration of dopamine receptor blockers such as haloperidol or pimozide.

ELIMINATION DISORDERS

Functional Encopresis

Encopresis is defined as repeated passage of feces in places not culturally appropriate for that purpose (APA,

1994). It is considered primary if a child was never fully toilet trained and secondary if the problem begins after effective training. Functional encopresis is considered to exist only after medical causes such as fecal incontinence, lactase deficiency, thyroid disease, hypercalcemia, and Hirschsprung's disease have been ruled out. It is more common in boys than girls.

Isolated occurrences of encopresis may happen when a sibling is born (as part of an overall regression reaction) or when a child is visiting a strange house or new school and is too shy to ask for the bathroom. It can occur in school because a teacher may not allow children to use a bathroom when they wish or because some school bathrooms may be occupied.

Encopresis is categorized as a mental health disorder because it can be a manifestation of a poor parent–child relationship. In a few instances it occurs because of extreme constipation. Hard bowel movements cause anal fissures. Because it hurts to move the bowels, children avoid bowel movements, leading to chronically distended rectums. They are then no longer able to sense when they need to defecate, so involuntary defecation occurs. This is a distressing condition for children because other children in school can detect the odor of a bowel movement on their clothing.

Assessment

To document encopresis, take a careful history of the condition, including the number of bowel accidents and the times they occur. Investigate any stress factors on the child. A physical examination that includes a rectal examination should be done to establish whether there is proper anal sphincter control. Therapy is based on the apparent cause.

Therapeutic Management

The administration of 1 to 6 tablespoons of mineral oil daily for 2 or 3 months will often soften stools so that bowel movements are not painful. Children on long-term mineral oil therapy generally are given water-soluble forms of vitamins A, D, and K, because these vitamins tend to be removed from the gastrointestinal tract with the mineral oil. Arranging to have children attempt to evacuate their bowels about two times daily (in the morning and after dinner) may create "habit" periods for them. Allowing children adequate time to sit on the toilet or encouraging them to take the time to do so may be helpful. Some children may be "too busy" to stop and go to the bathroom. If children evacuate their bowels before they leave for school in the morning, they are less likely to experience encopresis and embarrassment in school.

Emphasize to parents that children should not be punished for encopresis. Encourage them to pay as little attention as possible to bowel accidents and give praise for days when encopresis does not occur.

Functional Enuresis

Functional enuresis is defined as repeated involuntary or intentional urination during the day or at night after children have attained or are at an age at which they should have attained control over bladder function, when no organic cause for the problem can be found (APA, 1994). Although stress may be a factor in occurrences of functional enuresis, its primary cause is unknown. Most children outgrow the problem by adolescence. Like functional encopresis, the most serious mental impairment associated with enuresis is related to the child's feelings of failure with each occurrence and associated rejection by peers, parents, or other caregivers. All this contributes to a lowered sense of self-esteem. The problem and associated nursing diagnoses are described in more detail in Chapter 45. A similar problem is daytime urinary frequency, or the need to void as many as 10 or more times an hour. This also is associated with anxiety and fades with increased coping ability (Watemberg & Shaley, 1994).

OTHER PSYCHIATRIC DISORDERS AFFECTING CHILDREN

Childhood Depression

Children and adolescents both have depressive episodes similar to those experienced by adults (Harrington & Clark, 1998). The incidence ranges from 0.3% for pre-schoolers to 14% in adolescents. Depression is becoming an increasing concern in our society because the escalating suicide rate among children and adolescents has become a major societal problem. A child is considered to be depressed when five or more of the following symptoms exist for more than 2 weeks: loss of interest or pleasure, significant weight loss or gain, depressed mood, insomnia, psychomotor agitation, feelings of worthlessness or excessive or inappropriate guilt, diminished concentration, recurrent thoughts of death, and suicidal ideation (APA, 1994). Because these symptoms are easily missed, a history should be taken from the child as well as from the parents. Depression can be differentiated from "normal" sadness when children report they cannot remember the last time they felt happy or had a good time (**anhedonia**) (Figure 33-3). Children who are depressed need treatment to prevent their depression from

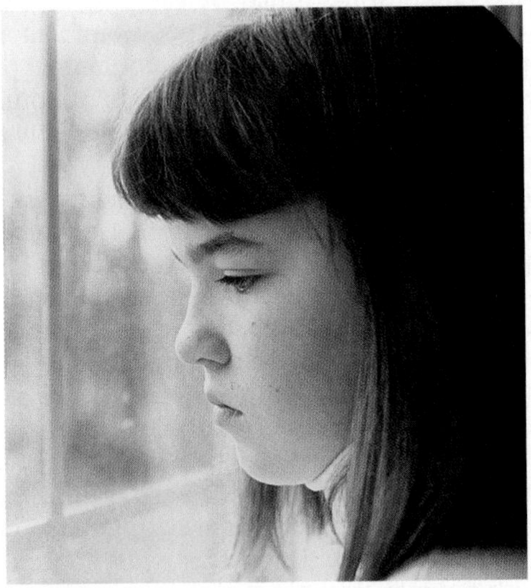

FIGURE 33.3 A school-aged girl showing signs of detachment and depression.

worsening. Counseling to discuss problems is necessary. Tricyclic antidepressants, monoamine oxidase inhibitors, second-generation antidepressives, and lithium carbonate are all used in treatment. In addition to these pharmacologic approaches, family or individual counseling may be necessary to help the child regain self-esteem and the family to understand the level of depression that has occurred. Attempted suicide as a result of depression is discussed in Chapter 12.

Childhood Schizophrenia

Schizophrenia is actually a group of disorders of thought processes characterized by the gradual disintegration of mental functioning (APA, 1994). It is a devastating mental illness that usually strikes at a young age in adolescence or young adulthood. Symptoms during childhood are usually undifferentiated or ill defined.

Over the years there has been a great deal of debate about the cause of schizophrenia. For a long time it was hypothesized that schizophrenia resulted solely from an impaired parent–child relationship. Current research, however, indicates that there is as much a genetic as an environmental basis for this disorder. It may well be that a combination of predisposing genetic factors that produce chemical reactions in combination with poor parent–child communication is responsible for the development of the disorder. The influence of the family on the course of the illness has been the subject of intense research over the past 20 years. Some family environments—for example, those with high **expressed emotion,** or frequent, intense expression of emotion and a critical attitude—have been categorized as those most likely to cause relapse in children with schizophrenia discharged from hospitals. Neurologic studies have shown a linkage between schizophrenia and temporolimbic disease or frontal lesions.

Children with schizophrenia experience hallucinations (hear or see people or objects that other people cannot). They are not responsive (have a **flat affect**) and may withdraw so completely that they are stuporous (**catatonia**). Although schizophrenic manifestations may occur suddenly following a major stress in a child's life (such as rejection by a boyfriend or girlfriend), subtle signs of mental illness have usually been present for some time.

A diagnosis of a psychotic disorder of this extent is a shock to parents. Fortunately, therapy with modern antipsychotic drugs is effective in reducing children's hallucinations and bizarre thinking. Drugs that may be prescribed include trifluopromazine, chlorpromazine, and prochlorperazine. Parents need help to support a child during a long period of therapy. Many children who are diagnosed as having schizophrenia in childhood will continue to have mental illness as adults. Continuing support and long-term follow-up are essential (Marshall, 1998).

KEY POINTS

Both cognitive impairment and mental health disorders pose long-term care concerns for children and their families.

Cognitive impairmemt still carries a stigma in many communities, although less so than previously. Parents may have a more difficult time accepting this diagnosis in their child than they would a physical illness. Help parents to gain the insight that cognitive impairment occurs in a proportion of infants in every population and having a child with this merely reflects a chance occurrence.

Most children who are cognitively challenged benefit from early schooling. Urge parents to enroll children in early education and intervention programs.

Mental health disorders often begin subtly in children, often first manifested as a behavior problem in school. Assess thoroughly any child referred for disruptive behavior in class for the possibility that he or she has a serious mental health problem.

Infantile autism is a pervasive developmental disorder that has a syndrome of behaviors, including fascination with movement, impairment of communication skills, and insensitivity to pain.

A number of disruptive behavior disorders, such as attention deficit hyperactivity disorder (ADHD), may occur in childhood. Such children may be treated with methylphenidate hydrochloride (Ritalin) to reduce the hyperactivity and allow them to achieve better in school and interact better at home.

Eating disorders seen in childhood include pica, rumination, anorexia nervosa, and bulimia. All of these disorders can lead to loss of weight and electrolyte imbalances if left unrecognized and untreated.

Tic disorders (e.g., Tourette's syndrome) are abnormalities of semi-involuntary movement thought to result from dysfunction of the basal ganglia.

Encopresis is the repeated passage of feces in places not culturally appropriate for that purpose. Therapy is both physiologic and psychological.

Schizophrenia may occur in childhood. This usually presents as disorganized behavior. Long-term therapy is necessary. Children who are depressed are at high risk for committing suicide. They need thorough assessment and close observation to be certain this does not happen.

CRITICAL THINKING EXERCISES

1. Todd is the second grader you met at the beginning of the chapter diagnosed with ADHD. His parents feel "at their wits' end" because his attention span is so short and his behavior so disruptive. What suggestions could you make to his parents to help him adjust better to the family routine?
2. A 3-year-old with cognitive impairment is critically ill with pneumonia. It is difficult to believe that her mother did not recognize sooner how ill the child was becoming and bring her sooner for care. Why would a parent have reacted this way?

3. You are asked to teach a health class to a group of seventh-grade girls. The topic is eating disorders. Develop a teaching plan for this class and include suggestions for possible written handouts to be distributed to the class.
4. The parents of an adolescent tell you that he seems increasingly depressed, so much so that he sleeps almost all day on weekends. Does this adolescent need a referral, or is he simply demonstrating usual adolescent behavior? What questions would you want to ask to be able to tell?

REFERENCES

American Psychiatric Association. (1994). *Diagnostic and statistical manual of mental disorders* (4th ed.). Washington, DC: American Psychiatric Association.

Calabrese, E. J., Stanek, E. J., James, R. C., & Roberts, S. M. (1997). Soil ingestion: a concern for acute toxicity in children. *Environmental Health Perspectives, 105*(12), 1354.

Chaney, C. A. (1995). A collaborative protocol for encopresis management in school-aged children. *Journal of School Health, 65*(9), 360.

Department of Health and Human Services. (1995). *Healthy people 2000: midcourse review.* Washington, DC: DHHS.

Gary, F., & Kavanagh, C. K. (1991). *Psychiatric mental health nursing*. Philadelphia: Lippincott.

George, L. (1997). The psychological characteristics of patients suffering from anorexia nervosa and the nurse's role in creating a therapeutic relationship. *Journal of Advanced Nursing, 26*(5), 899.

Happe, F., & Frith, U. (1996). The neuropsychology of autism. *Brain: Journal of Neurology, 119*(4), 1377.

Harrington, R., & Clark, A. (1998). Prevention and early intervention for depression in adolescence and early adult life. *European Archives of Psychiatry and Clinical Neuroscience, 248*(1), 32.

Jankovic, J. (1997). Tourette syndrome: phenomenology and classification of tics. *Neurologic Clinics, 15*(2), 267.

LeBlanc, L. A. et al. (1997). Comparing methods for maintaining the safety of a child with pica. *Research in Developmental Disabilities, 18*(3), 215.

Leekman, J. F. et al. (1997). Tic disorders. *Psychiatric Clinics of North America, 20*(4), 839.

Marshall, L. (1998). Eating disorders. In M. Boyd & M. Nihart. *Psychiatric nursing: contemporary practice.* Philadelphia: Lippincott-Raven.

St. Dennis, C. & Synoground, G. (1996). Pharmacology update: methylphenidate. *Journal of School Nursing, 12*(1), 5.

Walsh, B. T., & Devlin, M. J. (1998). Eating disorders: progress and problems. *Science, 280*(5368), 1387.

Ward, N. I. (1997). Assessment of chemical factors in relation to child hyperactivity. *Journal of Nutritional and Environmental Medicine, 7*(4), 333.

Watemberg, N., & Shaley, H. (1994). Daytime urinary frequency in children. *Clinical Pediatrics, 33*(1), 50.

Weeks, A., & Laver-Bradbury, C. (1997). Behavior modification in hyperactive children. *Nursing Times, 93*(47), 56.

SUGGESTED READINGS

Ardito, M. et al. (1997). Delivering home-based case management to families with children with mental retardation and developmental disabilities. *Journal of Case Management, 6*(2), 56.

Batal, H., et al. (1998). Bulimia: a primary care approach. *Journal of Women's Health, 7*(2), 211.

Field, T. (1996). Attachment and separation in young children. *Annual Review of Psychology, 47*(1996), 541.

Flakierska-Praquin, N., et al. (1997). School phobia with separation anxiety disorder: a comparative 20- to 29-year follow-up study of 35 school refusers. *Comprehensive Psychiatry, 38*(1), 17.

Gorman, M. (1998). Anorexia nervosa. *American Journal of Nursing, 98*(5), 16.

Griffiths, P. & Burns, J. (1997). Continence: a clean sweep . . . childhood encopresis. *Nursing Times, 93*(30), 64.

Rapin, I. (1997). Autism. *New England Journal of Medicine, 337*(2), 97.

Ricchini, W. (1998). For your patients: recognizing eating disorders. *Advance for Nurse Practitioners, 6*(4), 25.

Robertson, M., & Stern, J. S. (1997). The Gilles de la Tourette Syndrome. *Critical Reviews in Neurobiology, 11*(1), 1.

Workman, C. G., & Prior, M. (1997). Depression and suicide in young children. *Issues in Comprehensive Pediatric Nursing, 20*(2), 125.

Nursing Care of the Family in Crisis: Abuse and Violence in the Family

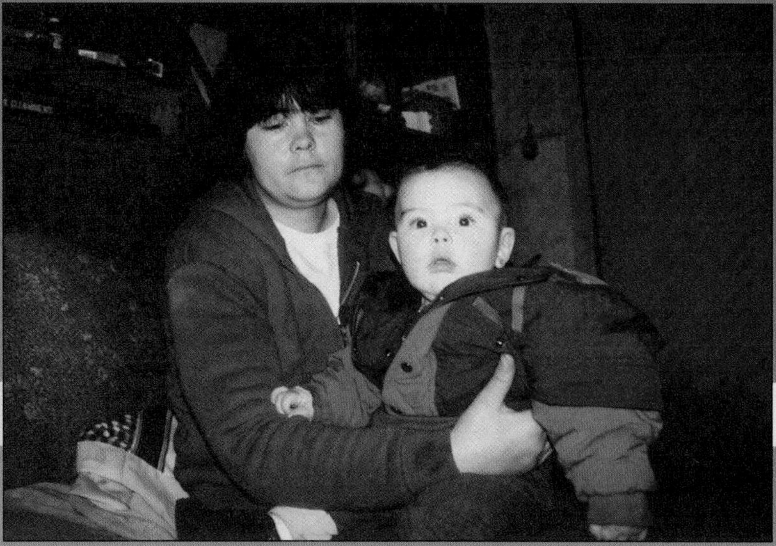

34

CHAPTER

Key Terms

- abuse
- battered child syndrome
- disorganization phase
- domestic abuse
- failure to thrive
- incest
- learned helplessness
- mandatory reporters
- molestation
- Munchausen syndrome by proxy
- pedophile
- permissive reporters
- rape trauma syndrome
- reorganization phase
- shaken baby syndrome
- silent rape syndrome

Objectives

After mastering the contents of this chapter, you should be able to:

1. Discuss the types of abuse seen in families and the theories explaining their occurrence.
2. Assess a physically or emotionally abused family.
3. Formulate nursing diagnoses related to the abused family.
4. Develop appropriate outcomes for an abused family.
5. Plan nursing care for the abused family, such as ways to role model better parenting.
6. Implement nursing care for the family in which abuse occurred.
7. Evaluate outcomes for effectiveness and achievement of care.
8. Identify National Health Goals related to the abused family that nurses can be instrumental in helping the nation achieve.
9. Identify areas related to care of the abused family that could benefit from additional nursing research.
10. Analyze ways that nurses can be instrumental in preventing family abuse.
11. Integrate knowledge of family abuse with nursing process to achieve quality child health nursing care.

Marie is a 3-year-old you see in an emergency room. Her mother tells you that Marie fell off a swing in the back yard. Marie has a broken forearm, a broken rib and multiple bruises on her chest and back. You notice in her chart that Marie was seen in the same emergency room a month ago for a burn on the palm of her hand. When you mention to her mother that Marie's injuries seem extreme for a simple fall, her mother says, "Marie isn't very pretty. I guess she's also clumsy." You suspect Marie may be a victim of child abuse. What questions would you want to ask to determine if this is so?

In previous chapters, you learned about normal growth and development of children. In this chapter, you'll add information about the effect on children when abuse in a family occurs. This is important information because it builds a base for prevention of other abuse.

After you've studied the chapter, turn to the Critical Thinking Exercises at the end of the chapter to help sharpen your skills and test your knowledge.

The increasing incidence of abuse in families is a growing concern in the United States. Abuse is associated with stress and has been linked to the inability of the family to handle external and internal stressors. Accordingly, abuse in the family is rarely an isolated event but rather an indication of how much the family needs care overall.

Abuse, defined as the "willful injury by one person of another" by the researchers who first identified the phenomenon (Helfer & Kempe, 1987), takes many forms—child abuse, which can be physical or emotional and includes neglect and sexual abuse; wife battering or other forms of domestic violence; and maltreatment of the elderly. Maternity, child health, and family nurses need to be especially observant for signs of possible family abuse and prepared to handle this highly emotional and complex problem objectively. It is important, first and foremost, to ensure the safety of the victim, but this must be done with sensitivity to the importance of maintaining and improving overall family functioning.

Abuse has long-term consequences because children from abusive families may become abusive parents themselves. It may lead to a post-traumatic stress disorder. National Health Goals related to child abuse are shown in the Focus on National Health Goals.

FOCUS ON NATIONAL HEALTH GOALS

Abuse of children is a national health disgrace and a national health concern. A number of National Health Goals address this issue:

- Increase to at least 30 the number of states in which at least 50% of children identified as neglected or physically or sexually abused receive physical and mental evaluation with appropriate follow-up as a means of breaking the intergenerational cycle of abuse.
- Reverse to less than 25.2/1000 the rising incidence of maltreatment of children younger than 18 years, specifically, reduce physical abuse to 5.7/1000, sexual abuse to 2.5/1000, emotional abuse to 3.4/1000 and neglect to 15.9/1000 (DHHS, 1995).

Nurses can be instrumental in helping the nation achieve these goals by educating parents about how to parent more effectively and identifying children in school or health care agency settings who have been abused or neglected. Additional nursing research would be helpful for the following questions: Can potentially abusing parents be identified on postpartum units and helped to avoid this? What counseling is necessary for adolescents who have been abused to help them be successful parents? What are the most helpful nursing interventions to use with parents when a child who has been abused is admitted to the hospital?

NURSING PROCESS OVERVIEW

for Care of the Family in Crisis

Assessment

Nurses are often the first people to identify symptoms of possible family abuse because they are often the first to see a child undressed at a health care visit and recognize significant bruising; they are often the person in whom a pregnant woman or child confides about the problem (see Assessing the Child for Signs of Abuse). When abuse in any form is suspected, it is essential to get as full a picture as possible. When child abuse is suspected, talking with parents first, without the child, and then interviewing the child may help to uncover inconsistencies in parents' explanations.

Nursing Diagnosis

Nursing diagnoses associated with abuse should address both the physical and emotional results of abuse:

- Pain related to burn on hand
- Risk for injury related to previous abuse
- Risk for violence, directed at others, related to admitted poor self-control
- Altered parenting related to high level of stress
- Ineffective family coping as manifested by child abuse related to alcohol use by father
- Self-esteem disturbance related to rape

Outcome Identification and Planning

Planning must center first on ensuring the safety of the abused family member and minimizing the effects of trauma. Long-term planning includes helping an abused family member find safe refuge and reestablishing self-esteem through a self-help or advocacy program. Teaching *empowerment,* or the ability to take charge of one's life, is particularly important for older children and women in abusing families.

Implementation

The most important intervention related to family abuse is prevention. Nurses can do much in all settings to promote healthy patterns of childrearing and ways of handling family stress. They can be particularly observant for families who seem to be at risk for abusive behavior. When instances of abuse are uncovered, role modeling is an intervention that can help parents who are ignorant about their children's needs and child behavior. Lecturing is not a useful intervention with any instance of abuse, but supportive education can be extremely valuable.

The following organizations are helpful for referral:

Parents Anonymous
520 South Lafayette Park Place
Suite 316
Los Angeles, CA 90057

National Committee for Prevention of Child Abuse
332 South Michigan Avenue
Suite 1600
Chicago, IL 60604-4357

National Association of State Victims of Child Abuse Laws (VOCAL)
P.O. Box 1314
Orangevale, CA 95662

Women Against Rape
P.O. Box 02084
Columbus, OH 43202

Outcome Evaluation

Nurses are mandatory reporters of child abuse; identifying and reporting this problem is a legal responsibility and an important nursing action. Outcome criteria should focus on specific measures of improved interaction:

- Parent holds baby appropriately and maintains good eye contact.
- Parent admits to losing control with children at home and voices desire to undergo counseling for problem.
- Parent states she has the Crisis Center telephone number by the telephone; parent will call for help if she feels under threat by partner.
- Adolescent states she is able to continue to think of herself with high self-esteem in spite of rape by stepbrother.
- Parent attends monthly meetings of Parents Anonymous.

CHILD ABUSE

As many as 25 to 27 of every 1000 children are reported yearly as being victims of child abuse. As many as 1000 children die every year from abuse. **Battered child syndrome,** a term used by the original researchers in the field to describe victims of severe abuse (Helfer & Kempe, 1987), is one of the leading causes of childhood death and disability. About 10% of all children seen in hospital emergency departments for traumatic injuries (more than 1 million children annually) are victims of abuse. Child abuse is not limited to young children. A major reason that runaway youths leave home is that they have been abused.

Because parenting is not an easy task and good parenting is not an automatic or truly instinctive ability, children in every community are injured because of abuse. Such abuse may be physical (the child is beaten or burned) or neglect (the child is not fed, clothed, supervised properly, or offered medical care or educational opportunities). Abuse may also be psychological or emotional. A number of women who threatened the health of a fetus by drug abuse have been viewed by the courts as child abusers.

ASSESSING the Child for Signs of Abuse

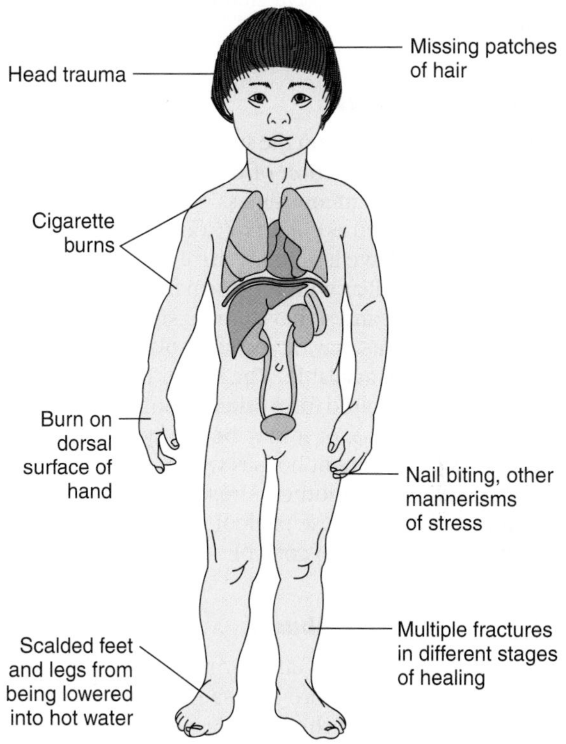

Abuse not only places a child at immediate risk but can also lead to long-term effects. Physically abused children are found to be more angry, noncompliant, and hyperactive than others; they may demonstrate poor self-control and low self-esteem. Children whose parents do not interact with them (emotional abuse) are more withdrawn and have a flatter affect than others. Children who suffer sexual abuse have long-term effects of depression, guilt, and difficulty enjoying sexual relations at the same levels as others. Because the abusive family is a disrupted one, children often have undiagnosed medical problems, such as anemia, otitis media, lead poisoning, and sexually transmitted diseases.

In addition, when children reach adulthood and begin parenting, they may rear their children in basically the same way as they were reared. A concern is that parents who themselves received little love or were abused as children never form a basic sense of trust and so grow into nonloving and abusing parents unless there is effective intervention.

Theories of Child Abuse

The most commonly accepted theory as to why child abuse occurs is that a special triad of circumstances is present or that three factors are generally operating (Helfer & Kempe, 1987):

- A parent has the potential to abuse a child.
- A child is seen as "different" in some way in the parent's eyes.
- A special event or circumstance brings about the abuse.

Parents Who Abuse

Parents who abuse seem, on the surface, little different from others. Only a small fraction of them (probably less than 10%) have a history of mental illness. Many of these parents, however, were abused as children (Coohey & Braun, 1997). Such parents may have less self-control than other parents. They may be unfamiliar with the normal growth and development of children and so have unrealistic expectations of a child. These parents may be socially isolated, with no support people readily available. The isolation may be by distance (a parent separated from other people in a farmhouse miles from neighbors), or it may be the type that exists in communities of apartment houses where neighbors do not routinely speak to one another. Abuse is strongly associated with excessive parental use of alcohol, a substance that removes inhibitions and self-control.

Children Who Are Abused

Abused children are viewed as somehow "different" by parents. They may be more or less intelligent than other children in the family; they may have been unplanned. They may have a birth defect; they may have an attention span deficit. Because the child is perceived as somehow different, a good parent–child relationship does not develop. This is most likely to happen with children who are born prematurely or who have an illness at birth, because they are kept from parents or separated from them by special nurseries or equipment for the first weeks of life, which is when normal bonding occurs.

Special Circumstance: Stress

A third factor in child abuse is stress, which may be a response to an event that would not necessarily be stressful to an average parent. It might be something as common as a blocked toilet, an illness in the family, a lost job, a landlord asking for the rent, or a rainstorm that canceled a planned activity. Child abuse crosses all socioeconomic levels because stress occurs at all levels. Stress generally has a greater impact when people do not have strong support people around them. Families whose internal support system is faulty or who have not formed outside support systems are apt to be families with a higher incidence of abuse.

During a health crisis, parents unable to deal with stress may not show the usual degree of compassion for children's degree of pain or offer to comfort. They may appear more concerned with how the injury affects them than how it affects the child: "This makes me look like a bad parent," not "I should have been more careful."

To prevent abuse, the child may assume a role reversal with the parent or become the comforting, solacing person. These children recognize very early in life that when a parent is upset, they will be hurt. They learn to comfort the parent and reduce the parent's stress and anxiety, thereby avoiding the hurt. The nurse should assess for this during a child health crisis; who is comforting whom?

> WHAT IF? What if you see a 4-year-old with severe burns in an emergency room who keeps telling her mother that everything is all right and that it wasn't the mother's fault, even though the mother reported that she spilled scalding coffee on the child? Is this a typical sign of abuse?

Reporting Suspected Child Abuse

State laws generally identify two types of responsibility in reporting child abuse: **mandatory reporters** and **permissive reporters.** Nurses are included in the mandatory category in most states; this means they *must* report suspected child abuse when they identify it. Failure to do so could result in a fine or possible loss of nursing licensure. The fact that the information was given in a confidential interview does not free the nurse from this responsibility.

All health care institutions and agencies have protocols on how the reporting should be handled. It is important to learn the protocol required in your particular agency, community, and state. After an official reporting of child abuse to an official child protection agency, a health care agency has the right, in most instances, to hold the child for 72 hours for protection to give an appointed caseworker time to investigate if abuse has occurred. Following the 72 hours, a court proceeding will determine whether a child should be returned to the parent's care. Because child abuse is a crime, the health care record of the child can be subpoenaed and displayed in court. Be certain when charting regarding child abuse that you make specific and factual notes (observations, not interpretations). Record conversations with parents in exact quotes when possible. Photographs of physical abuse aid the strength of the testimony of abuse, so these are usually ordered.

A second provision in most states is protection from having a lawsuit brought against a health care provider for reporting suspected abuse that is then proved false. This means it is better to err on the side of reporting suspected abuse rather than not reporting it, from both a child safety and a legal perspective. When abuse is officially reported, parents should be told that child abuse is suspected, because open lines of communication with parents are important to protect the child and to arrange counseling help for the parents.

> ✔ CHECKPOINT QUESTIONS
>
> 1. Are most parents who are child abusers mentally ill?
> 2. What is the triad that makes abuse possible?

Physical Abuse

Physical abuse is the action of a caregiver that causes injury to a child. It is commonly revealed by burns or head and hand injuries (see the Nursing Care Plan).

Nursing Care Plan

THE CHILD WHO HAS BEEN ABUSED

A 3-year-old boy is brought into the emergency department by his mother. "He got into the bathtub and burned himself."

Assessment: 3-year-old male dressed in wool coat and cap carried in by mother. Outside temperature 80°F. Mother's boyfriend present and protesting the removal of the child's clothing for examination. "It's too cold in here for that." Odor of alcohol noted on boyfriend's breath.

On examination, superficial burns noted on lower extremities up to midcalf. Partial-thickness burns noted on plantar aspects of both feet. Area moist with some blistering apparent. Further examination reveals four circular lesions resembling cigarette burns on right arm; large 4-cm ecchymotic area on both buttocks and anterior left thigh. Sharp, pointed, triangular-shaped blistering and inflamed area noted on back of left hand. Mother states circular lesions are "mosquito bites"; mark on hand is a "birthmark." Child remained passive while being examined but drew back when mother's boyfriend approached.

Mother divorced. Boyfriend lives with mother and child in one-bedroom apartment. Mother works as a waitress in a local restaurant from approximately 4 P.M. to 12 A.M. four nights a week. The physician approaches the mother and suggests that the child may have been beaten and burned. She states, "What can I do? My boyfriend is nice enough to watch him while I work."

Nursing Diagnosis: Fear related to repeated episodes of abuse and its effects

Outcome Identification: Child will demonstrate signs of increased comfort.

Outcome Evaluation: Child expresses fears verbally and through play; interacts with caregivers appropriately; demonstrates positive age-appropriate coping behaviors.

Interventions	Rationale
1. Approach the child in a calm manner and provide consistent caregivers for the child.	1. Approaching the child calmly and providing consistent caregivers help to foster a trusting relationship and minimize the child's exposure to stress.
2. Demonstrate acceptance of the child. Offer praise for positive behaviors.	2. All children have a need for acceptance. Praise for positive behaviors helps to reinforce the behaviors and promote the child's self-esteem.
3. Explain all procedures and treatments in language the child can understand.	3. Explanation in the child's terms helps to alleviate additional stress and anxiety associated with the experience.
4. Encourage the child to talk about what happened and incorporate the use of therapeutic play.	4. Talking and therapeutic play help the child express his feelings.
5. Reassure the child that he was not the cause of the abuse.	5. Because of their egocentric thinking, children often assume that they are responsible for maltreatment.
6. Make appropriate child abuse referral to keep child separate from abusing adult.	6. This is both a legal and child protective action.

Nursing Diagnosis: Ineffective family coping, disabling, related to situational stressors

Outcome Identification: The mother will demonstrate a beginning ability to arrange a caring family environment for child.

Outcome Evaluation: Parent identifies contributing factors to abusive situations; verbalizes existence of problem and need for assistance; uses community resources; demonstrates nurturing behaviors toward the child.

(continued)

Interventions	Rationale
1. Institute safety precautions for the child as appropriate. Anticipate the need for removing the boyfriend and/or child from the home environment.	1. Safety is essential for preventing further trauma. Removal is necessary to prevent probable future injury.
2. Approach the mother in an accepting, nonjudgmental, concerned manner. Inform her about notifying the appropriate agency about the abuse as required by law.	2. An accepting, nonjudgmental, concerned atmosphere helps to foster a sense of trust necessary for future interventions and action. Nurses are legally mandated to report child abuse.
3. Assess the situation for evidence of possible contributing factors, and assist mother in discussing events that preceded the incident. Stress her responsibility for making her home safe for her child.	3. Child abuse reflects a family in crisis and in need of help. Discussing difficulties and events in a controlled environment provides a safe outlet for emotion and also helps to increase awareness of the problem.
4. Explore her expectations of the child, listening for any complaints about him. Observe her responses and attitudes toward the child.	4. Exploration and observation provide clues to understanding possible influences on the mother's behavior.
5. Assist mother to view herself as responsible for her own and her child's safety.	5. Accepting responsibility is the first step in initiating change.
6. Review the typical growth and development of a child. Point out positive parenting behaviors, such as bringing the child in for care.	6. Review of normal growth and development helps to provide information and clarify any misconceptions that may have contributed to the abusive situation. Reinforcing positive parenting behaviors promotes feelings of accomplishment and self-esteem.
7. Take time to talk with the mother away from the child, focusing total attention on her.	7. Taking time away from the child to talk allows the mother to be the focus of attention, helping to meet her needs.
8. Explore with the mother about how she responds to frustration. Caution her not to discipline the child when angry.	8. Exploration may help identify the responses that may contribute to abuse. Disciplining when angry increases the risk for violence.
9. Role model appropriate parental behavior. Involve the mother in the child's care as appropriate. Supervise her care as necessary.	9. Role modeling provides the mother with objective examples of behaviors to follow, helping to promote more effective parenting skills. Involvement in care promotes active participation and opportunities for teaching and practicing these skills.
10. Offer praise and reinforcement for sound decision making on childrearing practices demonstrated.	10. Praise and reinforcement for positive behaviors enhances self-esteem.
11. Empathize with the mother about the difficulties associated with single-parent families. Refrain from blaming.	11. Empathy aids in fostering acceptance and trust. Blaming only serves to further deflate the mother's self-esteem.
12. Emphasize alternative age-appropriate methods for discipline.	12. Alternative methods for discipline reduce the risk for violent behavior, enhancing family functioning and promoting the esteem of all family members.
13. Arrange for referrals to appropriate community resources such as hotlines, crisis centers, and parent groups to assist the mother. Refer to social services.	13. Community resources provide additional support and help reduce possible stress. Social services can assist the mother with measures to reduce situational stressors, such as finances and child care.
14. Encourage the boyfriend to seek counseling for abusive behavior.	14. A demonstrated change in behavior is necessary before the boyfriend should return to the family unit.

Assessment

Interview. Always ask parents to account for any injury to a child's body. It is important to remember, however, that most childhood injuries are from accidents caused by the child's inability to distinguish safe situations from dangerous ones or because parents overestimate their child's ability to do such things as lighting a fire to burn trash or using a saw in a wood project. Most toddlers have a number of ecchymotic spots on their legs from bumping into tables or chairs. Some childhood diseases, such as leukemia or purpura, begin with easy bruising. Children with osteogenesis imperfecta will have frequent broken bones as a natural consequence of their disease. Because of inadequate fact finding in these instances, false reports do occur. This can lead to severe stress on a family that has been falsely accused and can interfere with the relationship between parents of an ill child and health care personnel who will then give care to the child (see Focus on Cultural Competence).

When a child has been physically abused, the injury is usually out of proportion to the history of the injury given by the parent (Figure 34-1). The parent may report, for example, that the child was playing underneath the coffee table when he reared up quickly and hit his head, sustaining a large hematoma and temporary loss of consciousness, or that an infant "rolled off the couch" and now has two broken arms. In other instances, the parents may give conflicting stories or can give no reason for the injury ("He woke up from his nap and couldn't move his arm; I don't know what could be wrong").

When questioned about the injury, abused children often repeat the parent's story; this loyalty to parents seems misplaced, but they may fear further beatings or simply believe that living with such parents is better than not having anyone. Ask about behavior problems in school or abnormal behavior, such as constant water drinking, because the constant stress under which these children live can result in this type of manifestation.

It is often difficult to remain emotionally uninvolved and not grow angry when talking to the parents of an abused child. Emotional involvement is not constructive, however; it rarely helps the parents to change, and it may cause them to avoid seeking health care in the future, leaving the child totally unprotected.

Always assume that the parents have done the best they could under the circumstances in which they found themselves. The fact that they have brought the child for care may mean they are seeking help; this may be their way of saying, "Help me; I don't want this to happen again." Child abuse is rarely an isolated phenomenon. Often the mother is also a victim and needs as much help and protection as the child.

Physical Examination. When children are examined at both well or ill child health care visits, be certain they are fully undressed so that their entire body can be observed during the course of the visit. Plot height and weight on a standard graph because these may be delayed in neglected children.

FOCUS ON CULTURAL COMPETENCE

There are some health practices that can be confused with child abuse. Coin-rolling, for example, a type of massage to draw illness out of the body used by Asians, leaves bruises on the back similar to those that would appear on a child who has been struck. Coin-rolling involves heating a coin and then vigorously rubbing it over the body, leaving red welts. Being aware of a practice such as coin-rolling aids understanding of the meaning of illness to parents and prevents false reports of child abuse.

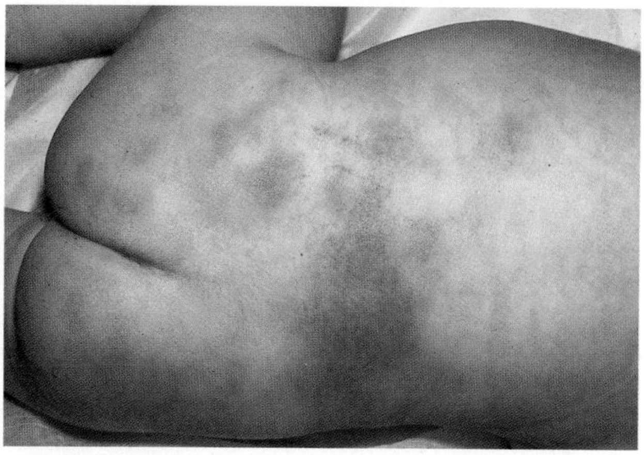

FIGURE 34.1 Large bruises on a child's body. With this type of injury, carefully assessing the history of the accident would be appropriate.

A number of injuries in children clearly signal child abuse. Children who are beaten with electrical cords, belts, or clotheslines have peculiar circular and linear lesions (Figure 34-2*D*). Children beaten with a belt buckle have additional curved lacerations from the imprint of the buckle; few other weapons produce such contusions. Abrasions or ecchymotic areas on the wrists or ankles may be present from a child being tied to a bed or against a wall (Figure 34-2*C*). Most parents protect their children's hands carefully, but children who are abused have a higher incidence of hand injury than others.

Burns or scalds occur frequently in abused children (Figure 34-2*B*). The peak age at which children accidentally burn themselves is 2 years; that of burns related to abuse is 3 years. When children burn their hand by accident, they usually burn the palm; burns from abuse are often on the dorsal surface. Scalding with hot water may be seen. A child placed in a tub of hot water, buttocks first, often has no burn in the center of his buttocks because they touched the tub; a ring of burns causing a "hole in the doughnut" effect appears around this. Young children do accidentally step into bathtubs containing water that is hot enough to burn. When this happens, however, the child usually falls forward and so also has burns on the hands and splash marks on the chest or face. When a child is lowered into scalding water as punishment, only the feet and the skin up to the knees are scalded.

Cigarette burns (see Figure 34-2*A*) are a common finding on the bodies of physically abused children. A fresh cigarette burn causes a blister that resembles the scab of impetigo or pediculosis; differentiation at this stage is often difficult. Impetigo lesions, however, heal without scarring. Cigarette burns and pediculosis heal with a definite circular scar.

Human bites or chunks of hair pulled off the scalp may be present. Head injury is common. Infants can suffer what has been termed **shaken baby syndrome** (Alexander & Smith, 1998). Repetitive, violent shaking of a small

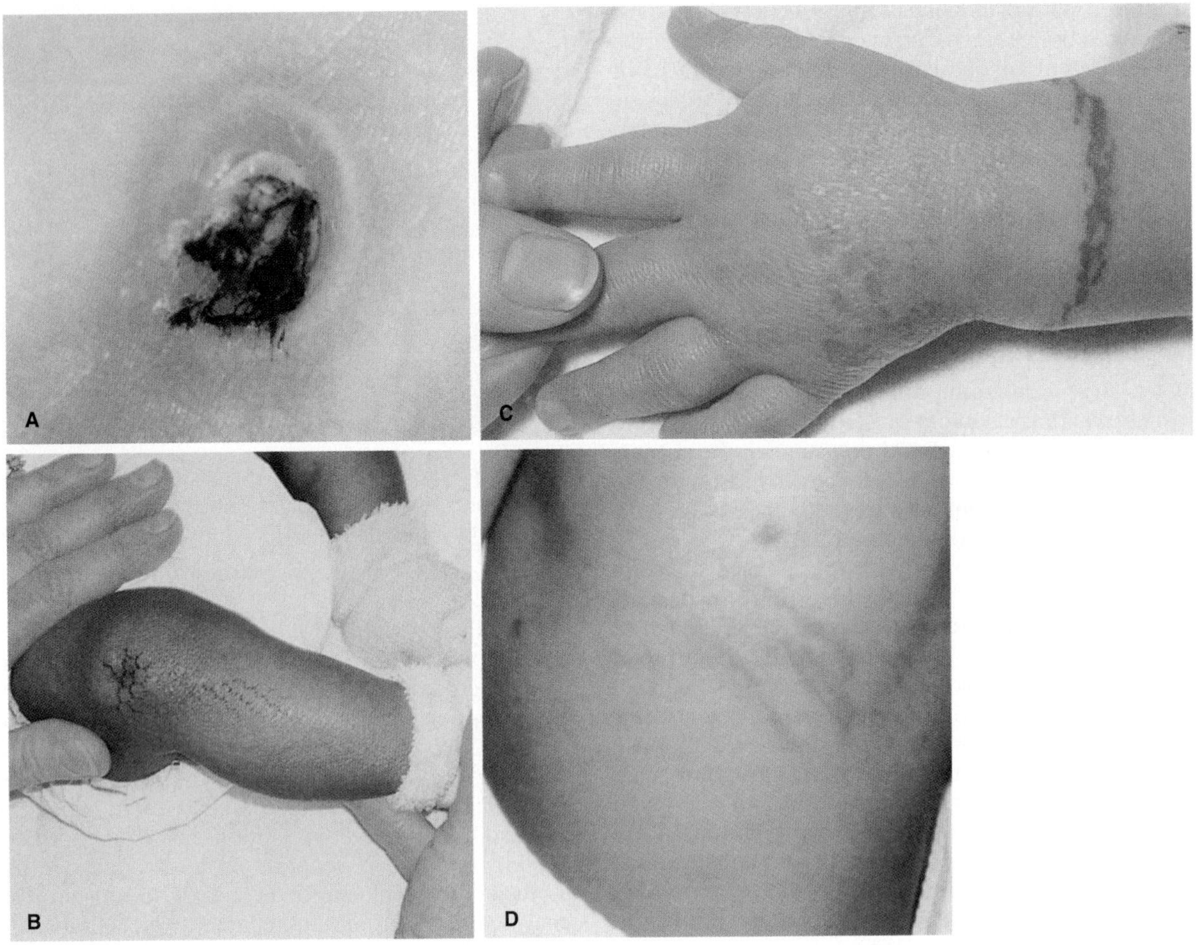

FIGURE 34.2 (**A**) Cigarette burn on child's foot. (**B**) Branding injury showing imprint of radiator cover. (**C**) Rope burn with edema and skin breakdown from being tied to crib rails. (**D**) Imprint marks from beating with a looped electrical cord.

infant by the arms or shoulders causes a whiplash injury to the neck, edema to the brain stem, retinal hemorrhages, and, potentially, a halt in respirations. In extreme instances, the infant may suffer brain hemorrhage and die (Duhaime et al, 1996). This is a particularly insidious form of child abuse because the damage inflicted on the infant is not readily apparent. Increased use of computed tomography scans and magnetic resonance imaging helps to detect these internal symptoms.

Broken bones are another frequent finding (Van Winckel et al, 1997). Children who are preschool age and younger generally do not fall far enough in normal accidents to break bones; a broken bone at this age suggests the child was thrown or struck so hard that the bone broke. Common findings include multiple fractures in different stages of healing, a single fracture with multiple bruises, rib or occipital fractures, and metaphyseal-epiphyseal injuries. Bones are not always broken if a child is shaken roughly, but the periosteum is torn, so the x-ray reveals a strange haziness along both sides of the bone shaft. Tibial torsion (twisting) is often seen (Figure 34-3). Deliberate poisoning is yet another form of child abuse. This usually occurs in a child younger than 2½ years.

Listen to children while they are being examined. If they did not hear the parent's explanation of the accident, they may say something that is not consistent with the parent's explanation of the accident. They may cry little in response to a painful procedure, such as an injection, because they are not used to receiving comfort for pain. They may draw back from an examiner more than the average child would because they are afraid of adults. These are very subjective observations, however, because children react in different ways to the fear involved in a recent injury.

NURSING DIAGNOSES AND RELATED INTERVENTIONS

Nursing Diagnosis: Risk for injury related to documented abuse by parent

Outcome Identification: Child will not experience further abuse for lifetime.

Outcome Evaluation: Child has no further physical injuries identifiable as being inflicted by abusing parent.

Prevent Further Abuse. Ideally, when child abuse is discovered, it would be optimal if the abuser's behavior could be changed and the family kept intact. In reality, once child abuse has been discovered, the child must usually be removed from the home so that no more abuse occurs. Even so, it is impossible to reverse the damage that has been

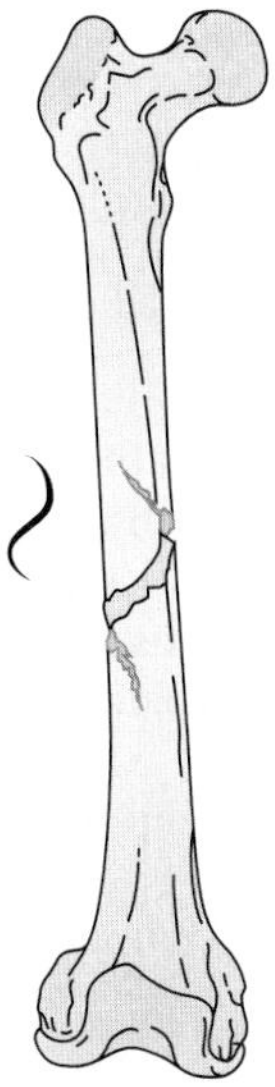

FIGURE 34.3 A spiral fracture around the bone is caused by a wrenching force and is frequently associated with child abuse.

done to the child's sense of trust and self-esteem. The goal of health providers with child abuse, therefore, must be prevention (Box 34-1). Because many child abusers were abused themselves, stopping child abuse in any one generation helps prevent it in the next.

Identifying parents who are potential abusers is a necessary step in prevention. Some parents can be identified as potential child abusers during pregnancy. Listen carefully to the way pregnant women or their partners talk about the child they are expecting. The parent who is overly concerned about the physical appearance or sex of the child ("This had better be a girl" or "He'd better not have his father's nose") may have difficulty accepting a child who does not meet these predetermined expectations. Listen for a parent who is concerned about "not letting children get the upper hand" or who says a child "had better be good." This parent may be conveying worry about how he or she will act when the child is "bad."

A parent may also be identified as a potential child abuser during the early postpartum period. All parents do not immediately bond or react warmly to their newborns. They may tentatively touch or pick up their infants. Be aware of parents who do not touch their infant within 24 hours or makes disparaging remarks about the child's appearance. Risk factors during pregnancy and the early postpartum period are shown in Box 34-2.

Parents may also be identified as potential abusers during health maintenance visits for the infant. By the time a baby is brought to a health care agency for an initial health maintenance visit, a good parent–child interaction should have begun. Listen for parents who say the baby is "nothing but trouble," "cries all the time," or "is bad." Ask new parents how it feels to be a new parent. "I'm enjoying it" is a different answer from "not what I expected" or "it's not much fun." Specific observations to make during postpartum and pediatric health care checkups are summarized in Box 34-3.

Helping parents to seek assistance from adequate support people is another necessary step in prevention. Home visits and clubs of abusing parents, such as Parents Anonymous, can be highly effective in establishing crisis intervention lines so that parents can reach out for help in time of crisis. Interventions that appear promising are home visiting, family counseling, and therapy.

BOX 34.1

MEASURES TO PREVENT CHILD ABUSE

1. Advocate courses for students in high school on parenting and growth and development of children.
2. Help children learn problem-solving techniques so they are not overwhelmed by mounting problems as adults.
3. Foster high self-esteem in children so they are not dependent on others but are self-assertive (they will not become a passive observer to battering).
4. Help parents with responsible reproductive life planning so children are desired.
5. Help parents locate support people in their community, such as Parents of Retarded Citizens or church or social contacts.
6. Teach children to verbalize their problems and to seek help for problems so they do not mount to overwhelming proportions.
7. Role model caring ways with children for parents.
8. Identify children who may be viewed as special in some way by parents (those separated at birth, premature, physically disabled).
9. Identify parents who were abused as children, and offer specific help to them to break a chain of child abuse.
10. Advocate joining Parents Anonymous as an effective support group for parents who may be potential abusers.

Another nursing responsibility aimed at preventing child abuse is helping young parents learn more about normal growth and development of children and how to be better parents (Figure 34-4). Courses in high school that describe sound parenting and review normal growth and development of children and the responsibility involved in parenting are important measures in preventing child abuse. Classes conducted in high-risk prenatal settings might have an impact.

Provide Consistent Care and Support for the Abused Child. A major nursing role in caring for an abused child is supplying a consistent, caring, adult presence for the abused child or furnishing a relationship that the child has never enjoyed.

Use a primary or case management type of nursing care assignment with abused children to offer them consistency and the security of a one-to-one relationship. Many abused children are not used to playing for their own enjoyment but only to the point that a parent wants to play a game; they watch you carefully for signs that you approve of their behavior. They are not used to such activi-

BOX 34.2

WOMEN AT HIGH RISK FOR POTENTIAL CHILD ABUSE OR NEGLECT THAT CAN BE IDENTIFIED IN THE PREGNANT OR POSTPARTUM PERIOD

1. Mother has had frequent changes of address in the year before delivery (more than 2 changes of address in the previous 12 months).
2. Mother has had past or present psychiatric treatment.
3. Likely incompetence of mother as a parent is seen because of apparent emotional problems.
4. Likely incompetence of the mother as a parent is seen because of apparent lack of intellectual ability.
5. Mother has unrealistic expectations of the new child.
6. Mother refused (or dropped out of) prenatal classes.
7. Mother changed her decision regarding adoption of the child.
8. A previous child was abused or neglected.
9. Mother suffered parental violence or neglect as a child.

(Egan, T. G., et al. [1990]. Prenatal screening of pregnant mothers for parenting difficulties. *Social Science and Medicine, 30,* 289; with permission.)

ties as sitting quietly and rocking or talking. Be careful when asking questions to imply that any answer is all right, or they will supply what they think you want to hear rather than the truth. (A question such as, "That feels better, doesn't it?" will be followed by an instant "yes" even though the child feels no improvement in symptoms.)

Evaluate and Promote Family Health. Nurses can be instrumental in helping evaluate whether a child would be safe in the parent's care in the future. When parents who are suspected child abusers visit in the health care facility setting, be certain they are given the same welcome and orientation to the facility and procedures as other parents. When caring for such a child, point out positive characteristics about the child or growth and development markers he or she has reached and realistic expectations of the age because lack of knowledge of normal growth and development may have contributed to the abuse.

For many parents, the response to a charge of child abuse is anger. For others, it is relief; now an unwanted child will be taken away from them. In some families, one of the parents is the abuser; the other is a victim also. The diagnosis of abuse may force the passive partner to make some important decisions about whether he or she wants to continue a marriage or a relationship with the abusive partner. These are not easy decisions to make; if decision making of any kind were easy for this parent, the circumstances probably would never have reached the point where child abuse occurred.

BOX 34.3

OBSERVATIONS TO BE MADE AT POSTPARTUM AND PEDIATRIC CHECKUPS TO DETECT CHILD ABUSE

1. Does the mother have fun with the baby?
2. Does the mother establish eye contact (direct *en face* position) with the baby?
3. How does the mother talk to the baby? Is everything she expresses a demand?
4. Are most of her verbalizations about the child negative?
5. Does she remain disappointed about the child's sex?
6. What is the child's name? Where did the name come from? When was the child named?
7. Are the mother's expectations for the child's development far beyond the child's capabilities?
8. Is the mother very bothered by the baby's crying? How does she feel about the crying?
9. Does the mother see the baby as too demanding during feedings? Is she repulsed by the messiness? Does she ignore the baby's demands to be fed?
10. What is the mother's reaction to the task of changing diapers?
11. When the baby cries, does she or can she comfort him or her?
12. What was (is) the husband's and/or family's reaction to the baby?
13. What kind of support is the mother receiving?
14. Are there sibling rivalry problems?
15. Is the husband jealous of the baby's drain on the mother's time and affection?
16. When the mother brings the child to the physician's office, does she become involved and take control over the baby's needs and what is going to happen (during the examination and while in the waiting room)? Or does she relinquish control to the physician or nurse (e.g., undressing the child, holding him or her, allowing the child to express fears)?
17. Can attention be focused on the child in the mother's presence? Can the mother see something positive for her in that?
18. Does the mother make nonexistent complaints about the baby? Does she describe to you a child that you do not see at all? Does she call with strange stories, such as the child has stopped breathing, changed color, or is doing something "on purpose" to aggravate the parent?
19. Does the mother make emergency calls for very small things?

(Kempe, C. N. [1976]. Approaches to preventing child abuse. *American Journal of Diseases of Children, 130,* 941, with permission.)

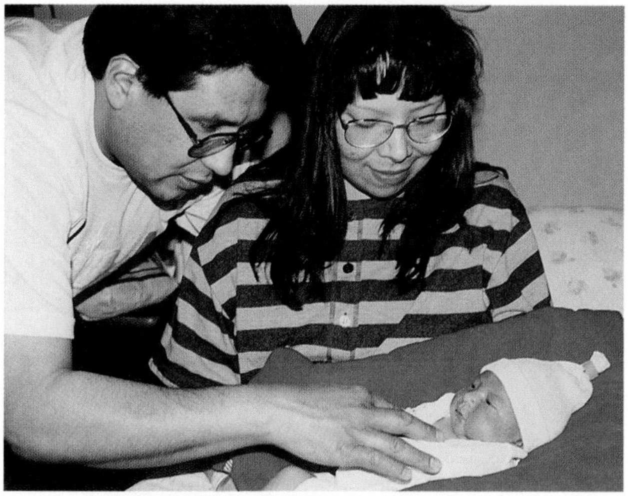

FIGURE 34.4 Teaching that all children have unique characteristics helps to prevent child abuse. Here, new parents explore the already noticeable unique aspects of their newborn.

Praise abusing parents for the things they do well; take time to talk to them away from the child so that your total attention is focused on them. Be certain they are referred for counseling.

Sometimes a child is removed temporarily from a home following child abuse, then returned to the home later when the stress that led to abuse has been removed. Such children need careful follow-up, as parents may revert to an abuse pattern if stress should occur again.

If a child has to be removed permanently from a parent's care, the foster family should visit before discharge from the hospital to make the change less frightening for the child. Children being removed from their parents in this way can feel an acute sense of loss and may grieve for the nonabusing parent or siblings very much. An abused child may also grieve for the abusing parent, especially if the child is convinced that he or she was responsible for the abuse and that the parent really was not to blame.

Evaluation of nursing goals for abused children must include not only whether they are physically safe, but also whether they are developing self-esteem so that they can become adults who do not need role reversal with their children. It should include whether the abuser received counseling and changed his or her behavior.

✔ CHECKPOINT QUESTIONS

3. What is shaken baby syndrome?
4. What is the national organization dedicated to helping potential abusers avoid abusing?

Physical Neglect

Physical neglect is a more subtle form of abuse than physical abuse but can be just as damaging to a child's welfare. A neglected child might appear unwashed, thin, and malnourished or be dressed without mittens, a coat, or shoes in cold weather. In some families, no one has a warm coat to wear or receives enough food because there is no money for these things; that is different from the family in which parents do have these things, but the children or this particular child does not. This type of abuse may be missed by teachers because, never seeing the other members of the family, they believe that all are dressed poorly.

In a health care setting, the difference between one child's care and other family members may be more noticeable. Not bringing a child for immunizations or not seeking early medical care for an infection are other examples of neglect. Not requiring a child to attend school, deliberately keeping a child out of school without setting up a home school program, or allowing a child to go unsupervised after school may also be interpreted as neglect.

Neglect may be willful, or it may occur if parents simply do not realize the normal needs of a child. Such parents need guidance from health care personnel.

Psychological Abuse

Psychological abuse includes constant belittling or threatening, rejecting, isolating, or exploiting the child. Psychological neglect is the absence of positive parenting. Children who are psychologically abused are likely to have difficulty becoming emotionally confident adults. Emotional abuse is the most difficult form of abuse to detect because it may occur only in the home, and its effects, although severe, may be subtle; however, it can be every bit as damaging to the child as physical abuse.

The parent who uses only negative terms to describe a child may be psychologically abusing a child. Be sure to include enough growth and development questions during a health assessment to reveal this, and observe parent–child interaction to determine whether this interaction is positive and healthy or negative and potentially unhealthy.

Munchausen Syndrome by Proxy

Munchausen syndrome by proxy refers to a parent who repeatedly brings a child to a health care facility reporting symptoms of illness when, in fact, the child is well (Bosch, 1997). The parent might report a history, such as seizures, excessive sleepiness, or abdominal pain. The child undergoes extensive diagnostic procedures or therapeutic regimens needlessly. Two classic findings of the syndrome include: 1) the symptoms are not easily detected by physical examination, only by history and 2) symptoms are present only when the abuser is providing care and disappear when care is provided by another person. The parent may deliberately inflict injury on the child (e.g., giving a laxative to induce diarrhea or slowly poisoning the child with a prescription drug). The parent is usually someone with some degree of medical knowledge and tends to stay with the child constantly, offering to give the majority of care. This can be very deceptive because wanting to stay and give care is also the hallmark of a very conscientious and caring parent. Because this syndrome reveals distorted perceptions on the part of the parents, it is almost always necessary to remove the children from the home to protect them.

Failure to Thrive (Reactive Attachment Disorder)

Failure to thrive is a unique syndrome in which an infant falls below the third percentile for weight and height on a standard growth chart or is falling in percentiles on a growth chart. This condition can be divided into two categories: syndromes with organic causes, such as cardiac disease, and syndromes with nonorganic causes that occur because of a disturbance in the parent–child relationship, resulting in maternal role insufficiency. Sometimes both physical and emotional factors play a role in failure to thrive (Steward & Garvin, 1997).

The nonorganic and mixed types can be considered a form of child neglect, although they represent a very complex interplay between parent and child. In many instances, the parent feels little emotional attachment to the child and may have a history of frequent moves and little family support. Often a parent is not offering enough food (parents are not aware of the cues their infants are giving them when they need more food or do not have enough concern for the children to feed them properly). Some infants are offered sufficient food, but the emotional deprivation they sense makes them so lethargic that they do not eat enough. A child may contribute to the poor parenting interaction by being an irritable, fussy, colicky, or difficult-temperament child. In some instances, the child may have neurologic dysfunction from a birth injury and may not respond as a normal child. The mother may have interpreted this lethargic behavior as lack of response to her and so did not carry out her half of the interaction adequately. Failure to thrive must be taken seriously because it can lead to cognitive impairment in the child (Mackner, Starr, & Black, 1997).

Assessment

All children should be weighed at routine health assessments, and their weight should be compared with standard growth curves so that children who are failing to thrive can be identified. Because of little parent–child interaction, there may be accompanying motor and social developmental delays present.

Take a detailed pregnancy history. In many instances, a breakdown in the development of parenting began in the prenatal period. A pregnancy that was unplanned or not accepted; a boyfriend or husband who left during the pregnancy; the death of a close friend or parent; an economic catastrophe, such as loss of a job; or a long distance move during pregnancy are all situations that can cause parenting to develop inadequately after pregnancy.

On physical examination, these infants generally demonstrate some typical characteristics:

- They may appear lethargic and have poor muscle tone, a loss of subcutaneous fat, or skin breakdown (Figure 34-5).
- They do not resist the examiner's manipulation as will the average infant.
- If emotionally deprived, they rock on all fours excessively, as if seeking stimulation.
- They may be more reluctant to reach out for toys or initiate human contact than the average infant.

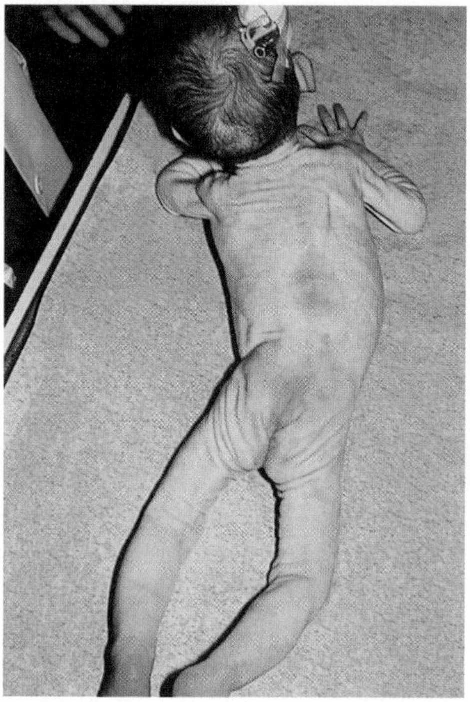

FIGURE 34.5 The child with failure to thrive experiences a loss of subcutaneous fat, muscle wasting, and skin breakdown.

- They stare hungrily at people who approach them as if they are starved for human contact. Some health care personnel experience an uneasy feeling when caring for these infants, because this eye contact is so intense.
- By the second month of life, they demonstrate little cuddling or conforming to being held.
- They achieve developmental milestones in the prone position (such as lifting the head and chest and following an object with the eyes) by the third or fourth month, but show delays in other behaviors that should appear in later months (such as sitting erect, pulling to a standing position, crawling, and walking).
- They demonstrate markedly delayed or absent speech because of the lack of interaction.
- They demonstrate diminished or nonexistent crying.

With advanced failure to thrive, the child's physical condition may be extremely poor; he or she may be nearing acidosis from starvation. If an upper respiratory infection develops, the child's resistance to infection may be so low that it could result in death.

Therapeutic Management

With rare exceptions, children with failure to thrive need to be removed from the parent's care for evaluation and therapy. If admitted to a hospital, studies other than routine admission blood work and urinalysis are usually delayed to avoid submitting these understimulated children to needless pain.

Severe failure to thrive in the early months must be treated rigorously, or it may lead to permanent neurologic damage or leave a child cognitively challenged because of protein deficits and interference with brain metabolism. Infants are placed on a diet appropriate for their ideal weight (the weight they would have been normally for the age). Gaining weight rapidly on this diet is diagnostic that their presenting illness was nonorganic failure to thrive.

NURSING DIAGNOSES AND RELATED INTERVENTIONS

A nursing diagnosis commonly used with children who fail to thrive is Altered nutrition, less than body requirements related to lack of desire to eat or parental neglect regarding nutritional needs. In addition, Altered parenting related to disturbance in parent–child bonding is often appropriate. A care plan designed for the family must be realistic. Parents cannot be made instantly to form a bond with their children, particularly if this lack of bonding has gone on for some time (Hutcheson et al., 1997). On the other hand, one should never give up hope that this will happen. With the proper support and guidance over time and when obstacles to bonding are removed, a healthy child–parent relationship could still develop.

Nursing Diagnosis: Altered nutrition, less than body requirements related to inadequate intake secondary to emotional deprivation

Outcome Identification: Child will take in adequate nutrients for growth by 24 hours.

Outcome Evaluation: Child shows interest in bottle feedings; child is able to establish a regular eating pattern; child begins to increase weight.

Ensure Adequate Nutrition. Keep a careful record of intake and output so that the number of calories being consumed every day is accurate. Assess stools for pH and reducing substances (glucose) to be certain the child is absorbing nutrients. If a stool tests positive for glucose on a Clinistix test or has an acid pH (less than 5.5), it suggests that carbohydrates are not being absorbed.

Evaluate how well the infant sucks or is able to take food from the spoon and swallow. Record any symptoms, such as pulling up the legs or crying after eating, that would suggest gastrointestinal discomfort.

Nurture the Child. Because children with failure to thrive are suffering from emotional deprivation, they need effective "parenting" from nurses who care for them. This does not mean that everyone who passes the crib should stop and play with them for a few minutes. It means that a member of the nursing team should be chosen to be the child's "parent" during the hospital stay (a primary nursing or case management pattern of assignment). It is important that this person be able to spend time rocking, giving a leisurely bath, talking, exposing to toys, and "parenting" the child rather than just giving routine care. Be certain that the person chosen for this role accepts the role and understands that interaction with the child must be active. Passive rocking without talking to the child or paying attention to him or her, for instance, may be no different than the parents' care (see Managing and Delegating Unlicensed Assistive Personnel).

Support and Encourage the Parents. Encourage parents of children with failure to thrive to visit as much as possible while the child is hospitalized; without encouragement, these parents may visit little or not at all. When they do visit, they should feed the child if they want and interact with him or her as they choose. People cannot change their emotional feelings about other people overnight. Telling them that they ought to pick up the baby more or hold him or her more while feeding is ineffective and may only increase the parents' feelings of inadequacy. Giving some suggestions about how the baby tries to communicate with them might be more effective. "Do you know what I think he's trying to say when he stops sucking like that? I think he's saying he's ready to be burped." Pointing out the infant's ability to respond to the parent may be helpful. "Look how he turns his head at the sound of your voice. He recognizes you."

Occasionally, a parent is so distraught by such factors as the illness or death of an older child or relative that he or she is simply unaware of how much energy is being drained by these events. These parents quickly can become good parents to a deprived child as soon as they realize what has been happening. More often, however, the disturbance in a parent–child interaction began so long before or is so great that a parenting bond cannot be established at this point. If the infant is discharged with the parents, parents will need effective follow-up in the months to come to see that they maintain parenting at an acceptable level. There is a very thin line between the child who fails to thrive and one who is abused. Some of these children need to be placed in foster homes for their own safety and to ensure that they receive adequate care.

Evaluation and Follow-Up. Failure to thrive is easy to correct from a physiologic standpoint. When given proper food in a caring environment, the infant usually gains weight rapidly. Adequate follow-up to ensure that the emotional and physical needs continue to be met is a much bigger problem—so big that the answer to the problem of infants who fail to thrive lies not in treatment but in prevention. Parents who may be at risk for poor parenting need to be identified during pregnancy so they can have close follow-up in the postnatal period. At health maintenance visits, secure careful, thoughtful pregnancy histories to elicit information about the psychosocial events that could lead to parenting breakdown. Some parents may need "respite" care for their children when they are overwhelmed by the task of parenting. They may need extended counseling to prevent parenting breakdown. Nurses can be instrumental in all phases of this care.

MANAGING AND DELEGATING UNLICENSED ASSISTIVE PERSONNEL

Unlicensed assistive personnel may be assigned the care of children with failure to thrive in a hospital setting. Be certain that when caring for these children, they understand it is important not to just feed them, but to interact with them to provide for them the type of loving relationship they have never experienced.

✔ **CHECKPOINT QUESTIONS**

5. What behaviors are forms of psychological abuse?
6. What are two classic findings of Munchausen syndrome by proxy?
7. What is the definition of failure to thrive?

SEXUAL ABUSE

Sexual abuse may be broadly defined as any sexual contact between a child and an adult. Adolescents and older children may also be perpetrators. Sexual abuse involves the coercion of dependent, developmentally immature children and adolescents in sexual activities that they do not fully comprehend, to which they are unable to give informed consent, or that violate the social taboos of family roles (Helfer & Kempe, 1987). There may be as many as 360,000 cases of sexual abuse a year in the United States. Although the victims are usually girls, the reporting of male abuse is increasing.

Sexual abuse is physically and emotionally destructive; it leaves children unable to trust others, and they have a sense of ambivalence to intimacy and an overall sense of worthlessness. Children should be taught at an early age that their bodies are their own and to report anyone who tries to touch them in a way they do not like (Figure 34-6).

Meagan's Law requires legal authorities to report when a sexual abuser moves into a neighborhood. Parents need to be aware of this law and insist that it be enforced. If they are aware that a former sexual abuser lives near them, they need to take appropriate precautions to protect their child's safety.

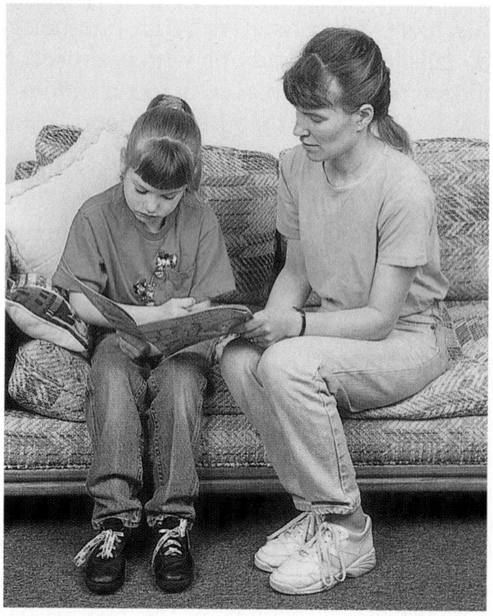

FIGURE 34.6 Teach children that their bodies are their own and that they have to give permission before anyone can touch them.

Molestation

Molestation is a vague term that includes "indecent liberties," such as oral-genital contact, genital fondling and viewing, or masturbation (Haywood et al, 1996).

A **pedophile** is an adult who seeks out children for sexual gratification. In contrast to a rapist, whose crime is violent, the pedophile may be very gentle and limit the involvement to molestation. Such a person is usually a man who suffered sexual abuse as a child and repeatedly selects children who are of the same age at which his abuse occurred. The relationship may involve people with either homosexual or heterosexual orientations. Many pedophiles take photos or videotapes of their activities with children to use for sexual gratification at a later date.

Rehabilitation of pedophiles is difficult because they are fixated emotionally at a childhood level (seeing themselves as children, they do not perceive relationships with children as wrong). Listen carefully to children who report that someone enjoys photographing them; ask children to describe what they mean by someone "touching" or "feeling" them to detect this type of abuse.

WHAT IF? What if a child told you he does not like to stay with a neighbor after school because the neighbor does "funny things"? Would you be concerned? What additional questions would you want to ask him or her?

Incest

Incest is sexual activity between family members. It often involves an older man and a young girl, although it may involve an older woman and younger boy, brother or sister, or same-sex partners. It may involve foster, adopted, and stepchildren. Incest is a deviation from the norm and is so strongly viewed as such by most people that incest taboos are common to most cultures.

Incest causes a great deal of guilt and loss of self-esteem in the abusing and the abused person (Waldman et al., 1997). The abuser is aware that this act is not culturally approved and still is unable to end the relationship; the victim recognizes this act as wrong yet is unable to resist the older person's advances. It is unlikely that other members of the family do not suspect that something wrong is occurring. This leads to guilt and feelings of worthlessness for not being able to protect the child.

Pornography and Prostitution

Pornography is the photographing by any media of sexual acts involving children or the distribution of such material. Child prostitution is arranging or participating in sexual acts with children. Both of these phenomena are demeaning to children. Child prostitution carries the physical risks of sexually transmitted disease and violence, the same as adult prostitution.

Assessment

Signs of sexual abuse are shown in Empowering the Family. The number of reported incidents of sexual abuse rep-

EMPOWERING THE FAMILY: Signs of Sexual Abuse

- A child verbally reports sexual activity with an adult.
- A child has an awareness of sex and sexual vocabulary that is beyond age expectations.
- A child engages in sexual expression with dolls.
- A child younger than 15 years is pregnant.
- A child has perineal, vaginal, or anal inflammation.
- A child has vaginal tears or anal fissures.
- A child has a sexually transmitted disease.
- Symptoms of increased anxiety, such as sleep disturbance, development of tics, nail biting, or stuttering are present.
- A child has a change in school performance, develops a school phobia, or is truant.
- A child expresses fear of being left alone with a certain adult.
- A child develops vague abdominal pain or acting-out behavior.

resents only a small portion of the actual number. Sexual abuse may be revealed on health history (e.g., a young girl worrying that she is pregnant); it may be revealed by a child's abnormal anxiety for a parent to return home from a hospitalization or anxiety about being left with a particular individual in the family (see Enhancing Communication). Young children who are submitted to this type of relationship often have extremely low self-esteem and may envision that they are so "bad" that they deserve to be treated this way.

Allowing young children to play with anatomically correct dolls is a common way of determining whether or not sexual abuse is occurring. Use of such dolls is controversial because there is a concern that without a common protocol for their use, overinterpretation of the child's actions could result. The average reaction of a preschooler or young school-age child who has not been abused is to undress the dolls, giggle for a moment or two about how they look, and then redress or put them aside. The child who is involved in an incestuous relationship makes the dolls perform a sexual act, such as placing the male doll's penis in the female doll's mouth. Asking the child to draw a picture of what happened may also be an effective way of revealing abuse.

WHAT IF? What if a stepbrother rapes his younger sibling? Because they are not blood relatives, is this incest?

Therapeutic Management

Sexual abuse, like physical abuse, is required to be reported. The perpetrator will then be interviewed by the police because this is a criminal offense. It is important that this information be collected in such a way that the adult's rights are respected and the testimony is therefore admissible in court.

Both the adult and child involved in a sexual abuse relationship need psychological counseling—the child to improve self-esteem and the adult to channel sexual expression to less destructive outlets. Improvement is most apt to occur if parents can admit that the abuse has been occurring. To improve the child's self-esteem, it is im-

ENHANCING COMMUNICATION

Cecily is a 4-year-old who is seen at a pediatric clinic for vulvovaginitis. You notice that on history taking, she uses a number of 4-letter words to describe where it hurts.

Less Effective Communication

Nurse: Mrs. Holly? Cecily seems to know some words that are unusual for a 4-year-old.
Mrs. Holly: She gets that from watching cartoons on TV.
Nurse: Cartoon characters don't usually use the words Cecily uses.
Mrs. Holly: We're proud she's advanced for her age.
Nurse: Okay. I just want you to know I think her vocabulary is advanced. Here is the medicine to apply to her bottom.

More Effective Communication

Nurse: Mrs. Holly? Cecily seems to know some words that are unusual for a 4-year-old.
Mrs. Holly: She gets that from watching cartoons on TV.
Nurse: Cartoon characters don't usually use the words Cecily uses.
Mrs. Holly: We're proud she's advanced for her age.
Nurse: Using words with sexual connotations doesn't necessarily mean her vocabulary is advanced. It means she most likely keeps company with an adult who talks to her that way.
Mrs. Holly: That's probably her uncle. He babysits for us once a week.
Nurse: Does Cecily mind staying with him?
Mrs. Holly: A free baby sitter doesn't happen every day.
Nurse: Let's talk some more about Cecily's vocabulary. Especially in light of her infection.

It is often very difficult for families to face the fact that a family member could be guilty of child sexual abuse. In these instances, it is necessary to pursue the subject, rather than let yourself be distracted, to help a parent examine what could be happening.

portant that the adult in the relationship admit the fault is all his or hers. Follow-up care is best done by one of the people who sees the child initially so that he or she does not have to recount the incident to strangers again and again. Whether therapy for sexually transmitted diseases or protection against pregnancy needs to be initiated should be considered.

Parents may need as much counseling as the child so that they can help the child to work through feelings about this situation. In many instances, the offender is a family member, such as an uncle, stepfather, or older brother. Often the relationship has been occurring for some time before it is reported. The parents may feel guilty that they allowed the family member access to the child or did not listen to the child's protestations that she did not like to be alone with this family member. If incest involves a parent, it may be extremely difficult for the parents to continue to relate to each other effectively enough to help the child. All children should be taught some simple rules to help them avoid sexual abuse (see Box 11-1 in Chapter 11).

RAPE

Rape is sexual activity that occurs under actual or threatened force of one person by another. *Forcible rape* is defined legally in most states as intercourse or penetration of a body orifice by a penis or other object. *Statutory rape* is sexual activity with a person under the age of consent (in most states, younger than 18 years) and is considered to have occurred in spite of the apparent willingness of the underage person. *Sexual assault* is used to refer to other forced sexual acts, such as oral-genital or anal-genital intrusion (see Focus on Nursing Research).

A growing phenomenon being reported today is "date rape," in which an individual forces a date or casual friend into having coitus despite a voiced unwillingness. The increasing misuse of flunitrazepam (Rohypnol), a drug easily dissolved in a drink, has led to a rise in date rape (see Chapter 12). It may be very difficult for the victim of date rape to find a sympathetic ear because her companion insists he meant no harm—he simply didn't believe her.

Both rape and sexual assault represent deviant behavior; they are crimes of violence, not acts of passion (Haddix-Hill, 1997). They lack the components of privacy and mutual consent, which are elements of "normal" sexual behavior. Both rape and sexual assault are degrading and dehumanizing and leave the victim feeling completely helpless. Both adolescent girls and boys should be informed about ways to prevent rape (including date rape) (see Box 12-4 in Chapter 12).

Rape has increasingly occurred during the last decade, although it is difficult to determine its actual incidence because so many rapes are unreported. It is believed, however, that the incidence of rape may be as high as one woman in five. Many women want to avoid the secondary, but no less severe, trauma associated with reporting rape. It is hoped that in the future, more sensitive treatment, both socially and professionally, will help to narrow this gap so that more victims of rape can receive the immediate treatment and follow-up care so essential to a complete recovery.

The average rape victim is an adolescent girl, although victims can be any age, and they can be male (Scarce, 1997). In more than half of reported rapes, the rapist is a stranger to the victim, although rapists frequently commit the act in the neighborhood in which they reside. Based on arrest data, the average rapist is a young adult man with a background of aggressive behavior. His motivation generally relates to expressions of power or anger; sexual satisfaction does *not* appear to be a dominant motive. An excessive amount of alcohol intake often precedes rape. Rape tends to be a repetitive, planned activity rather than an isolated event.

FOCUS ON NURSING RESEARCH

How Likely Are Women to Resist Sexual Assault?

For this study, 334 college women were asked whether they thought that if they were about to be sexually assaulted, they would resist the assault. Twenty-one percent of the women surveyed stated that they had been sexually assaulted. Twenty-two percent of the sample said they were "very likely" to resist sexual assault by a stranger with a weapon; 52% would resist a stranger without a weapon. Although the vast majority of the sample had changed their lifestyles to prevent a sexual assault, less than 20% of those surveyed had ever taken a self-defense class. The researchers suggest the need for an increase in the number of women taking self-defense classes and a need to revise young adult women's ideas about resisting sexual assault.

Easton, A. N. et al. (1997). College women's perceptions regarding resistance to sexual assault. *Journal of American College Health, 46*(3), 127.

Assessment

Many rape victims demonstrate immediate physical and emotional symptoms that can last for weeks. The symptoms describe what has been termed **rape trauma syndrome** and generally occur in two stages: disorganization and reorganization. In the immediate **disorganization phase,** victims feel a combination of humiliation, shame and guilt, embarrassment, anger, and vengefulness. They feel that their lives have been completely disrupted by the crisis and that they were unable to protect themselves from the assault. They may tremble from fear and may be in great pain from perineal lacerations. They are apt to start visibly at the sound of anyone approaching or touching them. They need gentle, sympathetic support people with them in the days following the event to allow them to feel safe. They may have nightmares of the attack occurring again. This immediate stage of disruption and disorganization generally lasts about 3 days.

The second stage of rape trauma syndrome, termed **reorganization,** may last for months or years. Many rape victims continue to report recurring nightmares, perhaps sexual dysfunction, and continuing inability to relate to men or face new and surprising situations. They may continue to have a great deal of difficulty discussing the rape.

Many rape victims, trying to outlive this personal offense, change their residence at great sacrifice to finances and lifestyle. If not offered constructive counsel, victims may still feel guilt or shame when thinking about the rape as long as 20 to 30 years later.

When victims do not report rape and thus receive no counseling, symptoms indicative of **silent rape syndrome** can result. When the subject of rape is mentioned, people with silent rape syndrome may grow increasingly emotionally disturbed; it may be evident in their history that they altered their behavior toward men at a certain point in life and perhaps began to resist actions, such as going outside or being alone in a house, after that time. This can be devastating to their ability to maintain employment or remain independent. They need counseling as much as the person who reported a rape.

Emergency Care

Although most large city police forces have special officers assigned to investigate rape charges, victims can be confused and further traumatized by police officers who imply that they provoked the attack or could have at least done more to resist or prevent it. This increases the victim's feeling of shame and degradation. It may be especially harmful to adolescents because people they have been taught to respect have no concept of the degree of fright they have experienced or the strength of their attackers. Health care providers generally are the second group of people victims see following an attack, and they need to be extremely cautious that they do not show any of the same callous behavior.

Most health care agencies where many rape victims are seen have a rape trauma team with specially educated counselors to talk to the victims immediately following the rape and to offer long-term counseling as needed. Nurses serve as important members of such teams and may provide primary care following rape. Any nurse should be able to offer emergency support, because it might be a long time before a specifically designated staff member arrives, and such services are not available in every community.

Because rape is a crime, the hospital chart of a rape victim is often displayed as part of a court procedure. For the victim to bring charges against the attacker, information concerning appearance and history need to be detailed in the hospital chart, so it is important that statements in a chart are accurate and unbiased. When recording a history, quote the victim's exact words whenever possible. Describe the victim's physical appearance carefully, including the presence and location of injuries, such as bruises, lacerations, teeth marks, or abrasions, and the condition of clothing. Ask if the victim bathed or washed before coming for care because this can obscure evidence and obliterate the presence of sperm. Ask if a woman was menstruating or using a tampon. The force of penis penetration with rape can cause a tampon to tear through the posterior vaginal wall into the abdominal cavity, causing an extreme loss of blood. Photographs should be taken as necessary to document the extent of injuries. Any clothing that is ripped or stained should be considered to be evidence of violent assault and should not be discarded.

Following this preliminary observation, a gynecologic or anal examination will be done to evaluate the physical condition of the victim and to document that rape occurred. This is done by recording the existence of any vaginal or perineal lacerations and aspiration of sperm or acid phosphate from the vagina or rectum. Acid phosphate is a substance that is not normally present in vaginal or rectal secretions but is present in semen. The presence of acid phosphate is extremely important if the male is infertile or sterile, because sperm may not be present. Its presence is the best proof that rape occurred. A vaginal and anal culture for gonorrhea and a Pap test are also taken. Blood will be drawn for a pregnancy test and a VDRL for syphilis. Prophylactic administration of antibiotics against gonorrhea and syphilis will be given. If a woman is not menstruating, she may be given oral contraceptives to avoid pregnancy. Victims may have a baseline blood sample drawn for human immunodeficiency virus (HIV) status.

Be certain during emergency care to offer privacy. Many people may want to ask the victim questions, including police officers or detectives, the victim's family, a rape trauma team, and the examining physician or nurse practitioner. Describing the experience is good, but lack of privacy during a perineal examination demonstrates little more concern for self-esteem than the attacker provided. Many female victims are uncomfortable with a male physician examining them after rape because they are temporarily fearful of men. It is helpful if a female nurse remains with the victim during this time, although a male nurse can be equally supportive because it is not the male-female contrast that a victim is seeking as much as an aggression versus caring contrast. Table 34-1 summarizes common tests and procedures for emergency care of rape victims.

Legal Considerations

Nurses working in emergency departments may be asked to testify in court as to the victim's appearance following the assault, although the documentation in the chart is generally all that is necessary. Many victims, especially adolescents, do not press charges against their assailants because they were too frightened or unable at the time to observe the assailant's appearance; therefore, they are unable to identify him later, or they are afraid that by naming him in court, he will return and kill them. Whether victims follow through with a legal action or not is their choice, but the incidence of rape might be reduced if rapists were aware that they are not apt to escape without a penalty for their crime. Taking the rapist to court may be the opportunity and appropriate time for victims to "fight back" and therefore not be as helpless as they were during the attack.

NURSING DIAGNOSES AND RELATED INTERVENTIONS

Nursing Diagnosis: Rape-trauma syndrome related to recent rape

Outcome Identification: Victim will demonstrate adequate coping behavior and eventually return to precrisis level of functioning.

Outcome Evaluation: Victim is able to discuss what happened to and intense feelings about the crime; victim voices ability to go forward with life.

TABLE 34.1 Common Specimen Procedures Following Rape*

PROCEDURE	PURPOSE
Oral washing	Client rinses mouth with 5 mL sterile water; collected in test tube. Analyzed for blood group antigens or sperm of attacker.
Fingernail scraping	Scrape under all of client's fingernails, and place scrapings in envelope. Analyzed for blood, skin, and clothing fibers of attacker.
Blood VDRL, HIV and HBsAg	Draw blood for antibody titer for syphilis, human immunodeficiency virus, and hepatitis B.
Blood typing	Client's blood is typed to differentiate it from attacker's type.
Pregnancy test	Either blood or a urine specimen may be obtained. Vaginal examination should be completed before woman voids.
Hair samples	Both scalp and pubic hairs of client (about 10) are removed for comparison with attacker's and placed in envelope.
Vaginal smear	Vagina is swabbed with dry applicator and smeared onto slide. Allow to dry for analysis of sperm.
Gonococcus smear	Cervix, vagina, rectum are cultured (also throat is cultured if oral coitus was attempted).
Vaginal washing	5 mL of sterile saline is placed in vagina and aspirated. Analyzed to detect sperm and acid phosphate.
Skin washings	Touch any dried stain of blood or semen on skin or clothing with a moistened cotton swab; drop into test tube. Analyzed for attacker's blood and semen.
Clothing care	Place any clothing stained or torn into a paper bag. Evidence of violent attack.

* Label all specimens carefully as to where they were obtained for medical therapy and legal evidence.

One of the major needs of any victim following a violent act is to talk about what happened. A person who can describe an incident begins to "put a fence around" or "contain" the event. This process brings the event down from "something terrible that has happened," a situation that leaves a person with a continuing high anxiety level, to "this specific thing has happened," a situation that allows the traumatic event to be examined and handled. Something that is concrete and describable is rarely as frightening as "something out there." This also applies to rape.

Ask the victim to describe the incident to you with an introduction such as, "Most people find it helps to talk about what happened to them." Table 34-2 lists areas to explore with victims to help them reduce the incident to a size they can begin to handle.

Victims should be given the number of a counseling service to telephone before they leave an emergency department. Because genital bruising may not be apparent until 24 hours after the rape, they may be asked to return for a reexamination the next day so this can be documented. Syphilis will not be apparent for up to 6 weeks in serum, so they should return for a repeat VDRL at that time. They may be advised to return in 6 weeks for HIV testing also. Be certain that victims have a support person to accompany them home and that they are aware that if their distress becomes acute, they can return as needed to the health care facility

TABLE 34.2 Areas to Explore in Rape Counseling

AREA	CONSIDERATIONS
The event	Where did the attack occur? What was happening at the time? This information is important for the victim to discuss and work through; otherwise, any time she is in similar circumstances again, she may have uncontrollable fears related to the attack. Walking home from school or waiting for an elevator in a public building are everyday actions that she will do often during her life. If she was raped in these circumstances, she can be assured that she was acting sensibly and that the rape was not her fault.
The assailant	Allowing an adolescent to review the description of the rapist may help her to realize that she may react in negative ways in the future to a man with the same build or description. The man may have approached her with a simple gesture, such as a hand on her shoulder. Others will perform this gesture again. She must work through her revulsion to handle it when it occurs in friendly circumstances.
The conversation	Describing the conversation with the rapist helps the adolescent to convince herself that she did not provoke the attack.
Details of the assault	Describing the actual assault is extremely difficult for most adolescents, but doing so allows them to work through it. Until they can describe the attack or the sexual act to which they had to submit, they may have difficulty in performing these same acts with persons of their choice.
Resistance to the assault	Many adolescents do not struggle during an assault because they realize that it could result in further harm to them. If someone asks them what they did to try to fight off the assailant, adolescents may feel again that they provoked or agreed to the attack. Reassure them that no action was probably the best action and the reason they are still alive. To improve self-esteem, counsel adolescents that rape is a violent crime and that usually the strength of an attacker is far too great for any female to resist effectively.

for additional care or counseling. Inform them about any local support groups that may provide follow-up counseling for victims of rape. One such organization, Women Against Rape, is active in many communities.

Nursing Diagnosis: Ineffective family coping, disabling, related to recent rape of family member

Outcome Identification: Victim's partner and family will develop adequate coping mechanisms to be able to support victim.

Outcome Evaluation: Partner or other family members are able to express their feelings about the rape to health care provider; they state confidence in their ability to support rape victim.

In many instances of rape of a woman, the victim's usual sexual partner has difficulty being a support person to her because he has as much difficulty dealing with the occurrence of rape as she does. Not infrequently, a relationship that was meaningful before the rape will deteriorate as a result of a sexual partner seeing the victim as now "soiled" or mistakenly believing that the victim was somehow responsible for the trauma or actually enjoyed the experience. In other instances, a usual sexual partner may become so overprotective following the incident (not allowing the victim to go out alone any longer; checking on her constantly) that she is not free to maintain her identity. The man may be so filled with vengefulness and anger that he cannot effectively relate to her without his anger surfacing toward her as well as toward the attacker. Parents of a young adolescent may feel this same way. Counseling for the victim's partner or family may help them to be truly supportive (Box 34-4).

BOX 34.4

GOALS OF CRISIS INTERVENTION FOR FAMILIES OF RAPE VICTIMS

- Helping the family to express openly their immediate feelings in response to a rape as a shared life crisis
- Helping the family to be supportive of and reassuring to the victim
- Helping the family work through immediate practical matters and initiate problem-solving techniques
- Helping the family develop cognitive understanding of what the rape experience actually means to the victim and to the family
- Explaining the possibility of future psychological and somatic symptoms that characterize a rape trauma syndrome and what the family can do to minimize these symptoms
- Activating qualities characteristic of healthy family functioning during the impact and resolution phases of the shared crisis
- Educating the family about rape as a *violent crime,* not a sexually motivated act, and eliminating focus on the victim's guilt or responsibility
- Eliminating the family's sense of guilt for not protecting the victim by assuring them that they could not have anticipated or prevented the rape
- Discouraging violent, destructive, or irrational retribution toward the rapist (under the guise of being on the victim's behalf) by encouraging a sharing of feelings of helplessness, sadness, hurt, and anger
- Encouraging discussion of the sexual relationship between partners; suggesting that the man let the victim know (a) that his feelings have not changed (when this is true) and that he still sexually desires her, (b) that he will wait for her to approach him, and (c) that sex therapy is available if they have difficulties that persist and want assistance in reestablishing normal sexual relations
- Explaining the possibility of sexually transmitted disease and pregnancy that may result from a rape, the preventive care necessary for the victim and spouse or boyfriend, and the follow-up care indicated
- Explaining that early crisis intervention often prevents long-term problems in resolving the crisis and that to seek counseling at this time does not imply mental illness (specify that crisis intervention usually lasts for 3–6 hours during the first few weeks post-rape)
- Referring the family for direct counseling when members' shared responses to the crisis interfere with their ability to cope adaptively
- Providing factual data, resource lists for counseling, and follow-up care *in writing* (because highly stressed persons do not hear or recall information verbally communicated)
- Letting families know that some decisions, such as whether to prosecute the rapist or move to a safer residence, can be postponed while more immediate needs, such as medical care, are taken care of. (This action helps the family (1) set priorities and organize decisions about what has to be done now and (2) gain emotional distance from the urgency and confusion felt during a crisis state to permit sound decision making later.)
- Identifying how the family has handled crises in the past and encouraging members to use adaptive coping mechanisms for this crisis
- Encouraging contact with persons identified as supportive to the family and offering to contact such persons
- Assigning a primary nurse to spend time talking with the family in the emergency department waiting room while the victim receives medical care
- Allowing time for thoughts and feelings in a decision-making process
- Using empathic listening to convey understanding of the family's feelings and concerns
- Asking if the nurse can check back with the family the next day to see how they are getting along and answer any questions they may have

CHECKPOINT QUESTIONS

8. What is a pedophile?
9. Is rape a crime of passion or violence?

DOMESTIC ABUSE

Domestic abuse is abuse by a family member against other individuals living in a household (i.e., spouses, children, parents, or grandparents). The fact that spousal abuse and child abuse may both exist in a family strengthens the necessity for nursing care to be family centered so that both these situations can be identified and halted. Children raised in such a family learn that violence is an acceptable method of managing aggression and perpetuate it to the next generation.

Like child abuse, this transcends all ethnic and social groups. If it appears to be more prevalent in the lower socioeconomic classes, it is because families at this level are more visible to service organizations and law enforcement officials. When wife battering occurs in middle or upper class houses, wives are often too embarrassed to let people know and keep the violence hidden longer.

Theories About Domestic Abuse

Violent family situations can be divided into two groups: those in which violence preceded the marriage or children and those in which the violence developed following the marriage or children. In the first and most frequently appearing group, although a woman may be the offender, violence is usually brought into the family by a man with a history of violence. His violence-prone characteristics usually erupt early in the courtship and grow progressively worse. He uses violence to handle any conflict and provokes a pervasive feeling of powerlessness in people around him. Such men usually have a history of early and prolonged exposure to family violence as children; alcohol is frequently associated with the expression of violence.

Spouses in the first group react to their situation in three phases (Table 34-3). During stage I, a light level of abuse, referred to as the *impact phase,* the woman uses denial as a defense mechanism. If she does not end the relationship at this point, abuse grows more frequent and more violent (by not stopping it, the woman is indirectly giving it permission to continue). During this second stage, she can no longer deny that the violence is occurring. At the same time, she cannot stop it because the violence is not provoked by her; she is only a convenient recipient of poorly controlled violent behavior. She is forced to use coping mechanisms, such as becoming very obedient and cooperative and doing everything her husband asks, in a desperate effort to reduce the violence. This phase is termed *psychological infantilism* or **learned helplessness.** The level of abuse can continue until the woman is being almost constantly physically abused (stage III). A fetus is in danger if abuse of a pregnant woman occurs at this stage. During this stage, the woman is forced to become isolated; she sinks into hopelessness and depression. She has difficulty seeking help because she is unable to believe that outside people might want to help her.

TABLE 34.3 Levels of Spouse Abuse

LEVEL	DESCRIPTION
I	Abuse is occasional; consists of slapping, punching, kicking, verbal abuse. Contusions occur.
II	Abuse is becoming more frequent; beatings are sustained and cause fractures, such as a broken jaw or rib fracture.
III	Abuse is even more frequent, perhaps daily. A weapon, such as a gun, baseball bat, or broom handle, may be used. Permanent disability or death from injuries, such as intracranial hemorrhage or concussion, may occur.

For women in the second violent family situation, violence occurs as a last resort when all other attempts at communication have failed. The behavior of one partner threatens the psychological defenses of the other, and each projects his or her feelings and shortcomings onto the other. Such a situation, however, is not typical of spouse abuse. In most instances, battered women marry husbands who bring violence into the family (Brookoff et al, 1997).

Assessment

When any type of abuse against an individual family member is identified, it is important to investigate further for evidence of abuse against other family members. Asking about the possibility of spouse abuse should be a priority with any woman seen for trauma. As many as 20% to 25% of women seen in emergency departments for trauma have been battered. Common injuries suffered by abused women are burns, lacerations, bruises, and head injury. Asking all women at physical examinations to account for any bruise they have helps detect this. Asking them if they are ever concerned about their safety or well-being helps detect emotional abuse (Limandri & Tilden, 1996).

Therapeutic Management

It may be difficult to understand how adults can tolerate abuse against themselves or their children. It is important, however, not to blame the victims. Hopelessness and powerlessness are consequences of continual abuse. Battered and emotionally abused individuals are often immobilized by a sense of guilt: They feel that if they were better people, their partners would not resort to beatings or verbal badgering. Because victims may have no access to money and no skills to earn any, they need a great deal of support to be able to leave their partners. Even if they have a skill and have supported themselves in the past, their self-esteem may be so low that they no longer believe they are able to put the skill to use. As the abuse becomes more violent, they may be afraid that their abusers will follow and kill them and their children if they leave. Other extended family members may be unwilling to shelter the victims for fear of being included in the violence. An important role for nurses is helping an abused family find a shelter where they can feel safe. Treatment for abusers needs to be scheduled, but safety is the first priority.

CHECKPOINT QUESTIONS

10. What is a prime reason that battered women do not seek help early in an abusive relationship?
11. What should be the first responsibility for nurses when domestic abuse is suspected?

KEY POINTS

At least 10% of children seen for traumatic injury received their injury from child abuse. A high suspicion for abuse should be present when burns, head injury, or rib fractures are present or when the history of the accident seems out of context for the injury.

Child abuse may exist in many forms. It may be physical, emotional, or sexual and may encompass neglect and abuse.

In infants, a "shaken baby syndrome" results in retinal or intracranial hemorrhage. Babies with this syndrome may appear groggy or unresponsive in an emergency department.

A triad of a "special parent, special child, special situation" is characteristic of the family in which child abuse occurs.

Failure to thrive is a syndrome in which an infant falls below the third percentile for weight and height on a standard growth chart. It is associated with a disturbance in the parent–child relationship.

Children who comfort parents in emergency settings may just be sensitive children, or they may be demonstrating "role reversal," a behavior characteristic of abused children.

In families in which a child is abused, the mother may also be a victim of abuse. Ask enough questions at health care visits to be certain that this problem does not exist as well.

Child abuse is legally reportable. Nurses can initiate reporting as an independent action or through their health agency's referral network.

Methods to prevent abuse in which nurses can actively participate include teaching about the expected growth and development of children, educating teenage parents for parenting roles, and teaching "empowerment," or a sense that children and adults have control of their own lives.

Sexual abuse of children can be prevented by teaching children to recognize abnormal advances and to know it is right to speak out about wrongs against them.

Abuse is a family, not an individual, problem. Therapy must include all family members to be effective.

Rape is a crime of violence, not of sexual intent. Rape victims need both short-term and long-term counseling.

CRITICAL THINKING EXERCISES

1. Marie is the 3-year-old you met at the beginning of the chapter. Although her mother told you that Marie fell from a swing, Marie has a broken forearm, a broken rib, and multiple bruises on her chest and back. Her mother tells you, "Marie isn't pretty. I guess she's also clumsy." What questions would you want to ask to determine if Marie has been abused?
2. You weigh a baby at a well child conference and discover that the infant's weight is below the second percentile on a standardized growth chart. What questions would you want to ask the mother to see if you can account for this? What particular areas would you want to assess on a physical examination?
3. A 4-year-old is seen in an ambulatory clinic for a purulent vulvovaginitis. A culture reveals this is from gonorrhea. What questions would you want to ask the child to determine how she contracted this? Suppose her parents are influential people in your community. Would this influence what questions you ask?

REFERENCES

Alexander, R. C., & Smith, W. L. (1998). Shaken baby syndrome. *Infants and Young Children, 10*(3), 1.

Bosch, J. J. (1997). Munchausen syndrome by proxy. *Journal of Pediatric Health Care, 11*(5), 252.

Brookoff, D. et al. (1997). Characteristics of participants in domestic violence: Assessment at the scene of domestic assault. *Journal of the American Medical Association, 277*(17), 1369.

Coohey, C., & Braun, N. (1997). Toward an integrated framework for understanding child physical abuse. *Child Abuse & Neglect, 21*(11), 1081.

Department of Health and Human Services. (1995). *Healthy people 2000: Midcourse review*. Washington, DC: DHHS.

Duhaime, A. C. et al. (1996). Long-term outcome in infants with the shaking-impact syndrome. *Pediatric Neurosurgery, 24*(6), 292.

Easton, A. N. et al. (1997). College women's perceptions regarding resistance to sexual assault. *Journal of American College Health, 46*(3), 127.

Haddix-Hill, K. (1997). The violence of rape. *Critical Care Nursing Clinics of North America, 9*(2), 167.

Haywood, T. W. et al. (1996). Cycle of abuse and psychopathology in cleric and noncleric molesters of children and adolescents. *Child Abuse and Neglect, 20*(12), 1233.

Helfer, R. E., & Kempe, R. S. (1987). *The battered child.* Chicago: University of Chicago Press.

Hutcheson, J. J. et al. (1997). Risk status and home intervention among children with failure-to-thrive: follow-up at age 4. *Journal of Pediatric Psychology, 22*(5), 651.

Limandri, B. J., & Tilden, V. P. (1996). Nurses' reasoning in the assessment of family violence. *Image: The Journal of Nursing Scholarship, 28*(3), 247.

Mackner, L. M., Starr, R. H., & Black, M. M. (1997). The cumulative effect of neglect and failure to thrive on cognitive functioning. *Child Abuse and Neglect, 21*(7), 691.

Scarce, M. (1997). Same-sex rape of male college students. *Journal of American College Health, 45*(4), 171.

Steward, D. K., & Garvin, B. J. (1997). Nonorganic failure to thrive: a theoretical approach. *Journal of Pediatric Nursing, 12*(6), 342.

Van Winckel, M. et al. (1997). Radiological case of the month: battered child syndrome. *Archives of Pediatrics and Adolescent Medicine, 151*(6), 621.

Waldman, T. L. et al. (1997). The adult personality of childhood incest victims. *Psychological Reports, 80*(2), 675.

SUGGESTED READINGS

Bryk, M., & Siegel, P. T. (1997). My mother caused my illness: The story of a survivor of Munchausen by proxy syndrome. *Pediatrics, 100*(1), 1.

Edgar, C. (1997). Surviving workplace trauma. *Lamp, 54*(8), 15.

Elliott, M. et al. (1995). Child sexual abuse prevention: what offenders tell us. *Child Abuse and Neglect, 19*(5), 579.

Janikowski, T. P., Bordieri, J. E., & Glover, N. M. (1997). Client perceptions of incest and substance abuse. *Addictive Behaviors, 22*(4), 447.

Ledray, L. E., & Netzel, L. (1997). DNA evidence collection. *Journal of Emergency Nursing, 23*(2), 156.

Lopez, R. F., & Schumann, L. (1997). Clinical health problem: Failure to thrive. *Journal of the American Academy of Nurse Practitioners, 9*(10), 489.

Mahony, C. (1997). Babies, bruises and black eyes. *Nursing Times, 93*(51), 14.

Mitchell, M. K. (1997). Domestic violence: teaming communities with providers for effective intervention. *Advanced Practice Nursing Quarterly, 2*(4), 51.

Patterson, M. M. (1998). Child abuse: assessment and intervention. *Orthopaedic Nursing, 17*(1), 49.

Rivara, F. P. et al. (1997). Alcohol and illicit drug abuse and the risk of violent death in the home. *Journal of the American Medical Association, 278*(7), 569.

Ruzicka, M. F. (1997). Predictor variables of clergy pedophiles.

Nursing Care of the Family Coping With Long-Term or Fatal Illness

35

CHAPTER

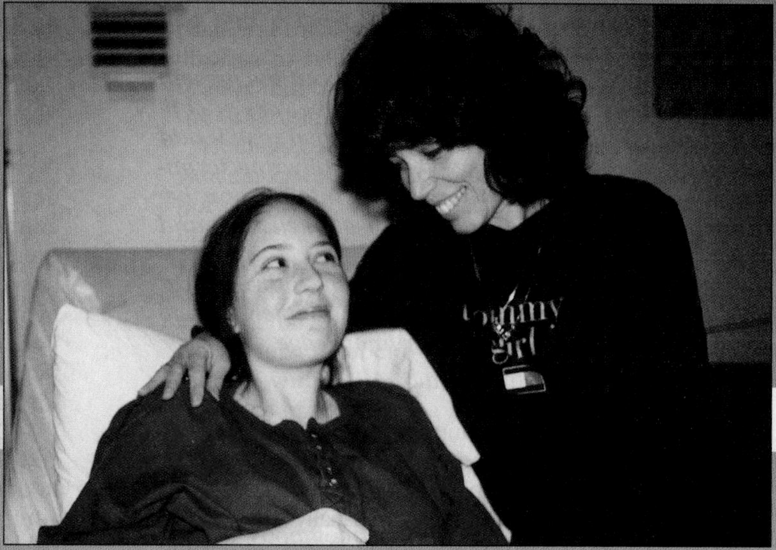

Key Terms

- **anticipatory grief**
- **death**
- **grief process**
- **vulnerable children**

Objectives

After mastering the contents of this chapter, you should be able to:

1. Describe common concerns of parents of children with a long-term or fatal illness.
2. Assess adjustment of the child and family with a long-term or fatal illness.
3. Formulate nursing diagnoses for the child with a long-term or fatal illness.
4. Identify outcomes for the child with a long-term or fatal illness.
5. Plan nursing care for the child with a long-term or fatal illness.
6. Implement nursing care for the child with a long-term or fatal illness.
7. Evaluate outcome criteria to be certain that nursing goals established for care were achieved.
8. Identify National Health Goals related to children with long-term or fatal illnesses that nurses could be instrumental in helping the nation achieve.
9. Identify areas related to care of the child with a long-term or fatal illness that could benefit from additional nursing research.
10. Use critical thinking to analyze ways that nursing care of the child with a long-term or fatal illness can be more family centered.
11. Integrate knowledge of long-term and fatal illness in children with nursing process to achieve quality child health nursing care.

- Parents state realistic plans for their child regarding school placement.
- Parents state they have been able to deal with their grief over child's diagnosis to maintain normal family functioning.
- Parents state they are able to cope with present stressors.
- Child states he or she is aware illness is chronic but thinks of himself or herself as a person able to accomplish many things in life.

THE CHILD WITH A DISABILITY OR CHRONIC ILLNESS

Because families have different resources and everyone reacts to situations differently, each child with a long-term illness or disability and his or her family need to be assessed for the potential to cope and provide necessary care. Through such assessment, appropriate interventions to help the family adapt can be started early in the course of the illness.

The Parents' Adjustment

Grief Reaction

Parents can be expected to experience a **grief process** or regulated steps in grieving when they are told their child will be disabled or is fatally ill (Kübler-Ross, 1969). Table 35-1 summarizes the stages of a grief reaction. Most parents with a disabled child never arrive at a full stage of acceptance; for parents with a fatally ill child, this may come only with the child's death.

During the first period of grief (shock or denial), parents are unable to plan past short-term goals (learning to change a dressing or which pills to give each day). Trying to establish long-term goals at this point (what type of school the child will attend, the vocations that are open to him or her) is useless because it all must be done again when parents are truly ready to look this far ahead. During the stage of anger, parents may be unwilling to learn (the whole thing is so unfair; planning is asking too much of them; how can they trust you? If you were really helpful, you would cure their child). This is a time of waiting also; the nurse should hold back advice until parents are more ready to accept it. During the bargaining stage of grief, parents are still not ready for planning. If their bargain is fulfilled (let their child be able to walk, and they will spend the rest of their life doing good), the plans they make now would have to be modified later.

During the next stage of grief—depression—parents are ready to make plans but need a great deal of help in planning. Be careful in working with people who are depressed that you do not totally plan for them rather than with them. Many parents of disabled children have low self-esteem (they believe if they were really good people, they would have had a normal child). This makes them feel that your suggestions must be better than any they could make. After they return home, however, they are the people who must live with these plans and so should participate in making them. Young adults with disabilities show an above-average incidence of depression, probably from the chronic stress of the disability on their life, part of which occurs from poor planning.

Some parents need guidance in making plans to prevent them from becoming so self-sacrificing that they ignore the needs and wishes of a marriage partner and other children (they will spend every waking moment with the ill child). Being a martyr is a way of easing guilt, a part of grief bargaining, a way of proving that they are equal to others—perhaps even the best parents in the entire world. These parents need time to talk about possible reasons why they feel they must push themselves in this manner. Perhaps they can find a middle-of-the-road approach to a child's care that allows time for all family members. Helping them plan a respite from the care of a sick child, such as an evening out while a babysitter cares for the child, is a part of this (Coyne, 1997).

WHAT IF? What if you arrange for a parent to spend an afternoon shopping so she can have some respite time away from an ill child and she spends the time cleaning her kitchen cupboards instead? Is this a good use of respite time?

By the time a disabled child is of school age, parents should begin to make some concrete plans as to who will care for the child when they die. This is very difficult for parents; it asks them to contemplate their own death (something that people rarely want to do) and the vulnerability of children when it occurs. They might consult

TABLE 35.1 Stages of Grief

STAGE	PARENTS' REACTION	DESCRIPTION
1	Denial	Parents have difficulty realizing what has occurred. They ask, "How could this have happened?"
2	Anger	Parents react to the injustice of being singled out this way. They say, "It isn't fair this is happening."
3	Bargaining	Parents attempt to work out a "deal" to buy their way out of the situation. They say, "If my child gets well, I'll devote the rest of my life to doing good."
4	Depression	Parents begin to face what is happening. They feel sad and unprotected.
5	Acceptance	Acceptance is being able to say, "Yes, this is happening, and it is all right that it is happening." With a child with long-term illness, parents may never reach this stage but will always remain in the chronic sorrow of the depression stage.

(Modified from Kübler-Ross, E. [1969]. *On death and dying.* New York: Macmillan; with permission.)

with family members about guardianship and with a lawyer to help them write a will that will provide future caretaking and economic support for the disabled child.

Factors Influencing Parental Adjustment

Certain circumstances appear to increase parents' difficulty in adjusting to a disabling or long-term illness in their child. These are the degree and timing of the disability, the experience of the parents, and the availability of support people.

Degree of Disability. The seriousness of a disability obviously affects the ability of parents to adjust. A child who needs total care will require a much more radical readjustment of parents' lives than will a child who only needs additional speech therapy for an hour a day. In most instances, the parents' perception of the child's disability is as important as the child's condition (Figure 35-1). A parent who envisioned a son as someday being an Olympic runner, for example, may perceive a son with congenital hip dysplasia as having a serious disability. A parent whose mental image of the child is that of a lawyer doing mainly desk work may not view the hip problem as a serious illness.

Many parents are not aware of the mental image that they carry of their child, an image that began to form the moment the woman realized she was pregnant. Hidden desires are often revealed if you ask parents, "If things could have been different, what kind of person would you have liked your child to be?" A parent who answers, "a kind person" can still have that wish fulfilled, no matter what the degree of disability. A parent who says "I always assumed my child would take over my business some day" may have some major mental adjusting to do.

Whether the disability is noticeable (spastic cerebral palsy) or not noticeable (controlled seizures) can make a difference in how parents adjust to the illness. A mother who takes her child with cerebral palsy shopping (a child who walks unsteadily and knocks over a display) may hear other shoppers say, "Wouldn't you think a mother would watch her child more carefully?" On days that her child wears long leg braces, however, shoppers' comments are more apt to be "Poor little thing. Isn't it wonderful that his mother brings him shopping with her?" She is happy to have signals (leg braces) that announce her child is different and cannot be held to standards for other children. Other parents might be more grateful that a child's disability is not a visible one—it makes the illness easier for them to accept.

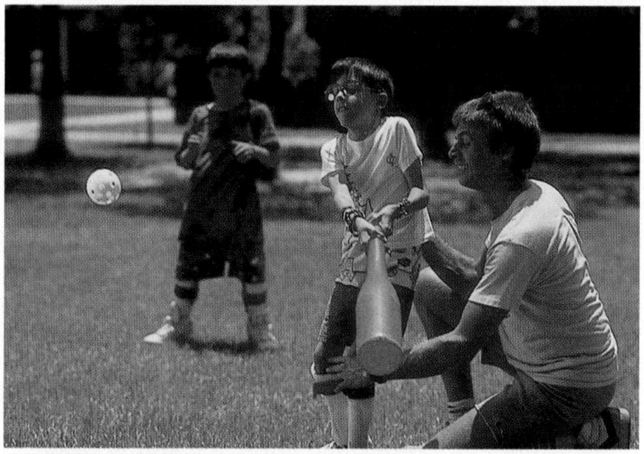

FIGURE 35.1 A parent's perception of a child's disability is important to how well the family adjusts. Often it is easier to accept a disability that allows for greater functioning in everyday activities.

Onset of the Illness. Whether a condition is apparent at birth (e.g., a myelomeningocele) or occurs at a later time (the child is struck by a car at school age) may make a difference in the parents' ability to adjust. For most parents, never having had a well child makes the child's illness easier to accept.

Effect of Parental Experience. First-time parents may have more difficulty caring for a disabled child than older, more experienced parents because all phases of parenting are more difficult for them. Because of inexperience, first-time parents could have difficulty evaluating how much activity a child needs or what toys are appropriate. On the other hand, first-time parents, because they have no preconceived opinions, may be more flexible than other parents. A young parent who has just this one child may have more time to spend in a daily exercise program than does a parent with five children.

Availability of Support People. The family that has few close friends and lives some distance from relatives is apt to have more difficulty adjusting to illness in a child than will the family that has close support people. People who have secondary support systems in the community, such as an organization for parents of disabled children or a local church or synagogue, usually do better than parents without these resources. People who are able to use health care resources effectively adjust more easily than those who are not able to do so. Ability to use health care resources depends on a number of factors:

- The availability of transportation (It is difficult to take a child in a 50-lb cast on a bus.)
- Whether the parent speaks the same language as health care providers (It is frustrating to go for care and be unable to make your needs known.)
- The financial situation and insurance coverage (It is frustrating to be told you need to see a specialist when you have no money or your health coverage does not pay for one.)
- How helpful health care providers have been in the past (If the best advice that has been given the parents up to this point has been, "Take your baby home and treat him as near normally as possible," parents may not see health care providers as a source of useful information or help.)

Life Events. A child's disability generally appears to be more acute at times the child would normally reach developmental milestones: at 12 months, when the baby should be taking his or her first step and is not; 6 years, when the child should begin school; first communion or bar mitzvah; time for a driver's license; or voting age. When the child does not reach these milestones, parents are reminded of the disability in a particularly painful way.

TABLE 35.2 Factors That Make It Easier for Parents to Adjust to a Child's Long-Term Illness

FACTOR	RATIONALE
Support people are available.	Caring for a child is a series of crises during which support people become very important.
A strong marital bond exists between the parents.	A marriage partner can serve as the strongest support person.
A good relationship exists between the child's parents and their parents.	The parents (because they had good care) have a firm sense of trust and the ability to give care to another.
The child is other than the first-born.	The parents have had practice parenting.
The family lives close to shopping, schools, and transportation.	The family is not isolated.
The family has a strong religious faith.	Secondary support systems are important in times of stress.
The parents were told of the child's disability as soon as possible.	Handicap is easier to accept if parents never thought of the child as totally well.

Factors that indicate that a family will probably be able to adjust to caring for a disabled child are summarized in Table 35-2.

The Ill or Disabled Child's Adjustment

The child's reaction to a disability or long-term illness is strongly influenced by the family's response. Family reactions may range from overprotectiveness to rejection and from denial to acceptance. The child's adjustment may also be influenced by peers and other support people, such as school personnel or health care providers. Social exclusion, discrimination, and physical barriers make it difficult for the child to adjust to a disability or long-term illness. On the other hand, inclusion in school and social activities, acceptance by peers and support people, and the ability to function as normally as possible help the child adjust.

The child's ability to cope with a disability or chronic illness is further influenced by personal attitude and temperament, self-concept, age and development, understanding of the condition, and degree of the disorder. As the child grows and life situations change, the child's ability to cope may improve or worsen. For example, an adolescent with a disability may become more optimistic about her condition because she is successfully working at her first job, or a child may become angered by his deteriorating condition because he is suddenly confined to a wheelchair.

Nursing interventions to help the child better adjust include encouraging optimal growth and development (see Chapters 8–12), promoting self-care activities, enhancing self-esteem, preventing social isolation, providing health teaching, and aiding families in the acceptance of the child's condition.

The Siblings' Adjustment

Siblings' reactions to a chronically ill or disabled child may be influenced by a number of factors; however, their reactions are most profoundly affected by the reactions and perceptions of the parents. Siblings of a chronically ill or disabled child may react with jealousy, anger, hostility, resentment, competition, guilt, or withdrawal. The siblings may feel that they take second place to the child who needs more care. These reactions are common when parents focus most of their attention on the ill or disabled child, allow the health problem and treatment to disrupt family life significantly, or grant the ill or disabled child special privileges and minimal discipline.

On the other hand, the siblings may react with acceptance, care, concern, or cooperation. Such reactions are common when parents set aside time each day for special activities with the well siblings (playing a table game or walking in the park with them; teaching a child to sew), carefully explain the condition and the necessity for special care, include the siblings in the care of the ill or disabled child, provide the siblings with respite from care of the ill or disabled child, and establish realistic rules for all family members (Williams, 1997).

At any one time, the siblings may experience a mixture of these feelings. For example, if Joe's parents must take his sister to chemotherapy during his swim meet, Joe may feel resentment that his parents missed the meet and yet sadness that his sister could not compete in the meet as well.

The Nurse and the Chronically Ill or Disabled Child

To help parents and children with a chronic illness or disability, it is important to be familiar with the child's condition and the possible complications that could occur. Over a period of years, parents become experts on the care of a child with a particular condition (see Enhancing Communication). This makes them apt to grow impatient with health care providers who appear to be unaware of things that they know. When young children are admitted to a hospital for care, review with parents on admission their typical way of carrying out a procedure so that you can continue to care for their child in the same way. As the child grows older, do this with the child. On the other hand, be available to show a parent or the child an easier way to do something if it seems appropriate. Frankly admitting to parents, "You're more familiar with the care of Jennifer than I am; you'll have to teach me some things," is a refreshing approach and not only allows parents to feel confidence in you (you are honest), but also increases their self-esteem (they are knowledgeable people).

ENHANCING COMMUNICATION

Samuel is a 1-year-old who was born with a number of congenital anomalies. He is admitted to the hospital for a second-stage revision of a colostomy. Although his abdominal skin was free of erythema on admission, 4 hours later, you notice it is reddened, and Samuel cries when you touch the irritated skin.

Less Effective Communication

Nurse: Look at Samuel's skin. It looks terrible.
Mrs. Circuso: I think that's from the adhesive tape.
Nurse: Oh, I don't think so. I tape this way all the time.
Mrs. Circuso: I never use it. Even on myself.
Nurse: Well, it usually works really well. I'll ask the doctor what she recommends.

More Effective Communication

Nurse: Look at Samuel's skin. It looks terrible.
Mrs. Circuso: I think that's from the adhesive tape.
Nurse: Oh, I don't think so. I tape this way all the time.
Mrs. Circuso: I never use it. Even on myself.
Nurse: Why is that?
Mrs. Circuso: Because it always causes such a reaction.
Nurse: Of course, that makes perfect sense. I should have asked you earlier what you thought was causing the problem.

It is easy to believe that a fellow nurse who has spent a great deal of time caring for a child has become an expert in the child's care. It is often more difficult to remember that a parent can easily become this type of expert too. Asking parents for their input not only can simplify care, but also adds to the parents' feeling of self-esteem, improving their parenting.

It is also important to be familiar with community resources for disabled children to be of help. Advising parents to see a dentist who specializes in caring for children with cerebral palsy when there is no one of that description less than 200 miles away not only is not helpful advice, but is actually destructive. It raises expectations in parents that cannot be met—accentuating, not solving, a problem.

Sometimes parents of disabled children do not comply well with instructions or do not keep health care appointments consistently. This failure to comply usually is related to their adjustment to the illness. As long as denial, anger, bargaining, or depression is functioning (and there is rarely a parent who has successfully moved completely through these stages of grief to acceptance), coming for health care or evaluation is a major demand on parents. Each visit is more of a reminder of the child's illness than a time of reassuring health assessment (Hutton, 1997).

Developmental Tasks

Children with disabilities often do not meet developmental milestones on schedule; achieving developmental tasks can be very difficult. When you are helping parents teach a child with a disability a developmental task, such as toilet training or using a spoon, it is good for them to break the task down into its component parts (e.g., reach for the spoon; grasp it; move it toward you; push it under the chosen food; lift it toward the mouth). This allows parents to appreciate that they are asking the child to do a task that encompasses 20 or more coordinated motions. Helping them learn this technique allows them to be patient in teaching all tasks in future years.

Caring for a chronically ill child is never easy. Support from interested health care personnel at all stages of the process is of great importance to the parents' acceptance of their child's illness. Ways to help children with disabilities achieve developmental tasks are discussed in Chapters 8 to 12. These include exposing them to normal events during a hospitalization (Figure 35-2).

Education

Children with a long-term disability often need provision for special education programs or at least for special hours of individualized instruction. Most of these children benefit from preschool programs, which may need adjustment to accommodate them. Children with a long-term disability miss school more often than do their classmates in a normal school setting because of health supervision visits, so they are likely to fall behind unless special plans to keep them with their school group are made. By federal law (Public Law 99-457, Education of the Handicapped Amendment), a school system must provide educational opportunities in the least structured setting possible beginning with preschool. You may have to be a strong child advocate to see that the best educational program available is being provided for a child.

Home Care

Most children with a chronic illness receive care at home today; planning for this care is discussed in Chapter 15. Caring for the disabled child and for siblings must be discussed. Ways to involve the family in community activi-

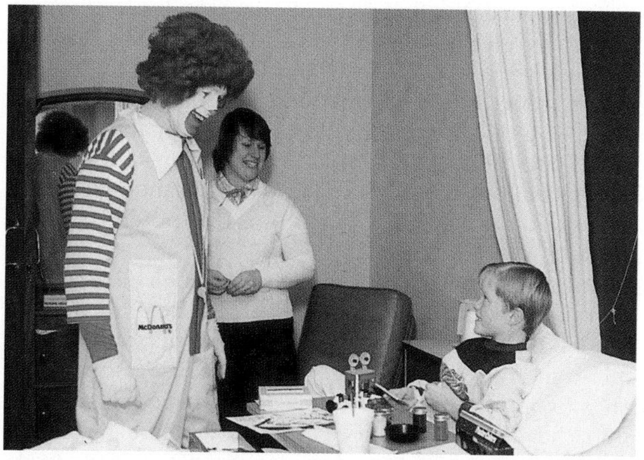

FIGURE 35.2 Ronald McDonald, a familiar face to many children, visits a young boy with a long-term illness. This helps him keep active and in touch with usual events during hospitalization.

ties are important. Children as young as preschool age are aware that a disabled child is "different" and may not choose him or her as a playmate. Some chronically ill children are latchkey children (see Chapter 11) after school; assessing whether this poses problems for care is very important. Preparing a child for puberty can be challenging as the child realizes some areas of life, including sexuality, may be limited (Hinds, 1997).

✔ CHECKPOINT QUESTIONS

1. What are the stages of a grief reaction?
2. Should you encourage a child with a long-term illness to attend a regular or special classroom?
3. How can parents help siblings better accept a chronically ill or disabled child?

THE CHILD WHO IS TERMINALLY ILL

Caring for a dying child is one of the hardest tasks in nursing. Most people are raised to accept the fact that elderly people die, but they have also lived a long life. Most people can accept the death of middle-aged people with the same philosophy—they experienced at least a portion of their life. It is often more difficult to accept the death of children because they have had so little opportunity to live. It can be so difficult to work though your own feelings about a child's dying that you have difficulty caring for the child or supporting the parents.

Family Grief Responses

Each family reacts in a unique way to the diagnosis of terminal illness in a child. This is often strongly influenced by culture (Gates, 1995). Being aware of the usual grief response that occurs in anticipation of the child's death helps in recognizing a response as grief and supporting a family through this very difficult period.

Denial

A parent's usual reaction to a diagnosis of fatal illness in a child is denial, the first stage of grief (see Table 35-1). Although people are aware that children die, most proceed through life thinking, "it will not happen to my child." When it does, they respond with disbelief or denial. The likelihood of this response is enhanced by the fact that many fatal illnesses, such as brain tumor or leukemia, begin insidiously. ("How can a few black-and-blue marks on a child's arms be the symptoms of a potentially fatal disease?")

How the parents handle this initial disbelief has a great deal to do with their relationship with health care personnel. If they have trusted health care personnel up to this point, they may be able to accept a diagnosis without questioning any further. If they do not have this relationship, they may feel the need to obtain a second diagnosis. This often involves considerable expense, but for many parents, it is a necessary step in moving past this first reaction. Parents who feel a need for a third, fourth, or fifth opinion may be having an unusually difficult time resolving a "surely not me" response. They need a factual explanation of why it is certain their child has this disease, such as a copy of the blood report or the pathologist's biopsy report. They need time to talk about how they feel. Only when people can grasp that the illness is definitely present can they begin to accept that the child's disease will ultimately prove fatal.

During a stage of denial, parents' actions may be inappropriate to the child's condition. They may talk of an "upset stomach from the flu" when the child is vomiting blood or "his cold" when the child has cystic fibrosis. It is easy to view such denial as a step that should be hurried (parents cannot begin to deal with the problem as long as they deny that there is a problem). This is true, but neither can they deal with a problem when it hurts as much as this does. Denial is a temporary pain reliever and is a necessary step on the way to acceptance.

Anger

Parents can be expected to enter a stage of anger soon—a change from "Surely not me" to "It's not right that it's happening to me." When parents are angry about a diagnosis, they may be unable to direct their anger appropriately. They may find themselves angry with the child (scolding him or her for crying during a painful procedure). One parent may be angry with the other parent (criticizing him or her for reckless driving or for eating a fattening food for lunch). They may be angry with you (for not answering the child's light immediately). They may be angry with the medical, x-ray, laboratory, and dietary staff or with the entire health care delivery system. It can be difficult to react to this kind of angry attack because it seems unjustified (after all, you came as soon as you could). Be certain that your first reaction is not to be angry in return. This could result in your staying away from the child's room for the rest of the day, resisting being submitted to that kind of unfair criticism again, and therefore not meeting the child's basic need to have support people around him or her.

A more therapeutic reaction is to accept this angry response as the stage of grief that it is and respond accordingly: "I'm sorry it seemed to take me so long to answer your call bell, but you seem angry about more than just the light. Would it help to talk about it?"

Parents' reactions to the anticipated death of a child will depend to a great extent on their experience with death in the past and the meaning of this child to them. Because grandparents live longer today, for some parents, fatal illness in a child is their first contact with death. Another influencing factor is that different children mean different things to parents. A child born to them at a happy time in life can represent all that is good and happy in their life. Loss of this child could also mean loss of all the joy the child represents.

When you ask grieving parents to talk, therefore, they may talk not about the child, but about how they felt when a parent died, how hard their job is for them, or how they feel their marriage is failing. This is part of grief: gathering resources, reworking stress from the past, and arming themselves to face stress in the near future. Parents often receive support from other parents on the hospital unit whose children also are terminally ill. They are helped by seeing parents of other children adjusting to approaching death—or if not adjusting, at least functioning in what passes for a normal manner.

Bargaining

Bargaining is an intermediate step in grief, a time when parents try to correct what is happening by making a bargain to be better people (a change from "This isn't right" to "I can make it right"). They vow to be better people or function in a different way in exchange for their child's life. When parents realize that bargaining is ineffective, they are at a very low point: They have been let down not only by health care providers, but also by the superior power with whom they tried to bargain. They may need more support when bargaining fails than at any other point.

Depression

When parents have passed through stages of denial, anger, and bargaining, a further step occurs: developing awareness of the true meaning of what is happening, with accompanying depression. This is a change from "I can make it not happen" to "It is happening." An emotion such as crying is the most common sign that this stage has been reached. Parents may ask more questions about care, procedures, or medications than before. Be careful that you do not interpret this questioning as criticism. Parents are asking why a child must have continuous dialysis not to criticize care, but because this is the first time they are fully aware of its serious implication.

Parents may work through the expected loss of a child by talking about their plans for the child, the kind of child he or she was, or how the child was doing in school. They may suddenly shower him or her with expensive gifts or trips. They may have a great deal of difficulty leaving the child after visiting hours. On the surface, this reaction appears to be a step backward (they were accepting the diagnosis so well; now they seem demanding and overwhelmed by it). Actually, this is the first time they have actually begun to appreciate the diagnosis and what it means.

At about this stage, parents need to think about preparing other children in the family for the death of the sibling. Siblings may need to visit the dying child to be assured that death is not as frightening and horrible as they believed. If they are not allowed to visit, they may interpret this as proof that death is such a horrible sight that they are not allowed to be exposed to it rather than that visiting is against the hospital rules.

Some children feel responsible for the death of a sibling. They may have wished the child dead so that they could have a room all by themselves or so they could have her bicycle. They were told not to wrestle with the ill sibling, and they did anyway. These children need assurance that wishing for something does not make it come true and that the sibling's death is uncontrollable. It will happen no matter what they or their parents did or will do.

Acceptance

The acceptance stage of the grief process is resolution that the child will die (a change from "This is happening" to "It's all right that this is happening"). Few parents reach this stage by the time of the child's death; grief work will need to continue for years past the time of the death.

Parental Coping Responses

Throughout the stages of grieving, parents will be developing important coping mechanisms to see them through this crisis. They may have already learned to cope positively with their child's illness and treatment measures, but the determination of death requires additional adjustments. Promoting the development of positive coping strategies while being sensitive to the unique needs of each family member is an important nursing responsibility. It may be difficult to determine when a coping strategy is truly helpful or when it has become maladaptive. For instance, seeking information is generally a very useful strategy for parents with ill children. Knowing what to expect reduces anxiety. Some parents, however, continue this procedure past the point at which information is helpful to them. They may believe that if they look hard enough, they'll discover a way to cure their child (prolonged denial), or they may "overintellectualize" their child's illness and impending death in an effort to block feelings of sadness.

Problem solving is always an effective coping strategy as long as parents are being realistic about which problems they can solve. Seeking and using the support of others, including health care providers and families with similar needs, is another positive strategy to encourage by providing the names of support groups or individual families (with their permission) who have gone through similar experiences. You may also need to help parents who are not comfortable accepting the help of others learn how to do so or simply learn how to feel comfortable expressing their feelings to others.

Assuring parents that their child will be kept comfortable and will not die in pain can be extremely comforting (McQuillan & Finlay, 1996). Parents may also be able to cope by searching for the meaning of their child's impending death in philosophical, spiritual, or religious terms. For these parents, body organ donation may be a meaningful way to give themselves some solace that their child will in some way continue to live. The Focus on Nursing Research provides insight into the type of support parents need to cope better with a dying child.

Anticipatory Grief

If a child dies suddenly, the parents' grief response begins only with the actual death. Most parents, however, have some warning that death is expected, so they begin a preparatory or **anticipatory grief** phase in which they gradually incorporate the reality of their child's fate into their thoughts. Such anticipatory mourning prepares parents for their child's death and saves them the abrupt, devastating, intolerable grief reaction that comes to parents whose child dies suddenly from trauma, such as a car accident, or from sudden infant death syndrome (see the Nursing Care Plan).

Although anticipatory grief does not shield the parents from experiencing renewed grief once their child has died,

Nursing Care Plan

THE FAMILY OF A CHILD WHO IS DYING

An 8-year-old female diagnosed with an inoperable brain tumor is receiving hospice care at home.

Assessment: 8-year-old female with history of brain tumor treated with radiation therapy and chemotherapy without results. Child considered terminal. Parents requesting no further treatment. "She's been through so much already. We wanted her to die at home with her family around her."

Child cachexic. Physiologic parameters deteriorating. Skin cool, damp, and mottled. Pulse rate 32 and weak; respirations 8. Rattling sounds noted from chest. Responsive only to deep pain stimuli. Parents and siblings (10-year-old brother and 6-year-old sister) at bedside.

Nursing Diagnosis: Anticipatory grieving related to impending death of the child

Outcome Identification: Family members demonstrate ability to cope with child's death.

Outcome Evaluation: Family members express feelings about anticipated death; demonstrate positive coping mechanisms.

Interventions	Rationale
1. Stay with the family and sit with them quietly if they prefer not to talk; allow them to cry. Arrange for visit by clergy if desired.	1. Staying with the family demonstrates caring and concern for their well-being and wishes and offers support. A visit by clergy provides the family with spiritual support.
2. Inform the family about what to expect. Explore their expectations and clarify any misconceptions.	2. Providing information helps to ease the family's fears and anxiety of the unknown.
3. Provide for the child's comfort, including positioning, turning, changing linens, applying lotion to her skin, moistening her lips, and alleviating any pain. Allow family members to provide care as desired without forcing them.	3. Providing comfort to the child is comforting to the family. Allowing family participation in care provides them with some sense of control over the situation, decreasing their feelings of powerlessness.
4. Allow family members to express their feelings. Listen to them and support their reactions, acknowledging their grief.	4. Expression of feelings provides a safe outlet for emotions. Listening, supporting, and acknowledging their grief helps to validate the family's feelings and promote trust.
5. Assist siblings with understanding the events and explore their perceptions. Allow them opportunities to express their feelings verbally, through stories, writing, or drawing pictures.	5. Siblings of dying children often experience a wide range of feelings, such as guilt, anger, jealousy, and fear. Children may have difficulty expressing their feelings verbally. Story telling and pictures are effective methods for expression.
6. Provide the family with opportunities to review special memories or experiences with the child.	6. Reviewing memories and special experiences provides a positive method for coping with grief.
7. Assist family with making arrangements for what to do when the child dies and afterward (if not already accomplished).	7. Assistance with planning provides support and aids in grieving, allowing for time to be spent with the child rather than on arrangements.
8. Maintain frequent contact with the family through phone calls and visits. Make sure that the family has the telephone number to contact with any questions, problems, or concerns.	8. Frequent contact with the family provides them with emotional and physical support.
9. If not already accomplished, initiate referral to community organizations as appropriate.	9. Community organizations provide for ongoing support.

FOCUS ON NURSING RESEARCH

What Type of Support Do the Parents of a Dying Child Need?

Two nurse researchers attempted to answer this question by interviewing 12 parents of 8 children who died either in the hospital or at home of various types of cancer. Three needs of parents were identified: (1) the need to have the child recognized as special while retaining as much normality within the child's and family's lives as possible; (2) the need for caring and connectedness with health care professionals; and (3) the need to retain responsibility for parenting their dying child.

This is an important study for nurses because it stresses how important it is for health care providers to help families maintain as near normal a lifestyle as possible while caring for a child who is dying. It gives direction to nurses to include parents in day-to-day care so they can maintain their parenting role.

James, L., & Johnson, B. (1997). An international account: the needs of parents of pediatric oncology patients during the palliative care phase. *Journal of Pediatric Oncology Nursing, 14*(2), 83–95.

it can be a very useful process for them to work through. A danger of anticipatory grief is that a parent may reach the acceptance stage of the grief process too far in advance of the child's death. If this happens, parents may accept the child's death so thoroughly that they begin to treat the child as if he or she had already died. They stop visiting. When they do visit, they may spend most of their time visiting other children on the unit or sitting in the waiting room talking to other parents. When once they spent time comforting their child, now they may fail to rock or touch the child as much. They may "clean out" the child's room and throw out or give away toys. Gradually they are drawing back from emotional attachment to shield themselves from the abrupt, stabbing pain that death will bring.

Children need a great deal of support if this happens, just as they did during the initial denial stage. Parents cannot help that the grief process did not time itself to coincide exactly with the child's death. They need understanding and not criticism for this reaction.

For some parents, when the child actually dies, the event may be anticlimactic. They have anticipated death so long that when it does occur, they cannot believe that it has actually happened. They may be so used to thinking constantly about their child's needs and having their child dependent on them that they do not know what to do. Some parents are reluctant to leave the hospital this final time. Leaving with the child's possessions is the step that will make the death real.

The Vulnerable or Fragile Child Syndrome

When anticipatory grief proceeds so effectively that parents begin to think of a youngster as already dead and then the child does not die, parents may find that their grief reaction was so complete that they are unable to reverse it; they cannot view the child as they did before. They begin to treat him or her in a cold and unfeeling way—as if the child were not really there but actually did die. Such children are termed **vulnerable or fragile children**. They may develop behavior problems as they grow older (acting-out behavior, such as temper tantrums, stealing in school, shoplifting as adolescents), as if to say, "Notice me: I am not dead." They require skilled counseling so that they can feel secure and learn to react effectively with others.

CHECKPOINT QUESTIONS

3. What stage of grief is apt to be most difficult for parents?
4. What is the purpose of anticipatory grief?

Children's Reactions to Impending Death

Children's reactions to death are strongly influenced by previous experiences and family attitudes. If children have little or no exposure to death, it can be a strange and frightening phenomenon. This is often the case when children are reared without pets or older relatives, forbidden to visit a dying relative, excluded from the rites of death, or discouraged from discussing the death of a loved one. To help ease the fear of death, encourage parents to maintain an open attitude, even if it is painful or uncomfortable. Children's reactions to death are also influenced by their stage of development and cognitive ability. Children's ability to understand death and steps families can take to help their children cope with death are shown in the Empowering the Family box.

Infants and Toddlers

Infants and toddlers are certainly too young to appreciate death except as the loss of a person who cared for them and the presence of a void in their life. If such a loss interferes with the development of a sense of trust, its implications for the child's ability to achieve warm, close relationships could last a lifetime.

Preschoolers

Preschoolers learn about the concept of death when a pet dies or they discover a dead bird or mouse. They envision death as temporary, however, and appear to have little of the adult's fear of it. This casualness toward death is sometimes interpreted as callousness (the first response of a child who is told that his brother has just been killed in an automobile accident is to ask if he can have his brother's radio). This happens because he thinks of his brother as being gone only for a short time, making this a chance to take advantage of his property. This concept is strengthened by children's cartoons, in which characters frequently are killed and then immediately revive and go on with the story.

Because preschoolers fear separation greatly, they are stunned by the death of a parent. If children grasp the

EMPOWERING THE FAMILY: Guidelines to Help Children Cope With Death

- Infants undoubtedly have no understanding of their impending death. Important points for caring for an infant who is dying are to keep him or her comfortable and secure and to remain nearby to prevent loneliness and insecurity.
- Toddlers, likewise, do not understand death. Even though a close relative or friend may have died, they are unable to relate this with what is about to happen to them. Toddlers like routine, so allowing them opportunities to make choices and providing consistent care are the most important measures for them.
- Preschool children probably envision death as a long sleep. This makes them much more afraid of separation than of the thought of dying. Urge parents or family members to spend time with them.
- Early school-age children understand death as separation but tend to view the separation as temporary. Over 9 years of age, children are able to realize that death is final. They still, however, are not as fearful of death as they are sad at the thought of being away from parents and frightened as to how they will manage without parents. Answer questions about death honestly (no one knows what it is really like but because it happens to everyone, it must not be anything to be fearful of). It is important to praise children for accomplishments to help them maintain their self-esteem so they can face this coming change.
- Adolescents have adult concerns and understanding of death. They may ask if it will be painful; they may feel angry about all that they will miss in life by dying. They may be concerned that they will need to answer for past ill deeds after death. Providing time and opportunities for them to ask and talk about death is important to help them work through a coming change. Allowing them to continue usual activities as much as possible helps them maintain self-esteem.

concept that they are dying, their major worry might be that they will be alone and separated. These children may need someone to stay with them constantly to assure them that they are not alone.

School-Age Children

School-age children begin to have additional experience with death, so their knowledge of it as a final measure increases. They may think of it, however, as something that happens only to adults. Talking to children about death can be a school nurse's responsibility (Schonfeld, 1996). Children's books tend to deal only shallowly with the subject, although many books that deal specifically with death are available to children (Box 35-1). As children near 8 or 9 years, they begin to appreciate that death is permanent. It is the same feeling they experienced when their parents left them at camp or went away for a weekend, but this time the separation will be permanent.

Most children of school age are aware of what is happening to them when their disorder has a fatal prognosis. They may learn from other children on the unit ("Are you the kid who's dying?"), from their parents' strange responses to questions, or from overhearing snatches of conversation about reports or physical findings. Children, however, are accustomed to meeting new situations—starting school, visiting a museum for the first time, boarding an airplane for the first time—and they cope with these experiences very well, as long as they know that someone they care about will be there to support them. Dying can be viewed in this same light as another new experience for them. They are able to cope with it well if they know that there will be someone with them. If the parents become unable to relate to a child this age because of their grief, the nurse may need to fill the gap (Figure 35-3).

Many children associate death with sleep (perhaps that was the explanation they were given for a grandparent's death), so they may be afraid to fall asleep without someone near them. They may need to have you sit with them while they fall asleep (if necessary, take patient charts to work on so you have the time to sit with them). The child may need the light left on (the better for you to work by) because he or she may associate death with darkness, not with naptime. Often the child who is dying is moved to the end of the hallway, away from the nurse's station. This frees the room for a child who needs frequent procedures (a justifiable move in terms of efficiency). Unfortunately, it may further isolate a child who needs support and the child's parents, who also need your support and your presence nearby. Advocate as necessary for continued interaction with a child who is dying.

BOX 35.1

BOOKS ABOUT DEATH FOR CHILDREN

Breebaart, J., & Breebaart, P. (1993). *When I die, will I get better?* New York: P. Bedrick Books.

Brown, L. K. (1996). *When dinosaurs die: a guide to understanding death.* Boston: Little, Brown.

Liss-Levenson, N. (1995). *When a grandparent dies: a kid's own remembering.* Woodstock, VT: Jewish Lights.

Tott-Rizzuti, K. (1992). *Mommy, what does dying mean?* Pittsburgh: Dorrance.

Weitzman, E. (1996). *Let's talk about when a parent dies.* New York: Rosen Group.

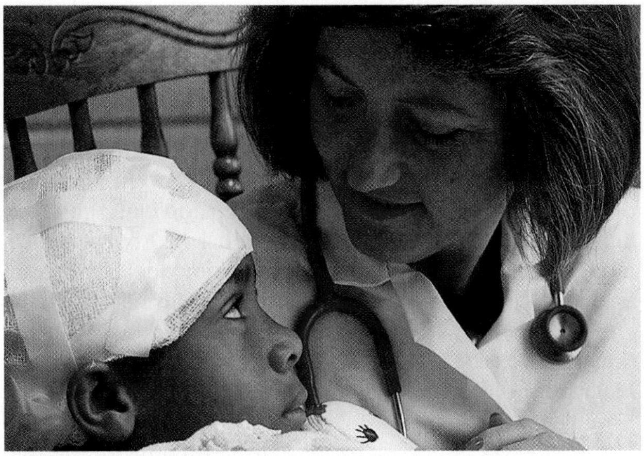

FIGURE 35.3 Primary nurse or one-to-one nursing relationships help children with long-term illnesses not to feel deserted.

Adolescents

Although adolescents have an adult concept of death, they also may feel immune to death. Driving at high speeds and walking along the ledges of high cliffs reflect this judgment. They may deny symptoms for longer than usual because they believe it is impossible that anything serious could be happening to them. They appreciate time provided for discussion of how they view death and ways they contributed to their family even though they are dying young. Continuing to participate in their typical activities helps them maintain a sense of control.

Environment for Death

The environment in which children die can influence their acceptance and their family's acceptance of death.

The Hospital

A few children who need a great deal of physical care (have a new tracheotomy, need lung ventilation) may remain in a hospital for care because their family does not have the skill, energy, or money to care for them at home. In a hospital setting, be certain that visiting hours are extended to parents and other family members so that a child is not left alone when he or she needs people around the most. Be certain the child has opportunities to maintain contact with peers.

The Home

Most children today are not kept in the hospital past the time it is determined that therapy is no longer effective. Many families prefer that a child die at home surrounded by family and familiar possessions rather than in a hospital. Time spent talking about arrangements—such as whom they should contact if the child suddenly becomes more ill than usual, how they will manage periodic checkups, or how they will purchase medicine or supplies—is important preparation for home care. Assess how the family will schedule its time to have some leisure periods free so they can balance the care of the ill child in their lives.

Home care can be an extremely satisfying experience both for the child who is dying and for the family, as long as safeguards exist for protecting the caregivers' health and for providing good care for the child. This is discussed further in Chapter 15.

The Hospice

In 1967, St. Christopher's Hospice in London was opened as a facility for people who wanted to die in a homelike setting while still under skilled professional care. Most large communities today have similar hospice settings, although places for children are still not available in many communities. In a hospice, friends and family are allowed unlimited visiting; even younger children and pets can visit. Children are invited to bring possessions that have importance to them. They are urged to choose the degree of pain relief they want. Strong analgesia is often used to make a child pain free (a criticism of hospice care is that this level of analgesia slows respiratory rates and actually hurries death).

A basic philosophy of hospice care is that death is an extension or part of life, not a separate entity; thus, it can be accepted—not with separate or awkward rituals but with the same warm concern as other situations in everyday life. For many children, hospice care will be furnished as part of home care so that they are not separated from their families.

Preparation for a Nursing Role With Dying Children and Their Families

Caring for dying clients can be an emotionally draining experience (Davies et al., 1996). Although it is best that nursing assignments be consistent so a child has meaningful support, for everyone there is a point at which he or she may need a respite from caring for a certain child or help in offering support for the parents. This is not admitting weakness but recognizing humanness and a sense of compassion that interferes with client need. Humanness and compassion should be keystones of professional nursing; they are not qualities for which one needs to apologize.

Self-Awareness

Before you can offer support to children in any circumstance, you need to be aware of your own reactions and feelings. Thus, to offer support to a child who is dying, it is helpful to examine how you feel about caring for someone who is dying.

Fear. Fear is a natural response to death because the phenomenon is new and strange. To overcome this fear, put it into perspective. In nursing, you care for many people who have illnesses and experiences you will never have; thus, caring for people with experiences beyond your own is not really strange but almost routine in nursing.

People who have never seen someone die are often afraid that the moment of death will be terrifying to watch. Death usually occurs gently, however, with body functioning gradually lessening until it stops in a pain-free, quiet manner. People who have been declared dead and were then resuscitated by heroic measures report that death was not frightening but involved a feeling of exceptional calm and comfort; a number of people have said afterward that they wished they had been allowed to die rather than be called back to their body because death seemed so appealing.

Failure. Some health care professionals find themselves drawing back from care of dying children because death symbolizes failure to them. This can make children feel as if they have failed—they have not been able to keep their body from dying despite everyone's best efforts.

Remind yourself that death is the ultimate outcome for everyone. At the point that death becomes unpreventable, the only failure that can exist is the failure of health care professionals to help a child achieve death with dignity and consideration and free of guilt that he or she has failed caregivers (Buss, 1998).

Grief

Nursing care is so intense that the relationship formed may be closer than you realize until the child is diagnosed as having a terminal illness or dies; only then do you feel the depth of the relationship. Because nurses and staff can develop such close bonds with terminally ill children, they may experience profound grief when the children die or no longer require their care (see Managing and Delegating Unlicensed Assistive Personnel). The grief that accompanies caring for dying children can be broken down into the same stages of grief experienced by the children themselves when they learn that they are dying.

Denial. There is a danger that a nurse who is in a stage of denial may care for children without mentioning that they have more than a simple illness. This includes omitting the use of such common expressions as, "How are you this morning?" to avoid having to hear the answer. Denial may be so extensive that you avoid going into a child's room unless you have an important procedure to do. This is confusing and lonely for children, because they miss the normal exchange of conversation and contact.

MANAGING AND DELEGATING UNLICENSED ASSISTIVE PERSONNEL

One of the most difficult aspects of caring for children with long-term illnesses or terminal care is letting-go of them when their condition improves so they are no longer ill or when their condition worsens and they die. Be certain that unlicensed personnel know not to continue a relationship past health agency discharge unless they are specifically asked by the family to do so. Unless they do let go this way, the family cannot experience a sense of competency in the care of their now well child. Help unlicensed assistive personnel to let go of a child who dies through a period of grieving and acceptance. Health care providers can have a difficult time establishing relationships with new children if they are still grieving for a former one.

Nurses sometimes change professions following the loss of a child to whom they felt close because they are unwilling to submit themselves to that level of hurt again.

Anger. Anger may be intense when a young child dies because the death seems so unfair. People who are angry have difficulty offering effective care. The person may perceive himself or herself as giving thorough, comforting care but is actually inflicting pain with sharp, abrupt movements. Anger clouds judgment for decisions, such as which analgesic would be best to administer. Dying children cannot approach angry caregivers or ask questions; they are left alone and perhaps feel guilty that they have caused this anger. Anger is always destructive.

WHAT IF? What if, while caring for a terminally ill child for an extended time, you notice yourself making poor judgments in your personal life (not following through on projects, spontaneous buying)? Could this be an expression of anger?

Bargaining. Caregivers begin to bargain for life just as children do. A statement such as "If Tommy just makes it through the weekend while I'm off, I'll spend all my extra time with him next week" is a bargaining statement. Statements of this kind are easy to overlook in your coworkers or yourself. Listening for them helps you to evaluate when a fellow worker is having difficulty caring for a particular patient and perhaps needs to change assignments. Hearing yourself say them should alert you that you are more involved with a child than you perhaps realize. You need to talk to someone about your feelings or ask for help. Remember that when bargaining fails, people reach their lowest point in grief. Recognizing bargaining statements in yourself helps you to be prepared for the depression that will follow.

Depression. Nurses who enter this phase may be ineffective caregivers, because depressed people are poor problem solvers (everything becomes a crisis). Nurses may make unwise decisions in their personal lives (e.g., drop out of a night school course, file for divorce) because they cannot effect good problem solving.

Depression is doubly destructive because when you are depressed, your reasoning processes are so slowed that you lose the ability to recognize that depression is the problem. When caring for a child who is expected to die, monitor your usual behavior to see if you are following your usual pattern. If irregularities occur (sleeping a great deal, not sleeping, loss of appetite), assess whether depression has overwhelmed you. When depressed, try to make no major decisions for at least a week to give your perspective time to change, or you may find later that you have made an unwise, irreversible decision.

Acceptance. The average person can reach a stage of acceptance in grief because he or she is subjected to few true losses in a lifetime. As a nurse on a unit where many terminally ill children come for care, you may find yourself facing loss or death repeatedly. Therefore, a stage of acceptance may never be reached. A caregiver who cannot reach a stage of acceptance is left in a stage of depression and cannot function.

To achieve a stage of acceptance, you may need to modify what it is you are accepting. You cannot accept the unfairness of death in children, but you can accept your ability to offer care that gives death dignity and compassion. Do not compensate for being unable to feel good by not feeling. This is a dangerous attitude because it also blocks your ability to feel happiness, love, and trust. You may need to ask for a temporary change of assignment to reestablish your perspective. You may need to concentrate on self-esteem therapy for yourself (doing something special for yourself, such as taking an evening to do nothing but meet your own needs).

Caring for the Dying Child

A child may live for days, weeks, or even months in a "dying phase." Attentive physical and emotional care is essential to the child's maintaining a sense of security and positive self-esteem during this time. It is also essential to the grieving process for both the child and the child's family. Frequent and substantive communication is a major part of providing this care. Children, like their parents, need the opportunity to talk about their fears and feelings about death. Practicing good communication skills when providing any care (e.g., when administering pain medication, starting intravenous lines, or providing basic comfort measures, such as a bath) will help to establish a trusting relationship with a child, making the child feel more comfortable about sharing feelings with you (Figure 35-4). Box 35-2 provides some specific guidelines about communicating with the child who is dying.

The Child's Family

For many children, terminal illness involves a series of hospital admissions interspersed with ambulatory care or home visits. Parents need time during these visits to talk about the problems they are having, not only with physical care (Should the child attend regular school? Could he come on vacation? How many times a day are they supposed to give the immunosuppressant?), but also about how it feels to live with a child who is dying (Are they having any difficulty answering the child's or siblings' questions?). Although many parents are reluctant to tell a child that he or she is dying, this is probably the soundest course once the child can see that his or her condition is deteriorating. There is often less anxiety in knowing what is happening than in hearing people whispering or spelling out words around you.

If the child experiences an exacerbation of the disease, parents may again begin an anticipatory grief reaction: anger, bargaining, depression, acceptance. The process will be cut short by improvement, only to begin again at the next exacerbation. Parents of a child being admitted

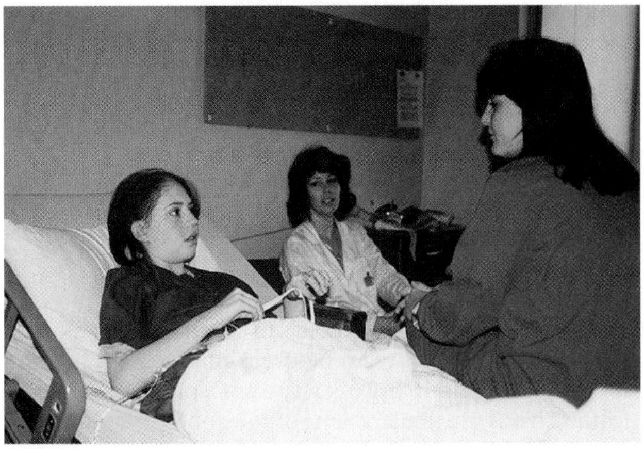

FIGURE 35.4 Good communication skills help build a trusting relationship, allowing the child to share feelings about being terminally ill.

BOX 35.2

APPROACHES TO COMMUNICATING WITH DYING CHILDREN

1. Children who are dying need stimulation in as near normal a way as possible. Continue active conversation to provide this.
2. Use moments of silence therapeutically. Such moments occur normally just as speech occurs normally. Do not feel you have to chatter to fill quiet intervals.
3. Use the words *death* and *dying* as appropriate in conversation. Trying to avoid a word makes interchanges awkward. Statements such as "These flowers are dying," "That's a dead-end job," or "I'm dying to try that" may make it acceptable for the child you are caring for to voice for the first time what is happening to him or her—"I'm dying, too; let me tell you about dead-ending."
4. Preserve dying children's defenses. If they are using denial or bargaining, do not try to push them to the next step of grieving by confrontation. Children will move on to the next step when they are psychologically ready.
5. Many children assume that they will die at night. Therefore, night is "owned" by the dying. A child may talk more freely at night about fears or an unfulfilled life ambition than during the day. Children may also be more frightened at night and enjoy having someone sit beside them until they fall asleep.
6. Be supportive, not trite. A statement such as "All of us are dying" is true but not helpful. A supportive statement, such as "This must be hard for you," is better.
7. Be aware that not all people's beliefs are the same as yours. A statement such as, "God works in mysterious ways" may explain death for you but can be little comfort to a family who does not envision that as true. A statement such as, "I believe God made some children die early to teach us to appreciate life" may evoke an angry response, such as, "Who could believe in a God like that?" rather than be comforting.

to the hospital for the 12th time for leukemia, therefore, may be in the same stage of grief as the parents whose child's leukemia is newly diagnosed.

When they are seen for health supervision visits, parents should be asked how other children in the family are managing. Often other children live with relatives so that the parents are free to spend a great deal of time visiting at the hospital or hospice. The parents may need reminding that although the dying child does need a lot of their time, other children find this illness in a sibling even more baffling than do the parents. When the ill child dies, siblings need active support to help them grieve (Ruden, 1996).

The Onset of Death

As death nears in children, physiologic changes, such as slowed metabolism, decreased cell oxygenation, and cell dysfunction, begin to occur.

Stroke volume of the heart decreases, so the power to circulate blood is reduced. The child's skin feels cool and appears mottled or cyanotic because blood can no longer be pushed to distal sites. Just before death, blood will begin to pool in the dependent body parts, making them appear purple. As circulation fails, absorption of a drug from a muscle becomes virtually impossible; an emergency drug would need to be administered intravenously to have an effect.

As peripheral circulation fails, less heat is lost from the body, and the temperature rises. The child's body may compensate for this by increased perspiration to increase heat loss through evaporation. This makes the child's skin feel cool and damp. You may need to change linens frequently because of the increased moisture on the skin. Because perfusion of distal body parts is impaired, turn children slowly to allow their circulation system to accommodate to the change in position.

Slowed respiration leads to increased secretions in the lungs and the appearance of rales (the crackling sound of air being pulled through fluid in alveoli). To compensate for a few minutes of very slow respirations, a child may take a number of quick or extremely deep inhalations periodically. Be certain the child's chest is not compressed so he or she has optimal lung expansion to do this.

A decrease in muscular function leads to severe weakness and fatigue. More and more, a child maintains the exact position in which you placed him or her. As the throat muscles become lax, the possibility of aspiration increases. Assess children carefully for an intact gag reflex before offering oral fluid. If the gag or swallowing reflex is impaired, position children on their side to allow saliva to drain from the mouth and prevent aspiration. An often-noticed phenomenon is constant hand movement—picking at bedclothes, for example—that probably represents the loss of upper centers of voluntary muscular control. Neurologically, deep reflexes, such as the Achilles, begin to fade.

As children near death, they begin to demonstrate a lessened level of consciousness, although they may remain perfectly alert until seconds before death. Vision apparently blurs because children tend to turn toward a light. Touch seems to remain intact because children often quiet to a gentle stroking of the arm or shoulder; they grasp your hand meaningfully as if touch is appreciated and felt. Hearing remains intact. You may need to remind family members and, on occasion, other health care personnel of this. Continue to explain procedures to unconscious children as if they were conscious because they undoubtedly do hear you. Never make any comment in their presence that you would not make if they were alert. Continue to use the same gentle touch and nonverbal communication motions, such as holding a hand or brushing hair from the forehead, as if children were fully conscious. They may be fully aware of your actions even though they can give no indication of it.

Digestion slows as total body metabolism slows. Constipation due to poor bowel tone and decreased peristaltic action will occur. The abdomen may become distended from intestinal flatus. Dehydration with dry mucous membranes and conjunctivae will occur unless an intravenous supplement is begun. Mouth dryness will lead to cracking and secondary infection and pain; prevent this by frequent cleaning of the mucous membrane with clear water and applying Vaseline to the lips. If eye conjunctivae appear dry, ask a physician to prescribe moistening eye drops; keep any crusting at eyelids washed away so that optimal vision is possible.

Keep skin surfaces from rubbing against one another by using supportive pillows and good positioning. Keep skin free from urine or feces from incontinence; this prevents painful decubitus ulcers from developing (normally not a major concern in children, but a concern here because of the lessened peripheral blood perfusion). Assess for pain (thrashing or moaning), and relieve this through appropriate comfort measures.

Documentation of Death

Defining when death occurs is controversial and involves both legal and ethical issues. Signs of death in a child not on ventilatory or mechanical assistance are the same as in adults:

- Absence of respirations
- No audible heart sounds by stethoscope
- No pulse by palpation
- No apparent blood pressure
- Absence of body movement or reflexes
- Dilated, fixed pupils

Death is officially determined by unreceptivity and unresponsivity; no spontaneous muscular movement or breath; no reflex response; and a flat electroencephalogram—again, the same as in adults.

Organ Donation

Parents may be asked by their physician or a specifically designated transplant team before a child's death to grant permission for body organs to be transplanted following death. This is particularly important for liver and kidney transplants because it is difficult to transplant adult size organs into children. If parents make the decision to allow organ donation, mark this information on the child's care plan in a conspicuous place, and alert the physician about the decision. When death does occur, the child's body will be maintained by a life-support system until a proper recipient for the body organ to be transplanted is located. The donation of body organs may help parents accept their child's death more easily, because they can feel their child has helped another person live.

After Care

Before beginning any after care with a child following death, check with family members to see if they want to spend a few minutes with the child or if there are any religious rites they want to complete before the body is prepared for the morgue. This is necessary for some parents to be able to comprehend that death has really occurred. Some people have special prayers they want to say; others want to say a final, private goodbye. Check that the child's bed and room look neat and clean before you ask family if they would like to spend some time in the room, particularly if a final resuscitation attempt resulted in blood-soaked sponges or scattered equipment.

Remain in the room with the family in case they need your support, but be unobtrusive. Some parents fear touching a child's body after death, but touch is a strong and intimate communication technique that a family member may appreciate being shown how to use. Role model touching by holding the child's hand or brushing hair away from the forehead as if the child were still alive. Some parents may seem unable to leave the room or to let go of the child's hand. You may need gradually to separate their hands, saying something such as, "I'll always remember Molly the way she was when I first met her—so full of life and always laughing. I'm sure that's how you'll always remember her, too." This helps parents begin to accept the fact that, in more than a physical sense, it is time to let go.

As a rule, crying is helpful for parents. You may need to tell them that it is all right to cry. On the other hand, do not interpret a lack of tears as a lack of feeling. Crying is not everyone's response to death. It is not unprofessional for nurses to cry at a child's death. A parent's warmest memory of a hospital experience may be that a nurse cried as she said goodbye to his or her child—the implication being that the child made an impact on people other than family.

> **FOCUS ON CULTURAL COMPETENCE**
>
> The way that death is viewed and the manner in which people express grief differ greatly across cultures. Some people are very expressive with grief; some are very restrained. The manner in which a child's body is handled after death also differs. Muslims, for example, forbid organ donations or transplants. Autopsies are not usually approved because it is important that children be buried quickly after death. Cremation is not permitted. Being aware that grief is expressed differently by different cultures allows for better understanding of parents' concerns and reactions during a child's fatal illness.

Autopsy Permission

If a child's death is a result of homicide, suicide, death within 24 hours after a hospital admission, suspected harmful death, or death in an institution or home where the child was not under a physician's care, an autopsy is required by law; parents have no input as to whether one is done. In other instances, it would be helpful to medical programs or research if an autopsy could be done, but parents must sign permission for this. Parents may refuse to allow autopsy permission for a child, thinking of their action as protecting the child from any more hurt or out of religious convictions (see Focus on Cultural Competence). Autopsies advance medical science, so they should be done if at all possible; on the other hand, parents do have every right to refuse permission without being made to feel guilty for their actions.

> **CHECKPOINT QUESTIONS**
>
> 5. With dying, what is the last sense lost?
> 6. Why is donation of liver and kidney from children so important?

KEY POINTS

Children with chronic illnesses need continual reassessment because, like all children, their needs change as they grow older. Larger doses of medicine will become necessary; such things as additional muscle strengthening exercises may be necessary.

Factors that make it easier for parents to accept chronic illness in a child include the presence of support people and being told about the disability at as young an age as possible.

Chronic illness in a child is often most difficult for parents to accept at what would have been the child's "milestones" of development. Extra support for both the parents and child may be necessary at these times.

Help children to do as much care for themselves as possible within the limits of a chronic illness. This empowers them to be as independent as possible.

Children are about 9 years old before they are able to understand the meaning of death and that it is permanent.

Children and parents are apt to need help to face a fatal diagnosis in the child. Urge parents and the child to ask for help to see them through this very difficult time in their lives.

CRITICAL THINKING EXERCISES

1. Charlie is the 3-year-old with leukemia you met at the beginning of the chapter. His parents tell you Charlie's disease has put them through a great deal of strain. What is a reason they would let him get so ill with pneumonia before they brought him for care?
2. The parents of a newborn with a myelomeningocele are both 40 years old and live on a farm; finances are tight, and they have no health insurance. Two grown children have expressed resentment at their parents being forced to spend so much time and money on a disabled child. How would you help this family? Do they have risk factors that might make adjusting to a disabled child more difficult than usual?
3. A 10-year-old in your care has an inoperable brain tumor. His parents have been told that he has only 6 more months to live. You notice the parents in the waiting room of the hospital comforting a set of parents whose child was just hit by a car and killed instantly; you hear them say that losing a child suddenly is better than what they are experiencing. Why do you think the parents feel this way? How could you help them with their feelings?
4. An adolescent with leukemia wants to donate his corneas for transplant if he should die. His parents think this is totally wrong and say they will not allow it to happen. How would you counsel this family?

REFERENCES

Buss, M. K. et al. (1998). The preparedness of students to discuss end-of-life issues with patients. *Academic Medicine, 73*(4), 418.

Coyne, I. (1997). Chronic illness: The importance of support for families caring for a child with cystic fibrosis. *Journal of Clinical Nursing, 6*(2), 121.

Davies, B. et al. (1996). Caring for dying children: nurses' experiences. *Pediatric Nursing, 22*(6), 500.

Department of Health and Human Services. (1995). *Healthy people 2000: midcourse review.* Washington, DC: DHHS.

Gates, E. (1995). Culture clash: The nursing care of dying children from cultural backgrounds that are different from the nurse's. *Nursing Times, 91*(7), 42.

Hinds, P. S. et al. (1997). Decision making by parents and healthcare professionals when considering continued care for pediatric patients with cancer. *Oncology Nursing Forum, 24*(9), 1523.

Hutton, N. (1997). Special needs of children with chronic illnesses. In K. B. Johnson & F. A. Oski (Eds.), *Oski's essential pediatrics.* Philadelphia: Lippincott-Raven.

James, L., & Johnson, B. (1997). An international account: the needs of parents of pediatric oncology patients during the palliative care phase. *Journal of Pediatric Oncology Nursing, 14*(2), 83.

Kübler-Ross, E. (1969). *On death and dying.* New York: Macmillan.

McQuillan, R., & Finlay, I. (1996). Facilitating the care of terminally ill children. *Journal of Pain & Symptom Management, 12*(5), 320.

Ruden, B. M. (1996). Bereavement follow-up: An opportunity to extend nursing care. *Journal of Pediatric Oncology Nursing, 13*(4), 219.

Schonfeld, D. J. (1996). Talking with elementary school-age children about AIDS and death: principles and guidelines for school nurses. *Journal of School Nursing, 12*(1), 26.

Williams, P. D. (1997). Outcomes of a nursing intervention for siblings of chronically ill children: a pilot study. *Journal of the Society of Pediatric Nurses, 2*(3), 127.

SUGGESTED READINGS

Broughton, B. K., & Lutner, N. (1995). Chronic childhood illness: a nursing health-promotion model for rehabilitation in the community. *Rehabilitation Nursing, 20*(6), 318.

Burke, S. O. et al. (1997). Stress-point intervention for parents of repeatedly hospitalized children with chronic conditions. *Research in Nursing and Health, 20*(6), 475.

Carroll, M. L., & Griffin, R. (1997). Reframing life's puzzle: support for bereaved children. *American Journal of Hospice and Palliative Care, 14*(5), 231.

Chambliss, C. R., & Anand, K. J. (1997). Pain management in the pediatric intensive care unit. *Current Opinion in Pediatrics, 9*(3), 246.

Frey, M. (1996). Behavioral correlates of health and illness in youths with chronic illness. *Applied Nursing Research, 9*(4), 167.

Graves, C., & Hayes, V. E. (1996). Do nurses and parents of children with chronic conditions agree on parental needs? *Journal of Pediatric Nursing, 11*(5), 288.

Reichenbach, M. B. (1996). Promoting normalcy in chronically ill children. *Orthopaedic Nursing, 15*(1), 37.

Ruppert, E. S. et al. (1998). The Prescribed Pediatric Center: A medical day treatment program for children with complex medical conditions. *Infants and Young Children, 10*(3), 19.

Scribano, P. V., Baker, M. D., & Ludwig, S. (1997). Factors influencing termination of resuscitative efforts in children: a comparison of pediatric emergency medicine and adult emergency medicine physicians. *Pediatric Emergency Care, 13*(5), 320.

Sterling, Y. M., Peterson, J., & Weekes, D. P. (1997). African-American families with chronically ill children: oversights and insights. *Journal of Pediatric Nursing, 12*(5), 202.

Appendix A

COMPOSITION AND INGREDIENTS OF INFANT FORMULAS

FORMULA	CALORIES (Per oz)	CALORIES (Per mL)	PROTEIN	FAT	CARBOHYDRATE	COMMENTS
Cow's milk	20	.67	80% casein, 20% whey	Butterfat	Lactose	
Enfamil 20[†]	20	.67	40% casein, 60% whey	45% soy, 55% coconut oils	Lactose	
Enfamil premature	20	.67	40% casein, 60% whey	40% MCT oil, soy and coconut oil	Corn syrup solids, lactose	Premature infants
Human milk	21	.70	40% casein, 60% whey	Human milk, fat	Lactose	
Isomil	20	.67	Soy protein	Coconut and soy oils	Corn syrup solids and sucrose	For cow's milk protein or lactose intolerance
Isomil SF	20	.67	Soy protein	Coconut and soy oils	Corn syrup solids	For cow's milk protein, lactose, or sucrose intolerance
Lofenalac	20	.67	Processed casein hydrolysate to remove most of the phenylalanine	Corn oil	Corn syrup solids and modified tapioca starch	For phenylketonuria (PKU), low in phenylalanine
MJ 3232A[‡]	20	.67	Casein hydrolysate	MCT oil	Tapioca starch, mono- and disaccharide free	Management of disaccharidase deficiencies
Nursoy	20	.67	Soy protein	Coconut, safflower, and soybean oils	Sucrose	For cow's milk protein or lactose intolerance
Nutramigen	20	.67	Casein hydrolysate	Corn oil	Corn syrup solids, modified corn starch	Use for sensitivity to intact milk protein, or for lactose intolerance
Portagen	20	.67	Sodium caseinate	88% MCT oil, 12% corn oil	Corn syrup sucrose	Use in fat malabsorption states, lactose intolerance (liver disease)
Pregestimil	20	.67	Casein hydrolysate with added L-cystine, L-tyrosine, L-tryptophan	60% corn oil, 40% MCT oil	Corn syrup solids, modified tapioca starch	Suitable for many malabsorption syndromes

(continued)

FORMULA	CALORIES (Per oz)	(Per mL)	PROTEIN	FAT	CARBOHYDRATE	COMMENTS
Prosobee	20	.67	Soy protein isolate and methonine	Soy oil, coconut oil	100% corn syrup solids (glucose polymers)	Use for lactose and cow's milk protein intolerance; sucrose intolerance; galactosemia
RCF			Soy protein isolate	Coconut and soy oils	None	Contains no carbohydrates
Similac 20†	20§	.67	Nonfat cow's milk	Coconut and soy oils	Lactose	
Similac 24LLBW	24	.80	Nonfat cow's milk	MCT oil, coconut and soy oils	Lactose and corn syrup solids	Dilute initial feedings. For premature infants with fluid intolerance
Similac PM 60/40	20	.67	Casein and whey (60/40 ratio whey/casein)	Coconut and soy oil	Lactose	(Ca:P=2:1) For infants predisposed to hypocalcemia; low salt content
Similac special care	20	.67	60% whey, 40% casein	MCT oil soy oil coconut oil	50% lactose 50% corn syrup solids	Premature infants Ca:P-2:1
Similac whey plus iron	20	.67	60% whey, 40% casein	Coconut, and soy oils	Lactose	
SMA 20	20	.67	Nonfat cow's milk, demineralized whey	Coconut safflower and soybean oils	Lactose	Low salt content
SMA Preemie	24	.80	60% whey, 40% casein	MCT oil coconut and soy oils	Lactose and glucose polymers	Premature infants

* Precentage of calories supplied
† Also comes with iron (12 mg/L)
‡ Mixed as 81 g diet powder plus 59 g added carbohydrate per quart
§Varies with amount carbohydrate added
|| Ernst JA, et al. (1983). Vapor pressure method as determined by manufacturers method. *Pediatrics* 72, 350.
(Rowe P, (ed.) (1987). *The Harriet Lane handbook* (ed 11). Chicago: Year Book Medical Publishers, p. 338.
Values listed were provided by manufacturers except where indicated otherwise.)
(Oski, F. A., et al. [1994]. *Principles and practice of pediatrics* [2nd ed.]. Philadelphia: J. B. Lippincott, pg. 540–541.

Appendix B

DRUG EFFECTS IN LACTATION

Adrenergics	Parenteral *epinephrine* (Adrenalin) is excreted in breast milk; the status of other adrenergic bronchodilators is not known. *Albuterol* (Proventil, Ventolin) had tumorigenic effects in animals; if considered necessary, breast-feeding should be discontinued. Oral drugs used as nasal decongestants (*e.g., pseudoephedrine* [Sudafed], others) are contraindicated in nursing mothers because of higher than usual risks to infants from sympathomimetic drugs.
Analgesics	*Acetaminophen* (Tylenol) is excreted in breast milk in low concentrations. No adverse effects have been reported, and it is probably the analgesic-antipyretic drug of choice for nursing mothers. Salicylates (*e.g., aspirin*) are excreted in breast milk in small amounts. Adverse effects on nursing infants have not been reported but are a potential risk. Narcotic analgesics such as *meperidine* (Demerol) are excreted in breast milk, but amounts may not be enough to cause adverse effects in the nursing infant. Some authorities recommend waiting 4 to 6 h after a dose before nursing. *Alfentanil* (Alfenta) should probably not be given. Significant amounts were found in breast milk 4 h after a dose.
Angiotensin-Converting Enzyme (ACE) Inhibitors	*Captopril* (Capoten) is excreted in breast milk, but effects on the infant are unknown. It is not known whether *enalapril* (Vasotec) or *lisinopril* (Prinivil, Zestril) is excreted in breast milk. In general, nursing is not recommended while taking these drugs.
Antianginal Agents (Nitrates)	Safety for use in the nursing mother has not been established.
Antianxiety and Sedative-Hypnotic Agents (Benzodiazepines)	*Diazepam* (Valium) and other benzodiazepines should generally be avoided. They are excreted in breast milk and may cause lethargy and weight loss in the infant. The drugs and their metabolites may accumulate to toxic levels in neonates because of slow drug metabolism.
Antiarrhythmics	When these agents are required for a nursing mother, breast-feeding should generally be discontinued. *Quinidine* (Quinaglute), *disopyramide* (Norpace), and *mexiletine* (Mexitil) are excreted in breast milk; it is unknown whether *procainamide* (Pronestyl, Procan), *lidocaine* (Xylocaine), and *flecainide* (Tambocor) are excreted. There is a potential for serious adverse effects on infants.
Antibiotics	*Penicillins* are excreted in breast milk in low concentrations and may cause diarrhea, candidiasis, or allergic responses in nursing infants. *Cephalosporins* are excreted in small amounts and may alter bowel flora, cause pharmacologic effects, and interfere with interpretation of culture reports with fever or infection. *Aztreonam* (Azactam) is excreted in small amounts; discontinuing breast-feeding temporarily is probably indicated. It is unknown whether *imipenem/cilastatin* (Primaxin) is excreted. The aminoglycosides *netilmicin* (Netromycin) and *streptomycin* are excreted in small amounts. Because these drugs are nephrotoxic and ototoxic, the immature kidney function of neonates and infants should be considered. *Tetracyclines* are excreted in breast milk and should be avoided. *Sulfonamides* are excreted and generally contraindicated. They may cause kernicterus in the neonate and diarrhea and skin rash in the nursing infant. *Erythromycin* is excreted and may become concentrated in breast milk. No adverse effects on nursing infants have been reported. However, the potential exists for alteration in bowel flora, pharmacologic effects, and interference with fever workup. *Nitrofurantoin* (Macrodantin) is excreted in very small amounts. However, safety for use in nursing mothers has not been established, and infants with glucose-6-phosphate deyhydrogenase (G-6-PD) deficiency may be adversely affected. *Clindamycin* (Cleocin) is excreted. Breast-feeding is probably best discontinued if the drug is necessary, to avoid potential problems in the infant. *Cinoxacin* (Cinobac) and *norfloxacin* (Noroxin) are probably excreted, and there is a potential for severe adverse effects in nursing infants. Depending on the mother's need for the drug, either the drug or breast-feeding should be discontinued. *Isoniazid* (INH) and *rifampin* (Rifadin) are excreted in breast milk, and nursing infants should be observed for adverse drug effects. *Trimethoprim* (Proloprim, Bactrim) is excreted and may interfere with folic acid metabolism in the infant.

(continued)

Anticholinergics	*Atropine* and others are excreted and may cause infant toxicity or decreased breast milk production. Safety for use is not established.
Anticoagulants	*Heparin* is not excreted in breast milk; *warfarin* (Coumadin) is excreted, but some evidence suggests no harm to the nursing infant. More data are needed, and heparin is preferred if anticoagulant therapy is required.
Anticonvulsants	*Phenytoin* (Dilantin) and other hydantoins are excreted and may cause serious adverse effects in nursing infants. The drug or breast-feeding should be discontinued. *Phenobarbital* is excreted in small amounts and may cause drowsiness in the infant.
Antidepressants	Tricyclic antidepressants such as *amitriptyline* (Elavil) and others are excreted in small amounts; effects on nursing infants are not known. Other antidepressants have not been established as safe for use.
Antidiabetic Drugs	*Insulin* does not enter breast milk and is not known to affect the nursing infant. However, insulin requirements of the mother may be decreased while breast-feeding. Oral agents *chlorpropamide* (Diabinese) and *tolbutamide* (Orinase) are excreted in breast milk; the status of other sulfonylureas is unknown. There is a potential for hypoglycemia in nursing infants.
Antidiarrheals	*Diphenoxylate* (Lomotil) and *loperamide* (Imodium) should be used cautiously during lactation; effects on the nursing infant are unknown.
Antiemetics	Although information is limited, most of the drugs (*e.g.*, phenothiazines such as *promethazine* [Phenergan] and antihistamines such as *dimenhydrinate* [Dramamine]) are apparently excreted in breast milk and may cause drowsiness and possibly other effects in nursing infants. Antihistamines used for antiemetic effects also may inhibit lactation. *Metoclopramide* (Reglan) is excreted and concentrated in breast milk; it should be used cautiously, if at all.
Antihistamines	$Histamine_1$ receptor antagonists such as *diphenhydramine* (Benadryl) may inhibit lactation by their drying effects and may cause drowsiness in nursing infants. For most of the commonly used drugs, including over-the-counter allergy and cold remedies, little information is available about excretion in breast milk or effects on nursing infants. $Histamine_2$ receptor antagonists such as *cimetidine* (Tagamet) and *ranitidine* (Zantac) are excreted in breast milk. *Famotidine* (Pepcid) was excreted in animals, but it is not known whether it is excreted in human breast milk. It is generally recommended that either the drug or nursing be discontinued.
Antihypertensives	Beta-adrenergic blocking agents should generally be avoided by nursing mothers. *Propranolol* (Inderal) and *metoprolol* (Lopressor) are excreted in low concentrations; *acebutolol* (Sectral) and its major metabolite are excreted; it is unknown whether *nadolol* (Corgard) and *timolol* (Blocadren) are excreted. *Methyldopa* (Aldomet) is excreted; effects on nursing infants are unknown. It is unknown whether *hydralazine* (Apresoline) is excreted; safety for use is not established. *Captopril* (Capoten), *clonidine* (Catapres), *guanabenz* (Wytensin), and *guanfacine* (Tenex) are not generally recommended because information about effects on nursing infants is limited. Calcium channel blocking drugs should not be given to nursing mothers. *Verapamil* (Calan) and *diltiazem* (Cardizem) are excreted in breast milk.
Antimanic Agent	*Lithium* is excreted in breast milk and reaches about 40% of the mother's serum level. Infant serum and milk levels are about equal. If the drug is required, nursing should be discontinued.
Antipsychotic Drugs	Little information is available considering the extensive use of these drugs. *Chlorpromazine* (Thorazine) and *haloperidol* (Haldol) have been detected in breast milk in small amounts. Safety has not been established.
Antithyroid Drugs	Nursing is contraindicated for clients on the antithyroid drugs *propylthiouracil* and *methimazole* (Tapazole).
Beta-Adrenergic Blocking Agents	See ***Antihypertensives.***
Bronchodilators (Xanthine)	*Theophyline* (Theo-Dur) enters breast milk readily; use in caution.
Calcium Channel Blocking Agents	See ***Antihypertensives.***
Corticosteroids	*Prednisone* (Deltasone), *dexamethasone* (Decadron), and others appear in breast milk and could suppress growth, interfere with endogenous corticosteroid production, or cause other adverse effects in nursing infants. Advise mothers taking pharmacologic doses not to breast-feed.
Digitalis	*Digoxin* (Lanoxin) is excreted. However, infants receive very small amounts, and no adverse effects have been reported.
Diuretics	If diuretic drug therapy is required, nursing mothers should discontinue breast-feeding. Thiazide diuretics such as *hydrochlorothiazide* (HydroDIURIL) and the loop diuretic

(continued)

	furosemide (Lasix) are excreted in breast milk. It is unknown whether *bumetanide* (Bumex) and *ethacrynic acid* (Edecrin) are excreted. Little information is available about potassium-sparing diuretics, such as *amiloride* (Midamor), *triamterene* (Dyrenium, Dyazide, Maxide), and *spironolactone* (Aldactone). They are not recommended for use.
Laxatives	*Cascara sagrada* is excreted in breast milk and may cause diarrhea in the nursing infant. It is not known whether *docusate* (Colace) is excreted.
Nonsteroidal Anti-inflammatory Drugs	Most of the drugs, such as *ibuprofen* (Motrin, Advil), are excreted in breast milk, and nursing is not recommended. However, occasional use of therapeutic doses is probably acceptable.
Thyroid Hormones	Small amounts are excreted in breast milk. The drugs are not associated with adverse effects on nursing infants but should be used with caution in nursing mothers.

(From Abrams, A. C. [1998]. *Clinical drug therapy* [5th ed.]. Philadelphia: Lippincott.)

Appendix C

TEMPERATURE AND WEIGHT CONVERSION CHARTS

Conversion of Pounds to Kilograms

POUNDS	0	1	2	3	4	5	6	7	8	9
0	—	0.45	0.90	1.36	1.81	2.26	2.72	3.17	3.62	4.08
10	4.53	4.98	5.44	5.89	6.35	6.80	7.25	7.71	8.16	8.61
20	9.07	9.52	9.97	10.43	10.88	11.34	11.79	12.24	12.70	13.15
30	13.60	14.06	14.51	14.96	15.42	15.87	16.32	16.78	17.23	17.69
40	18.14	18.59	19.05	19.50	19.95	20.41	20.86	21.31	21.77	22.22
50	22.68	23.13	23.58	24.04	24.49	24.94	25.40	25.85	26.30	26.76
60	27.21	27.66	28.12	28.57	29.03	29.48	29.93	30.39	30.84	31.29
70	31.75	32.20	32.65	33.11	33.56	34.02	34.47	34.92	35.38	35.83
80	36.28	36.74	37.19	37.64	38.10	38.55	39.00	39.46	39.91	40.37
90	40.82	41.27	41.73	42.18	42.63	43.09	43.54	43.99	44.45	44.90
100	45.36	45.81	46.26	46.72	47.17	47.62	48.08	48.53	48.98	49.44
110	49.89	50.34	50.80	51.25	51.71	52.16	52.61	53.07	53.52	53.97
120	54.43	54.88	55.33	55.79	56.24	56.70	57.15	57.60	58.06	58.51
130	58.96	59.42	59.87	60.32	60.78	61.23	61.68	62.14	62.59	63.05
140	63.50	63.95	64.41	64.86	65.31	65.77	66.22	66.67	67.13	67.58
150	68.04	68.49	68.94	69.40	69.85	70.30	70.76	71.21	71.66	72.12
160	72.57	73.02	73.48	73.93	74.39	74.84	75.29	75.75	76.20	76.65
170	77.11	77.56	78.01	78.47	78.92	79.38	79.83	80.28	80.74	81.19
180	81.64	82.10	82.55	83.00	83.46	83.91	84.36	84.82	85.27	85.73
190	86.18	86.68	87.09	87.54	87.99	88.45	88.90	89.35	89.81	90.26
200	90.72	91.17	91.62	92.08	92.53	92.98	93.44	93.89	94.34	94.80

Conversion of Pounds and Ounces to Grams for Newborn Weights

	OUNCES															
POUNDS	*0*	*1*	*2*	*3*	*4*	*5*	*6*	*7*	*8*	*9*	*10*	*11*	*12*	*13*	*14*	*15*
0	—	28	57	85	113	142	170	198	227	255	283	312	430	369	397	425
1	454	482	510	539	567	595	624	652	680	709	737	765	794	822	850	879
2	907	936	964	992	1021	1049	1077	1106	1134	1162	1191	1219	1247	1276	1304	1332
3	1361	1389	1417	1446	1474	1503	1531	1559	1588	1616	1644	1673	1701	1729	1758	1786
4	1814	1843	1871	1899	1928	1956	1984	2013	2041	2070	2098	2126	2155	2183	2211	2240
5	2268	2296	2325	2353	2381	2410	2438	2466	2495	2523	2551	2580	2608	2637	2665	2693
6	2722	2750	2778	2807	2835	2863	2892	2920	2948	2977	3005	3033	3062	3090	3118	3147
7	3175	3203	3232	3260	3289	3317	3345	3374	3402	3430	3459	3487	3515	3544	3572	3600
8	3629	3657	3685	3714	3742	3770	3799	3827	3856	3884	3912	3941	3969	3997	4026	4054
9	4082	4111	4139	4167	4196	4224	4252	4281	4309	4337	4366	4394	4423	4451	4479	4508
10	4536	4564	4593	4621	4649	4678	4706	4734	4763	4791	4819	4848	4876	4904	4933	4961
11	4990	5018	5046	5075	5103	5131	5160	5188	5216	5245	5273	5301	5330	5358	5386	5415
12	5443	5471	5500	5528	5557	5585	5613	5642	5670	5698	5727	5755	5783	5812	5840	5868
13	5897	5925	5953	5982	6010	6038	6067	6095	6123	6152	6180	6209	6237	6265	6294	6322
14	6350	6379	6407	6435	6464	6492	6520	6549	6577	6605	6634	6662	6690	6719	6747	6776
15	6804	6832	6860	6889	6917	6945	6973	7002	7030	7059	7087	7115	7144	7172	7201	7228

Conversion of Fahrenheit to Celsius

CELSIUS	FAHRENHEIT	CELSIUS	FAHRENHEIT	CELSIUS	FAHRENHEIT
34.0	93.2	37.0	98.6	40.0	104.0
34.2	93.6	37.2	99.0	40.2	104.4
34.4	93.9	37.4	99.3	40.4	104.7
34.6	94.3	37.6	99.7	40.6	105.2
34.8	94.6	37.8	100.0	40.8	105.4
35.0	95.0	38.0	100.4	41.0	105.9
35.2	95.4	38.2	100.8	41.2	106.1
35.4	95.7	38.4	101.1	41.4	106.5
35.6	96.1	38.6	101.5	41.6	106.8
35.8	96.4	38.8	101.8	41.8	107.2
36.0	96.8	39.0	102.2	42.0	107.6
36.2	97.2	39.2	102.6	42.2	108.0
36.4	97.5	39.4	102.9	42.4	108.3
36.6	97.9	39.6	103.3	42.6	108.7
36.8	98.2	39.8	103.6	42.8	109.0

$(°C) \times (9/5) + 32 = °F$

$(°F - 32) \times (5/9) = °C$

Appendix D

GROWTH CHARTS

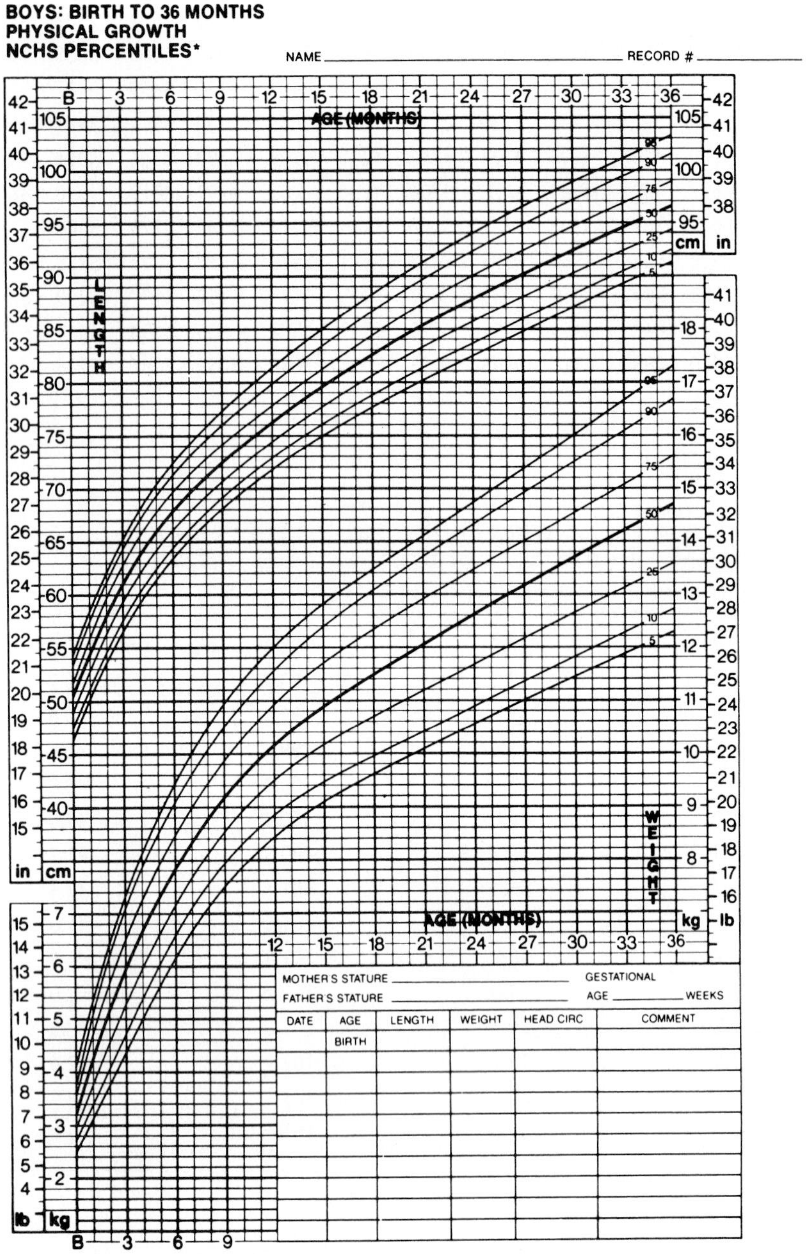

Source: *Adapted from Hamill, P. V. V., et al. (1979). Physical growth: National Center for Health Statistics percentiles.* American Journal of Clinical Nutrition, 32, *607. Data from the Fels Research Institute, Wright State University School of Medicine, Yellow Springs, OH. Courtesy of Ross Laboratories.*

GIRLS: BIRTH TO 36 MONTHS
PHYSICAL GROWTH
NCHS PERCENTILES*

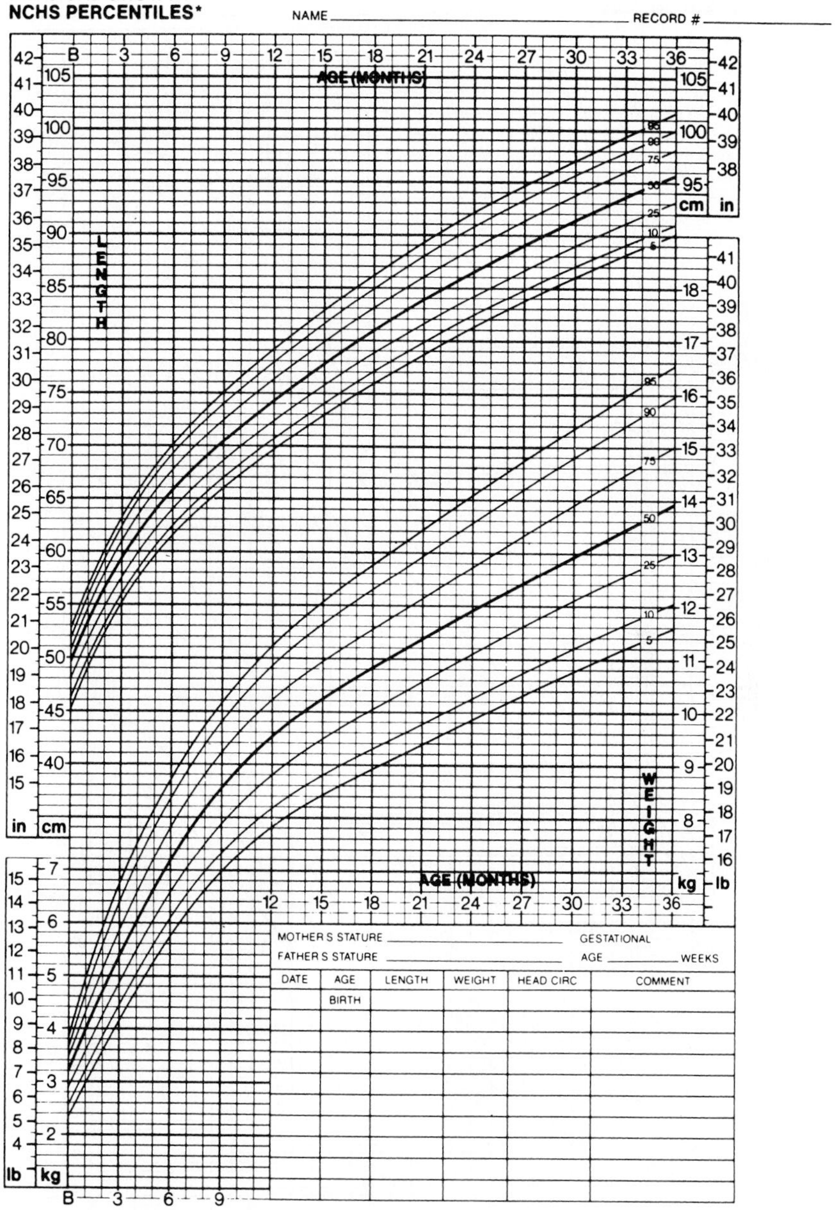

Source: *Adapted from Hamill, P. V. V., et al. (1979). Physical growth: National Center for Health Statistics percentiles.* American Journal of Clinical Nutrition, 32, *607. Data from the Fels Research Institute, Wright State University School of Medicine, Yellow Springs, OH. Courtesy of Ross Laboratories.*

BOYS: 2 TO 18 YEARS
PHYSICAL GROWTH
NCHS PERCENTILES*

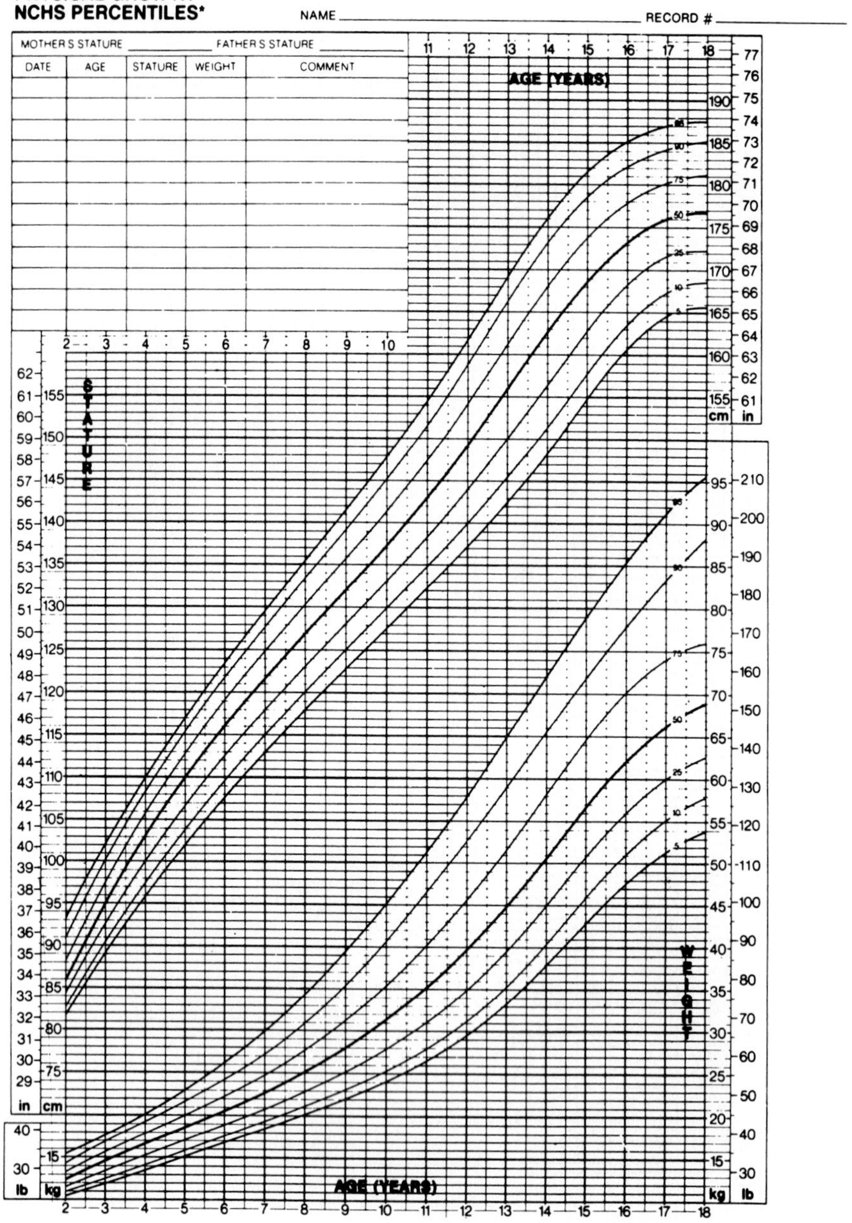

Source: *Adapted from Hamill, P. V. V., et al. (1979). Physical growth: National Center for Health Statistics percentiles.* American Journal of Clinical Nutrition, 32, *607. Data from the Fels Research Institute, Wright State University School of Medicine, Yellow Springs, OH. Courtesy of Ross Laboratories.*

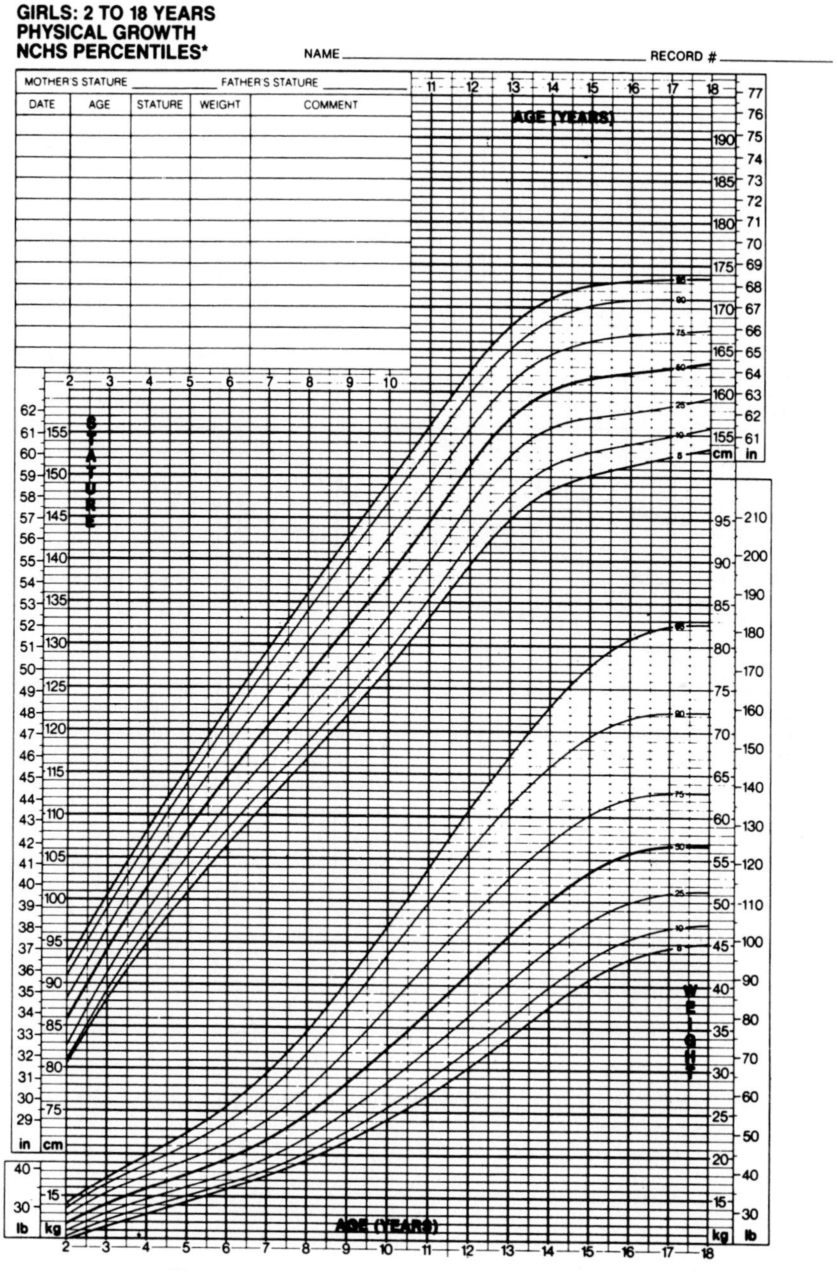

Source: *Adapted from Hamill, P. V. V., et al. (1979). Physical growth: National Center for Health Statistics percentiles.* American Journal of Clinical Nutrition, 32, *607. Data from the Fels Research Institute, Wright State University School of Medicine, Yellow Springs, OH. Courtesy of Ross Laboratories.*

HEAD CIRCUMFERENCE: GIRLS

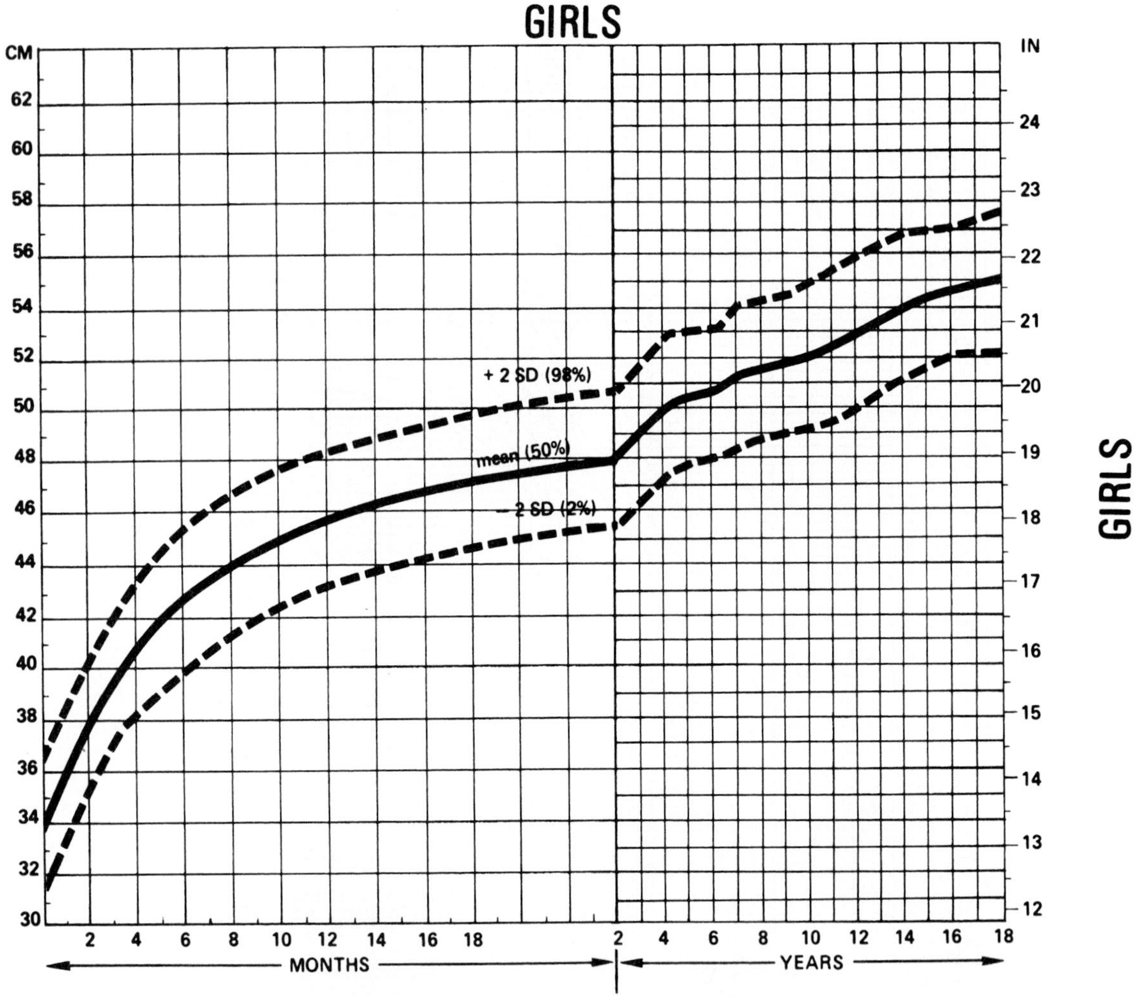

Source: *Nellhaus, G. (1968). Composite international and interracial graphs.* Pediatrics, 41, *106. Copyright American Academy of Pediatrics 1968.*

HEAD CIRCUMFERENCE: BOYS

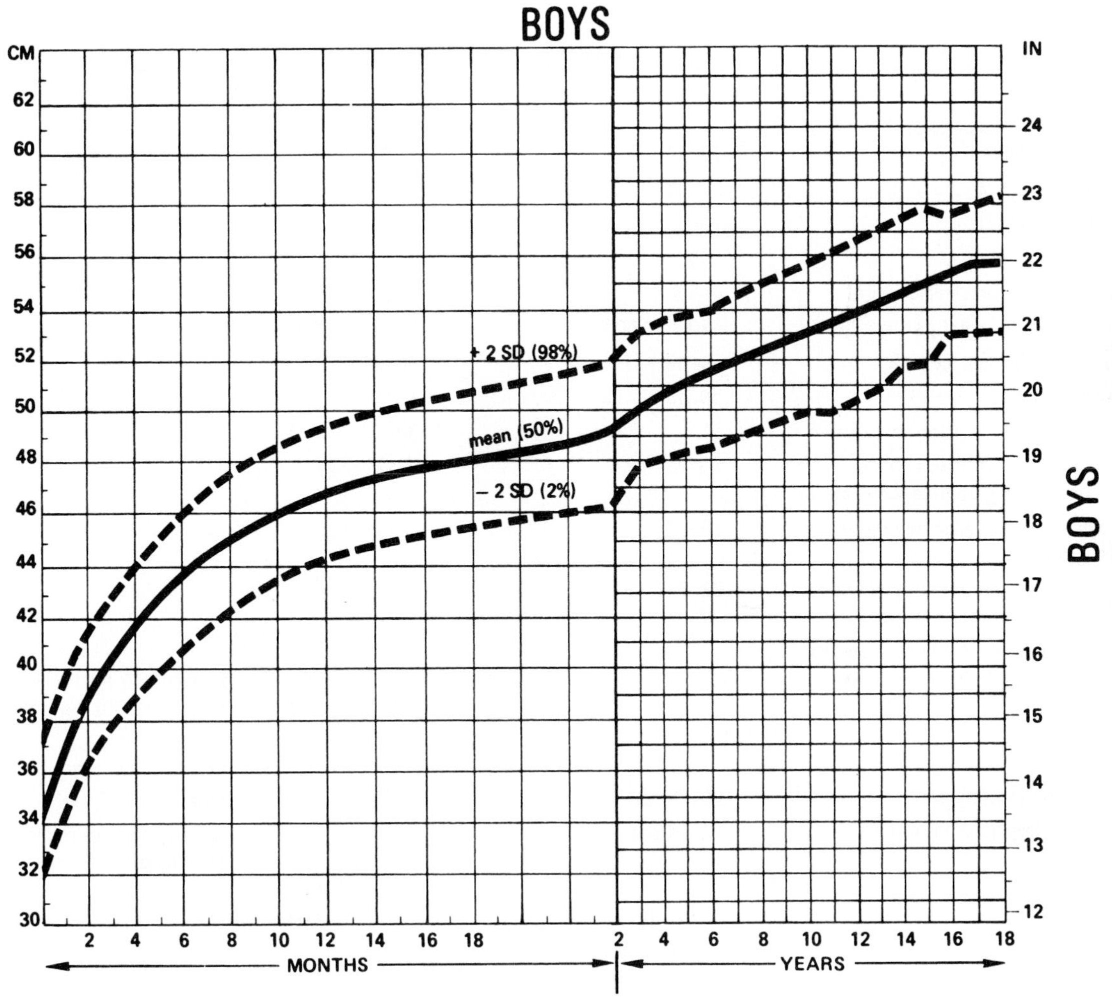

Source: *Nellhaus, G. (1968). Composite international and interracial graphs.* Pediatrics, 41, *106. Copyright American Academy of Pediatrics 1968.*

Appendix E

STANDARD LABORATORY VALUES

PREGNANT AND NONPREGNANT WOMEN

VALUES	NONPREGNANT	PREGNANT
Hematologic		
Complete Blood Count (CBC)		
Hemoglobin, g/dL	12–16*	11.5–14*
Hematocrit, PCV, %	37–47	32–42
Red cell volume, mL	1600	1900
Plasma volume, mL	2400	3700
Red blood cell count, million/mm^3	4–5.5	3.75–5.0
White blood cells, total per mm^3	4500–10,000	5000–15,000
Polymorphonuclear cells, %	54–62	60–85
Lymphocytes, %	38–46	15–40
Erythrocyte sedimentation rate, mm/h	≤	30–90
MCHC, g/dL packed RBCs (mean corpuscular hemoglobin concentration)	30–36	No change
MCH (mean corpuscular hemoglobin per picogram)	29–32	No change
MCV/μm^3 (mean corpuscular volume per cubic micrometer)	82–96	No change
Blood Coagulation and Fibrinolytic Activity†		
Factors VII, VIII, IX, X		Increase in pregnancy, return to normal in early puerperium; factor VIII increases during and immediately after delivery
Factors XI; XIII		Decrease in pregnancy
Prothrombin time (protime)	60–70 sec	Slight decrease in pregnancy
Partial thromboplastin time (PTT)	12–14 sec	Slight decrease in pregnancy and again decrease during second and third stage of labor (indicates clotting at placental site)
Bleeding time	1–3 min (Duke) 2–4 min (Ivy)	No appreciable change
Coagulation time	6–10 min (Lee/White)	No appreciable change
Platelets	150,000 to 350,000/mm^3	No significant change until 3–5 days after delivery, then marked increase (may predispose woman to thrombosis) and gradual return to normal
Fibrinolytic activity		Decreases in pregnancy, then abrupt return to normal (protection against thromboembolism)
Fibrinogen	250 mg/dL	400 mg/dL
Mineral and Vitamin Concentrations		
Serum iron, μg	75–150	65–120
Total iron-binding capacity, μg	250–450	300–500
Iron saturation, %	30–40	15–30
Vitamin B_{12}, folic acid, ascorbic acid	Normal	Moderate decrease

(continued)

PREGNANT AND NONPREGNANT WOMEN *(continued)*

VALUES	NONPREGNANT	PREGNANT
Serum protein		
Total, g/dL	6.7–8.3	5.5–7.5
Albumin, g/dL	3.5–5.5	3.0–5.0
Globulin, total, g/dL	2.3–3.5	3.0–4.0
Blood sugar		
Fasting, mg/dL	70–80	65
2-hour postprandial, mg/dL	60–110	Under 140 after a 100-g carbohydrate meal is considered normal
Cardiovascular		
Blood pressure, mm Hg	120/80‡	114/65
Peripheral resistance, dyne/s · cm^{-5}	120	100
Venous pressure, cm H_2O		
Femoral	9	24
Antecubital	8	8
Pulse, rate/min	70	80
Stroke volume, mL	65	75
Cardiac output, L/min	4.5	6
Circulation time (arm-tongue), sec	15–16	12–14
Blood volume, mL		
Whole blood	4000	5600
Plasma	2400	3700
Red blood cells	1600	1900
Plasma renin, units/L	3–10	10–80
Chest x-ray studies		
Transverse diameter of heart	—	1–2 cm increase
Left border of heart	—	Straightened
Cardiac volume	—	70-mL increase
Electrocardiogram	—	15° left axis deviation
V_1 and V_2	—	Inverted T-wave
kV_4	—	Low T
III	—	Q + inverted T
aVr	—	Small Q
Hepatic		
Bilirubin total	Not more than 1 mg/dL	Unchanged
Cephalin flocculation	Up to 2+ in 48 h	Positive in 10%
Serum cholesterol	110–300 mg/dL	↑ 60% from 16–32 weeks of pregnancy; remains at this level until after delivery
Thymol turbidity	0–4 units	Positive in 15%
Serum alkaline phosphatase	2–4.5 units (Bodansky)	↑ from week 12 of pregnancy to 6 weeks after delivery
Serum lactate dehydrogenase		Unchanged
Serum glutamic-oxaloacetic transaminase		Unchanged
Serum globulin albumin	1.5–3.0 g/dL	↑ slight
	4.5–5.3 g/dL	↓ 3.0 g by late pregnancy
A/G ratio		Decreased
α_2-globulin		Increased
β-globulin		Increased
Serum cholinesterase		Decreased

(continued)

PREGNANT AND NONPREGNANT WOMEN *(continued)*

VALUES	NONPREGNANT	PREGNANT
Leucine aminopeptidase		Increased
Sulfobromophthalein (5 mg/kg)	5% dye or less in 45 min	Somewhat decreased
Renal		
Bladder capacity	1300 mL	1500 mL
Renal plasma flow (RPF), mL/min	490–700	Increase by 25%, to 612–875
Glomerular filtration rate (GFR), mL/min	105–132	Increase by 50%, to 160–198
Nonprotein nitrogen (NPN), mg/dL	25–40	Decreases
Blood urea nitrogen (BUN), mg/dL	20–25	Decreases
Serum creatinine, mg/kg/24 hr	20–22	Decreases
Serum uric acid, mg/kg/24 hr	257–750	Decreases
Urine glucose	Negative	Present in 20% of gravidas
Intravenous pyelogram (IVP)	Normal	Slight to moderate hydroureter and hydronephrosis; right kidney larger than left kidney
Miscellaneous		
Total thyroxine concentration	5–12 μg/dL thyroxine	↑ 9–16 μg/dL thyroxine (however, unbound thyroxine not greatly increased)
Ionized calcium		Relatively unchanged
Aldosterone		↑ 1 mg/24 hr by third trimester
Dehydroisoandrosterone	Plasma clearance 6–8 L/24 hr	↑ plasma clearance tenfold to twentyfold

* At sea level. Permanent residents of higher levels (e.g., Denver) require higher levels of hemoglobin.
From Bobak IM, et al. (1995). *Maternity nursing* (2th ed.). St Louis: C. V. Mosby.
† Pregnancy represents a hypercoagulable state.
‡ For the woman about 20 years of age.
10 years of age: 103/70.
30 years of age: 123/82.
40 years of age: 126/84.

INFANTS AND CHILDREN

The following reference values for laboratory tests represent guidelines only, since the reference range from one institution to the next will vary, depending on the laboratory method used. To simplify the interpretation of laboratory results reported in International System (SI) units, conversion factors (from SI to conventional units) are provided. SI base units are the gram (g), the liter (L), and the mole (mol). Other abbreviations used throughout this table are listed below.

SI Prefixes

FACTOR	PREFIX	SYMBOL
10^{3}	kilo	k
10^{-1}	deci	d
10^{-2}	centi	c
10^{-3}	milli	m
10^{-6}	micro	μ
10^{-9}	nano	n
10^{-12}	pico	p
10^{-15}	femto	f

Abbreviations

Cl	confidence interval
d	day
F	female
h	hour
Hb	hemoglobin
M	male
MCHC	mean corpuscular hemoglobin concentration
MCV	mean corpuscular value
mEq	milliequivalent
min	minute
RBC	red blood cell
s	second
SD	standard deviation
U	unit
WBC	white blood cell
yr	year

Blood

TEST	SI REFERENCE RANGE	CONVERSION FACTOR	CONVENTIONAL UNITS REFERENCE RANGE
Adrenocorticotropic hormone (ACTH)	Cord: 130–160 ng/L 1st week: 100–140 Adult 0800 h: 25–100 1800 h: <50		Cord: 130–160 pg/mL 1st week: 100–140 Adult 0800 h: 25–100 1800 h: <50
Alanine aminotransferase (ALT)	<1 yr: 5–28 U/L >1 yr: 820		Same as SI
Albumin	35–50 g/L		3.5–5.0 g/dL
Aldolase	Newborn: <32 U/L Child: <16 Adult: <8		Same as SI
Aldosterone	Newborn: 0.14–1.66 nmol/L 1 wk–1 yr: 0.03–4.43 1–3 yr: 0.14–1.66 3–5 yr: <0.14–2.22 5–7 yr: <0.14–1.39 7–11 yr: 0.14–1.94 11–15 yr: <0.14–1.39	nmol/L × 36.1 = ng/dL	Newborn: 5–60 ng/dL 1 wk–1 yr: 1–160 ng/dL 1–3 yr: 5–60 ng/dL 3–5 yr: <5–80 5–7 yr: <5–50 7–11 yr: 5–70 11–15 yr: <5–50
Alkaline phosphatase	Infant: 150–400 U/L 2–10 yr: 100–300 11–18 yr (M): 50–375 11–18 yr (F): 30–300 Adult: 30–100		Same as SI
α_1-antitrypsin	2–4 g/L		200–400 mg/dL
α-fetoprotein	Fetal: peak of 2–4 g/L Cord: <0.05 g/L >1 yr: <30 µg/L		Fetal: 200–400 mg/dL Cord: <5 >1 yr: <30
Ammonia nitrogen	9–34 µmol/L	µmol/L × 1.4 = µg/dL	13–48 µg/dL
Amylase	Newborn: 5–65 U/L >1 yr: 25–125		Same as SI
Androstenedione	Child: 0.17–1.7 nmol/L Adult (M): 2.4–5.2 Adult (F): 2.7–8.0	nmol/L × 28.7 = ng/dL	Child: 5–50 ng/dL Adult (M): 70–150 Adult (F): 76–228
Angiotensin-converting enzyme	<670 nmol · L^{-1} · S^{-1}	nmol · L^{-1} · S^{-1} × 0.06 = nmol/mL/min	<40 nmol/mL/min
Anion gap [Na – (Cl + HCO_3)]	7–14 mmol/L		7–14 mEq/L
Aspartate amino-transfer (AST)	<1 yr: 15–60 U/L >1 yr: ≤20 U/L		Same as SI
Bicarbonate	<2 yrs: 20–25 mmol/L >2 yrs: 22–26 mmol/L		<2 yrs: 20–25 mEq/L >2 yrs: 22–26
Bilirubin (total)	*Preterm* / *Full term* Cord: <34 / <34 µmol/L 0–1 d: <137 / <103 1–2 d: <205 / <137 3–5 d: <274 / <205 Thereafter: <34 / <17	µmol/L × 0.05848 = mg/dL	*Preterm* / *Full term* Cord: <2 / <2 mg/dL 0–1 d: <8 / <6 1–2 d: <12 / <8 3–5 d: <16 / <12 Thereafter: <2 / <1
Bilirubin (conjugated)	0–3.4 µmol/L	µmol/L × 0.05848 = mg/dL	0–0.2 mg/dL
Calcium (ionized)	1.12–1.23 mmol/L	mmol/L × 4 = mg/dL	4.48–4.92 mg/dL
Calcium (total)	Preterm <1 wk: 1.5–2.5 mmol/L Term: <1 wk: 1.75–3 Child: 2–2.6 Adult: 2.1–2.6	mmol/L × 4 = mg/dL	6–10 mg/dL 7–12 8–10.5 8.5–10.5

(continued)

Blood *(continued)*

TEST	SI REFERENCE RANGE	CONVERSION FACTOR	CONVENTIONAL UNITS REFERENCE RANGE
Immunoglobulin E	Newborn: 0–24 µg/L 6–12 yr: 0–480 Adult: 0–960		Newborn: 0–10 U/mL 6–12 yr: 0–200 Adult: 0–400
Insulin, fasting	3–23 mU/L		3–23 µU/mL
Iron	Newborn: 20–48 µmol/L 4–10 mo: 5.4–12.5 3–19 yr: 9.5–27.0 Adult: 13.0–33.0	µmol/L × 5.587 = µg/dL	Newborn: 110–270 µg/dL 4–10 mo: 30–70 3–10 yr: 53–119 Adult: 72–186
Iron-binding capacity	Newborn: 10.6–31.3 µmol/L Thereafter: 45–72	µmol/L × 5.587 = µg/dL	Newborn: 59–175 µg/dL Thereafter: 250–400
Lactate	Venous: 0.5–2.0 mmol/L Arterial: 0.3–0.8	mmol/L × 9.01 = mg/dL	Venous: 5–18 mg/dL Arterial: 3–7
Lactate dehydrogenase	Newborn: 160–1500 U/L Infant: 150–360 Child: 150–300 Adult: 100–250		Same as SI units
Lactate dehydrogenase isoenzymes		*Fraction of total* LD 1 (heart): 0.24–0.34 LD 2 (heart, RBCs): 0.35–0.45 LD 3 (muscle): 0.15–0.25 LD 4 (liver, muscle): 0.04–0.10 LD 5 (liver, muscle): 0.01–0.09	
Lead	<1.16 µmol/L	µmol/L × 20.7 = mgm/dL	<24 gmg/dL

Lipids	**95th %ile values—mmol/L (mg/dL)**				**5th %ile values—mmol/L (mg/dL)**	
	VLDL (Cholesterol)		*LDL (Cholesterol)*		*HDL (Cholesterol)*	
	M	*F*	*M*	*F*	*M*	*F*
5–9 yr:	0.47 (18)	0.62 (24)	3.34 (129)	3.62 (140)	0.98 (38)	0.93 (36)
10–14 yr:	0.57 (22)	0.59 (23)	3.41 (132)	3.52 (136)	0.96 (37)	0.91 (35)
15–19 yr:	0.67 (26)	0.62 (24)	3.36 (130)	3.49 (135)	0.80 (31)	0.91 (35)
			mmol/L × 38.61 = mg/dL			

TEST	SI REFERENCE RANGE	CONVERSION FACTOR	CONVENTIONAL UNITS REFERENCE RANGE
Luteinizing hormone	Prepubertal: <5 IU/L Adult (M): 3.9–18 Adult (F): 2.0–22.6		Prepubertal: <5 mIU/L Adult (M): 3.9–18 Adult (F): 2.0–22.6
Magnesium	0.75–1.0 mmol/L	mmol/L × 2 = mEq/L	1.5–2.0 mEq/L
Methemoglobin	<46 µmol/L	µmol/L × 0.0065 = g/dL	<0.3 gdL
Osmolality	285–295 mmol/kg		285–295 mOsm/kg
Phosphorus	Newborn: 1.36–2.91 mmol/L 1 yr: 1.23–2.00 2–5 yr: 1.13–2.20 Adult: 0.97–1.45	mmol/L × 3.097 = mg/dL	Newborn: 4.2–9.0 mg/dL 1 yr: 3.8–6.2 2–5 yr: 3.5–6.8 Adult: 3.0–4.5
Phytanic acid	<0.003 fraction of total serum fatty acids		<0.3% of total serum fatty acids
Potassium	<10 days: 3.5–6.0 mmol/L >10 days: 3.5–5.0		<10 days: 3.5–6.0 mEq/L >10 days: 3.5–5.0
Progesterone	*Males* Prepubertal: 0.35–0.83 nmol/L Adult: 0.38–0.95	nmol/L × 0.314 = ng/mL	 0.11–0.26 ng/mL 0.12–0.30
	Females Prepubertal: <0.95 Pubertal stage II: <1.46 III: <1.91 IV: 0.16–41.34		 ≤0.30 ≤0.46 ≤0.60 0.05–13.0

(continued)

Blood *(continued)*

TEST	SI REFERENCE RANGE	CONVERSION FACTOR	CONVENTIONAL UNITS REFERENCE RANGE
	Follicular: 0.06–2.86 Luteal: 19.08–95.40		0.02–0.9 6.0–30.0
Prolactin	Newborn: <200 μg/L Adult: <20 μg/L		Newborn: <200 ng/mL Adult: <20 ng/mL
Protein, total	Preterm: 40–70 g/L Term newborn: 50–71 1–3 mo: 47–74 3–12 mo: 50–75 1–15 yr: 65–86		Preterm: 4.0–7.0 g/dL Term newborn: 5.0–7.1 1–3 mo: 4.7–7.4 3–12 mo: 5.0–7.5 1–15 yr: 6.5–8.6
Pyruvate	0.03–0.10 mmol/L	mmol/L × 8.81 = mg/dL	0.3–0.9 mg/dL
Renin	Adults: 0.30–1.14 $ng \cdot L^{-1} \cdot S^{-1}$	$ng \cdot L^{-1} \cdot S^{-1} \times 3.6$ = ng/mL/h	Adults: 1.1–4.1 ng/mL/h
Sodium	135–145 mmol/L		135–145 mEq/L
Somatomedin C	0–2 yr: 220–1000 IU/L 3–5 yr: 270–1600 6–10 yr: 370–2100 11–12 yr: 450–2800 13–14 yr: 1100–4000 15–17 yr: 1000–2900 Thereafter: 460–1500		0–2 yr: 0.22–1.00 U/mL 3–5 yr: 0.27–1.60 6–10 yr: 0.37–2.10 11–12 yr: 0.45–2.80 13–14 yr: 1.10–4.00 15–17 yr: 1.00–2.90 Thereafter: 0.46–1.50
Testosterone, free	Prepubertal: 2.08–13.19 pmol/L Adult (M): 48.6–201 Adult (F): 6.94–25		Prepubertal: 0.06–0.38 ng/dL Adult (M): 1.40–5.79 Adult (F): 0.20–0.73
Testosterone, total	Prepubertal: 0.35–0.70 nmol/L Adult (F): 0.8–2.6 Adult (M): 9.5–30		Prepubertal: 10–20 ng/dL Adult (F): 23–75 Adult (M): 275–875
Thyroid-stimulating hormone (TSH)	Cord 0–17.4 μU/L 1–3 days: 0–13.3 Thereafter: 0–5.5		Cord: 0–17.4 mIU/mL 1–3 days: 0–13.3 Thereafter: 0–5.5
Thyroxine (T_4), total	Cord: 95–168 nmol/L <1 mo: 90–292 1 mo–1 yr: 93–213 1–5 yr: 94–194 5–10 yr: 83–172 10–15 yr: 72–151 Adult: 55–161	nmol/L × 0.0775 = μg/dL	Cord: 7.4–13.0 μg/dL <1 mo: 7.0–22.6 1 mo–1 yr: 7.2–16.5 1–5 yr: 7.3–15.0 5–10 yr: 6.4–13.3 10–15 yr: 5.6–11.7 Adult: 4.3–12.5
Thyroxine (T_4), free	9–22 pmol/L	pmol/L × 0.0777 = ng/dL	0.7–1.7 ng/dL
Transferrin	Newborn: 1.30–2.75 g/L Adult: 2.20–4.00		Newborn: 130–275 mg/dL Adult: 220–440
Triglycerides	**Normal Upper Limits—mmol/L (mg/dL)** *Male* 0–4 yr: 1.12 (99) 5–9 yr: 1.14 (101) 10–15 yr: 1.41 (125) 15–19 yr: 1.67 (148)	*Female* 1.26 (112) 1.19 (105) 1.48 (131) 1.40 (124) mmol/L × 88.55 = mg/dL	
Triiodothyronine (T_3)	Cord: 0.23–1.16 nmol/L <1 mo: 0.49–3.70 1 mo–1 yr: 1.70–4.31 1–5 yr: 1.62–4.14 5–10 yr: 1.45–3.71 10–15 yr: 1.28–3.31 Adult: 1.08–3.14	nmol/L × 65.1 = ng/dL	Cord: 15–75 ng/dL <1 mo: 32–240 1 mo–1 yr: 110–280 1–5 yr: 105–269 5–10 yr: 94–241 10–15 yr: 83–215 Adult: 70–204
Triiodothyronine resin uptake	0.25–0.35		25%–35%

(continued)

Blood (*continued*)

TEST	SI REFERENCE RANGE	CONVERSION FACTOR	CONVENTIONAL UNITS REFERENCE RANGE
Urea nitrogen	2–7 mmol/L	mmol/L × 28 = mg/dL	5–20 mg/dL
Uric acid	120–420 µmol/L	µmol/L × 0.0169 = mg/dL	2–7 mg/dL
Vitamin A	Newborn: 1.22–2.62 µmol/L Child: 1.05–2.79 Adult: 1.05–2.27	µmol/L × 28.65 = mg/dL	Newborn: 35–75 µg/dL Child: 30–80 Adult: 30–65
Vitamin B_6	14.6–72.8 nmol/L	nmol/L × 0.247 = ng/mL	3.6–18 ng/mL
Vitamin B_{12}	96–579 pmol/L	pmol/L × 1.355 = pg/mL	130–785 pg/mL
Vitamin C	11.4–113.6 µmol/L	µmol/L × 0.176 = mg/dL	0.2–2.0 mg/dL
Vitamin D_3 (1,25 dihydroxy)	60–108 pmol/L	pmol/L × 0.417 = pg/mL	25–45 pg/mL
Vitamin E	11.6–46.4 µmol/L	µmol/L × 0.043 = mg/dL	0.5–2.0 mg/dL
Zinc	10.7–22.9 µmol/L	µmol/L × 6.54 = µg/dL	70–150 µg/dL

Hematology

	HB (g/dL)		HEMATOCRIT (%)		MCV (fL)		MCHC (g/dL RBC)			WBC (1,000/mm³)		PLATELETS (1,000/mm³)
AGE	***Mean***	***-2 SD***	***Mean***	***-2 SD***	***Mean***	***-2 SD***	***Mean***	***-2 SD***	RETICULOCYTE (%)	***Mean***	***95% CI***	***Mean (Range)***
Term (cord blood)	16.5	13.5	51	42	108	98	33.0	30.0	3.0–7.0	18.1	9.0–30.0	290
1–3 days	18.5	14.5	56	45	108	95	33.0	29.0	1.8–4.6	18.9	9.4–34.0	192
2 weeks	16.6	13.4	53	41	105	88	31.4	28.1		11.4	5.0–20.0	252
1 months	13.9	10.7	44	33	101	91	31.8	28.1	0.1–1.7	10.8	5.0–19.5	
2 months	11.2	9.4	35	28	95	84	31.8	28.3				
6 months	12.6	11.1	36	31	76	68	35.0	32.7	0.7–2.3	11.9	6.0–17.5	
6–24 months	12.0	10.5	36	33	78	70	33.0	30.0		10.6	6.0–17.0	(150–300)
2–6 years	12.5	11.5	37	34	81	75	34.0	31.0	0.5–1.0	8.5	5.0–15.5	(150–300)
6–12 years	13.5	11.5	50	35	86	77	34.0	31.0	0.5–1.0	8.1	4.5–13.5	(150–300)
12–18 years (M)	14.5	13.0	43	36	88	78	34.0	31.0	0.5–1.0	7.8	4.5–13.5	(150–300)
12–18 years (F)	14.0	12.0	41	37	90	78	34.0	31.0	0.5–1.0	7.8	4.5–13.5	(150–300)

Urine

TEST	SI REFERENCE RANGE	CONVERSION FACTOR	CONVENTIONAL UNITS REFERENCE RANGE
Aminolevulinic acid	8–53 μmol/d	μmol/d × 0.131 = mg/d	1–7 mg/d
Calcium	<0.1 mmol/kg/d	mmol/d × 40 = mg/d	<4 mg/kg/d
Copper	<0.6 μmol/d	μmol/d × 63.7 = gmg/d	<40 μg/d
Coproporphyrin	<300 nmol/d	nmol/d × 1.527 = μg/d	<200 μg/d
Cortisol, free	70–340 nmol/d	nmol/d × 0.362 = μg/d	25–125 μg/d
Creatinine	Infant: 71–177 μmol/kg/d Child: 71–194 Adolescent: 71–265	μmol/kg/d × 0.113 = mg/kg/d	Infant: 8–20 mg/kg/d Child: 8–22 Adolescent: 8–30
Cystine	40–260 μmol/d	μmol/d × 0.12 = mg/d	5–31 mg/d
Dehydroepiandrosterone (DHEA)	<5 yr: <0.3 μmol/d 6–9 yr: <0.7 10–15 yr: <1.4 Adult (M): <8.0 Adult (F): <4.2	μmol/d × 0.288 = mg/d	<5 yr: <0.1 mg/d 6–9 yr: <0.2 10–15 yr: <0.4 Adult (M): <2.3 Adult (F): <1.2
Epinephrine	<55 nmol/d	nmol/d × 0.183 = μg/d	<10 μg/d
Fluoride	<50 μmol/d	μmol/d × 0.019 = mg/d	<1 mg/d
Homovanillic acid (HVA)	*mmol/mol/creatinine* 1–12 mo: 0.75–21.7 1–2 yr: 2.5–14.3 2–5 yr: 0.43–8.4 5–10 yr: 0.31–5.6 10–15 yr: 0.15–7.4 15–18 yr: 0.31–1.24	mmol/mol creatinine × 1.61 = μg/mg creatinine	*μg/mg creatinine* 1–12 mo: 1.2–35.0 1–2 yr: 4.0–23.0 2–5 yr: 0.7–13.5 5–10 yr: 0.5–9.0 10–15 yr: 0.25–12.0 15–18 yr: 0.5–2.0
Metanephrines	*mmol/mol/creatinine* <1 yr: 0.001–2.64 1–2 yr: 0.15–3.09 2–5 yr: 0.20–1.72 5–10 yr: 0.25–1.55 10–15 yr: 0.001–0.38 15–18 yr: 0.03–0.69	mmol/mol creatinine × 1.74 = μg/mg creatinine	*μg/mg creatinine* <1 yr: 0.001–4.6 1–2 yr: 0.27–5.38 2–5 yr: 0.35–2.99 5–10 yr: 0.43–2.70 10–15 yr: 0.001–1.87 15–18 yr: 0.001–0.67
Norepinephrine	<590 nmol/d	nmol/d × 0.169 = μg/d	<100 μg/d
Osmolality	50–1200 μgmol/kg		50–1200 mOsm/kg
Oxalate	110–440 μmol/d	μmol/d × 0.088 = mg/d	10–40 mg/d
Porphobilinogen	0–8.8 μmol/d	μmol/d × 0.226 = mg/d	0–2 mg/d
Potassium	25–125 mmol/d (varies with diet)		25–125 mEq/d
Pregnanetriol	<7.4 μmol/d	μmol/d × 0.3365 = mg/d	<2.5 mg/d
Protein	10–140 mg/L		1–14 mg/dL
Steroids: 17-hydroxycorticosteroid	Prepubertal: 2.76–15.5 μmol/d Adult (M): 11–33 Adult (F): 11–22	μmol/d × 0.3625 = mg/d	Prepubertal: 1–5.6 mg/d Adult (M): 4–12 Adult (F): 4–8
Steroids: 17-ketosteroids	<1 mo: ≤6.9 μmol/d 1 mo–5 yr: <1.73 6–8 yr: 3.47–6.9 Adult (M): 21–62 Adult (F): 14–45	μmol/d × 0.2884 = mg/d	<1 mo: <2 mg/d 1 mo–5 yr: <0.5 6–8 yr: 1–2 Adult (M): 6–18 Adult (F): 4–13
Uric acid	1.48–4.43 mmol/d	mmol/d ×169 = mg/d	250–750 mg/d
Vanilylmandelic acid (VMA)	*mmol/mol/creatinine* 1–6 mo: 1.71–9.71 6–12 mo: 1.14–8.57 1–5 yr: 1.14–5.71 5–10 yr: 0.86–4.00 10–15 yr: 0.57–3.43 >15 yr: 0.57–3.43	mmol/mol creatinine × 1.75 = μg/mg	*μg/mg creatinine* 1–6 mo: 3–7 6–12 mo: 2–15 1–5 yr: 2–10 5–10 yr: 1.5–7 10–15 yr: 1–6 >15 yr: 1–6

Cerebrospinal Fluid

CELL COUNT RANGE
Preterm: 0–25 WBC × 10^6 cells/L (57% polymorphonuclears) Term: 0–22 WBC × 10^6 cells/L (61% polymorphonuclears) Child: 0–7 WBC × 10^6 cells/L (0% polymorphonuclears)

	CELL COUNT PERCENTILES								
	Total WBC			***Polymorphonuclears***			***Monocytes***		
	25%	***50%***	***75%***	***25%***	***50%***	***75%***	***25%***	***50%***	***75%***
<6 wk	0.50	2.57	5.16	0	0	2.42	0	0.83	2.71
6 wk–3 mo	0.34	1.86	3.75	0	0	0.66	0	0.96	2.78
3–6 mo	0.00	1.11	2.31	0	0	0.40	0	0.43	1.64
6–12 mo	0.41	1.47	3.25	0	0	0.52	0.03	0.93	2.32
>12 mo	0.00	0.68	1.82	0	0	0	0	0.25	1.45

TEST	SI REFERENCE RANGE	CONVENTIONAL UNITS REFERENCE RANGE
Glucose	Preterm: 1.3–3.5 mmol/L Term: 1.9–6.6 Child: 2.2–4.4	Preterm: 24–63 mg/dL Term: 34–119 Child: 40–80
Protein	Preterm: 0.65–1.50 g/L Term: 0.20–1.70 Child: 0.05–0.40	Preterm: 65–150 mg/dL Term: 20–170 Child: 5–40
Pressure	<200 mm H_2O	<200 mm H_2O

(Rowe, P. C. [1994]. Laboratory values. In F. A. Oski, et al. [Eds.] *Principles and practice of pediatrics* [2nd ed.]. Philadelphia: J. B. Lippincott.)

Appendix F

PULSE, RESPIRATION, AND BLOOD PRESSURE VALUES

Pulse Rate at Various Ages

AGE	RANGE	AVERAGE
Newborn	70–170	120
1–11 months	80–160	120
2 years	80–130	110
4 years	80–120	100
6 years	75–115	100
8 years	70–110	90
10 years	70–100	90

	GIRLS		BOYS	
	Range	***Average***	***Range***	***Average***
12 years	70–110	90	65–105	85
14 years	65–105	85	60–100	80
16 years	60–100	80	55–95	75
18 years	55–95	75	50–90	70

Variations in Respirations with Age

AGE	RATE PER MINUTE
Newborn	40–90
1 year	20–40
2 years	20–30
3 years	20–30
5 years	20–25
10 years	17–22
15 years	15–20
20 years	15–20

Normal Blood Pressure for Various Ages

AGE	SYSTOLIC (MEAN ± 2 SD)	DIASTOLIC (MEAN ± 2 SD)
Newborn	80 ± 16	46 ± 16
6 months–1 year	89 ± 29	60 ± 10*
1 year	96 ± 30	66 ± 25*
2 years	99 ± 25	64 ± 25*
3 years	100 ± 25	67 ± 23*
4 years	99 ± 20	65 ± 20*
5–6 years	94 ± 14	55 ± 9
6–7 years	100 ± 15	56 ± 8
8–9 years	105 ± 16	57 ± 9
9–10 years	107 ± 16	57 ± 9
10–11 years	111 ± 17	58 ± 10
11–12 years	113 ± 18	59 ± 10
12–13 years	115 ± 19	59 ± 10
13–14 years	118 ± 19	60 ± 10

* The point of muffling is shown as the diastolic pressure.

Average Blood Pressure in Adult American Females

		WHITE WOMEN		BLACK WOMEN	
	Age	***Average (mm Hg)***	***SD***	***Average (mm Hg)***	***SD***
Systolic	Under 20	111.0	13.7	112.7	13.2
	20–29	116.9	13.8	119.1	14.7
	30–39	121.4	16.3	128.1	20.2
	40–49	129.3	19.6	138.3	22.8
Diastolic	Under 20	69.3	9.8	70.0	10.1
	20–29	73.7	7.2	75.4	9.7
	30–39	76.9	10.7	82.0	13.0
	40–49	80.6	11.6	86.9	13.9

SD = standard deviation.
(Adapted from Stamler, J, et al. [1976]. Hypertension screening of one million Americans. *Journal of the American Medical Association, 235,* 2299. Copyright © 1976, American Medical Association.

Appendix G

CARE MAPS

Name: ______________________________

This care path is a guideline and is not intended to create a standard of care. This guideline may be modified based on individual patient's needs.

	Consults Date	Proced/Tests Date	Pt/Family Ed Date	Routine visits	Meds Date	Other Date	Initials
Pre-conception	MD RD, prn RN, prn MSW, prn	PAP, breast exam Hx/family hx screen for Sickle cell, TaySach prn	Wellness ed. Nutrition Self br. exam Abstain from Tob, ETOH, etc	Yearly and prn	PNV FeSO-4 Folic Acid		
Week 1-8	MD RD RN MSW	Preg test, prn Initial labs HIV, prn Sickle cell, prn	Given prenatal handbook Additional info:	1/Mo. First 32 Weeks, and prn	PNV FeSO-4		
Week 8-12	MD RD, prn RN, prn MSW, prn	PAP, breast exam DNA probe Urine tox.					
Week 12-16	MD RD, prn RN, prn MSW, prn	Order MSAFP to be done in weeks 15-17					
Week 16-20	MD RD, prn RN, prn MSW, prn	Order U/S to be done in weeks 18-22	Refer to childbirth/ VBAC class				
Week 20-24	MD RD, prn RN, prn MSW, prn	Order 1 hr GTT, H&H ~24 weeks	Epidural class Breastfeed or bottle				
Week 24-28	MD RD, prn RN, prn MSW, prn	GBS 28 weeks, prn	Additional info.		(Rhogam 28 weeks prn)		
Weeks 28-32	MD RD, prn RN, prn MSW, prn		S/Sx PTL				
Weeks 32-36	MD RD, prn RN, prn MSW, prn	Vag exam at 36 wks if ctx	S/Sx labor	Bi-monthly		NST, prn Fetal/pelvic index, prn	
Weeks 36-40	MD RD, prn RN, prn MSW, prn			Weekly til del.			
Week 40-del.	MD RD, prn RN, prn MSW, prn						
Postpartum	MD RD, prn RN, prn MSW, prn	PAP, breast exam	Care of self PP (care of infant) Family planning Wellness	(2 wks for C/S) 6 weeks	(Rhogam prn) (Rubella prn)		

Patient Problems Identified:

PATIENT INDENTIFICATION

CARE PATH: Obstetric Prenatal
Care Path Code: 080

ST. JOHN'S MERCY MEDICAL CENTER, ST. LOUIS, MO

Name: ______________________________

This care path is a guideline and is not intended to create a standard of care. This guideline may be modified based on individual patient's needs.

Prob. #		Day 1/Day of Admission Date:	LOS Day _____ Date:	LOS Day _____ Date:	LOS Day _____ Date:
	ADL	☐ Bedrest ☐ BR/BRP ☐ Wheelchair ☐ Bedside commode ☐ Shower ☐ Up ad lib	☐ Bedrest ☐ BR/BRP ☐ Wheelchair ☐ Bedside commode ☐ Shower ☐ Up ad lib	☐ Bedrest ☐ BR/BRP ☐ Wheelchair ☐ Bedside commode ☐ Shower ☐ Up ad lib	☐ Bedrest ☐ BR/BRP ☐ Wheelchair ☐ Bedside commode ☐ Shower ☐ Up ad lib
	Assessment / Monitor	Maternal assessments: ☐ VS q 4 hours ☐ VS q 4 hours while awake ☐ VS q shift ☐ VS BID Vaginal bleeding Uterine activity Membrane status Vaginal discharge Fetal assessments: ☐ FHR q 4 hours ☐ FHR q shift ☐ Fetal kick counts (DFMR)	Maternal assessments: ☐ VS q 4 hours ☐ VS q 4 hours while awake ☐ VS q shift ☐ VS BID Vaginal bleeding Uterine activity Membrane status Vaginal discharge Fetal assessments: ☐ FHR q 4 hours ☐ FHR q shift ☐ Fetal kick counts (DFMR)	Maternal assessments: ☐ VS q 4 hours ☐ VS q 4 hours while awake ☐ VS q shift ☐ VS BID Vaginal bleeding Uterine activity Membrane status Vaginal discharge Fetal assessments: ☐ FHR q 4 hours ☐ FHR q shift ☐ Fetal kick counts (DFMR)	Maternal assessments: ☐ VS q 4 hours ☐ VS q 4 hours while awake ☐ VS q shift ☐ VS BID Vaginal bleeding Uterine activity Membrane status Vaginal discharge Fetal assessments: ☐ FHR q 4 hours ☐ FHR q shift ☐ Fetal kick counts (DFMR)
	Consults	☐ Perinatal CNS ☐ House officers ☐ NICU staff ☐ Social Services ☐ Pastoral Services	☐ Perinatal CNS ☐ House officers ☐ NICU staff ☐ Social Services ☐ Pastoral Services	☐ Perinatal CNS ☐ House officers ☐ NICU staff ☐ Social Services ☐ Pastoral Services	☐ Perinatal CNS ☐ House officers ☐ NICU staff ☐ Social Services ☐ Pastoral Services
	Procedures/ Tests	Laboratory tests: ☐ CBC ☐ CRP ☐ 24 hour urine ☐ UA for proteinuria Perinatal Center: ☐ NST ☐ Modified BPP	Laboratory tests: ☐ CBC ☐ CRP ☐ 24 hour urine ☐ UA for proteinuria Perinatal Center: ☐ NST ☐ Modified BPP	Laboratory tests: ☐ CBC ☐ CRP ☐ 24 hour urine ☐ UA for proteinuria Perinatal Center: ☐ NST ☐ Modified BPP	Laboratory tests: ☐ CBC ☐ CRP ☐ 24 hour urine ☐ UA for proteinuria Perinatal Center: ☐ NST ☐ Modified BPP
	Treatments	________ ________ ________ ________ ________	________ ________ ________ ________ ________	________ ________ ________ ________ ________	________ ________ ________ ________ ________
	Meds/Vs	☐ Prenatal vitamins ☐ Refer to Medication Administration Record	☐ Prenatal vitamins ☐ Refer to Medication Administration Record	☐ Prenatal vitamins ☐ Refer to Medication Administration Record	☐ Prenatal vitamins ☐ Refer to Medication Administration Record
	Nutrition	Regular Diet ________ ________	Regular Diet ________ ________	Regular Diet ________ ________	Regular Diet ________ ________
	Pt. /Family Education	Purpose and course of tx S&S PTL	Purpose and course of tx S&S PTL	Purpose and course of tx S&S PTL	Purpose and course of tx S&S PTL
	Discharge Planning	Appropriate to clinical and social situation Ongoing reinforcement	Appropriate to clinical and social situation Ongoing reinforcement	Appropriate to clinical and social situation Ongoing reinforcement	Appropriate to clinical and social situation Ongoing reinforcement
	Spiritual/ Psycho/Social/ Emotional Needs	Assess support system Assess family separation anxiety Assist in dealing with high-risk pregnancy Make available information on Pastoral Services Evaluate spiritual needs and respond as appropriate PRN Provide significant sacraments and rituals as requested	Assess support system Assess family separation anxiety Assist in dealing with high-risk pregnancy Assist in developing coping skills Evaluate spiritual needs and respond as appropriate PRN	Assess support system Assess family separation anxiety Assist in dealing with high-risk pregnancy Assist in developing coping skills Evaluate spiritual needs and respond as appropriate PRN	Assess support system Assess family separation anxiety Assist in dealing with high-risk pregnancy Assist in developing coping skills Evaluate spiritual needs and respond as appropriate PRN
Multidisciplinary Team Signatures		________ ________ ________ ________	________ ________ ________ ________	________ ________ ________ ________	________ ________ ________ ________

Patient Problems

1. Potential preterm birth
2. Vaginal bleeding
3. Stress related to high-risk pregnancy
4. Stress related to family separation

CARE PATH: Antepartum Complications
Code 089

ST. JOHN'S MERCY MEDICAL CENTER, ST. LOUIS, MO

PATIENT IDENTIFICATION

Name: ______________________________

This care path is a guideline and is not intended to create a standard of care. This guideline may be modified based on individual patient's needs.

Prob. #		Intrapartum	0-4 Hours Date:	4-8 Hours Date:	8-12 Hours Date:	12-24 Hours Date:
3	ADL	Bedrest or ambulation as tolerated	Bedrest or ambulation as tolerated	Up ad lib (assist PRN)	Up ad lib (assist PRN)	Up ad lib (assist PRN)
3	Assessment Monitor	Perinatal Unit admission assessment Ongoing assessments PRN	Immediate postpartum assessments VS Q 15" until stable, then Q 4h VS are WNL	VS Q 4h, VS are WNL Postpartum checks Q 4h - are WNL Assess mother/infant attachment	VS Q 4h, VS are WNL Postpartum checks Q 4h - are WNL Assess mother/infant attachment	VS Q 4h, VS are WNL Postpartum checks Q 4h - are WNL Assess mother/infant attachment
1,2, 4	Consults	Perinatal CNS Anesthesia PRN House officer PRN Resolve PRN NICU staff PRN	→ → → →	Lactation consultant PRN Social Service PRN/ WIC PRN	Lactation consultant PRN Social Service PRN/ WIC	Lactation consultant PRN Social Service PRN/ WIC
3	Procedures/ Tests	Hct PRN	Assess Rubella Titer status Assess need for Rhogam		Rhogam screen PRN	
1	Treatments	External EFM Internal EFM PRN	Ice to perineum Cath PRN	Ice to perineum Cath PRN Supportive bra PRN	Ice to perineum Cath PRN Supportive bra PRN Sitz bath PRN	Ice to perineum Supportive bra PRN Sitz bath PRN
1,2	Meds/IVs	Pain medication IV or IM PRN Alternative D_5 LR/LR when in active labor PRN Epidural/Pudendal/ Pericervical Pitocin augmentation PRN	Pain medication PRN Tucks PRN Anusol PRN Pitocin 20u IV then D/C	Pain medication PRN Tucks PRN Anusol PRN Stool softener PRN	Pain medication PRN Tucks PRN Anusol PRN Stool softener PRN	Pain medication PRN Tucks PRN Anusol PRN Stool softener PRN Rhogam PRN Rubella vaccine PRN
1	Nutrition	Ice chips PRN	Tolerate PO fluids Regular diet	Adequate fluids Regular diet	Adequate fluids Regular diet	Adequate fluids Regular diet
2	Pt./Family Education	EFM Labor support coaching - encourage support person in role	Self peri care/safety issues Perineum care - comfort measures Mother/baby booklet Initiate bottle or breast-feeding Initiate infant care	Bath/cord care and baby care demo Self care reinforcement and demos Discuss normal involution, lochia, fatigue, activity levels, and nutritional needs.	→ → →	Breast pump if indicated
2	Discharge Planning	Mother/baby teaching form	Determine LOS Begin discharge instructions	Continue discharge instructions	→	Assess parent/infant interaction Assess need for home health follow-up Discharge instructions reviewed with mother and S.O.
2,4	Spiritual/ Psycho/ Social/ Emotional Needs	Support patient/S.O. Facilitate a positive childbirth experience	Assess maternal role strengths	Assist mother's transition through tasks of taking on maternal role	→	→
	Multi-disciplinary Team Signatures					

Patient Problems

1. Discomfort/pain
2. Learning needs
3. Potential for instability - postpartum
4. Potential alteration in coping related to childbirth

CARE PATH: VAGINAL BIRTH — DRG# 373

ST. JOHN'S MERCY MEDICAL CENTER, ST. LOUIS, MO

PATIENT IDENTIFICATION

Name: ____________________

This care path is a guideline and is not intended to create a standard of care. This guideline may be modified based on individual patient's needs.

Prob. #		Intrapartum	0-4 Hours Date:	4-8 Hours Date:	8-12 Hours Date:	12-24 Hours Date:
3	ADL	Bedrest or ambulation as tolerated	Bedrest PRN	Dangle x 1 Ambulate with assist PRN Chair/rocker PRN	→ →	→
1,3	Assessment Monitor	Perinatal Unit admission Ongoing assessments PRN	Immediate postpartum assessments VS q 15 min x4, q 30 min, then q 4 hr VS are WNL	Immediate postpartum assessments - are WNL Assess mother/infant interaction VS q 4hr while awake VS are WNL	Listen for bowel sounds → → VS are WNL	→ → → VS are WNL
1, 2, 4	Consults	Perinatal CNS Anesthesia PRN House officer PRN Resolve PRN NICU staff PRN	→ → → → →	→ → → → →	Lactation consultant PRN Social Service PRN WIC PRN	Lactation consultant Social Service, WIC PRN
3	Procedures/ Tests	CBC Type and screen	Assess Rubella Titer status Assess need for Rhogam	→ →	Rhogam screen PRN	
1, 3	Treatments	EFM IV Foley catheter Abdominal shave prep	Ice to incision Foley cath TCDB q 2 hr Peri acre q 4 hr I&O q shift x 48 hr	→ → → → →	→ → → Dressing removed PRN	Foley cath PRN → Peri care q 4 hr PRN → →
1, 3, 5	Meds/IVs	Epidural IVF - LR/D5LR	PCA/Epidural IV fluids Pitocin to IV Antiemetic PRN Antibiotics PRN Benadryl PRN	→ → → → →	→ → → → →	IV fluids PRN Pitocin PRN → → →
1, 2	Nutrition	NPO (as ordered for scheduled sections)	Ice chips PRN (sips and chips)	→	Clear liquids	Advance as tolerated
2, 4	Pt./ Family Education	EMF Explain procedures	Mother/Baby booklet Safety issues Pharmacologic and non-pharmocologic pain control and comfort measures Initiate breast feeding/ bottle feeding	Initiate infant care Normal involution, lochia, perineal care	Initiate self care	Reinforce self care with demos Baby/cord care demo Breast pump if indicated
2, 4	Discharge Planning	Mother/baby teaching form	Determine LOS	Begin discharge instructions	→	→ Assess parent interaction
2, 4	Spiritual/ Psycho/ Social/ Emotional Needs	Support patient/ significant other Facilitate positive childbirth experience	Assess maternal role strengths	Assist mother's transition through tasks of taking on maternal role	→	→
	Multi-disciplinary Team Signatures					

Patient Problems

1. Discomfort/pain
2. Learning needs
3. Potential for instability - postpartum involution
4. Potential alteration in coping related to childbirth
5. Potential for infection

PATIENT IDENTIFICATION

CARE PATH: CESAREAN BIRTH — DRG# 371

ST. JOHN'S MERCY MEDICAL CENTER, ST. LOUIS, MO

Care Path: Cesarean Birth - DRG #371

Prob. #		24-48 Hours Date:	48-72 Hours Date:
3	ADL	Encourage ambulation	Up ad lib
1, 3	Assessment Monitor	Bowel sounds are present Assessments BID are WNL Assess mother/infant interaction VS q 4 hr while awake VS are WNL	VS QID
1, 2, 4	Consults	Lactation consultant Social Service, WIC PRN	Lactation consultant Social Service, WIC PRN
3	Procedures/ Tests		H&H
1, 3	Treatments	Cath PRN I&O q shift x 48 hr Dressing removed PRN Supportive bra PRN	Staple removal PRN
1, 3, 5	Meds/IVs	PO analgesics PRN Pitocin PRN Antiemetic PRN Antibiotics PRN Benadryl PRN IV fluids PRN Rhogam PRN Rubella vaccine PRN Mylicon PRN Stool softeners PRN	Mylicon PRN Stool softeners PRN PO analgesic PRN Suppositories/laxatives PRN
1, 2	Nutrition	Advance as tolerated	Regular diet
2, 4	Pt./ Family Education	Breast pump if indicated	Self care and infant care return demos
2, 4	Discharge Planning	Discharge instructions Assess parent interaction Assess need for home health follow-up	Reinforce discharge instructions Assess parent interaction Assess need for home health follow-up
2, 4	Spiritual/ Psycho/ Social/ Emotional Needs	Assist mother's transition through tasks of taking on maternal role Encourage family and other support systems	Assist mother's transition through tasks of taking on maternal role
	Multi-disciplinary Team Signatures		

Name: ______________________________

This care path is a guideline and is not intended to create a standard of care. This guideline may be modified based on individual patient's needs.

Prob. #		Birth	0-4 Hours Date:	4-8 Hours Date:	8-12 Hours Date:	12-24 Hours Date:
1	ADL	Bedrest and position for holding	→	→	→	→
1,3	Assessment Monitor	Apgars Newborn assessment	Newborn assessment on admission and Q 8h VS, Respiratory status, skin color, and temp WNL Observation: check for maternal hepatitis surface antigen	Temp PRN and Q shift	→ Newborn assessment Q 8h VS WNL	→ →
1, 2, 3	Consults	NICU Team in attendance PRN	Orthopedics PRN Genetics PRN Infectious disease PRN	Orthopedics PRN Genetics PRN Infectious disease PRN	Orthopedics PRN Genetics PRN Infectious disease PRN	Orthopedics PRN Genetics PRN Infectious disease PRN
1, 2, 3	Procedures/ Tests	Cord blood PRN	Chemstrips PRN BP PRN O_2 sat PRN-O_2 sat WNL Attach security sensor Assess hepatitis titer	Chemstrips PRN		Metabolic screen
1-4	Treatments	Gastric lavage PRN	→ Initial newborn bath Cord care	Cord care Cath PRN Ultrasounds PRN Circumcision PRN and circ care	Cord care Cath PRN Ultrasounds PRN Circumcision PRN and circ care	Cord care Ultrasounds PRN Circumcision PRN and circ care Discharge weight
3	Meds/IVs	Illotycin ointment	Vitamin K IM		Hepatitis vaccine PRN	
2	Nutrition	Initiate breastfeeding	Continue breastfeeding Initiate formula feeding	→ Continue formula feeding	→ →	→ →
1-4	Pt./ Family Education	See Maternal Care Path				
1-4	Discharge Planning	See Maternal Care Path				Assess need for home health follow-up
1-4	Spiritual/ Psycho/ Social/ Emotional Needs	See Maternal Care Path				
	Multi-disciplinary Team Signatures					

Patient Problems

1. Alteration in body temperature
2. Alteration in nutritional requirements
3. Potential for infection
4. Alteration in skin integrity

PATIENT IDENTIFICATION

CARE PATH: NORMAL NEWBORN— DRG# 391

ST. JOHN'S MERCY MEDICAL CENTER, ST. LOUIS, MO

Care Path: Normal Newborn — DRG#391

Prob. #		Day 2 Date:				
1	ADL	Bedrest and position for holding				
1,3	Assessment Monitor	Temp PRN and Q shift VS WNL				
1, 2, 3	Consults	Orthopedics PRN Genetics PRN Infectious disease PRN				
1, 2, 3	Procedures/ Tests					
1-4	Treatments	Cord care Ultrasounds PRN Circumcision PRN and circ care Discharge weight				
3	Meds/IVs					
2	Nutrition	Continue breastfeeding Continue formula feeding				
1-4	PT./ Family Education					
1-4	Discharge Planning	Assess need for home health follow-up				
1-4	Spiritual/ Psycho/ Social/ Emotional Needs					
	Multi-disciplinary Team Signatures					

Name: ______________________________

This care path is a guideline and is not intended to create a standard of care. This guideline may be modified based on individual patient's needs.

Prob. #		Admission Day/Day 1 Date:	Day 2 Date:
4,5	ADL	Activity as tolerated.	→
1, 3 4	Assessment/ Monitor	Head to toe assessment per standard. VS q 4°. BP q shift. Accurate I&O. Daily wt.	→ → → → →
2, 4, 5, 6	Consults	Social Service consult within 24 hours of admission if appropriate.	→
1, 3, 4	Procedures/ Tests	Chem 6, UA. Consider stool for Rotovirus.	Follow up lab abnormalities.
	Treatments		
1, 4	Meds/IVs	Bolus IV IV fluids	↓ IV rate
1, 3	Nutrition	NPO→ Diet as prescribed.	Diet as prescribed - encourage fluids.
1, 2 6	Pt./ Family Education	Review care expectations with patient and family.	Review measures to prevent dehydration, signs & symptoms of dehydration.
4	Discharge Planning	Assess need for intervention necessary for discharge.	Discharge home if stable & tolerating PO.
6	Spiritual/ Psycho/ Social/ Emotional/ Develop-mental Needs	Provide information on Pastoral Services. Assess spiritual/emotional needs of patient & family as appropriate. Notify Child Life & assess individual needs for explanations & for coping.	Contact with faith community as requested. Intervention as needed based on spiritual/ emotional assessment. Provide sacraments, rituals as requested.
	Multi-disciplinary Team Signatures		

Patient Problems

1. Fluid volume deficit.
2. Knowledge deficit - hospital procedures.
3. Alteration in nutrition - less than both requirements.
4. Potential for comorbid condition.
5. Alteration in mobility.
6. Coping - ineffective, individual.

CARE PATH: Pediatric Gastroenteritis
Care Path Code: 096

ST. JOHN'S MERCY MEDICAL CENTER, ST. LOUIS, MO

PATIENT IDENTIFICATION

Name: ______________________________

This care path is a guideline and is not intended to create a standard of care. This guideline may be modified based on individual patient's needs.

Prob. No.		Day 1	Day 2	Day 3	Day 4	Day 5
5	ADL	OOB when stable	Up to chair. Up ad lib as tol.	Ambulate in hall TID.		
1,4	Assessment/ Monitor	Head to toe assessment per standards. VS Q 4°.				
3	Consults	Social Service evaluation within 24 hours of admission if appropriate.				
1,4, 5	Procedures/ Tests		Gentamicin peak/ through level around 3rd dose.			
	Treatments	Turn, cough, breathe Q 2 hrs. Accurate I&O. Reinforce drsg., if drsg present. Straight cath/Foley cathether within 8 hrs. post-op if no void.	Daily dressing change as indicated.	→	→	→
	Meds/IVs	• IV antibiotics (as ordered) • PCA as indicated • Antipryetic • Anteimetic • IV fluids	DC PCA basal rate.	DC PCA ↓ IV fluid rate.	Heplock IV	
	Nutrition	NPO except ice chips	Clear liquids as tolerated.	Advance diet to regular for age as tolerated.	→	→
	Pt./ Family Education	Review care expectations with patient & family.				Review S/S infection, dehydration, diet. Activity limitations.
	Discharge Planning	Assess need for intervention necessary for discharge.				Home medications. Wound care.
	Spiritual/ Psycho/ Social/ Emotional/ Developmental Needs	Provide information on Pastoral Care Services. Assess spiritual/ emotional needs of patient & family. Notify Child Life & assess individual needs for explanations & coping.	→ →	→ →		
	Multi-disciplinary Team Signatures					

Patient Problems

1. Potential for instability post-op
2. Fluid volume deficit
3. Coping - ineffective/individual
4. Potential for comorbid condition
5. Alteration in mobility
6. Knowledge deficit for caregiver
7. Potential for acute pain

PATIENT IDENTIFICATION

CARE PATH: Pediatric Appendectomy with Complications
Care Path Code: 119

ST. JOHN'S MERCY MEDICAL CENTER, ST. LOUIS, MO

Name: ______________________________

This care path is a guideline and is not intended to create a standard of care. This guideline may be modified based on individual patient's needs.

Problem Number		Time: 0-1 Hour Pre-Procedure	Time: 1-3 Hour Post Procedure	Time: 3 Hour → Extended Post Procedure
1, 3	ADL	Up as tolerated.	Bedrest until awake and alert.	Up ad lib with supervision.
1, 3	Assessment/ Monitor	Head to toe assessment per standard. VS Q 4 hours	Head to toe assessment HR, RR, BP, & O_2 Sat. Q 15 min. until pt. returned to baseline functioning.	
	Consults	Consult Pediatrician/Radiologist for sedation orders as indicated.		
1, 2	Procedure	MRI/CT Labs as ordered.		
1	Treatments	Transport to NRI/CT with pulse oximeter and ambu bag		
1, 3	Meds/IVs	Place heplock.	D/C IV Resume home meds	
2	Nutrition	NPO	Clear liquids - Advance to regular diet.	
1, 2, 3	Pt./ Family Education	Review care expectations with patient & family.	Post sedation/procedure teaching	⟶
1, 2, 3	Discharge Planning	Assess need for intervention necessary for discharge.	D/C when awake and alert	⟶
1	Spiritual/Psycho/ Social/Emotional/ Developmental Needs	Notify Child Life and assess individual needs for explanations & for coping. Provide information on Pastoral Services as indicated.	⟶	⟶
	Multidisciplinary Team Signatures			

Patient Problems

1. Knowledge Deficit: invasive procedure
2. Alteration in fluid/nutrition
3. Alteration in level of consciousness

PATIENT IDENTIFICATION

CARE PATH: Pediatric MRI/CAT Scan
Care Path Code: 098

ST. JOHN'S MERCY MEDICAL CENTER, ST. LOUIS, MO

Name: ______________________________

This care path is a guideline and is not intended to create a standard of care. This guideline may be modified based on individual patient's needs.

Prob. No.		Day 1 Admission Day Date: __________	Day 2 Date: __________	Day Date: __________
5, 4	ADL	Activity as tolerated	Activity as tolerated	
1	Assessment/ Monitor	Head to toe assessment per standard VS Q 4 h. BP q shift I&O q shift Daily wts	Head to toe assessment per standard VS Q 4 h. BP q shift I&O q shift Daily wts Reassess need for SaO2 monitoring	Head to toe assessment per standard VS Q 4 h. BP q shift I&O q shift Daily wts VS prior to discharge
4	Consults	Childlife consult	Childlife consult	Physician consult considered if patient not improved (i.e., pulmonary)
4, 1	Procedures/ Tests	CXR (P.P.D. if ordered) Chem 6, CBC, BC	Check C&S results Follow up lab abnormalities	Check C&S results Consider CXR if patient not improved
4	Treatments	See Respiratory Therapy protocol (R.T. to evaluate pulmonary toilet, O2 [sat], bronchodilator) O2 PRN	Respiratory Therapy (see R.T. protocol for patient education) O2 PRN/O2 sat BID/PRN	Discontinue O2/protocol
4, 2	Meds/IVs	I.V. antibiotics (administered within 4 hours after admission) I.V. fluids	I.V. antibiotics - reassess Consider change to I.V. heplock	I.V. antibiotics - reassess and consider switch to oral antibiotics Discontinue I.V. heplock Prescription for home meds
2	Nutrition	Diet as prescribed Encourage fluids	Diet as prescribed Encourage fluids	Diet as prescribed Adequate fluid intake
3, 1	PT./ Family Education	Review care expectations with patient and significant other R.T. to introduce patient education regarding disease process, norms, irritants and therapies	Continue R.T. education per protocol Patient education concerning medication, activities, and nutritional needs	Reinforce patient education and assess understanding Discharge outcomes reviewed with family
3, 5	Discharge Planning	Social Service evaluation within 24 hours of admission if appropriate	⟶ PRN conference with multidisciplinary team	Evaluate need for home equipment (nebulizer), home health care Discharge home if stable and to oral antibiotics Instructions on P.P.D. reading and report to primary physician if done
	Spiritual/Psycho/ Social/Emotional Needs	Provide information on Pastoral Services	Assess spiritual/emotional issues of patient and family as appropriate Contact with faith community PRN Patient care conference PRN Provide sacraments, rituals as requested	Intervention as needed based on spiritual/emotional assessment Patient care conference PRN Provide sacraments/rituals as requested
Multidisciplinary Team Signatures				

Patient Problems

1. Gas exchange impaired - ineffective breath pattern
2. Fluid volume deficit
3. Coping - ineffective/individual
4. Potential for comorbid condition
5. Alteration in mobility
6. Knowledge deficit of caregiver

PATIENT IDENTIFICATION

CARE PATH: Pediatric Pneumonia
Care Path Code: 030

ST. JOHN'S MERCY MEDICAL CENTER, ST. LOUIS, MO

Name: ______________________________

This care path is a guideline and is not intended to create a standard of care. This guideline may be modified based on individual patient's needs.

Prob. #		Day before OR	Day of OR Date:	Post-op Day 1 Date:	Post-op Day 2 Date:	Post-op Day 3 Date:
4	ADL	Activity as tolerated	Bedrest	Bedrest	Bedrest - lower extremities Chair - upper extremities	Bedrest - lower extremities Chair - upper extremities
2	Assessment/ Monitor		Neuro, circulatory, Resp. Post-op: Bleeding will be absent or controlled, N/V will be controlled No iatrogenic complications or return to OR will occur Post-op diagram done by MDs	Circulatory, VS q 4h Ketamine (BCI/PICU) - Cardiac monitor, SpO_2, VS q 5 min. during change, suction set-up SpO_2 will be maintained at >90%	Circulatory, VS q 4h Ketamine (BCI/PICU) - Cardiac monitor, SpO_2, VS q 5 min. during change, suction set-up	Circulatory, VS q 4h Grafts will be intact, adherent and vascularized No S/S of infection, pressure, shearing noted
	Consults					
2	Procedures/ Tests	CBC and Chem 6 Consider T&X	CBC post-op Chem 6 post-op Consider transfusion if H&H < 10/30	CBC Chem 6	CBC Chem 6	
1	Treatments	Dressing change OD or BID with AgSD PT/OT during change Ememas for buttock or thigh grafts/donors Consent forms (per MD)	Pre-op: Ce layons to op areas AgSD to remaining wounds Shave, prep donors Splints, Cerous, AgSD to OR Post-op: I&O per foley, cerous soaks q 2h until AM drsg. change	Ketamine dressing change: (BC/PICU) wet to dry AgSD sandwich dressings to new grafts AgSD to nongrafted, unhealed areas AgSD or op site to donors PT/OT for ungrafted areas Splints at all times	Ketamine changes: (BC/PICU) wet to dry sandwich to grafts AgSD to donors and unhealed nongrafted areas BID change - evaluate PT/OT for ungrafted areas Splints at all times	Begin removing staples in grafts AgSD to margins and unhealed areas BID change - evaluate PT/OT for ungrafted areas Splints at all times
2, 3	Meds/IVs	Routine meds IV access, heplock Obtain transfusion order if H&H <10/30	Pre-op on call Antibiotic Anesthesia meds as ordered Post-op antibiotic and pain tx Patient reports pain <4 on 1-10 scale IV or D5LR or LR	Ketamine (BC/PICU) Antibiotic Pain meds Patient reports pain <4 on 1-10 scale Continue IV fluids	Ketamine (BC/PICU) Pain meds Patient reports pain <4 on 1-10 scale Heplock IV	Routine meds Pain meds PRN Patient reports pain <4 on 1-10 scale D/C IV after drsg. change
1, 6	Nutrition	Hi-cal shakes Patient instructed on changing nutritional needs	NPO before OR Post-op → gradually advance to hi-cal hi-pro diet, shake	NPO after midnight before Ketamine Hi-cal hi-pro diet after drsg. changes Cal. count	NPO for Ketamine Previous diet after drsg. changes Cal. count	Patient intake will be >85% of estimated caloric/protein requirements Hi-cal diet, shakes Cal. count

Care Path: Tangenital Excision Split Thickness - DRG 458

Prob. #		Day before OR	Day of OR Date:	Post-op Day 1 Date:	Post-op Day 2 Date:	Post-op Day 3 Date:
6	Pt./ Family Education	Pre-op teaching re: STSG Post-op care: Bowel prep IV, NPO Ce soaks Activity Splints Ketamine change (BC & PICU only) Pt. will be instructed on post-op pain management	Reinforce post-op care Splints as indicated	Reinforce post-op course	Reinforce graft healing, splinting activity	Patient/caregiver communicates understanding of injury, treatment and projected goals
	Discharge Planning					Patient identifies appropriate "home" caregiver and discharge needs Start any Home Health referrals
5, 6	Spiritual/ Psycho/ Social/ Emotional Needs	Social Service consult at time of adm to determine needs during hospitalization and community resource referrals Activity Therapy assess. Provide Pastoral Care info.			Pastoral Care to evaluate spiritual needs of patient/family as needed	Social Service to continue discharge planning with community agencies
Multidisciplinary Team Signatures						

Patient Problems

1. Alteration in skin integrity
2. Potential for instability after injury/procedeure
3. Alteration in comfort/pain
4. Alteration in mobility - loss of function/scarring
5. Alteration in self-image - disfigurement/scarring
6. Knowledge deficit

PATIENT IDENTIFICATION

CARE PATH: Tangential Excision Split Thickness Skin Graft (Minor Procedure) - DRG 458 / Code 035

ST. JOHN'S MERCY MEDICAL CENTER, ST. LOUIS, MO

Page 2 - Excision Split Thickness Skin Graft (Minor Procedure)

Prob. #		Post-op Day 4 Date:	Post-op Day 5 Date:	Post-op Day 6 Date:	Post-op Day 7 Date:	Post-op Day 8 Date:
4	ADL	Chair - lower extremities NWB BRP - upper extremities	Chair - lower extremities NWB Ambulate - upper extremities	Chair - lower extremities WBAT (ace wraps when up) AD LIB - upper extremities	Ambulatory	Ambulatory, patient performing ADLs
2	Assessment/ Monitor	Circulatory, VS q 4h Grafts will be intact, adherent and vascularized	VS q 8h	VS q 8h	Routine VS	Donor site shows progressive healing and absence of infection
	Consults					
2	Procedures/ Tests				CBC Chem 6	
1	Treatments	Remove any remaining staples AgSD to margins, unhealed areas BID change - evaluate PT/OT for ungrafted Splints on at all times	Poss tub Trim grafts AgSD to margins, unhealed areas BID - evaluate PT/OT, evaluate for temp., pressure garments, Initiate AROM Splinting at HS	Poss tub AgSD to margins, unhealed areas BID - evaluate Dept. tx - PT/OT (upper ext.) Splinting HS	Poss tub AgSD to margins, unhealed areas BID - eveluate PT/OT - Dept. tx, obtain v.o. for pressure garments	PT/OT Discharge Booklet
2, 3	Meds/IVs	Routine meds, pain meds PRN Patient reports pain <4 on 1-10 scale	Routine meds, pain meds PRN Patient reports pain <4 on 1-10 scale	Routine meds, pain meds PRN Patient reports pain <4 on 1-10 scale	Routine meds, pain meds PRN Patient reports pain <4 on 1-10 scale	Routine meds If discharged, send meds for pain control at home
1, 6	Nutrition	D/C calorie count Hi-cal diet Shakes	Hi-cal shake diet	Hi-cal shake diet	Hi-cal shake diet	Hi-cal shake diet
6	Pt./ Family Education	Patient/caregiver communicates understanding of injury, tx, and projected goals	Patient/caregiver communicates understanding of injury, tx, and projected goals	Family caregiver to view wound care.	Family / S.O. participate in wound care, PT/OT discharge teaching.	Patient/caregiver independent with wound and skin care, home exercise program and S/S infection
	Discharge Planning					Home if applicable Home Health if applicable SNF if applicable Patient/caregiver identifies available support systems
5, 6	Spiritual/ Psycho/ Social/ Emotional Needs	As STSG heals, evaluate patient/family adjustment to trauma	Continue follow-up with psych, chaplain, Social Service and Activity Therapy	Continue follow-up with psych, chaplain, Social Service and Activity Therapy	Obtain post-hospitalization appointments or consults if needed.	
Multidisciplinary Team Signatures						

Appendix H

STANDARD PRECAUTIONS

Use Standard Precautions, or the equivalent, for the care of all patients. *Category IB**

A. Handwashing

(1) Wash hands after touching blood, body fluids, secretions, excretions, and contaminated items, whether or not gloves are worn. Wash hands immediately after gloves are removed, between patient contacts, and when otherwise indicated to avoid transfer of microorganisms to other patients or environments. It may be necessary to wash hands between tasks and procedures on the same patient to prevent cross-contamination of different body sites. *Category IB*

(2) Use a plain (nonantimicrobial) soap for routine handwashing. *Category IB*

(3) Use an antimicrobial agent or a waterless antiseptic agent for specific circumstances (eg, control of outbreaks or hyperendemic infections), as defined by the infection control program. *Category IB* (See Contact Precautions for additional recommendations on using antimicrobial and antiseptic agents.)

B. Gloves

Wear gloves (clean, nonsterile gloves are adequate) when touching blood, body fluids, secretions, excretions, and contaminated items. Put on clean gloves just before touching mucous membranes and nonintact skin. Change gloves between tasks and procedures on the same patient after contact with material that may contain a high concentration of microorganisms. Remove gloves promptly after use, before touching noncontaminated items and environmental surfaces, and before going to another patient, and wash hands immediately to avoid transfer of microorganisms to other patients or environments. *Category IB*

C. Mask, Eye Protection, Face Shield

Wear a mask and eye protection or a face shield to protect mucous membranes of the eyes, nose, and mouth during procedures and patient-care activities that are likely to generate splashes or sprays of blood, body fluids, secretions, and excretions. *Category IB*

D. Gown

Wear a gown (a clean, nonsterile gown is adequate) to protect skin and to prevent soiling of clothing during procedures and patient-care activities that are likely to generate splashes or sprays of blood, body fluids, secretions, or excretions. Select a gown that is appropriate for the activity and amount of fluid likely to be encountered. Remove a soiled gown as promptly as possible, and wash hands to avoid transfer of microorganisms to other patients or environments. *Category IB*

E. Patient-Care Equipment

Handle used patient-care equipment soiled with blood, body fluids, secretions, and excretions in a manner that prevents skin and mucous membrane exposures, contamination of clothing, and transfer of microorganisms to other patients and environments. Ensure that reusable equipment is not used for the care of another patient until it has been cleaned and reprocessed appropriately. Ensure that single-use items are discarded properly. *Category IB*

F. Environmental Control

Ensure that the hospital has adequate procedures for the routine care, cleaning, and disinfection of environmental surfaces, beds, bedrails, bedside equipment, and other frequently touched surfaces, and ensure that these procedures are being followed. *Category IB*

G. Linen

Handle, transport, and process used linen soiled with blood, body fluids, secretions, and excretions in a manner that prevents skin and mucous membrane exposures and contamination of clothing, and that avoids transfer of microorganisms to other patients and environments. *Category IB*

H. Occupational Health and Bloodborne Pathogens

(1) Take care to prevent injuries when using needles, scalpels, and other sharp instruments or devices; when handling sharp instruments after procedures; when cleaning used instruments; and when disposing of used needles. Never recap used needles, or otherwise manipulate them using both hands, or use any other technique that involves directing the point of a needle toward any part of the body; rather, use either a one-handed "scoop" technique or a mechanical device designed for holding the needle sheath. Do not remove used needles from disposable syringes by hand, and do not bend, break, or otherwise manipulate used needles by hand. Place used disposable syringes and needles, scalpel blades, and other sharp items in appropriate puncture-resistant containers, which are locat-

ed as close as practical to the area in which the items were used, and place reusable syringes and needles in a puncture-resistant container for transport to the reprocessing area. *Category IB*

(2) Use mouthpieces, resuscitation bags, or other ventilation devices as an alternative to mouth-to-mouth resuscitation methods in areas where the need for resuscitation is predictable. *Category IB*

I. Patient Placement

Place a patient who contaminates the environment or who does not (or cannot be expected to) assist in maintaining appropriate hygiene or environmental control in a private room. If a private room is not available, consult with infection control professionals regarding patient placement or other alternatives. *Category IB*

* *Category IB.* Strongly recommended for all hospitals and reviewed as effective by experts in the field and a consensus of HIC-PAC based on strong rationale and suggestive evidence, even though definitive scientific studies have not been done.

(From Guideline for isolation precautions in hospitals developed by the Centers for Disease Control and Prevention and the Hospital Infection Control Practices Advisory Committee [HICPAC], January 1996.)

ANSWERS TO CHECKPOINT QUESTIONS

CHAPTER 1

1. Promotion and maintenance of optimal family health to ensure cycles of optimal childbearing and childrearing
2. Family-centered care better provides for holistic care.
3. Two other requirements of a profession are that members set their own standards and monitor their practice quality.
4. A philosophy of cost containment in reference to health care has greatly influenced all types of nursing care.
5. The leading causes of neonatal mortality are prematurity, low birth weight, and congenital anomalies.
6. The infant mortality rate is the health statistic most commonly used for international comparison.
7. The Family Medical Leave Act supports family-centered care by mandating that employers with 50 or more employees provide a minimum of 12 weeks unpaid, job-protected leave to employees who meet a set criterion, so the employees may care for a newborn, an ill family member, or a personal illness.
8. Empowerment of healthcare consumers has become increasingly important due to the influence of managed care and focus on cost containment and a strengthened focus on health promotion and disease prevention.
9. Family nurse practitioners are able to care for the entire family, so form long-term and comprehensive relationships with families.
10. The pediatric nurse practitioner serves as primary health caregiver or as the sole health care person the parents and child see at all visits.

CHAPTER 2

1. The number of nuclear families has decreased due to the increase in divorce, single-parenthood, and remarriage as well as acceptance of alternative life styles.
2. A single-parent family offers a child a special parent–child relationship as well as more opportunity for self-reliance and independence.
3. Homosexual partners may not receive health care because they may lack health insurance coverage.
4. Small families have fewer child care requirements; however, they also have less experience in childrearing.
5. Children from countries with inadequate health supervision may have a greater risk of illnesses such as hepatitis B and intestinal parasites, as well as growth retardation.
6. Shorter hospital stays put the responsibility for providing and maintaining health care on the family. Parents may have to provide care that used to be given only in the hospital.
7. A genogram is a diagram that shows family structure, history, and member roles, usually through several generations. An ecomap is a diagram of family and community relationships.
8. The Family APGAR is a screening tool of the family environment.
9. If adequate public transportation is not available, the patient will have trouble making appointments and may be unable to receive follow-up care or health maintenance.

CHAPTER 3

1. A cultural more is the expected or usual values of a particular group.
2. Stereotyping is the expectation that people will act in a characteristic manner without regard to individual characteristics.
3. Cultural competence is the integration of cultural elements to enhance communication and work effectively with people.
4. Touch can be a comforting gesture, but it may also be uncomfortable or culturally unacceptable.
5. Time orientation can interfere with health care if the orientation of the family is different from the health-care provider. For example, if extensive rehabilitation is required, a family that is past oriented may have difficulty coping with the future planning necessary.

CHAPTER 4

1. Implantation, or contact between the growing structure and the uterine endometrium, occurs approximately 8 to 10 days after fertilization.
2. Embryo
3. Two arteries and one vein
4. Amnion and chorion
5. About 24 weeks' gestation
6. IgG

7. Several factors influence the amount of damage a teratogen can cause. These include the strength of the teratogen, timing of the teratogenic insult, and the teratogen's affinity for specific tissue.
8. Cocaine, particularly its crack form, causes maternal vasoconstriction, compromising placental blood supply and so interfering with the fetal nutrient supply. Its use is associated with spontaneous abortion, preterm labor, meconium staining, limb defects, and intrauterine growth retardation.
9. A phenotype is a person's outward appearance; a genotype is the actual gene composition.
10. 23
11. Autosomal recessive inheritance disorder
12. Only a part of the chromosome needs to be affected for a disorder to occur.
13. During meiosis of the ovum
14. Any person who is concerned about the possibility of transmitting a disease to his or her children should have access to genetic counseling for advice on the inheritance of disease. The timing of genetic counseling is important. The ideal time is before the first pregnancy. Couples who seek counseling after a first affected child is born need counseling before a second pregnancy occurs.
15. First, the individual or couple being counseled needs a clear understanding of the information provided. This principle applies to the first pregnancy and any future pregnancies. Second, it is never appropriate for any health care provider to impose his or her own values or opinions on others. Couples need to be made aware of all the options available to them, to think about these options and make their own decisions.
16. Anovulation may occur from a genetic abnormality such as Turner's syndrome (hypogonadism) in which there are no ovaries to produce ova. Turner's syndrome (45XO) is marked by a webbed neck, short stature, sterility, and possible cognitive impairment.
17. Children with Down syndrome usually have some degree of cognitive impairment, but the impairment can range from that of an educable child (intelligence quotient [IQ] of 50 to 70) to one who is profoundly affected (IQ less than 20).

CHAPTER 5

1. The newborn loses 5 to 10% of birth weight (6 to 10 oz) during the first few days after birth.
2. The head circumference is usually 34 to 35 cm (13.5 to 14 inches) in a mature newborn. A mature newborn with a head circumference greater than 37 cm or less than 33 cm (14.8 and 13.2 inches, respectively) should be carefully investigated for neurologic involvement, although occasionally a newborn will fall within these limits and still be perfectly normal.
3. Newborns lose heat by four separate mechanisms: convection, conduction, radiation, and evaporation. Convection is the flow of heat from the body surface to cooler surrounding air. Conduction is the transfer of body heat to a cooler solid object in contact with the baby. Radiation is the transfer of body heat to a cooler solid object not in contact with the baby. Evaporation is loss of heat through conversion of a liquid to a vapor.
4. The first breath of a newborn is initiated by a combination of cold receptors, a lowered PaO_2 (PaO_2 falls from 80 mm Hg to as low as 15 mm Hg), and an increased $PaCO_2$ ($PaCO_2$ rises as high as 70 mm Hg). A first breath requires a tremendous amount of pressure (about 40 to 70 cm H_2O).
5. The most accurate method of eliciting the Moro reflex is to hold newborns in a supine position and allow their heads to drop backward an inch or so. They abduct and extend their arms and legs. Their fingers assume a typical "C" position. They then bring their arms into an embrace position and pull up their legs against their abdomen (abduction). The reflex simulates the action of someone trying to ward off an attacker, then covering up to protect himself. It is strong for the first 8 weeks of life and fades by the end of the 4th or 5th month, when the infant can roll away from danger.
6. Acrocyanosis is a normal phenomenon in the first 24 to 48 hours after birth.
7. Milia disappear by 2 to 4 weeks of age as the sebaceous glands mature and drain.
8. Polydactyly is the term for the presence of extra digits.
9. The five areas that are assessed with Apgar scoring are heart rate, respiratory rate, muscle tone, reflex irritability, and color.
10. A Dextrostix heel-stick reading of less than 40 to 45 mg/100 mL of blood suggests hypoglycemia.
11. The newborn's mouth should be suctioned for mucus by a bulb syringe as soon as the head is born.
12. The umbilical cord falls off between the 7th to 10th days of life.
13. Erythromycin ointment
14. A 1-month-old infant requires 110 to 120 calories per kilogram of body weight (50 to 55 kcal/lb) every 24 hours to provide an adequate amount of food for maintenance and growth.
15. Cow's milk contains casein, which is large, tough, and difficult to digest.
16. In a newborn 30 to 35% of body weight is extracellular fluid. The fluid requirements for a new-

born is 150 to 200 mL/kg (2.5 to 3.0 oz/lb) per 24 hours.

17. The position that is considered the best for bubbling an infant is to hold the baby in a sitting position on the lap, then lean the child forward against one hand, with the index finger and thumb supporting the head. This position provides head support, yet leaves the other hand free to pat the baby's back.
18. Women may breastfeed for varying lengths of time. Some do it for 1, 2, or 3 months, then wean the child from breast to bottle. Many continue until the child is 6 to 12 months of age and then wean directly to a small cup or glass. Some continue to breastfeed until the child is preschool age.
19. It is important that a newborn formula have iron added to ensure that the newborn receives enough of this to prevent iron-deficiency anemia.
20. An 8-lb newborn requires 20 to 24 ounces of fluid a day (8 × 2.54 to 3 oz).
21. Two physiologic risks of bottle propping are aspiration and otitis media.

CHAPTER 6

1. If a newborn fails to spontaneously draw in a first breath, the nurse's first action should be to suction the infant's mouth and nose with a bulb syringe and rub the newborn's back to see if skin stimulation initiates respirations.
2. Do not suction for longer than 10 seconds at a time to avoid removing excessive air from an infant's lungs.
3. Good lung expansion
4. 40 cm H_2O pressure for the first time
5. You should depress the sternum of the newborn when performing closed cardiac massage approximately ½ to ¾ inch (1 or 2 cm).
6. 35.5° to 36.5°C (95.9° to 97.7°F)
7. Kangaroo care
8. Through non-nutritive sucking with a pacifier at feeding times
9. The two most common viruses transmitted to the newborn in utero are cytomegalovirus and toxoplasmosis.
10. Increased hematocrit level and increased total amount of red blood cells (polycythemia)
11. Small-for-gestational-age newborns are at higher risk for problems with maintaining body temperature than the average newborn because they lack subcutaneous fat.
12. Some large-for-gestational-age infants have difficulty establishing respirations at birth because of birth trauma. Increased intracranial pressure from birth of the larger-than-usual head may lead to pressure on the respiratory center. This, in turn, causes a decrease in respiratory function. A diaphragmatic paralysis may occur due to cervical nerve trauma as the head is bent laterally to allow for birth of the large shoulders. This prevents active lung motion on the affected side. If the infant had to be delivered by cesarean birth, transient fluid can remain in the lungs and interfere with effective gas exchange.
13. The infant is an inexperienced newborn, so sucking may not be effective enough for the infant to obtain an adequate supply of milk.
14. The preterm infant is unable to initiate effective respirations as quickly as the mature infant.
15. 40 to 100 mL/kg/day
16. 115 to 140 kcal/kg/day
17. Immature nervous system
18. First immunizations are given to preterm infants at chronological age.
19. Surfactant deficiency
20. The rationale for administering pancuronium to infants on ventilators is to increase pulmonary blood flow and abolish spontaneous respiratory action. Doing so allows mechanical ventilation to be accomplished at lower pressures, because there is no normal muscle resistance to overcome. The possibility of pneumothorax is reduced, while PaO_2 is increased.
21. Transient tachypnea of the newborn typically resolves within 72 hours of life.
22. The measures that could be used to stimulate the infant with apnea are gently shaking the infant or flicking the sole of the foot.
23. The peak age of incidence for SIDS is between 2 weeks and 1 year.
24. An alarm sounds on an apnea monitor when the neonate experiences a period of apnea of 20 seconds or more or a decreased heart rate below 80 bpm.
25. The maternal and fetal blood types most commonly associated with ABO incompatibility are maternal type O and fetal type A blood.
26. Use of phototherapy is the first method of choice for treating hemolytic disease of the newborn.
27. The nurse would typically expect bleeding from hemorrhagic disease of the newborn to occur on days 2 to 5 of life.
28. The cause of retinopathy of prematurity is exposure to a high concentration of oxygen.
29. Beta-hemolytic, group B streptococcal infection
30. Acyclovir and vidarabine
31. To prevent serum glucose from falling too low
32. The average time of onset for withdrawal symptoms for the heroin-addicted neonate is 24 to 48 hours after birth. However, in some cases they may not appear for up to 10 days.

33. Two characteristic facial features of the neonate with fetal alcohol syndrome are short palpebral fissures and a thin upper lip.

CHAPTER 7

1. Growth is generally used to denote an increase in physical size or a quantitative change, whereas development is used to denote an increase in skill or the ability to function (a qualitative change).
2. Neurologic and lymphoid tissue grow most rapidly during early childhood.
3. Freud defines libido as instinctual drives within an individual.
4. The toddler who consistently responds to questions with "no" is learning autonomy.
5. The best toys to promote a sense of initiative are those that provide the opportunity and freedom to initiate motor play, such as bikes, paints, and modelling clay.
6. The adolescent must develop a sense of identity.
7. The preschool child is using assimilation when he tells you his broken leg wants to get fixed.
8. The preschool child is using intuitive thought.
9. The stage of moral reasoning in school-age children is often termed the "nice" stage because they engage in actions because they are nice rather than necessarily right.
10. Kohlberg's theory of moral development is often criticized for being male-oriented.

CHAPTER 8

1. 100 to 120 beats per minute
2. Infants have a greater percentage of extracellular fluid (35% of body weight) compared with the 20% in adults.
3. Ventral suspension, prone, sitting, and standing
4. Approximately 8 months
5. 10 months
6. Two words plus ma-ma and da-da
7. Binocular vision
8. 6 to 8 weeks
9. At approximately 8 months
10. Around 10 months of age
11. Aspiration
12. Up to approximately 2 months
13. At approximately 6 months of age
14. Infant cereal
15. Approximately 12 months
16. By establishing some schedule of consistent activity with a consistent caregiver
17. Turning away from or spitting out tastes they don't enjoy
18. Unclear but may be related to overfeeding, swallowing too much air, or using formula too high in carbohydrates
19. Putting the infant to bed with a bottle containing sugar water, formula, milk, or fruit juice; which causes tooth decay

CHAPTER 9

1. Lordosis of the spine is common during the toddler years.
2. Toddlers have distended abdomens because their abdominal muscles are not yet strong enough to support abdominal contents.
3. The 2-year-old child should master two-word, noun–verb, simple sentences.
4. The typical play pattern of toddlers is parallel play (side-by-side individual play). They enjoy toys they can manipulate and like active, stimulating play.
5. The most common source of lead poisoning is lead paint, which the toddler chews, sucks, or eats from objects such as window sills, walls, or furniture.
6. It is not generally recommended that fat be restricted from the diet of a child under age 2.
7. In order to toilet train the child must have control of rectal and urethral sphincters. A good way to know that the child's development has reached this point is to wait until the child is able to walk well independently.
8. Although toddlers can sit well, it is not safe to leave them in a bathtub unsupervised.
9. Parents can best eliminate the toddler's extreme negativism by limiting the number of questions asked and providing him or her with an opportunity to make choices.
10. "Time out" is a technique of teaching children that actions have consequences. Parents select a non-stimulating area, and the child must quietly remain there for a specified amount of time.

CHAPTER 10

1. Height and weight gain during the preschool years is minimal.
2. Rarely do new teeth develop during this time. Most children have all their deciduous teeth by age 2½.
3. A 3-year-old uses about 900 vocabulary words.
4. If children do not develop a sense of initiative, they may face new situations with a sense of guilt.
5. Preschoolers outgrow their car seats when they reach 40 lbs. Because preschoolers may be too small for regular seat belts, a booster seat is the safest method to restrain the child.

6. A child who ingests food from all pyramid groups does not need additional supplements.
7. Night grinding is a way to release tension, allowing the child to fall asleep. Children who grind their teeth extensively may have anxiety to a greater degree than the average child.
8. Relating time and space to something the child knows, such as meals, television shows, or a friend's house, is an effective method to minimize separation anxiety.
9. An imaginary friend is normal as long as the imaginary friend does not interfere with other relationships.
10. Bringing a gift for older siblings helps ease sibling rivalry.
11. A parent who is bothered by masturbation might instruct the child to masturbate in private, explaining that some things are done in some places and not in others. The parent should not call unnecessary attention to the act as this can increase anxiety and cause increased activity.
12. Respiratory and gastrointestinal infections are frequent in children attending child care or preschool settings.
13. Broken fluency is a developmental phenomenon that normally fades at the end of the preschool period.

CHAPTER 11

1. Swelling of rapidly growing lymphatic tissue fills the narrow tube of the appendix, trapping fecal material; this can lead to inflammation.
2. Frontal sinuses develop at about age 6.
3. Supernumary nipples enlarge with puberty as they are affected by estrogen and androgen.
4. Boys begin to experience nocturnal emissions with puberty as seminal fluid is produced.
5. A 9-year-old gang is typically of the same sex, has a secret code or name, and excludes someone.
6. Boy and Girl Scouts provide constructive activities and strengthen a sense of autonomy. They encourage children to complete small projects, frequently helping to build a sense of industry.
7. Learning class inclusion leads to collecting.
8. Fairness is a step in moral development.
9. A type A school lunch supplies one-third of a child's RDA.
10. Children need additional exercise because school is basically a sit-down activity.
11. If children eat candy, they should eat a type of candy that dissolves fast so it remains in contact with the teeth for only a short time.
12. After it has been established that the child with school phobia is free from illness, he or she should be encouraged to attend school. Counseling for the whole family and addressing a potential conflict are also recommended.

CHAPTER 12

1. Growth ceases during adolescence due to closure of the epiphyseal lines of long bones.
2. Apocrine sweat glands are responsible for adolescent body odor.
3. Testosterone is the hormone that influences male facial hair development at puberty.
4. Menarche is the term for the first menstrual period. The beginning of breast development is called thelarche.
5. The four tasks adolescents must achieve to gain a sense of identity are accepting their changed body image, establishing a value system or what kind of person they want to be, making a career decision, and becoming emancipated from their parents.
6. Early adolescents often dress and act alike; this allows them to establish a sense of identity, because they are not excluded from the group. Knowing who they are not is one step in discovering who they are.
7. Parents who suspect their children are sexually active should make sure that they are knowledgeable about safer sex practices.
8. The final stage of cognitive development is the state of formal operations, which involves the ability to think in abstract terms and use the scientific method to arrive at conclusions.
9. Formal reasoning doesn't deter adolescents from shoplifting because some teens have difficulty envisioning a department store or a large corporation as capable of suffering economic loss from stealing.
10. The leading cause of death among adolescents is accidents, most commonly those involving motor vehicles.
11. The three minerals most apt to be deficient in an adolescent diet are iron, calcium, and zinc.
12. Girls taking tetracycline are apt to develop candidal vaginitis.
13. The danger of a very-low-calorie diet for obese adolescents is that such a diet provides insufficient protein and may be deficient in vitamins, potentially leading to inadequate nitrogen balance and, in turn, impaired growth.
14. Sexual identity or gender is the inner sense a person has of being male or female, which may be the same as or different from biologic gender.
15. The effects of Rohypnol are drowsiness, impaired motor skills, and amnesia.
16. It is recommended that an adolescent have well-established menstrual cycles for at least 2 years before beginning oral contraceptives to reduce

the risk of causing permanent suppression of pituitary-regulating activity and to prevent halting of the preadolescent growth spurt.

17. In addition to preventing pregnancy, condoms are the best method to prevent STDs.
18. Four factors that contribute to the rising rate of teenage pregnancy are the earlier age of menarche in girls, an increase in the rate of sexual activity among teenagers, a lack of knowledge about (or failure to use) contraceptives, and a desire by young girls to have a child.
19. Two major reasons why adolescents seek prenatal care late are denial of the pregnancy and also to protect the pregnancy—if she doesn't tell anyone, no one can suggest that she terminate it.
20. Two common complications associated with adolescent pregnancy are cephalopelvic disproportion and postpartal hemorrhage.
21. The young adolescent is at a higher risk for postpartal hemorrhage because it may be secondary to the overdistention of a not yet fully developed uterus, or it can result from perineal or cervical lacerations, which are usually deeper in the adolescent because of the infant's size in relation to the girl's body.
22. Al-Anon is the organization to use for referral of children of alcoholics.
23. Chronic inhalation of cocaine can cause ulceration in the mucous membranes of the nose.

CHAPTER 13

1. Leading questions supply their own answers.
2. Six areas to explore regarding the chief concern are duration, intensity, frequency, description, associated symptoms, and actions taken.
3. Important areas to consider when eliciting a day history are play, sleep, hygiene, and eating habits.
4. It is important to ask for a family health history because some diseases are inherited.
5. A health history should conclude with "Is there anything more we should know about your child?" or "Is there anything I didn't mention that you want to ask about?"
6. Four techniques used in physical assessment are inspection, palpation, percussion, and auscultation.
7. Blood pressure is included as part of a routine assessment at age 3 years.
8. On a standardized scale all weights between the 10th and 90th percentile are considered normal.
9. The following factors should be assessed during an examination of the skin: temperature, color, texture, turgor, and presence of any lesions.
10. The red reflex is elicited by shining a flashlight or ophthalmoscope light into the pupil.
11. Normal ear alignment is determined when a line drawn from the inner canthus of the eye through the outer canthus and then to the ear touches the top of the ear pinna.
12. When a child has epiglottitis the gag reflex should not be elicited.
13. Edema, erythema, wrinkling, retraction, or dimpling of the skin suggest that a tumor is growing in the deeper layers of breast tissue.
14. Pulmonary heart valves are heard best at the second left intercostal space.
15. Routine scoliosis screening should begin at age 12 years.
16. The preschool E chart is a good type of eye chart for cognitively impaired or non-English-speaking children.
17. Normal conversation is approximately 50 to 60 dB.

CHAPTER 14

1. Shortened length of stays and minimized hospital admissions have dramatically changed health teaching by making the window for teaching very narrow.
2. Three types of learning include cognitive, psychomotor, and affective learning.
3. During the school-age years, learning capability is concrete.
4. Motivation to learn or to appreciate how their life will be improved through learning may affect children's emotional readiness to learn. Some factors such as exhaustion, pain, low self-esteem, or distaste for a certain aspect of care must be resolved before children are emotionally ready to learn.
5. Five minutes is the typical attention span of a preschooler.
6. Careful assessment is needed to determine whether formal or informal teaching is the best format for a given situation.
7. Peer learning not only improves knowledge but may improve attitude and motivation to learn. Children may be more comforted by other children's experiences or may be more willing to accept the advice or solutions of a peer.
8. Trying to modify beliefs or values by behavior modification is unethical.
9. Playing board games is a good technique for school-age children.
10. Children do tend to listen to mass media messages if the messages are attention-getting and brief.

CHAPTER 15

1. School-age children understand quite a bit about the workings of major body parts. Early grade-school children are able to name the functions of the heart, lungs, and stomach.
2. Newborns are more likely to lose a devastating amount of body water with diarrhea or vomiting

because their total body water is composed of approximately 40% of extracellular water and, in turn, much less water is stored in the cells.

3. Useful techniques in preparing preschoolers for hospitalization include allowing the child to bring transitional objects, reading books about hospitalization, and playing or acting out hospitalization and procedures.
4. Height and weight should be measured on hospital admission to determine overall growth and allow for determination of surface area.
5. According to Robertson, the first stage of separation anxiety is protest.
6. As a rule home care is more cost-effective than hospitalization.
7. A box or additional pillows can be placed under the mattress to elevate the head of a regular bed to a gatch position.
8. To encourage a sense of trust in infants, maintain a schedule as close to their normal routine as possible. To promote a sense of autonomy in ill toddlers and a sense of initiative in preschoolers, allow them to make choices about their care. To promote a sense of industry in school-aged children, explain to them about specific procedures and involve them as much as possible in the actual care. To promote a sense of identity in adolescents, help them to participate as much as possible in as many activities as they did before and encourage them to maintain self-care activities and good hygiene.
9. Children accept smaller, fuller glasses of fluid more readily.
10. To ensure that a hospital crib is safe, be sure that side rails are in good repair, fully raised at all times and secured; push bedside stands and tables away from the crib so that the child cannot climb over the rail and use the stand or table as a step down; be sure crib caps are used for small children.
11. Sleepwalking occurs during NREM sleep, probably during the deepest part of stage IV.
12. Children with sensory deprivation lose the ability to make decisions and become easily confused or depressed.
13. Caregivers can make television watching more interactive by playing along with game shows or children's programs such as "Sesame Street" or discussing the characters and plots of a particular show.
14. A cylinder 1 inch in diameter is the most dangerous size for a toy because it totally occludes the trachea if it is aspirated.

CHAPTER 16

1. Schoolage children can worry that they will fail a "test," a worry that places unnecessary stress on them.
2. A mummy restraint should be used when a young child needs to be temporarily immobilized.
3. Radioactive iodine will destroy the thyroid if it is not blocked from entering the gland.
4. Endoscopy is direct visualization of the gastrointestinal tract by a fiberoptic tube passed through the mouth. Bronchoscopy is direct visualization of the larynx, trachea, bronchi, and alveoli by a fiberoptic tube passed through the nose or mouth.
5. The blood pressure cuff should be no more than two thirds and not less than half the length of the upper arm.
6. A tympanic thermometer registers in about 2 seconds.
7. The fingertip and the heel are both appropriate sites for obtaining a capillary puncture and heel.
8. A 24-hour urine should be timed from the time of the discard urine.
9. Perineal pressure is applied during suprapubic aspiration in girls to block the urethra.
10. To use a nomogram, draw a line from the child's height to the child's weight. The point at which it crosses the middle line is the child's surface area.
11. Ear drops should be given at room temperature; cold drops can cause pain.
12. The preferred administration site for an intramuscular injection in an infant is the quadriceps muscle of the anterior thigh.
13. Automatic rate infusion pumps, fluid chambers, and mini-droppers are safety devices to ensure the proper rate of fluid during intravenous fluid therapy.
14. Intraosseous transfusions are used in emergencies when it is difficult to establish usual IV access or in a child with such extensive burns that the usual sites for intravenous infusion are not available.
15. A nasogastric tube in an infant is measured from the bridge of the nose to the earlobe to a point halfway between the xiphoid process and the umbilicus.
16. A TPN solution contains approximately twice the amount of glucose normally administered in an intravenous solution, which may cause dehydration as the body tries to reduce the amount of glucose recognized by the kidneys as excessive by eliminating it.
17. An enema catheter in an infant should be inserted 1 inch.
18. Parents should give acetaminophen rather than aspirin for children's fever because aspirin has been associated with the development of Reye's syndrome.

CHAPTER 17

1. Diffuse body movements; tears; high-pitched, sharp, harsh cry; stiff posture; lack of play; fisting; and guarding are frequent physical findings of infants in pain.

2. To assess pain accurately, use the toddler's terminology.
3. Children are often more adept at imagery because their imaginations are less inhibited.
4. With substitution of meaning the child places another, often fantastic meaning on a painful procedure. With thought stopping, the child stops an anxious thought by replacing it with a realistic positive thought.
5. A child's pain management program can include both pharmacologic and non-pharmacologic methods.
6. IM routes are used infrequently with children because they are associated with pain on administration and produce great fear in children.
7. Conscious sedation provides an analgesia.
8. Epidural analgesia does not lead to spinal headache.

CHAPTER 18

1. Cleft lip is more prevalent in males.
2. A child with cleft palate repair should not use a straw because it could tear the suture line.
3. Before surgery, feeding a child with cleft lip is a problem because the infant has difficulty maintaining suction and is at an increased risk for aspiration.
4. The chief danger of tracheoesopheal fistula is aspiration from seepage of fluid from the esophagus into the lungs.
5. The most important consideration in care of the child with omphalocele at birth is protecting the sac from rupturing.
6. Low intermittent nasogastric suction is used for newborns because higher pressure can break down the stomach lining.
7. The most common site for intestinal obstruction in the infant is the duodenum.
8. The best preoperative position for an infant with a diaphragmatic hernia is with the head elevated or turned so the compressed lung is down.
9. Taping a coin on a newborn's umbilicus to reduce an umbilical hernia can actually cause intestinal obstruction or bowel strangulation.
10. It is important for parents to perform rectal dilatation after surgical repair of an imperforate hernia.
11. Changes with increased cranial pressure include increased blood pressure and temperature and decreased pulse and respirations.
12. After a shunting procedure the infant's bed should be flat or only slightly raised (approximately 30 degrees).
13. A meningocele sac should be kept moist to keep it from drying and rupturing.
14. Surgery is performed to repair a neural tube defect as soon as possible after birth, usually within 24 hours.
15. Syndactyly describes the condition in which two fingers are fused.
16. Passive stretching exercises and encouraging the infant to look in the direction of the affected muscle are important measures to teach parents of a child with a torticollis.
17. Developmental hip dysplasia is best assessed by assessing for hip abduction.
18. The affected hip is abducted and externally rotated.
19. The presence of only streak gonads (small; nonfunctional gonads) results in sterility.
20. The muscles of children with Down syndrome are unusually relaxed, often described as a "rag-doll" appearance.

CHAPTER 19

1. The frontal sinuses and the sphenoidal sinuses do not develop until 6 to 8 years of age.
2. After age 2, foreign bodies more often lodge in the right bronchus.
3. Tachypnea is often the first indicator of airway obstruction.
4. Wheezing is heard most noticeably on expiration when an obstruction is in the lower trachea or bronchioles.
5. Two noninvasive methods for measuring oxyhemoglobin saturation include pulse oximetry and transcutaneous oxygen monitoring.
6. Tidal volume (TV) denotes the amount of air inhaled or exhaled.
7. Vaporizers providing a warm mist can seriously scald children if accidentally pulled over on them.
8. Instruct children to inhale rather than blow out against the mouthpiece of an incentive spirometer.
9. Gloves should be worn when suctioning a tracheostomy.
10. Covering the opening with a gauze square tied to the child's neck like a bib is a good method to keep crumbs out of a tracheostomy.
11. A capnometer measures the amount of CO_2 in inhaled or exhaled breaths.
12. Pancuronium (Pavulon) may be administered to abolish spontaneous respiratory activity.
13. Children with choanal atresia develop signs of respiratory distress at birth or immediately after they quiet and attempt their first breath.
14. Infants should not be prescribed acetylsalicylic acid (aspirin) because of its association with Reye's syndrome.
15. The palatine tonsils are typically involved with tonsillitis.

16. Subtle signs of post-tonsillectomy bleeding include an increasing pulse rate, frequent swallowing, throat clearing, and a feeling of anxiety.
17. The most effect treatment for laryngitis is for children to rest their voice for at least 24 hours, until the inflammation subsides.
18. Never attempt to directly visualize the epiglottis directly with a tongue blade or obtain a throat culture unless a means of providing an artificial airway is readily available.
19. A series of five back blows followed by five chest thrusts is considered the most effective method for dislodging an aspirated foreign body in infants.
20. Bronchiolitis is most often seen in children younger than age 2 years, with the highest incidence in winter and spring.
21. Wheezing is the most common presenting symptom in children with asthma.
22. A short-acting beta 2-agonist such as albuterol is the chief medication given for an acute asthma attack.
23. Children with chronic illness, those who have had a splenectomy, or those who are immunocompromised should receive a pneumococcal vaccine.
24. A semi-Fowler's position generally allows for the best lung expansion.
25. Miliary tuberculosis refers to tuberculosis that has spread to other parts of the body.
26. A level greater than 60 mEg/L chloride in sweat is diagnostic of CF.

CHAPTER 20

1. Infants with heart disease generally have tachycardia and tachypnea.
2. Organic heart murmur denotes a heart murmur resulting from heart disease.
3. Blood tests help to support the diagnosis of heart disease or to rule out anemia or clotting defects.
4. Routine blood pressure screening begins at age 3 years.
5. Because anemia stresses the heart, an iron supplement is generally given to an infant with congenital heart disease.
6. Children with congenital heart defects need prophylactic antibiotic therapy before oral surgery because streptococcal organisms generally present in the mouth are often involved in infectious endocarditis.
7. Assess pulse and blood pressure every 15 minutes after cardiac catheterization.
8. Cardiac arrhythmias may result from the mechanical action of the catheter having touched the conduction nodes of the heart.
9. After cardiac surgery; children should be encouraged to cough and deep breath to prevent pooling of secretions in the respiratory system.
10. Post perfusion syndrome is most apt to occur 3 to 12 weeks after surgery.
11. Children tend to develop hypervolemia after cardiac surgery because of increased production of aldosterone and an increase in antidiuretic hormone secretion.
12. The drug most commonly prescribed for anticoagulation therapy is sodium warfarin.
13. Acute rejection of a transplanted heart occurs in about 7 days.
14. With atrial septal defect, blood flow is from left to right.
15. Indomethacin is used to treat patent ductus arteriosus.
16. With total anomalous pulmonary venous return, blood must be shunted across a patent foramen ovale or patent ductus arteriosus to reach the left side.
17. The four defects that present with tetralogy of Fallot include pulmonic stenosis, ventricular septal defect, dextroposition of the aorta, and hypertrophy of the right ventricle.
18. To strengthen heart contractility, digoxin is commonly prescribed.
19. In the child receiving furosemide, the nurse should be alert for hypokalemia.
20. Rheumatic fever occurs as a result of a group A beta-hemolytic streptococcus infection.
21. During the first stage of Kawasaki disease, the primary manifestation is high fever that does not respond to antipyretics.
22. Administration of ampicillin or amoxicillin before ear, nose, throat, tonsil, or mouth surgery or childbirth helps prevent infectious endocarditis.
23. An abdominal bruit is suggestive of renal vascular disease.
24. Accurate measurement of LDL requires a 12-hour fasting period before blood sampling.
25. The most frequent effect of cardiomyopathy is severe dilation of the left or both ventricles, which impairs systolic function and leads to heart failure.
26. Respiratory failure is the most frequent cause of cardiac arrest.
27. A 1:5 ratio of ventilation to compression is used for resuscitation of an infant.

CHAPTER 21

1. Macrophages are responsible for engulfing, ingesting, and neutralizing a pathogen.
2. Two types of lymphocytes produced by bone marrow are type T and B cell lymphocytes.
3. Maternal transmission of HIV by placental spread is the most common cause for childhood HIV.
4. HIV-positive children are begun on prophylactic TMP-SMZ for *Pneumocystis carinii.*

5. Contact dermatitis indicates a type IV hypersensitivity.
6. Skin testing is done to isolate an antigen to which a child is sensitive.
7. Epinephrine is the first-line drug to treat anaphylaxis.
8. Angioedema occurs where skin is loosely bound by subcutaneous tissue such as the eyelids, hands, feet, genitalia, and lips.
9. Food allergy probably causes atopic dermatitis in infants.
10. In infants, atopic dermatitis affects flexor surfaces of extremities and dorsal surfaces of wrists and ankles.
11. Food allergies are usually treated with elimination diets.
12. Patch testing is used to identify the allergen of contact dermatitis.

CHAPTER 22

1. Incubation, prodromal, illness, and convalescence are the four stages of an infectious disorder.
2. Reservoir, portal of exit, means of transmission, portal of entry, and susceptible host are five components of the chain of infection.
3. Children receive DTaP at 2, 4, and 6 months and between 15 and 18 months.
4. Children should receive varicella immunization any time after their first birthday, usually between 12 to 18 months, and at 11 to 12 years of age if they do not have a reliable history of immunization.
5. The hallmark of roseola is the appearance of a rash immediately after the sharp decline in fever.
6. A discrete, pink-red, maculopapular rash is typically the first sign of rubella noticed by parents.
7. Koplik's spots are found only with rubeola.
8. The four stages of chickenpox lesions are (1) macula, (2) papule, (3) vesicle, and (4) crust.
9. Swelling of mumps is typically located at the parotid gland, just in front of the earlobe.
10. Children with infectious mononucleosis are at risk for splenic rupture upon abdominal palpation.
11. Beta-hemolytic streptococci group A are responsible for scarlet fever.
12. Staphylococci are often the organisms involved in food poisoning episodes in summer months.
13. Massive cell necrosis and inflammation is the result of exotoxin production by diphtheria bacilli.
14. Complications of pertussis include pneumonia, atelectasis, and emphysema.
15. Helminthic infections are transmitted by unclean foods and hands.
16. *Candida albicans* is responsible for thrush.

CHAPTER 23

1. The two major forms of white blood cells are granulocytes and agranulocytes.
2. Megakaryocytes is the term used to denote immature platelets.
3. In children the preferred aspiration sites for bone marrow are the iliac crest and spines.
4. All potential donors are typed for human leukocyte compatibility.
5. The formation and development of white blood cells, platelets, and red blood cells are all affected by aplastic anemia.
6. Iron chelation therapy is needed for hypodermoclysis, which is the result of many long-term transfusion of packed red cells.
7. Ferrous sulfate is the drug of choice to improve red cell formation and replace iron stores.
8. For absorption of vitamin B_{12} from the intestine, an intrinsic factor must be present in the gastric mucosa.
9. The medical treatment of choice for congenital spherocytosis is generally splenectomy at approximately age 5 to 6 years.
10. Children with sickle cell anemia need more fluid during the summer months.
11. Parietal and frontal bossing change the shape of the skull, upper teeth protrude, the base of the nose may broaden and flatten.
12. With autoimmune acquired hemolytic anemia, laboratory findings reveal that the red cells are extremely small and round, resembling hereditary spherocytosis.
13. Henoch-Schonlein syndrome is often associated with allergies.
14. Salicylates should be avoided in children with ITP because they interfere with blood clotting by preventing the aggregation of platelets at wound sites.
15. The coagulation component factor VIII is deficient in hemophilia A.
16. With even minor abrasions, children with hemophilia must have bleeding controlled by administration of factor VIII.

CHAPTER 24

1. Interstitial fluid accounts for a greater percentage of body weight in infants than in adults.
2. With isotonic dehydration, the body initially compensates by a shift of interstitial fluid into the blood vessels.
3. The major cation of the extracellular fluid is Na^+.
4. The major cation of intracellular fluid is K^+.

5. Although NPO status for a child experiencing vomiting is determined by age, an average of 3 to 6 hours should be sufficient.
6. The two primary causes of diarrhea are viral and bacterial invasion of the gastrointestinal tract.
7. A metabolic acidosis is present with severe diarrhea.
8. Salmonella may be the causative organism if a child develops diarrhea after eating raw eggs.
9. An elevated prone position for 1 hour is the best position after feeding for a child with gastrointestinal reflux.
10. Vomiting almost immediately after feeding that grows increasingly forceful until it is projectile is associated with pyloric stenosis.
11. Fiberoptic endoscopy is the most reliable diagnostic test to confirm peptic ulcer disease.
12. Bowel or stomach perforation, blood loss anemia, and intestinal obstruction are three complications of peptic ulcer disease.
13. Hepatitis A and hepatitis E are transmitted through fecally contaminated water.
14. Hepatitis D is most responsible for fulminant hepatitis.
15. With bile duct obstruction, absorption of fat and fat-soluble vitamins is poor.
16. Children with esophageal varices are at high risk for rupture of varices, which can lead to a large quantity of blood loss.
17. Hypoglycemia is a danger of liver transplant because glucose levels are regulated by the liver, and transplanted organs may not function efficiently at first.
18. Currant jelly–like stools are present with intussusception.
19. Volvulus develops during fetal life between approximately 6 and 10 weeks.
20. Signs of NEC usually appear in the first week of life.
21. The point of sharpest pain is often one-third of the way between the anterior superior iliac crest and the umbilicus (McBurney's point).
22. Steatorrhea; deficiency of fat-soluble vitamins A,D,K, and E; malnutrition; and a distended abdomen are the four most common symptoms of celiac disease.
23. Gluten must be restricted in a child with celiac disease.
24. A low-residue diet is usually ordered for the child with aganglionic megacolon.
25. The cause of inflammatory bowel disease is probably an alteration in immune system response or an autoimmune process.

CHAPTER 25

1. A nephron is the major functioning unit of the kidneys.
2. Creatinine in urine remains constant regardless of the amount of protein in the diet.
3. The presence of UTI is established by urine culture.
4. Cystoscopy is a difficult procedure for many children because it is painful and requires them to lie still for the procedure.
5. To empty urine from a continent urinary reservoir, the parent or child catheterizes the abdominal urethra three or four times daily.
6. The meatus may be near the glans, midway back or at the baseof the penis in the child with hypospadias.
7. *Escherichia coli* is the organism that most commonly causes UTIs.
8. After recurrent UTIs, children are prescribed a prophylactic antibiotic for 6 months.
9. UTI is a common symptom associated with vesicoureteral reflux.
10. Enuresis is found more commonly in boys.
11. Orthostatic proteinuria is spilling of albumin into the urine when the child stands upright.
12. Acute glomerulonephritis is characterized by a sudden onset of hematuria and proteinuria.
13. Four characteristic symptoms of nephrotic syndrome include (1) proteinuria, (2) edema, (3) low serum albumin, and (4) hyperlipidemia.
14. Oliguria is one of the first symptoms noted with acute renal failure.
15. Children with chronic renal failure are generally placed on low-protein, low-phosphorus diets.

CHAPTER 26

1. Precocious puberty occurs more often in females than males.
2. Girls have until 17 years of age before they are said to have delayed puberty.
3. Males with undescended testes are at high risk for testicular cancer and infertility.
4. The first symptom of testicular torsion is severe scrotal pain.
5. Endometriosis leads to dysmenorrhea because displaced endometrial tissue bleeds and sloughs the same as intrauterine endometrium.
6. Child abuse should be suspected in a young child with vulvovaginitis.
7. Yes. Breast implants are placed in back of breast tissue.
8. Yes. Breast cancer could exist concurrently with fibrocystic breast condition.

9. Candidiasis vaginal infection typically presents with a white, cheese-like discharge, redness, and itching.
10. Gonorrhea is a serious STD because it can lead to infertility in both sexes.

CHAPTER 27

1. Following arginine or insulin testing, children may develop severe hypoglycemia.
2. It may be embarrassing to have to take an intranasal medication at school.
3. The most serious effect of congenital hypothyroidism is cognitive impairment.
4. Children with hyperthyroidism are often unable to write or speak clearly, they may have hand tremors, and they also may be unable to sit still during class.
5. Girls who have adrenogenital syndrome at birth are born with masculinized genitalia; the clitoris is enlarged to look like a penis.
6. Aldosterone regulates sodium so the child becomes dehydrated quickly.
7. Children most frequently develop type I diabetes mellitus.
8. Typical symptoms of hypoglycemia are nervousness, weakness, sweating, and tremors.
9. The chief symptom of latent tetany is jitteriness from neuromuscular irritability.
10. Children with glycogen storage disease are unable to break down stored liver glycogen into glucose.

CHAPTER 28

1. To test for graphesthesia (ability to recognize a shape that has been traced on the skin), ask a preschooler to close his eyes and then trace first a circle, then a square on the back of his hand; ask him if the shapes are the same or different. For the older child, trace a number, for example, 8, 3, 0, and 1, and ask the child to identify each one.
2. Cranial nerve XI (accessory)
3. Deep tendon reflexes diminish in intensity with decreasing level of consciousness.
4. The intraventricular catheter monitoring method is considered the most accurate.
5. The four types of cerebral palsy are spastic, dyskinetic (athetoid), ataxic, and mixed.
6. Contractures can be prevented with the use of partial leg braces and passive and active exercises. These exercises can be incorporated into play activities.
7. Meningeal irritability is assessed by positive Brudzinski's and Kernig's signs.
8. Children with meningitis are placed on droplet precautions for 24 hours after the start of antibiotic therapy to prevent infection transmission.
9. Enteroviruses are the most frequent cause of encephalitis.
10. Reye's syndrome generally occurs after a viral infection such as varicella (chickenpox) or an upper respiratory infection. Research has identified an association between the use of acetylsalicylic acid (aspirin) and nonsteroidal antiinflammatory agents (NSAIDs) during the viral infection, with the onset of Reye's afterward.
11. The antitoxin for botulism is rarely given to infants because it is made from a horse serum base and can cause a hypersensitivity reaction.
12. A partial seizure with motor signs begins in the fingers and spreads to the wrist, arm, and face.
13. Absence seizures can usually be demonstrated in children by asking them to hyperventilate and count out loud. If they are susceptible to such seizures, they will breathe in and out deeply, possibly 10 times, stop and stare for 3 seconds, then continue to hyperventilate and count, unaware that they paused.
14. Seizures increase at puberty, possibly resulting from glandular changes or sudden growth and the need for an increased medicine dosage, or they may result in part from adolescent rebellion against prescribed medication routines.
15. Breath-holding is a phenomenon that occurs in young children when they are stressed or angry. The child breathes in and, because he is upset, does not breathe out again, or else breathes out and then does not inhale again. As brain cells become anoxic, the child becomes cyanotic and slumps to the floor, momentarily unconscious. With loss of consciousness, the child begins breathing again. With a tamper tantrum, a child deliberately attempts to hold his breath and pass out.
16. Loss of autonomic nervous system function would occur during the second recovery phase.
17. Spasticity results from the loss of upper level control or transmission of meaningful innervation to the lower muscles.
18. The cervical and thoracolumbar areas of the spine are the ones most likely to sustain injury.

CHAPTER 29

1. Children with myopia need corrective (concave) lenses to enable them to see at a distance.
2. Nystagmus is seen in children with vision-impairing lesions, such as congenital cataracts, and also occurs as a neurologic sign when there is a lesion of the cerebellum or brain stem.
3. Ptosis may be congenital (frequently hereditary and bilateral) or acquired (generally unilateral), such as a result of injury to the third cranial nerve (neurogenic) or to the lid or levator muscle.

4. A cover test or Hirschberg's test will reveal strabismus.
5. Foreign bodies such as sand or dirt that are loose on the conjunctiva can be removed by irrigation with a sterile normal saline solution or by gentle wiping with a well-moistened, sterile, cotton-tipped applicator after the eyelid is everted.
6. Immediate treatment with corticosteroids and antibiotics has significantly reduced the incidence of sympathetic iritis and need for enucleation.
7. For the infant with congenital glaucoma, the cornea appears enlarged, edematous, and hazy. The infant may have tearing, pain, and photophobia.
8. Vomiting increases intraocular pressure, which could injure the suture line.
9. Children are legally blind if their vision is less than 20/200 on a standard eye chart or their peripheral vision is less than 20 degrees.
10. Sound is a major way in which visually impaired children experience their environment.
11. Serous otitis media is a result of chronic otitis media.
12. It is important to assess for cholesteatoma because, if untreated, it can lead to mastoiditis, meningitis, and possibly facial nerve paralysis.

CHAPTER 30

1. Increase in the length of long bones occurs at the cartilage segment (the epiphyseal plate).
2. Electromyography studies the electrical activity of skeletal muscle and nerve conduction using needle electrodes inserted into muscle masses.
3. A window may be placed in a dried cast if an infection, usually identified as a hot spot on the cast surface, is suspected.
4. With crutches, weight bearing is by the arms.
5. Children may have bowlegs as part of normal development (seen most commonly in 2-year-olds).
6. Treatment of Legg-Calvé-Perthes disease requires a long period of therapy.
7. Osteomyelitis in older children is most often caused by *Staphylococcus aureus.*
8. Synovitis most commonly occurs in the hip joint of children.
9. Scoliosis may be functional (caused by a secondary problem) or structural (a primary deformity).
10. Following spinal instrumentation surgery, the child should be log-rolled.
11. Surgical correction is generally necessary when the degree of curvature is greater than 40 degrees.
12. NSAIDS are the drugs of choice for treating JRA.
13. Myasthenia gravis involves an interference with acetylcholine at the synaptic junctions, leading to symptoms of progressive muscle weakness.
14. Duchenne's disease is the most common form of muscular dystrophy.

CHAPTER 31

1. In children ages 5 to 9 years, the most frequent types of accidents include motor vehicle accidents, bicycles, drowning, burns, and accidents involving firearms.
2. The Poison Prevention Packaging Act of 1970 has decreased the incidence of childhood poisonings.
3. A simple linear skull fracture occurs commonly in the lambdoid suture line.
4. Subdural hematoma is venous bleeding into the space between the dura and arachnoid membrane, occurring when head trauma lacerates minute veins in this area. The collection of blood generally is bilateral. Epidural hematoma is bleeding into the space between the dura and the skull, occurring when head trauma is severe. Subdural hemorrhage is generally venous bleeding, but epidural hemorrhage is usually a result of rupture of the middle meningeal artery and therefore is arterial bleeding. It usually is intense and causes rapid brain compression.
5. A head injury is the most common cause of a coma.
6. A Glasgow coma score of 10 indicates moderate trauma.
7. Air under the diaphragm on abdominal x-ray suggests intestinal or gastric rupture.
8. The spleen is the most frequently injured organ in abdominal trauma.
9. Very young children display a mammalian diving reflex when they plunge under cold water.
10. Prophylactic antibiotic therapy may be used after a near-drowning episode to prevent pneumonia and additional airway interference.
11. With caustic poisoning, vomiting should not be induced because the corrosive substance will burn as it comes up just as it did going down.
12. Acetylcysteine is the antidote for acetaminophen poisoning.
13. A chelating agent is used to remove lead from soft tissue and bone and thus eliminate it in the urine.
14. Children can be poisoned by insecticides (1) by accidental ingestion or (2) through skin or respiratory tract contact when playing in an area that has recently been sprayed with one.
15. A swallowed chicken bone would be removed by esophagoscopy.
16. Sudden warming will increase the metabolic rate of cells. Without adequate blood flow to the area

because of still-present vasoconstriction, additional damage will occur.

17. A second-degree burn involves the entire epidermis.
18. Because nerves have been burned, third-degree burns are not painful.

CHAPTER 32

1. When a tumor has metastasized, it has spread from its primary location to a distant site.
2. Stage II disease implies that cancer cells cannot be totally removed by surgery.
3. Chemotherapeutic agents cause nausea and vomiting because they attack fast-growing cells, such as the cells lining the stomach.
4. Two common side effects of vincristine are constipation and loss of sensation in the fingers.
5. First signs commonly seen in the child with leukemia are fever, bruising, nosebleeds, and fatigue.
6. In children with leukemia and central nervous system involvement, methotrexate is administered intrathecally (into the spinal cord).
7. The incidence of Hodgkin's disease is highest in adolescents.
8. The first sign of Hodgkin's disease is usually a painless, enlarged lymph node.
9. Parents may dismiss the vomiting that occurs with brain tumors because it is not accompanied by nausea.
10. Straining at stool increases intracranial pressure.
11. The first usually reported symptom of osteosarcoma is bone pain.
12. Children waiting for surgery for Ewing's sarcoma should not bear weight on the affected leg.
13. An important nursing responsibility for children waiting for surgery for Wilms' tumor is to prevent abdominal palpation in the child.
14. A common finding in children with retinoblastoma is a white pupil.

CHAPTER 33

1. The four categories of cognitive impairment are mild, moderate, severe, and profound.
2. Children with an IQ of 45 can learn to talk and communicate, but they have only poor awareness of social conventions. They can learn some vocational skills during adolescence or young adulthood and to take care of themselves with moderate supervision. They are unlikely to progress beyond the second-grade level in academic subjects. As adults, they may be able to contribute to their own support by performing unskilled or semiskilled work under close supervision in a sheltered workshop setting. They may learn to travel alone to familiar places. They need supervision and guidance when in stressful settings.
3. To reach optimal level of functioning, areas such as the care setting, health maintenance needs, education, self-care activities, and preparation for adulthood must be addressed.
4. Assessment findings may include social isolation, stereotyped behaviors, resistance to change in routine, abnormal responses to sensory stimuli, insensitivity to pain, inappropriate emotional expressions, movement disturbances, poor speech development, and specific, limited intellectual problems.
5. The three major characteristics of ADHD are inattention, impulsivity, and hyperactivity.
6. Problems with sequencing interfere with the child's concept of before and after.
7. Methylphenidate hydrochloride (Ritalin) is often used to treat ADHD.
8. Therapy for children with conduct disorders focuses on modifying the home environment and training in social and problem-solving skills.
9. Separation anxiety occurs slightly more frequently in girls.
10. Iron deficiency anemia is commonly associated with pica.
11. Anorexia nervosa may occur in boys, but occurs most often in girls.
12. Bulimia refers to recurrent binge eating and purging, while anorexia nervosa is an intense preoccupation with food creating a feeling of revulsion to the point of excessive weight loss.

CHAPTER 34

1. No. As few as 10% of child-abusing parents are mentally ill.
2. The triad of child abuse is special parent, special child, and special circumstance.
3. Shaken baby syndrome is caused by an adult severely shaking a child, causing a whiplash injury to the neck, edema to the brain stem, and typical retinal hemorrhages.
4. Parents Anonymous is the national organization to help child abusers.
5. Psychological abuse includes constant belittling or threatening, rejecting, isolating, or exploiting the child.
6. In Munchausen syndrome by proxy, symptoms are those that are not easily detected by physical exam and occur only when the abuser is present.
7. Failure to thrive is defined as a child with weight and height below the third percentile.
8. A pedophile is an adult who seeks out children for sexual gratification.
9. Rape is a crime of violence.

10. Battered women do not seek help early in an abusive relationship because they are using denial as a defense mechanism.
11. The safety of the abused family is the priority.

CHAPTER 35

1. A grief reaction consists of the stages of denial, anger, bargaining, depression, and acceptance.
2. If at all possible, children with chronic illnesses should attend regular classrooms.

3a. Parents can help siblings by setting aside time for activities with them, as well as explaining the illness and procedures and including them in the care of the ill child.

3b. The stage of depression is apt to be the most difficult for parents as it is the first time they really face what is happening.

4. Anticipatory grief can blunt the hurt of the child's death.
5. The last sense lost with dying is hearing.
6. Organ donations of livers and kidneys from children are important because it is difficult to transplant adult organs into children.

INDEX

Page numbers followed by f indicate figures; those followed by t indicate tables.

C

G

O

T

U

W

X

Y

Z

Photo Credit List

Unit 1 Opener: © Barbara Proud
Unit 2 Opener: © Sharon Guynup
Unit 3 Opener: photo by Melissa Olson
Unit 4 Opener: courtesy of A.I. duPont Institute, Children's Hospital, Wilmington, DE
Unit 5 Opener: © Caroline Brown, RNC, MS, DEd

Chapter 1 Opener: photo by Melissa Olson
Fig. 1-1: © B. Proud
Fig. 1-4: © Caroline Brown, RNC, MS, DEd
Fig. 1-5: © B. Proud
Fig. 1-6: © B. Proud

Chapter 2 Opener: photo by Danielle DiPalma
Fig. 2-1: photo by Melissa Olson
Fig. 2-6: photo courtesy of Briar Bush Nature Center, Abington, PA

Chapter 3 Opener: © Caroline Brown, RNC, MS, DEd
Fig. 3-1: © Kathy Sloane
Fig. 3-2: © Caroline Brown, RNC, MS, DEd
Fig. 3-4: © Jeff Greenberg/Science Source/Photo Researchers

Chapter 4 Opener: © Petit Format/Nestle/Science Source/Photo Researchers
Fig. 4-4: © Petit Format/Nestle/Science Source/Photo Researchers
Fig. 4-10: AB: © NMSB/Custom Medical Stock Photo
Fig. 4-11: A © Barbara Proud
Fig. 4-11: B © SPL/Custom Medical Stock Photo

Chapter 5 Opener: © Caroline Brown, RNC, MS, DEd
Fig. 5-1: photo by Melissa Olson
Fig. 5-3 A-E: photo by Keith Cotton, from Weber, J. and Kelley, J. [1998], *Health Assessment in Nursing.* Philadelphia: Lippincott-Raven Publishers.
Fig. 5-3 F, G: © Caroline Brown, RNC, MS, DEd
Fig. 5-4: A-D: from *"Variations and Minor Departures in Infants,"* courtesy of Mead Johnson
Fig. 5-5: © Caroline Brown, RNC, MS, DEd
Fig. 5-6: © Caroline Brown, RNC, MS, DEd
Fig. 5-7: © Billy E. Barnes/Stock Boston
Fig. 5-8A,B: © Bob Daemmrich/Stock Boston
Fig. 5-10: © Caroline Brown, RNC, MS, DEd
Fig. 5-11: photo by Keith Cotton
Fig. 5-14: photo by Melissa Olson, with permission of Chestnut Hill Hospital, Philadelphia, PA
Fig. 5-15: © B. Proud
Fig. 5-16: © Caroline Brown, RNC, MS, DEd
Fig. 5-17: © Caroline Brown, RNC, MS, DEd
Fig. 5-18: © Caroline Brown, RNC, MS, DEd

Chapter 6 Opener: © Caroline Brown, RNC, MS, DEd
Fig. 6-1: © Caroline Brown, RNC, MS, DEd
Fig. 6-3A, B: © Caroline Brown, RNC, MS, DEd
Fig. 6-4: © Caroline Brown, RNC, MS, DEd
Fig. 6-5: © Caroline Brown, RNC, MS, DEd
Fig. 6-6 A-J: © Caroline Brown, RNC, MS, DEd
Fig. 6-7: © Caroline Brown, RNC, MS, DEd
Fig. 6-8: © Caroline Brown, RNC, MS, DEd
Fig. 6-9: photo courtesy of Respironics/Healthdyne Technologies, Marietta, GA
Fig. 6-10: © Caroline Brown, RNC, MS, DEd
Fig. 6-11: © Caroline Brown, RNC, MS, DEd

Chapter 7 Opener: photo courtesy of Mark and Lynn Sharroot
Fig. 7-1: © B. Proud
Fig. 7-3: © Bob Kramer
Fig. 7-4: photo courtesy of Michael and Joanie Russell
Fig. 7-5: photo by Melissa Olson

Chapter 8 Opener: © Caroline Brown, RNC, MS, DEd
Fig. 8-2 A,B: © Caroline Brown, RNC, MS, DEd
Fig. 8-3A: © Custom Medical Stock Photo
Fig. 8-3B: © B. Proud
Fig. 8-4: photo by Melissa Olson
Fig. 8-5: photo courtesy of Robert and Jenifer Segar
Fig. 8-6: © B. Proud
Fig. 8-7: © Lauberman/Science Source/Photo Researchers
Fig. 8-8: photo by A.J. Olson
Fig. 8-9: © B. Proud
Fig. 8-10: © B. Proud
Fig. 8-11: photo by Melissa Olson
Fig. 8-12: photo by Melissa Olson
Fig. 8-13: photo by Melissa Olson
Fig. 8-14: photo by Melissa Olson
Fig. 8-15: © Caroline Brown, RNC, MS, DEd
Fig. 8-16: photo by Melissa Olson
Fig. 8-17: photo courtesy of Siu Ling Chen
Fig. 8-18: photo by Melissa Olson
Fig. 8-19: photo by Melissa Olson
Fig. 8-20: photo by Melissa Olson
Fig. 8-21: © K.L. Boyd, DDS/Custom Medical Stock Photo

Chapter 9 Opener: photo by John Olson
Fig. 9-1 A: © Michael Levin
Fig. 9-1 B: © B. Proud
Fig. 9-2: © B. Proud
Fig. 9-3: photo by Melissa Olson
Fig. 9-4: photo by Melissa Olson
Fig. 9-5: © David J. Sams/Stock Boston
Fig. 9-6: © B. Proud
Fig. 9-7: © B. Proud

Chapter 10 Opener: photo by Melissa Olson
Fig. 10-1: © B. Proud
Fig. 10-2: photo by Melissa Olson
Fig. 10-3: photo by Melissa Olson
Fig. 10-4: © B. Proud
Fig. 10-5: © B. Proud
Fig. 10-6: © Taeke Henstra/Science Source/Photo Researchers

Chapter 11 Opener: © B. Proud
Fig. 11-1: courtesy of Janet Weber
Fig. 11-3: © B. Proud
Fig. 11-4: photo by Melissa Olson
Fig. 11-5: © Stephen Frisch/Stock Boston
Fig. 11-6: photo by Melissa Olson
Fig. 11-7: photo courtesy of USDA Photo
Fig. 11-8: photo by Melissa Olson, with permission of Dynamic Modern Dentistry, Glenside, PA
Fig. 11-9: © Jose Carillo/Stock Boston

Chapter 12 Opener: photo by Melissa Olson
Fig. 12-3: photo by Melissa Olson
Fig. 12-4: © B. Proud
Fig. 12-5: © Billy Barnes/Stock Boston
Fig. 12-6: from Sauer, G.C. and Hall, J.C. [1996], *Manual of Skin Diseases, 7th ed.* Philadelphia: Lippincott-Raven Publishers.

Chapter 13 Opener: © Lesha Photography
Fig. 13-1: © B. Proud
Fig. 13-2: © B. Proud
Fig. 13-3: © B. Proud
Fig. 13-4: © B. Proud
Unnumbered Fig. NP 13-1 A: photo by Keith Cotton
Unnumbered Fig. NP 13-1 B: © B. Proud
Fig. 13-5 A,B: photos by John Gallagher, with permission of Wyncote Family Medicine, Wyncote, PA
Fig. 13-6: photo by Keith Cotton
Fig. 13-7: © Lesha Photography
Fig. 13-9: © B. Proud
Fig. 13-12: © Lesha Photography
Fig. 13-15: © B. Proud
Fig. 13-19: © B. Proud
Fig. 13-21: © B. Proud
Fig. 13-22: © B. Proud
Fig. 13-23: © NMSB/Custom Medical Stock Photo
Unnumbered Fig. NP13-2 A,B: © B. Proud
Fig. 13-24 A,B: © Lesha Photography
Fig. 13-24 C,D: photos by John Gallagher, with permission of Wyncote Family Medicine, Wyncote, PA
Fig. 13-28: photo by John Gallagher, with permission of Wyncote Family Medicine, Wyncote, PA
Fig. 13-29: © Lesha Photography

Chapter 14 Opener: © Caroline Brown, RNC, MS, DEd
Fig. 14-1: © SPL/Custom Medical Stock Photo
Fig. 14-2: © B. Proud
Fig. 14-3: © Lesha Photography
Fig. 14-6: © B. Proud
Fig. 14-7: © B. Proud

Chapter 15 Opener: © Sharon Guynup
Fig. 15-1: © Bob Kramer
Fig. 15-2: © Bob Kramer
Fig. 15-3: © Bob Kramer
Fig. 15-4: © Susan Leavines/Science Source/Photo Researchers
Fig. 15-5: © B. Proud
Fig. 15-6: © Lesha Photography
Fig. 15-7: © John Meyer/Custom Medical Stock Photo
Fig. 15-8: © B. Proud
Fig. 15-9: © Lesha Photography
Fig. 15-12: © B. Proud
Fig. 15-13: © Daemmrich/Stock Boston

Chapter 16 Opener: © B. Proud
Fig. 16-2: © John Watney/Science Source/Photo Researchers
Fig. 16-3: © Bachmann/Stock Boston
Fig. 16-4 A: © Alexander Tsiaras/Science Source/Photo Researchers
Fig. 16-4 B: © Richard T. Nowitz/ Science Source/Photo Researchers
Fig. 16-5: © Simon Fraser/Department of Radiology, RVI, Newcastle/SPL/Science Source/Photo Researchers
Fig. 16-6: Larry Mulvehill/Science Source/Photo Researchers
Fig. 16-7 A,B: © B. Proud
Fig. 16-8: © B. Proud
Fig. 16-9: © B. Proud
Fig. 16-10 B: photo courtesy of Leica Microsystems, Inc., Deerfield, IL

Fig. 16-14: © Lesha Photography
Fig. 16-15: © B. Proud
Fig. 16-16: © B. Proud
Fig. 16-17 B: photo by John Gallagher, with permission of Wyncote Family Medicine, Wyncote, PA
Unnumbered Fig. NP 16-2: © Lesha Photography
Fig. 16-19: © Caroline Brown, RNC, MS, DEd
Fig. 16-20:© Caroline Brown, RNC, MS, DEd
Fig. 16-21 B: © Lesha Photography
Fig. 16-22: © Lesha Photography
Fig. 16-23: photo by Danielle DiPalma
Fig. 16-24: © Caroline Brown, RNC, MS, DEd
Fig. 16-25 B: © Will and Deni McIntyre/Science Source/Photo Researchers
Fig. 16-27: © Caroline Brown, RNC, MS, DEd

Chapter 17 Opener: © Lesha Photography
Fig. 17-1: © Lesha Photography
Fig. 17-4: photo by John Gallagher, with permission of Wyncote Family Medicine, Wyncote, PA
Fig. 17-5: © Lesha Photography
Fig. 17-6: © Caroline Brown, RNC, MS, DEd

Chapter 18 Opener: © Caroline Brown, RNC, MS, DEd
Fig. 18-2: © Biophoto Associates/Science Source/Photo Researchers
Fig. 18-3 A,B: photos courtesy of Medela, Inc., McHenry, IL
Fig. 18-6: © Ansary/Custom Medical Stock Photo
Fig. 18-9: © SIU/Science Source/Photo Researchers
Fig. 18-11: © Joseph R. Siebert, PhD/Custom Medical Stock Photo
Fig. 18-13: © NMSB/Custom Medical Stock Photo
Fig. 18-14: © Alexander Tsiara/Science Source/Photo Researchers
Fig. 18-15: © M. Grecco/Stock Boston
Fig. 18-16: © JPD/Custom Medical Stock Photo
Fig. 18-17 A: © Jim Stevenson/SPL/Science Source/Photo Researchers

Chapter 19 Opener: © Caroline Brown, RNC, MS, DEd
Fig. 19-4: © Caroline Brown, RNC, MS, DEd
Fig. 19-6 A,B: © Lesha Photography
Fig. 19-8: © Caroline Brown, RNC, MS, DEd
Fig. 19-9 A,B: © Lesha Photography
Fig. 19-10: © Caroline Brown, RNC, MS, DEd
Fig. 19-11: © Steve Woit/Stock Boston
Fig. 19-12 A,B: © Lesha Photography
Fig. 19-13 B: © Frank Siteman/Stock Boston
Fig. 19-14: © Caroline Brown, RNC, MS, DEd
Fig. 19-16: © Lesha Photography
Fig. 19-17: © Lesha Photography
Fig. 19-20: © Lesha Photography
Fig. 19-21 A,B: © Lesha Photography

Chapter 20 Opener: © Caroline Brown, RNC, MS, DEd
Fig. 20-3: © Hough/Custom Medical Stock Photo
Fig. 20-4: © Lesha Photography
Fig. 20-5: © Caroline Brown, RNC, MS, DEd

Chapter 21 Opener: from Zitelli, B.J. and Davis, H.W. [1997], *Atlas of Pediatric Physical Diagnosis, 3rd ed.* St. Louis: Mosby-Year Book, Inc.
Fig. 21-4: © SIU/ Biomed Communications/Custom Medical Stock Photo
Fig. 21-6: from Sauer, G.C. and Hall, J.C. [1996], *Manual of Skin Diseases, 7th ed.* Philadelphia: Lippincott-Raven Publishers
Fig. 21-7: © Beckman/Custom Medical Stock Photo

Chapter 22 Opener: © Dr. P. Marazzi/SPL/Science Source/Photo Researchers
Fig. 22-4: © SPL/Custom Medical Stock Photo
Fig. 22-5: © NMSB/Custom Medical Stock Photo
Fig. 22-6: © Martin/Custom Medical Stock Photo
Fig. 22-7: © Dr. P. Marazzi/SPL/Science Source/Photo Researchers
Fig. 22-8: © Dr. P. Marazzi/SPL/Science Source/Photo Researchers
Fig. 22-9: © Dr. H.C. Robinson/SPL/Science Source/Photo Researchers
Fig. 22-10 B: © Morris Huberland/Science Source/Photo Researchers
Fig. 22-11: © Dr. P. Marazzi/SPL/Science Source/Photo Researchers
Fig. 22-12: © Dr. P. Marazzi/SPL/Science Source/Photo Researchers
Fig. 22-13: © Larry Mulvehill/ Science Source/Photo Researchers
Fig. 22-14: photo courtesy of Stuart Starr, MD, The Children's Hospital of Philadelphia
Fig. 22-15: © SPL/Science Source/Photo Researchers
Fig. 22-16: © Custom Medical Stock Photo

Chapter 23 Opener: photo by Melissa Olson
Fig. 23-3: from Zitelli, B.J. and Davis, H.W. [1997], *Atlas of Pediatric Physical Diagnosis, 3rd ed.* St. Louis: Mosby-Year Book, Inc.
Fig. 23-4: from Zitelli, B.J. and Davis, H.W. [1997], *Atlas of Pediatric Physical Diagnosis, 3rd ed.* St. Louis: Mosby-Year Book, Inc.

Chapter 24 Opener: © Gary Wagner/Stock Boston
Fig. 24-3: © Larry Mulvehill/ Science Source/Photo Researchers
Fig. 24-6: from Zitelli, B.J. and Davis, H.W. [1997], *Atlas of Pediatric Physical Diagnosis, 3rd ed.* St. Louis: Mosby-Year Book, Inc.
Fig. 24-9; Fig. 43-4: from Zitelli, B.J. and Davis, H.W. [1997], *Atlas of Pediatric Physical Diagnosis, 3rd ed.* St. Louis: Mosby-Year Book, Inc.
Fig. 24-12: Fig. 43-4: from Zitelli, B.J. and Davis, H.W. [1997], *Atlas of Pediatric Physical Diagnosis, 3rd ed.* St. Louis: Mosby-Year Book, Inc.

Chapter 25 Opener: photo courtesy of Karen M. Polise, MSN, RN, Division of Nephrology, The Children's Hospital of Philadelphia
Fig. 25-4: photo courtesy of Karen M. Polise, MSN, RN, Division of Nephrology, The Children's Hospital of Philadelphia
Fig. 25-5: photo courtesy of Karen M. Polise, MSN, RN, Division of Nephrology, The Children's Hospital of Philadelphia
Fig. 25-7 A,B: photos courtesy of Karen M. Polise, MSN, RN, Division of Nephrology, The Children's Hospital of Philadelphia
Fig. 25-11: photo courtesy of Karen M. Polise, MSN, RN, Division of Nephrology, The Children's Hospital of Philadelphia
Fig. 25-13: from Zitelli, B.J. and Davis, H.W. [1997], *Atlas of Pediatric Physical Diagnosis, 3rd ed.* St. Louis: Mosby-Year Book, Inc.

Chapter 26 Opener: © B. Proud
Fig. 26-1: photo by Melissa Olson

Chapter 27 Opener: © Lesha Photography
Fig. 27-2: © David/NMSB/Custom Medical Stock Photo
Fig. 27-3: from Zitelli, B.J. and Davis, H.W. [1997], *Atlas of Pediatric Physical Diagnosis, 3rd ed.* St. Louis: Mosby-Year Book, Inc.
Fig. 27-6: © Lesha Photography
Fig. 27-7: © Lesha Photography
Fig. 27-8: © Lesha Photography
Fig. 27-9: © Lesha Photography

Chapter 28 Opener: © B. Proud
Fig. 28-3 A,B: © Lesha Photography
Fig. 28-4 A,B: © B. Proud
Fig. 28-8: © Lois Silver/Custom Medical Stock Photo
Fig. 28-9: © B. Proud
Fig 28-10 A-D: photos by John Gallagher
Fig. 28-14: photo courtesy of Sue Moses
Fig. 28-15: © Elisa Peterson/Stock Boston

Chapter 29 Opener: © Bob Daemmrich/Stock Boston
Fig. 29-3: from Tasman, W. and Jaeger, E.A. [1996], *Wills Eye Hospital Atlas of Clinical Ophthalmology.* Philadelphia: Lippincott-Raven Publishers.
Fig. 29-5: from Tasman, W. and Jaeger, E.A. [1996], *Wills Eye Hospital Atlas of Clinical Ophthalmology.* Philadelphia: Lippincott-Raven Publishers.
Fig. 29-9: © Bob Daemmrich/Stock Boston
Fig. 29-10: © Stephen Frisch/Stock Boston

Chapter 30 Opener: © Caroline Brown, RNC, MS, DEd
Fig. 30-2 A,B: © Shout Pictures/Custom Medical Stock Photo
Fig. 30-3: © CC Studio/SPL/Photo Researchers. Inc.
Fig. 30-5 A-C: © Will and Deni McIntyre/Science Source/Photo Researchers
Fig. 30-8: © BSIP/Custom Medical Stock Photo
Fig. 30-9: © Gary Wagner/Stock Boston
Fig. 30-13 A: SIU Biomedical Communications/Custom Medical Stock Photo
Fig. 30-14: © Aaron Haupt/Science Source/Photo Researchers
Fig. 30-15: © Caroline Brown, RNC, MS, DEd
Fig. 30-17: photo courtesy of A.I. duPont Institute, Children's Hospital, Wilmington, DE

Chapter 31 Opener: © Christopher Brisco/Science Source/Photo Researchers
Fig. 31-6: © Caroline Brown, RNC, MS, DEd
Fig. 31-7 A,B: radiographs courtesy of Dr. Jerald P. Kuhn, Children's Hospital, Buffalo, NY
Fig. 31-10 A: © Dr. P. Marazzi/SPL/Science Source/Photo Researchers
Fig. 31-10 B: © NMSB/Custom Medical Stock Photo
Fig. 31-11: © Dr. Michael English/Custom Medical Stock Photo
Fig. 31-12: © Dr. P. Marazzi/SPL/Science Source/Photo Researchers
Fig. 31-13: © Kathy Sloane/Science Source/Photo Researchers
Fig. 31-14: © CC Studio/SPL/Photo Researchers. Inc.
Fig. 31-15: © Dr. P. Marazzi/SPL/Science Source/Photo Researchers

Chapter 32 Opener: © SPL/Custom Medical Stock Photo
Fig. 32-2: © Caroline Brown, RNC, MS, DEd
Fig. 32-3: © SIU Biomedical Communications/Custom Medical Stock Photo
Fig. 32-5: © Caroline Brown, RNC, MS, DEd

Chapter 33 Opener: © Custom Medical Stock Photo
Fig. 33-1: © Richard Hutchings/Science Source/Photo Researchers
Fig. 33-2: © B. Proud
Fig. 33-3: © Caroline Brown, RNC, MS, DEd

Chapter 34 Opener: © Caroline Brown, RNC, MS, DEd
Fig. 34-1: © Biophoto Associates/Photo Researchers
Fig. 34-2 A-D: from Zitelli, B.J. and Davis, H.W. [1997], *Atlas of Pediatric Physical Diagnosis, 3rd ed.* St. Louis: Mosby-Year Book, Inc.
Fig. 34-4: © Caroline Brown, RNC, MS, DEd
Fig. 34-5: from Zitelli, B.J. and Davis, H.W. [1997], *Atlas of Pediatric Physical Diagnosis, 3rd ed.* St. Louis: Mosby-Year Book, Inc.
Fig. 34-6: © Lesha Photography

Chapter 35 Opener: © Caroline Brown, RNC, MS, DEd
Fig. 35-1: © Bachman/Science Source/Photo Researchers
Fig. 35-2: © Bob Kramer
Fig. 35-4: © Caroline Brown, RNC, MS, DEd

Child Health Nursing *Self-Study CD-Rom Instructions*

SYSTEM REQUIREMENTS

A PC-compatible computer with a CD-Rom drive along with an Intel 386 or better processor
Windows 3.1 or later
4 Megabytes of RAM (minimum); but recommend 8 MB RAM on Windows 95
8 Megabytes of RAM (minimum); but recommend 12 MB RAM minimum on Windows 95
3 Megabytes of available hard disk space.

INSTALLATION

Installing *Child Health Nursing* for Windows:

1. Start up Windows.
2. Insert the *Child Health Nursing* CD-Rom into the CD-Rom drive.
3. From the Program Manager's File Menu, choose the Run command (for windows 95, click Start . . . Run).
4. When the Run dialog box appears, type d:\setup (or whatever drive your CD-Rom is using) in the Command Line box. Click OK or press the Enter button.
5. The *Child Health Nursing* installation process will begin. A dialog proposing the directory "CHNSG" on the drive containing Windows will appear. If the name and location are correct, click OK. If you want to change this information, type over the existing data, then click OK.
6. When the *Child Health Nursing* setup routine is complete, a new group called *"Child Health Nursing"* will appear on your desktop.
7. Start the *Child Health Nursing* self-study program by double-clicking on its icon.

CHILD HEALTH NURSING SELF-STUDY PROGRAM

Child Health Nursing contains approximately 200 questions that review the content covered in *Child Health Nursing.*

This is not a timed test. Take your time; consider the questions and the possible answers carefully.

The Main Menu screen allows you to select which unit you would like to review. To begin a unit test, choose Start Test for that unit. To continue a test that you have already begun, choose Resume Test. To restart the test and erase your results from a previous test, choose Restart Test. To review the answers you have given and compare them with the correct answers, choose Answers.

When you choose Start Test, Resume Test, Restart Test, or Answers, the test and the program's Toolbar will appear.

CHILD HEALTH NURSING'S TOOLBAR

The Toolbar contains a series of buttons that provide direct access to all test program functions. When you move the cursor over a button, an explanation of its function displays in the Status Bar, which is immediately above the Toolbar.

To get help at any time during the test, choose the Program Help button. Program Help reviews basic functions of the program.

Answer each question by clicking on the oval to the left of an answer selection or by selecting the appropriate letter on the keyboard (e.g., A, B, C, D, etc.). When an answer is selected, its oval will darken. If you change your mind about an answer, simply select that choice, by mouse or keyboard, again.

To register your answer selection and proceed to the next question, click on the Right arrow button or press Return.

After taking the test and receiving your score, you may review your answers by clicking on the Answers button on the Main Menu screen.

If you are unsure about an answer to a particular question, the program allows you to mark it for later review. Flag the question by clicking on the Mark button. To review all marked questions for a test, click on the Table of Contents button, which is immediately to the right of the Mark button.

The Table of Contents window lists every question included on the test and summarizes whether it has been answered, left unanswered, or marked for later review. Click on an item in the Table of Contents window, and the program will move to that test question.

Use the Arrow buttons to move to the first, previous, next, or last question.

At any time during the test or when you are finished taking the test, click on the Stop button. If you wish, you may return to the session at a later time without erasing your existing answers by clicking on the Resume Test button on the Main Menu.

After taking a test, view the correct answer for each test question by using the Answers button on the Main Menu. This will take you back to the test, but you will not be able to modify the answers you have given. Click on the Q/A button (to the right of the Stop button), and a window will pop up explaining the correct answer to the question. (The Q/A button will only appear when you are in the "Answers" section of the test.) You may also wish to use the Table of Contents button to show you which questions you marked for review.

To exit the *Child Health Nursing* program, click the Quit button on the Main Menu.